P9-DZM-588

Nursing Alert

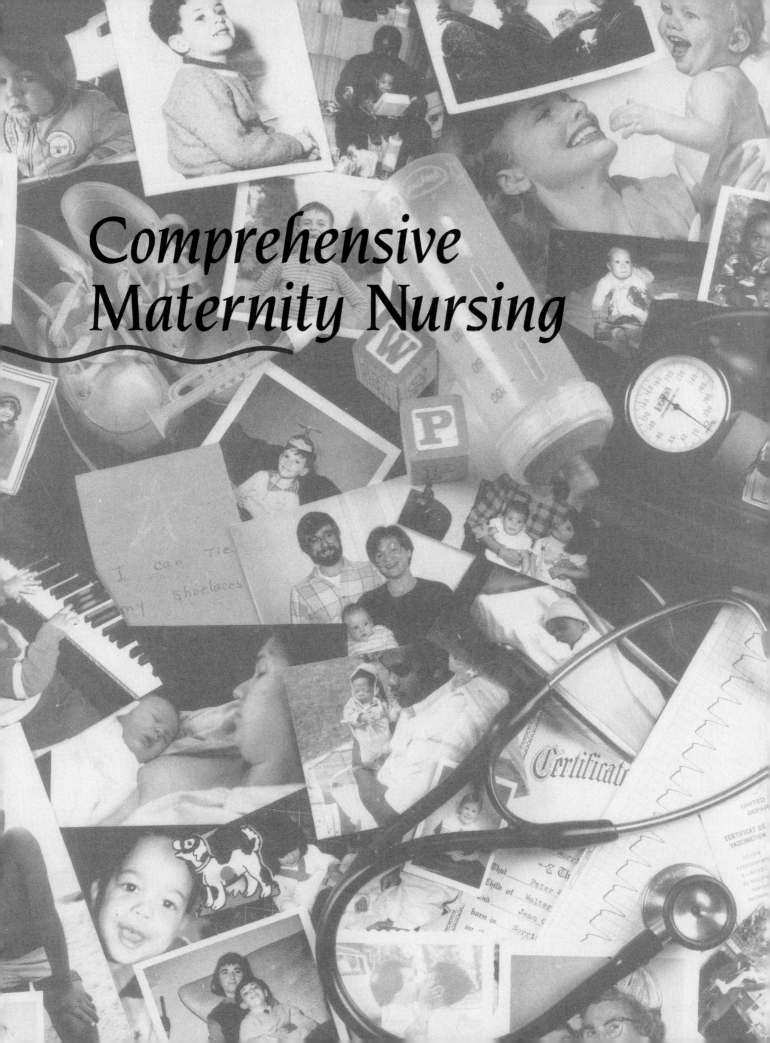

Comprehensive Maternity Nursing

Comprehensive Maternity Nursing

Nursing Process and the Childbearing Family

SECOND EDITION

Katharyn Antle May
R.N., D.N.Sc., F.A.A.N

Associate Professor and Chairperson
Department of Family and Health Systems
  Nursing
Vanderbilt University School of Nursing
Nashville, Tennessee

Associate Clinical Professor
Department of Family Health Care Nursing
University of California, San Francisco

Laura Rose Mahlmeister
R.N., Ph.D.

Associate Professor
School of Nursing
University of San Francisco,
San Francisco, California

Many illustrations by Childbirth Graphics, Ltd., Rochester, New York

J.B. LIPPINCOTT COMPANY   Philadelphia

Grand Rapids   New York   St. Louis   San Francisco
London   Sydney   Tokyo

Acquisitions Editor: *David P. Carroll*
Developmental Editor: *Eleanor Faven*
Project Editor: *Lorraine D. Smith*
Copy Editors: *Toby M. Troffkin, Cristina E. Russo*
Indexer: *Helene Taylor*
Art Director: *Susan Hess Blaker*
Designer: *Doug Smock*
Production Manager: *Carol A. Florence*
Production Coordinator: *Pamela Milcos*
Compositor: *Progressive Typographers*
Printer/Binder: *Murray Printing Co.*
Cover Printer: *Lehigh Press*
Photographic Collages: *Walter Plotnick*

Second Edition

6 5 4 3 2

Library of Congress Cataloging-in-Publication Data

Comprehensive maternity nursing: nursing process and the childbearing family/[edited by] Katharyn Antle May, Laura Rose Mahlmeister; many illustrations by Childbirth Graphics, Ltd. — 2nd ed.
    p.   cm.
    Includes bibliographical references.
    ISBN 0-397-54733-1
    1. Obstetrical nursing. I. May, Katharyn A. II. Mahlmeister, Laura Rose.
    [DNLM: 1. Obstetrical Nursing. 2. Perinatology — nurses' instruction. WY 157 C737]
RG951.C66   1990
610.73'67 — dc20
DNLM/DLC   89-14587
for Library of Congress   CIP

The following figures have been illustrated and copyrighted by Childbirth Graphics, Ltd., P.O. Box 20540, Rochester NY 14602-0540:

5-1; 5-2; 5-4; 5-5; 5-6A; 5-7; 5-8; 5-9; 5-10; 5-11; 5-12; 5-13; 5-14; 5-15; 5-16; 5-17; 5-18; 5-19; 5-20; 5-21; 5-22; 6-1; 6-2; 6-3; 6-4; 6-5; 6-6; 6-7; 6-8; 6-9; 6-10; 6-11; 7-1; 7-2; 8-1; 8-3; 8-4; 8-7; 8-8; 8-9; 13-1; 13-2; 13-5; 14-2; 14-3; 14-4; 14-5; 14-6; 14-7; 14-8; 16-1; 16-2; 16-3; 16-4; 17-2; 17-5; Breast Self Examination (Ch. 18); 19-1; 19-2; 19-3; 21-3; 21-4; 22-1; 22-2; 22-3; 22-4; 22-5; 22-6; 22-7; 22-8; 22-9; 22-10; 22-11; 22-12; 22-13; 22-14; 22-15; 22-17; 22-18; 23-5; 24-4; 24-11; 24-12; 24-18; 25-1; 25-4; 25-7; 25-8; 26-1; 26-2; 26-3; 26-6; 26-7; 27-2; 27-3; 28-1; 28-2; 28-3; 28-4; 28-5; 28-6; 28-7; 28-9; 28-10; 28-12; 28-13; 28-14; 29-1; 30-1; 30-2; 30-3; 30-4; 30-5; 30-6; 31-19; 31-20; 32-3; 32-4; 32-7; 32-8; 32-9; Heelstick (Ch. 32); 32-10A; 32-10B; 32-11; 32-12; 32-13; 32-14; 37-4; 37-5; 37-6; 37-7; 37-10; 37-13

Contributors

Paulette Converse Avery, R.N., M.S.

Assistant Professor
Samuel Merritt College of Nursing
Oakland, California

Toni Ayres, R.N., Ed.D

Lecturer
Department of Family Health Care Nursing
University of California, San Francisco

Lecturer
Department of Counseling
San Francisco State University
San Francisco, California

Jeanette M. Broering, R.N., M.S.

Assistant Clinical Professor
Department of Family Health Care Nursing and
Division of Adolescent Medicine
University of California, San Francisco

* Designates coauthorship

Linda L. Chapman, R.N., D.N.Sc.

Assistant Professor
Samuel Merritt College of Nursing
Oakland, California

29 Nursing Care of the Family in the
      Postpartum Period*

Nancy Donaldson, R.N., D.N.Sc.

Associate Director of Nursing
Director for Nursing Research
University of California, Irvine Medical Center
Orange, California

36 Individual and Family Adaptation in the
      Fourth Trimester

Yolanda Gutierrez, M.S., R.D.

Assistant Clinical Professor
Department of Family Health Care Nursing
University of California, San Francisco

15 Maternal Nutrition in Pregnancy

37 Maternal and Infant Nutrition in the
      Fourth Trimester

Gina Jensen–Hill, C.N.M., M.S.

Nurse Midwifery Service
Obstetrics and Gynecology Faculty Practice
University of California, San Francisco

30 Postpartum Complications*

Lisa K. Mandeville, R.N., M.S.N.

Administrative Coordinator, Maternal–Fetal Division
Vanderbilt University Medical Center
Nashville, Tennessee

17 Assessment of Fetal Well-being*

Joan Marks, M.S.

Director, Human Genetics Program
Sarah Lawrence College
New York, New York

9 Genetics and Genetic Counseling*

Alice Nakahata, R.P.T., M.A., A.C.C.E.

National Teacher Trainer, ASPO/Lamaze
Childbirth Educator
Co-owner and Producer, Bay Area Birth Education
  Series (BABES), Inc.

21 Preparation for Childbirth*

Jean D. Neeson, R.N.C., M.S.N., N.P.

Director, Women's Health Nurse Practitioner Program
Associate Clinical Professor
Department of Family Health Care Nursing
School of Nursing
University of California, San Francisco

Associate Clinical Professor
Department of Community and Family Medicine
School of Medicine
University of California, San Diego

  5 Normal Reproductive Anatomy and
      Physiology
  8 Family Planning and Contraception
  9 Genetics and Genetic Counseling*
10 Adolescent Sexuality and Childbearing*
13 Physiologic Adaptations in Pregnancy
14 Fetal Development

Ellen Olshansky, R.N., D.N.Sc.

Assistant Professor
Department of Parent–Child Nursing
University of Washington
Seattle, Washington

  7 Fertility and Infertility

* Designates coauthorship

Kathryn Patterson, Ph.D., C.N.M.

Perinatal Nurse
Tokos Medical Corporation
San Francisco, California

Linda C. Robrecht, C.N.M., M.S.

Nurse Midwifery Service
Obstetrics and Gynecology Faculty Practice
University of California, San Francisco

Deanna Sollid, R.N., M.S., A.C.C.E.†

Audiovisual Consultant
Department of Family Health Care Nursing
University of California, San Francisco
Co-owner and Producer, Bay Area Birth Education
  Series (BABES), Inc.

Nan H. Troiano, R.N., M.S.N.

Assistant in Obstetrics–Gynecology, Maternal–Fetal
  Division
Regionalization Coordinator
Vanderbilt University Medical Center
Nashville, Tennessee

Francene Weatherby, R.N.C., Ph.D.

Assistant Professor
University of Oklahoma College of Nursing
Oklahoma City, Oklahoma

---

*Designates coauthorship
†Deceased

Reviewers

Patricia A. Beezer, M.S., R.N.

Instructor
Department of Nursing
Rhode Island College
Providence, Rhode Island

Rose B. Cannon, R.N., M.N.

Assistant Professor
School of Nursing
Emory University
Atlanta, Georgia

Elizabeth Gilbert, R.N., M.S.

Associate Professor
College of Nursing
Grand Canyon University
Phoenix, Arizona

Kristine Henderer, R.N., Ed.D.

Assistant Professor
School of Nursing
University of Portland
Portland, Oregon

Susan A. Johnson, R.N.C., M.S.N.

Assistant Professor
Tri-College University Nursing Program
Concordia College
Moorhead, Minnesota
and North Dakota State University
Fargo, North Dakota

Judy Wright Lott, A.R.N.P., M.S.N.

Assistant Professor
College of Nursing
University of Florida
Gainesville, Florida

Deborah Narrigan, M.S.N., C.N.M.

Assistant Professor
Department of Family and Health Systems Nursing
Vanderbilt University
Nashville, Tennessee

Judith C. Peters, R.N., M.S.

Associate Professor of Parent/Child Nursing
School of Nursing
Loma Linda University
Loma Linda, California

Ruth Slocum, R.N., M.N., C.N.M.

Assistant Professor
Cedarville College
Cedarville, Ohio

Karen Stolte, R.N., Ph.D.

Professor
College of Nursing
University of Oklahoma
Oklahoma City, Oklahoma

Special Acknowledgments

Deborah Jones, R.N., M.S.N.

Perinatal Nurse Specialist
Tokos Medical Corporation
Nashville, Tennessee

Labor and Delivery Staff Nurse
Baptist Hospital
Nashville, Tennessee

Consultation on Nursing Care Plans, Chapters 32, 34

Diane M. Joyce, R.N.C., M.S.N.

Staff Nurse, Neonatal Intensive Care Nursery
Vanderbilt University Medical Center
Nashville, Tennessee

Consultation on Nursing Care Plans, Chapter 34

Lisa Lommel, R.N.C., M.S., M.P.H.

Assistant Clinical Professor
Department of Family Health Care Nursing
University of California, San Francisco

Consultation on Chapter 10

Carla Wicklein Metz, R.N.C., M.S.N., N.N.P.

Clinical Nurse Specialist/Neonatal Nurse Practitioner
T.C. Thompson Children's Hospital
Chattanooga, Tennessee

Consultation on Nursing Care Plans, Chapters 32, 34

Laurie Scott, R.N., M.S.N.

Staff Nurse, HCA West Side Hospital
Nashville, Tennessee
Graduate Student, Vanderbilt University School of
  Nursing
Nashville, Tennessee

Consultation on Nursing Care Plans, Chapter 18

M. Colleen Stainton, R.N., D.N.Sc.

Associate Professor
Faculty of Nursing and Faculty of Medicine
Department of Obstetrics and Gynecology
University of Calgary
Calgary, Alberta, Canada

Contribution of photographs; consultation on photographic art

Deborah Stumpf, R.N., M.S.N.

Staff Nurse, Perinatal Service
Metropolitan General Hospital
Nashville, Tennessee

Consultation on Nursing Care Plans, Chapter 28

Preface

Health care is not static. It is a rapidly developing and expanding field where application of new knowledge, new diagnostic and monitoring equipment, and new pharmaceuticals and biologicals is employed to give newborns a greatly improved chance for life and to extend to the elderly a healthier and more productive life. Today's professional nurse is learning to work smarter rather than harder and is acquiring new understanding of the physical mechanism that is the human body, its vulnerability to insult (injury/disease), and the principles that underlie health promotion and disease prevention.

Many new issues involving pregnancy and childbearing have also arisen. The controversy surrounding abortion has assumed new dimensions; the ethics of life support for incompletely developed infants are being debated; women, many of them upwardly mobile, have decided to have a career first and then children while they are still on the safe side of 35; adolescents, many of them single, choose to carry their babies to term and raise them themselves; and drug abuse and AIDS have changed the outcome of neonatal health. In all of these, the role of the maternity nurse assumes new importance.

Each new edition of a textbook offers its authors and contributors opportunity to provide factual as well as conceptual updating. New editions consolidate the latest findings and explore new ideas. This second edition of *Comprehensive Maternity Nursing* is dedicated to the new professional nurse who is acquiring superior knowledge and skills, is challenged by the needs of the profession, and whose dedication to patients enriches the meaning of the word "care" in the phrase "health care." The new professional nurse welcomes an ever-expanding role as a primary member of what is soon to become a 21st century health care team. The advent of a new millenium presages more responsibility and greater professional development in the field of nursing. The contemporary nurse is challenged to advance the profession as it strives to meet the needs of a new century and a new society.

This text provides not only the basic knowledge required for safe, effective, and sensitive nursing care but also the technical and scientific information necessary to equip the student to understand and evaluate the consequences of that care. Unit One lays the groundwork for the text, emphasizing the place of maternity nursing within the larger health care system and the nursing profession as a whole. Unit Two discusses the psychosocial, physiologic, and genetic parameters of human reproduction and the areas of sexuality, fertility, and genetics as important to clinical nursing care in the prenatal and interconceptual periods. Unit Three builds on bases outlined in the previous chapters and emphasizes the physiologic processes that prepare the woman's body to support the growing fetus; the development of the fetus from conception; the family's adaptation to the many changes pregnancy brings; nutrition as a primary factor influencing the quality of fetal outcome; the teaching and counseling of the expectant family; and common pregnancy-related medical problems. This unit helps prepare the nurse to assess, diagnose, intervene, and counsel during pregnancy. Unit Four emphasizes a family-centered physiologic approach to nursing care and gives the student detailed knowledge of current practices in preparation for childbirth, the process of labor and birth, and the basis of nursing care in low-risk, moderate-risk, and high-risk situations. Unit Five encompasses the critical transitions experienced by mother, newborn, and family in the first hours, days, and months after birth. Nursing support of individual and family health is a major theme.

Chapters are designed to provide sequential, programmed progress in understanding and proficiency from both theoretical and practical standpoints. Each chapter is free standing, with its subject matter clearly delineated so that the chapter content represents a clinical resource. A completely new chapter on adolescent sexuality and childbearing has been added to this edition. Adolescents face rising problems with pregnancy and the threat of sexually transmitted diseases (STDs); nurses must learn ways of caring for adolescents and their problems in a compassionate, nonjudgmental manner. Up-to-date information on HIV is presented throughout the book.

Tables, displayed extracts, illustrations, and photographs have been carefully selected to enhance specific elements within the text. Displayed extracts have been further strengthened with many new additions related to family considerations, legal/ethical considerations, nursing alerts, nuring research, related research, and self-care teaching.

As nursing authors, we were faced with the question of which pronoun to use when referring to the nurse. We have chosen to use "she." We hope the small but growing number of male colleagues in nursing understand that this reflects not a sexist attitude but the need for clear, nondistracting language in a textbook such as this.

We are pleased to share our philosophy and approach to maternity nursing with you — that it is a privilege to assist, to counsel, and to care for expectant mothers, fathers, and their families, and to share in the wonder of the birthing process.

Katharyn Antle May, R.N., D.N.SC., F.A.A.N.
Laura Rose Mahlmeister, R.N., Ph.D.

Foreword from the First Edition

In a society where values, rules, and practices concerning childbirth are changing rapidly, women and their families seek guidance from many sources. However, women rely on maternity nurses to provide specific, accurate, and appropriate information about what they should expect and request from the health care system, and about what choices they have regarding their own care. Consumers of maternity care are understandably confused by the fact that practices vary from setting to setting and from health professional to health professional. Consumers are also beginning to recognize that they will likely need a well-informed and expert guide if they are to receive the type of care they need and have a right to expect. Maternity nursing has long provided expert physical and emotional care to childbearing women and their families. However, the changing health care system now requires a new aspect of nursing practice, one that emphasizes efficiency and effectiveness in the use of new technology without sacrificing the family-centered, sensitive, supportive care that women and their families need and increasingly demand.

Comprehensive Maternity Nursing is an innovative maternity nursing text that provides a framework for this type of nursing practice. The book's orientation toward the present and future enables the student to sense the rapidity with which society and maternity care practices are changing and to make judgments accordingly. Recognizing the need and desire of families to assume more responsibility for their own health, the authors have placed a strong emphasis on nursing's role in health promotion and self-care during the childbearing year. The authors also draw from current knowledge about the family unit and emphasize that maternity care is truly family care and that choices in maternity care should be family choices.

Major trends in the wider field of nursing are reflected in this text. Nursing diagnoses for various aspects of maternity care are included throughout the text and with nursing care plans. Nursing practice is described in clear, concise language, with an eye toward minimizing unnecessary intervention and optimizing the health of the woman and her family. Key concepts of adaptation and development are used to organize knowledge drawn from the wider field of human studies, all with the explicit goal of promoting optimal individual and family health during the childbearing year.

Comprehensive Maternity Nursing provides a fresh, invigorating approach to nursing care of the family during pregnancy, childbirth, and the postnatal period. It reflects the growing, dynamic nature of scientific nursing practice with attention to healing and holism, a combination important in all areas of care, but nowhere more so than in the care of childbearing families.

Ramona T. Mercer, R.N., Ph.D., F.A.A.N.
Professor Emerita
Department of Family Health Care Nursing
University of California, San Francisco

Quick Reference Contents

Contents

Unit Five   ADAPTATION IN THE POSTPARTUM PERIOD

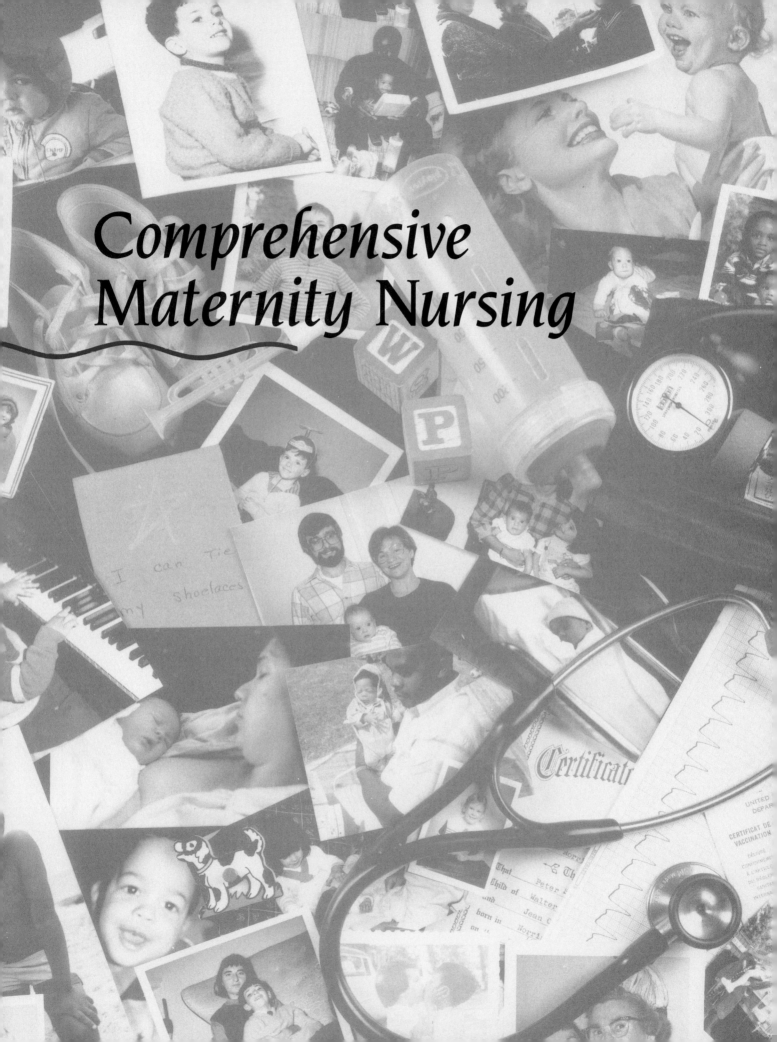

Comprehensive Maternity Nursing

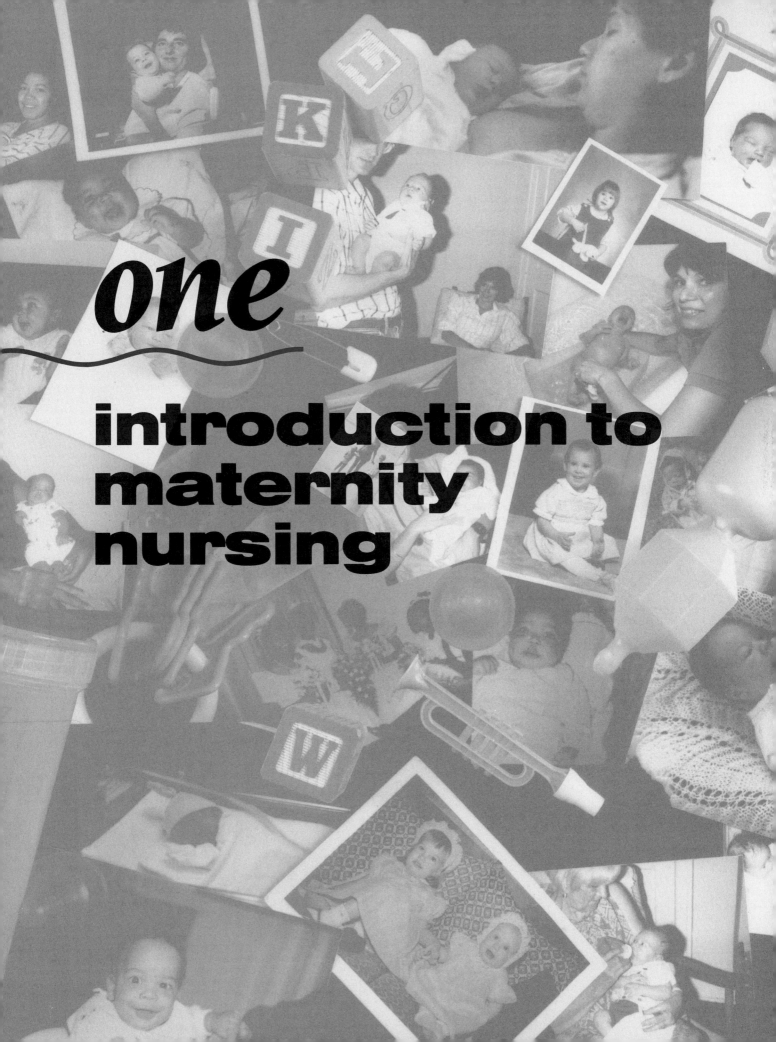

one

introduction to maternity nursing

1
contemporary maternity care

LEARNING OBJECTIVES

After studying the material in this chapter, the student should be able to

- Outline historical trends affecting the development of maternity care in the United States

- Discuss current rates of maternal and infant mortality in the United States and identify major factors contributing to those rates

- Identify social and economic trends affecting the current organization of maternity care

- Describe some advances in medical technology in the field of maternity care and discuss the ethical questions associated with the use of that technology

KEY TERMS

Birth rate

Infant mortality rate

Maternal mortality rate

Morbidity rate

Neonatal period

Neonatologist

Nurse midwife

Perinatal period

Perinatologist

Postpartum period

The knowledgeable maternity nurse understands the evolution of health care patterns and the influence of a variety of factors on contemporary delivery of maternal–child health care. Awareness of changing trends also helps the nurse anticipate how those trends will affect personal practice and, ultimately, the well-being of childbearing families.

HISTORICAL PRACTICES IN MATERNITY CARE

Usually women have cared for other childbearing women throughout much of human history. Birth practices in ancient cultures of the world that did not develop written language and relied only on oral transmission of knowledge have been lost or can be reconstructed only by examining current "primitive" practices (Goldsmith 1984). The roots of maternity care in the Western world are also ancient; the first recorded obstetric practices are found in Egyptian records dating back to 1500 B.C. Practices such as vaginal examination and the use of birth aids are referred to in writings from the Greek and Roman empires, but much of that information was lost in the Dark Ages. Advances in medicine made during the Renaissance in Europe led to the modern "scientific" age of obstetric care.

Significant discoveries and inventions by physicians in the 16th and 17th centuries set the stage for scientific progress. Such inventions include the obstetric forceps, which were first devised by Peter Chamberlen (1560–1631) and modified by William Smellie (1697–1763). François Mauriceau (1637–1709) noted that puerperal or "childbed" fever was an epidemic disease, like others that plagued the European countries. This laid the groundwork for Semmelweis, who, in the 19th century, concluded that puerperal fever was spread by contamination from the hands of physicians who were caring for many women without observing elementary hygienic procedures. The early work of physicians and scientists in Europe is reflected in such common terms in contemporary practice as *Hegar's sign* (softening of the lower segment of the uterus during pregnancy) and *Nägele's rule* (a method for calculating estimated due dates).

Maternity Care in America, 1700–1950

When colonists came to North America, they brought traditional English birth practices, including attendance by other women during childbirth and the "lying-in period" of several weeks. The less crowded environment in America, the relative absence of epidemic disease, and the more healthful and plentiful food sources resulted in

healthier women with more successful pregnancies and births. Beliefs about high maternal mortality during childbirth among colonial women are exaggerated. Maternal deaths related to childbirth were relatively rare, and women had children over an extended period. The average age at first birth was 22 years, and births typically occurred every 2 to 3 years until conception was no longer possible. However, child mortality was high, and colonial families in which seven or eight children were born were likely to see two or three die before the age of 10. This mortality rate was still lower than that in England, however. A child in the colonies had a 75% to 85% chance of surviving to 21 years of age, whereas in London one sixth of all recorded deaths occurred among children under the age of 6 years. (Wertz 1977).

Midwifery Care

Birth practices were largely the province of midwives — women who were experienced in attending births and who had many children of their own. Midwives usually were taught by apprenticeship to other midwives and sometimes were sanctioned and given semiofficial status by local religious leaders, who testified to their good character and their abstention from such heretical practices as witchcraft. In the English tradition, midwives were regarded not as part of the medical establishment but as a separate profession with a unique social role. In some cases, the midwife might also be a "doctoress," one skilled in herbal remedies and practical care of the ill and injured. Formal training and licensure for "doctoring" in America were not required until the mid-19th century.

The Emergence of the Obstetrician

Physicians and male midwives began to replace midwives after 1800. Interestingly, they did so more rapidly in America than in England, perhaps because "magical" influences or rituals surrounding birth were common in England, and tended to keep physicians away from attendance at births, but were rare in America. Another factor was the increasing number of men who received medical education in Europe and returned to America to practice after 1750. These doctors brought a knowledge of scientific advances not available to American midwives and were eager to establish a professional practice with some status in society. Despite the fact that physician or male midwife practice was not superior to midwife practice in the majority of births, and might even have been inferior in some cases, doctors and male midwives came to be regarded as more able birth attendants and were increasingly sought after by middle- and upper-class families.

Trained doctors remained rare for some time, and for a short period, both midwife practice and physician practice were common in America. Midwives were still called for uncomplicated births, and physicians were called in for complicated deliveries. Some physicians established schools of midwifery with the intention of supporting this model of collaborative practice. However, few women applied for training and large numbers of men came, so the new profession of male midwifery got off to a rapid start. This may have been because early schools were profit-making enterprises and were not government-supported, unlike schools of midwifery in Europe. Women were likely not to be able to afford training and may have resisted the notion of being trained by men about practices already known to women. Also, the Victorian beliefs about appropriate activities for women were beginning to be felt at this time, which soon restricted women's opportunities for participation in training programs of any kind.

The increasing numbers of men being trained as midwives reinforced the existing trend toward training men as physicians. By the late 19th century, midwifery had been absorbed into medical training as a specialty all doctors could practice. The increasing popularity of analgesia for childbirth, introduced by Simpson in 1847 with his use of chloroform, also contributed to the consolidation of physician control over most maternity care. Midwife attendance at birth among the middle class virtually disappeared by the late 1800s; this set the stage for the next major change in maternity care in America, the shift from home to hospital birth in the early 20th century.

The Shift to Hospital Care for Childbirth

Prior to 1900, less than 5% of births in the United States took place in hospitals. Only destitute or very ill women were cared for in "lying-in" hospitals. Crowded conditions, lack of skilled nursing care, and the predominance of patients already at risk for illness contributed to high morbidity and mortality among postpartal women and their infants. Hospital policies and procedures, such as use of surgical aseptic techniques for all procedures and routine separation of mothers and infants with the establishment of traditional newborn nurseries, were developed to minimize the risk of infection on obstetric services. Hospitals developed training programs for nurses, which ensured an acceptable level of nursing care. However, students supervised by graduate nurses assumed the nursing care of hospitalized patients while most graduate nurses provided in-home "private duty" nursing as an employee of a family and were only occasionally employed by a physician.

With the increasing organization of medicine in the United States came many changes in the American way of birth. Hospitals, built in part with an influx of federal funds, opened and provided a centralized setting for physician practice. Legislation was passed in many states in the early part of the 20th century outlawing midwifery

practice in the belief that hospital-based physician care was superior. This, compounded by the economic pressures of the Great Depression of the 1930s and the resulting sharp decline in the birth rate, caused a decline in the practice of in-home delivery and "private duty" nursing for childbearing women.

The hospital setting provided support for the physician's increasingly technological approach to obstetrics, and it gradually became the setting of choice for childbirth. Advances in analgesia and anesthesia increased safety and comfort for many women. Advances in operative and life-support techniques allowed intervention for mothers and infants not dreamed possible at the beginning of the century. However, maternal and infant mortality rates declined slowly, primarily because of preventable public health problems, such as poor nutrition, infectious diseases, and ignorance.

These high rates of maternal and infant mortality among indigent women, many of whom were immigrants concentrated in cities, were the impetus for the first federal involvement in maternity care. The Sheppard-Towner Act of 1921 provided funds for state-managed programs in maternal-child health. However, despite evidence that maternal and infant mortality declined sharply under these programs, the bill was repealed in 1930, primarily because of opposition from organized medicine. Other charitable programs were also providing services to indigent women and children, and two of these gave rise to nurse-midwifery in the United States in the 1930s. The Maternity Center Association was founded in 1918 in New York City to provide care to poor women and children and began training public health nurses in midwifery in 1932. The Frontier Nursing Service, established in 1925 by Mary Breckinridge to provide care for families in a remote area of Appalachia, began training nurse midwives shortly before World War II. Nurse midwives became primary-care providers for many impoverished families during the 1930s, a pattern that continues today.

Federal involvement in maternal-child health continued during the Depression; a national commission determined that maternal-child health services should be a federal priority, and in 1935, Title V of the Social Security Act was amended to provide funding for maternal-child health programs. Title V programs targeted those most in need and gave rise to today's programs, such as Maternal and Infant Care (MIC) projects, which emphasize comprehensive prenatal and infant care in public clinics.

By the 1950s, the practice of obstetrics in the United States was controlled by physicians, with nurse-midwifery practice concentrated only in indigent populations. The hospital was the predominant setting for childbirth, and virtually all nurses caring for childbearing families were employed by hospitals. By 1970, more than 90% of births in the United States were attended by physicians and occurred in hospitals.

The Evolution of Maternity Nursing

The movement away from home birth to hospital birth required the presence of skilled nursing staff on obstetric wards. In the years before World War II, obstetric nursing was focused on acute care and the prevention of communicable diseases. As was true in nursing in general, obstetric nursing was a highly restricted role characterized by deference to the physician, a lack of autonomy, and an almost religious dedication to work. Initially, obstetric nursing services were organized to provide care across all areas — labor and delivery, postpartum, and nursery — and much obstetric care was provided by family physicians ("general practitioners") throughout the 1950s and 1960s. As time went by, however, specialization in both medicine and nursing increased.

Specialty organizations in maternity nursing emerged, first the Nurses' Association of the American College of Obstetricians and Gynecologists in 1969 and later the Division of Maternal – Child Nursing within the American Nurses Association. The establishment of clinical journals within maternity nursing, such as the *Journal of Obstetric, Gynecological and Neonatal Nursing* in 1972 and *MCN — American Journal of Maternal-Child Nursing* in 1976, reflected the evolution of the specialty. This specialization was further consolidated by the practice of nurses working in large federally funded maternal and child health programs and by the establishment of training programs for nurse practitioners in women's health care in the 1960s. In the hospital setting, intensive neonatal care emerged as a subspecialty in both medicine and nursing, and specialty organizations and clinical journals now exist in perinatal care and neonatal care.

CURRENT ORGANIZATION OF MATERNITY CARE

The developments in the early 20th century in obstetrics and nursing contributed directly to the way maternity health care is organized and delivered today. Antenatal or prenatal care is delivered largely in outpatient settings, such as clinics and private practices. Birth care is still predominantly delivered by obstetrician-gynecologists and nurses in hospital settings although certified nurse midwives practice in most states and manage the care of low-risk and moderate-risk women throughout pregnancy, birth, and the interconceptional period. The rate of home births in the United States is estimated to be less than 10%. Some nurse midwives attend home births for low-risk women in settings where hospital transfer and admission provisions have been made. Physicians who attend unplanned home births are still rare. Lay (or empiric) midwives practice in some states, in most cases

without a standardized program of study and without certification or licensure, and account for a small number of home births.

Patterns of Maternity Care Delivery

The hospital settings in which maternity care is delivered in the United States have changed significantly in recent years. Changes include the development of alternative birth centers, birth rooms, rooming-in units, and mother – baby units as alternatives to the more traditional labor and delivery, postpartum, and newborn units. Lengths of hospitalization for childbirth have decreased dramatically, from a routine 10-day stay during the 1950s to the current routine hospitalization of 3 days or less for mothers and infants without complications. Postnatal care is usually given on an outpatient basis, with routine follow-up of a normal newborn at about 2 weeks of age, and follow-up care for the mother at 4 to 6 weeks after delivery. Settings that provide routine home-visit follow-up for families after birth are not common. Routine home visits are usually provided as part of an early discharge (within 24 hours of birth) program for low-risk mothers and infants or through a public health nursing department for mothers and infants seen to be at high risk for problems in the postpartum period.

Financial and Geographic Influences

The family's ability to pay for care may have a profound impact on the type of maternity care they receive. Private-care providers, such as physicians and nurse midwives, generally practice on a fee-for-service basis and are eligible to receive payment from health insurance plans, often called third-party payers; nurse practitioners in some areas do not receive *direct* third-party payment but may be reimbursed through a physician practice. *Health maintenance organizations,* or prepaid health plans, usually offer a range of comprehensive maternity care services and may utilize nurse midwives and nurse practitioners to a greater extent to deliver primary care to childbearing families. Services provided by public agencies, such as public health departments, clinics, county and city hospitals, and teaching hospitals, often utilize interdisciplinary health care teams to provide care for socioeconomically disadvantaged "multiproblem" families. Such agencies and institutions depend in large part on federal and state funds to pay costs.

Where women and their families live also directly affects the type of maternity care they are likely to receive. Private-care providers, particularly physicians, tend to be concentrated in urban areas rather than in rural or remote areas. This maldistribution of physicians and other primary-care providers has been a major concern of health planners since the early 1970s. Families in remote regions may have no primary-care provider available nearby and often travel long distances for hospital care. Metropolitan areas have a wide variety of services available to those able to pay for care. Those in lower socioeconomic groups, especially in inner-city areas, often are limited to care at a city or county hospital because of state and federal reimbursement regulations. In many areas of the country, private providers are reluctant to provide care to women receiving state or federal health and welfare support because the level at which the professional is reimbursed is much lower than the level of reimbursement from private insurance and often does not cover the complete cost of treatment. This restricts even further the options for maternity care available to poor women and their families and concentrates high-risk populations at public institutions.

Maternal and Infant Mortality

Health care is often evaluated by examining numerical data on mortality and morbidity in a given population. In maternity care, statistics such as birth rate, maternal and infant mortality, and birth weight are major indicators of health (Table 1 – 1).

Birth Rate

Birth rate is reported as the number of live births per 1000 in population. Birth rates and death rates in the United States are presented in Figure 1 – 1. Birth rates steadily declined from peaks in the 1950s to a low in 1975 – 1976 and have shown small increases since that time. There has been a steady increase in the number of first births to women over 30 years of age, probably reflecting larger numbers of "baby-boom" children who are delaying their families for financial reasons. Birth rates are typically higher for nonwhites than whites in the United States (see Table 1 – 1).

Birth Weight

Birth weight is an important indicator in maternity care, since low birth weight is associated with higher infant mortality. The average birth weight for infants born in the United States in 1980 was 3360 g (7 lb 7 oz). A birth weight of less than 2500 g is considered to be *low birth weight*. Low birth weight is more common among nonwhites, teen-agers, and women over 40 years of age. In 1980, low birth weight infants accounted for 6.8% of all births, a rate that has remained almost unchanged since 1976.

Table 1 – 1 **Summary of Maternal and Infant Health Indicators in United States, 1960 – 1985**

	1960	1970	1975	1980	1985
Birth Rate					
(Number of live births per 1000 in population)					
Total	23.7	18.4	14.6	15.9	15.8
White	22.7	17.4	13.8	14.9	14.8
Black	31.9	25.3	20.7	22.1	21.1
Maternal Mortality					
(Maternal deaths per 100,000 live births from complications of pregnancy, childbirth, and the puerperium)					
Total	37.1	21.5	12.8	9.2	7.9
White	26.0	14.4	9.1	6.7	5.1
Black	103.6	59.8	31.3	21.5	22.2
Neonatal Mortality					
(Infant deaths per 1000 live births prior to 28 days old, exclusive of fetal deaths [20 weeks of gestation to delivery])					
Total	18.7	15.1	11.6	8.5	7.0
White	17.2	13.8	10.4	7.5	6.1
Black	27.8	22.8	18.3	14.1	12.1
Infant Mortality					
(Infant deaths from birth to 1 year of age per 1000 live births)					
Total	26.0	20.0	16.1	12.6	10.6
White	22.9	17.8	14.2	11.0	9.3
Black	44.3	32.6	26.2	21.4	18.2

U.S. National Center for Health Statistics: Health – United States, 1987. Washington, DC, US Government Printing Office, 1987

Recent Trends

There have been significant improvements in health outcomes for mothers and infants in the last 50 years, particularly in the last decade. Estimated *maternal mortality,* expressed as number of maternal deaths per 100,000 live births, has declined steadily in the United States from 21.5 in 1970 to 7.9 in 1985 (see Table 1–1).

However, improvements are slower in the *infant mortality rate,* which is expressed as the number of deaths under 1 year of age per 1000 live births. Between 1950 and 1977, infant mortality dropped from 30 to 14 deaths per 1000 live births. In 1985, the infant mortality rate was estimated to be 10.6. Figure 1–2 shows this decline.

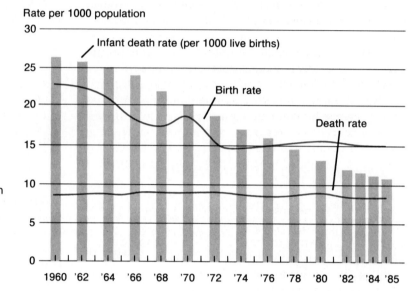

Figure 1–1. Birth and death rates in the United States, 1960–1985. (National Center for Health Statistics: Health-United States, 1987. U.S. Government Printing Office, 1987)

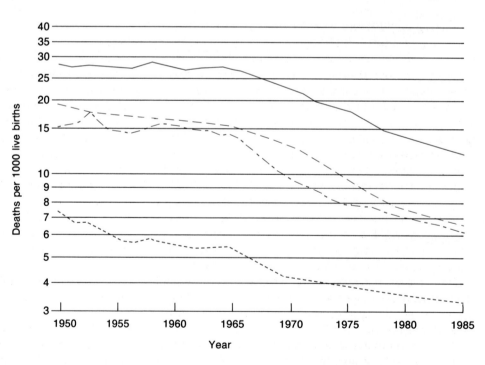

Figure 1–2. Infant mortality rates in the United States, 1950–1985. (National Center for Health Statistics, Health-United States, 1987. U.S. Government Printing Office, 1987)

—————— Black neonatal

– – – – White neonatal

–·–·–·– Black postneonatal

-------- White postneonatal

However, even this decreased rate placed the United States 15th in infant mortality worldwide. Nearly two-thirds of the infant deaths in the United States are related to low birth weight; other contributing factors are congenital anomalies and sudden infant death syndrome. About 10% of infant deaths occur in the first day after birth and about 70% in the neonatal period (the first 28 days after birth).

The comparatively unfavorable infant mortality rate in the United States also in part reflects the fact that health care is nationalized in many Western European countries, increasing the accessibility of early prenatal care. In the United States, early prenatal care and prenatal education, prevalent in middle-class groups, still do not consistently reach poor women and families who are most in need. The United States also compares unfavorably with other developed countries in regard to adolescent childbearing, with rates double that of such countries as France, Germany, and the United Kingdom (Allen Guttmacher Institute 1987; Miller 1987).

The infant mortality rate has fallen in recent decades in all nations, but relative rankings for the United States have worsened, suggesting that other nations are doing a better job at meeting the needs of childbearing families. Indeed, concern is growing in the United States that services available to women and children are inadequate and that barriers to early prenatal care for those most in need are increasing (American Nurses Association 1987).

Further, there is particular concern about rising rates of low and very low birth weight infants among blacks in the United States (Institute of Medicine 1985). A 1983 survey of 45 cities showed that infant death rates, traditionally higher among blacks than whites, are increasing disproportionately in the black population. In 32 cities surveyed, the black infant death rate was more than 50% higher than the white rate, and in 15 cities, the infant death rate among blacks was double that among whites. This racial gap in infant survival is thought to be primarily due to rises in the rate of low birth weight infants born to black women. Among 32 cities surveyed, half showed an increase in the incidence of low birth weight among black infants during 1980. Teen-age pregnancies, at particular risk for low birth weight infants, are increasing more rapidly among blacks than whites. Poverty is the salient factor here, rather than race; two thirds of black women and three fifths of teen-agers giving birth in the United States each year are living at or below the poverty level (Alan Guttmacher Institute 1987).

Statistics on maternal and infant mortality show that those who are least able to afford private care have the worst obstetric and neonatal outcomes. This raises a serious question about the continued investment of financial resources in the development of high technology designed to save infants who otherwise would die, when poor maternal and infant health status results in part

from socioeconomic need. To some extent, however, recent declines in maternal and infant mortality are a result of research advances and the development of technology to diagnose and treat complications of childbearing early. Developments in the new fields of neonatology and perinatology have saved lives of mothers and infants who only 25 years ago would not have survived. Remaining challenges in maternity care will be to reduce the rates of late or absent prenatal care and to reduce low birth weight and related problems, especially among racial and ethnic minority groups. Nationwide objectives for pregnancy and infant health care by the year 1990 are shown in the display on page 10, Public Health Objectives for Pregnancy and Infant Health in the United States by the Year 1990. It is likely that only two of these objectives, reduced infant mortality and neonatal mortality for all races, will have been met.

Emergence of High-Risk Specialties

Since the 1960s, two new medical specialties, neonatology and perinatology, have profoundly affected the organization and delivery of maternity care.

Neonatology and Perinatology

Neonatology, the medical care of newborns, especially those at high risk in the neonatal period, has emerged as a distinct subspecialty in pediatrics. This became possible in large part because of research that produced technological innovations in life support and life function monitoring in the neonate. As the research and practice base of the specialty grew, a range of levels of neonatal care developed, such as transitional care, special care, and intensive care nurseries. Nursing responsibilities in the monitoring and care of high-risk and sick neonates expanded as the scope of medical treatment increased. Today, neonatal care is a truly interdisciplinary effort, including contributions of nurses, physicians, respiratory therapists, pharmacists, laboratory scientists, social service workers, and clergy. Some 330,000 newborns are cared for in neonatal intensive care units across the United States, most commonly for conditions associated with low birth weight and prematurity.

The field of *perinatology,* a hybrid of neonatology and obstetrics, emerged in response to research on the treatment of the mother and fetus before and during childbirth. A major impetus to the development of perinatology as a subspecialty was provided by advances in our ability to monitor fetal status. These advances include electronic fetal monitoring, amniocentesis, therapy to treat preterm labor, and, most recently, fetal therapy, including fetal surgery. As perinatology grew, once again nursing responsibilities for the monitoring and care of high-risk obstetric patients grew. Now many hospitals

Public Health Objectives for Pregnancy and Infant Health in the United States by the Year 1990

Improved Health Status

1. By 1990 the national infant mortality rate (deaths for all babies up to 1 year of age) should be reduced to no more than 9 deaths per 1000 live births.
2. By 1990 the neonatal death rate (deaths for all infants up to 28 days old) should be reduced to no more than 6.5 deaths per 1000 live births.
3. By 1990 the perinatal death rate should be reduced to no more than 5.5 per 1000.
4. By 1990 no county and no racial or ethnic group of the population (*e.g.,* black, Hispanic, American Indian) should have an infant mortality rate in excess of 12 deaths per 1000 live births.
5. By 1990 the maternal mortality rate should not exceed 5 per 100,000 live births for any county or for any ethnic group (*e.g.,* black, Hispanic, American Indian).

Reduced Risk Factors

6. By 1990 low birth weight babies (less than 2500 g) should constitute not more than 5% of all live births.
7. By 1990 no county and no racial or ethnic group of the population (*e.g.,* black, Hispanic, American Indian) should have a rate of low birth weight infants (prematurely born and small-for-age infants weighing less than 2500 g) that exceeds 9% of all live births.
8. By 1990 the majority of infants should leave hospitals in car-safety carriers.

Increased Public – Professional Awareness

9. By 1990, 85% of women of childbearing age should be able to choose foods wisely (state special nutritional needs of pregnancy) and understand the hazards of smoking, alcohol, pharmaceutical products, and other drugs during pregnancy and lactation.

Improved Services – Protection

10. By 1990 virtually all women and infants should be served at levels appropriate to their need by a regionalized system of primary, secondary, and tertiary care for prenatal, maternal, and perinatal health services.
11. By 1990 the proportion of women in any county or racial or ethnic group (*e.g.,* black, Hispanic, American Indian) who obtain no prenatal care during the first trimester of pregnancy should not exceed 10 percent.
12. By 1990 virtually all newborns should be screened for metabolic disorders for which effective and efficient tests and treatments are available (*e.g.,* PKU and congenital hypothyroidism).
13. By 1990 virtually all infants should be able to participate in primary health care that includes well child care; growth development assessment; immunization; screening, diagnosis, and treatment for conditions requiring special services; appropriate counseling regarding nutrition, automobile safety, and prevention of other accidents such as poisonings.

Department of Health and Human Services: Promoting health/preventing disease: Public Health Service implementation plans for attaining the objectives for the nation: Pregnancy and infant health. Public Health Reports (Suppl), September – October, 1983

have antenatal or high-risk perinatal units in addition to the more traditional labor and delivery units.

Use of the terminology to describe areas related to these new specialties tends to be inconsistent. The term *perinatal* technically refers only to the period from 28 weeks of pregnancy through the first 28 days after birth. However, because the field of perinatology focuses typically on the *high-risk* mother and fetus/infant, the term is sometimes used to connote "high-risk" as well. For example, many graduate nursing programs prepare "perinatal clinical nurse specialists," yet the degree of concentration on high-risk nursing care varies from program to program. A hospital may employ a "perinatal nurse clinician" when, in fact, the maternity care in that facility is primarily for low-risk mothers and infants. The terms *perinatal health care* and *perinatal nursing* are increasingly used instead of *obstetric* or *maternity care* and *obstetric* or *maternal – newborn nursing.*

Regionalization of Perinatal Health Care

The emergence of the high-risk specialties of neonatology and perinatology in medicine, and the resulting growth in nursing responsibilities, led to dramatic changes in the organization of health care for mothers and infants. The trend toward regionalization of maternal and newborn care began in the 1960s as an effort to meet the needs of sick newborns. At that time, only a few institutions had the expert staff and facilities needed for intensive neonatal care. Professional groups and health planning agencies drafted long-term plans for regional perinatal care, and between 1975 and 1980, eight regions in the country developed perinatal networks.

Regionalized perinatal care is a network of relationships between hospitals providing care to mothers and newborns. Centers are designated as Level I (primary or entry-level care), Level II (moderate-risk care), or Level III (tertiary or high-risk care). Patients are referred and transported, if need be, between centers for the level of care needed. Another aspect of regionalization provides for closing low-volume obstetric units and establishing and maintaining specialized training for medical and nursing staff. Regionalization began as a means to ensure widespread access to the rapidly developing high technology care available at only a few centers. Now, however, as the costs of health care continue to climb, regionalized perinatal care is seen as a means to minimize duplication of services and keep costs down.

Some groups concerned with maternal and infant health believe that regionalized perinatal care as currently organized has overemphasized tertiary care and weakened (or, at best, underemphasized) primary care. They point out that referral for "stepped-down" care — that is, referral from intensive to intermediate care — is infrequent. This may reflect overuse of intensive care units, and it results in higher overall health care costs, crowded referral centers, and increased family stress. The overriding goal of regionalized care is to decrease the number of mothers and infants at risk and to ensure access to the appropriate level of care. Critics point out that current practice seems to be aimed at reducing risk by providing high-risk intervention to normal mothers and infants, even though there is no evidence that doing so improves outcomes among these patients. They argue that the emphasis in a regionalized system of perinatal care should be at the primary level, where such important aspects of care as prevention, health education and maintenance, continuity of care, and a family-centered approach can be implemented.

Implications for Nursing Practice

Some believe that the deficiencies of the current high-risk emphasis in care can be countered by focusing on humanistic concerns, preventive practice, and the use of effective, less expensive, and less technologically oriented models of care (Jacox 1988). John Naisbitt, a futurist, pointed out in his book *Megatrends* (1982) that as technology increases, so does the need for intensive human contact. He suggests that a "high-tech/high-touch" philosophy is required and specifically cites nursing as an example of that combination of high technology expertise and intensive human caring.

These needed aspects of care are what nursing has historically provided. The practice of nurse midwifery exemplifies this holistic, health-oriented, family-centered approach to maternity care. However, traditional nursing practice in maternity care has been fragmented to a large extent, preventing the nurse from caring for mothers and infants together throughout the childbirth experience. Some suggest that nursing has been too quick to adopt the language and philosophy of high technology as well as the responsibility for managing the high technology of high-risk birth. As a result, nurses are beginning to lose their ability to assess patients using noninvasive methods (such as auscultation, palpation, and observation) and have failed to develop nursing strategies to prevent and treat undesirable patient conditions. Holistic care contends that the major nursing objective in the care of mothers and infants should be to keep childbirth and infancy as normal as possible by concentrating attention on discovering how to maximize factors that favor good physical and emotional health.

Although nurses have recently examined ways to minimize the negative effects and maximize the positive effects of such procedures as cesarean birth and electronic fetal monitoring, they have not yet taken responsibility for discovering how to *prevent* the need for such intervention. An outstanding example of the power of proactive nursing research and practice can be seen in the work of some pioneers in maternity nursing. Claire Andrews and Joyce Roberts, (1983), both nurse midwives, conducted important early research on the effects of maternal position and ambulation on uterine efficiency and on the position of the fetus in the maternal pelvis during labor. This research developed knowledge that enables the nurse to alter the course of labor and birth directly without using invasive means. The findings of these studies are discussed in Unit IV, Childbirth.

The need for control of health care costs in maternity care, the need for caring and expert nurses to counteract the increasingly technological approach to medical care, and the recent expansion of nursing research both in scope and in depth combine to give nurses the opportunity to make a significant contribution to improving the quality of care delivered to mothers, infants, and families. Another trend has had an equally strong impact on the current organization of maternity care in the United States and will continue to influence care in the future: the family-centered birth movement.

The Family-Centered Birth Movement

A recent trend in maternity care that in some ways has competed with the trend toward increasing technological intervention is one that will be called here the *family-centered birth movement*. This trend is discussed in greater detail in Chapter 2. However, in order to understand how maternity care came to be organized as it is today, one should remember that many of the practices we now may take for granted in maternity nursing, such as early parent–neonate contact and the participation of fathers in birth and prenatal education classes, were relatively rare only 25 years ago.

Consumerism in Maternity Care

In the late 1950s, inspired by the writings of Lamaze, Dick–Read, and others, a coalition of consumers, health care professionals, and childbirth teachers recognized that standard practices in obstetric care did not acknowledge birth as a normal family event and that some practices were frankly unnecessary and unsafe for normal healthy mothers and infants. These activists began to press for changes in standard obstetric practices. The first practices to be challenged were the routine use of analgesics and anesthesia for childbirth and the routine exclusion of fathers from labor and delivery units.

This movement, known in its early days as the *natural childbirth movement,* grew in strength and popularity and began to include more health professionals and concerned laypeople through the 1960s. Several specialty organizations were formed from the original grass roots coalition, including ASPO/Lamaze and the International Childbirth Education Association. The major strategy was to educate expectant parents in prepared childbirth classes about their rights as patients and about the range of practices in low-risk obstetric care and to encourage parents to ask for the type of birth care they wanted, within the limitations of safety. The movement relied heavily on knowledgeable consumers demanding family-centered birth care for themselves and for others.

This proved to be remarkably successful, and changes in obstetric care happened quickly. By the early 1970s, prepared childbirth was a relatively accepted practice in the United States, routine use of anesthesia in childbirth was on the decline, and attendance by fathers at labor and birth was becoming commonplace in many areas of the country. These groups, with growing support from such professional groups as the American College of Nurse Midwives, went on to focus attention on other aspects of obstetric health care where changes were needed. They continue to be the major forces behind the establishment of procedures permitting early extended parent–newborn contact, the expansion of available nurse midwifery services, and the creation of alternative birth centers.

Implications for Nursing Practice

The family-centered birth movement has had a dramatic impact on maternity nursing practice, especially in such areas as managing safe care of the newborn without routine parent–infant separation, supporting the father during the birth event, and individualizing care of the laboring woman rather than following routine types of labor care. By and large, the changes brought about by the family-centered birth movement are consistent with the values and goals of nursing in general. This trend is of enough importance that Chapter 2 has been devoted to an in-depth discussion of family-centered maternity nursing.

THE CHANGING CONTEXT OF MATERNITY CARE

The creative event of childbirth has entered an era of dramatic change — for the participants and for the health care system itself. This time of transition in the human life cycle, when two people become parents and when a family is born, has recently been caught up in a revolution in maternity care.

The elements of this revolution are many. The social structure and function of the family are changing; the needs of individual families are changing; the technology of obstetrics is changing; the management of childbirth is changing; professional attitudes about childbearing are changing; outcomes of birth are changing; and, indeed, the entire marketplace in which women give birth is changing.

Social Trends Influencing Maternity Care

Patterns of maternity health care delivery are changing rapidly in response to a number of current social trends in the United States. The most important factors influencing health care of childbearing families are current economic conditions, technological advances and the ethical problems they present, issues of professional accountability and liability, and changes in sex-role expectations and family size. The nurse must be knowledgeable about these factors because they directly affect the delivery of maternity nursing care now and in the future.

Economic Conditions

During the last two decades the United States has experienced a threefold increase in the cost of health and medical care. Various strategies have been tried and have failed to control this explosive cost increase. As costs have soared, the number of people forced to rely on state or federal assistance for health care has risen dramatically. Cutbacks in services may result in increasing complications and less favorable obstetric outcomes among poor women. A cycle then results in which infant and mothers who are at high risk because of poverty conditions require intensive medical services that, in the long run, result in higher health care costs. These and other economic conditions are directly affecting the delivery of maternity care and the practice of nursing in this arena.

Cost Containment.   Cost containment is becoming a major concern in the field of maternity care. Although maternity services in hospitals typically break even or lose money, they are regarded as "loss leaders" — that is, as services that may not pay for themselves but that draw other kinds of revenue into the hospital. For example, the increased use of pediatric care facilities, intensive care units, operating rooms, or diagnostic units may cover any losses incurred in the short term. Some characteristics of maternity care as currently delivered are receiving special attention with a view to containing costs.

Costs of High Technology.   The costs of operating intensive care units, especially neonatal intensive care units, are extremely high. The budget for a neonatal intensive care unit with 20 beds may run as high as $1.7 million per year, half of which may be spent for nursing personnel. Hospital costs to the patient's family, excluding physicians' fees, may run as high as $10,000 per week. Neonatal care has already become more expensive than such adult services as coronary artery bypass surgery. The skyrocketing costs of maternal–neonatal intensive care may result in stricter regulation of the establishment and utilization of such units and certainly will increase the pressure toward regionalization of perinatal care.

Unnecessary Use of Intensive Care Units.   Recent studies of utilization of neonatal intensive care units indicates that the costs may be high because of unnecessary referrals. One study found that as many as 50% of the admissions to a neonatal intensive care unit were full-term newborns being admitted for "observation." This may reflect patterns of medical education, where physicians are trained to rely on high-technology settings in teaching centers and continue to do so in private practice. There is also a tendency for institutions to fill intensive care unit beds because the reimbursement rates from insurance carriers are higher for care given in neonatal intensive care units than for similar care in normal newborn nurseries.

These high costs are passed on to consumers through direct billing, higher insurance rates, and a further escalation in health care costs. The *primary* service delivered in maternal and neonatal intensive care units is highly skilled *nursing* care. Therefore, nurses should participate in evaluations of the cost effectiveness and appropriate utilization of intensive care units (Fig. 1–3).

Prospective Payment.   One major strategy for controlling health care costs has been the proposal to change payment for care by federal sources to a prospective basis, meaning that a certain level of reimbursement is agreed on in advance for a particular type of care, regardless of the *actual* costs for a given patient. This strategy was designed first for Medicare reimbursement and was in place by 1987; most insurance companies adopted a similar reimbursement system.

One way the level of reimbursement for care is determined is by *diagnosis-related groups* or DRGs. Hospitals or care providers are reimbursed at a particular rate for care delivered to all patients in a given DRG. One major complaint about DRGs is that these categories do not adequately recognize the intensity of the nursing care

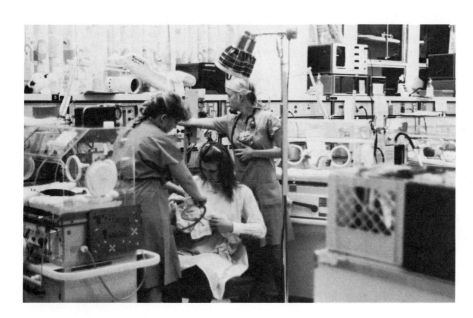

Figure 1–3. Nurses caring for a mother and her infant in a neonatal intensive care unit. (Photo: Teresa Rodriguez)

needed; nursing care is combined with other institutional costs rather than being treated as a separate budget item. The DRG system is being examined by nursing experts, and alternative systems that more accurately account for nursing care will certainly be developed.

Since the major thrust of the DRG system is for Medicare reimbursement, the trend toward prospective payment is less pronounced in maternity care. Although little information is available as yet from institutions where maternity care costs are calculated by such a system, there are some predictable implications. Prospective payment for maternity care is certain to pressure providers to shorten hospital stays, prevent complications early, and emphasize self-care and health promotion activities. Prospective payment for maternity care may also stimulate interest in alternative ways of providing care by utilizing more types of care providers and less technology-intensive settings for care.

Reimbursement for Nursing Services.   Recent economic changes in the health care arena have made reimbursement for nursing services a popular topic of debate within and outside the profession. In most hospitals, nursing services have been lumped together in a category with other miscellaneous services and considered part of the institution's routine operating costs. Since 1968, as operating budgets for hospitals have increased, the percentage of hospital expenses spent for nursing salaries has steadily decreased. However, nursing services are an income-generating function in hospitals, since third-party payers reimburse specifically for nursing services. For this reason, the true cost and cost effectiveness of inpatient nursing services have been difficult to determine.

There are some areas of nursing practice, such as primary care, where costs and outcomes attributable to nursing care can be easily isolated. Nurse midwifery has consistently been shown to deliver care equal to or of higher quality than physician care at a lower cost (Jacox 1988). Nurse midwives have for some time been eligible to receive direct third-party reimbursement in most states. Some nurse practitioners in women's health are now also eligible for direct third-party reimbursement. These mechanisms allow for evaluation of the cost effectiveness of primary care delivered by nurse specialists. However, similar developments in inpatient settings are just beginning. Many institutions are now exploring ways to organize cost accounting so that the cost effectiveness of inpatient nursing services can be more precisely examined, and in some areas, clinical nurse specialists are receiving payment on a fee-for-service basis. Reimbursement for nursing services is seen by many nurse leaders as an essential step in documenting the major contribution nursing makes in health care and in legitimizing nursing roles.

Technological Advances

The context of maternity care is also changing rapidly in response to advances in medical technology. The technology of maternity care has developed dramatically in the last 15 years, beginning with the widespread introduction of electronic fetal monitoring and amniocentesis and continuing with the advent of ultrasonography, *in vitro* fertilization, and, most recently, fetal surgery. Each of these technological advances has significantly affected the delivery of maternity care.

Electronic Fetal Monitoring

The widespread use of *electronic fetal monitoring* began in the early 1970s in the United States. Electronic fetal monitoring can detect fetal heart rate abnormalities that may signal fetal distress *in utero*. It can detect problems earlier, and unlike auscultation alone, it graphically displays the fetal heart rate and uterine activity. However, the widespread use of electronic fetal monitoring has been linked to the rising incidence of cesarean deliveries and other maternal and fetal complications, such as maternal infection and scalp tissue trauma in the infant from electrode placement. The quality of clinical decisions based on electronic fetal monitoring data depends greatly on the expertise of the clinician and on whether or not other fetal assessment techniques are available to verify information gained by electronic monitoring. Electronic fetal monitoring also tends to interfere with maternal mobility during labor, which may indirectly contribute to longer and more difficult labors. Furthermore, by the mid-1980s, a series of randomized clinical trials failed to demonstrate clear-cut advantages of electronic fetal monitoring in low-risk labor and birth, although its usefulness in situations where the fetus is known to be at risk is widely recognized. See Chapter 25 for further discussion of electronic fetal monitoring.

Amniocentesis

Amniocentesis is a procedure in which amniotic fluid is collected so that fetal status can be assessed. Fetal cells in the fluid can be screened for genetic abnormalities, and fetal lung maturity can be determined with chemical tests. The procedure, which has a fetal mortality risk of 1% to 2%, has become more common since the development of ultrasonography, which allows a precise location and visualization of the placenta and the fetus. Amniocentesis has provided the means whereby parents can know if a fetus has certain genetic abnormalities, such as Down syndrome, Tay–Sachs disease, or neural tube defects. The procedure also allows for precise determination of fetal lung maturity; this information is critical in the treatment of preterm labor and in decision making about timing of delivery when maternal or fetal health is in jeopardy. See Chapters 9 and 17 for further discussion of amniocentesis.

Chorionic Villus Sampling

Chorionic villus sampling (CVS) is a procedure, first used in the late 1960s, to sample fetal tissue directly for genetic testing. CVS will probably largely replace other procedures for genetic assessment of the fetus, since it detects a larger number of disorders than is possible with amniotic fluid studies; risks of the two procedures are comparable. In addition, the procedure can be done earlier in pregnancy. Results of CVS are available more rapidly than with other procedures, with results available within 72 hours, while a complete chromosomal study requires 7 to 10 days (compared to 2–4 weeks for amniocentesis). CVS is likely to expand the range of genetic screening available during pregnancy dramatically and will probably replace amniocentesis as a genetic screening procedure in the near future. See Chapter 9 for further discussion of chorionic villus sampling.

Ultrasonography

Ultrasonography or *ultrasound* is the first apparently safe technology for visualizing the fetus *in utero*. Ultrasonography makes possible the diagnosis of conditions such as multiple gestation, ectopic pregnancy, and certain congenital anomalies. It also permits a more precise determination of fetal size and gestational age, pattern of fetal growth, and placental location and permits confirmation of fetal position *in utero*. The precise visualization of the fetus under ultrasound has permitted the rapid expansion of the use of amniocentesis at reduced risk and the use of intrauterine treatments, such as intrauterine exchange transfusion and fetal surgery. However, the effects of ultrasound on the fetus are still being investigated and questions about the long-term safety of the procedure are being raised. See Chapters 9 and 17 for further discussion of ultrasonography.

In Vitro *Fertilization and Germ Cell Banks*

Advances in laparoscopic surgical techniques and in cell technology have permitted *in vitro* fertilization in humans. The first documented "test tube" baby was born in 1978. *In vitro* fertilization usually involves the harvesting of a mature ovum from a women who is otherwise unable to conceive, often because of fallopian tube obstruction. The ovum is fertilized *in vitro* with sperm from the woman's partner, transferred to her uterus, and allowed to implant. The practice of germ cell banking, or storage of sperm or ova, is also emerging as an option for people who wish to ensure the availability of their germ cells for future use. This practice has both legal and medical implications. In 1984 a court in Australia was asked to decide if the frozen fertilized ova of a couple killed in a plane crash had legal claim to the couple's estate, since the couple had intended to proceed with implantation. *In vitro* fertilization also makes possible the use of surrogate mothers for gestation and birth, an alternative to adoption for couples who are fertile (*i.e.,* are producing ova and sperm) but for some reason are themselves unable to conceive and bear children.

Fetal Surgery

Fetal surgery is one of the newest technological advances in the field of reproductive medicine and is available at a few tertiary care centers in the United States. Experimental work led to the first clinical applications of fetal surgery in 1981 (Inturrissi 1985). Fetal surgery was made possible by advances in ultrasonography, which allowed diagnosis of fetal abnormalities that usually resulted in severe neonatal pathology and death but that could be corrected by surgical intervention. Abnormalities that currently are amenable to fetal surgery are urinary tract obstructions, which disrupt fetal development and, when left untreated, are incompatible with life. Abnormalities that are potentially treatable by fetal surgery include obstructive hydrocephalus and congenital diaphragmatic hernia. This advance in treatment has created new demands for nursing expertise and has focused increased attention on the needs of families for whom emerging technologies offer new hope for successful childbearing (Inturrissi 1985).

Ethical Dilemmas

Each of these advances in technology opens up new opportunities for saving and enhancing the quality of life. However, each also presents risks to the provision of safe, humane care and creates ethical dilemmas with which all care-providers, perhaps especially the nurse, must grapple. Although ethical dilemmas confront nurses in all fields, the juxtaposition of life and death that is characteristic of birth highlights moral questions with which professionals and consumers must deal. The issue of abortion is one that has troubled thoughtful people for centuries and is still being debated. The new technologies emerging in the field of reproductive medicine create new ethical dilemmas and seem to raise more questions than they answer.

Nurses in maternity care are likely to be involved in caring for individuals and families who will be directly affected by these advances in technology and by the legal and ethical concerns they raise. Nurses must consider the implications of the care they deliver. The individual nurse must identify those areas in which she should not practice because of her ethical beliefs. However, the nurse must also distinguish between true ethical positions and personal preferences and must avoid imposing her value system on others when she has no compelling reason to do so.

Abortion

Perhaps the most widely recognized ethical dilemma facing the maternity nurse is the issue of induced abortion, and few issues are argued as hotly on the American scene. Induced abortion is the termination of pregnancy by expulsion of the fetus prior to 28 weeks of gestation, a limit arbitrarily established as the point at which a fetus might reasonably be expected to survive outside the uterus. The ethical problems center primarily on two issues: when the fetus can be said to be alive and human, and thus deserving of protection by the state, and the conflict between maternal and fetal rights. The debate about whether and when a fetus may be considered a human life is an ancient one and is not likely to be resolved. The ''pro-life'' and ''pro-choice'' factions are opposed along those two points: ''pro-life'' advocates claim that a fetus is alive and human and that abortion therefore constitutes killing, and ''pro-choice'' advocates contend that, regardless of the status of humanness accorded to a fetus prior to viability, a woman has the right to control what happens to her body.

Recent legal decisions and legislative actions have *not* established or refuted the moral permissibility of abortion. Legal actions taken to date have prevented individuals and states from interfering with a woman's action based on her personal convictions. In 1973 the Supreme Court, in its *Roe v Wade* decision, set aside all restrictive state laws governing abortion. The decision stated that in the first trimester a woman was free to have an abortion if she so desired, and the states were free to restrict abortion only in the second and third trimesters. The *Danforth v Planned Parenthood* decision in 1976 established that a husband's consent is not legally required for abortion. The legal situation was clouded by the controversial Hyde Amendment, which was added to the Social Security Act to prevent the use of Medicaid funds for abortions, even those deemed medically necessary.

The nurse is often the caretaker most involved with women either deciding about or undergoing induced abortion. The Nurses' Association of the American College of Obstetricians and Gynecologists specified guidelines for its members on nursing rights and responsibilities in 1972, and the American Nurses' Association's Code for Nurses speaks to the professional responsibility of the nurse in this regard. Both statements stipulate that although the nurse may be personally opposed to abortion, she may not as a professional impose her beliefs in her care of patients or in interactions with other professionals and may not ethically refuse to render postabortion care or to assist with an abortion procedure in cases where the woman's life is clearly endangered. Nurses have the right to refuse to assist in the performance of abortions without

the threat of coercion in their workplace. They also have the responsibility to inform agencies in which they work of their attitudes in this regard.

Sex Selection and Genetic Engineering

The techniques of amniocentesis and *in vitro* fertilization pose ethical questions about the consequences of unnatural manipulation of human reproduction. Amniocentesis for the specific purpose of sex determination is possible now, although the number of elective abortions for sex selection is probably quite low. Anmiocentesis for determination of specific desired genetic traits will be possible in the near future. Some question whether *eugenics,* the intentional selection of desired genetic traits for reproduction, may be the next step and point out that the elimination of even defective genes from the human gene pool has evolutionary implications that we do not yet fully understand. *In vitro* fertilization and embryo transplantation present even greater opportunity for genetic manipulation, since the genetic material of the fertilized ovum could potentially be altered.

These techniques also raise serious questions about the effect on individuals and families. What are the risks involved? It will take many years of research and many offspring to determine the long-term effects of *in vitro* fertilization on the children. As long as these procedures remain costly and complicated, they are likely to be limited to a very few patients. On what basis shall access to this technology be decided? Do all men and women have a right to procreation, regardless of the cost of the techniques necessary to achieve it? What are the psychological and social implications of sex selection of offspring, of *in vitro* fertilization using gametes from outside the marital dyad, or of surrogate childbearing? What will be the legal and social status of offspring resulting from these techniques? These questions have yet to be answered, yet they will have significant implications.

Passive Euthanasia and Care of Neonates With Defects

Another ethical dilemma facing health care providers is the care of neonates with defects. The issue centers on the quality and sanctity of life. When should medical technology be used to keep an infant alive? One distinction sometimes discussed is the distinction between ordinary and extraordinary means of preserving life. However, given the pace of technological development, this distinction can be hard to make. Many medical procedures now regarded as commonplace were once considered extraordinary measures.

The dilemma is compounded by the fact that some infants who have little or no hope for any meaningful quality of life, or who are born with a condition that is itself terminal, can be sustained for long periods with intensive care. When should treatment be initiated and terminated? Who should decide? An incident in 1982 highlighted these questions. An infant was born with Down syndrome and a gastrointestinal defect that required treatment if the infant was to survive. The parents decided to withhold treatment; media attention resulted, and eventually the Department of Health and Human Services (DHHS) responded with the so-called Baby Doe regulations, which stipulated that any facility that withheld life-saving treatments from infants with serious defects would lose federal financial assistance. These regulations also required that a sign to that effect be posted in all neonatal units and established a 24-hour telephone hotline for the reporting of violations. These regulations were strongly opposed by health care professionals as arbitrary and unnecessary. The regulations were eventually withdrawn, but the question remains: in the case of an infant with a serious defect, how much should we intervene? Who decides?

The costs of intervention are high. Neonatal intensive care is among the most expensive types of care available. The long-term costs of supporting children who have survived but are left with overwhelming mental and physical handicaps are great. The strain on families is severe and contributes to high levels of family disruption and divorce. The nurse is intimately involved in caring for such infants, assisting in emergency procedures, initiating resuscitation, following orders not to resuscitate, providing ongoing care to critically ill infants, and caring for the parents and families. Regrettably, there are many questions and very few clear answers. The nurse working in this field must be sensitive to the ethical questions she faces. Nursing responsibility includes participating in decision making and assisting other professionals and families in making the best decision possible under difficult circumstances (Fig. 1 – 4).

Professional Accountability and Liability

A factor directly affecting the arena of maternity care is the increased attention to professional accountability and liability in health care. The nurse, as a professional, is accountable for her actions and can be held liable if she performs in a careless, uninformed, or unprofessional manner that places the patient at risk, even if she was following a physician's order. Physicians, and increasingly nurses, are finding that their professional practice is open to scrutiny and may be legally challenged by consumers of health care. Current maternity care takes place in a social context in which medical miracles and medical malpractice are equally commonplace.

In some cases, consumers expect the "perfect" birth and infant, and when the unexpected happens, they look to the courts for redress. This practice leads to "defensive" health care, in which procedures are done not because of the patient's needs but out of fear of potential litigation should something go wrong. The nurse must be aware of this aspect of contemporary health care and recognize that accountable and safe nursing practice rests on a sound knowledge base, responsible communication and documentation of care, and concerned action in the patient's best interest. Chapter 4 discusses this issue in more detail. Throughout this text, ethical and legal considerations in maternity nursing practice will be highlighted.

Changing Sex Roles and Family Structures

Changes in sex-role expectations and family structures in the United States are also contributing to the changing

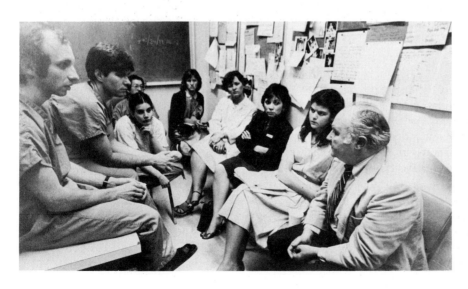

Figure 1 – 4. A team of physicians, nurses, social workers, and an ethicist discuss difficult neonatal care decisions in "ethics rounds." (Courtesy of University of California, San Francisco. Photo: Paul Fusco)

context of maternity care. Middle-class and upwardly mobile men and women are choosing to have smaller families and to delay childbearing until they are better established financially. More women are entering the work force, staying in it longer, and returning to work sooner after childbirth. More than half of American women in families with children under 5 years of age are employed outside the home. Such factors as increasing incidence of separation and divorce, the lack of high-quality, affordable child care, and the changing expectations of women create role strain for many parents.

On the other hand, changes in sex-role expectations have positive effects as well. Men and women may choose to become single parents or to remain childfree, options that were not socially acceptable for many adults a decade or two ago. Women are pursuing careers in demanding professions and achieving rewarding family lives. Men have become more involved in pregnancy and childbirth in recent years. Although the vast majority of primary caretakers of small children are still mothers, the number of fathers taking increased responsibility for daily child care and home management duties is on the rise. In some areas of the country, the nurse working in a well-baby clinic may meet the father bringing an infant in for routine health care as often as the mother.

This rapid change in family functions and sex-role expectations is particularly apparent in the changing patterns of health care delivery to childbearing families. Such practices as the routine separation of parents and infant and the exclusion of the father from childbirth and early parenting have given way to practices that focus on family needs during childbirth and emphasize the normal, natural aspects of childbearing. Chapter 2 focuses on family-centered maternity care and the nurse's central role in delivery of that care. Family considerations are of major importance in maternity nursing practice and will be highlighted throughout this text.

THE FUTURE OF MATERNITY CARE

We have seen how social trends have had a dramatic impact on the context of maternity care and how nursing practice is influenced by these trends. The future certainly holds more technological development, more discoveries that save life and enhance the quality of life, and more developments in medical and health care that hold potential for harm as well as for good. However, the fact that the recent technological explosion in maternity care has been balanced by the trend toward family-centered, health-oriented care is a hopeful sign.

Nursing has played a key role in the provision of safe and humane maternity care, and its contributions are still underestimated by many. Nurses will need to become more involved in shaping care and in setting directions for the health care system of the future. The maternity care system of the future will need to be health-oriented. It should allow us to acknowledge childbirth as a major event in people's lives and in the most important institution in our society, the family. In the next chapters, we will see why nursing is a crucial component in contemporary care and in the maternity care of the future.

CHAPTER SUMMARY

Recent developments in technology, including electronic fetal monitoring, fetal surgery, and neonatal intensive care have dramatically changed maternity care and have saved and prolonged lives that only 25 years ago would have been lost. Maternal mortality has been reduced, but infant mortality related to low birth weight continues at unacceptably high levels, especially among poor people and minority groups. The changing economic picture in health care has affected services to families. Prospective payment and direct reimbursement for nursing services offer opportunities to deliver more cost-effective care. However, high costs and unnecessary use of neonatal intensive care units conflict with the need for low-cost but effective prenatal care. Emerging technologies have created ethical questions with which consumers and professionals must struggle. Along with the trend toward increasing technological sophistication in maternity care, there is an equally strong trend toward family-centered care. The role of the nurse in contemporary maternity care is central to the welfare of families, and nurses must take more active leadership positions in shaping the maternity care system of the future.

STUDY QUESTIONS

1. Identify three historical trends in the United States that have directly affected the current organization of maternity care; discuss the nature of their influence.

2. Define the terms *maternal mortality rate, infant mortality rate,* and *low birth weight.* How do infant mortality rates in the United States compare to those in other industrialized countries? List some possible reasons for this.

3. List some national priorities in maternity care that were to be implemented by 1990. Why have these been identified as priorities? How many do you think have been reached?

4. What are DRGs? What effect might they have on the delivery of maternity care?
5. List three major technological advances in maternity care. Identify the ethical questions that arise with the use of these technologies.

REFERENCES/BIBLIOGRAPHY

Alan Guttmacher Institute: Financing Maternity Care in the US. New York, Alan Guttmacher Institute, 1987

American Nurses' Association: Access to Prenatal Care: Key to Preventing Low Birthweight. Kansas City, MO, American Nurses Association, 1987

Andrews C: Changing fetal position. J Nurse Midwifery 25:7, 1980

California State Department of Consumer Affairs: Pregnant Women and Newborn Infants in California: A Deepening Crisis in Health Care. Sacramento, 1982

Goldsmith J: Childbirth Wisdom from the World's Oldest Societies. New York, Congdon and Weed, 1984

Hughes D, Johnson J, Simons J, Rosenbaum S: Maternal and Child Health Data Book. Washington, DC, Childrens' Defense Fund, 1986

Institute of Medicine: Preventing Low Birthweight. Washington, DC, National Academy Press, 1985

Inturrissi M, Perry S, May K: Fetal surgery: Parental responses, nursing implications and the role of the clinical nurse specialist. J Obstet Gynecol Neonatal Nurs 14:271, 1985

Jacox A: The OTA report: A policy analysis. Nurs Outlook 35(6):262, 1988

Miller A: Maternal Health and Infant Survival. Washington, DC, National Center for Clinical Infant Programs, 1987

Naisbitt J: Megatrends. New York, Warner Books, 1982

Roberts J, Mendez–Bauer C, Wodell D: The effects of maternal position on uterine contractility and efficiency. Birth 10(4):243, 1983

Wertz R, Wertz D: Lying-in: A History of Childbirth in America. New York, Free Press, 1977

SUGGESTED READINGS

American Nurses' Association: Access to Prenatal Care: Key to Preventing Low Birthweight. Kansas City, MO, American Nurses' Association, 1987

Holleran C: Nursing beyond national boundaries: The 21st century. Nurs Outlook 36(2):72, 1988

Maglacas A: Health for all: Nursing's role. Nurs Outlook 36(2):66, 1988

Miller A: Maternal Health and Infant Survival. Washington, DC, National Center for Clinical Infant Programs, 1987

2 family-centered maternity care

LEARNING OBJECTIVES

After studying the material in this chapter, the student should be able to

- Define family-centered maternity care

- Discuss the major principles underlying the philosophy of family-centered maternity care

- Describe common components of a comprehensive program of family-centered maternity care

- Identify strategies for change and sources of resistance in the provision of maternity care

- Discuss the nurse's role in establishing and maintaining family-centered maternity care for childbearing families

KEY TERMS

Birthing room

Early extended parent–infant contact

Free-standing birth center

In-hospital (alternative) birth center

Rooming-in

Family-centered maternity care is defined as "the delivery of safe, quality health care while recognizing, focusing on, and adapting to both the physical and psychosocial needs of the client-patient, the family, and the newly born. The emphasis is on the provision of maternity/newborn care that fosters family unity while maintaining physical safety" (Interprofessional Task Force on Health Care of Women and Children 1978). Most health care organizations (medicine, nursing, hospital, and public health associations) in the United States and Canada have formally recognized that family-centered maternity care is essential to the provision of good obstetric care.

This consensus among professional organizations is meaningless unless this philosophy is put into practice. The effectiveness of family-centered maternity care ultimately rests on the commitment of individual professionals as they interact with the families in their care. In fact, the important difference between traditional obstetric care and family-centered maternity care is *attitudinal*. Family-centered care is based on supporting the integrity of the family and individualizing care to promote individual and family health; thus, it is possible in every setting and for every patient and family, regardless of physical setting or patient characteristics. In many areas of the United States, certain components of family-centered maternity care (such as father participation in birth and early extended parent–infant contact) have already been implemented and are now part of standard maternity care. In other areas, progress has been slower.

It is especially significant that aspects of family-centered care are still rarely available to women who are at risk for or who develop complications during childbearing or who are likely to be at increased psycho-social risk, that is, poor, young, single or nonwhite. The rationale has been that safety demands more traditional approaches to obstetric care when medical intervention is necessary. However, if professionals are committed to the values of family-centered care, it would seem that taking steps to counteract stress with supportive family-oriented care would be even more important when intensive medical intervention is needed. Those families that are designated "high-risk" may need the benefits of supportive, individualized care the most. Much change is still needed to institute care that treats birth as a family event rather than a medical emergency. Nursing has participated in making many changes and must now provide leadership in working with consumers to implement safe, high-quality family-centered maternity care.

Nurses have much at stake in this effort because family-centered maternity care is, in essence, the fullest expression of professional nursing practice with childbearing families. Childbirth is, in most cases, a normal event in the lives of women and their families. The goal of maternity nursing must be to preserve health and to support families through the transition of pregnancy and childbirth. To do this, the individual nurse must be knowledgeable about the nature and goals of family-centered maternity care. This chapter outlines the philosophy of family-centered maternity care and identifies the major components of that care. Family-centered maternity care is a major emphasis in maternity nursing. This approach to maternity care provides the basis for the discussion of the role of the nurse in maternity care presented in Chapter 3.

THE PHILOSOPHY OF FAMILY-CENTERED MATERNITY CARE

Those who provide family-centered maternity care treat each family with dignity, as individuals. Their philosophy is expansive and inclusive, and its foundation is the concept that informed families can make wise decisions about their own care. All policies are designed to promote the maximum health, safety, and welfare of mother, baby, and other family members while enhancing their childbearing experience. Care-giving and parenting skills are taught to mothers and fathers so that they gain confidence in their ability to care for their new baby. Strengthening their inner resources enables them to parent, and that is what childbirth is: the beginning of parenting, the beginning of a family.*

Family-centered maternity care reflects an underlying philosophy about the nature of childbirth and of families. This philosophy is consistent with the holistic, person-centered perspective of nursing in general and easily forms the basis for nursing practice in maternity care. However, the family-centered perspective is not limited to nursing care but should extend to physician and midwife care and to all professionals who come in contact with childbearing families. The following principles are central to the philosophy of family-centered maternity care.

The family is capable of making decisions about care during the childbearing period, given adequate information and professional support. This principle requires care providers to enter into a partnership with the family, rather than assuming the role of an "authority" on which the family becomes dependent. Patient education is essential, and families are included in discussions about care and in decision making.

---

* McKay S, Phillips C: Family Centered Maternity Care. Rockville, MD, Aspen Publications, 1984. Reprinted with permission of Aspen Systems Corporation.

In the majority of cases, childbirth is a normal, healthy event in the life of a family. This principle focuses the professional's attention on maintaining the health of the client and family during the child-bearing cycle. Pregnancy and birth are viewed as states of health that may require preventive or supportive care, rather than as illness states that must be "treated." Health maintenance cannot occur without the active participation of the family members themselves, so the professional must emphasize patient teaching and self-care activities.

Childbirth is the beginning of a new set of important family relationships. This principle requires the professional to organize care in a way that enhances positive interactions among parents, the infant, and other family members and minimizes strain on family resources. The professional's concern extends beyond physical needs in recognition of the fact that health also has social and psychological dimensions.

Basic Components of Family-Centered Maternity Care

Several national reports have identified the provision of family-centered maternity care as a high priority in the field of maternal and child health. Among the most important of these reports is the *Joint Position Statement on Family Centered Maternity/Newborn Care in Hospitals* by the Interprofessional Task Force on Health Care of Women and Children (made up of representatives of the American Academy of Pediatrics, the American College of Obstetricians and Gynecologists, the American Nurses' Association, the Nurses' Association of the American College of Obstetricians and Gynecologists, and the American College of Nurse Midwives). Nurses should be familiar with this report. McKay and Phillips (1984), two nursing authorities on family-centered care, summarize the major points as follows:

- Hospitals should offer childbirth preparation classes for both mothers and fathers, including education on the role of men at birth.
- Fathers should be included during the entire birth process.
- Hospitals should provide homelike birthing rooms that can be used instead of standard delivery rooms, if the family so chooses. Birthing rooms should contain informal furnishings and bear little resemblance to a surgical facility.
- Hospitals should consider an end to restrictions on young children visiting their mothers and newborn siblings in the hospital.
- Hospitals should develop programs for discharge of mothers as soon after birth as possible so that the

family can quickly return to the more psychologically secure atmosphere of the home.

The usual features of a comprehensive family-centered birth program and traditional obstetric care are listed in the accompanying display.

Usual Features of Comprehensive Family-Centered Birth Care and Traditional Obstetric Care

Family-Centered Care

Prenatal and parent education classes

Family participation in labor, birth, and the postpartum period, including
- Attendance by the father or a support person during labor and birth
- Unrestricted family visitation
- Sibling participation in birth

Presence of support person at complicated or cesarean birth, if circumstances permit

Use of a homelike birth room

Flexible policies regarding "routine" procedures

Postbirth recovery without routine transfer of family

Early extended parent–infant contact

Flexible rooming-in policy

Family involvement in special neonatal care unit, including transport of mother and newborn, if necessary

Early postbirth discharge with close follow-up

Traditional Care

Separation of woman from family during labor or birth to promote asepsis or to protect against legal liability

Transfer from labor room to delivery room for actual birth

Restriction of maternal activity during labor

Routine use of medication, episiotomy, or other procedures

Use of lithotomy position for delivery

No support person present for complicated or cesarean delivery

Early transfer of newborn to nursery without provisions for parent–infant contact

Restriction of newborn feedings and other activities to a set schedule

Restriction of sibling and family visitation in postbirth period

Restrictive policies regarding rooming-in

No postbirth home follow-up

Routine postpartum check no sooner than 6 weeks after birth

Rationale for Family-Centered Maternity Care

Early research on family-centered maternity care attempted to show that this type of care has long-term psychological benefits for the mother, father, neonate, and family. Findings on *long-term* psychological benefits, such as better parenting and more nurturant, loving family relationships, have been inconclusive. This is not surprising, given the complexity of the factors that influence individual and family health. However, one fact is clear from evaluation research: families are pleased with family-centered maternity care, and there is evidence of some important *short-term* gains. Supportive family-centered care may contribute to more personal satisfaction in the birth experience, more positive relationships between mother, father, and newborn in the first 2 months of life, and more parental confidence about their ability to care for their newborn.

The philosophy of family-centered maternity care is now widely accepted in most areas of the country, at least in principle, and many institutions and clinicians have made great strides in implementing this philosophy in their care. The following section surveys some current trends in family-centered maternity care.

CURRENT TRENDS IN FAMILY-CENTERED MATERNITY CARE

Trends in maternity care tend to spread unevenly across the United States, with changes being readily adopted in some areas and strongly resisted in others. However, practices that are characteristic of family-centered care have become widely known and have some broad acceptance among care-providers and parents. Some of the more important of these practices will be discussed briefly here. These aspects of care will be discussed in more depth in later chapters.

Birth Options and Alternatives

Parents and professionals often describe aspects of family-centered care as *options* or *alternatives*. This reflects the underlying philosophy that families have the right to make some choices for themselves in relation to the pregnancy and birth care they receive. The nurse should realize, however, that practices that are unexamined and that therefore may be unsafe cannot be legitimate options in the hospital setting. The nurse is responsible for assessing the possible risks and benefits of birth practices and for advising families of the known risks.

However, many options can be managed safely in the hospital setting if the nurse objectively evaluates the safety needs and takes steps to ensure that they are met. The nurse should recognize that resistance to change in routine practices is sometimes based on habit or a desire to control events rather than on actual risks to the patient. The nurse must keep in mind the goal of a healthy mother, baby, and family and individualize care toward that goal.

Family Participation in Birth

One of the most widely recognized trends in family-centered maternity care has been the dramatic change in the level of family participation in pregnancy and childbirth. Attendance by the father at prenatal classes and birth, a rare occurrence only 25 years ago, has become commonplace in most parts of the country (Fig. 2–1). Along with this change has come increasing interest in active involvement of other family members, such as grandparents and siblings.

Participation by Fathers in Vaginal and Cesarean Births. The role of the father is changing, and men are taking a more active participatory role in the birthing and upbringing of their children. The trend is for more active participation and involvement by fathers in the birth process. During labor the father can lend physical and emotional support to his laboring partner. This active involvement has become the norm in many hospitals and birthing centers today. Many childbirth classes now offer support classes for men to discuss their own needs and concerns during pregnancy and birth. Fathers are usually prepared for this support role in prenatal classes. However, even "unprepared" fathers can provide effective support to their laboring partners.

Unfortunately, the father's labor coach role in childbirth has been overemphasized at the expense of recognizing that labor and birth are significant events for the father in his own right. Fathers respond to childbirth in a variety of ways. Some fathers participate willingly, and actively support their partners with little assistance from the nurse. Others find this role difficult and prefer to be more passive bystanders during the event (May 1982). Even a "prepared" father may feel inadequate in the role of labor support person and may lack knowledge about specific ways to increase his partner's comfort. Supporting the father in the role in which he appears to be most comfortable is the primary responsibility of the nurse. This underscores the need for the nurse to be aware of the distinct individual needs of fathers experiencing the pregnancy, labor, and birth.

During the past decade participation by fathers at cesarean births has also become commonplace in some parts of the country. During the procedure the father is able to support the mother by being with her throughout

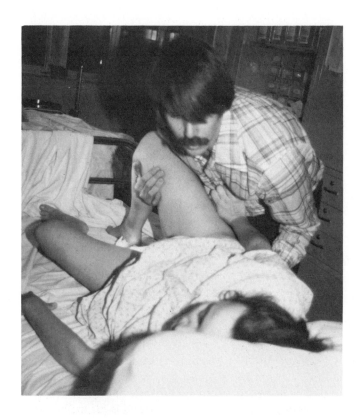

Figure 2-1. Participation by fathers in labor and birth has become an important part of the childbirth experience for many families. (Courtesy of John B. Franklin Maternity Hospital, formerly Booth Maternity Center, Philadelphia, PA)

the operation and often enjoys holding and showing the baby to the mother for the first time. Aside from supporting the mother, fathers may also experience personal satisfaction and an increase in self-esteem from participating in a cesarean birth (May and Sollid 1984). However, resistance to attendance by fathers at cesarean births is widespread among physicians and hospital administrators. The opposition stems in part from concerns about the emotional distress fathers might experience during emergency procedures and about possible lawsuits brought by fathers who observe events in the operating room. This opposition continues despite the fact that such incidents are extremely rare and remain undocumented in health care literature.

"Support People" for Labor and Birth. A major feature of family-centered maternity care is the presence of a supportive person, who can be the father, another family member, a friend, or a trained labor support person, often a childbirth educator or an experienced nurse. The effects of a supportive companion on the progress of labor and birth have been documented. One report on Guatemalan women found that women who labored in the presence of a supportive companion, called a *doula*, had much lower complication rates than women who labored alone (Sosa et al. 1980). The report suggests that the presence of a support person reduces the mother's anxiety, thus reducing the secretion of stress hormones or catecholamines. Catecholamines are believed to impair

uterine blood flow, which may result in disruption of labor and can contribute to fetal distress. The importance of a supportive companion can also be seen in mothers' reports of their birth experiences. Women consistently report that caring support contributes directly to a positive birth experience (Young 1982).

Participation by Siblings. Family participation in birth has recently been extended to siblings. Since 1976 numerous hospitals in the United States have allowed participation by siblings at birth, responding to consumer demand for this option (Fig. 2-2). A family's decision to include a child at the birth is often based on cultural attitudes, the parents' desires, and the support (or lack of it) by health care providers (Murphy 1988). Parents who want to involve the sibling in childbirth see birth as a family event and feel that excluding the older child detracts from family unity.

Some proponents of sibling participation feel that family bonding is increased and sibling rivalry may be lessened when the older child is present at the birth. Although studies have not conclusively proved this, no studies have documented harmful effects of sibling participation. However, careful and thorough preparation of siblings who are going to be present at labor and birth is extremely important, and evidence of preparation of the sibling is required in many settings before the sibling can participate in the birth.

Classes offered by providers, hospitals, and childbirth

groups to prepare children for birth and for becoming a big sister or brother are becoming common in many parts of the country. Such classes, usually taught by nurses, help prepare children for the birth by showing visual aids, including birthing dolls, cord clamps, and other delivery equipment, along with a hospital tour to familiarize the child with the birth environment. Parents are also given information on the changes they can expect in the older child once the new baby arrives.

New Settings for Childbirth

Family-centered maternity care also includes options in the actual setting for childbirth. The establishment of alternative childbirth settings is perhaps the most dramatic of the changes in American obstetrics in recent years.

In-Hospital Birth Centers.   Since 1976 in-hospital birth centers have opened in hospitals throughout the

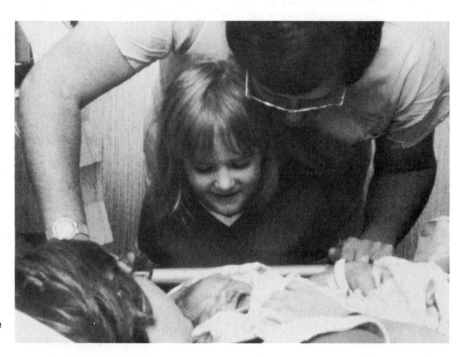

Figure 2–2. Participation by siblings in childbirth is gaining in popularity across the United States. (Photo: BABES, Inc.)

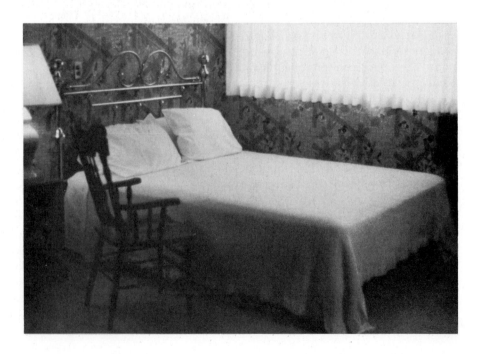

Figure 2–3. A birth center room in the hospital setting. (Photo: BABES, Inc.)

United States. These centers were developed in response to the home birth movement and because of pressure from consumers to humanize care during childbirth. In-hospital birth centers consist of suites of birthing rooms, usually staffed independently from the hospital maternity unit. The rooms have homelike furnishings, and equipment is stored out of sight (Fig. 2–3). Facilities may also develop individual birthing rooms within a conventional maternity unit for the same purpose. The family usually labors, delivers, and recovers in the same room. Because of this special care, most birth centers have a policy that only mothers with a normal or low-risk pregnancy and labor may use the birth center. Centers also must have criteria by which decisions can be made about keeping the mother in the birth center or transferring her to the conventional labor and delivery unit if complications develop in labor. Most in-hospital birth centers provide for early postbirth discharge (within 24 hours), and many provide in-home follow-up care. Some of the advantages and disadvantages of in-hospital birth centers are listed in the accompanying display.

Freestanding Birth Centers.   Freestanding (or out-of-hospital) birth centers, such as John B. Franklin Maternity Hospital and Family Center (formerly Booth Maternity Center) in Philadelphia and The Birth Place in Palo Alto, California, were designed for families who want to participate actively in their own prenatal care and who are expecting a normal labor and delivery. Low-cost, comprehensive care is provided by a staff of nurse midwives, physicians, and nurses to families choosing a more home-like environment in which to labor and deliver. Back-up obstetric care at a nearby hospital and arrangements for referral and transport to that facility are essential to a safe and successful center. Unlike hospital birth centers, a freestanding center is an adaptation of the home rather than a modification of the hospital. As with other types of birth centers, early postbirth discharge is routine, and nursing follow-up in the home is often provided.

The Single-Room Maternity System.   A new development in the 1980s was the single-room maternity system. This system was proposed as an alternative to the traditional maternity unit/in-hospital birth center arrangement that is now common in hospitals and will serve both low-risk and high-risk families. This type of unit has a central service area containing all the equipment necessary for the entire hospital stay. This area is surrounded by single rooms, including a birthing bed, bathroom facilities, and nursery equipment. In emergencies all necessary equipment can be brought into the birth room from the central service core. Mothers deliver in the birthing bed, and cesarean deliveries may be done in an adjoining operating suite. A primary-care nurse is assigned to the family throughout their hospital stay.

This system eliminates multiple transfers because the mother labors, gives birth and recovers in the same room and is discharged from it. The infant is also assessed and cared for in this room. Some of the advantages of this type of unit are listed in the display on page 28, Advantages of the Single-Room Maternity Cluster Unit. This cluster system emphasizes both safety and family-centered care. The use of the primary-care nurse, responsible for nursing care of the family from admission to discharge, is also an important element of this system.

Home Births.   In the past 2 decades the number of home births increased in certain areas of the United States, particularly in California (Fig. 2–4). This trend is concurrent with the increased use of obstetric technology and appears to be a direct result of consumers' perception that technology is overused in childbirth. Approximately 3% of births nationwide occur at home; this figure may be low, because not all home births may be reported as such. The reasons most frequently given for choosing a home birth are the desire to have family and friends close by during and after birth, a view of pregnancy and birth as normal events and thus out of place in a hospital, the desire to have more control over the experience, and the desire to give birth in familiar surroundings (McClain 1981). Women choosing home birth often are aware of

---

Advantages and Disadvantages of In-hospital Birth Centers

Advantages

Family togetherness with no parent–infant separation

Continuity of care by one set of providers throughout the birth and postbirth period

Noninterventionist approach to care; holistic focus on wellness

Lower cost than conventional maternity units

Pleasant environment conducive to relaxation

Immediate availability of obstetric emergency care should complications occur

Early discharge (within 24 hours) after birth

Minimal transfer between hospital units of mother or infant

Increased family control over decisions about the birth experience

Disadvantages

Lack of encouragement from professionals to use birth centers

Disappointment if transfer out of the center is necessary

Over-restrictive or unrealistic admission and transfer criteria

Advantages of the Single-Room Maternity Cluster Unit

Advantages for the Family

Decreased disruption of the physical and emotional aspects of childbirth

Increased opportunity to establish rapport with nursing personnel

No separation of mother, support person, and infant

Reduced risk of injury and infection because multiple transfers are avoided

Reduced hospital costs because equipment and services are consolidated

Advantages for Nursing Staff

Greater involvement with family during the birth process

Closer and more continuous contact with patient

Fewer communication problems because of fewer transfers, less duplication of paperwork

Less time spent in unit maintenance and clean-up

Increased potential for job satisfaction

Advantages for the Physician or Nurse Midwife

Greater involvement with family

Potential for increased patient load and revenue

Increased ease in care-giving because patients are clustered in one location

Decreased potential for liability from patient injury or infection

Increased opportunities for parent education

More cost-effective care

Adapted from Fenwick L, Dearing R: The Cybele Cluster: A Single Room Maternity Care System for High- and Low-Risk Families. Spokane, Cybele Society, 1981

the social and physical risk involved but consider the risks of hospitalization to be more serious (McClain 1981).

Families deciding to have a home birth need to be well informed and knowledgeable about the need for a skilled care-giver. Birth attendants may include a physician, a certified nurse midwife, or a lay (or empiric) midwife. Lay midwives usually do not complete a specified educational program and learn their skills through apprenticeship to another midwife. Certified nurse midwives complete a standardized educational program and are licensed to practice in most states. Physicians are generally opposed to home births, and many refuse to provide back-up med-

ical and hospital admission services for families who choose a home birth. However, in some areas of the country, nurse midwives are now receiving more support from obstetricians and are obtaining hospital admitting privileges and negotiating collaborative arrangements for delivering care.

The major necessities for a successful and safe home birth are

- Careful prenatal assessment to rule out potential risk factors
- A skilled birth attendant experienced in home birth
- Effective and accessible hospital care should complications arise

Women who choose home births must be in a low-risk category, have adequate prenatal care, and have immediate access to a hospital setting should complications occur in either mother or infant. This is usually provided for by certified nurse midwives or lay midwives working in collaboration with a physician for back-up services and hospital admitting privileges. Unfortunately, some physicians and health care facilities who are opposed to home birth actively prevent such collaboration or act punitively toward patients who must be admitted after attempting a home birth. Early research findings on home births are difficult to interpret because of apparent bias in some studies. However, there is no evidence that home birth presents increased risk to low-risk mothers or their infants when compared with hospital births. Complication rates in home births attended by nurse midwives and physicians are generally lower than complication rates in the hospital setting. This is what one would expect, since home birth services would generally be offered only to women at low obstetric risk.

Changing Birth Practices

Some practices in the actual care delivered during labor and birth are also characteristic of family-centered maternity care. Most family-centered settings provide for ambulation during labor, flexibility in maternal position for the actual birth, and discussion and negotiation with the woman and her partner regarding "routine procedures." These aspects are discussed in detail in Chapters 21–24. Other options that are associated with family-centered maternity care include gentle birth practices and extended parent–newborn contact.

Nonviolent or Gentle Birth Practices

Certain birth practices known as nonviolent or gentle birth practices have become popular since the publication in 1975 of *Birth Without Violence* by Frederick Leboyer, a French physician. In this book, Leboyer described how he believed traditional birth practices can cause psychological trauma to the neonate and outlined certain practices to minimize that trauma. These procedures include

- Low, indirect lighting in the birth room
- Minimal talking or noise during birth
- Gentle handling and massage of the neonate immediately after birth
- Minimal stimulation of the neonate unless absolutely necessary

- Placement of the neonate on the mother's abdomen immediately after birth
- Postponement of cord clamping until after pulsation has ceased
- Immersion of the neonate in a warm water bath (Fig. 2-5)

These steps are intended to provide the newborn with a more peaceful entry into a new world. Although not all of these steps are possible or practical with each birth, many

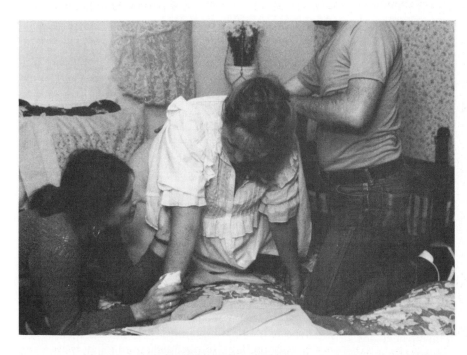

Figure 2-4. A home birth: mother laboring in a comfortable kneeling position with father and nurse midwife providing support. (Photo: BABES, Inc.)

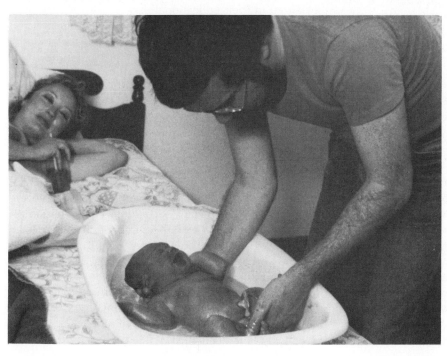

Figure 2-5. The father gives the newborn a warm Leboyer bath after birth at home. (Photo: BABES, Inc.)

can be taken to reduce the stimuli that bombard the neonate without compromising safe care. While the advantages of these steps have not been scientifically substantiated, many can be considered "risk-free" in a normal birth and may be comforting to parents and neonates.

Extended Early Parent–Infant Contact

During the 1950s and 1960s new parents were routinely separated from each other and from their infants during the hospital stay. This separation was done primarily because of concerns about infection control and partly because the large amounts of medications during labor and birth reduced the responsiveness of both mothers and infants to some extent.

With the advent of family-centered maternity care, early parent–infant contact is becoming standard in most settings. Early contact may have benefits for the infant as well as the parents. During the first hour after birth, and again for periods over the first days of life, the infant is particularly alert and is able to take in much more stimulation than was once thought possible. Further, some researchers suggest that parents are more receptive to their infants immediately after birth and that contact during this time facilitates the acquaintance process. This process has become popularly known as *parent–infant bonding* (Klaus and Kennell 1981).

However, it is also important to recognize that humans are remarkably adaptable. If early parent–infant contact is not possible because of maternal or neonatal complications, parents should be reassured that they can make up for this lack of contact and that their relationship need not be affected by short periods of necessary separation. In situations where neonatal intensive care is required, parent–infant contact is still encouraged, and fathers may have early contact with their baby until the mother is sufficiently recovered to see her infant herself.

Early Mother–Infant Discharge

Families have become more knowledgeable about childbirth, and many now prefer to return home within 24 hours after delivery. Hospitals and birth centers frequently encourage early discharge when adequate postbirth follow-up care is available. Some clinics, birth centers, and hospitals arrange for the primary-care nurse to visit the family during the first 3 days at home. Others request parents to return to the birth setting for assessment during that time or rely on telephone follow-up for assessment of the family's progress.

Nursing responsibilities in the hospital setting include a thorough assessment of the family's resources and appropriate referral for postbirth follow-up if early discharge is chosen. During postbirth follow-up, the nurse assesses the physical condition of mother and infant and also assesses how well the family is adapting in the early postpartum period. Not only can the nurse make a more accurate assessment of the family situation in the home, but she also has a unique opportunity to provide anticipatory guidance and support during those first weeks at home with a newborn. (See Chapter 36 for further discussion of this topic.)

DYNAMICS OF CHANGE IN MATERNITY CARE

The change toward family-centered maternity care was stimulated in large part by consumer demand and by the efforts of dedicated childbirth educators, nurses, physicians, and activists who saw that such changes were needed. As the birth rate continues to slow in the United States, there is increasing competition to attract childbearing populations for health care. More facilities advertise attractive birthing rooms and prenatal education programs.

However, if the motivation for such change is *only* financial, there is the risk that only lip service will be paid to the philosophy of family-centered care. Restrictive policies may continue in a more attractive physical setting. As stated before, the major difference between family-centered maternity care and traditional obstetrical care is *attitudinal.* If providers' attitudes do not change, the care they deliver will not change. Providers must be prepared to *support* childbearing families, not *control* them.

This is sometimes difficult because providers are often socialized in their educational experiences to view their care from an illness perspective and to rely only on methods that have been "proved scientifically sound." For this reason, providers and families sometimes have very different beliefs and values about maternity care. Unless providers consider the social and emotional aspects of birth care as well as the physiologic aspects, families will continue to experience frustration and dissatisfaction.

Achievements in Family-Centered Care

Considerable progress has been made in achieving some of the goals of family-centered care. Policies restricting participation by fathers in childbirth have been eliminated in many facilities. Many institutions have established or plan to establish alternative birth centers. The demand for nurse midwifery services continues to increase as nurse midwives establish themselves in practice across the country. More physicians are willing to discuss with women and their partners whether "routine procedures" are needed.

Areas Where Change Is Needed

In some areas a need for change persists, and new problems will arise as the technology of obstetric care continues to evolve. Some facilities continue to restrict the presence of support people during labor or allow only fathers to be in attendance. Such policies result in decreased levels of emotional support for many women during labor and birth. Family visitation is still restricted in some settings, despite evidence that family visitation on postpartum units does not result in higher infection rates. Fathers are often separated from their partners during administration of regional anesthesia and during cesarean childbirth, times when women frequently report that they needed their partner's support most. Nurse midwives in many parts of the country continue to face staunch opposition from obstetricians when applying for hospital privileges, despite evidence that nurse midwifery can provide high-quality, less expensive maternity care for most childbearing families.

Family-centered care is still restricted in large part to "normal" childbearing. Women who have or are at risk for complications in childbearing are often "risked out" of family-centered options, because some feel that the mother's care can only be safely managed in traditional ways. Sometimes, however, the safety problems can be overcome more easily than the attitudes of the professionals. Some settings have recognized this, such as the Family-Centered Birth Program at University of California, San Francisco. That program was designed to accommodate moderate-risk and some high-risk obstetric patients in homelike birth rooms and shows that, if family-centered care is valued, intensive monitoring and intervention during childbirth can be provided safely while still individualizing care and emphasizing family support (May and DiTolla 1984).

To make further progress, consumers and concerned providers will need to collaborate in planning and implementing care more effectively than ever before. Nursing can provide leadership in these efforts, because the goals of professional nursing practice—the diagnosis and treatment of human responses to actual and potential threats to *health*—are consonant with the needs of childbearing families.

IMPLICATIONS FOR NURSING CARE

Nursing has been at the forefront in acknowledging that people, whenever possible, should be actively involved in their own health care. This is particularly evident in nursing practice in maternity care. Nurses currently provide many of the direct services most valued by families, in-cluding primary care giving, prenatal education, sibling preparation, and midwifery. As stated before, the philosophy and practices of family-centered maternity care reflect the fullest development of the nursing role. The role of the nurse in maternity care involves education, care giving, patient advocacy, and the planning and implementation of changes in maternity services. All of these activities are essential aspects of family-centered care. In fact, history shows that the family-centered birth movement has influenced and has been influenced by the evolution of maternity nursing as a specialty. Nurses are now actively contributing to changes in care by developing and evaluating innovation through clinical practice and research. The quality of birth care in the future depends in large part on how well nurses continue to contribute to this quiet revolution in maternity care.

The Evolving Role of the Nurse

As childbirth practices continue to evolve and as technology becomes more complex, the nurse needs to be a

NURSING RESEARCH

Nurses' Responses to Family-centered Care

A descriptive study was conducted to determine what changes nurses report in maternity care and in their practice as a result of the trend toward more family-centered care. Sixty maternity nurses from ten hospitals in the midwestern United States were interviewed. Nurses reported that patients are better informed about what to expect than they were only a few years ago but now expect "ideal" care. However, patients are increasingly older or younger than in the past, and many are at high risk. Nurses reported more job satisfaction because of family-centered practices but noted that these changes increase their workload, especially in the areas of "traffic management" and patient teaching. Some conflicts arise with inadequate time for teaching in the postpartum period and the need to care for all family members instead of just mothers or babies. Further, some conflicts arise with physicians who are not supportive of the nurses' independent judgments or of family-centered care. The authors suggest that increased workload, sicker patients, less time to give care, and lack of interdisciplinary support contribute to nursing job stress but that nurses are committed to giving family-centered care despite these factors.

Stolte K, Myers S: Nurses' responses to changes in maternity care. Birth 14(2):82, 1987

NURSING RESEARCH

Effects of Sibling Visitation on Newborn Infection Rates

A recent study was conducted to determine if a sibling visitation program on a postpartum unit resulted in higher incidence of infection in the newborns. Signs and symptoms of infection at 7 and 14 days of life were assessed in 38 term infants who had direct contact with their older siblings and an adult, in 30 infants who had contact only with an adult visitor but who had older siblings at home, and in 25 infants without siblings at home who had contact only with an adult visitor during the postpartum hospital stay. Results indicated no increase in frequency of signs and symptoms of infection in newborns who had direct contact with their older siblings. However, a system for monitoring siblings for signs of infection must be instituted whenever sibling visitation is permitted. Nurses are responsible for instructing siblings and parents on handwashing and other precautions while visiting the newborn, and for instructing parents how to assess their children for infection.

Solheim K, Spellacy C: Sibling visitation: Effects on newborn infection rates. J Obstet Gynecol Neonatal Nurs 17(1):43, 1988

specialist and needs to be proficient at a high level of skilled nursing. Concurrently, the consumer is demanding a more humane and family-centered philosophy in maternity care, and the nurse must respond with caring, compassion, and concern for family needs. All of these changes require the professional nurse to apply a holistic approach in her nursing practice and offer her a unique opportunity to utilize the full range of her nursing skills.

Rarely is the nurse so intimately involved with families as during the critical passage into parenthood. The quality of her care during the hospital stay contributes directly to how poorly or how well families begin that transition. However, in the practice of family-centered nursing, the nurse's role also extends into the postbirth period. The nurse can act as a liaison with other community resources helpful to new parents, such as parenting and counseling services, breast-feeding assistance, well-baby services, and parent education and support groups. Because new families are so vulnerable during this transition period, the nurse's support or lack of support will be long remembered with praise or with frustration and anger, depending on her actions.

CHAPTER SUMMARY

Family-centered maternity care is individualized maternity care that focuses on the physiologic, psychological, and social needs of individuals and families during the childbearing year. Family-centered care is a major trend in contemporary obstetric care and has the support of most professional groups concerned with maternal and child health. The underlying philosophy of family-centered maternity care emphasizes the right of the woman and her family to make decisions about their own care, the normal nature of childbirth as a family event, and the importance of birth as the beginning of parent–infant and sibling relationships that extend over a lifetime.

Major components of family-centered maternity care are comprehensive parent education; individualized care during labor and birth in a humane, comfortable setting; and emphasis on education and support to help the parents to effectively take care of the newborn. Much progress has been made in the last two decades, but the increasing importance of technology in maternity care requires continued attention to the emotional and social components of childbearing. The overall goals of maternity nursing practice closely parallel the goals of family-centered maternity care, and nursing will need to take the lead in further establishing family-centered care as the standard practice of the 1990s.

STUDY QUESTIONS

1. What is family-centered maternity care? Why did it evolve? What are the benefits and risks of family-centered care?
2. List three principles that underlie the philosophy of family-centered maternity care. Why are these principles especially important in nursing care?
3. Define and describe the following components of family-centered maternity care:

    Early extended parent–infant contact
    Presence of a support person during labor
    Alternative birth centers
    Birthing rooms
    Gentle birth techniques
    Father participation

4. What special nursing responsibilities arise when trends in birth practices change? What must the nurse consider when parents request new or unusual types of care?
5. What are possible sources of resistance to changes in maternity care? What strategies can the nurse use to

help establish and maintain family-centered practices?

REFERENCES/BIBLIOGRAPHY

Interprofessional Task Force on Health Care of Women and Children: Joint position statement on the development of family-centered maternity and newborn care in hospitals. Chicago, Interprofessional Task Force on Health Care of Women and Children, 1978

Klaus M, Kennell J: Parent – Infant Bonding. St. Louis, CV Mosby, 1981

Leboyer F: Birth Without Violence. New York, Knopf, 1975

May K: The father as observer. MCN 7(5):319, 1982

May K, DiTolla K: In-hospital alternative birth centers: Where do we go from here? MCN 9(1):48, 1984

May K, Sollid D: Unanticipated cesarean birth: From the father's perspective. Birth 11(2):87, 1984

McClain C: Women's choice of home or hospital birth. J Fam Pract 12:1033, 1981

McKay S, Phillips C: Family Centered Maternity Care. Rockville, Md., Aspen Publications, 1984

Murphy S: A study of sibling relationships in the perinatal period. Doctoral dissertation, University of California, San Francisco, 1988

Sosa R, Kennell J, Klaus M et al: The effect of a supportive companion on perinatal problems, length of labor and mother – infant interaction. N Engl J Med 303:597, 1980

Young D: Family-centered principles, programs and teamwork. In Young D: Changing Childbirth. Rochester, NY, Childbirth Graphics, 1982

SUGGESTED READINGS

Burst H: The influence of consumers on the birthing movement. Top Clin Nurs 5(3):42, 1983

Norr K, Nacion K: Outcomes of postpartum early discharge, 1960 – 1986: A comparative review. Birth 15(1):2, 1988

Shearer E, Shiono P, Rhoads G: Recent trends in family-centered maternity care for cesarean-birth families. Birth 14(3):135, 1987

Vestal K: A proposal: Primary nursing for the mother-baby dyad. Nurs Clin North Am 17(1):3, 1984

3 the professional nurse in maternity care

LEARNING OBJECTIVES

After studying the material in this chapter, the student should be able to

- List the major nursing roles in contemporary maternity care and the type of educational preparation required for each

- Identify characteristics of a profession that nursing currently exhibits or is striving to develop

- Describe five major aspects of professional practice in nursing

- List some functions of specialty organizations and name those that are important in maternity nursing

- Discuss some major impediments to the full development of professional nursing practice in maternity care

- Identify factors that will have a dramatic effect on maternity nursing in the future

KEY TERMS

Accountability

Professionalism

Standards of nursing practice

Nursing has evolved from an era of dependence on the physician early in this century to a new age of interdependence and autonomy. Maternity nurses are actively engaged in redefining their own practice and refocusing their roles as collaborative ones with medicine and other disciplines in the health care arena. Maternity nurses are increasingly recognizing their responsibility and accountability for their own practice and their potential power to make needed changes in the delivery of health care to childbearing families.

This chapter gives an overview of the nature of nursing in general and of maternity nursing as a specialty within the larger profession. The scope of maternity nursing and the roles of nurses in the field are outlined. The importance of professional organizations and standards of practice are highlighted. Finally, some future trends in maternity nursing are outlined, as well as some impediments to professional nursing practice in maternity care.

THE NATURE OF PROFESSIONAL NURSING

Whether nursing is in fact a profession or an occupation is a matter of some debate. Some generally agreed upon characteristics of a profession are the following:

- It is organized to provide unique services.
- It has an identified body of knowledge on which services are based.
- It requires standardized education at the university level.
- It maintains self-regulated professional standards.
- It entails individual responsibility and accountability for practice.
- It engenders independent functioning and career commitment.
- It provides socially valued and compensated services.

Although nursing has made progress in all of these areas, much is yet to be achieved. Many believe that nursing is an *emerging* profession and that progress will accelerate in the future. Professionalism in nursing is increasing, and the growth in the number of nurses with advanced preparation will further that trend. Many nurses, including the authors, are optimistic about the future of nursing. We are also of the opinion that some of the best examples of professional nursing can be seen in the specialty of maternity nursing, including the practice of nurse midwives and advanced clinical specialists. We believe that the use of the term *professional* is appropriate, and so we refer to *professional nursing* throughout this text.

Definition of Maternity Nursing

Nursing has been defined as the diagnosis and treatment of human responses to actual and potential health problems (American Nurses Association 1983). The field of maternity nursing is devoted to the delivery of care to childbearing families and, as explained in Chapter 2, is based on a family-centered approach to care. Thus, maternity nursing can be defined as the diagnosis and treatment of the responses of childbearing women, their families, and their newborn infants to actual or potential health problems.

Kathryn Barnard (1982), a leading nurse researcher in the field of maternal–child nursing, identified the following aspects of the nurse's role as having particular importance in the health care of childbearing and childrearing families:

- Providing comfort and therapy in the presence of illness or disability, such as the birth of a high-risk infant
- Caring for people during periods of transition, such as pregnancy and childbirth
- Playing a major role as health educator for childbearing and childrearing families
- In the inpatient setting, regulating the environment on the patient's behalf, monitoring, and surveillance

THE SPECIALTY OF MATERNITY NURSING

Maternity nursing is usually seen as extending from conception through the first 3 months after birth. There is a logical overlap and collaboration with the field of pediatric nursing, and, in fact, the term *maternal–child health* is still used to refer to the field overall.

The term *maternity nursing* has been used since World War II to refer to the nursing care of childbearing women and their families. The term clearly implies that the mother is the primary recipient of care but encompasses the needs of the newborn and the expanding family. The more traditional term *obstetric nursing* is still common and reflects the obvious link with the medical speciality of obstetrics. That term itself is an interesting one. The root of the word *obstetric* is the Latin verb *obstare*, meaning "to stand beside." The noun *obstetrix* referred to a woman who stood by during labor. The term *obstetrics* has been used only since the turn of the century. Before that time, that branch of medicine was called *midwifery*, a term still used in England.

As mentioned in Chapter 1, the term *perinatal nursing* came into use in the early 1970s in response to the development of the field of perinatal medicine. There continues to be some inconsistency in the use of the term, which sometimes is used to refer only to the care of the woman and the fetus/neonate and at other times implies a high-risk focus as well. In any event, perinatal nursing is emerging as a subspecialty within the larger field of maternity nursing.

The Scope of Maternity Nursing

In the field of maternity nursing, the range of roles available to nurses is wide. This in part reflects the fragmentation of maternity care that exists in many settings. It also reflects the continued evolution of the role of the nurse midwife and the more recent development of the clinical specialist and primary-care nurse practitioner roles. Increasingly, the scope of practice in this field is based on university education and is responsive to rapidly changing delivery system needs.

Nurse Clinicians in Inpatient Maternal and Newborn Care

Nurses in clinical practice in hospital settings may have a variety of educational preparation, depending on the requirements of their institution. Although entry-level positions may be available in labor and delivery and newborn care, often these positions require an internship or an extended orientation period because of the specialized nature of nursing practice in those areas.

Many facilities maintain separate nursing staff for labor and delivery, for postpartum care of the mother, and for newborn care. Separating the care of the mother and infant into these arbitrary "phases" can cause problems in the delivery of comprehensive and well-organized nursing. The nurse, depending on the unit in which she works, may not have contact with family members and may not see the woman or her family for more than brief periods during the hospital stay. Staffing arrangements such as this may contribute to nurses' perceiving themselves as specializing in one area or another.

The division between maternal and newborn nursing care has also widened to some extent since the emergence of neonatology as a medical subspecialty. Many newborn nurseries are now linked administratively with pediatrics and neonatal intensive care units. Under these circumstances nurses may regard themselves more as neonatal nurses with less responsibility for direct care of the mother. In contrast to this arrangement, other facilities have implemented "mother–baby units," in which nurses assume primary care of mothers and their newborns in the postbirth period. The primary-care nurse is assigned to be responsible for the care of a woman and her family from admission through postbirth follow-up and may even have prenatal contact with the family. This arrangement emphasizes comprehensive nursing care, allows for greater continuity of care, and encourages the nurse to maintain a range of clinical skills across settings (Fig. 3–1).

The Clinical Nurse Specialist

The clinical specialist is a registered nurse who has completed a master's degree program in nursing designed to provide in-depth content in reproductive health and expertise in planning, supervision, and delivery of nursing care to families during the childbearing period.

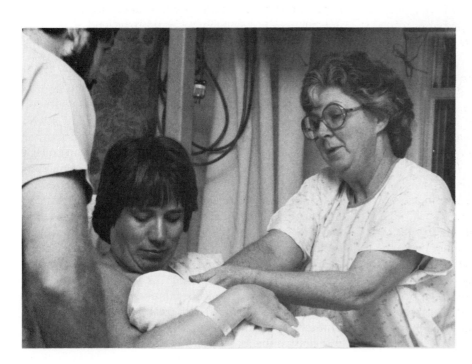

Figure 3–1. A labor and delivery nurse giving immediate postbirth care to the new family. (Photo: BABES, Inc.)

Major functions of the clinical nurse specialist are consultation, patient and staff education, and coordination and delivery of nursing care to families requiring intensive nursing support. The scope of this type of advanced clinical practice may be seen in the ANA Standards of Practice for the Perinatal Nurse Specialist (see the display on page 40). The clinical nurse specialist is often based primarily in the inpatient setting but can work across settings to facilitate continuity of care. She may also have primary responsibility for patient education programs, such as prenatal and parenting classes and support groups. The clinical specialist may carry a caseload of patients with particular health problems or may work exclusively with high-risk patients and their families (Fig. 3–2).

The Women's Health Nurse Practitioner

The women's health nurse practitioner is a registered nurse with advanced clinical preparation in the provision of primary care to women. This clinical preparation may be obtained in a certificate program or as part of a master's degree in nursing. Graduate programs are more in-depth and often prepare the nurse to function as a clinical nurse specialist with nurse practitioner skills. In most cases, nurse practitioners must attend programs that meet state requirements in order to be licensed to practice as a nurse practitioner. Nurse practitioners in women's health conduct comprehensive health assessments and manage normal prenatal, postbirth, and gyne-

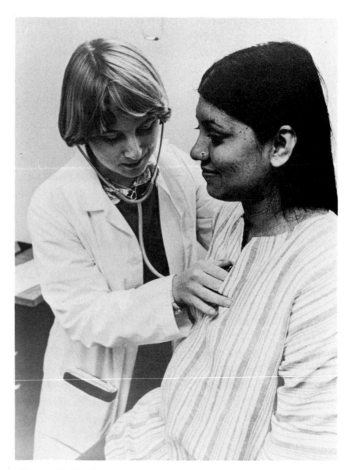

Figure 3–3. A nurse practitioner completing a prenatal health assessment. (Courtesy of University of California, San Francisco. Photo: Richard Brooks)

cologic care in collaboration with physicians and nurse midwives. They diagnose and treat common problems and refer patients to physician care according to established protocols (Fig. 3–3).

The Certified Nurse Midwife

Certified nurse midwives are registered nurses who have completed a program of study at the certificate or master's degree level recognized by the American College of Nurse Midwifery and a certification examination conducted by that organization. Certified nurse midwives are prepared to deliver normal gynecologic care as well as primary care to women during pregnancy and childbirth and to women and their newborns during the postbirth period (Fig. 3–4). Certified nurse midwives manage labor and birth, prescribe, and may perform certain medical and surgical procedures (such as local anesthesia and episiotomy) within the scope of nurse midwifery practice. Certified nurse midwives also collaborate with physicians in the care of patients with complex health problems. If prepared at the master's degree level, they may function

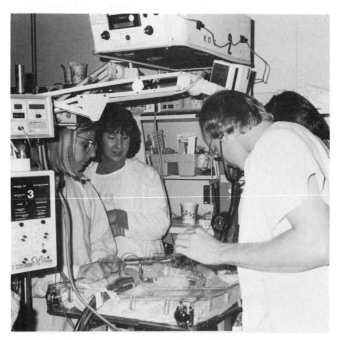

Figure 3–2. The maternity clinical specialist consults with staff in the neonatal intensive care unit about the newborn of one of her high-risk patients. (Photo: Colleen Stainton)

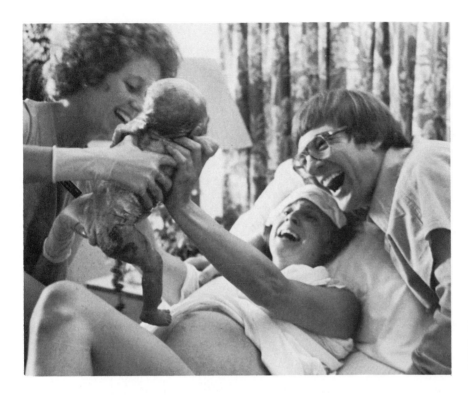

Figure 3–4. A nurse midwife in attendance at childbirth. (Courtesy of St. Luke's/Roosevelt Hospital Center, New York)

as clinical specialists in addition to their nurse midwifery practice.

Thus, the scope of nursing practice in maternity care demonstrates at least partial attainment of professional status, as reflected in the provision of unique services needed by society and increasingly common preparation at the university level. Another element of professional status is widespread recognition of professional standards of practice (see the display, page 41).

Recognition of Standards of Practice

Professional nursing practice is characterized by its recognition and knowledge of standards of practice in a given field. The overall scope of nursing practice is determined in large part by Nurse Practice Acts in each state. However, because practice usually changes more rapidly than legislation, the scope of nursing practice is also governed by community standards, such as those established in work settings as policies and procedures or those stated by the Joint Commission on Accreditation of Hospitals (JCAH). Usually these are the standards to which the nurse is *legally* held.

Specialty organizations also establish standards that are specific to particular areas of nursing practice. In maternity nursing, standards of practice with which the nurse should be familiar are the American Nurses' Association Standards of Maternal–Child Health Nursing Practice (1983), the ANA Standards of Practice for the Perina-

tal Nurse Specialist (1985), and the Nurses' Association of the American College of Obstetricians and Gynecologists (NAACOG) Standards of Obstetric, Gynecologic and Neonatal Nursing (1986). The major points of the ANA standards are listed in the display on page 41. Most institutions have copies of the NAACOG standards. The student should read and become familiar with these standards.

Involvement in Professional and Specialty Organizations

An important aspect of professional practice is participation in professional organizations. Professional organizations evolve in part because professions by their nature must be *self-regulating* to a large extent. Only members themselves have the knowledge to determine the level of expertise necessary for competent practice. Professions regulate access to professional training, have considerable control over licensure requirements, and are responsible for establishing standards for the education and practice of their members. These functions in nursing are carried out by the American Nurses' Association, its constituent state associations, and the National League for Nursing.

Most professions also have specialty organizations that serve similar functions within a well-defined area of practice. Specialty organizations are necessary in most cases because the scope of knowledge in a profession is too

Major Points of ANA Standards of Practice for the Perinatal Nurse Specialist

Standard I: Data Collection

The nurse assesses the childbearing family to identify risk factors, educational needs, care needs, referral needs, and transport needs.

Standard II: Diagnosis

The nurse uses nursing diagnoses and accepted perinatal classification system diagnoses to express conclusions supported by recorded assessment data and current scientific premises.

Standard III: Planning

The nurse establishes a plan of care for the childbearing family based upon nursing diagnosis that includes specific goals and interventions delineating nursing actions unique to that family's needs.

Standard IV: Intervention

The nurse implements interventions based on the developed plan of nursing care.

Standard IV-A: Physiological and Interpersonal Intervention

The nurse implements specific physiological and interpersonal therapeutic interventions that promote perinatal health care.

Standard IV-B: Patient Education and Support

The nurse develops and participates in education programs to assist clients and families in achieving optimal family development.

Standard IV-C: Perinatal Transport

The nurse participates in the organization and implementation of perinatal (maternal and neonatal) transport programs.

Standard V: Evaluation

The nurse evaluates client and family responses to nursing interventions and evaluates specific programs in order to provide for the revision of the data base, nursing diagnoses, nursing care plans, and program development.

Standard VI: Collaboration

The nurse collaborates with nurses and other professionals in providing care to perinatal families.

Standard VII: Education

The nurse contributes to the educational and professional development of colleagues.

Standard VIII: Community Service

The nurse promotes standards for perinatal care in the community.

Standard IX: Research

The nurse improves the quality of perinatal nursing through scientific inquiry.

Standard X: Professional Development

The nurse assumes responsibility for personal professional development.

American Nurses' Association, Council of Perinatal Nurses: Standards of Practice for the Perinatal Nurse Specialist. Kansas City, American Nurses' Association, 1985

broad across the entire field for effective communication and implementation of appropriate standards. The nursing specialty organizations pertinent to maternity care are the Nurses' Association of the American College of Obstetricians and Gynecologists and the American College of Nurse-Midwifery.

The individual nurse has a responsibility to join and participate in professional and specialty organizations for several reasons. First, these organizations set standards for education and practice. The practicing nurse has a responsibility to be knowledgeable about that process and to participate in it. Second, professional and specialty organizations are responsible for assisting nurses to up-

date and extend their professional knowledge and skills. Each organization has a program of professional continuing education, and most publish newsletters and professional journals — both important ways in which nurses can continue their own education.

Career Commitment and Innovative Practice

Another characteristic of a profession is the extent to which it engenders career commitment and independent, innovative functioning. The various well-differentiated

Major Points of ANA Standards of Maternal – Child Health Nursing

Standard I: The nurse helps children and parents attain and maintain optimum health.

Standard II: The nurse assists families to achieve and maintain a balance between the personal growth needs of individual family members and optimum family functioning.

Standard III: The nurse intervenes with vulnerable clients and families at risk to prevent potential developmental and health problems.

Standard IV: The nurse promotes an environment free of hazards to reproduction, growth and development, wellness, and recovery from illness.

Standard V: The nurse detects changes in health status and deviations from optimum development.

Standard VI: The nurse carries out appropriate interventions and treatment to facilitate survival and recovery from illness.

Standard VII: The nurse assists clients and families to understand and cope with developmental and traumatic situations during illness, childbearing, childrearing, and childhood.

Standard VIII: The nurse actively pursues strategies to enhance access to and utilization of adequate health care services.

Standard IX: The nurse improves maternal and child health nursing practice through evaluation of practice, education, and research.

American Nurses' Association: Standards of Maternal and Child Health Nursing Practice. Kansas City, MO, American Nurses' Association, 1983

roles available to nurses in maternity care, that is, clinician, nurse specialist, nurse practitioner, or certified nurse midwife, are evidence of the growing trend toward modes of full professional practice. In addition, innovative practice roles are developing in response to consumer and health care system needs.

Nurse Consultants

The increasing specialization found in maternity nursing is also giving rise to the need for nurse consultants, experts in a particular area of practice who establish a private practice to provide consultation to agencies on a fee-for-service basis. For example, nurses are more frequently called upon to provide expert review of materials and to act as expert witnesses regarding potential professional liability issues. Other expert nurses consult with corporations who are developing equipment or products to be used in patient care, or are paid as speakers at continuing education meetings. Still others establish themselves as consultants to publishers of textbooks or periodicals on perinatal health issues. All of these roles require considerable clinical expertise as well as specialized skills and experience necessary for the consultative role itself.

Innovations in Clinical Nursing Services

Much of maternity nursing involves providing services to individuals who are healthy and are attempting to prevent health problems during pregnancy and childbirth. Indeed, the strong emphasis on health promotion, self-care, and patient teaching has contributed to the emergence of the private practice role in nursing. While nurse midwives and nurse practitioners have historically practiced in collaborative arrangements with physicians and other health professionals, some are now choosing to concentrate on an aspect of their practice that is more independent, such as providing prenatal or breastfeeding education or counseling persons who have concerns about their fertility.

The options for independent practice for nurses employed in inpatient settings have been more limited. One of the most common ways for maternity nurses to establish an independent practice is through childbirth education. They may teach classes in a particular hospital setting as an independent contractor or may teach in the community on a fee-for-service basis.

However, some unique independent practice arrangements have also developed around the country. Maternity nurses have established group practices to provide one-to-one postpartum recovery care and home-visit follow-up for families desiring early postbirth discharge. The nurses share on-call time and are paid on a fee-for-service basis. Other nurses have established themselves in private practice to do sibling preparation for childbirth, offering group and private classes for families wanting to teach their older children about childbirth. Clinical specialists have set up practices in collaboration with obstetricians to provide childbirth education, postbirth home follow-up, and parent support groups on a fee-for-service basis.

The field of maternity nursing will continue to change in response to the changing social context of childbirth and maternity care. Many changes in the field will reflect changes in the nursing profession overall. These trends will likely include increasing pressure for cost-effective care under prospective payment systems and greater interest within nursing in innovative practice, accompanied by mounting resistance from other professions as competition for clients in health care increases.

Innovative practices by maternity nurses are important to the future development of the specialty. Nurses have for too long undervalued their contribution to health care and underestimated their ability to provide services beyond the usual nursing roles and practice settings. However, as nurses work to develop and strengthen their clinical practice base, there are some impediments to full professional practice that will continue to confront them.

CHALLENGES IN PROFESSIONAL NURSING PRACTICE

By and large, the problems that constrain maternity nursing practice are the ones facing the entire profession: the difficulty of demonstrating the actual cost and value of nursing care in the hospital setting; the ongoing struggle to establish and maintain nursing in a decision-making position in planning and implementing health care delivery; the problem of recruiting intelligent, career-minded individuals into the field despite relatively low pay and low status; and the challenging, often extremely difficult working conditions.

Physician Oversupply and Maldistribution

Some problems seem to be more clearly focused in the field of maternity nursing. One such issue is the projected oversupply of physicians in metropolitan areas while rural areas continue to be underserved in terms of prenatal and obstetric care (Rhodes 1986a). This will have an impact on the scope of nursing practice with childbearing families. Will this problem mean changes in certified nurse midwife and nurse practitioner practice in maternity/women's health? The answer is likely yes, since physician resistance to nursing roles in primary health care is increasing already in metropolitan areas where professionals tend to concentrate and where competition for clients is most acute. In recent years, certified nurse midwives have experienced discrimination in obtaining hospital admitting privileges, and attempts have been made to limit the scope of their practice through legislative changes sponsored by organized medicine in several states.

The crisis in liability insurance (described later in this chapter) has meant that many already underserved populations continue to lose physician providers. A 1985 survey showed that 12.3% of the members of the American College of Obstetricians and Gynecologists had stopped providing obstetric care because of the increasing liability risk, with some individual states showing a dropout rate as high as 21%. However, despite the fact that provision of perinatal services by Certified Nurse Midwives (CNMs) and Nurse Practitioners (NPs) remains a logical solution, resistance from individual physicians and from organized medicine still limits nurses practicing in these roles to a significant degree (Jacox, 1987; National Commission to Prevent Infant Mortality 1988).

Will the physician oversupply in some regions mean that some services now regarded as nursing functions will be absorbed by medicine? Possibly. The next 20 years will be critical in the field, and outcomes will depend in large part on how well nurses demonstrate the value and cost-effectiveness of their practice. Individual nurses will need to document and communicate clearly their unique contributions to the health care needs of childbearing families. Collectively, nursing must continue its legislative activities and consolidate its position in a collaborative rather than a subordinate role with medicine.

Sexism in the Health Care System

A lingering problem facing nurses is the impact of sexism. Sexism is especially evident in maternity care because not only nurses but also clients are usually female. Clearly, some of the more restrictive practices in obstetrics during the 1940s and 1950s reflected the general view of women as dependent and unable to make decisions about their own care. Organized medicine, like other professions, adopted a sexist ideology growing out of the Victorian Age. This ideology persists in subtle ways to this day.

Many of the most obvious expressions of sexism in maternity care have been eliminated as family-centered care has gained acceptance. However, the nurse can observe lingering problems in the way women are treated as consumers in the health care system. When a woman has a somatic complaint, is the assumption more easily made that her problem is "emotional" or "stress-related"? Would the same assumption be made if the patient were male? Would the provider's assumption be communicated to the patient in the same way? Do hospitals continue to restrict support persons for birth to the "father of the baby"? What if the woman has chosen to be a single parent? What if she wants someone who would be more supportive, such as a woman friend, to be with her during the birth?

There are also obvious examples of sexism in the interactions of health care *providers* in maternity care. Some come not from medicine, but from within nursing itself. In one court case, a hospital claimed that it was inappropriate for male nurses to work in labor and delivery. The rationale given was that although the woman chooses her obstetrician, she has no control over nurses giving care and that the services of a male nurse in labor and delivery would violate the privacy of the patient. The hospital's claim was upheld, despite testimony on behalf of the plaintiff, a male nurse who had requested assignment in labor and delivery, that female nurses give care to male patients in all other settings without prior patient selection, that male obstetricians frequently not of the woman's own choosing give intimate care, and that poor women have never had freedom of choice about the sex of providers giving care (Greenlaw 1981).

An appeal was lost in this case, but the logic of the decision raises some disturbing questions. Is it appropriate to restrict the access of male medical and nursing students to training in obstetric care or to restrict providers of a certain race because they would not be of the patient's choosing? Clearly, this decision and its implications pose a serious impediment to professional nursing and perpetuate the paternalism that has characterized the health care system's treatment of women and of nursing in general (Greenlaw 1981). Maternity nurses have an excellent vantage point from which they can identify and work to change problems such as this one as they confront patients and colleagues from all disciplines.

Complexity in Ethical Decision Making

Ethical decision making is, at times, exceedingly complex in maternity care, especially around dilemmas that technological advances in reproduction, genetics, and perinatology pose for families and care-providers. Unfortunately, such advances often occur faster than clinicians can develop guidelines for their appropriate application. The ethical implications of such advances become especially important for the nurse, since, by and large, it is the nurse who spends the most time with families facing difficult decisions.

Because of this increasing complexity in decision making on ethical issues, there has been much attention devoted to this topic in the clinical literature. One recurring theme in the literature focuses on the issue of maternal versus fetal rights (Rhodes 1986c). The concept of the fetus as a patient separate from the mother has emerged with the technology to assess fetal well-being and to treat fetal conditions. Probably the most difficult cases arise when a mode of therapy becomes an accepted practice, and a woman refuses it. In recent years several court cases have resulted in court-ordered cesarean deliveries to protect a potentially viable fetus over the mother's objections to the surgery.

These cases have been controversial for two main reasons. First, it is clear that fetal life and well-being do not exist independently of the mother. Second, forced medical treatment of the fetus against the mother's wishes requires that she become a patient against her will, and if she is a competent adult, that is generally not acceptable legally or ethically. It is unclear how far the courts will go to protect the viable fetus over the objection of the mother, and no case has yet required a mother to submit to surgical intervention to protect a fetus before viability.

However, the very standard of viability is likely to change, as technological advances move from experimental treatment to standard of care with increasing rapidity (Rhodes 1986c).

Ethical analysis of enforced fetal therapy will probably continue to be a pressing issue in perinatal care for some time to come and will focus on an estimation of risks and benefits to both fetus and mother. For instance, the following are some questions that must be asked:

- How certain or uncertain are the potential benefits to the fetus and the mother?
- How great are the potential benefits?
- What risks are involved for fetus and mother?
- Of what magnitude are those risks?

Aumann (1988) states that simplistic approaches to ethical decision making, that is, emphasizing fetal rights, women's rights, parental desires, or health care providers' capabilities alone, are inadequate in perinatal nursing and that a variety of factors may be relevant in any particular situation.

However, regardless of the inescapable complexity and difficulty of such decisions, it is imperative that the professional nurse collaborate with others to ensure that sound decision making is applied in solving ethical problems. This requires that the nurse acquire a working knowledge of clinical ethics and the ability to recognize ethical dilemmas and, further, that the nurse take an ethical stance in relation to practice and act based on that stance (Archer–Duste 1988). A full discussion of clinical ethics is beyond the scope of this text; however, ethical issues in maternity nursing care will be highlighted throughout.

Litigation and Professional Liability

Professional liability is defined as responsibility for acts of negligence; in health care more specifically, liability concerns the provision of substandard care that results in patient injury. Individual liability includes acts of omission and commission, that is, both failing to do something that should have been done as well as doing something incorrectly or outside of accepted standards of care. The employer may also be liable for employee negligence, even if the employer is without fault in the particular situation in which harm is claimed. Thus, most litigation involving patient claims of injury will name nurses and physicians as well as the hospital itself.

The nurse is liable for her own acts, committed either alone or with others; the nurse is generally not liable for the acts of others in which she was not involved. However, again, many lawsuits name both nurses and physicians, either because the cause of the injury is unclear or because both participated in the actions which the patient claims caused the injury. In obstetric nursing, joint actions are common, especially in emergency situations where assessments and interventions happen very quickly (Styles 1982).

The issue of professional liability has become especially important in nursing in recent years. Until the 1970s nurses were rarely named in litigation. However, the nursing literature and behaviors in the workplace now reflect concerns about the significant legal risk faced by obstetric nurses, especially those practicing in labor and delivery.

Nurses working in labor and delivery are at special risk for litigation for several reasons. First, most lawsuits are based on a claim that the infant has sustained severe birth injury and will require long-term care. Second, most cases center on a claim that substandard care *caused* this injury. Cause and effect are often difficult to prove, but even evidence of substandard care unrelated to the injury may lead to a decision against the care provider. Finally, labor and delivery nurses are especially vulnerable because of the frequent unavailability of physicians. The labor and delivery nurse must collect and communicate information to the physician, who then uses it to decide about medical care; often the time frame between first observation of worrisome signs and actual harm to mother or fetus is very short. Thus, the labor and delivery nurse must be skilled at monitoring, interpreting, and communicating information as well as acting promptly on that information (Rhodes 1986b; Styles 1982).

Certain elements of nursing practice are especially critical and therefore are likely to be susceptible to legal challenge if a claim is later brought against the nurse and/or the birth attendant. These critical nursing errors, which consistently appear in cases that come to litigation, are listed in the accompanying Nursing Alert and are discussed briefly below.

A key legal expectation of the professional nurse is the ability to foresee harm to the patient. Thus, the initial history and examination must be complete so that the nurse may identify risk factors that will influence the process of ongoing nursing care. The nurse must assess the patient's immediate status and recognize situations that require additional action, including communication with the birth attendant. The nurse is legally responsible for initiating and maintaining timely and effective communication regarding the patient's status. This responsibility includes provision of critical information to enable the birth attendant to make reasonable judgments and making requests for assistance specific.

Documentation of patient status and the care rendered is another nursing responsibility with critical legal implications. The patient record is regarded as the only valid record of events from a legal standpoint. The chart must provide evidence that the nurse maintained standards of

NURSING ALERT

Critical Nursing Errors in Cases Involving Litigation

The following nursing errors are found consistently in chart reviews of cases involving charges of professional malpractice:

- Incomplete initial history and physical examination
- Failure to observe and take appropriate action
- Failure to communicate changes in the patient's condition
- Incomplete and/or inadequate documentation
- Failure to use/interpret fetal monitoring appropriately

These errors or omissions may seem unimportant and may not be proved to directly contribute to injury to the patient but may cast enough doubt about clinical care that a judgment against the professional will result.

Chagnon L, Easterwood B: Managing the risks of obstetrical nursing. MCN 11(5):303, 1986

practice in her own care and that policies and procedures were followed. This requires the nurse not only to document problems but also to document what actions were taken to resolve those problems and the effectiveness of those actions.

Appropriate use and interpretation of fetal monitoring has become a central element in contemporary obstetrical nursing practice. There continues to be concern about the widespread use of electronic fetal monitoring in low-risk situations where benefits have not been demonstrated. However, in the presence of any risk factor, continuous fetal monitoring is standard practice, and the nurse is responsible for maintaining appropriate surveillance and for interpreting data on fetal heart rate accurately. This aspect of practice is discussed in detail in Chapter 25.

The most effective way to avoid professional liability in nursing practice on an individual level is through careful, critical assessment of clinical care against recognized standards. At the institutional level, the process of "risk management" involves setting up standards of practice, standards for professional training, and policies and procedures that are designed to reduce or eliminate the chances of patient injury.

However, these measures have clearly not been sufficient, and the rising incidence of litigation in obstetric care in recent years has caused nationwide concern about the economic and human costs of malpractice and liability. Indeed, obstetrics has become one of the three specialities most susceptible to malpractice litigation. This explosion in litigation against care providers has been recent: 80% of all medical malpractice cases in United States history have been filed since 1975. Almost three quarters of all the obstetrician/gynecologists in the United States have been sued, and nearly 30% have had three or more suits filed against them (Nurses' Association of The American College of Obstetricians and Gynecologists 1987). One especially unfortunate result of the malpractice crisis has been the rising cost of liability insurance and its effects on access to obstetrical care (National Commission to Prevent Infant Mortality 1988).

All obstetrical care providers have been affected by extreme increases in liability insurance rates. Unfortunately, this fact has led to unwillingness on the part of some physicians to provide maternity services because of the risk of lawsuits. The low reimbursement rates for Medicaid patients is hastening the departure of physicians from obstetric practice. Even though some states have increased Medicaid payments for maternity, nearly all are still below usual charges and insurance payment rates. This gap in access to care cannot be filled readily by other providers, such as nurse midwives and nurse practitioners, since they likewise are saddled with increasing insurance costs and cannot practice without a collaborative arrangement with a physician.

A few states have enacted legislation aimed at alleviating problems of affordability and availability of liability insurance and of access to maternity care for low-income groups. Examples of such actions include creating state funds to help pay liability insurance premiums for obstetrical care providers who practice in underserved areas and requiring the state government to cover malpractice awards against providers in public clinics. Other states are considering reducing the period of time within which malpractice suits must be brought, known as the statute of limitations; in some states, the statute of limitations begins to apply only when the child reaches the age of majority (usually 18), thus extending the threat of liability over many years (National Commission to Prevent Infant Mortality 1988).

Thus, the nurse who cares for childbearing families must accept the fact that increased risk of malpractice litigation is, for the near future, part of her professional life. Maternity nursing, especially labor and delivery care, requires absolutely current knowledge and understanding of assessment, monitoring, and treatment modalities as well as of identification of risk factors and signs of impending complications. As Rhodes (1986b) states, "the nurse's expertise is the ultimate protection against liability for negligence." A full discussion of legal issues in perinatal nursing is beyond the scope of this text; however, such issues will be highlighted throughout.

THE FUTURE OF MATERNITY NURSING

A multitude of factors is likely to directly affect the future of maternity nursing. The accompanying display highlights factors that are considered driving forces in the future of health care. Projections suggest that the health care delivery system will continue to change in response to profit and cost-containment incentives. The gap between technological developments and the resources to pay for them will continue to increase. The number of underserved will increase, and women and dependent children will continue to be overrepresented in that group.

The future of maternity nursing is likely to include increasing numbers of nurses based outside of the hospital. Nurse specialists will move across settings with clients, although there will continue to be a need for highly technically skilled professional nurses in tertiary settings. The maternity nurse's role in health education and preventative care will expand, especially in providing care to underserved populations (Sullivan et al. 1987).

Forces Impacting the Health Care Delivery System in the Future

Shifting payment systems
Government intervention in cost containment
Increasing competition among health care providers
Technology explosion
Increasing interest in self-help and wellness
Increased supply of physicians
Reduced ability of organizations to provide levels of uncompensated care
Expanded knowledge base related to health and illness
Ethical concerns about technological advances and limited resources
Increasing numbers of educated consumers
Increased complexity of patient needs and severity of patient conditions
Increased numbers of nurse leaders with advanced education
Continued business and industry concern related to health care costs and insurance benefits
Declining pool of college applicants

National Commission on Nursing Implementation Project: A Projection of the Immediate Future in Health Care. Unpublished paper, 1986

However, pressures of cost-containment and the continuing nursing shortage will strain resources in the short term and may compromise standards of practice, especially in facilities serving the poor. Technological advances in high-risk perinatal care will place maternity nurses on the challenging cutting edge of clinical ethics in the areas of fetal therapy and genetics. Escalating malpractice concerns will abate somewhat as governmental actions help to moderate liability risks. Concerns about competition and a shrinking middle-class population will continue to fuel opposition to nurse midwifery and nurse practitioner practice from some quarters in organized medicine.

Research in nursing will enter the mainstream of health sciences, and investigators in maternal–child nursing will lead the way in many areas. Family well-being and the promotion of health during the childbearing years will be a major focus of scientific work. Clinical trials testing the effectiveness of nursing interventions will be conducted on a regular basis. Findings will accumulate to form a well-organized scientific base for practice and will demonstrate the value of nursing services to the childbearing population (Sullivan et al. 1987).

The future of maternity nursing is a challenging and rewarding one. It requires creativity, adaptability, a thirst for knowledge, and a commitment to improving human health by serving the needs of families at a critical transition point: pregnancy and childbirth. The following quotation succinctly describes the present and future role of the maternity nurse in the provision of health care: "Providing health care means articulation with the client in a way that maximizes communication and preservation of personhood in a collaborative effort. That we have not achieved this is obvious. That we can is the challenge" (Hawkins and Higgins 1981).

CHAPTER SUMMARY

The role of the professional nurse in maternity care is complex and challenging, constantly evolving in response to societal needs and expectations, to changes in the health care delivery system, and to technological advances and the ethical dilemmas they bring. The expectations of professional practice include self-regulation, the establishment of standards of education, and the adoption of high levels of individual responsibility and accountability. The opportunities in the field have enabled nurses to create new and innovative careers as nurse specialists and consultants. However, many challenges face professional nurses in the field, including maldistribution of care-providers, sexism, ethical dilemmas and the malpractice litigation crisis. Despite these challenges

the future will require that nurses find new and creative ways to ensure access to high-quality nursing services for all who need them and, by doing so, help protect the health and well-being of the next generation.

STUDY QUESTIONS

1. What are the major roles in which nurses function in maternity care? What types of educational preparation are required for each?
2. What are some characteristics of a profession? Give examples of ways in which nursing is demonstrating those characteristics?
3. Name the specialty organizations that are important in maternity nursing. What functions do they have?
4. Identify five journals that would be important for the maternity nurse to read on a regular basis and explain your rationale.
5. Why is ethical decision making an essential aspect of contemporary maternity nursing? What guidelines describe the nurse's responsibility in ethically difficult patient care situations?

REFERENCES/BIBLIOGRAPHY

American Nurses Association: Standards of Maternal-Child Health Nursing Practice. Kansas City, MO, American Nurses Association, 1983

Archer–Duste H: Clinical ethics: A mandate for nursing. J Perinat Neonatal Nurs 1(3):49, 1988

Aumann G: New changes, new choices: Problems with perinatal technology. J Perinat Neonatal Nurs 1(3):1, 1988

Barnard K: Maternal–child health nursing: A perspective on service, research and training. Zero to Three: Bulletin of the National Center for Clinical Infant Programs 2(4):1, 1982

Greenlaw J: Delivery rooms: For women only? Law Med Health Care 28(Dec):29, 1981

Hawkins J, Higgins L: Maternity and Gynecological Nursing. Philadelphia, JB Lippincott, 1981

Institute of Medicine: Preventing low birthweight. Washington, DC, National Academy Press, 1985

Jacox A: The OTA report: A policy analysis. Nurs Outlook 35(6):262, 1987

National Commission to Prevent Infant Mortality: Malpractice and Liability: An Obstetrical Crisis. Washington, DC, 1988

Nurses' Association of the American College of Obstetricians and Gynecologists: Professional Liability Series. Washington, DC, 1987

Rhodes A: Malpractice suits: Implications for obstetric nurses. MCN 11(3):203, 1986a

Rhodes A: Maternal vs. fetal rights: Implications for nurses. MCN 11(4):243, 1986b

Rhodes A: Liability for the actions of others. MCN 11(5):315, 1986c

Styles M: On Nursing. St. Louis, CV Mosby, 1982

Sullivan T, Lee J, Warnick M, Green L, et al: Nursing 2020: A study of nursing's future. Nurs Outlook 35(5):233, 1987

SUGGESTED READINGS

Andrews L: Legal and ethical aspects of new reproductive technologies. Clin Obstet Gynecol 29(1):190, 1986

Ashley J: Hospitals, Paternalism and the Role of the Nurse. New York, Teachers College Press, 1976

Jacox A: The OTA report: A policy analysis. Nurs Outlook 35(6):262, 1987

Nosek J: Ethics (Special issue). J Perinat Neonatal Nurs 1(3), 1988

Sullivan T, Lee J, Warnick M, Green L, et al: Nursing 2020: A study of nursing's future. Nurs Outlook 35(5):233, 1987

4 conceptual foundations of maternity nursing

LEARNING OBJECTIVES

After studying the material in this chapter, the student should be able to

- Discuss the advantages of using a conceptual framework in clinical practice

- Explain the concept of adaptation and why adaptation theory may be a useful perspective from which to view childbearing families

- Explain the nursing process and its relationship to the nursing care plan

- List nursing diagnoses that may be applicable to the care of childbearing families

- Differentiate nursing diagnoses and collaborative problems

- Explain why teaching is such an important element of maternity nursing care

- Explain the importance of communication and documentation in professional practice

KEY TERMS

Theoretical or conceptual framework

Adaptation

Nursing diagnosis

Collaborative problem

As an emerging health care profession, nursing shares responsibility for the promotion of human health. As discussed in Chapter 3, characteristics of professions on a large scale, such as recognition of standards of practice and self-regulation through involvement in professional and specialty organizations, must therefore also apply to nursing. Other characteristics of professional status address the knowledge base common to a professional group and the organizing frameworks within which these professionals practice.

This chapter focuses on the use of an identifiable knowledge and theory base, the use of a systematic approach to practice, and the documentation of practice in maternity nursing care. Although many elements addressed in this chapter are common to all fields of nursing, some have particular importance in the care of childbearing families.

KNOWLEDGE AND THEORY BASE

Nursing practice is based on knowledge and theory about how humans respond to actual or potential threats to health. This knowledge base and the theories that organize it are constantly changing. Change is part of scientific and professional practice because new knowledge is continually being developed and old methods are continually being reexamined in light of new knowledge. The development of new knowledge in health care is especially dramatic, and health care professionals must update their knowledge base continually. The nurse is accountable for maintaining and updating her knowledge base through continuing study and professional education and for evaluating her own learning needs in relation to her practice setting. As noted in Chapter 1, the scientific advances related to obstetric and perinatal care are proceeding at such a dramatic pace that keeping abreast of the latest developments is a challenge to every professional.

The knowledge and theory base for maternity nursing encompasses the physiologic, psychologic, developmental, and social aspects of childbearing in the context of the family. "Family" may be defined in many ways. However, from a nursing perspective, care must be based on the patients' definitions of family—that is, on whom they identify as most significant in their lives—and not on some "objective" definition.

The knowledge base required for maternity nursing is broad. In the process of giving maternity care, the nurse may interact with people of all ages, from a variety of cultures, and of varying educational backgrounds and expectations, since family units vary in all those ways.

Because the knowledge base required for caring for childbearing families is so broad, it is essential that the professional nurse have a way of organizing this knowledge and of looking at families and the health challenges they face in a systematic fashion. The following section discusses the importance of conceptual frameworks and theories in nursing, emphasizing adaptation as a useful organizing principle in maternity care.

Use of Conceptual Frameworks and Theories

A professional discipline operates from a body of knowledge that is developed and organized in such a way that it can be utilized by its practitioners. Such bodies of knowledge are usually defined by commonly accepted views or perspectives. Often these perspectives are seen in conceptual frameworks and theories used in practice. These perspectives change over time as the field develops and more knowledge is generated.

For example, medicine has historically operated from a rather narrow biological perspective on health and illness. This view emphasized the physical sciences and concentrated on biophysical methods of diagnosis and treatment of illness. This perspective has been quite successful in stimulating research and opening new frontiers of treatment. However, as chronic conditions and diseases of lifestyle become the dominant health threats, other perspectives integrating behavioral and psychologic explanations of illness have begun to gain acceptance in medicine.

Nursing is a young, still rapidly evolving field, and its knowledge base is just beginning to be developed and organized. There is still no one guiding perspective in nursing, although much progress has been made in recent years with a widely accepted definition of nursing and with the identification of *person, health, environment,* and *nursing* as the major domains of interest for nursing. The process of knowledge development in nursing is well under way, and conceptual frameworks and theories are increasingly utilized in nursing practice as a way to help organize necessary knowledge and orient it toward patient problems.

The terms *conceptual framework* and *theory* simply refer to the organizing tools available to the professional. A conceptual framework is defined as a global view of phenomena of interest in a field. A conceptual framework includes *concepts,* which are mental images or ideas, and a set of statements that show how these concepts are linked together. Individual nurses, as they become expert in their practice, often develop their own conceptual frameworks or their own way of looking at patients and families. An example of how a conceptual framework can be used in maternity nursing is shown in the accompanying display. Another example of a conceptual framework that is useful in practice can be found in Chapter 36,

Advantages of Using a Conceptual Framework to Guide Clinical Practice: An Example

Nurse A is a good maternity clinician and reads articles on such topics as sibling visitation and breast-feeding in order to keep informed about advances in her field. She has found that most new mothers, if given a little reassurance and some basic tips on baby care, can feed and care for their babies fairly well when they return home after delivery.

Nurse B is also a good clinician. However, she bases her practice not only on her experience but also on a conceptual framework she has developed. Within this framework, each mother–baby pair is viewed as a unique puzzle, and the various ways in which their personalities, temperaments, and behaviors fit together are analyzed.

Consequently, in helping new mothers feed and handle their babies in the hospital, Nurse B not only gives these mothers basic information and reassurance but also spends time pointing out to them the unique infant behaviors (cues) and maternal responses that she has observed. In addition, Nurse B asks mothers to discuss their own observations about how their babies react to feeding and handling. She helps new mothers to respond to their babies as unique individuals and to recognize when they have done a good job.

Mothers who are under the care of Nurse A and Nurse B may not seem to behave that differently while in the hospital, but after discharge differences may begin to appear. When a new or unexpected situation arises, such as an infant crying bout, mothers under the care of Nurse B may be more confident and better able to understand their babies' responses and interpret their babies' needs than the mothers under the care of Nurse A. Although both Nurse A and Nurse B provide good care to new mothers, Nurse B's use of a conceptual framework gives her care something extra.

Advantages of Using a Conceptual Framework

Nurse A	Nurse B
(Does not use a conceptual framework)	(Uses a conceptual framework)
Knows current facts about practice	Knows current facts about practice and organizes these facts into a meaningful framework
Teaches standard parent education	Teaches standard parent education but adapts this teaching to her conceptual framework of "mother–baby puzzles"
Gives each mother the facts and skills she needs to know to care for her baby	Gives each mother the facts and skills she needs to help her understand and respond to her baby's unique needs
Teaches mothers what to do in standard situations	Teaches mothers the skills of observation that are relevant to both standard and unexpected situations

Avant K, Walker L: The practicing nurse and conceptual frameworks. MCN 9:87, 1984. Copyright 1984, American Journal of Nursing Company. Reprinted with permission.

focusing on family adaptation in the period after the birth of an infant.

A theory can be thought of as a more specific and a better-defined version of a conceptual framework. A theory is also made up of concepts linked together by statements, but concepts in a theory are well-defined, specific, and usually measurable in some way. In addition, the relationships between concepts in a theory are more precisely and systematically stated. This allows theories to be tested and refined through research, while conceptual frameworks are usually too general and their concepts too vaguely defined to be tested scientifically.

Adaptation: An Organizing Perspective

Throughout this text, *adaptation* is used as an organizing perspective on the childbearing family. Adaptation theory is a widely accepted perspective in psychology and has provided the basis for work on stress and coping, crisis intervention, and other widely recognized areas of research and practice. Nurse theorists have proposed and tested nursing models based on adaptation theory (Roy 1976; Johnson 1980). This text uses a conceptual framework focusing on adaptation (St. Louis University 1979) as a way to help organize the broad and varied knowledge base needed to provide nursing care to childbearing families.

Adaptation is defined here as the capacity to modify behavior and to change the environment, when necessary, to meet needs; as such, adaptation is a basic characteristic of life. Adaptation is an active process of maintaining optimum conditions over time in relationship to constantly changing demands.

Adaptation occurs in individuals and families and involves physiologic, psychologic, sociocultural, and spiritual dimensions. Most life changes require adaptation in most or all dimensions simultaneously. The quality of adaptation is a function of the nature of the stimulus and the dimensions it impacts as well as of the individual's capacity for change.

The particular characteristics of individual adaptation express the person's uniqueness; thus, human adaptation is endlessly variable. Depending on the resources available to the individual, adaptive responses can be adequate or inadequate, functional or dysfunctional. Health, illness, and survival depend upon the quality of adaptation that is possible for the individual or family. Health implies functional or effective responses that result in a dynamic equilibrium, characterized by maximum potential for living and wholeness. Illness implies dysfunctional or ineffective responses that result in disequilibrium, characterized by reduced potential for living and distress.

To some extent, the individual determines what stimuli will be attended to, the mode of adaptation, and the pace of change. However, in general, the greater the number of changes occurring in a given period of time, the more difficult it is for the individual to adapt. Even when the outcome of adaptation is positive, the process itself may be stressful. Previous successful adaptation is likely to expand the individual's repertoire of adaptive responses and contribute to more flexibility and enhanced ability to meet future demands. In contrast, inability to adapt effectively further reduces the individual's resources and compromises well-being, making future adaptation even more difficult.

Adaptation in the Childbearing Family

For several reasons, as will be discussed in succeeding chapters, adaptation is an especially useful organizing perspective when considering the childbearing family. Childbearing and early child rearing are normally periods of concentrated and sometimes intense physiologic and psychologic change. The pregnant woman must adapt to hormonal changes followed by pronounced physical and emotional changes as pregnancy progresses. Her partner must also adjust to the woman's changes, as well as to the new expectations and pressures of becoming a father. The experience of pregnancy also touches other family members who must accept the reality of the expected child and the role changes that will result.

The process of birth and recovery is also a sequence of complex physiologic and physical adaptations for both mother and newborn. Just as pronounced are the necessary adaptations of mother, father, and newborn during the first 3 months after delivery: the parents learn to interpret and respond to the infant's cues and to integrate the parental role into their lives while maintaining other

roles; the infant begins to master early communication skills and integrate physical and emotional development into a coherent whole.

The concept of adaptation is a useful organizing perspective not only for clinical practice but also for research and scholarship in maternity nursing. Most of the nurse scientists whose work appears in the Suggested Readings for this chapter, and which will be discussed further in upcoming chapters, have made substantial contributions to knowledge about childbearing families through research that has included elements of adaptation theory.

Research and Scholarship

Another attribute of a profession is vigorous activity by its members in the field of research and scholarship. Research and scholarship are essential to any profession because these activities build and renew the knowledge base from which its members operate. Research is defined here as the systematic collection, analysis, and reporting of new information, while scholarship is defined as the systematic study, evaluation, and utilization of existing information. Until recently, most of the knowledge taught in maternity nursing was knowledge "borrowed" from other disciplines. However, as more nurses prepare to engage in research and scholarship, that trend is changing.

While large-scale nursing research projects require additional preparation in research methods at the graduate level, nurses in clinical practice are in the best position to identify pressing nursing care problems and to observe and document effects of different types of nursing care. Nurses in practice can also make a significant contribution to the field by systematic analysis and reporting of effects of nursing care in single cases. This is needed because the profession is only beginning to describe and categorize nursing problems or diagnoses. Published case studies enable clinicians to compare interventions and outcomes and to share knowledge that would otherwise not be communicated outside one particular setting. This type of communication and comparison of practice adds to the accumulation of nursing knowledge and enables nurses to develop and test solutions to clinical problems much more rapidly than does practicing in isolation.

Nurses in maternity care are beginning to focus concerted attention on problems in clinical practice. There has been a dramatic increase in emphasis on scholarship and organized research efforts, as staff nurses are encouraged to incorporate new knowledge into clinical care and nurses in clinical leadership positions in many teaching hospitals are expected to engage in clinical research. Specialty journals now publish scholarly clinical and research articles regularly. Nursing organizations are identifying priority research problems facing nurses in clinical

Research Priorities in Perinatal Nursing

Nurses' Association of the American College of Obstetricians and Gynecologists (NAACOG), the specialty organization of obstetric, gynecologic, and neonatal nurses, established the following research priorities in 1988 which identify areas of particular significance to the specialty, such as the nursing process, interventions, and outcomes of care:

Maternity Nursing

- Prenatal care
- Low birth weight
- Human immunodeficiency virus (HIV)-positive mothers and infants
- Adolescent pregnancy and pre-pregnancy counseling/ care
- Drug and other substance abuse during pregnancy
- Stressors and their effects during pregnancy
- Utilization of care by pregnant population

Women's Health Nursing

- Prevention of sexually transmitted diseases (STDs) in women, particularly the prevention of HIV/acquired immunodeficiency syndrome (AIDS); and care and support of women and families with STDs
- Psychosocial and physical experience of women in midlife and later years
- Behavioral and environmental factors influencing the health of minority women, including ethnic and cultural minorities and social minorities, such as the homeless and other vulnerable groups
- Women's adaptations to multiple roles and related health outcomes

- Impact of reproductive technology and reproductive pharmacology on women's health over the life span

Neonatal Nursing

- Low birth weight infants and infants in families known to experience high rates of disease, dysfunction, and death
- Promotion of growth and development in all settings, including the hospital and the home
- Short- and long-term consequences of care and parenting
- Evaluation of current and evolving models of home care in terms of quality of patient outcomes and cost of care

The Professional Role of Nurses in Delivery of Care

- Context of nursing practice, including constraints and support in the professional environment and effects of malpractice
- Factors affecting recruitment, retention, and attrition
- Alternative educational pathways and new roles for nurses providing care
- Description of role and scope of current nursing practice in various settings
- Dissemination and utilization of research findings

---

practice (see the accompanying display) and setting aside funding for important studies focusing on priority problems.

The process of knowledge generation is especially exciting in maternity care because the scope of needed knowledge is broad and multifaceted. Throughout this text, nursing research will be highlighted to acquaint the student with current work in the field.

SYSTEMATIC APPROACH TO PRACTICE

In addition to the utilization and generation of an organized knowledge and theory base, a profession is expected to foster a systematic approach to practice. In nursing this is best exemplified by the use of the nursing process as an agreed upon standard of practice and by the

use of the more recent development of diagnostic categories specific to nursing. The following section addresses the nursing process, emphasizing elements that will be utilized throughout the text.

The Nursing Process

Systematic practice in the care of patients and their families can be seen in the use of the nursing process and its written form, the nursing care plan. The *nursing process,* the application of the problem-solving process in clinical nursing care, is the way in which nurses ensure that patient problems are systematically assessed and treated. The nursing process focuses the nurse's attention on a logical progression of decisions and actions aimed at resolving specific patient problems. The steps in the process are to assess the patient's status and to identify problems, to plan and implement appropriate nursing care, and to evaluate the effectiveness of that care. The process is circular, with initial assessment, intervention,

Overview of the Nursing Process

Assessment

- Collect data
- Validate data
- Organize data
- Identify patterns

Diagnosis

- Analyze data
- Formulate nursing diagnoses
- Identify collaborative problems

Planning/Implementation

- Set priorities
- Establish goals
- Determine interventions
- Document the plan of care
- Continue data collection
- Perform nursing interventions
- Document nursing care
- Maintain current plan of care

Evaluation

- Establish outcome criteria
- Evaluate goal achievement
- Identify variables affecting goal achievement
- Modify/terminate plan of care

and evaluation leading to adjustments in care and reassessment of the patient's status.

The *nursing care plan* is the detailed written form of the nursing process. The care plan documents the identified patient problem, the planned intervention and expected outcomes, and the techniques for evaluating the effectiveness of the care. Nursing care plans may also be broken down in a variety of ways, but the underlying principles remain the same. The care plan enables the nurse to communicate the plan of care to others, to document the care delivered, and to evaluate the effectiveness of her care against specified criteria, called *expected outcomes*.

Use of the nursing process in maternity nursing is identical to its use in other areas of nursing. However, nurses practice in a wide variety of settings in maternity care. The pace of movement through the process and the type of information available to the nurse will vary from setting to setting and in accordance with the nature of the patient problems with which she deals.

For instance, during labor and delivery, the process of assessment, intervention, and evaluation may occur over periods of only minutes as the mother's physiologic status and behavioral patterns change. At birth, nursing assessment and intervention may appear to be nearly simultaneous as the nurse assists the neonate in establishing respiration. The labor and delivery nurse usually has access to the patient's prenatal record and can often directly observe interactions among family members as she assesses the mother's status. The labor and delivery nurse often sees immediate results of her care. However, she typically has contact with the family for a period of only hours and may not have the opportunity to evaluate long-term outcomes of her care.

In an outpatient setting, such as prenatal clinic or a home-visit follow-up program, a nurse may have contact with the mother and sometimes with family members over weeks or months. Her clinical problem solving will stretch over repeated contacts. She may not see immediate results of her intervention but may see movement toward long-term goals over time. The clinic or home-visit nurse typically has access to the complete patient record but may not have many opportunities to observe family interaction.

Other nurses working in more specialized clinics, such as antenatal assessment units where amniocentesis or ultrasound tests are done, will have only single contacts with mothers and their families. Their nursing assessments may be focused on a particular identified problem, and they may depend heavily on written data collected by others. Nurses in such specialized settings must rely on information in the patient record to evaluate the effectiveness of their care.

The steps in the nursing process may be named or broken down slightly differently in other texts. The terminology used throughout this text is as follows:

- Assessment
- Diagnosis
- Planning and Implementation
- Evaluation

Assessment

Assessment of patient status is the initial step in nursing care. *Assessment* includes data collection and analysis. The nurse first collects data in a variety of ways.

- Completion of a nursing history
- Interview and observation
- Measurement of vital signs and physiologic indicators

- Review of medical record
- Use of standardized assessment tools

Standardized assessment tools are becoming available to maternity nurses to assess the needs of childbearing women and their families in a variety of ways. Usually these assessment tools are first used in research and then are demonstrated to be useful in planning and delivering clinical nursing care. Some commonly used assessment tools in maternity care are listed in Table 4–1.

Diagnosis

The nurse analyzes data obtained through assessment and identifies patient problems, which may be thought of as health needs for which the patient sees no ready solu-tion without expert assistance, that may require nursing or medical care. This process is called *diagnosis,* and the conclusions the nurse draws may include nursing problems that the nurse may appropriately treat as well as possible medical problems that must be referred to a physician for care.

The classification of nursing problems into diagnostic categories began in 1973 with the First Conference on Nursing Diagnosis, and the work continues to the present. Diagnostic categories in nursing are seen as an important step toward standardization of assessments and the establishment of a common terminology related to patient needs and appropriate nursing care.

Nursing Diagnoses

As recommended by Carpenito (1987), the term *nursing diagnosis* will be used throughout this book to refer to a specific statement of a problem that the nurse can legally identify and for which the nurse can order definitive

Table 4–1   **Examples of Assessment Tools Useful in Maternity Nursing**

Tool	Purpose	Description
1. Maternal–Fetal Attachment Scale (parent self-report)	Measures aspects of maternal attachment to fetus A paternal version has been developed and tested	Contains 33 written scales focusing on differentiation of self from fetus, interaction with fetus, attribution of characteristics to fetus, giving of self, and role taking
2. Apgar Scoring System	Allows quick, comprehensive evaluation of neonate's immediate adaptation to birth process and extrauterine life Indicates extent to which newborn requires more vigorous management or resuscitation	Rates five components (heart rate, respiratory effort, muscle tone, reflex irritability, and color) on a scale from 0–2 Ratings are done at 1 and 5 minutes after birth Scores of 0–3 reflect severe distress; 4–6, moderate distress; and 7–10, mild or absent distress
3. Brazelton Neonatal Behavior Assessment Scale (BNBAS; completed by professional)	Assesses social/interactive behavior of newborns from birth to 1 month May be used to examine early individual differences in infants Has been used in nursing as a strategy for teaching parents about newborn capabilities	Examination guide contains 27 reflex items, 27 behavioral response items, and ratings of infant's predominant states, need for stimulation, and self-quieting activities. Typical exam requires 30 minutes Training is necessary to establish skill in evaluation
4. Neonatal Perception Inventories (NPI; parent self-report)	Measures maternal perception of newborn, comparing a hypothetical "average" baby with perception of own baby Based on assumption that mothers ideally will rate their own newborn better than average	Written scale asks for rating of own baby and average baby on six characteristics: sleeping, feeding, spitting up, elimination, crying, and predictability of behavior. Useful in combination with other assessment of maternal–newborn relationship
5. Home Observation Measurement of Environment (HOME, birth–3 years; completed by professional)	Identifies aspects of environment that enhance development of infants	Observation of 1 hour in home on six subscales focusing on maternal responsiveness and organization of physical (especially play) environment

References for additional information:
(1) Cranley M: Development of a tool for the measurement of maternal attachment during pregnancy. Nurs Res 30:281, 1981
(2–5) Humenick S: Analysis of Current Assessment Strategies in the Health Care of Young Children and Childbearing Families. Norwalk, CT, Appleton-Century-Crofts, 1982

NURSING RESEARCH

intervention to maintain the health state or reduce, eliminate, or prevent alterations. The following selected nursing diagnoses (part of the list approved June 1988 by the North American Nursing Diagnosis Association) are of particular use to the nurse in maternity care:

Nursing Diagnoses Related to Mother, Father, Family

- Anxiety
- Bowel elimination, altered: constipation
- Breast-feeding, ineffective
- Comfort, altered: pain
- Coping, family: potential for growth
- Coping, family: ineffective, compromised
- Decisional conflict
- Fatigue
- Fear
- Grieving, anticipatory
- Grieving, dysfunctional
- Health maintenance, altered
- Infection, potential for
- Injury, potential for
- Knowledge deficit
- Nutrition, altered: less than body requirements more than body requirements
- Parenting, altered: actual/potential
- Self-concept disturbance
- Sexuality patterns, altered
- Urinary elimination, altered patterns of

Nursing Diagnoses Related to the Neonate

- Body temperature, altered, potential
- Bowel elimination, altered: diarrhea
- Comfort, altered: pain
- Respiratory function, potential altered
- Infection, potential for
- Injury, potential for
- Nutrition, altered: less than body requirements more than body requirements
- Tissue integrity, impaired: actual/potential

Collaborative Problems

The diagnostic phase of the nursing process may yield both nursing diagnoses and collaborative problems, as shown in Figure 4–1. Collaborative problems are physiologic complications that are or may be present in conjunction with pathology or as a result of treatment.

The following is a statement of a collaborative problem:

- Potential complication: Sepsis

When the nurse is monitoring for a cluster of complications, the problem may be stated as follows:

- Potential complication of circumcision: Hemorrhage, Hypothermia

Nurses anticipate and monitor for the onset and status of collaborative problems and work with medicine and other disciplines for definitive treatment of collaborative problems.

Differentiation

Carpenito (1990) differentiates between nursing diagnoses and collaborative problems, as illustrated in Figure 4–2. Both types of problems may require specific nursing

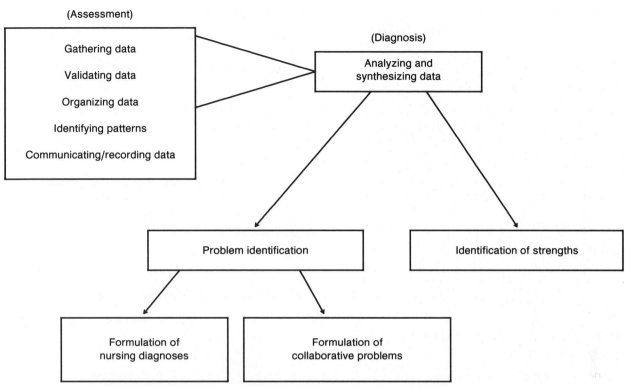

Figure 4–1. The diagnostic phase of the nursing process, resulting in formulation of either nursing diagnoses or collaborative problems. (Alfaro R: Nursing Diagnosis and the Nursing Process: A Step-by-Step Guide, 2nd ed. Philadelphia, JB Lippincott, 1990)

Differentiating Nursing Diagnoses From Other Client Problems

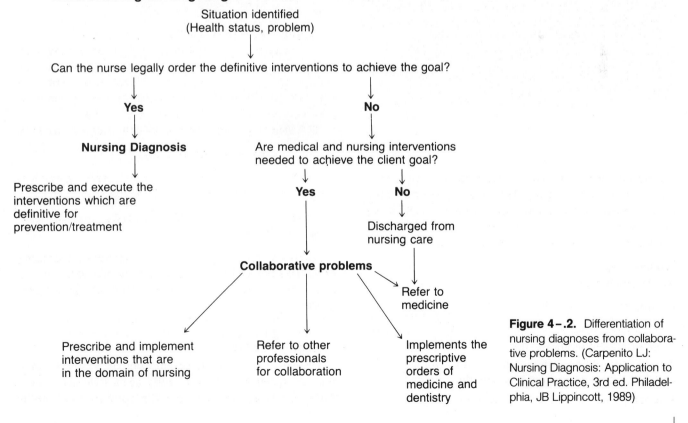

Figure 4–.2. Differentiation of nursing diagnoses from collaborative problems. (Carpenito LJ: Nursing Diagnosis: Application to Clinical Practice, 3rd ed. Philadelphia, JB Lippincott, 1989)

Nursing Diagnoses in Maternity Nursing

Nursing diagnoses have three components:

Title

The title offers a concise description of the patient's actual, potential, or possible state of health and often reflects a change of status by use of the words "impaired," "alteration," or "deficit."

Actual: Problem is present.

Potential: Problem may occur, and monitoring is indicated.

Possible: Problem may be present, and more data are needed to establish patient status.

Example

Alteration in nutrition: less than body requirements

Fear:

Potential alteration in family processes:

Etiologic/Contributing Factors

These are factors that appear to be causing or contributing to the patient's problem. Since the actual causes of patient problems are not always known with certainty, the words "related to" are used. This points out a relationship between the patient problem and the factors listed but does *not* state a *causal* relationship. When etiologic/contributing factors are unknown, that can be stated.

Example

Alteration in nutrition: less than body requirements related to morning nausea and vomiting

Fear: related to possible need for cesarean birth

Potential alteration in family processes: related to birth of a family member

Defining Characteristics

Defining characteristics are a list of signs and symptoms that have been observed in the patient. Lists of defining characteristics appear in guides to nursing diagnoses; however, not all defining characteristics need be present in a particular patient in order to use a diagnosis in that patient's care.

Example

Alteration in nutrition: less than body requirements related to morning nausea

Defining characteristics:

- 16 weeks' gestation
- Weight loss of 2 lb

Fear: related to possible cesarean birth

Defining characteristics:

- Expressed feelings of loss of control
- Increasing questioning about birth

Potential alteration in family processes: related to birth of a family member

Defining characteristics:

- Expressed concerns about meeting emotional/physical needs of members
- Expressed concerns about sources of help

Common Errors in Nursing Diagnosis

Nursing diagnoses are *not*:

Medical diagnoses, such as diabetes mellitus

Treatments, such as fetal monitoring or cesarean birth

Diagnostic studies, such as sonography

Nursing diagnoses should *not*:

Make judgmental statements or assertions that may have legal implications.

Examples of Incorrect Nursing Diagnoses

Potential alteration in parenting due to mother's low IQ

Fear related to father's illegal immigration status

---

intervention. Throughout this text, nursing diagnoses and collaborative problems (usually in the form of *Potential complication: [specify]*) will be discussed for specific groups of patients and will form the bases of nursing care plans. Priorities for any particular patient must be determined by the conditions, the nurse, and the client. The nursing care plans throughout this text will list patient problems for a class of patients in order by clinical priority.

Planning and Implementation

Planning for nursing care requires the nurse to set priorities among the range of patient problems she may have identified. The patient's condition dictates which problems have immediate priority and which ones can be dealt with later. For example, in life-threatening situations the nurse limits assessment and intervention to obtaining data necessary for emergency intervention. More complete assessment is delayed until the patient is physiologically stable. When a patient is in acute physical or psychologic distress, the nurse assesses the cause of the distress and then takes action to reduce the stressor before attempting further assessment.

In most maternity nursing situations, the patient is not in a life-threatening situation or in acute distress. For this reason, the maternity nurse must be particularly careful to involve the patient in setting priorities and planning for her own care. Outside the narrow range of life-threatening situations, the nurse may find Maslow's (1943) hierarchy of human needs useful in identifying the patient's priorities for nursing care. This hierarchy organizes needs into five levels: physiologic needs, safety needs, and the needs for love, self-esteem, and self-actualization. Physiologic and safety needs are seen as basic. Maslow theorized that the person will be preoccupied with and motivated by unmet basic needs. His or her attention will be focused on those basic needs until they are met. As needs are met, the person's attention and behavior are gradually reorganized, and a new, higher need will emerge.

During pregnancy many patients and families will experience the needs to feel safe, to maintain the integrity of the love relationship, and to maintain a positive self-image during the dramatic changes childbearing creates in the family system. Priorities for nursing care will depend in large part on the *patient's* perception of her situation. The plan of care will likely focus on providing information and counseling the woman about ways to meet her needs for love and self-esteem. During childbirth the woman's needs may be focused more at the physiologic and safety levels. The patient's perceptions of her needs may be unclear or difficult to express, and the nurse must rely on her assessment skills to establish priorities for nursing care. The plan of care during this time will *first* be directed at maintaining physiologic integrity and providing for safety needs, then at needs for love and security as provided by family members.

An essential aspect of planning care is the establishment of *expected outcomes*. Expected outcomes express what is to be accomplished within a specified time period. Expected outcomes are derived from the problems identified in the diagnostic phase and will be used to evaluate the effectiveness of care on an ongoing basis. Expected outcomes of care must be stated in such a way that a third party could determine whether or not they match the actual outcomes. Throughout this text, expected outcomes for common patient problems will be specified in relation to nursing care and will be listed in related nursing care plans for particular groups of patients.

The nurse is responsible for documenting specific patient problems, interventions, and expected outcomes for each problem. This plan of care is usually communicated to colleagues through verbal and written reporting. Some institutions have standardized care plans for groups of patients; the nurse then individualizes these based on her assessment of patient needs.

Once a plan of care is established, the nurse implements the plan through interventions directed at priority nursing diagnoses and/or collaborative problems. Effective nursing intervention requires the nurse to have an accurate understanding of underlying physiologic and psychosocial principles and to have skills in monitoring and observation, in administering physical care and comfort measures, and in communicating clearly and sensitively with childbearing women and their families.

Patient Teaching for Self-Care

Most childbearing women are healthy and simply require assistance in managing their own health through the normal psychologic and physical transition of pregnancy, childbirth, and postbirth recovery. A nursing intervention of major importance during pregnancy is *teaching for effective self-care*. Teaching women and their families how to care for themselves effectively is a nursing responsibility. The nurse must understand principles of adult learning and use them in her patient teaching.

The nurse plans and implements teaching based on the following considerations:

- Patient/family learning needs
- Principles of teaching/learning
- Physical and psychologic condition of patient/family
- Sociocultural factors

**Teaching for Effective Self-Care:
Principles of Adult Learning**

Learning may be defined as a change in behavior.

Learning requires activity on the part of the learner.

Learning is directly affected by the physical and social environment.

Learners ultimately learn what *they* actively desire to learn.

Learners are motivated when they understand and accept the purpose of the learning situation.

Learners are motivated when they can see the usefulness of the learning in their own terms.

Gorman A: Teachers and Learners in the Interactive Process of Education. Boston, Allyn and Bacon, 1969

Guidelines for Effective Patient Teaching

- Determine the individual learning needs of each patient on the basis of an assessment of her knowledge and concerns.
- Set priorities. Consider what is most important for your patient to learn and how much time is available to teach it, then teach the most important information first.
- Provide a comfortable environment. This may mean ensuring privacy and communicating to the patient that you are interested in her and are willing to listen and answer her questions.
- Allow the patient the opportunity to absorb the teaching. If possible, review the teaching later in the day or the next day to see how much was remembered and to answer any questions.
- Use simple terminology. Be sure the patient understands the words you use and remember that many medical and nursing terms may be new to the patient.
- Reinforce your teaching with visual aids. Many facilities have audiovisual aids that can supplement or replace some direct patient teaching. Printed materials are always helpful, since they can augment teaching or provide additional information. However, printed materials must be at an appropriate reading level and in suitable language.
- Include the family in teaching whenever possible. Family members need most types of information just as much as the mother does.
- Always document your teaching. Charting the patient teaching you have done provides documentation of the care the patient has received and alerts other staff members to continuing learning needs.

Patient/Family Learning Needs. The unique learning needs of the patient and family must be clearly identified in order for teaching to be effective (Fig. 4–3). The nurse should not assume that all families want or need the same information. Each family member brings a wealth of life experiences to the process of childbearing. The nurse who teaches in rote fashion without consideration of individual differences will not adequately meet patients' learning needs.

Principles of Teaching/Learning. Major principles of teaching/learning are used by the nurse in patient teaching. The patient's existing knowledge level should be identified before teaching starts. The nurse should create a physical and emotional climate conducive to learning and should offer positive feedback and support. Demonstrations of specific self-care tasks should be pro-

vided. Perhaps most important, the nurse should be able to recognize signs of readiness for learning and make full use of teaching opportunities.

Physical/Psychologic Conditions. Teaching for effective self-care and discharge teaching must take physical and emotional conditions into account. The presence of pain, physiologic disturbance, fatigue, or worry will affect the family member's ability to learn. A crisis situation, such as an unexpected complication, will greatly diminish the family's ability to assimilate information, and information may have to be repeated two or three times before it is taken in.

The length of contract the nurse has with the family will also determine the extent and depth of teaching that is possible. Short prenatal visits may preclude in-depth teaching in some settings. Shortened hospital stays have the same effect. In these situations the nurse must identify and cover essential points of information and establish ongoing follow-up with family members so that their teaching needs can be met.

Sociocultural Factors. Education, financial status, religious beliefs, and ethnic background are factors the nurse must take into account before patient teaching is begun. It is essential that the nurse convey her recognition of and respect for family values and belief systems. Knowledge of the family members' educational levels will guide the nurse in teaching approaches and the selection of appropriate instructional materials. The nurse should also have knowledge of the family's economic resources in order to make appropriate recommendations for supplies and equipment.

The nurse must recognize the learning needs of the father and other family members. Although she may have only limited contact with the father or spouse, he needs emotional support and skillful teaching during the child-

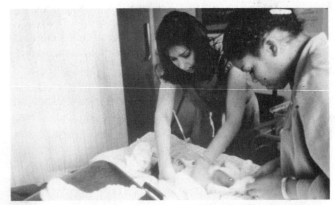

Figure 4–3. Nurse–parent teaching. The nurse provides valuable teaching about newborn care and parenting as she assists parents in bathing and changing their newborn for the first time. (Photo: Kathy Sloane)

bearing year. Many men have little or no experience with childbearing and are especially nervous about their ability to care for a small infant. The nurse can utilize specific strategies to help the father feel more comfortable and to encourage him to express his own learning needs. The nurse should avoid focusing exclusively on the woman and should become familiar with common learning needs of other family members so that teaching can be planned for and implemented when opportunities arise.

Evaluation

Once interventions have been implemented, the nurse must evaluate the effects of her intervention with the patient by comparing the expected outcomes with outcomes actually observed. Nursing evaluation of actual outcomes may then result in a reassessment and adjustment in the plan of care or in a refocusing on other identified problems if care has been successful.

As a professional, the nurse is also accountable for examining the effectiveness of her care and for exploring ways in which care can be improved. *Quality assurance programs,* in which records are audited and actual care is evaluated against standards of care, are one mechanism that nurses use to examine the quality of care. *Clinical research* is another way in which nurses examine their own practice, either by testing the effectiveness of care or by generating new knowledge on which care can be based.

DOCUMENTATION OF EFFECTS OF NURSING CARE

Documentation of practice is basically the process of communication at three levels: communication between the nurse and the patient about nursing care, communication between the nurse and her colleagues, and communication between the nurse and the wider community. Effective communication allows the consumer or the wider community to hold the professional nurse accountable for her practice and allows knowledge to accumulate within the profession in a way that leads to improvement in care.

Communication and Accountability in Nursing Practice

If documentation of practice did not exist, consumers and society at large would have to rely on the individual professional's determination of her own effectiveness. For professionals who are always ethical and objective in their evaluation of their practice, this system would work well enough, but it would not protect society from professionals without such high standards. Without communication among professionals through scientific publications and meetings, knowledge would accumulate very slowly. Improvements in care would be discovered more by trial and error than by inquiry based on established knowledge. The benefits of one nurse's discoveries would be unavailable to other nurses who might effectively use that knowledge.

Each of these levels of communication—nurse–patient, nurse–colleague, and nurse–community—are important in maternity nursing. Failure on any level will diminish the effectiveness of nursing care. Whether the consequences are short-term for one particular patient or

LEGAL/ETHICAL CONSIDERATIONS

Documentation of Discharge Teaching and Legal Liability

The nurse is faced with the task of completing an ever-expanding discharge teaching plan for parents within a contracting time frame. Parent education is ideally begun in the antepartum period, but it is the nurse's responsibility at the time of discharge to ensure that essential elements of infant care and safety have been reviewed and that parents have demonstrated competency in basic infant care skills. This challenge arises in a period when parents are increasingly willing to litigate when they believe that negligence on the part of health professionals has resulted in the injury or death of their infant.

Documentation of all aspects of discharge planning and teaching is critical to ensure that no important aspect of parent teaching is overlooked; it constitutes a legal record for use by the health care facility if a lawsuit is instigated. Although the discharge plan is always individualized, utilizing a formal checklist or teaching plan assists the clinician to use her time efficiently. It is also essential in today's litigious climate to retain a written record of the areas of infant care and safety that were covered.

Parents should also be provided with written materials that review and reinforce the teaching plan and with the phone numbers of important resources. If a language barrier is identified, a translator should be used and, whenever possible, educational materials should be given to the family in their primary language. These actions will enhance the quality of the discharge plan and reduce legal risks for the practitioner.

of longer duration for the community as a whole will depend on where the failure occurs.

Nurse–Patient Communication

Communication between nurse and patient is basic in nursing practice. Through communication the nurse builds a trusting relationship with patients and assists them in meeting their own health needs. Principles of therapeutic communication in maternity care are the same as those needed in other areas of nursing. However, the philosophy of family-centered maternity care requires the nurse to communicate not only with the woman but also with her family members, often in situations where they feel uncertain or fearful and need increased support.

Communication between the nurse and the patient also reflects the extent to which the nurse considers the patient an individual who controls her own health and who can make decisions about her own care. If the nurse believes this, then she must provide complete explanations for decisions that have to be made and must work with the woman and her family to set priorities for their care.

The issue of *informed consent* is an especially important one in relation to labor and birth care. The woman (and her support person, if applicable) should be informed about the need for any procedure — why it is done, its adverse reactions (if any), and any reasonable alternatives — before the procedure is begun. Then the woman's verbal or written consent must be obtained. Only in extreme emergencies can failure to obtain informed consent be justified (Trandel–Korenchuk, 1982).

Nurse–Colleague Communication

Communication between the nurse and her colleagues is of the greatest importance to the safety and overall effectiveness of medical and nursing care. This communication occurs in a variety of ways: team meetings, patient rounds, staff reports, and care plans. However, the most important way of documenting care and communicating to others is the patient's *medical record*. The medical record should include all pertinent information on the patient's condition and should outline the care that is planned or has been implemented and the effects of that care.

The content of hospital records may vary depending on state regulations. Accreditation bodies may require that specific types of information appear in any medical record.

Although in most respects charting in maternity nursing is similar to charting in other settings, some specialized types of record keeping are used in labor and delivery because of the rapid, time-limited changes that occur with labor and birth. Unit IV, Adaptation in the Intrapartal Period, includes samples of labor records now in use.

Usually the patient record is the major communication mechanism between medical and nursing staff. Consequently, clear, concise, and complete nursing records are absolutely essential to safe and effective health care. Nursing observations should be charted carefully, communicating what was seen and, if appropriate, what was inferred. For example, the entry "patient appears comfortable" is meaningless: it communicates no factual information. However, the entry "patient up to bathroom $\times 2$ without assistance, refused pain medication, and states she is comfortable" gives useful information about the patient's condition and the nursing care that has been given.

Nursing care plans are also a means of communication among colleagues. Care plans are important because nursing has 24-hour accountability for care of patients, and communication must occur among several nurses who will be involved in a particular patient's care. The care plan should be comprehensive and detailed so that any nurse in the setting can utilize the care plan to organize her care, even if she has not had previous contact with that patient. This is especially important in maternity

NURSING RESEARCH

Congruence Between Intershift Reports and Patients' Actual Conditions

After listening to 57 intershift reports on 19 different units of an 800-bed metropolitan teaching hospital, the actual patient condition was verified and compared by an investigator with the information communicated during report. Of 2952 items of patient status communicated in report and verified later, the overall congruence (or agreement) rate was 70%, with rates on individual units ranging from 50% to 98.3% congruence.

The overall rate of omission of important information was 11.7%, with the most common omission being in the category of intake and output. The overall incongruency rate (information in report different from actual patient condition) was 12.3%, with the most common errors having to do with intravenous infusion site and rate.

This study suggests that work overload may be an important variable in determining the accuracy of intershift reporting. Nurses need to verify patient condition before assuming responsibility for care, and to institute procedures to safeguard against inaccurate reporting of patient status.

Richard J: Congruence between intershift reports and patients' actual conditions. Image 20(1):4, 1988

Information Required in Hospital Patient Records by Accreditation Bodies

Identification information

Evidence of appropriate informed consent or indication of the reason for its absence

Medical history

Report of physical examination

Diagnostic and therapeutic orders

Observations of the patient's condition

    Progress and nursing notes

    Reports of all procedures and tests and their results

Conclusions

    Provisional diagnoses

    Associated diagnoses

    Clinical resume

    Autopsy reports

Greenlaw J: Documentation of patient care: An often underestimated responsibility. Law Med Health Care 29:172, 1982

are apparent. However, until recently, many nurses were not actively involved in making these changes, even though many aspects of family-centered care fell within the scope of nursing practice. It is possible that if nursing had been more in touch with consumer views about birth care, there would have been less conflict and more rapid progress in establishing family-centered care.

Today, as nurses assume more responsibility for planning and delivering comprehensive family-centered birth care, they often are in close communication with consumers and community groups about the effectiveness and acceptability of the care they receive. This will be increasingly important as cost-containment measures and the shrinking childbearing population cause increased competition in the field.

However, it is as important for the nurse to inform consumers about health care as it is for nurses to listen to consumers' views. Nurses have traditionally valued and been involved in health education, both in one-to-one interaction with patients and in community health education programs. Nurses are often very effective health educators, in part because of their comprehensive view of health and human needs. Nurses could increase their effectiveness in health education by taking advantage of opportunities to communicate through television, radio, and print media features on health.

nursing, where hospitalizations are usually short and much patient teaching must be done before discharge.

The nurse also has a responsibility to communicate with colleagues in her specialty area and the profession as a whole about problems in clinical practice. The major mechanism for this communication is through nursing journals and other publications. This may not seem to be of great importance to students or novice nurses, but without scholarly communication, nurses could not be effectively educated and the profession could not advance its knowledge base. Nurses in clinical practice can contribute directly to the shared knowledge base by publishing in the nursing literature. Until now, nurse educators and researchers have been much more active in this type of communication. However, clinicians are in an *ideal* position to contribute valuable nursing knowledge and should consider this an important activity.

Nurse – Community Communication

Nurse – community communication involves exchange of information with consumers. Again, this may not seem particularly pressing to the student or novice nurse, who often focuses more on aspects of direct patient care. However, nurse – community communication has important long-term consequences, particularly in the field of maternity care. As described in Chapter 2, the effects of consumer activism in American maternity care

CHAPTER SUMMARY

Maternity nursing is based on elements of professional practice: an identifiable knowledge and theory base, a systematic approach to practice, agreed upon standards of practice, documentation of clinical practice, and participation in and support of professional and specialty organizations.

The *knowledge and theory base* of maternity nursing encompasses the physiologic, emotional, social, and cultural aspects of childbearing within the context of the family, and individual and family responses to alterations in health status during the childbearing year. A *systematic approach to nursing practice* is reflected in the nursing process, which focuses attention on assessment of patient problems, appropriate nursing intervention, and evaluation of the effectiveness of that intervention. *Documentation of clinical practice* includes communication at several levels: between the nurse and the patient and her family, between the nurse and her colleagues, and between the nurse and the wider community of consumers and professionals. Therapeutic interaction and an emphasis on teaching for effective self-care are important concerns in nurse – patient communication. Safety and continuity of care are important goals in nurse – colleague communication; the nurse must give careful attention to clear and complete nursing records. Nurse–community communication is not a major element of clinical care but has long-range implications for the perception of nursing services by consumers and for the advancement of knowledge in the field.

As the field of maternity nursing changes, new patterns of practice are evolving, such as independent nursing practice and increasing use of conceptual frameworks or models to guide practice. Many challenges lie ahead as the birth rate declines and as nursing as a predominantly female profession comes to grips with the remaining barriers to full professional practice. Maternity nursing has been and continues to be a microcosm of the larger profession with all its problems, satisfactions, and rewards.

STUDY QUESTIONS

1.   Discuss what is meant by each of the following terms as they relate to professional nursing practice and why each is important:

    Identifiable knowledge and theory base
    Systematic approach to practice
    Documentation of practice

2.   What are the advantages of using a conceptual framework to guide clinical practice? Why is adaptation a useful organizing perspective for maternity care?

3.   Explain the difference between a nursing diagnosis and a collaborative problem. What are the elements in a complete nursing diagnosis? What is each element designed to communicate?

4.   List some characteristics of adult learners and explain how they might influence the process of patient teaching. Why is it essential that patient teaching be documented?

5.   Why is nurse–community communication especially important in the field of maternity nursing?

REFERENCES/BIBLIOGRAPHY

Carpenito L: Nursing Diagnosis: Application to Clinical Practice, 3rd ed. Philadelphia, JB Lippincott, 1990

Johnson D: The behavioral system model for nursing. In Riehl J, Roy C (eds): Conceptual Models for Nursing Practice, 2nd ed. New York, Appleton-Century Crofts, 1980

Maslow A: A theory of human motivation. Psychol Rev 5:370, 1943

Roy C: Introduction to Nursing: An Adaptation Model, 2nd ed. Englewood Cliffs, NJ, Prentice-Hall, 1987

St. Louis University: Adaptation: A Theoretical Base for Nursing. St. Louis, MO, 1979

Trandel–Korenchuk D: Informed consent: Client participation in childbirth decisions. J Obstet Gynecol Neonatal Nurs 11:379, 1982

SUGGESTED READINGS

Gillis C, Highley B, Roberts B, Martinson I: Toward a Science of Family Nursing. Menlo Park, CA, Addison-Wesley, 1989

Hanson S, Bozett F: Dimensions of Fatherhood. Beverly Hills, CA, Sage Publications, 1985

Lederman R: Psychosocial Adaptation in Pregnancy. Englewood Cliffs, NJ, Prentice-Hall, 1984

Mercer R: First-time Motherhood: Experiences from teens to forties. New York, Springer Publishers, 1986

Rubin R: Maternal Identity and the Maternal Experience. New York, Springer–Verlag New York, 1984

Stevens KA: Nursing diagnoses in wellness childbearing settings. J Obstet Gynecol Neonatal Nurs 17(5):329, 1988

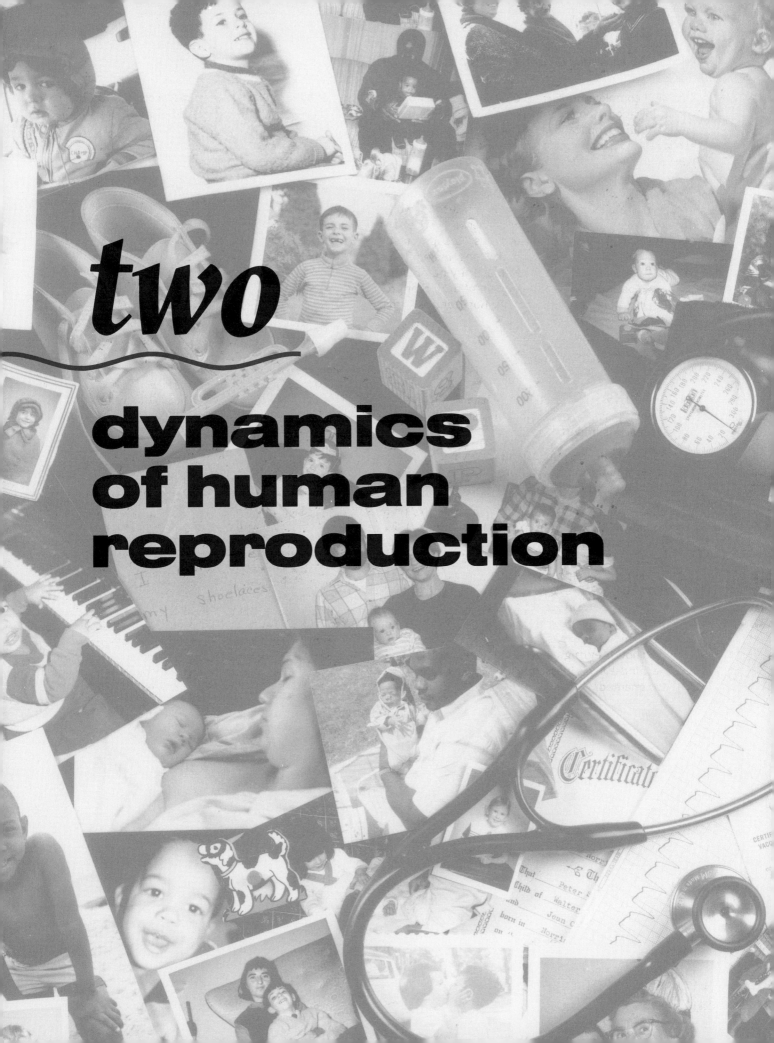

two

dynamics of human reproduction

5 normal reproductive anatomy and physiology

LEARNING OBJECTIVES

After studying the material in this chapter, the student should be able to

- Describe the differentiation process in fetal development

- Demonstrate a basic understanding of the male and female reproductive tracts

- Identify the structures making up the male internal and external genitalia and understand their function

- Identify the structures making up the female internal and external genitalia and understand their function

- Discuss the importance of testosterone to normal male generative function

- Identify the major female hormones and their functions

- Discuss the menstrual cycle and identify phases of the cycle and their dominant hormones

KEY TERMS

Climacteric

Copulation

Endometrial cycle

Gonad

Gonadotropins

Hot flash

Invagination

Menarche

Menopause

Menstrual cycle

Menstruation

Morphology

Oocyte

Oophorectomy

Osteomalacia

Osteopenia

Osteoporosis

Ovarian cycle

Ovulation

Puberty

Somatic

Spermatogenesis

Steroidogenesis

Stroma

Vacuole

Vasocongestion

For most men and women, human reproductive function is something that comes "naturally." For nurses working with women and their families, however, knowledge of male and female anatomy and confidence in dealing with the sensitive issues surrounding reproduction are directly related to successful interactions with individuals in the home or health care setting. These two prerequisites, knowledge and confidence, are essential to successful counseling in human reproduction but may take time and patience to obtain. The first step is to learn the reproductive system well and use opportunities as they arise to share information and answer questions openly. Teaching adolescents about reproduction is a special challenge to the nurse but provides a special satisfaction when they respond positively and show interest and understanding.

Women may be less knowledgeable than men about their sexual anatomy since their organs are concealed.

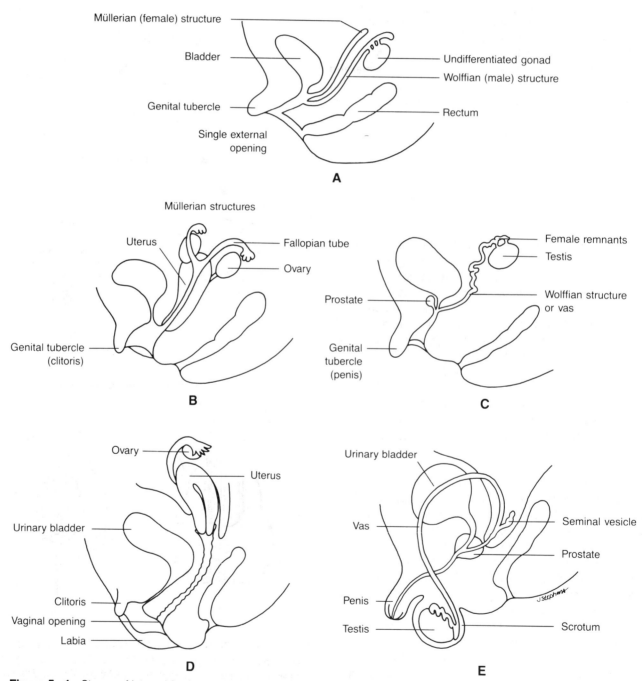

Figure 5–1. Stages of internal fetal sex differentiation. (Adapted from Masters W, Johnson V: Human Sexual Response. Boston, Little, Brown & Co, 1966) (Childbirth Graphics)

They also may be less comfortable about discussing their sexual anatomy than men and reserve their questions for close friends or health care providers. The nurse, in her role as health promoter, is the ideal person to dispel the myths and misinformation perpetuated by uninformed sources.

There is not one system in the human body that is not affected in some way by the sex hormones. Although all body systems are exposed to the sex steroids, the male and female generative organs are controlled by them. The ebb and flow of hormones plays an important role in sexual activity. For conception to occur, hormone levels must be sustained at a critical level in the female.

This chapter presents the anatomy of the male and female reproductive systems, discussing the external and internal structures and their function. Since the function of these organs is almost totally controlled by the hormonal system, the hormones of both sexes and their importance in maintaining a normal reproductive tract are discussed.

SEXUAL DIFFERENTIATION

Although biologically (that is, genetically), sex is determined at conception, for the first 6 weeks of gestation, the conceptus remains sexually undifferentiated, meaning that its anatomy is neither male nor female. In the fifth and sixth weeks of pregnancy, two primitive gonads form. The gonads are considered *bipotential,* meaning that they can differentiate into either testes or ovaries. Two paired primitive duct systems form in both male and female embryos at this time, the *müllerian* ducts and the *wolffian* ducts, as shown in Figure 5–1.

Basically, each reproductive structure in one sex corresponds to a similar structure in the other sex. This is true in part because reproductive structures in both sexes are homologous, that is, they rise from the same embryonic tissue.

The primitive gonads will develop into testes when *H-Y antigen* (controlled by the Y chromosome) is present. Without the H-Y antigen, the primitive gonads will always develop into ovaries. Fetal androgen must continue to be present in the appropriate amounts and at the right times for the further development of the male structures from the wolffian ducts. The testes will be formed by the eighth week if the embryo is male and will produce two chemicals: *müllerian duct inhibiting substance* and *androgens.* Müllerian duct inhibiting substance causes the müllerian ducts (or female duct system) to shrink and nearly disappear. The androgens, which are hormones that cause masculinization, consist of testosterone and dihydrotestosterone. Testosterone stimulates the development of the wolffian ducts into the epididymis, vas deferens, sem-

inal vesicles, and ejaculatory ducts. Dihydrotestosterone stimulates the development of the penis, scrotum, and prostate gland.

The differentiation of the primitive gonads into ovaries does not depend on hormones. The ovaries develop about the 12th week of embryonic life, and the müllerian duct system forms the uterus, fallopian tubes, and inner third

A. Before sixth week (undifferentiated)

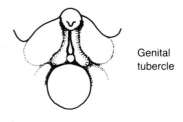

Genital tubercle

B. Seventh to eighth week

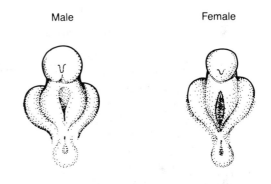

Male   Female

C. Twelfth week (fully developed)

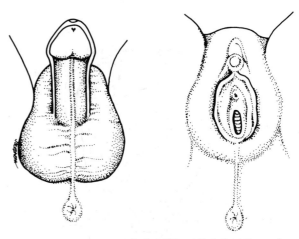

Figure 5–2. Three stages in the differentiation of the male and female external genitalia. *(A)* The undifferentiated stage appears during the second month of gestation. *(B)* The differentiated stage occurs about the third month of gestation. *(C)* The fully developed stage at birth. (Childbirth Graphics)

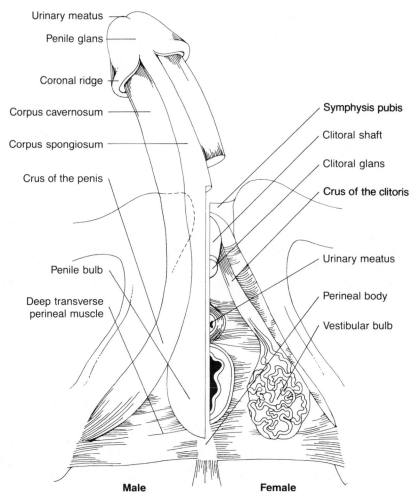

Urinary meatus
Penile glans
Coronal ridge
Corpus cavernosum
Corpus spongiosum
Crus of the penis
Penile bulb
Deep transverse perineal muscle

Symphysis pubis
Clitoral shaft
Clitoral glans
Crus of the clitoris
Urinary meatus
Perineal body
Vestibular bulb

Male   **Female**

Figure 5–3. Clitoral and penile structures. This drawing allows comparison of the placement and size of clitoris and penis. Note that the vestibular and penile bulbs are similar in size. The crura of the penis and clitoris are also similar in size, shape, and anchoring site. The pelvic bones of the female are slightly larger than those of the male. The pendulous portion of the penis is vastly larger than its homologue, the clitoral shaft and glans. (After Sherfey MJ: The Nature and Evolution of Female Sexuality, 2nd ed. New York, Random House, © 1972)

of the vagina. The wolffian duct system in the female shrinks into tiny remnants, since the high levels of testosterone needed to stimulate its growth are not present.

The external genitals begin to differentiate between the 7th and the 14th week of development. There is a slight amount of testosterone in the female embryo,

which develops the clitoris, vulva, and vagina. In the male, testosterone causes the shaft of the penis to form by the growing together of the folds that would develop into the labia minora in the female (Fig. 5–2).

The genital tubercle develops into the glans of the clitoris in the female and the glans of the penis in the male.

Table 5–1   **Sexual Development in the Fetus**

	Characteristic	Male	Female
Fertilization	Chromosomal complement	X Y	X X
6th week	Gonadal development	Testes	Ovaries
	Androgen level	High	Low
8th week	Internal ducts		
	wolffian	Form vas deferens and associated glands	Degenerate
	müllerian	Degenerate	Form vagina, uterus, and fallopian tubes
12th to 14th week	External anatomy		
	Genital tubercle	Forms glans of penis	Forms glans of clitoris
	Labioscrotal folds	Form scrotum and lower shaft of penis	Form major and minor labia

The adult form of these homologous organs is shown in Figure 5–3. The labioscrotal swellings become the outer vaginal lips of the female and the scrotum in the male. Thus, by the 12th to 14th week of gestation, the biologic sex of the fetus has been fairly well established, as shown in Table 5–1.

STRUCTURE AND FUNCTION OF THE MALE REPRODUCTIVE SYSTEM

Organs of the male reproductive system include the testes, or male gonads, which produce sperm; ducts that store or transport sperm; accessory glands that produce secretions constituting the semen; supporting structures; and the penis. The three major functions of the male reproductive system are spermatogenesis, performance of the male sex act, and hormonal regulation of the male reproductive functions. Structures of the male reproductive system are illustrated in Figure 5–4.

Male Reproductive Structures

External Male Genitalia

- Penis
- Scrotum

Internal Male Genitalia

- Testes (gonads) and seminiferous tubules
- Ductal system
  Epididymis
  Ductus deferens (vas deferens), seminal vesicles, and ejaculatory duct
  Urethra
- Accessory glands
  Prostate gland
  Bulbourethral glands

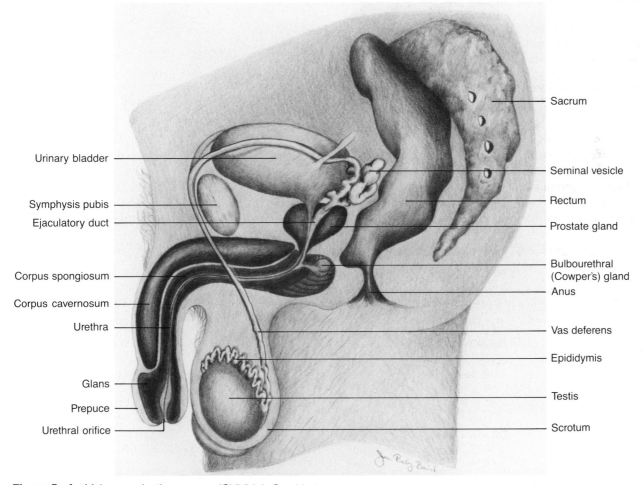

Figure 5–4. Male reproductive organs. (Childbirth Graphics)

External Male Genitalia

Penis

The *penis,* the male copulatory organ, serves to deliver semen into the female reproductive tract. It is elongated, pendant, and consists of a shaft attached anteriorly and laterally to the pubic arch and a glans located at its distal end. Essential parts of the organ are three cylindrical columns of cavernosa, or erectile bodies, and the urethra that passes through its median body.

The erectile columns that make up the bulk of the penis are two lateral *corpora cavernosa* and a single *corpus spongiosum* (see Fig. 5–3). The corpora cavernosa are surrounded by an outer longitudinal layer and an inner circular layer of dense fibrous connective tissue called the *tunica albuginea.* This sheath of tissue controls the distention of the erectile tissue beyond a certain point.

The two corpora cavernosa are separated by a layer of fascia and form the anterior portion of the penis.

The corpus spongiosum, similar to its neighboring bodies, surrounds the urethra and is in the median posterior position. The urethra within the corpus spongiosum remains patent during sexual excitement to allow passage of semen during ejaculation. Extending beyond the lower borders of the corpora cavernosa, the corpus spongiosum becomes the glans penis at its distal end.

Supported by fibrous connective tissue, the structure of the penis contains no adipose tissue and is covered by loose skin. The skin at the neck of the penis behind the glans folds back on itself and forms a cufflike, movable *foreskin,* or *prepuce* (Fig. 5–5). Surgical removal of the foreskin is called *circumcision.* The skin of the glans is hairless, and its surface contains many highly sensitive nerve papillae.

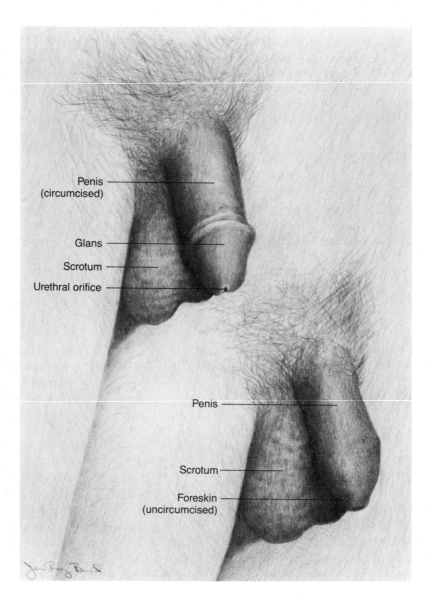

Figure 5–5. External male genitalia, circumcised and uncircumcised. (Childbirth Graphics)

Sensory impulses to the glans penis are highly organized. Sexual sensations pass through the pudendal nerve, the sacral plexus, the sacral portion of the spinal cord, and up the spinal cord to unidentified areas of the cerebrum. Areas adjacent to the penis also aid in stimulation of the sex act. Signals are also sent to the spinal cord from stimulation of the anal epithelium, the scrotum, and perineal structures. (See Chapter 6 for the neurologic bases of the male sexual response.)

Erectile Tissue

Internally, the cavernous bodies consist of a spongelike meshwork of lined spaces (venous sinusoids) that receive and drain blood through the afferent arteries and efferent veins. These vessels remain collapsed when the penis is flaccid but become turgid with blood when sexual excitement occurs, causing pressure on the fibrous sheets of the corpora cavernosa. The trapping of blood within the cavernous bodies causes the penis to become stiff and erect. After ejaculation has occurred and sexual excitement subsides, the arteries contract, draining blood from the cavernous bodies and leaving the penis flaccid. This process is called *detumescence.* Blood supply to the penis is primarily supplied by the internal pudendal artery and is drained by veins of the same name. See Chapter 6 for a summary of the male sexual response cycle.

Scrotum

The *scrotum* is formed by the invagination of loose skin and fascia originating from the lower abdominal wall. It appears externally as a pouch of skin separated by a median ridge known as the *raphe.* Secretions emanating from the sebaceous glands in the scrotal skin produce a distinctive odor. The skin is also more darkly pigmented than that surrounding it and has a sprinkling of scattered hairs.

During fetal life the skin and subcutaneous fascia were the only epidermal layers that invaginated from the abdominal wall to construct the scrotal sac. To form the covering of the spermatic cord, the remaining layers of the abdominal wall were penetrated by the testes and their ducts, vessels, nerves, and muscle tissue as they journeyed from the abdominal cavity into the scrotum during the seventh fetal month. The point where these structures penetrate the abdominal wall is weakened, predisposing men to inguinal hernias.

The subcutaneous fascia of the scrotal wall is made up of involuntary muscle fibers called the *tunica dartos.* In the presence of cold, these muscles contract, causing shrinking and wrinkling of the wall. This mechanism draws the scrotum closer to the body when additional warmth is needed. The testes contained within the scrotum cannot produce sperm if the testes are maintained at body temperature; for this reason the testes are de-scended into the scrotum, where a cooler temperature is maintained. Men who have jobs that require long hours of sitting, such as truck drivers, or who wear tight pants or frequently use a hot tub may experience temporary infertility due to the inhibition of spermatogenesis by excessive heat.

Internal Male Reproductive Organs
Testes (Gonads) and Seminiferous Tubules

Internally, the scrotum is divided into two sacs by a septum. Each sac contains a single testis. The *testis* is a solid, ovoid organ about 4 cm long and weighing approximately 100 g. It is covered by a thick, fibrous, whitish-appearing coat called the *tunica albuginea.* It is from the fibrous coat that septa pass into the interior of the testis, dividing it into about 250 lobules *(lobuli testis).* The septa converge on the posterior border of the testis, where blood vessels, nerves, and the ductus deferens enter and exit. This area is called the *mediastinum testis.*

Each lobule contains one to three *seminiferous tubules,* the essential structures of the testes (Fig. 5–6). When unraveled, each tube is about 60 cm long. On the inner surface of the tunica albuginea, loose connective tissue enters to fill the spaces between the seminal tubules. Contained in this tissue are Leydig's cells, which make up the endocrine-secreting tissue that produces testosterone. Cells lining the tubules are also sperm-producing (spermatogenic).

Spermatogenesis

Beginning at an average age of 13 years and continuing throughout life, spermatogenesis occurs in all seminiferous tubules, resulting from stimulation by the anterior pituitary gonadotropin hormones. Testosterone, one of these hormones, is produced by the Leydig's cells within the seminiferous tubules and is responsible for stimulating the formation of mature, functional sperm.

The first stage of spermatogenesis begins with the growth of spermatogonia into enlarged cells called *spermatocytes.* The spermatocyte then divides by the process of meiosis, in which no new chromosomes are formed but separation of chromosomal pairs occurs. Two *spermatids* are formed, each containing 23 chromosomes. After several weeks of maturing in the epididymis, the spermatids become *spermatozoa,* or mature sperm.

At all stages of germinal cell division and in the final conversion of spermatocytes into spermatozoa, the developing spermatozoa are in contact with Sertoli's cells. These cells are essential in providing a special environment in which the germinal cells develop. They secrete fluid that bathes the germinal cells; provide fluid within the seminiferous tubule that contains nutrients for the developing and newly formed spermatozoa; and secrete

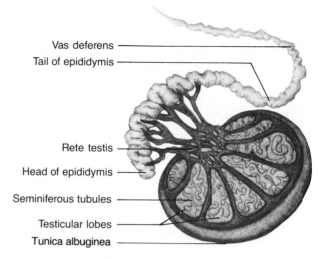

Vas deferens
Tail of epididymis

Rete testis
Head of epididymis
Seminiferous tubules
Testicular lobes
Tunica albuginea

A

Figure 5–6. *(A)* Structure of the testis and epididymis (Childbirth Graphics) with *(B)* a cross section of a seminiferous tubule.

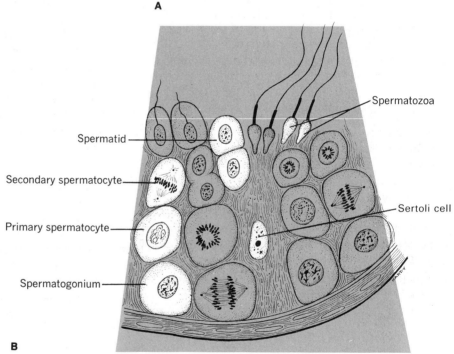

Spermatozoa

Spermatid

Secondary spermatocyte

Sertoli cell

Primary spermatocyte

Spermatogonium

B

müllerian duct inhibiting factor, a hormone that inhibits formation of fallopian tubes in the male during fetal sexual differentiation. The entire period of spermatogenesis from germinal cell to sperm takes approximately 75 days.

A mature sperm consists of a head, neck, and tail. Chromosomal material is contained in its head and neck, and the tail contains the contractile mechanism for self-propulsion. On the front portion of the sperm is the *acrosome,* which contains substances that facilitate the entry of the sperm into the ovum. The centrioles are aggregated in its neck, and the mitochondria that contain the cell's source of energy are arranged in a spiral in its body (Fig. 5–7).

A long tail, an outgrowth of one of the centrioles, ex-

tends beyond the body of the sperm. Provided with energy by the mitochondria, the tail projects the sperm forward when it is released into the female genital tract. As the tail waves back and forth and moves spirally near its tip, a snakelike propulsion projects the sperm forward at the speed of 20 cm per hour.

Although some sperm are stored in the epididymis, most are stored in the vas deferens and its ampulla. Sperm maintain their fertility for several months when stored within the body. With normal sexual activity, prolonged storage does not occur. With excessive sexual activity, sperm may be stored for no longer than 4 hours. Sperm that have been ejaculated and remain at body temperature live only 24 to 72 hours. When semen is

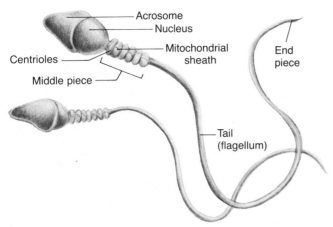

Figure 5-7. Structure of the sperm. (Childbirth Graphics)

stored at low temperatures, the sperm will survive for several weeks; when frozen at temperatures below −100° C sperm have been preserved for years.

Semen

Ejaculated *semen,* the discharge from the male urethra after orgasm, is composed of fluids from the vas deferens, seminal vesicles, prostate, and mucous glands. Fluid from the seminal vesicles makes up the bulk of semen (60%) and helps to dilute the sperm, which would otherwise have impaired motility due to their sheer numbers. This fluid is the last to be ejaculated and serves to wash sperm from the ejaculatory duct and urethra. The semen's milky appearance derives from the prostatic fluid, while its mucoid consistency comes from secretions of the seminal vesicles and mucous glands.

The average *p*H of the combined semen is alkaline at 7.5.

Ductal System

Epididymis. The *epididymis* is a small, oblong body located beside the posterior surface of the testis. It consists of a convoluted tube 13 to 20 feet in length and terminates at its lower pole into the ductus deferens. It constitutes the beginning of the excretory duct of each testis and stores sperm within it. The sperm are maintained within it for 3 weeks as they mature and become motile.

Ductus Deferens, Seminal Vesicles, and Ejaculatory Ducts. Located on the posterior border of the testis, the *ductus deferens* retraces the upward course through the abdominal wall that the testis took in its embryonic descent. It is a highly muscular channel that can be felt as a rigid, almost wirelike structure in the upper part of the scrotum.

Each ductus joins the spermatic cord through the in-

guinal canal and arches around the ureter to the posterior wall of the bladder. It is joined at this point by short ducts that originate at the *seminal vesicles.* The seminal vesicles are coiled and branched and produce a sticky secretion that provides a supportive medium in which sperm becomes more motile. The secretion also contains an abundance of fructose and other nutrients and large quantities of prostaglandin and fibrinogen. During ejaculation the seminal vesicles empty their contents into the *ejaculatory duct* after the sperm have emerged from the *vas deferens.* Not only does this fluid add bulk to the semen but it supplies nutrients to the sperm. It is postulated that prostaglandins aid fertilization by rendering the cervical mucus more receptive to sperm. Prostaglandins may also cause reverse peristaltic contractions of the uterus and oviducts, helping to move the sperm toward the ovaries.

Before entering the prostate, the ductus becomes enlarged into the terminal ampulla. In this area spermatozoa and tubal secretions are stored. Each ductus joins the short ducts of one of the seminal vesicles to form two ejaculatory ducts, both of which traverse the entire length of the prostate. In these ducts the sperm are mixed with seminal and prostatic secretions. If ejaculation does not occur regularly, spermatozoa degenerate, die, and are reabsorbed. After a period of abstinence, the first ejaculation may contain many deformed and degenerated sperm.

Ejaculation. When sexual excitement reaches a critical level, smooth and skeletal muscles of the male reproductive system contract and empty the semen into the urethra *(emission).* Then, by a series of rapid, rhythmic muscle contractions, the semen is forcefully expelled from the penis *(ejaculation),* and orgasm is experienced. During ejaculation the sphincter at the base of the bladder is closed—semen cannot enter the bladder, and urine cannot be expelled.

Urethra

The male *urethra* serves as a passage for both urine and semen. It extends from the bladder to the external urethral orifice and consists of three portions: the prostatic portion, which passes through the prostate and is the location where the ejaculatory and prostate ducts empty their fluids into the urethra; the membranous portion, which penetrates the urogenital diaphragm, where it is surrounded by the external urethral sphincter muscle; and the penile urethra, which passes through the spongy erectile body called the *corpus spongiosum* (see Fig. 5-4). Numerous urethral glands open into this area and are called the *urethral lacunae* (gland openings). At the glans, the bulbous anterior extremity, the corpus spongiosum flattens to form the *fossa navicularis.* The urethra widens at this point and terminates at its slitlike orifice, where semen or urine is passed.

Accessory Glands

Prostate. The prostate gland is fully developed before puberty, but its full growth is realized only after stimulation from testosterone. The prostate gland surrounds the neck of the bladder and the first 3 cm of the urethra (the tube through which urine and ejaculate are discharged to the outside). About the size of a chestnut, the prostate is a solid organ consisting of a median and two lateral lobes. It lies in front of the rectum and can be palpated for size, congestion, and nodularity through the rectal wall. It contains an inner layer of smooth muscle fiber that, when contracted, secretes a thin, opalescent fluid into the urethra. This fluid is alkaline and contains calcium, citric acid, and other substances. Its alkalinity may be important in counteracting the acidity of the secretions from the ductus and seminal vesicles. Sperm are optimally mobile in an alkaline *p*H of 6.0 to 6.5.

Bulbourethral Glands (Cowper's Glands). The two *bulbourethral glands* are the size and shape of a pea and are located in the urogenital diaphragm, which forms the floor of the pelvis. Ducts of the glands open into the posterior cavernous urethra. The fluid secreted by the glands is clear, viscous, and alkaline. Its alkalinity assists in neutralizing acidic female vaginal secretions, which would be detrimental to sperm survival. For a review of the passage of sperm through the male reproductive system, see Table 5–2.

Female Reproductive Structures

External Female Genitalia

- Vulva (pudenda)
- Mons pubis
- Clitoris
- Labia majora
- Labia minora
- Vestibule
  Urethral meatus
  Vaginal orifice and Skene's glands
  Bartholin's glands
- Perineum

Internal Female Genitalia

- Vagina
- Uterus
- Fallopian tubes
- Ovaries
- Supporting structure of the female pelvis
  Bony pelvis
  Perineum

Accessory Organs

- Breasts

Table 5–2   Passage of Sperm Through the Male Reproductive System

Organ	Function
Testes	• Produce spermatogenic cells
	• Produce testosterone
Seminiferous tubules	• Divide spermatocytes by meiosis
Epididymis	• Stores mature spermatozoa
	• Moves sperm along tract by smooth muscle action
	• Contributes secretions to seminal fluid
Ductus deferens	• Stores spermatozoa and tubal fluid in its ampulla
	• Carries spermatozoa to duct of seminal vesicle by muscular contraction
Seminal vesicles	• Contribute nutrient-laden secretions and prostaglandins to semen
	• Join ductus deferens to become ejaculatory duct
Ejaculatory duct	• Extends from junction of ductus deferens and seminal vesicles through prostate gland to prostatic urethra, carrying sperm
Bulbourethral glands (Cowper's glands)	• Secrete viscid alkaline fluid contributing to semen and deacidifying acidic vaginal environment
Prostatic urethra	• Counteracts acidity of semen by addition of alkaline secretions to increase sperm motility
Penile urethra (corpus spongiosum)	• Allows excretion of ejaculate to exterior
External urethral orifice	• Permits exit of semen

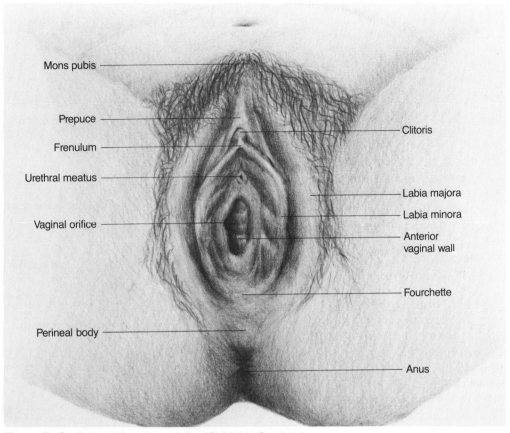

Figure 5-8. External female genitalia. (Childbirth Graphics)

STRUCTURE AND FUNCTION OF THE FEMALE REPRODUCTIVE SYSTEM

The female reproductive tract consists of the external genitalia, which include the vulva, mons pubis, labia majora, labia minora, the vestibule of the vagina and its related structures, and the perineum. Internal reproductive structures include the vagina, uterus, fallopian tubes, ovaries, and the supporting structures of the female pelvis, as shown in the shaded box, opposite page. The breasts are considered accessory organs.

External Female Genitalia

Vulva

Also known as the *pudenda, vulva* is the term used to designate all externally visible structures from the pubis to the perineum, as shown in Figure 5-8.

Mons Pubis

Also known as the *mons veneris,* the *mons pubis* is the fatty cushion that lies over the anterior symphysis pubis. After menarche, pubic hair grows over the mons pubis.

The characteristic distribution of this hair is called the *escutcheon.* The female escutcheon occupies a triangular area with a base formed at the upper margin of the symphysis and an apex formed of hair growing downward over the labia majora and thighs. In males the escutcheon is less circumscribed, with an apex at the umbilicus and hair growing downward over the thighs. This secondary sexual characteristic does not necessarily follow a textbook description. In oriental women pubic hair may be sparse and fine, while in black women it is coarse, thick, and curly. Many normal women have pubic hair growth that more resembles the male pattern, with upward growth on the abdomen and downward growth on the thighs.

Clitoris

The clitoris is a small, cylindrical, erectile body. It lies within the anterior portion of the vulva and projects between the upper branched lamellae of the labia minora, which form the prepuce that covers the clitoris. Consisting of a glans, a body (corpus), and two crura, it rarely exceeds 2 cm in length. As shown in Figure 5-9, the *glans* of the clitoris is a smooth, round bump. It is highly sensitive to touch, since it contains many nerve endings.

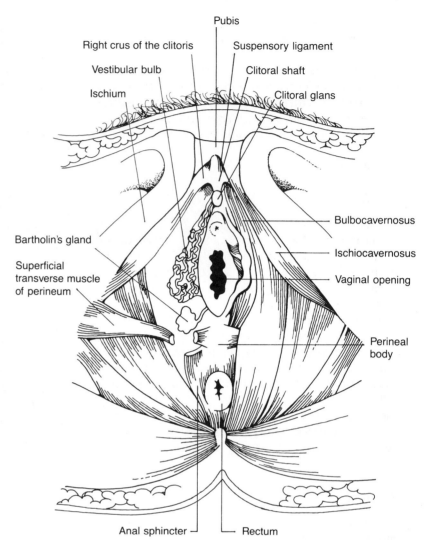

Figure 5–9. Perineal structures. The superficial tissues, including the clitoral hood, have been removed. The right crus is shown anchoring onto the pelvic bone, and the right vestibular bulb flanks the vagina. The crus is a ligamented extension of the corpus cavernosum; the bulb is a highly vascular sac that forms the internal portion of the corpus spongiosum. The muscle sheaths that cover these structures are pictured on the opposite side. The Bartholin's gland occasionally becomes infected, enlarged, and painful and interferes with sexual relations. (After Goldstein B: Human Sexuality. New York, McGraw-Hill, 1976) (Childbirth Graphics)

Erectile tissue and blood vessels lie just under the top layer of muscles. The erectile tissue is of two types: the firm tissue in the shaft and legs of the clitoris, and the more elastic tissue in the bulb that lies underneath the outer lips.

The glans has only one known function, which is to focus and accumulate sexual sensations. The clitoral hood often covers the glans, and observing the glans may be difficult unless the hood is retracted and the inner lips of the vagina parted.

The clitoris may vary considerably in size and shape, but these factors have little to do with the intensity of sexual arousal.

Labia Majora

The *labia majora* are two rounded folds of pigmented adipose tissue covered with skin that converge at the mons pubis and extend downward and backward to the posterior commissure. They measure 7 to 8 cm in length and 2 to 3 cm in width and taper at their lower borders. These tissue folds form the lateral boundaries of the vulva and are analogous to the scrotum in men.

The labia majora differ in appearance from woman to woman, depending on the amount of fatty tissue they contain. After puberty their outer surfaces become covered with curly, dark hair while their inner surfaces are smooth and hairless. In nulliparous women and in girls the labia are approximated and conceal the underlying structures. In multiparous women the labia become less full and remain separated. After menopause they shrink and may disappear.

Labia Minora

When the labia majora are separated, the *labia minora* are exposed. These two thin folds of skin are devoid of hair and subcutaneous fat but are richly supplied with blood vessels and sensitive nerve endings. Although not as sensitive as the clitoris, both the labia majora and the labia minora contain numerous genital corpuscles, major mediators of erotic sensation that contribute to overall sexual stimulation.

Lying within the labia majora, the labia minora extend posteriorly to the fourchette in nulliparous women and blend into the labia majora in multiparous women. Anteriorly, the labia minora converge into two lamellae (thin plates of skin). The lower plate is fused and forms the frenulum of the clitoris, while the upper pair form the clitoral prepuce.

Vestibule

The *vestibule* is an almond-shaped area, bordered by the labia minora, that extends from the clitoris to the posterior fourchette. Lying on either side of the vestibule beneath the mucous membrane are the *vestibular bulbs*. These structures are elongated masses of vascular, erectile tissue that connect with the clitoris and are homologous to the male corpus spongiosum, the erectile tissue surrounding the male urethra. In the posterior vestibule the area located between the posterior fourchette and the vaginal opening is called the *fossa navicularis*. This fossa is normally obliterated by childbirth and is only observable in nulliparous women.

The vestibule also contains the openings of six structures that drain into it: the urethra, the two Skene's ducts of the paraurethral glands, the vaginal orifice, and the two ducts of Bartholin's glands.

Urethra

The female urethra is about 4 cm long and courses downward and anterior to the bladder neck. It terminates in the vestibule of the vagina between the labia minora and about 2.5 cm posterior to the glans of the clitoris.

A spongy body of tissue surrounds the urethra, probably protecting it from direct pressure during sexual activity. The area is called the *urethral sponge*. Located in the urethral sponge are several glands called the *paraurethral glands* (Skene's glands), whose specific function is unknown.

The urethral meatus is characterized by a vertical slit 2 to 3 cm in length that appears puckered and lies just above the vaginal opening. On either side of the urethral meatus at approximately 5 and 7 o'clock are two small duct openings to the paraurethral (Skene's) glands. They are approximately 0.5 mm in diameter and may not be visible. These glands are sometimes involved when a gonorrhea or chlamydia infection is present.

Vaginal Opening and Hymen.   The opening to the vagina is located at the inferior portion of the vestibule and varies greatly in size and shape. The *hymen,* a fold of mucous membrane, partially covers the vaginal opening and marks the division between the external and internal

organs. In virgins it is often hidden by the labia minora. After the first sexual experience, the membrane is ruptured and the hymenal tags are visible at the vaginal opening. These are called *carunculae myrtiformes* (hymenal remnants). Variations in the hymen are shown in Figure 5-10. Folklore that treats the rupture, or absence, of a hymen as proof of lost virginity or sexual intercourse is fallacious. The hymen can be ruptured in vigorous physical activity or by use of tampons, or it may be congenitally absent.

An imperforate hymen is one that occludes the entire vaginal opening, causing retention and backup of menses in the vagina when menstruation begins at puberty. Pressure from the retained fluid is painful. Surgical opening of the hymen is a simple procedure and allows free flow of secretions and menstrual blood.

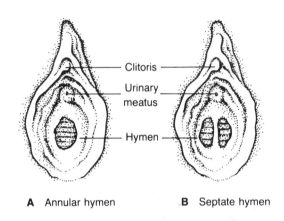

A Annular hymen   **B** Septate hymen

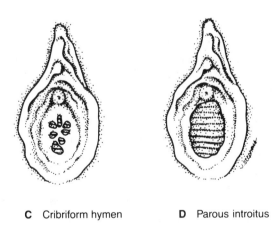

C Cribriform hymen   **D** Parous introitus

Figure 5-10. Variations in the hymen. *(A)* The annular hymen forms a ring around the opening of the vagina. *(B)* The septate hymen has one or more bands of tissue that cross the vaginal opening. *(C)* The cribriform hymen covers the vaginal opening but has many small perforations. *(D)* The parous introitus has small remnants of hymenal tissue left after a vaginal delivery. (Childbirth Graphics)

Bartholin's Glands. *Bartholin's glands* are 0.5 to 1.0 cm in diameter and are located in the lower vestibule, one on either side of the lateral margins of the vaginal orifice. Their ducts are 1.5 to 2.0 cm in length and secrete a clear, odorless mucus that originates from the gland. Normally, the Bartholin's gland and duct are not palpable, and a cystic swelling at the base of the labia majora most often indicates a cyst or abscess. This results from pyogenic organisms becoming trapped in the gland duct, occluding its lumen and causing the gland to become infected.

Perineum

The *perineum* is the region of the genital area that lies between the vulva and the anus. Anteriorly it is bounded by the symphysis pubis, laterally by the ischial tuberosities, and posteriorly by the coccyx. This area contains a complex structure of skin, muscles, fascia, blood vessels, nerves, and lymphatics. Support of this area is primarily provided by the urogenital and anal triangles.

Perineal Body. In obstetrics the *perineal body* is referred to as the perineum. The perineal body is composed of muscular structures that provide central support to the perineum. These structures include the levator ani, the bulbocavernous muscle, the superficial and deep perineal muscles, and the external anal sphincter. During delivery these structures are often lacerated. This area is covered in greater detail later in this chapter when the supporting pelvic structures are discussed.

Vessels and Nerves. The primary blood and nerve supply to the perineum is provided by branches of the internal pudendal artery and pudendal nerve. Their perineal branch of the posterior femoral cutaneous nerve and a branch of the ilioinguinal nerve are also important to the innervation of this area.

The blood and nerve supply to the vulva, also known as the urogenital triangle, is provided by branches of the internal pudendal artery and pudendal nerve. The perineal branch of the posterior femoral cutaneous nerve and a branch of the ilioinguinal nerve all provide cutaneous innervation to the mons pubis, the labia majora, and to most of the perineum.

Internal Female Reproductive Organs

The internal female reproductive organs are illustrated in Figure 5–11.

Vagina

The vagina serves three purposes. It is the excretory duct of the uterus, through which its excretions and men-

strual blood flow; it is the female organ of copulation; and it is the canal for the birth of an infant.

To accommodate these functions, the vagina is structured as a musculomembranous tube lined with transverse, corrugated mucosa called *rugae,* which are pliable and capable of marked distention during childbirth. Normally its walls lie close together with a small space between them. The anterior vaginal wall is 6 to 7 cm in length, and the posterior wall measures 7 to 10 cm.

At the *introitus,* or the vaginal opening, there is a perforated fold of pink mucous membrane called the hymen (see previous section on vaginal opening).

At its terminal end the circumference is attached to the uterine cervix. Its posterior wall is attached high on the posterior cervix, accounting for its additional length. As a consequence, a small, pouchlike area called the *posterior fornix* is formed beneath the cervix. Similar but smaller spaces surrounding the lateral and anterior vaginal attachments are called the *lateral* and *anterior fornices.* These areas provide access for vaginal palpation of the uterus and adnexa (area of the oviducts and ovaries), through their thin-walled tissues. The posterior fornix also provides surgical access into the peritoneal cavity called the *rectouterine pouch,* or the cul-de-sac of Douglas. Material can be obtained from this cul-de-sac for diagnostic purposes by aspiration or surgical incision through the vaginal wall. This procedure is called *culdocentesis* or *colpotomy.*

Anatomically, the vagina is located between the bladder and the rectum (see Fig. 5–11). The tissue separating the bladder from the vagina is called the *vesicovaginal septum,* and that separating it from the rectum is called the *rectovaginal septum.* These tissues are also important because manual palpation of the bladder and the rectum and ligaments is possible through their thin walls. It might be said that a fourth purpose of the vagina is to permit assessment of pelvic structures.

Vaginal Environment

The mucosa of the vaginal wall is lined with stratified squamous epithelium. This layer of cells, when stimulated by estrogen, maintains the normal acidic vaginal ecology. Maintenance of this ecology depends on a delicate physiologic balance of hormonal and bacterial action. Döderlein's bacilli, more commonly known as *lactobacilli,* are normal vaginal inhabitants. When estrogen is adequate, the squamous epithelium contains an adequate supply of glycogen, on which the lactobacilli thrive. A by-product of glycogen metabolism by the lactobacilli is lactic acid. This acid maintains the normal 4.0 to 5.0 *p*H acidic milieu of the vagina.

This cycle begins at menarche, when estrogen production is initiated, and ends at menopause, when estrogen production becomes inadequate to maintain menstrua-

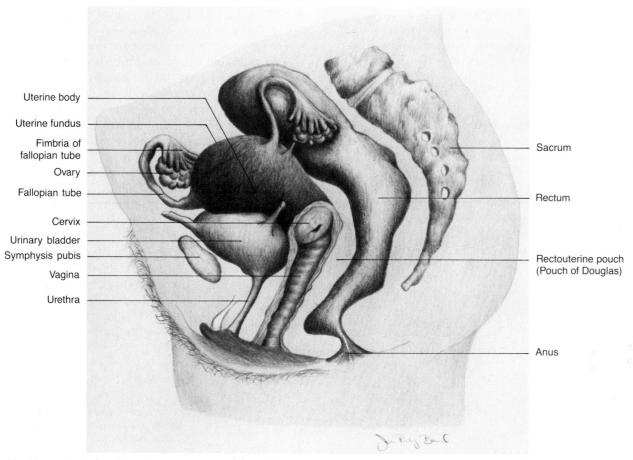

Uterine body

Uterine fundus

Fimbria of
fallopian tube

Ovary

Fallopian tube

Cervix

Urinary bladder

Symphysis pubis

Vagina

Urethra

Sacrum

Rectum

Rectouterine pouch
(Pouch of Douglas)

Anus

Figure 5–11. Internal female reproductive organs. (Childbirth Graphics)

tion. During the reproductive years this normal process is interrupted only by changes in the vaginal environment caused by infection, frequent douching, chronic illness, use of antibiotics that kill off the normal flora, poor hygiene, malnutrition, or debilitation. Pregnancy and oral contraceptive use alter hormone levels and may cause changes in the vaginal cycle that predispose some women to infection.

During pregnancy the vaginal rugae become more pliable in order to permit additional distention of the vaginal walls to accommodate delivery of the infant. Moreover, in preparation for childbirth the vagina becomes increasingly vascular and its walls grow thicker and longer. An increased amount of white vaginal discharge during the gestational period is normal.

Uterus

The normal *uterus* is a small, muscular organ (Fig. 5–12). It has the following functions:

To proliferate its lining (endometrium) once each month in anticipation of conception, and to shed its lining when conception does not occur (menstruation)

To provide a proliferated endometrium for the implantation of a fertilized ovum

To develop a placenta that will provide the means to nourish and support the developing fetus during pregnancy

To develop musculature that will not only protect the fetus but will contract during labor to expel the neonate

The nonpregnant uterus is located in the lower pelvis and lies between the urinary bladder anteriorly and the rectum posteriorly. Shaped like an inverted, flattened pear, its anatomical subdivisions include two major but unequal parts. The triangular upper portion of the uterus is called the *body* or *corpus,* and the lower portion is called the *cervix* (Fig. 5–13). The dome-shaped upper segment of the uterine body that is located between the insertion points of the fallopian tubes is called the *fundus uteri* or, more commonly, the *fundus.*

The uterine body is composed of three layers: an outer

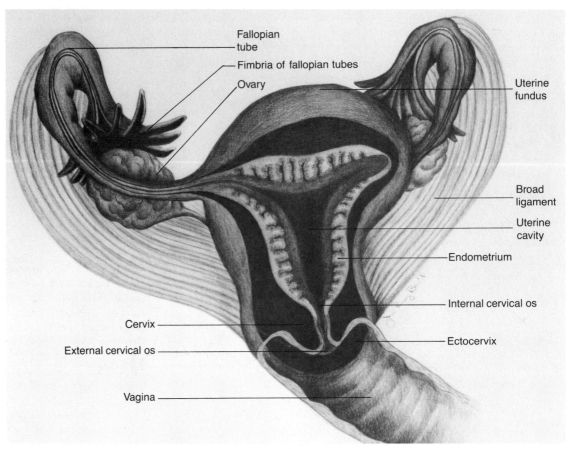

Figure 5-12. The uterus and broad ligament. (Childbirth Graphics)

covering of serous peritoneum; a thick middle layer of muscle fiber (myometrium), which makes up the bulk of the uterus; and an inner mucous layer of glands and supporting stroma attached to the myometrium, called the *endometrium*. The inner anterior and posterior surfaces of the uterus (or the endometrium) lie in close approximation and form a mere slit.

The axis of the uterus varies (Fig. 5-14). It normally forms a sharp angle with the vagina so that its anterior portion rests on the superior surface of the bladder. The uterine body is then in a horizontal plane when the woman is standing erect. A bend is created in the area of the isthmus, causing the cervix to face downward. In this position the uterus is said to be *anteverted*, the most

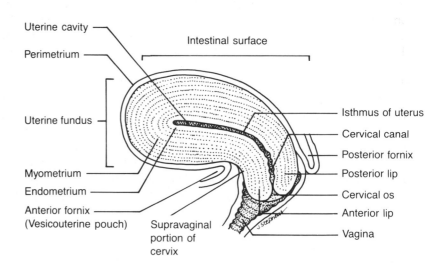

Figure 5-13. Cross section of the normal uterus. (Childbirth Graphics)

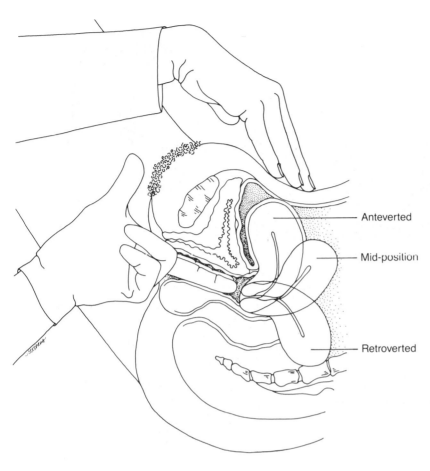

Anteverted

Mid-position

Retroverted

Figure 5–14. Rotation of the uterus. The anteverted uterine fundus rotates approximately 90° anterior to the long axis of the uterus and can be palpated by the abdominal band on bimanual examination. In the mid-position the long axis of the uterus lies in the same plane as the vagina and will not be palpable on bimanual examination. In the retroverted position the uterus rotates posteriorly to the long axis of the vagina and may be felt through the posterior fornix on bimanual examination or through the rectal mucosa on rectal examination. (Childbirth Graphics)

common uterine position. Other, less common normal positions include anteflexion, in which the uterus is flexed forward at the isthmus and bends upon itself; retroversion, in which the uterus bends backward upon itself; midline or military position, in which the uterus does not bend; and lateral version, in which the uterus bends to one side. The uterus is partially mobile, and although the cervix is fixed, the uterine body may move to the front or back. Uterine position may change depending on the position of the woman's body.

During pregnancy the primary site of uterine growth is in the myometrium. During the first half of pregnancy, there is a proliferation of new muscle fibers, and under the influence of estrogen, the myometrial cells increase to about 200 billion at term. During the latter half of pregnancy, the myometrium becomes hypertrophied, and its fibers increase over tenfold in length.

As gestation progresses, the uterine wall thins and becomes soft and easily compressible to accommodate fetal growth and movement. This process also makes possible palpation of the fetus through the uterine wall.

Isthmus

The *isthmus* is the area that lies between the uterine body and the cervix. This portion of the uterus is about 5

to 7 mm in length and lies above the internal os of the cervix. Its upper limit marks the lower boundary of the corpus; at its lower limit the isthmus marks the transition from its own mucosa to the mucous membrane of the endocervical canal at its internal os. The isthmus is shown in Figure 5–15 along with the comparative sizes of the uterus at different developmental stages.

The isthmus in its nonpregnant state is unimpressive, but during pregnancy it takes on special significance. As the uterus grows in pregnancy, the isthmus increases in length and becomes soft and compressible. One of the signs of early pregnancy, known as *Hegar's sign,* is the softening of the isthmus between the uterine body and the cervix. As pregnancy progresses, the isthmus expands to accommodate the growth of the uterus and gradually becomes incorporated into it. During labor the upper uterine segment (the corpus) is firm and hard, while the lower uterine segment (the isthmus) is distended and passive. This allows the lower segment and the cervix to dilate and expand during labor, while the upper segment contracts to push the fetus out.

Uterine Cervix

The *cervix* is the portion of the uterus that lies below the isthmus. The exterior portion of the cervix visible on

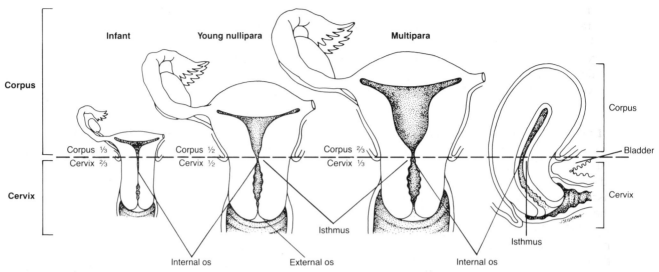

Figure 5-15. Comparative sizes of prepubertal, adult nonparous, and multiparous uteri, frontal and sagittal sections, and the changing proportions of the cervix and corpus. (Childbirth Graphics)

speculum examination is called the *portio vaginalis,* or the *ectocervix.* The external *cervical os* is located at the lower extremity of the ectocervix. Protruding from 1 to 3 cm into the vagina, the ectocervix will appear different in women, depending on their age, parity, and use of oral contraceptives. Normally, it is pink, but it may appear purplish during pregnancy and pale pink after menopause. It is approximately 2 to 3 cm in diameter in nulliparous women and 3 to 5 cm after vaginal delivery. Cervical tears are common during delivery, causing characteristic changes in its appearance.

Prior to childbirth, the cervical os is a small, regular opening. After childbirth the os becomes a transverse slit (sometimes described as fish-mouthed) that may even divide the cervix into anterior and posterior lips. Severe trauma to the cervix at the time of delivery may cause it to become irregular, nodular, or stellate.

The mucosa of the endocervical canal is lined with a single layer of columnar epithelium. Columnar cells are mucus-secreting and in the cervix produce a thick, tenacious, mucoid secretion. If for any reason a gland duct becomes occluded, causing its secretions to back up and be retained in the gland, nabothian cysts are formed. These are benign, smooth, small, round, yellowish cysts that are frequently seen on the cervix during speculum examination and require no treatment. The cervical secretion is one ingredient of the normal vaginal discharge. During pregnancy the cervical mucus forms a plug within the canal that effectively blocks bacteria and other substances from entering into the uterine cavity.

The ectocervix, or that portion of the cervix protruding into the vaginal canal, is covered with the same squamous epithelium that lines the vagina. Since the cervical canal is lined with columnar cells that extend to the cervical os, the point at which the squamous and columnar epithelium meet is called the *squamocolumnar junction* (Fig. 5-16). In the reproductive years this junction is located at the lower portion of the cervical canal. During pregnancy, and in women using oral contraceptives, the junction is located on the ectocervix and appears red, bumpy, and symmetrical. To the untrained eye it may appear eroded or abnormal because of the presence of exposed ducts of the columnar cells that open onto the cervix. This process is usually normal and is called *ectopy* (displacement) or *ectropian* (eversion of an edge or margin). This area is also called the transformation zone, since one type of cell is merging into another — that is, columnar into squamous. The squamocolumnar junction is significant because it is the location where cervical cancer usually begins. For this reason, when Pap smears are performed, cells must be retrieved from the squamocolumnar junction whether it is located inside the cervical os or on the ectocervix. Specimens received by the cytology laboratory without cells representative of the squamocolumnar junction are of little value for diagnosing early carcinoma, and the patient will have to return for collection of a second specimen.

Ligaments of the Uterus

The supportive ligaments that maintain the position of the uterus are those that extend from either side of the uterus, namely, the broad, round, and the uterosacral ligaments.

Broad Ligament. The broad ligament is a winglike transverse fold of peritoneum that arises from the floor of the pelvic cavity between the bladder and the rectum. It effectively divides the pelvic cavity into two compartments, anterior and posterior. The uterus lies within its median portion and is attached on either side. Its free border contains the fallopian tubes. The outer third portion of the broad ligament forms the suspensory ligament of the ovary, through which the ovarian vessels pass. The dense portion of the ligament is located laterally and is called the cardinal ligament, or transverse cervical ligament.

Round Ligament.   Arising below and anterior to the oviducts, the round ligaments extend from either side of the lateral portions of the uterus. Each is continuous with the broad ligament and extends downward to the inguinal canal. Passing through the inguinal canal, they terminate within the upper portions of the labia majora. During pregnancy these ligaments hypertrophy and become larger and longer. As the fetus grows and the uterus enlarges, these ligaments become stretched, causing discomfort to the pregnant woman. Round ligament pain is one of the most common complaints of pregnancy, and when the woman is unaware of its etiology, may be of concern to her. (See Chapter 5.)

Uterosacral Ligament.   The uterosacral ligaments attach to the cervix and encircle the rectum. These ligaments form the lateral boundaries of the rectouterine cul-de-sac (Pouch of Douglas) and support the uterus by the traction they exert upon the cervix posteriorly.

Fallopian Tubes

The fallopian tubes, or oviducts, convey the sperm entering the tube to the ova and convey the ova into the uterus by means of their ciliated lining. Extending from the superior angles of the uterine corpus to the region of the ovaries, each tube is 8 to 14 cm long, is covered with peritoneum, and has a lumen lined with mucous membrane. Each tube is divided into four portions:

1.   The interstitial portion within the uterine musculature, which travels upward and outward from the uterine cavity
2.   The isthmus, the narrow portion adjoining the uterus, which gradually passes into the ampulla
3.   The ampulla, which is wider and more tortuous and terminates in the infundibulum
4.   The infundibulum, a fimbriated, funnellike opening situated at the distal end of the oviduct that opens into the abdominal cavity. The infundibulum lies close to the fimbria ovarica, which is longer than other fimbriae and forms a shallow gutter to the

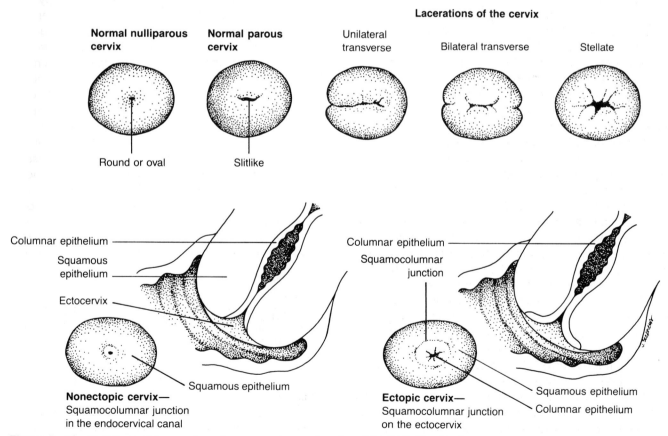

Figure 5–16. Variations of the cervix and squamocolumnar junction. (Childbirth Graphics)

ovary. These distal openings from each tube connect the pelvic cavity to the outside world. This means that they can become a source of danger when infection travels through the vagina, uterus, and fallopian tubes into the abdomen.

Thickness of the oviduct varies from 2 to 3 mm in diameter at the narrow isthmus to 5 to 8 mm at the widest portion of the ampulla. It has an outer longitudinal and an inner circular layer of smooth muscle tissue. Ciliated columnar epithelium lines the oviducts and, in combination with tubal contractions, is in large measure responsible for the movement of the ovum through the tube. When ovulation occurs, the tubal musculature and its suspensory ligament becomes increasingly active. They draw the ovary and the flaring end of the tube close together while the fimbriae sweep the ovum into the oviduct.

The fallopian tube is more than just a passageway for the fertilized ovum to reach the uterus. Its lumen must be patent (open) and wide enough to permit the ovum (the largest cell in the body) and the sperm to migrate through it, and the fluid contained in its interior facilitates the conditioning of the ovum for penetration by the sperm. For further discussion of conception and fetal development, see Chapters 7 and 14.

Ovaries

The *ovaries* are paired, almond-shaped organs that function to develop and produce ova and to secrete steroid sex hormones. Each ovary measures approximately 2.5 to 5.0 cm in length, 1.5 to 3.0 cm in breadth, and 0.7 to 1.5 cm in width and weighs approximately 4 to 8 g.

Lying on either side of the uterus on the lateral walls of the true pelvis, the ovaries are attached by a short fold of tissue called the *mesovarium* to the posterior broad ligament of the uterus. Between the folds of this structure the blood vessels and nerves pass to reach the hilus of the ovary. The ovaries are also attached by the ovarian ligament to the side of the uterus and, by the suspensory ligament, to the pelvic wall.

Covered by columnar epithelium, the mature ovary consists of a cortex and medulla. The *medulla,* the central portion of the ovary, is made up of supporting tissue (stroma), nerves, blood vessels, lymphatic tissue, and smooth muscle fibers. No ova or follicles are present in this central area.

The *cortex* is the outer ovarian layer. It is in this area that the ovarian and graafian follicles are located. Ovarian follicles in various stages of maturity are numerous during the follicular phase of the menstrual cycle (Fig. 5–17). When mature, the ova project into the surface of the cortex. They are then called *graafian follicles*. These follicles secrete the female hormone estrogen. It is the maturation of these follicles, particularly the follicle that is destined to ovulate, that produces the midcycle spurt of

estrogen necessary for ovulation to occur. The remaining follicles degenerate at the stage of development that they have achieved; this is called *follicular atresia.* Following ovulation the cells of the follicle that has ruptured undergo rapid increase in size and form a yellow body, the *corpus luteum.* The corpus luteum also produces small amounts of estrogen and large amounts of progesterone, the female hormone of the luteal, or second, phase of the menstrual cycle.

The Ovary Over the Life Span

During fetal life ovarian follicles are formed in the ovary in a complex series of events. The cycle of follicle formation, a variable degree of ripening of many oocytes, and atresia occur. These events are the same as those that occur during adult reproductive life, but full maturity, as evidenced by ovulation, does not take place.

At a point as early as 4 to 6 weeks of fetal life, the quiescent female ovary begins to synthesize small amounts of estrogen. By 6 to 8 weeks' gestation, the oogonia (the primordial cells from which oocytes originate) begin rapid mitotic multiplication and produce 6 to 7 million germ cells by 20 weeks' gestation. This astounding number of germ cells is the maximum number that the ovary will ever contain. During the female lifetime these numbers decrease, until 50 years later the store of germ cells becomes exhausted at menopause. The process of egg depletion by atresia begins at about 15 weeks' gestation, as maturation of the oocytes begins.

As a result of follicle maturation and atresia during fetal life, the total number of germ cells is reduced to 1 to 2 million by birth, a loss of 80% of the total number of oocytes (brain cells are the only other body cells that constantly decrease without being replenished). By puberty, germ cells number 300,000 to 400,000, still many more than are needed for future reproduction. During the next 30 to 40 reproductive years, these cells will become further depleted as menopause approaches. The typical monthly menstrual cycle of follicle maturation, ovulation, corpus luteum formation, and menstrual bleeding occurs approximately 400 times during the fertile years.

Beginning at about 38 to 40 years of age, ovulation decreases in frequency. The ovarian follicles that remain are less sensitive to gonadotropin stimulation and may not reach maturity. This means that less estrogen is being secreted as fewer follicles ovulate. As more cycles become anovulatory, the estrogen needed to stimulate growth of new follicles gradually diminishes until menopause ensues, at an average age of 51 years.

Pelvic Blood and Nerve Supply

The uterine artery supplies the major portion of blood to the uterus. It is a large vessel that runs anteriorly over the levator ani muscle to the base of the broad ligament. It

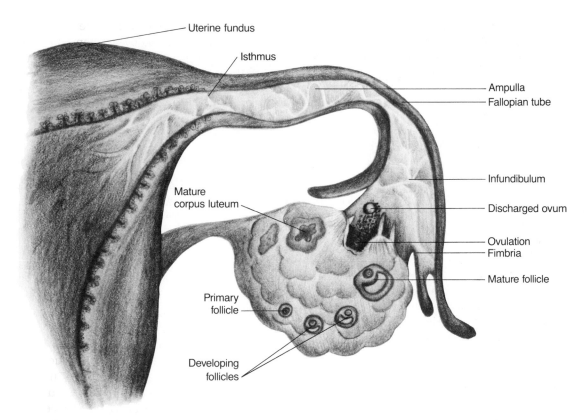

Figure 5–17. The ovary. In response to low levels of blood estrogen the hypothalamus releases FSH, initiating the maturation of an oocyte and increased estrogen production. FSH production decreases as estrogen levels rise and triggers the production of LH, which peaks rapidly and results in ovulation. Following ovulation the empty follicle remains in the ovary and develops into the corpus luteum, which takes over the production of estrogen, particularly progesterone. (Childbirth Graphics)

courses through the broad ligament and supplies branches to the vagina, uterus, and uterine tubes. It anastomoses with the ovarian artery. The internal pudendal artery passes through the pelvis, supplying blood to the perineal region.

Corresponding veins in the pelvic cavity form a large plexus before ending in the same branches as the arteries. These plexuses surrounding the reproductive organs are located in the subserous fascia. The ovarian vein ascends with the arteries and drains into the inferior vena cava and renal vein.

Nerves supplying the pelvis consist of somatic motor and sensory fibers that supply the muscles of the pelvic outlet and skin of the perineum. Pelvic viscera are innervated by autonomic plexuses that supply sympathetic and parasympathetic motor and visceral sensory nerves to the pelvic organs.

Supporting Structures of the Female Pelvis
Bony Pelvis

The *bony pelvis* is constructed for strength and stability and serves to transmit body weight to the lower extremi-

ties. In women it is especially adapted to childbearing. Its dimensions must be adequate to allow delivery of an infant. When any of its anterior, posterior, or transverse diameters are insufficient to permit passage of the largest diameter of the infant's head, cesarean delivery becomes necessary. Measurement to assess the size of the bony pelvis is usually done by vaginal examination and is called *pelvimetry.*

The pelvis, meaning "basin," is composed of four bones: two innominate bones, the sacrum, and the coccyx. The innominate bones result from the fusion of the ilium, the ischium, and the pubis, as shown in Figure 5–18. The sacroiliac joint fuses the sacrum to the iliac portion of the innominate bones posteriorly, and the symphysis pubis is joined anteriorly. The pelvis is divided into two parts by the linea terminalis, a plane that passes through the sacral promontory and the upper margin of the symphysis pubis. The false pelvis is that portion lying superior to the linea terminalis (also called the *pelvic brim*). The false pelvis varies in size among women and is not of obstetric significance. The true pelvis lies below the linea terminalis and is of special significance in parturition because it is the first bony canal through which the

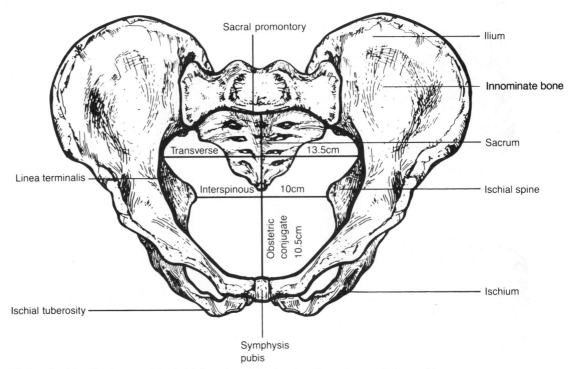

Sacral promontory

Ilium

Innominate bone

Sacrum

Transverse   13.5cm

Interspinous   10cm

Ischial spine

Obstetric conjugate 10.5cm

Linea terminalis

Ischium

Ischial tuberosity

Symphysis pubis

Figure 5-18. The bony pelvis. Adult female pelvis showing the anteroposterior and transverse diameters of the pelvic inlet and the interspinous (transverse) diameter of the midpelvis. Normally the obstetric conjugate is greater than 10 cm. (Childbirth Graphics)

infant must pass. Consisting of a part of the ilium, the ischium, the pubis, and the sacrum and coccyx, its bony wall is more complete than that of the false pelvis. Its superior border, the circumference of which marks the pelvic brim, is called the *inlet*. At its lower circumference, bordered by the tip of the coccyx and the ischial tuberosities and spines, lies the pelvic outlet. The ischial spines are of particular significance because the distance between them (10.5 cm) represents the shortest diameter of the pelvis. If the infant's head cannot pass through the ischial spines during delivery, a cesarean birth will be necessary. The rectum is housed posteriorly in the true pelvis, and the bladder is located anteriorly. The uterus and vagina are located between these two structures.

The pelvic cavity is a curved canal; when the body is in a standing position, the pelvis is in an oblique position relative to the trunk. The plane of the inlet of the true pelvis forms an angle of 60° with the horizontal plane. The anterior spine of the ilium is in the same vertical plane as the top of the symphysis pubis. The pubic arch in women is characteristically at a 90° to 100° angle that forms an arch under which the infant's head can easily pass.

Pelvic Planes and Diameters. Describing locations in the pelvis is difficult because of its peculiar shape, and variations in the shapes and planes of the pelvis are numerous. Since the size and shape of the individual pelvis are important to the mechanism of labor and its manage-

ment, awareness of these differences is important. For convenience, four imaginary flat surfaces crossing the pelvis at different levels are conventionally described (Fig. 5-19). These planes are (1) the plane of the pelvic inlet (or superior strait); (2) the plane of greatest dimensions; (3) the plane of least dimensions (midpelvis); and (4) the plane of the pelvic outlet (or inferior strait). The size and shape of the pelvic inlet (superior strait) determine the type of pelvis — gynecoid (normal), android, anthropoid, or platypelloid, as shown in Chapter 16.

Contents of the Bony Pelvis. The pelvis contains not only the pelvic organs but also the sigmoid colon, cecum, and ileum. The *sigmoid colon* continues into the pelvis as the rectum, which lies anterior to the sacral promontory. The uterus lies between the rectum and the bladder and divides the pelvis into two pouches, the rectouterine and the vesicouterine (Fig. 5-20). The *rectouterine pouch* (commonly known as the *cul-de-sac* [or pouch] *of Douglas* or the *posterior cul-de-sac*) is formed by the peritoneum that reflects from the rectum to the posterior wall of the uterus and vagina. In the *vesicouterine pouch* the peritoneum is reflected from the anterior–inferior surface of the uterus to the urinary bladder, as shown in Fig. 5-20.

The uterine body is normally bent anteriorly at a right angle to the vagina. The fallopian tubes extend laterally from the uterine fundus to the lateral pelvic walls, with

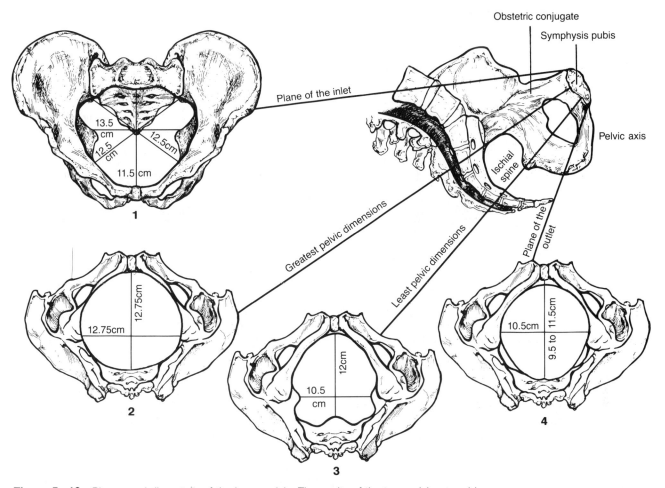

Figure 5-19. Planes and diameters of the bony pelvis. The cavity of the true pelvis resembles an obliquely truncated curved cylinder with its height greatest posteriorly. Note the curvature of the pelvic axis. (Childbirth Graphics)

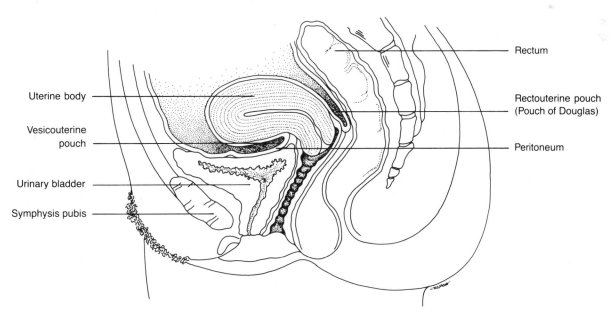

Figure 5-20. The rectouterine and vesicouterine pouches, showing their relation to the peritoneum in the female pelvis. The rectouterine pouch is of particular interest because it is through the vaginal wall adjacent to the ectocervix that culdoscopy allows visualization of the viscera of the pelvic cavity and culdocentesis may be performed to obtain secretions from the rectouterine pouch for therapeutic or diagnostic purposes. (Childbirth Graphics)

the almond-shaped ovaries attached to the broad ligament in close approximation. The ureters and round ligaments are also located on the lateral walls of the pelvic cavity. Fascia, numerous ligaments, muscles, blood vessels, and nerves help to support, nourish, and innervate all the organs located in the pelvic cavity.

Perineum

The *perineum,* the region between the thighs and the buttocks, is the most inferior portion of the trunk. Anteriorly, it is bounded by the pubic arch, laterally by the pubic and ischial rami, and posteriorly by the sacrum and coccyx.

Pelvic Floor Muscles

When the female pelvis is viewed from below, the center of the pelvic floor seems to project downward much like a funnel, with the anal canal at its center. The two levator ani muscles and the coccygeus muscle make up the pelvic floor, forming a figure eight around the vagina and anus. Since these muscles support the entire pelvic contents, they are of great importance (Fig. 5–21). The pubococcygeal muscle is constructed in such a way that it can expand enough for childbirth and contract

enough to keep the pelvis supported. However, the presence of the vaginal and anal openings in the muscle causes an inherent weakness in the muscular structure. During childbirth the pelvic floor muscles are stretched to their limit by passage of the infant and will never regain their previous strength or integrity. If tears occur during birth, even more damage can be done. Women who practice Kegel's exercises to strengthen these perineal muscles after childbirth may have better bladder and vaginal tone then those who do not (see Chapter 18 for an explanation of Kegel's exercises). Some protection may be afforded by these exercises against the weakening of urinary control in later years.

The urogenital diaphragm reinforces the perineum by surrounding the membranous portion of the urethra with ring-shaped fibers. The medial portion of the pelvic floor and the urogenital diaphragm jointly support the pelvic contents when a woman is standing erect. The urogenital diaphragm also provides fascia that fuses in the midline to fill the spaces between the medial border of the levator ani, where it binds the borders of the pubococcygeal muscles. Support of the urogenital diaphragm is supplied by the superficial transverse perineal, the bulbocavernosus, and the ischiocavernosus muscles.

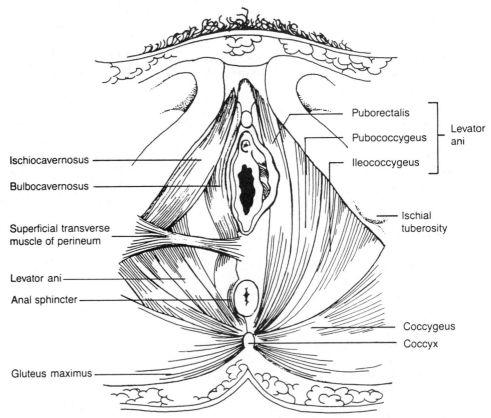

Figure 5–21. Muscles of the pelvic floor. Two of the three major muscle groups that form the floor of the pelvis are shown. The muscles on the right half are deep in the pelvis and form a hammock to help support the pelvic organs. This group is popularly known as the PC muscle. The most superficial muscles are pictured on the left. (Childbirth Graphics)

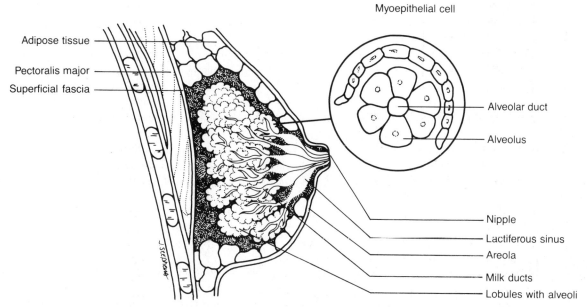

Myoepithelial cell

Adipose tissue

Pectoralis major

Superficial fascia

Alveolar duct

Alveolus

Nipple

Lactiferous sinus

Areola

Milk ducts

Lobules with alveoli

Figure 5–22. Breast structure and action of the myoepithelial cell during breast-feeding. Under the influence of prolactin, the alveoli secrete milk. When the baby begins to suck, oxytocin is released and causes the myoepithelial cells to contract and squeeze milk into the ducts during the "let-down" reflex. The milk flows into the lactiferous sinus, where it collects for immediate use by the infant. (Childbirth Graphics)

The levator ani and coccygeus muscles are innervated by the sacral plexus (third and fourth sacral nerves). All other perineal muscles are innervated by the perineal branch of the pudendal nerve. The blood supply to the perineum is provided by branches of the internal pudendal artery and vein.

Breasts

The appearance of the *breasts* (mammary glands) varies from woman to woman. Although the breasts are usually approximately equal in size, one may be slightly larger than the other. The size, shape, and symmetry of the breasts are largely influenced by heredity, hormone stimulation, and nutrition.

The female breasts are located in the superficial fascia of the pectoral region. They lie over the pectoralis major muscles and are attached to them by a layer of connective tissue. Normally, each breast extends vertically from the second to the sixth rib and laterally from the lateral sternal border to the axilla. The skin of the breasts is similar to that found on the abdomen. The areola surrounding the nipple has hair follicles around its border; in dark-haired, dark-skinned women the areola will appear dark brown, while in fair-skinned women it will appear pink.

Each breast consists of about 20 irregular lobes of secreting tissue, separated by adipose tissue. The amount of fatty tissue determines the size of the breast, but breast size has no relationship to the amount of milk produced from the lactating breast. Each lobe has one lactiferous duct that converges to the areola of the nipple. Alveoli are milk-secreting glands contained in each lobe. They appear as grapelike clusters with stems that terminate in the ducts. The alveoli and their adjacent ducts are surrounded by myoepithelial cells. These cells, shaped like quarter moons, are contractile and squeeze milk from the alveoli into a duct that forms a reservoir called the *ampulla,* or *lactiferous sinus,* as shown in Figure 5–22. The nursing infant must grasp the nipple and areola in its mouth in order to compress the ampulla and cause it to eject the milk that is stored behind it.

Breasts are present in rudimentary forms in infants, children, and men. In infancy both male and female mammary glands are underdeveloped and consist of a few rudimentary ducts lined by epithelium and surrounded by collagenous tissue. During puberty and adolescence the female produces increased amounts of estrogen, which causes the elongation of the mammary ducts and the growth of their epithelium. Fat and fibrous tissue surround the ducts, resulting in the increased size and firmness of the adolescent breast. The areola and nipple also increase in size and become pigmented.

Secondary mammary development occurs when ovulation begins, usually 1 to 2 years after menarche. The effect of progesterone from the luteal phase of the menstrual cycle causes formation of the mammary lobules. During each menstrual cycle, changes occur in the breasts as a result of the concentration of the female hormones estrogen and progesterone in the blood. These cyclical breast changes continue to occur for the remainder of the woman's reproductive years.

In preparation for milk production, marked changes occur in the breast during pregnancy and after parturition through a complex sequence of endocrine events. These changes are discussed in Chapter 13, and breast-feeding is discussed in Chapter 37.

HORMONAL CONTROL OF THE MALE AND FEMALE REPRODUCTIVE CYCLES

Hormones and Their Glands

A *hormone* is a substance released from special tissue into the bloodstream to travel to distant responsive cells, where it exerts its effects. Sex hormones are produced by the endocrine glands and are chemical compounds that produce profound physiologic effects in target organs of the reproductive system.

Neuroendocrinology is the study of hormones and the means by which the brain influences the timing, production, and amount of hormone secretions. The pituitary and the hypothalamus are primary structures, located in the brain, that are responsible for many of these functions.

Pituitary Gland

The *pituitary gland,* known as the *hypophysis,* is one of the most complex of all endocrine glands. It is a small, pea-shaped structure lying at the base of the brain that is connected to the hypothalamus by a system of blood vessels and nervous tissue fibers. The function of its hormones is to stimulate other endocrine glands to produce hormones that, in turn, stimulate the growth and maturation of tissue. Its role in sexual physiology is to secrete the gonadotropins, follicle-stimulating hormone (FSH) and luteinizing hormone (LH), which stimulate the sex organs, and a third hormone, prolactin, which is responsible for stimulating milk production in the female breast.

The pituitary gland consists of two lobes, the posterior lobe (neurohypophysis) and the anterior lobe (adenohypophysis). It is from the anterior lobe that the LH and FSH are produced, stimulated by gonadotropin-releasing hormone (GnRH) secreted by the hypothalamus, which reaches the pituitary through the hypophyseal portal venous system.

Hypothalamus

Even though the *hypothalamus* occupies only 0.3% of the brain, it receives sensory input from all portions of the central nervous system and performs many essential functions. It is responsible for regulating such body mechanisms as appetite, thirst, water conservation, sleep, autonomic response, and endocrine secretion. Neuroendocrine substances released from neural cells within the hypothalamus stimulate the secretion of growth hormone (GH), thyroid-stimulating hormone (TSH), adrenocorticotropic hormone (ACTH), and the gonadotropins FSH and LH.

Other neural cells within the hypothalamus have characteristics of both nerve and endocrine gland cells and respond to signals from the blood stream as well as neurotransmitters within the brain (neurosecretion).

Male Reproductive System

Testosterone is primarily responsible for the distinguishing characteristics of the masculine body. During fetal development the testes are stimulated by chorionic gonadotropin from the placenta to produce moderate amounts of testosterone. During childhood little testosterone is produced, and it is not until the age of 10 to 13 years that its production is greatly increased.

Beginning at puberty, the hypothalamus of the young male stimulates the pituitary gland to produce follicle-stimulating hormone (FSH) and luteinizing hormone (LH). The function of FSH is to stimulate the germ cells within the testes of the male to manufacture sperm, while the

---

Male Secondary Sexual Characteristics Produced by Testosterone

- Growth of the penis, scrotum, and testes until about age 20
- Prolific hair growth on the body, pubis, face, and chest. (Testosterone may cause a decrease of hair growth on the head if two factors contributing to baldness are present: a genetic predisposition to baldness and a genetic predisposition to the production of more than average quantities of androgenic hormones.)
- Deepening of the voice as a result of hypertrophy of the laryngeal mucosa and enlargement of the larynx.
- Thickening of the skin and the secretions of the sebaceous glands, which predisposes to acne.
- Increased muscular development as result of protein deposition in the tissue
- Thickening of the bones as a result of greater quantities of calcium being deposited in the bone matrix

function of LH is to stimulate the production of testosterone in the testes.

Testosterone is responsible for the development of the secondary sexual characteristics in the male that occur at puberty. It is unclear how testosterone causes these changes to occur. It is believed that testosterone stimulates increased production of protein in cells, and most particularly in "target cells," of the tissues responsible for development of the secondary sexual characteristics. This stimulus continues until approximately age 50, when it dwindles rapidly to become 20% to 50% of the peak value by age 80.

Testosterone and other male sex hormones secreted by the testes, in combination with steroids produced by the adrenal cortex, are collectively called *androgens*. Androgens produced by the adrenals are much less potent than testosterone and cannot duplicate its function.

Female Reproductive Cycle

Hormones associated with the female reproductive system serve three important and interrelated functions:

* Satisfaction of sexual desires
* Maturation of the reproductive organs

Female Hormonal System

The female hormone system consists of three separate hierarchies of hormones and activities.

Level 1

The hypothalamus secretes gonadotropin-releasing hormone (GnRH) to the pituitary in response to signals received from higher centers in the central nervous system or from the external environment. Rather than controlling the menstrual cycle, the hypothalamus responds to positive or negative feedback from the ovarian hormones.

Level 2

The anterior pituitary hormones, follicle-stimulating hormone (FSH) and luteinizing hormone (LH), are secreted to stimulate the ovary in response to stimulus from the GnRH of the hypothalamus.

Level 3

The ovarian hormones estrogen and progesterone are secreted in response to stimulation from FSH in the follicular phase and from LH in the luteal phase of the menstrual cycle.

* Preparation of the reproductive organs for conception, gestation, and childbirth

The pituitary gland monitors the levels of estrogen and progesterone secreted by the ovaries, and when blood levels of these hormones reach a certain concentration, they are "turned off" by the pituitary.

Whereas the neurohormone that controls the gonadotropins LH and FSH is called the gonadotropin-releasing hormone, the neurohormone that controls prolactin (the hormone involved in milk secretion) is the prolactin-inhibiting factor (PIF). Not only do these hormones affect the pituitary, but behavioral effects have been associated with several of the releasing factors. The hypothalamus is sensitive to information about emotional and stressful situations received from the environment by means of the nervous and circulatory systems. It is not uncommon for women to experience menstrual changes during disruptive periods of their lives. For instance, women who were in the military and were shipped to war zones overseas during World War II experienced long periods of amenorrhea or other types of menstrual dysfunction. When young women leave home to attend college or to seek employment, they may also experience menstrual problems. Young women at menarche usually experience a year of erratic, heavy, and unpredictable menstrual bleeding due to hypothalamic immaturity.

It was believed for many years that the hypothalamus was the "great regulator" of the hormonal system. This theory has been debunked during the past decade as scientific research has proved that the ultimate regulator of the female hormonal system is the ovary and, more specifically, that the growing follicle, destined to ovulate from the ovary and producing increasing amounts of estrogen, is in control.

The primary hormones of the female reproductive system include estrogen, progesterone, and the gonadotropins, FSH and LH (Table 5–3). These hormones, their sources, and their effects on the body are described in Table 5–4.

The interactions of the structures of the female hormonal system and their effects on the cyclical function of the generative system are extremely complex and are known as the hypothalamic-pituitary-ovarian system.

Menstrual Cycle

Menarche

Menarche refers specifically to the first menstruation and is not the same as puberty. *Puberty* is a term that describes the period of transition from childhood to maturity, in which menarche is one major event. In early menarche menses are usually anovulatory (no ovulation occurs) and may be irregular and heavy. This pattern usually continues for 12 to 18 months, after which normal

(text continued on page 96)

Table 5-3   **Female Hormones**

Hormone	Description
Estrogen	Hormone produced by ovarian follicles, corpus luteum, adrenal cortex, and placenta during pregnancy. It is associated with "femaleness." The three principle types are (a). Estrogen E_1 (estrone)—the estrogen of menopause, oxidized from estradiol. (It is the second most active type, with a relative potency of 10.) (b). Estradiol E_2—the estrogen of reproductive-age women and the most potent type (relative potency 100) (c). Estriol E_3—the estrogen of pregnancy, formed from estradiol and estrone in liver, uterus, placenta, and estrogen precursors from the fetal adrenal gland. (It is the least potent estrogen with a relative potency of 1.)
Progesterone	Hormone secreted by the corpus luteum of the ovary, adrenal glands, and placenta during pregnancy. It is the hormone of the luteal phase of the menstrual cycle and of pregnancy.
Gonadotropins (FSH and LH)	Hormones that, when stimulated by GnRH from the hypothalamus, are released from the anterior pituitary gland to stimulate follicular growth and development, growth of graafian follicle and production of progesterone
GnRH	Hormone that acts on the pituitary gland to release LH and FSH in response to feedback from the ovarian follicle destined to ovulate
Prolactin	Hormone produced by the pituitary gland, which, in association with estrogen and progesterone, stimulates breast development and formation of milk during pregnancy. (Stress of any kind can also stimulate prolactin release in the nonpregnant woman.)

Table 5-4   **Influence of Female Hormones on the Body and Menstrual Cycle**

Organ/System	Action of Estrogen	Action of Progesterone	Action of Gonadotropins
Uterus	• Increases excitability of myometrium • Causes proliferation of endometrium • Increases amount of cervical mucus and produces ferning and spinnbarkeit • Causes uterine growth in pregnancy	• Promotes secretory changes in endometrium • Decreases amount of cervical mucus and renders it impermeable to sperm • Causes loss of ferning • Promotes coiling of uterine arteries • Promotes deposition of glycogen in endometrium • Causes menstruation to occur when conception has not taken place • Reaches peak of activity one week after ovulation	• None
Fallopian tubes	• Influences activity of tubal musculature	• Decreases tubal contractility in later luteal phase • May be important to transport fertilized ovum into uterus	• None
Vagina	• Causes proliferation and cornification of vaginal epithelium • Maintains optimum acidic pH of 3.5–5.5 in vagina	• Causes change from cornified superficial cells to intermediate and basal cell predominance	• None

(continued)

Table 5-4   **Influence of Female Hormones on the Body and Menstrual Cycle**   (continued)

Organ/System	Action of Estrogen	Action of Progesterone	Action of Gonadotropins
Mammary glands	• Promotes development and growth of ductal system, gland buds, and nipples • Partially responsible for lobular and alveolar growth and deposition of fatty tissues • Promotes increased production of prolactin in pregnancy	• Promotes development of lobules and alveoli during pregnancy in preparation for lactation • Causes retention of subcutaneous fluid and swelling of breasts before menstruation	• None
Ovaries	• Interact with gonadotropins to stimulate growth of ovarian follicle and release of ovum • Produce estrogen • May be responsible for LH surge at menstrual midcycle	• Possibly involved in ovulation	FSH • Initiates and stimulates development of ovarian follicles • Promotes estrogen production and secretion by ovarian follicles LH • Causes final growth of graafian follicle • Causes steroidogenesis in conjunction with FSH • Stimulates ovary • Aids in formation of corpus luteum from ruptured follicle • Promotes production of progesterone by the corpus luteum
Skin	• Diminishes sebaceous activity of skin • Increases water content of skin	• May increase sebaceous activity of skin	• None
Cardiovascular system	• Increases blood flow • Increases amount of angiotensin, Factor V, and prothrombin in blood	• None	• None
Secondary sexual characteristics	• Responsible for female contours of fat deposition, and axillary and pubic hair	• Partially responsible for breast development	• None
Thermogenic activity		• Increases the basal body temperature about 0.4–0.6°C after ovulation, identifying luteal function. • Influences deposition of glycogen in endometrium to furnish nutrients for implantation and support of fertilized ovum	• None
Metabolism	• Causes sodium and water resorption from kidney tubules • Affects calcium metabolism and bone growth	• None	• None

cycles usually occur monthly. There is a correlation between mothers' and daughters' ages at menarche.

Age of menstrual onset in the United States has been declining steadily and is now between 9.1 and 17.7 years, with a mean of 12.8 years. Earlier menarche in this decade is possibly due to better nutrition and health care. Body weight has been suggested as a critical factor in the initiation of growth and the occurrence of menarche. Body weight of 48 kg and 17% body fat may reflect a required state of metabolism that initiates menarche. This hypothesis does not address the fact that there is no specific age or size at which a young woman can expect to experience menarche.

The usual sequence of events in growth initiation, lasting approximately 2 years, comprises thelarche (the beginning of breast development), pubarche (the beginning of the development of pubic hair), and finally, menarche. All major body systems are influenced by the beginning of estrogen secretion. Thus, this hormone plays an essential role in adolescent development.

Control of the reproductive cycle depends on constant release of GnRH; this in turn depends on the interaction of the releasing hormones, LH and FSH, and the ovarian hormones, estrogen and progesterone. Levels of these hormones are controlled by a feedback system that is positive (stimulatory) or negative (inhibitory), as shown in Figure 5–23.

The long feedback loop demonstrates efforts of blood levels of target organ hormones to stimulate the hypothalamus to increase the amount of releasing hormones, thus triggering the pituitary to increase production of FSH or LH. The short feedback loop indicates negative feedback of the gonadotropins on the pituitary secretion when their levels become too high and need to be lowered. This is accomplished by the inhibitory effects of GnRH in the hypothalamus.

Normal menstrual cycles indicate that this system is working harmoniously and that maturity of the hypothalamic pituitary–ovarian axis has been achieved. Any dysfunction in the absence of a physical anomaly indicates the disruption of one or more of the system's hierarchies. When birth control pills are used, the resulting high levels of circulating hormones shut down this system and inhibit ovulation.

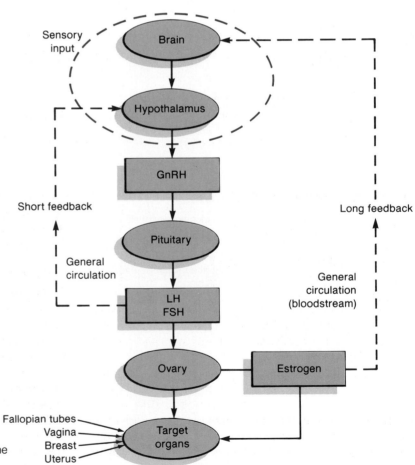

Figure 5–23. Diagrammatic representation of the neuroendocrine feedback mechanisms.

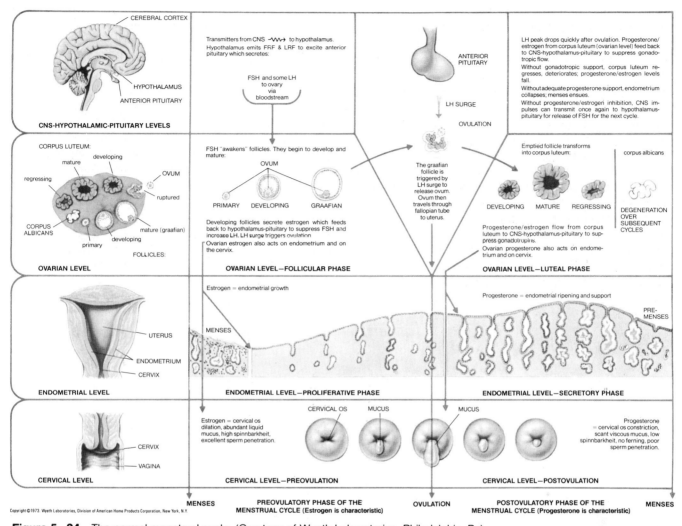

Figure 5-24. The normal menstrual cycle. (Courtesy of Wyeth Laboratories, Philadelphia, Pa)

Normal Menstrual Cycle

The *menstrual cycle* is a normal, predictable, and anticipated event that occurs regularly over the span of a woman's reproductive years. At menarche it signals the beginning of womanhood and fertility; at the other extremes of life, the absence of menstruation signals menopause and the end of fertility. *Menstruation* is defined as the bleeding and physiologic shedding of the uterine endometrium that occur at approximately monthly intervals from menarche to menopause.

The normal menstrual cycle is variable, and in the same person may vary in number of days from cycle to cycle.

The menstrual cycle can be considered as two interrelated cycles. One cycle takes place in the ovary and depends on the other, which is occurring simultaneously in the uterus. This unique mechanism cyclically affects the endometrium to get it ready for the development of the fertilized egg at the precise time of the month when the egg is present. The ovarian and menstrual cycles are summarized in Figure 5-24 and Table 5-5.

Ovarian Cycle

Follicular Phase. The ovarian phase of the menstrual cycle lasts from about the 4th to the 14th day of the cycle. During this 10-day phase, the cycle is under the influence of FSH secreted by the pituitary. Its function is to stimulate a number of ovarian follicles to grow, develop, and produce estrogen. Each follicle contains an egg cell (ovum), but only one is destined to mature fully and to ovulate. Other growing follicles are less receptive to FSH and estrogen stimulation and will have limited growth.

Although estrogen is secreted by all the growing follicles, the dominant follicle secretes the major portion. When the estrogen level is high, it is carried by the blood

Table 5-5   **Ovarian and Menstrual Cycle**

Follicular/Proliferative Phase (Estrogen Dominant)	Ovulation (Gonadotropin Surge)	Luteal/Secretory Phase and Menses (Progesterone Dominant)
Early Follicular Phase (Ovarian)— 2–6 Days • Rise in FSH levels, beginning day 24, due to estrogen decrease in previous luteal phase • Early growth of ovarian follicles *Advanced Follicular Phase (Ovarian)—7–16 Days* • Stimulation of graafian follicle by FSH • Continued follicular growth with increased production of estradiol, reaching a peak before ovulation • Stimulation by FSH and estradiol of rapid rise in LH production after day 10 (positive feedback) • Decline in FSH just prior to ovulation in response to increased estrogen from developing follicle (negative feedback) • Secretion of estradiol, primarily by follicle that will ovulate • Increase of preovulatory progesterone production to 2–3 ng/ml • Atresia of all but dominant ovarian follicle caused by androgen production late in phase *Proliferative Phase (Uterine)* • Estrogen stimulation, producing Proliferation of endometrium and myometrium Increased vascularity, vasodilation, and rhythmic contraction of uterine blood vessels Increased uterine motility in nonpregnant uterus in preparation for effect of progesterone after ovulation	• LH surge at midcycle requires Estradiol concentration over 200 mg/ml and exposure to estrogen for a minimum of 50 hours • Rupture of follicle, usually within 24 hours of LH peak • Ovulation (occurs only if mature follicle [adequate estrogen] is present) • Modest rise in FSH (may be necessary for normal corpus luteum development) • High gonadotropin levels, lasting only 24 hours • Precipitous drop in estrogen, probably due to luteinization of follicle • Shift from estrogen to progesterone dominance	*Luteal/Secretory Phase* • Initial sharp drop of estrogen (time from midcycle LH surge to menses is consistently about 14 days in 90% of women) • Plasma level of progesterone of 3 mg/ml produced, reliable evidence of ovulation at peak (8–9 days postovulation) • Formation of corpus luteum (CL) from follicle remnants after ovulation; synthesis by CL of androgens, estrogens, and progesterone • Stimulation by progesterone growth of endometrium, with coiling, enlargement, and spiraling of arteries in preparation for implantation of fertilized ovum • With fertilization, the CL is maintained and progesterone production reaches a plateau at 9–13 days after ovulation, implantation occurs 6–8 days after ovulation • Secretion of human chorionic gonadotropin by the implanting blastocyst (maintains steroidogenesis of CL until the 6th–10th week of gestation, when the placenta takes over) • Without fertilization, maintenance of CL is maintained by LH for 14 (±2) days Inhibition of LH secretion by high progesterone levels Decrease in estrogen production after degeneration stimulating FSH secretion • Degeneration, scarring, and eventual disappearance of the CL taking place over a 3-month period • Rise in FSH levels, beginning day 24, to stimulate early follicular development for the new cycle *Menstrual Phase* Menstruation, with sloughing off of the endometrium

stream to the pituitary gland, where it exerts a negative feedback effect on the hypothalamus. In turn, the hypothalamus signals the pituitary to inhibit its FSH production because the dominant follicle is producing high levels of estrogen. A progesterone surge after day 10 of the cycle stimulates the production of LH, which will suppress the lesser follicles while causing the graafian follicle (the dominant follicle) to mature. On day 14, with the aid of a progesterone spurt, a peak of LH causes the ovum to burst from the surface of the ovary, and ovulation has occurred (see Fig. 5–24.)

Because the number of days necessary for follicle maturation varies, it is the follicular phase of the cycle that causes variation in the length of menstrual cycles from month to month.

Ovulation.   Ovulation usually occurs 14 days before the beginning of the next menstrual cycle. The timing of ovulation is important because if conception is desired, the ovum must be fertilized within 1 to 2 days of ovulation while the sperm and ovum are still viable. For those couples not desiring pregnancy, it is important that contraception be used during the fertile period.

Ovulation can be detected in about 25% of women by lower abdominal discomfort on the side where ovulation has occurred. Called *mittelschmerz,* this pain may be caused by follicular fluid or blood released from the ruptured follicle, which irritates the peritoneum. Women who experience mittelschmerz may be at an advantage for planning pregnancy; however, this symptom may not occur during every cycle. Another method of determining ovulation is the daily use of a basal body temperature chart, which shows a shift of body temperature just before ovulation. Use of this method to determine time of fertility is discussed in Chapter 8.

Luteal Phase.   The luteal phase begins about the 15th day of the cycle and ends about the 28th. As a consequence of the midcycle LH surge that caused ovulation, estrogen levels fall sharply early in the luteal phase while the brief midcycle rise of progesterone initiates the precipitous drop of LH.

After the rupture of the graafian follicle and the release of the ovum, the cells of the empty follicle increase in size and fill with a yellow pigment called *lutein* to form the corpus luteum. Under the influence of LH, the corpus luteum begins to produce high levels of progesterone and low levels of estrogen. Capillaries contained within the central cavity of the corpus luteum fill with blood 8 to 9 days after ovulation, and vascularization of the cavity is complete. At this time blood levels of estrogen and progesterone have reached their peak. Progesterone counteracts the effects of estrogen and suppresses new follicular growth in the ovary.

If fertilization of the egg (conception) does not occur, the corpus luteum begins to decline about 10 days after ovulation. Levels of FSH begin to rise about day 26 to begin early follicular development in the ovary in preparation for the new cycle. The LH concentration becomes so low that it can no longer support the corpus luteum. As the corpus luteum degenerates, its production of estrogen and progesterone falls off rapidly, and these hormones reach their lowest level. As a result, the endometrium begins to shed and menstrual flow ensues.

When conception has occurred, the corpus luteum is maintained beyond 14 days by the presence of human chorionic gonadotropin (HCG), an LH-like hormone se-

creted by the implanting blastocyst. The function of HCG is to maintain the growing blastocyst until the placenta is sufficiently developed to take over production of estrogen and progesterone at about 6 to 10 weeks' gestation.

Endometrial (Uterine) Cycle
Proliferative Phase.   As the ovarian follicles are developing and producing increasing amounts of estrogen in the follicular phase, the uterine endometrium is growing and being reconstructed in preparation for ovulation and possible conception. Reconstruction occurs in response to the increasing estrogen secretion from the growing follicles. Endometrial glands are at first narrow, tubular, and lined with low columnar epithelial cells. These cells rapidly multiply by mitosis, stratify, and extend peripherally to line with neighbor glands, forming a continuous lining of the endometrial cavity. The *stroma,* or foundation tissue of the endometrium, develops, and spiral vessels form a loose capillary network beneath the epithelial membrane. Re-expanding after its menstrual collapse, the endometrium grows from 0.5 mm to between 3.5 and 5.0 mm in height. Growth of the stroma results not only from estrogen stimulation, but also from incorporation of ions, water, and amino acids. Tissue growth has occurred, but the major element in achieving endometrial height is stromal "reinflation."

Secretory Phase.   The secretory phase of the uterus occurs in conjunction with the luteal phase of the ovarian cycle to provide support for the growth of the early embryo. The endometrium is dependent on both estrogen and progesterone activity and has reached the height it achieved by the end of the proliferative phase just prior to ovulation. In preparation for implantation, gland growth becomes increasingly tortuous and the coiling of the spiral vessels is intensified. During the 7-day postovulatory period, glandular cells join together, forming large openings into the endometrial cavity. They appear to become exhausted, their lumina distended and cell surfaces fragmented (see Fig. 5–24). The stroma becomes increasingly edematous, and the spiral vessels are densely coiled and swollen. This readies the endometrium for implantation of the fertilized ovum.

When conception does not occur, HCG is not produced, the corpus luteum dies, and the levels of estrogen and progesterone fall. Hormone withdrawal causes the endometrium to become dehydrated and to shrink in height, the blood flow within the spiral vessels diminishes, the stromal cells disintegrate, and menstruation begins. Within 13 hours the height of the endometrium shrinks from 4.00 mm to 1.25 mm. Menstrual flow ceases in 3 to 4 days as a result of events that include prolonged vasoconstriction of the uterine stroma and vessels and healing of the glandular elements through the effects of the estrogen being produced in the newly forming follicles.

Menstruation. The length of the normal menstrual cycle is determined by counting from the first day of a period to the first day of menses the following month. Normally the menstrual cycle varies from 24 to 34 days, the average interval being 28 days. Duration of menstruation is variable, but 2 to 8 days is considered normal. In most women the duration of flow is usually consistent from cycle to cycle.

Blood loss during normal menstruation varies from spotting to heavy bleeding and may be as little as 30 ml or as much as 80 ml. More than 80 ml is considered excessive. Most blood loss occurs during the first 3 days of menstruation, so that heavy blood loss is usually not prolonged. Menstrual blood loss may be influenced by a variety of factors on any level of the system. These include, but are not limited to, general state of health, disease, psychic upset, medications, drug therapy or abuse, and anovulatory cycles.

Menstrual discharge contains not only blood but such substances as endometrial debris, prostaglandins, enzymes, cervical mucus, desquamated vaginal cells, and bacteria. Normally odorless, the menses emit a characteristic odor from action of bacteria on the discharge when perineal hygiene is less than optimum.

The usual clotting that occurs when bleeding is caused by a cut or other trauma does not occur with menstrual blood. Clotting is prevented during menses by a high level of fibrinolysin, a substance contained in the endometrium. If continued heavy bleeding is sustained, however, fibrinolysin may become depleted, causing clotting of menstrual blood.

Absence of Menstruation. In women who have been experiencing regular, normal menses, the absence of a period may come as a surprise. In sexually active women who use contraception but may have forgotten or ignored its use on one or more occasions, the lack of menstruation should come as no surprise. Women who use contraception carefully and consistently may attribute lack of menstruation to a physiologic problem. In sexually active women not using a birth control method, missed menses should be anticipated.

If a sexually active woman who is healthy and experiencing no temporary physical or emotional problems misses a menstrual period, pregnancy should be assumed until proven otherwise. When pregnancy has occurred, the embryo is well established before the woman even misses her first menstrual period. The physiologic events of pregnancy that occur unnoticed in the interim between the beginning of the last menstrual period and the woman's realization of a missed menses are swift and dramatic. The events surrounding conception are discussed in Chapter 7.

Menopause

Menopause and its effects on women is one of the least understood areas of health care and is still surrounded by myth and "old wive's tales," despite modern understanding of hormonal and physiologic change. Emotional factors and lack of appreciation of what symptoms really portend play major roles in understanding the physiologic process called menopause.

The *climacteric* is the term used to describe the period of approximately 15 years during which the woman's body is preparing itself for the cessation of menses. Climacteric means "rung of the ladder," a developmental stage in the life cycle of women. It is first seen when frequency of ovulation decreases, and ends with atrophy of the secondary sexual characteristics. Menopause is one milestone in the progression of the many physical and emotional events that occur during the transitional years from middle to old age.

The 1980 U.S. census reported that of the 116 million women in this country, 32 million were 50 years of age or older. The majority of these women had, or would shortly have, their final menstrual period. According to life expectancy tables, a woman aged 50 can expect to live approximately 28 more years, or one third of her life without ovarian function. Earlier in the 20th century menopause arrived as early as 35 to 40 years of age. Today, contributing factors to later onset of menopausal symptoms are related to better nutritional habits, planning for parenthood, less strenuous physical labor, and more and better health care.

Most women are in relatively good health during middle age and old age. They have few problems during the climacteric years. The transition from regular menstrual cycles to cessation of menstruation usually is characterized by gradual phasing out of menstrual periods over months, or as much as several years.

On a continuum, the physiologic events of the climacteric are divided into three phases: premenopause, menopause, and postmenopause. The frequency of ovulation begins to decrease in the mid-30s. This is the first evidence of the climacteric. Women are free of hormonal change symptoms until the late 40s when menstrual cycles may become erratic. The climacteric may be characterized over time by irregularities in the woman's menstrual pattern from light to heavy flow.

At birth a baby girl is endowed with all of the oocytes (eggs) she will ever have. During the reproductive years from menarche to menopause, the eggs are formed and ovulation occurs. However, the ovary is programmed to exhaust its numbers of ooyctes that have produced the major portion of estrogen during the woman's reproductive years. This loss of ovarian follicle function results in a substantial decrease of estrogen and, in turn, causes a change in the sex hormone output of the hypothalamus, pituitary, and adrenal glands. This dramatic decrease in circulating estrogen (estradiol), is considered the most significant endocrine change of menopause. The levels of luteinizing hormone (LH), and follicle stimulating hormone (FSH) are gradually elevated and peak at 2 to 3 years after menopause, resulting in a dramatic decline of circulating estrogen.

The amount and rate of estrogen loss has multiple effects on symptoms that women will experience.

- *Slow loss of estrogen.* Women experience minimal vasomotor symptoms, abnormal and prolonged uterine bleeding (that may cause iron deficiency anemia), and other possible problems resulting in bleeding such as fibroids, anovulatory bleeding, or malignancy. Slow, sustained loss of estrogen results in late menopause.
- *Normal or moderate estrogen loss.* With moderate estrogen loss women tend to experience mild, periodic flushes and less blood loss.
- *Rapid estrogen loss* means that the woman will experience intense vasomotor symptoms, more intense flushes, and, possibly, earlier menopause.

Elevated levels of both follicle stimulating hormone and luteinizing hormone work overtime to stimulate the ovary, and are seen as conclusive evidence of ovarian shut-down and resulting menopause.

Once menopause occurs and ovarian production of estrogen ceases, the postmenopausal ovaries and adrenals secrete the male hormone testosterone. Testosterone from both these sources is transported to peripheral fat deposits of women where, along with cholesterol, it is metabolized into estrone, a weak analog of estrogen. This process is known as peripheral conversion. The amount of available testosterone and the rate of peripheral conversion determine the amount of estrone produced. Women with more body fat will have more circulating estrone than women who are thin, and thus have a lower incidence of menopausal symptoms. As much as 10 times the amount of estrone may be found in very obese women. Estrone may figure in the well-known association between obesity and the development of endometrial cancer. The obese population is also prone to diabetes and high blood pressure.

It cannot be predicted who will experience menopausal symptoms. Eighty percent of women have one or more symptoms; 10% have such serious symptoms that they interfere with daily activities; 10% have no symptoms, and of the 80% to 90% of women who experience symptoms, only 30% will seek medical care.

Cumulative Effects of Aging and Hormonal Deficiency

Menopause and the aging process interrelate. With decreasing ovarian function and consequent loss of estro-

gen, all systems of the body are affected and changed. A change in adrenal secretions of androgens from an anabolic process to a catabolic process is manifested by a variety of physical and psychologic effects.

These changes result in a general loss of elasticity of the vulvar tissue; pubic hair becomes sparse and brittle; the labia minora disappear. The skin of the vulva becomes thin and easily traumatized, its thickness is five cell layers as compared to 20 layers during the reproductive years. This is a late occurrence at 70 to 80 years. The glans of the clitorus may atrophy and disappear beneath the prepuce. The introitus gradually constricts but happens less rapidly when the woman has regular intercourse. Supporting structures of the vagina lose their elasticity and tone, creating susceptibility to rectocele, cystocele, and uterine prolapse, especially during menopause. Decreased estrogen to the vagina reduces epithelial cell glycogen reducing its normal acidity and predisposing to infection. Bloody staining from the vagina and dyspareunia can occur from dryness or contraction of the vagina.

Changes in organ and connective tissue also occur. The endometrium of the uterus atrophies, the uterus shrinks

SELF-CARE TEACHING

The Menopausal Woman

The nurse can use these teaching points with the woman facing menopause.

- Menopause is a normal physiologic process; related discomforts are temporary.
- Verbalize your stresses and concerns with your health care worker.
- Focus on the positive elements of your life. Many activities can bring satisfaction and rewards.
- Avoid overwork and fatigue but practice daily exercise for your mental and physical health.
- Follow a diet adequate in foods from all major food groups, including a variety of fiber-rich foods to avoid constipation. Also include three to four daily servings of calcium-rich foods to prevent osteoporosis.
- If you smoke (especially if you are on estrogen replacement therapy), quit smoking.
- Hot flashes will decrease and probably stop within a year. To avoid or decrease hot flashes try wearing layered clothing (allowing removal of outer layers) and keep blankets to a minimum to maintain warmth without overheating.
- Even though your sexuality may change gradually, it should continue as a satisfying experience. Drugs that may decrease sexual desire include antihypertensives, antidepressants, antihistamines, and barbiturates.

in size and takes a position in the long axis of the vagina, with increasing retroversion due to diminished muscular support. The ovaries atrophy, follicles diminish, and decreased estrogen causes a gonadal response with marked elevation of FH and LH. There is atrophy of connective tissues and muscular supports of the vagina, urethra and rectum. Cystocele, urethrocele, and rectocele may occur due to lack of estrogen support and multiple stressors of time, such as pregnancy, labor, and instrumentation. There is atrophy of the breast acini and lobules and progressive involution from the periphery to the nipple. Atrophic changes occur in the urinary tract. These may cause dysuria, prolapse of the urethra (urethral caruncle), or stenosis of the external meatus; bacterial urethritis may result from increased amounts of residual urine; ascending infection into the bladder and symptoms of urinary frequency and dysuria; decreased fluid intake may lead to urine concentration and bacterial multiplication.

Vasomotor Instability. Probably the best known symptom of the climacteric is commonly called the "hot flash" or "hot flush." It occurs as a result of estrogen depletion; however, its etiology remains unknown. It is now accepted as a physiologic problem rather than a psychological one. The severity of this symptom provides a rough index of the degree and rapidity of estrogen depletion. The following are some of its symptoms:

- A warm (hot) feeling that begins in the chest and works its way up to the neck and face.
- The skin becomes very red, very like an extreme blush.
- Flushes can vary from an occasional warm flush to as many as 10 to 20 severe flushes per day that may last from a few minutes to half an hour.
- Profuse sweating may occur, followed by chilling.
- Sweating in conjunction with the flush may be more common at night and be so extreme that bedclothes become soaked.
- Heart palpitations may be noticed (in the absence of heart disease).
- Excitement or stress may bring on the symptoms.

Estrogen Replacement Therapy. In the 1970's estrogen replacement therapy (ERT) was questioned as a possible factor in endometrial cancer. However, after study and reevaluation, estrogen replacement is now in favor and is seen as a logical way of relieving menopausal discomforts. Not all women can take estrogen and patients must be carefully selected and monitored. Its use in selected, symptomatic patients is warranted under the following circumstances.

1. Severe vasomotor symptoms
2. Atrophic changes of the genitourinary tissue
3. Osteoporosis
4. Premenopausal surgical removal of the ovaries (oophorectomy)

THE AGING PROCESS IN WOMEN

Aging is a natural, basic, biologic process of all living organisms. It is a process that begins at birth. All organic creatures age — some rapidly; others more slowly. Aging is multidimensional. Basic genetics, life-style, diet, disease, injury, substance abuse, and environmental factors are all variables in the aging equation. The study of biologic mechanisms that cause aging is a science called gerontology.

Age-Related Physical Adaptations

The most apparent signs of the aging process in middle-aged and older women are physical changes. Menopause and the climacteric, discussed in the previous section, are a primary physical and hormonal change.

Adaptations in Body Composition

Women become shorter as they age, and lean body weight decreases. These changes increase in pace after age 50 when body muscle is replaced by fat. The body becomes softer, less firm, and weight generally increases. Tolerance for temperature change is also reduced. (Osteoporosis is discussed at the end of the chapter.)

Contraindications to Estrogen Replacement Therapy

Absolute

- Estrogen-dependent tumors
- History of known or suspected pregnancy
- Compromised liver function, as in acute liver disease
- Blood clotting disorders such as thrombophlebitis, myocardial infarction, vascular disease, or pulmonary embolism
- Stroke
- History of undiagnosed vaginal bleeding
- D.E.S. exposure (mother/daughter)
- Insulin-dependent diabetes mellitus

Relative

- Hypertension
- Endometriosis
- Gallbladder disease

Adaptations of the Skin

Changes in the composition of facial and body skin causes wrinkles and sagging due to loss of subcutaneous fat. Women who smoke are more susceptible to wrinkles than those who do not smoke. Abnormal pallor of the skin may indicate iron deficiency, or megaloblastic anemia (B_{12} or folic acid deficiency). One of three women aged 65 and older suffers from dermatoses and other skin disorders (Morrissey 1986). Hyperkeratoses, raised warts, flat black or brown warty areas on the head, neck, and trunk should be assessed for melanoma.

Adaptations of the Musculoskeletal System

Aging muscles lose their elasticity and power due to increased amounts of fibrous tissue that supplants muscle tissue. This process begins in the late 20's and as aging progresses, replaces muscle tissue with fat. Changes in body stamina and configuration occur and tissues become less firm. Back pain may result from loss of abdominal muscle tone that helps to support the upright position. Muscle cramps in the extremities at night, or after exercise are common. The cramps must be differentiated from claudication or arteriosclerosis obliterans. Changes in the spine such as bone brittleness and vertebral atrophy may result from osteoporosis. It is during and after the 50's that the most advanced state of bone loss commences. Between the ages of 65 and 75, arthritis becomes more common in women than men (Morrissey 1986).

Adaptations of the Cardiovascular System

Cardiac output decreases by 30% between the ages of 25 and 65 years (Morrissey 1986). Progressive loss of elasticity and an increase in calcium deposits in the arteries cause decreased distensibility of the blood vessels and may result in increased blood pressure. Cardiac pain that radiates and causes tightness in the chest may indicate angina. As compared to men aged 65 to 75 years, women are more likely to have severe high blood pressure and elevated cholesterol levels (Morrissey 1986).

Adaptations of the Genitourinary Tract

Urinary symptoms are common in older women and nocturnal frequency and incontinence is a stressful disability. The number of nephrons in the aging kidney are reduced and the functional capacity of the kidneys is decreased. Polyuria may result from unregulated diabetes or chronic renal failure. Dysuria may indicate the presence of a urinary tract infection. Renal insufficiency may be problematic when there are increased demands on renal function such as dehydration, infection, or congestive heart failure.

Adaptations of the Gastrointestinal System

Absorption, motility, and enzyme secretion are reduced in the intestines during aging. The weight of the liver is decreased by 20% after age 50, causing slowing of liver metabolism (Morrissey 1986). Difficulty swallowing (dysphagia) is a common complaint. It is an important symptom and its duration is useful in its diagnosis. Gastric production of hydrochloric acid is decreased with age, but should cause few problems. The incidence of hiatal hernia increases to 69% after age 70 (Morrissey 1986). Constipation is a frequent complaint and may be caused by lack of bulk food in the diet, lack of physical activity, chronic laxative ingestion, inadequate fluid intake, and chronic denial of the urge to defecate.

Adaptations in Endocrine Function

Significant changes in thyroid and pancreatic function may occur with aging. Primary hypothyroidism may occur in the elderly woman. It is accompanied by lethargy, constipation, cold intolerance, loss of hearing acuity, increased drying of the skin and, possibly, cardiomegaly. By age 70 and over, one half of the population have abnormal 1 to 2 hour postprandial glucose levels (Morrissey 1986). However, late onset diabetes does not cause the serious complications experienced in a younger population.

Adaptations in the Senses

As people age, there is deterioration of the senses of smell, taste, eyesight, and hearing.

Vision.   By age 65 approximately one half of all people have a visual acuity of 20/70 or less. Eyeglasses or contact lenses are worn by 92 of every 100 persons aged 65 or older. During the years 50 to 60 the lenses become more rigid and the pupil is less efficient (Morrissey 1986). The lenses begin to yellow and create deficiencies in color perception. Cataracts (opacity of the lens of the eye or its capsule or both), and glaucoma (an eye disease that increases intraocular pressure) can occur. The visual field decreases and there is need for more light in order to see. *Arcus senilis,* an opaque ring around the periphery of the cornea, is a normal variant in aging.

Hearing.   By the mid 20's hearing loss begins and tends to increase over the life span. Functional hearing loss is present in 55% of people over 65. These hearing problems include the lack of ability to detect the volume of sound and pitch. Many high-frequency sounds are lost about age 60. Distractions and sounds may make hearing difficult and cause decreased social interactions (Morrissey 1986).

Osteoporosis

Osteoporosis, called ''the silent epidemic,'' is the most common skeletal deficiency. It is the process of prolonged, excessive bone loss only partially replaced by new

Women at Risk for Osteoporosis

At risk for the development of osteoporosis are

- Women who have had an early menopause
- Women who have had surgical removal of their ovaries at a young age
- Women who have had a family history of osteoporosis
- White women (black women are at less risk because they have larger bones and great muscle mass)
- Women of British, European, Chinese, and Japanese ancestry
- Women of fair complexion and small body size
- Women with endocrine disorders such as hyperparathyroidism, hyperthyroidism, Cushing syndrome, kidney disease, diabetes, and rheumatoid arthritis
- Women who smoke cigarettes
- Women with poor eating habits that do not provide the calcium needed to meet the nutritional demands of healthy bones. (Should avoid use of caffeine and alcohol)
- Women who are immobilized for long periods
- Women with milk intolerance, allergies, or who are vegetarians

bone formation. Other forms of bone loss in women are osteopenia and osteomalacia. *Osteopenia* is a normal age-related reduction in bone loss and *osteomalacia* is the adult equivalent of rickets, in which a deficiency of calcium and phosphorus crystals in the collagen framework of the bone is caused by vitamin D deficiency. Loss of estrogen secretion in postmenopausal women is now recognized as a major factor in the development of osteoporosis. During the first 20 years after menopause, 75% or more of bone loss occurs because of estrogen deficiency (Notelovitz and Ware 1985). Bone loss begins as early as the 20s when trabecular (honey-coned interior) bone is lost from the vertebrae. After menopause, a woman will lose cortical (harder, outer covering) bone twice as fast as a man. By age 80, a woman will have lost 47% of her trabecular bone structure, while a man will have lost only 14% (Lund 1987).

Signs of osteoporosis may be detected by the woman, her family, or gynecologist. Loss of height, postural change, and back pain indicate crushing of spinal vertebrae. This occurs in women when working around the house, opening a sticky window, or bending down to pick up something from the floor. Back pain is immediate and severe, but may be ignored as a simple backache. Should incidences continue they may result in a permanently bent posture.

A more subtle sign of possible osteoporosis in elderly women is transparent skin on the backs of the hands due to lack of collagen (also a component of bone) in the outer layer of the skin. A recent study showed an 83% incidence of osteoporosis in these women (Lund 1987).

Bone mineral loss must be between 20% to 40% before bone mass reduction can be detected by x-ray filming. Using standard x-ray filming is a relatively crude method and presumes major bone loss as a prerequisite (Notelovitz and Ware 1985). With the introduction and use of single photon absorptiometry (SPA) in bone density measurement, it is now possible to screen for and confirm bone loss, indicating the need for nutritional supplementation, exercise therapy, or other treatment. SPA screening does not fully correlate with the trabecular content of the spine.

Single absorptiometry should be requested for younger patients who have hysterectomies or oophorectomies, or who are experiencing calcium depleting endocrine problems. Measurements using two photon energy sources of differing strength (dual photo absorptiometry) are more useful because direct measurements of the femoral neck and spine are possible. However, like the single-photon method, the dual-photon method does not discriminate between cortical and trabecular bone. Computed tomography (CT Scan), while expensive, is valuable in determining the extent of osteoporosis. It measures bone mineral while obtaining an image in either the axial or appendicular skeleton. It also has the ability to measure trabecular and cortical bone separately. The CT scanner is the only means available that can measure density of spinal trabecular bone at most risk for fracture (Lund 1987). When providing care to older women, the nurse should be cognizant of the importance of assessing the patient's risk for, and possible symptoms of, osteoporosis. When a family history of osteoporosis and other risks are identified the nurse should chart her findings and inform the physician. Additionally, she can discuss with the woman categories of risk that include, diet, exercise, estrogen therapy, smoking, and alcohol use.

Diet. If the woman's diet is poor and caffeinated drinks and coffee are her primary source of liquids, she risks calcium loss through urinary excretion and the high salt content of "junk foods" that are excreted along with calcium. More important, loss of calcium through excretion triggers the release of parathyroid hormone that, in turn, removes calcium from the bones in order to restore calcium balance in the circulation. Calcium intake sufficient for the needs of the body, including the bones, is necessary to replace lost calcium and to maintain bone strength. Developing good eating habits that includes a diet high in calcium, foods that are rich in all other nutrients, and sunshine exposure will provide the vitamin D that is needed for calcium absorption.

Nursing Research

Calcium Intake and Osteoporosis Risk Assessment

This descriptive study examined the daily calcium intake of 41 healthy women 25–35 years of age. Subjects were asked to complete a 3-day dietary recall. Thirty-one of the 41 subjects consumed an average 904 mg of calcium, considerably less than the level of 1250 mg needed to maintain a positive calcium balance. Thus, the majority of the women in this study were at increased risk for developing osteoporosis in later life.

Nurses must be aware of potential calcium deficiencies in younger women and stress the importance of adequate dietary intake to prevent problems in later life. Teaching strategies might include a list of common foods describing calcium content per serving. Nurses also must be aware that most women are uninformed about risk factors for osteoporosis.

Carter L: Calcium intake in young adult women: Implications for osteoporosis risk assessment. J Obstet Gynecol Neonatal Nurs 16(5): 301–308, 1987

Exercise.   Lack of appropriate exercise plays a significant role in the development of osteoporosis. In response to the stresses of the muscle-pull and weight-bearing that occur during exercise the bones grow larger and stronger. Women who do not exercise sufficiently experience an increased rate of bone loss.

Estrogen Therapy.   Estrogen replacement has a major positive impact on the risk of fractures in older women. With estrogen therapy there may be as high as a 50% to 60% decrease in arm and hip fractures. When estrogen is supplemented with calcium, there may be as much as an 80% reduction in vertebral compression fractures (Notelovitz 1985). In the absence of estrogen, calcium supplementation has little impact on compact bone (Notelovitz 1986).

Smoking.   Cigarette smoking is associated with earlier menopause and increased risk of osteoporosis. Blood levels of estrogen are lower in smokers than nonsmokers. The lower levels of estrogen in the smokers put them at higher risk for reduced bone density (Notelovitz 1986). It may not be the smoking *per se* that contributes to osteoporosis, but the life-style of the smoker herself. Also, lung function in the smoker is less efficient and may affect the woman's ability to exercise. There is an assumption that because smoking interferes with the general circulation,

it may have some effect on blood circulation to the bones (Notelovitz 1985).

Alcohol.   Calcium absorption through the intestines is impaired by alcohol use and may effect the ability of the liver to activate vitamin D. Vitamin D is an essential ingredient for the absorption of calcium. It is also likely that heavy alcohol consumption may compromise proper nutrition and exercise.

IMPLICATIONS FOR NURSING CARE

The nurse who will be providing health care to women in both obstetrical and gynecological settings must be not only equipped educationally but emotionally and philosophically as well.

Knowledge of male and female reproductive anatomy and physiology is essential. Without knowledge and understanding of these complex systems, it would be difficult to grasp the concepts of the normal menstrual cycle, fertility, contraception, or the important role of the maternal systems on the growth and development of the human fetus.

It is therefore incumbent upon the nurse to be fully informed of the diverse and complex systems that constitute women's reproductive capabilities. To do this she must stay abreast of new knowledge, technological advances, and scientific research that is related to women and their reproductive health.

CHAPTER SUMMARY

The nurse needs knowledge of the anatomy and physiologic functions of the reproductive system not only for a personal scientific base but also in order to teach women about their bodies.

Each reproductive structure in one sex corresponds to a similar structure in the other sex. During the first 4 or 5 weeks of pregnancy, all embryos are alike anatomically; sexual differentiation begins around the 6th week.

The male and female generative organs are controlled by the sex hormones. Primary in the complex system is the pituitary-hypothalamus axis. Testosterone is the primary male hormone, while the primary female reproductive hormones are estrogen, progesterone, and the gonadotropins, FSH and LH.

Both male and female reproductive systems are comprised of external and internal organs. Male external organs include the penis and scrotum, and the internal organs are testes and seminiferous tubules, the ductal system, and accessory glands, which include the prostate and bulbourethral glands. The female reproductive tract consists of the following external organs: vulva, mons pubis, labi majora and minora, vestibule of the vagina, and the perineum. Internal structures include the vagina, uterus, fallopian tubes, and ovaries. Breasts are accessory organs.

STUDY QUESTIONS

1. The reproductive structures of the male and female arise from the same embryonic tissue.
   (a) What term describes this similarity?
   (b) What chemical(s) are necessary for the development of male structures from the wolffian duct?
   (c) What chemical(s) are necessary for the development of female structures from the müllerian duct?
2. After six weeks gestation the conceptus becomes sexually differentiated.
   (a) What antigen must be present in order to produce a male child?
   (b) Name the substance that must be present in the male conceptus to complete development of the male embryo.
   (c) Name the male hormone that is most important in the development of secondary sexual characteristics at puberty.
3. At what average age does the male begin to produce functional spermatozoa?
4. For what reason are spermatozoa stored in the scrotum?
5. What structures are contained within the vestibule of the female genitalia?
6. Maintenance of the vaginal ecology is dependent upon a delicate balance of hormonal and bacterial action.
   (a) What is the single most important bacteria that assists in maintaining the normal acid environment of the vagina?
   (b) What hormone is essential to this process?
   (c) What is the normal vaginal *p*H, and how is it maintained?
   (d) Interruption of the vaginal *p*H may occur; list five possible causes.
7. What are the major functions of the uterus?
8. What is the major function of the fallopian tube?

REFERENCES/BIBLIOGRAPHY

Abraham SF, Beaumont PJV, Fraser IS, Llewellyn–Jones D: Body weight, exercise and menstrual status among ballet dancers in training. Br J Obstet Gynecol 89:507–510, 1982

Artal R, Wiswell RA: Exercise in Pregnancy. Baltimore, Williams & Wilkins, 1986

Artal R, Wiswell RA: The Effects of Exercise on the Menstrual Cycle. Baltimore, Williams & Wilkins, 1986

Coupey SM, Saunders DS: Physical maturation. In Lavery JP, Sanfilippo JS (eds): Pediatric and Adolescent Obstetrics and Gynecology. New York, Springer–Verlag, 1985

Federation of Feminist Women's Health Centers: A New View of a Woman's Body. New York, Simon & Schuster, 1981

Guyton AC: Textbook of Medical Physiology, 7th ed. Philadelphia, WB Saunders, 1986

Hacker NF, Moore JG: Essentials of Obstetrics and Gynecology. Philadelphia, WB Saunders, 1986

Lavery JP, Sanfilippo JD: Pediatric and Adolescent Obstetrics and Gynecology. New York, Springer-Verlag, 1985

Lund K: Osteoporosis. Calif Nurs Rev 37: July/August, 1987

Masters WH, Johnson V: Human Sexual Inadequacy. Boston, Little, Brown & Co, 1970

Morrissey S: Aging. In Griffith–Kenny J: Contemporary Women's Health: A Nursing Advocacy Approach. Menlo Park, Addison-Wesley, 1986

Notelovitz M: Osteoporosis: A decade's findings in prevention, diagnosis and treatment. The Female Patient 11(9): 49, 1986

Notelovitz M, Ware W: Stand Tall! Every Woman's Guide to Preventing Osteoporosis. Toronto: Bantam Books, 1985

Pauerstein CJ: Clinical Obstetrics. New York, John Wiley & Sons, 1987

Perke K, Schweiger U, Laessle R, Dickhout B et al: Dieting influences the menstrual cycle: Vegetarian vs. nonvegetarian diet. Fertil Steril 46(6):1083, 1986

Pritchard JA, MacDonald PC, Gant NF: Williams Obstetrics, 17th ed. East Norwalk, CT, Appleton-Century-Crofts, 1985

Speroff L, Glass RH, Kase NG: Clinical Gynecologic Endocrinology and Infertility, 3rd ed. Baltimore, Williams & Wilkins, 1989

SUGGESTED READINGS

Carter LW: Calcium intake in young adult women: Implications for osteoporosis risk assessment. J Obstet Gynecol Neonatal Nurs 16(5):301, Sept/Oct 1987

Coralli CH, Raisz LG, Wood CL: Osteoporosis: Significance, risk factors and treatment. Nurs Pract 11(9):16, 1986

Couch JE: Functional Human Anatomy, 4th ed. Philadelphia, Lea & Febiger, 1985

Cumming DC: The reproductive effects of exercise and training. Current Problems in Obstetrics, Gynecology, and Fertility 10(6):231, 1987

Dunn MM: Guidelines for the effective personal fitness prescription. Nurse Practitioners: The American Journal of Primary Care 12(9):9, September 1987

Eisenberg E: Menarche: The transition from childhood to womanhood. In Barns LA (ed): Advances in Pediatrics, Vol 31, pp 359–369. Chicago, Year Book Medical Publ, 1984

Goldfarb AF: What your patients need today. Contemporary OB/GYN Vol 20 (Special Issue), April 1987

Hammond MG: Monitoring ovulation. Contemporary OB/GYN (Special Issue), pp 59–68, September 1987

Hasselbring B, Greenwood S, Castleman M: Medical Self Care: Book of Women's Health: The Authoritative Guide For Taking Control of Your Own Well-Being. Garden City, NY, Doubleday, 1987

Marsiglio A, Holm K: Physical conditioning of the aging adult. Nurse Pract 13(9):33, 1988

Mattox JH: Normal menstruation. In Wilson JR, Carrington ER (eds): Obstetrics and Gynecology, 8th ed. St Louis, CV Mosby, 1987

Shangold MM: Factors affecting menstrual flow, Contemporary OB/GYN, 25(4):73, 1985

Shangold MM, Mirkin G: The adolescent athlete. In Lavery JP, Sanfilippo JS (eds): Pediatric and Adolescent Obstetrics and Gynecology. New York, Springer–Verlag, 1985

Wilson MA: Evaluating menstrual disorder—premenstrual syndrome, dysmenorrhea, amenorrhea. J Obstet Gynecol Neonatal Nurs 13(12):11, 1985

6 human sexuality

LEARNING OBJECTIVES

After studying the material in this chapter the student should be able to

- Discuss the concept of sexual health

- Discuss the changes that occur for both women and men during sexual response

- Explain the triphasic nature of the sexual response cycle

- Describe how pregnancy results in changes in sexual response in the areas of desire, arousal, and orgasm

- Identify issues of sexual concern for pregnant couples in all three trimesters and postpartum

- Discuss the basic guidelines for advising couples on the relative risks of intercourse during pregnancy and postpartum

- Offer specific suggestions to improve sexual problems for each stage of pregnancy and postpartum

KEY TERMS

Abstinence

Coitus

Cunnilingus

Dyspareunia

Extragenital

Libido

Masturbation

Myotonia

Orgasm

Orgasm restriction

Refractory period

Sexual health

Tonic contraction

Vasocongestion

Western cultural messages sometimes make it difficult to connect the image of parenthood with the idea of sexual desire and activity, since the Western cultural heritage is influenced by religious belief in the immaculate conception of the Madonna. Beliefs about sexual activity during pregnancy have ranged from complete prohibition to an absolute lack of restriction. The rationale and guidelines for these restrictions have been inconsistent.

Many patients want more information about sexual feelings and behaviors during pregnancy and the postpartum period but are reluctant to initiate the discussion with a direct question to the nurse or physician. Frequently, health professionals do not inquire about the patient's sexual concerns or questions because they lack the training to do so.

Both medical and nursing schools traditionally avoided including human sexuality in their curriculum. Progress is being made slowly, but along with a stronger emphasis on total patient care, medical and nursing programs are adding human sexuality to their curriculum. Still, there is little standardization about what is taught to medical and nursing students.

This chapter will acquaint health professionals with basic information about human sexuality, as a foundation for understanding how sexuality may be affected by childbearing. The chapter examines the ways in which the changes of pregnancy can inhibit or enhance sexual feelings and incorporates the most recent information on the sexuality of pregnant couples, the relative risks and advantages of sexual activity, and the ways in which the nurse can intervene with information, suggestions, and support.

SEXUAL HEALTH

The primary goal of health professionals caring for clients who may have sexual concerns needs to be the promotion of *sexual health*. Maddock (1975) states that sexually healthy individuals have

- A certain amount of cognitive knowledge about sexual phenomena

- A degree of self-awareness about their own attitude toward sex

- A well-developed usable value system that influences sexual decisions

- Some degree of emotional comfort and stability in relation to sexual activities in which they and others engage

Covington (1987) states that sexual health encompasses effective birth control, the avoidance of sexually transmitted viral and bacterial diseases, and recognition

RELATED RESEARCH

AIDS Knowledge and Sexual Behavior Change in Unmarried Adults

Over 400 unmarried adults living in a low-incidence city were interviewed concerning their knowledge about AIDS, HIV testing, their level of concern, and the extent of change in their sexual behavior. Sixty-five percent of the sexually active nonmonogamous adults reported having changed their behavior because of concern about AIDS; another 8% reported having been careful even prior to the epidemic. The most common changes were reducing the number of sexual partners (52%), and learning more about potential sexual partners (51%). Thirty-seven percent reported using condoms to minimize risk. The most important factor in whether or not behavior change occurred was the level of concern for self; the level of knowledge did not serve to differentiate between those who changed their behavior and those who did not.

Implications for health care are reflected in the extent to which this relatively well-educated population still was uninformed about the epidemic. Nearly 40% believed that HIV could be transmitted much like the common cold; one fourth of those interviewed believed HIV could be transmitted by sharing a drinking glass or living with someone who was infected. However, even though this population overestimated the degree of contagion of HIV, they clearly understood that sexual contact spreads HIV. These findings suggest that health professionals may need to assess an individual's concern for self in the face of a particular health threat, before attempting to motivate behavior change for disease prevention.

Keeter S, Bradford J: Knowledge of AIDS and related behavior change among unmarried adults in a low-prevalence city. American Journal of Preventive Medicine 4(3):146–148, 1988

of the numerous factors that may enhance or detract from the state of sexual well-being. According to the World Health Organization (1975), a state of sexual well-being includes freedom from fear, shame, guilt, false beliefs, and other psychological factors inhibiting sexual response and sexual relationships.

Developmental Aspects of Sexuality

The roots of shame, guilt, and false beliefs or, conversely, the instillation of positive reassurance that sexuality is healthy begins early in childhood. Children learn about their sexuality in infancy, when they are learning the names for parts of their bodies, particularly their genitals, and learning whether they are a boy or a girl.

The underlying message about the relative comfort or discomfort of a parent with the sex education of a child comes through to the child in a myriad of ways. How the family deals with nudity, masturbation, childhood sex play, explaining where babies come from, and preparation for the changes anticipated in puberty, will all give the child a certain attitude or belief about the possibility of asking further questions or bringing up sexual issues for discussion.

According to mental health professionals, by age 5, children should have a basic understanding of body parts and their functions and a general knowledge of where babies come from. Correct anatomical names should be used. They should have a firm idea of their own gender and an understanding of the concept of maleness and femaleness.

By ages 6 to 9, children need assurance that their bodies belong to them and that they have a choice in permitting or refusing physical affection. A child should never be forced to kiss relatives or family friends and they should be taught how to recognize and avoid sexual abuse.

By ages 9 to 12, children should know what body changes to expect at puberty and that each child develops at his or her own rate. They should understand the human reproductive system and how it works, including menstruation. They need to know that masturbation and "wet dreams" are a normal part of growing up and that there is a difference between being physically mature enough and emotionally mature enough for intercourse (Klein 1987).

Generally, adolescent cognitive development is a continuously maturing process that moves from concrete or literal thinking to abstract thinking. The concrete thinking of early adolescence (approximately ages 10 to 14) is here-and-now thinking and is related to what the adolescent has experienced in the past or is currently experiencing. The long-term consequences of actions may have little meaning to an adolescent who thinks concretely. Adolescents often do not use contraception to prevent pregnancy or condoms to prevent sexually transmitted diseases because they are unable to link the act of intercourse to the possibility of pregnancy or disease (Yoos 1987).

The health professional needs to use concrete concepts and language and to stress immediate results the adolescent can relate to. When discussing the need to prevent pregnancy at this stage, it is important to translate the more abstract ideas of pregnancy into the concrete changes it would cause in the adolescent's life (Proctor 1986).

By the ages of 12 to 14, adolescents should know about contraception, and there should be clarification of any misinformation about conception and contraception. Adolescents need to understand the advantages of avoiding too-early sexual activity and that human sexuality is a natural aspect of life (Klein 1987).

About the age of 15 or 16 years, the thinking process matures so the adolescent can begin to understand cause-and-effect relationships and can hypothesize a future option. These more mature abilities to integrate past, present, and future are relatively stable by late adolescence (approximately ages 17 to 21+). During times of stress or illness, many people revert to concrete thinking.

According to Erikson, the most important task of adolescence is identity formation. Part of achieving a growing, separate identity must include coming to recognize one's fertility. Acceptance of this aspect of sexuality is necessary to ensure responsible sexual behavior that includes the use of contraception. Early adolescents then, in the concrete-thinking stage, are the most difficult to influence in the use of contraception. If they do become pregnant, many will choose to keep their babies because they cannot project into the future. Sexuality in adolescence is further discussed in Chapter 10.

Sexual Identity

Sexual identity is composed of three parts: gender identity, gender role behavior, and sexual orientation (Moses and Hawkins 1982). Gender identity is the perceived internal sense of being a girl or a boy, and it is usually firmly established by age 4. Gender role behaviors are the behaviors that the culture typically assigns to a particular gender. Sexual orientation refers to how a person defines himself or herself, that is, as heterosexual, homosexual, or bisexual.

During early adolescence (ages 10 to 14), young people normally concentrate heavily on their relationships with their peers. They search for their own concept of normalcy through comparison with peers of the same sex. Sometimes same-sex friendships include homosexual experiences, and this seems to be a rather common psychosocial developmental experience (Rigg 1982).

By middle adolescence (ages 13 to 17), many young people start to be concerned about their sexual orientation, especially if they feel, or once felt, attracted to someone of the same sex. This is often called gay identification/confusion. Parents, health professionals, and society place undue concern on the issue of homosexuality at this stage, especially since it is normal for same-sex exploration to occur (Muscari 1987). The awkwardness of new heterosexual social and interpersonal relationships is not easily bridged, and thus there is continued need for same-sex comradeship and intimacies.

It is important to note here that adolescents often find it difficult to discuss their concerns with *anyone*. If they become too isolated or alienated from their peers and family, they may feel suicidal. It is therefore vitally important for health professionals to be alert to adolescents' concerns regarding sexual orientation. (Adolescent sexuality is further discussed in Chapter 10.)

Gender role behavior continues to be mastered throughout late adolescence and young adulthood. Sexual orientation is usually clearly defined by young adulthood; however, the negative sanctions against homosexuality often are enough of a barrier that gay or lesbian young adults may not choose to "come out" or openly enter into same-sex relationships until long after they acknowledge their sexual orientation to themselves.

Sexuality continues to evolve and change during the adult years, partly in response to psychological maturation and adaptation, and in part because of physiologic changes in the body with childbearing and aging. The following sections discuss the physiologic elements of human sexuality, and the specific changes in sexuality through the childbearing cycle.

SEXUAL PHYSIOLOGY

Embryonic and Infant Sexual Functioning

Male fetuses appear to have the capacity for intrauterine erection, as demonstrated by sonograph pictures. The erection is cyclical on a fairly regular basis (Calderone 1983). There has been no direct observation before birth of clitoral erection or vaginal lubrication in female fetuses; however, these are possible from birth onward (Langefeldt 1980). Fetuses also sometimes suck their thumbs, fingers, and toes, and thus it would seem that from the very beginning of a child's life, sexual capacity is an integral part of its being. The historic Kinsey research (1948) reported the capacity for orgasm in boys as young as 5 months and girls as young as 4 months. The following description is given by Kinsey:

> The orgasm in an infant or other young male is, except for the lack of an ejaculation, a striking duplicate of orgasm in an older adult . . . the behavior involves a series of gradual physiologic changes, the development of rhythmic body movements with distinct penis throbs and pelvic thrusts, an obvious change in sensory capacities, a final tension of muscles, especially of the abdomen, hips and back, a sudden release with convulsions, including rhythmic anal contractions — followed by the disappearance of all symptoms.

This phenomenon may be set in motion simply by pressing the thighs together, masturbation by hand, or pressing the genitals against a doll or blanket.

Adult Sexual Response Cycle

Masters and Johnson's Four-Phase Theory

In the 1950s, Dr. William H. Masters and Mrs. Virginia Johnson began laboratory observations of human sexual responses at the Reproductive Biology Research Foundation in St. Louis. The observations were made during masturbation, sexual intercourse, and "artificial coition" using a lighted camera in the vagina. Masters and Johnson (1966) described the response cycle they observed in terms of four phases: the *excitement* phase, the *plateau* phase, the *orgasm* phase, and the *resolution* phase. The phases are general descriptions and certainly vary from person to person and from experience to experience. Moreover, the transition from one phase to another is not always clearly demarcated.

Excitement Phase

The primary reaction to sexual stimuli is *vasocongestion,* meaning that more blood flows into an organ than flows out of it. The engorgement, or vasocongestion, may be triggered by direct physical stimulation, a sexually stimulating sight, or an erotic train of thought. The second reaction to sexual stimuli is *myotonia,* the contraction of various muscle fibers, muscles, and groups of muscles. The myotonia is evidenced by spasms in the hands and feet (carpopedal spasms), facial grimaces, and tensing of extremities or other body parts during orgasm. The physiologic changes that proceed through the sexual response cycle remain basically the same regardless of the type of stimulation used, such as manual stimulation by oneself or one's partner, oral-genital stimulation, penile-vaginal intercourse, fantasy, or, in some, breast stimulation.

In women the first sign of sexual excitation is vaginal lubrication, which occurs 10 to 30 seconds after sexual stimulation is begun. The vasocongestion of the spongy tissue surrounding the walls of the vagina appears to force fluid through the semipermeable membrane that lines the vagina. The lubrication looks like a sweating reaction. Bartholin's glands and the glands lining the cervix do not contribute any significant amount of fluid to the lubrication. The clitoral glans swells as the tissue engorges, and the clitoral shaft increases in diameter and elongates (Fig. 6–1). The clitoris actually becomes erect with sufficient stimulation and arousal.

Neither the size and location of the clitoris nor the amount of swelling is related to sexual responsiveness or to the ability to reach orgasm.

Other changes in the female genitals in the excitement phase include lengthening of the back of the vagina, raising of the cervix and uterus, and flattening and elevation of the labia majora. The labia minora also increase in size (Fig. 6–2).

Extragenitally, the nipples frequently become erect during this phase, the areolae become engorged, the

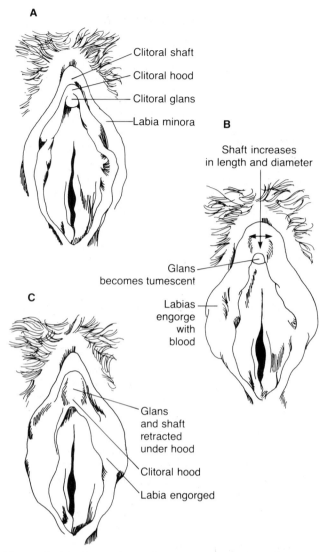

A

Clitoral shaft
Clitoral hood
Clitoral glans
Labia minora

B

Shaft increases
in length and diameter

Glans
becomes tumescent

Labias
engorge
with
blood

C

Glans
and shaft
retracted
under hood

Clitoral hood

Labia engorged

Figure 6-1. Clitoral changes during sexual arousal. *(A)* Unstimulated clitoris. *(B)* Excitement phase. *(C)* Plateau phase. The orgasmic phase is omitted because of lack of information. (After Goldstein B: Human Sexuality. New York, McGraw-Hill, 1976) (Childbirth Graphics)

veins of the breast become more obvious, and the breasts swell.

In men the first sign of vasocongestion is the penile erection (Fig. 6-3). The skin ridges of the scrotal sac smooth out and the scrotum thickens. The spermatic cords shorten, raising the testes toward the body. Nipple erections may occur.

For both men and women, especially in lighter-skinned people, the "sex flush," a maculopapular rash, may appear on the upper abdomen, spreading up toward the breasts. Pulse rate and blood pressure begin to rise as sexual arousal increases.

Plateau Phase

The plateau phase is characterized by a degree of sexual arousal that is much higher than the excitement phase and is lower than the threshold level required to trigger orgasm. In women the most prominent change is the formation of the orgasmic platform, which is an engorgement of the outer third of the vagina. The result is a narrowing of the vaginal opening. During intercourse the orgasmic platform grips the base of the penis. The uterus elevates further, moving the cervix out of the way, and there is further ballooning of the inner two thirds of the vagina. The clitoral glans is raised further away from the vaginal opening and appears to hide up under the hood. The clitoral shaft is shortened by as much as 50%. Lubrication of the vagina slows down, especially if the plateau phase is prolonged (Fig. 6-4).

In nulliparous women the labia minora change from pink to bright red just before orgasm. In parous women the color change is from bright red to deep wine. The swelling of the areola may mask the nipple erection, and the breasts may increase in size by 25% in women who have never breastfed. Breast swelling in women who have breastfed is not noticeable.

In men the plateau phase is characterized by an increase in the swelling of the coronal ridge, and the glans may deepen its reddish-purple color. The testes swell by about 50% to 100% over their unstimulated size, and they

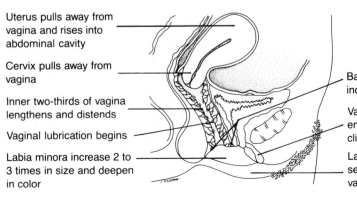

Uterus pulls away from vagina and rises into abdominal cavity

Cervix pulls away from vagina

Inner two-thirds of vagina lengthens and distends

Vaginal lubrication begins

Labia minora increase 2 to 3 times in size and deepen in color

Bartholin's glands: Vestibular bulbs increase in size

Vasocongestion or blood engorgement increases clitoral size 2 to 3 times

Labia majora flatten and separate away from vaginal opening

Figure 6-2. Female excitement stage. (Childbirth Graphics)

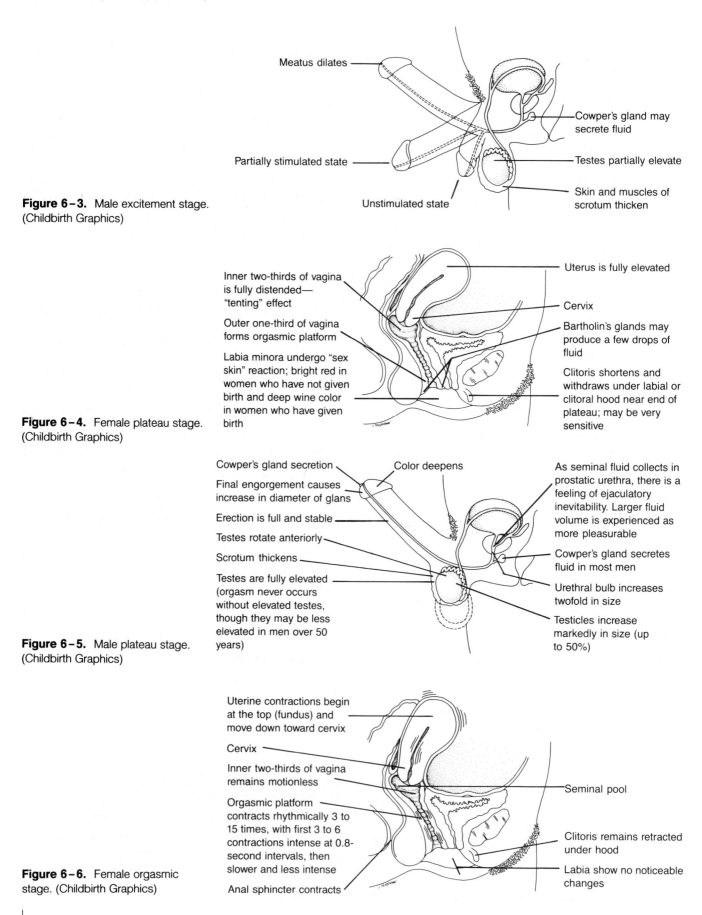

Figure 6–3. Male excitement stage. (Childbirth Graphics)

Meatus dilates

Partially stimulated state

Unstimulated state

Cowper's gland may secrete fluid

Testes partially elevate

Skin and muscles of scrotum thicken

Figure 6–4. Female plateau stage. (Childbirth Graphics)

Inner two-thirds of vagina is fully distended— "tenting" effect

Outer one-third of vagina forms orgasmic platform

Labia minora undergo "sex skin" reaction; bright red in women who have not given birth and deep wine color in women who have given birth

Uterus is fully elevated

Cervix

Bartholin's glands may produce a few drops of fluid

Clitoris shortens and withdraws under labial or clitoral hood near end of plateau; may be very sensitive

Figure 6–5. Male plateau stage. (Childbirth Graphics)

Cowper's gland secretion

Final engorgement causes increase in diameter of glans

Erection is full and stable

Testes rotate anteriorly

Scrotum thickens

Testes are fully elevated (orgasm never occurs without elevated testes, though they may be less elevated in men over 50 years)

Color deepens

As seminal fluid collects in prostatic urethra, there is a feeling of ejaculatory inevitability. Larger fluid volume is experienced as more pleasurable

Cowper's gland secretes fluid in most men

Urethral bulb increases twofold in size

Testicles increase markedly in size (up to 50%)

Figure 6–6. Female orgasmic stage. (Childbirth Graphics)

Uterine contractions begin at the top (fundus) and move down toward cervix

Cervix

Inner two-thirds of vagina remains motionless

Orgasmic platform contracts rhythmically 3 to 15 times, with first 3 to 6 contractions intense at 0.8-second intervals, then slower and less intense

Anal sphincter contracts

Seminal pool

Clitoris remains retracted under hood

Labia show no noticeable changes

114

are pulled up against the perineum. Often a small amount of a clear, preejaculatory fluid comes out of the male urethra, probably from Cowper's gland. This fluid may contain sperm, which is why coitus interruptus (pulling the penis out before ejaculation) is not a reliable form of birth control (Fig. 6–5).

For both men and women in the plateau phase, the sex flush may spread over the body, and muscle tension is increased both voluntarily and involuntarily. Breathing rates can increase to hyperventilation. Recorded heart rates range from 100 to 175 beats per minute. The increase in blood pressure is 20 to 60 mm Hg systolic and 10 to 20 mm Hg diastolic for women and 20 to 80 mm Hg systolic and 10 to 40 mm Hg diastolic for men.

Orgasm Phase

Orgasm is a reflex response to a stimulus that is sufficiently effective to reach the threshold level of arousal. The reflex can be thought of as similar to a sneeze. The blood causing the vasocongestion of the erectile tissue is forced back into the bloodstream by the contraction of muscles surrounding that tissue.

In women there is an initial contraction of the orgasmic platform and then, depending on the intensity of the orgasm, there may be anywhere from 3 to 15 contractions of the orgasmic platform at 0.8-second intervals (Fig. 6–6). Contractions of the uterus occur during this time, beginning at the top of the uterus and progressing down toward the cervix.

In men orgasm happens in two stages (Fig. 6–7). First there is an initial contraction of the smooth muscles of the internal organs: the tubuli epididymis, the vas deferens, the seminal vesicles, and the prostate gland. This initial contraction, called the *emission phase,* deposits seminal fluid into the prostatic urethra. This event has been labeled by Masters and Johnson as the "sensation of ejaculatory inevitability." The second phase, *ejaculation,* follows almost immediately and consists of rhythmic 0.8-second contractions of the ischiocavernous and bulbocavernous muscles at the base of the penis, the prostate gland, and perineal muscles. These contractions push the semen from the prostatic urethra through the penile urethra and outside the penis in a series of squirts.

Semen is made up of fluid from the prostate, the seminal vesicles, and the vas deferens and contains live spermatozoa from the testes. The seminal fluid is not propelled into the bladder because the internal sphincter of the neck of the bladder closes tightly during ejaculation. This also prevents urine from escaping from the bladder during orgasm.

For both men and women, there are extragenital changes at orgasm. The sex flush intensifies and is present in 75% of women and approximately 25% of men. Respiratory rates may be as high as 40 breaths per minute. Heart rates ranging from 110 to 180 beats per minute have been recorded. Blood pressure may elevate by 30 to 80 mm Hg systolic and 20 to 40 mm diastolic.

Historically, erotic novels had many references to fluid gushing from the vagina during orgasm, and this has probably promoted the myth that women ejaculate. After Masters and Johnson's laboratory study of sexual response, the conclusion was that female ejaculation did

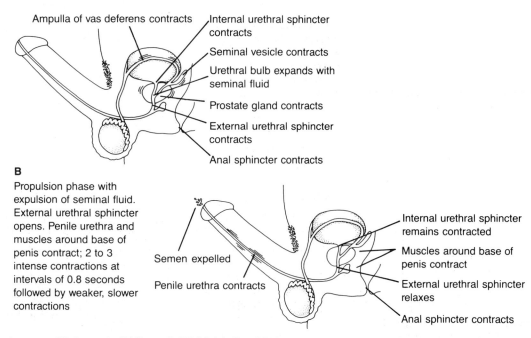

A

Emission phase with a build up of pressure caused by seminal fluid— the result of early contractions of internal sexual organs. Semen concentrates in urethral bulb of prostate

Ampulla of vas deferens contracts

Internal urethral sphincter contracts
Seminal vesicle contracts
Urethral bulb expands with seminal fluid
Prostate gland contracts
External urethral sphincter contracts
Anal sphincter contracts

B

Propulsion phase with expulsion of seminal fluid. External urethral sphincter opens. Penile urethra and muscles around base of penis contract; 2 to 3 intense contractions at intervals of 0.8 seconds followed by weaker, slower contractions

Semen expelled
Penile urethra contracts

Internal urethral sphincter remains contracted
Muscles around base of penis contract
External urethral sphincter relaxes
Anal sphincter contracts

Figure 6–7. Male orgasmic stage. *(A)* Stage 1. *(B)* Stage II. (Childbirth Graphics)

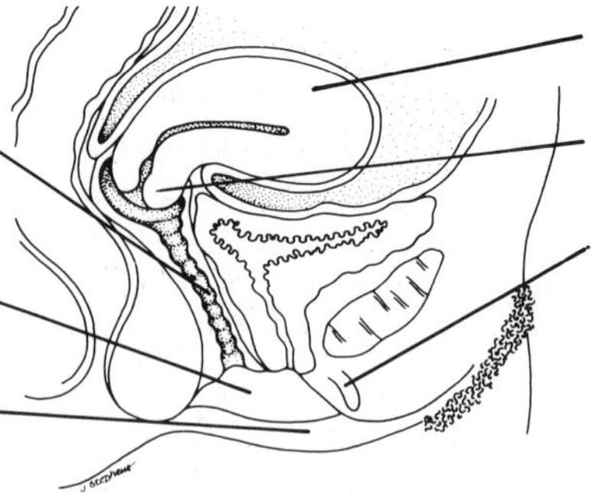

Vagina returns to unaroused state; outer one-third very quickly; inner two-thirds in 5 to 8 minutes

Labia minora lose color and erection in 10 to 15 seconds

Labia majora return quickly to unaroused state

Uterus returns to unaroused position

Cervix drops into seminal pool

Clitoris descends in 5 to 10 seconds to resting state, with complete resolution in clitoral shaft taking 5 to 30 minutes

Figure 6-8. Female resolution stage. (Childbirth Graphics)

not occur. A small number of women who have been studied recently appear to gush fluid from the urethral opening at the time of orgasm, and this phenomenon is particularly found in women with very strong pubococcygeal muscles (Perry and Whipple 1981). Laboratory analysis has not yet determined conclusively what this fluid is. It looks like neither urine nor vaginal lubrication. As yet, the percentage of women who are capable of this expulsion of fluid and the source of the fluid remain undetermined. Possibly, the paraurethral glands contribute, but this has not been documented.

Resolution Phase

The resolution phase is the return of the genital organs and body to the unaroused state. If there has been no orgasm, resolution takes longer because of lingering vasocongestion. If there has been considerable, prolonged excitement, the unrelieved vasocongestion may feel heavy or aching (Figs. 6-8 and 6-9) (Masters, Johnson, and Kolodny 1982).

In addition, the orgasm triggers the release of muscular tension throughout the body. The sex flush disappears, and a film of perspiration may cover the whole body or just the soles of the feet and palms of the hands.

In women the uterus moves back down into its unstimulated position, and the cervix dips into the seminal pool area. If semen has been deposited there, the sperm can then more easily travel into the uterus. The clitoris, inner and outer lips, and vagina resume their unstimulated size and positions.

In men there is first a rapid loss of erection, then the scrotum thins out, the testes descend, and there is a loss of testicular congestion. The initial changes for both men and women happen in the first 5 to 10 minutes. Final return to the unstimulated state may take 30 minutes.

The main difference between men and women during the resolution phase is that males have a *refractory period* and women do not. The refractory period is "a recovery time during which further orgasm or ejaculation is physiologically impossible" (Masters, Johnson, and Kolodny 1982). Thus, even with continued effective stimulation, the man is unable to go through the sexual response cycle until the recovery time is over. There may be a partial or full erection. The length of the refractory period varies from person to person and from experience to experience. The refractory period lengthens as the man gets older and if there are repeated ejaculations in a period of several hours (Masters, Johnson, and Kolodny 1982). One estimate of refractory time is from 10 to 45 minutes (Comfort 1972).

Women are capable of being multiorgasmic, meaning that they can repeatedly go through the response cycle to orgasm without the recovery time. In order to be multiorgasmic, women need consistently effective stimulation. This type of stimulation most frequently occurs with masturbation rather than intercourse. Several factors may contribute to this phenomenon: continued sexual stimulation during masturbation is relatively easy; there is not the distraction of having a partner present; and during masturbation, there is more frequent use of fan-

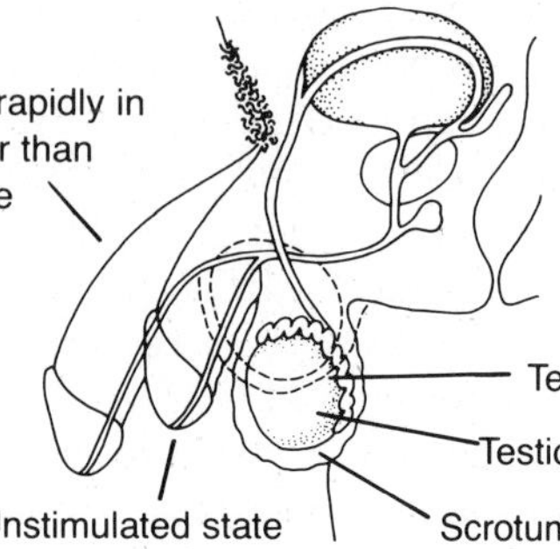

Penis decreases rapidly in size to 50% larger than unstimulated state

Testes descend

Testicular congestion is lost

Unstimulated state

Scrotum thins and folds return

Figure 6-9. Male resolution stage. (Childbirth Graphics)

tasy as compared with intercourse (Masters, Johnson, and Kolodny 1982). Thus, the actual percentage of women who experience multiple orgasms during a single sexual encounter is rather low. Kinsey reported a figure of 14%, and Athanasiou and associates reported that 16% of female readers of *Psychology Today* said they could have multiple orgasms during penile-vaginal intercourse (Crooks and Bauer 1983). This indicates only that multiple orgasms are possible, either through intercourse or through masturbation, but is no measure of female sexual adequacy. Women should not feel inadequate if they are not having multiple orgasms. Many women are satisfied by one orgasm during a sexual experience or even by having only occasional orgasms.

Men may also experience multiple orgasms, if the definition of having two or more climaxes within a short period of time is used. The period between orgasms is longer than for women and depends on the length of the refractory period.

For a summary of the sexual response cycle changes, see Table 6–1, page 118.

Kaplan's Triphasic Theory

The Masters and Johnson model has been a very useful tool for the descriptions of primarily genital sexual arousal physiology. Helen Singer Kaplan has suggested a model in which sexual response is made up of three phases: *desire, excitement, orgasm*. If we compare Kaplan's model with Masters and Johnson's, the orgasm phases are similar; Kaplan's excitement phase includes the excitement and plateau phases of Masters and Johnson, and desire is not included by Masters and Johnson. The Kaplan model is based on the fact that each phase is governed by a separate neurophysiologic system (Kaplan 1979). This separate neural circuitry explains the possibility of separate inhibition of each of the three phases and has contributed to the advancement of therapy for sexual dysfunctions and the further understanding of the physiology of sexual response.

Desire Phase

Desire (sex drive or *libido*) is similar to other drives in that it is governed by a system of neurotransmitters in the brain that either excite or inhibit it. When the system is activated, the person feels some degree of interest in sex, is open to sex, or may just feel vaguely restless. When the system is inhibited, a person is not interested in sex, is not open to sex, and becomes "asexual." The inhibitory and activating sex centers are known to be located in the limbic system, with nuclei in the hypothalamus and preoptic region.

The limbic system generates and regulates emotion and motivation. The sex centers are also probably connected to the pleasure and pain centers of the brain. Having sex stimulates the pleasure centers, and early research suggests that the neurons of the pleasure centers have chemical receptor sites for a brain-produced chemical called *endorphin*. Endorphin is a morphinelike chemical that causes euphoria and alleviates pain. There is the possibility of the elimination of pain through sexual arousal. On the other hand, the presence of pain—actual physical pain or the painful perception of a sexual object or situation as dangerous or destructive—can inhibit sexual desire. In the brain, pain has priority over pleasure, so that the perception of physical injury or the anticipation of injury focuses the individual on survival instead of sexual desire.

The sex centers are also probably connected to parts of the brain that store and retrieve memories and analyze experiences. Therefore, sexual desire is shaped by the knowledge of what will and what will not motivate a person toward a sexual experience. The sex centers in the brain are also connected to genital reflexes in such a way that when libido is activated, the genital responses of erection, lubrication, and orgasm occur easily. When there is inhibited libido, the threshold for genital reflexes is much higher, and it may take very intense stimulation to produce any arousal at all.

The exact effects of hormones on sexual desire have yet to be specifically determined. *Estrogen* is *not* currently known to enhance sexual desire in females, but its exact role in sexual arousal is not yet known. Estrogen does act on the vaginal walls to keep them elastic and lubricated. More is known about *testosterone* as the "libido hormone" in both genders. Although the exact mechanism is not known, absence of testosterone causes absence of sexual desire. Another hormone secreted in the brain, luteinizing hormone-releasing factor (LH-RF), may turn out to enhance sexual desire even in the absence of testosterone or when testosterone is ineffective.

Excitement Phase

The excitement phase is characterized by vasodilation and is activated by two centers in the spinal cord, one at S_2, S_3, and S_4 and one at T_{11}, T_{12}, L_1, and L_2 (Figs. 6–10 and 6–11). The activation of these two centers causes the arterioles of the genitals to dilate. The effect in men is to cause filling of the cavernous spaces of the corpora cavernosa. The dilation of the penile arteries is brought about by parasympathetic impulses from the spinal erection centers, which cause the muscles in the arterial walls to relax. The mechanism restricting penile outflow of blood is not clearly understood. Possibly, outflow of erectile blood is controlled by a sympathetic component, though erectile response is primarily parasympathetic.

In women the genital vasodilation produces generalized swelling of the labia and the tissues surrounding the vagina and lubrication. It is believed that this female re-

(text continued on page 120)

Table 6-1   **Summary of Sexual Response Cycle Changes**

General Physiologic Changes	Specific Changes in Women	Specific Changes in Men

Excitement Phase

Excitement phase occurs at the onset of arousal. The stimulation may be physical or psychic. Erotic feelings come through all senses—sight, feel, touch, smell, taste, hearing—and through thought or fantasy.

General Physiologic Changes	Specific Changes in Women	Specific Changes in Men
1. *Vasocongestion* (engorgement—more blood flows into the area than flows out of it) is the primary reaction to stimulation, regardless of technique.	1. *Vaginal lubrication* is the primary sign of the excitement phase. Lubrication is due to vasocongestion and occurs within 10 to 30 seconds of the onset of stimulation. Vaginal lubrication appears as a "sweating" reaction of vaginal lining. (Lubrication was previously thought to be produced by the uterus and Bartholin's glands. Masters and Johnson disproved this by observing lubrication in women with complete hysterectomies.)	1. *Erection of the penis* is the primary sign of the excitement phase. Erection is due to vasocongestion in the penis and occurs within a few seconds, regardless of the nature of the stimulation. A small penis may double in length. The lengthening is less marked in a large penis.
2. *Myotonia* (contraction of various muscle fibers, muscles, and groups of muscles) is the secondary reaction to stimulation, regardless of technique.	2. *Expansion of inner two thirds of vagina* occurs as phase is prolonged. (Back of vagina begins to balloon out 3.75 to 4.25 cm in width and 2.3 cm to 3.5 cm in length.)	2. *Enlargement of testicles* is owing to engorgement as phase is prolonged.
3. *Tachycardia.* Heart rate increases in direct proportion to rising tension, regardless of stimulation technique.	3. *Elevation of cervix and uterus* occurs as excitement phase is prolonged. Cervix is pulled up and out of the way.	3. *Elevation of testicles* is owing to shortening of spermatic cords that suspend the testicles in the scrotal sac.
4. *Blood pressure elevation* occurs in direct proportion to rising tension, regardless of stimulation technique.	4. *Engorgement of clitoral glans and clitoral shaft* occurs if phase is prolonged. Degree of swelling is not related to either sexual responsiveness or ability to achieve orgasm.	4. *Thickening, flattening, and elevation of scrotal sac* occurs as phase is prolonged.
5. *Respiratory rate increases* are slight in this phase.	5. *Separation and flattening of labia majora.* Changes in labia are heightened in multiparous women owing to increased engorgement.	5. *Erection of nipples* occurs inconsistently in men.
	6. *Engorgement of labia minora* occurs.	
	7. *Erection of nipples* occurs owing to contraction of nipple muscle fibers. Nipples may not erect simultaneously.	
	8. *Enlargement of breasts* begins if phase is prolonged. Areola begins to swell, and pattern of veins on surface of breast becomes more distinct.	
	9. *"Sex flush"* appears as maculopapular rash starting on abdomen and spreading over breasts. Time of appearance varies for different people in different phases.	

Plateau Phase

Plateau phase is a more advanced stage of arousal during which the person is actively engaged in sexual activity and stimulation, either alone or with a partner. The entire body is responding with increasing intensity and reaching toward a peak (orgasm).

General Physiologic Changes	Specific Changes in Women	Specific Changes in Men
1. *Vasocongestion.* Engorgement reaches its maximum level during plateau phase.	1. *Formation of the orgasmic platform.* The primary sign of plateau appears as engorgement and swelling of tissues surrounding outer third of the vagina. As a result of this final engorgement, the diameter of the vaginal opening is reduced. (If a penis is in the vagina at this time, the effect is actually a gripping of the base of the penis.) Appearance of the orgasmic platform does not necessarily mean orgasm is imminent.	1. *Expansion in diameter of coronal ridge* (at base of glans). The glans may deepen in color to a reddish purple hue.

(continued)

Table 6–1   **Summary of Sexual Response Cycle Changes** (continued)

General Physiologic Changes	Specific Changes in Women	Specific Changes in Men
2. *Myotonia.* Muscle tension in both involuntary and voluntary muscles reaches its maximum level.	2. *Full expansion of inner two thirds of vagina.* Back of the vagina is now widely ballooned.	2. *Enlargement of testicles* by up to 50% occurs.
3. *Tachycardia.* Recorded rates average from 100 to 175 beats per minute.	3. *Full elevation of cervix and uterus.*	3. *Elevation of testicles.* Testicles now rotate and are positioned in close contact with the perineum. This is a sign that orgasm is imminent.
4. *Blood pressure elevation.* Systolic pressure can rise 20 to 60 mm Hg and diastolic pressure can rise 10 to 20 mm Hg.	4. *Retraction of clitoris glans* occurs due to shortening of clitoral shaft. Glans seems to be hiding but is still responsive to stimulation.	4. *Secretion from Cowper's gland,* often called preejaculatory fluid. Small amounts of this clear fluid appear at the urethral opening. Live spermatozoa have been observed in this fluid.
5. *Respiratory rate.* Can become hyperventilation late in phase	5. *Engorgement of labia majora* continues to its fullest extent.	
	6. *"Sex skin"* appears in labia minora, late in plateau phase. The inner lips turn a deep red color. It is a sign of impending orgasm if effective erotic stimulation is continued.	
	7. *Full engorgement of areola.* The swelling can be so marked that it masks nipple erection.	
	8. *Increase in breast size.* Change is greater in women who have never breastfed.	
	9. *Sex flush* may be more prominent now.	
	10. Slight secretion from Bartholin's glands may occur.	

Orgasm Phase

Orgasm is considered the peak or climax of sexual arousal and is intensely pleasurable.

1. *Vasocongestion* is reversed by orgasm.	1. *Contraction of orgasmic platform* usually appears as an initial spasm followed by a series of rhythmic contractions at 0.8-sec intervals. The more intense the orgasm, the more contractions will follow.	1. *Ejaculation* takes place in two phases. During the first phase, fluid containing live spermatozoa and secretions from the prostate, seminal vesicles, and vas deferens begins to pool in the prostatic urethra as a result of a series of rhythmic contractions of those organs. This signals the stage of ejaculatory inevitability. During the second phase, rhythmic contractions of the urethral bulb and penis at 0.8-sec intervals propel the fluid out the end of the penis, since the internal sphincter of the bladder is tightly closed.
2. *Myotonia.* Muscles throughout the body tend to contract at orgasm. Face may be contorted, muscles of the neck, arms, and legs frequently contract in a spasm, gluteal and abdominal muscles are often contracted, and carpopedal spasms of the hands and feet may occur.	2. *Rhythmic contractions of uterus* begin at fundus and move like a wave down to the cervix. If orgasm is very intense, uterine contractions may be severe.	2. *Contraction of anal sphincter* at 0.8-sec intervals.
3. *Tachycardia.* Rates range from 100 to 180 beats per minute.	3. Orgasm occurs even in women with hysterectomies and women who have had the clitoris surgically removed.	
4. *Blood pressure elevation.* Systolic increase from 30 to 80 mm Hg, diastolic increase from 20 to 40 mm Hg.	4. *Contraction of anal sphincter* at 0.8-sec intervals.	

(continued)

Table 6–1   **Summary of Sexual Response Cycle Changes** (continued)

General Physiologic Changes	Specific Changes in Women	Specific Changes in Men
5. *Hyperventilation.* Rates of up to 40 breaths per minute.	5. External urethral sphincter may contract.	
	6. Cervical os may relax.	

Resolution Phase

The body begins to return to its preexcitement state. There is often a sense of calm and wellbeing.

1. *Vasocongestion.* Congested blood is released back into general circulation after orgasm. If there is no orgasm, reversal of vasocongestion may take a couple of hours.	1. *Disappearance of orgasmic platform* occurs rapidly.	1. *Refractory period.* During this period, the man is physiologically unable to initiate the sexual response cycle. He may feel subjectively aroused during this time and may still have a partial erection, but the pelvic organs need time for the sexual response mechanisms to become operational again. In some men, this period will be no longer than 10 minutes.
2. *Relaxation.* Muscles feel relaxed; body feels generally rid of tension.	2. Clitoris rapidly returns to normal position (5–10 sec).	2. Loss of erection occurs in two stages. During the first stage, 50% of the erection is rapidly lost. The second stage, the loss of the rest of the erection, occurs more gradually.
3. Respiratory rate, pulse rate, and blood pressure return to normal levels.	3. Sex flush rapidly disappears.	3. Testicles decrease in size and descend to their preexcited state.
4. Sweating reaction may occur in which body is covered with a thin film of moisture.	4. Vaginal walls relax (10–15 min).	
	5. Cervix and uterus descend to normal position. The cervix rests in a small depression in the vagina called the *seminal pool.*	
	6. Cervical os remains open for 20 to 30 minutes after orgasm.	
	7. Breast size and nipple erection decrease slowly.	
	8. Labia minora and labia majora return to normal color and position.	
	9. *Note:* Women have the capacity for multiple orgasms. That is, they can return to orgasm with continued or renewed effective erotic stimulation without dropping below plateau phase. The potential for orgasm is available until the point of exhaustion.	

Adapted from Masters W, Johnson V: Human Sexual Response. Boston, Little, Brown & Co, 1966

sponse is also primarily controlled by the *parasympathetic* nervous system.

The two spinal centers, T_{11} to L_2 and S_{2-4}, are believed to respond to different stimuli. The upper center responds to psychic stimuli (sight, sound, smell, taste, thought, emotion, and so on), while the lower center responds more to tactile input from the genitals. The lower center seems to be reflexive, not needing any input from the higher center to respond.

Control of excitement, then, can be enhanced or inhibited by the higher brain using psychic stimuli plus experiential factors, including memory.

Orgasm Phase

The orgasm phase is a genital reflex consisting of contractions of certain genital muscles. The sensory impulses that trigger orgasm enter the spinal cord at the sacral level through the pudendal nerve, and the efferent tract carrying the impulses away from the spinal cord is from T_{11} to L_2. The first phase of male orgasm, the emission phase, is

Figure 6–10. Neurologic bases of the female sexual response. (Childbirth Graphics)

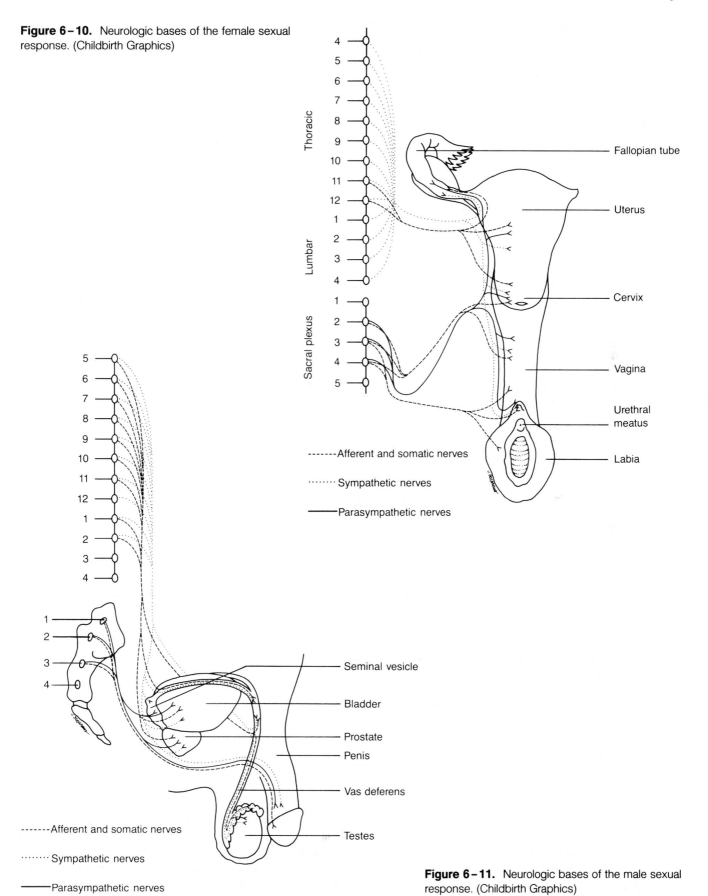

Thoracic
4
5
6
7
8
9
10
11
12

Lumbar
1
2
3
4

Sacral plexus
1
2
3
4
5

Fallopian tube

Uterus

Cervix

Vagina

Urethral meatus

Labia

------ Afferent and somatic nerves

.... Sympathetic nerves

——— Parasympathetic nerves

5
6
7
8
9
10
11
12
1
2
3
4

1
2
3
4

Seminal vesicle

Bladder

Prostate

Penis

Vas deferens

Testes

------ Afferent and somatic nerves

.... Sympathetic nerves

——— Parasympathetic nerves

Figure 6–11. Neurologic bases of the male sexual response. (Childbirth Graphics)

governed by the sympathetic nervous system. It is thought that there may be an as yet unidentified reflex center that controls the second part of the male orgasm as well as the female orgasm. Orgasm seems to be more under the voluntary control of the individual than arousal, through the connections between the spinal orgasm centers and the higher brain. This means that there is a physiologic mechanism for learned inhibition of orgasms (Kaplan 1979).

Theories of Orgasm

Three types of orgasms have been described by women since the work of Masters and Johnson (Francoeur 1982).

Tenting Type

This is the orgasm as described by Masters, Johnson, and Kaplan, in which the clitoris is the main source of erotic stimulation. The impulses travel by way of the pudendal nerve back to the sacral spinal center. Orgasm results from the buildup and discharge of muscle tension in the pubococcygeal muscle, and the orgasmic platform closes.

A-frame or Uterine Type

This is the orgasm described by Perry and Whipple, in which the urethral sponge (Grafenberg spot) next to the anterior wall of the vagina is stimulated and sends erotic impulses along the pelvic nerve to the spinal reflex center. The orgasm results from the buildup and discharge of muscle tension in the deeper muscles of the vagina. The uterus contracts and pushes down, and the orgasmic platform opens.

Blended Type

This orgasm is described as involving stimulation from both the clitoris and the urethral sponge (Grafenberg spot), sending nerve impulses that cross over both the pelvis and pudendal nerves.

The Source of Female Orgasm: Clitoral or Vaginal?

The controversy over whether females have orgasms from clitoral or vaginal stimulation has raged since Sigmund Freud postulated his theories on female sexuality. According to Freud, orgasms from clitoral stimulation were immature, whereas orgasms from vaginal stimulation (intercourse) were mature. Freud assumed that a woman could "transfer" her sexual focus from the clitoris to the vagina. As a result of this Freudian judgment, the sexual adequacy of a woman has been measured by whether or not she has an orgasm during intercourse. This belief is still widely held, but it is not supported by clinical research data. Masters and Johnson's (1966) laboratory studies demonstrated that an orgasm is an orgasm

regardless of the point of stimulation (clitoral, labial, vaginal, breast, or fantasy). Kinsey (1948) data showed that only 47% of married women reached orgasm in all or nearly all marital coitus after 20 years of continuous marriage. Later studies, such as Hite's (1977), suggest that the percentage of women who experience orgasm from penile-vaginal thrusting only may be as low as 30%. That figure is nearly doubled if additional clitoral stimulation is added during coitus. According to Kinsey, the orgasm rate for women during masturbation is 95%, which would suggest that for many women the stimulation during coitus is often ineffective in triggering orgasmic response. Masturbation is a highly reliable means of producing orgasm because effective stimulation is easily learned, and it is usually directed at the area with the most nerve endings (clitoris and labia). The vagina has fewer nerve endings, and pleasurable sensations are often felt as pressure on the congested tissues surrounding the vagina, rather than direct friction on the vaginal lining. The outer third of the vagina is more innervated than the inner two-thirds. Women ought to feel comfortable having their orgasms any way they can, and they should not feel pressured to live up to an unrealistic cultural standard.

Limits of Research Findings

The consideration of human sexuality as a science has not kept pace with the dramatic progress made in medical research in immunology, hemodialysis, brain surgery, respiratory illness, organ transplants, or cardiology. In today's world of technological sophistication and rapid accumulation of data, adequate sex research that would give us much-needed data on human sexuality is simply not available. There are few qualified researchers, money to support research in this field has been almost completely eliminated, and most of the sex research that has been done in the past has focused on men. The shortage of qualified faculty knowledgeable in sexual medicine precludes effective professional instruction in both sex education and research.

ADAPTATION TO SEXUALITY DURING PREGNANCY

Information on sexuality and pregnancy is limited. Studies of sexuality during pregnancy and in the postpartum period have produced conflicting data. Without further research, one can only say now that there appears to be a wide range of normal feelings, sexual desires, frequency of intercourse, sexual enjoyment, and sexual adjustment after the birth or during a medical complication with the pregnancy. Few studies have interviewed or questioned couples. Most have relied on the pregnant woman alone for information, and most used retrospective questionnaires. What does seem clear is that each couple is unique and that a multitude of factors affect the sexual relationship during pregnancy, such as the following:

- The sexual pattern before pregnancy, including frequency, enjoyment, comfort, and ability to communicate about sex
- The meaning of sex to each member of the couple (whether sex is viewed positively or negatively)
- The meaning of the pregnancy to each member of the couple and the experience of previous pregnancies, if any
- The woman's general state of health during pregnancy
- Any medical problems that may occur during the pregnancy
- The state of the couple's relationship
- Advice from physician or nurse regarding sex during pregnancy
- Whether the pregnancy is planned or accidental
- Fear of miscarriage or of hurting the fetus
- How the woman and her partner feel about the changes her body goes through

Sexual Response Cycle Changes

In pregnancy there is generally intensification of all phases of the female sexual response cycle except, perhaps, desire.

Desire Phase Changes

While there are numerous studies that document variations in sexual interest during pregnancy, basically they record general patterns that may have little to do with a particular couple. There are individual changes in interest that are influenced by countless factors that are difficult to document. The mother's physical status, comfort, and well-being are closely linked to her interest in sexual activity. Bing and Coleman (1977) described four typical patterns of interest in sex during pregnancy.

The first pattern showed a steady continuous increase in sexual interest that exceeds the baseline prepregnancy interest in sex and does not decline in the third trimester. Only a minority of the women surveyed by Bing and Coleman demonstrated this pattern.

Pattern 2 showed a decline in sexual interest in the first trimester, a relative increase in the second trimester and early third trimester, and a decreasing interest by the end of the third trimester. This general pattern is supported by studies by Masters and Johnson (1966) that found interest in the second trimester increasing to a higher level than before pregnancy. These studies also showed an increase in planning for a sexual encounter, increase in fantasies of

a sexual encounter, and increase in sexual dream content by the second trimester. Studies by Kenny (1971), Tolor and DiGrazia (1976), and Falicov (1973) also documented this pattern. However, the Falicov study shows that sexual interest in the second trimester does not go above prepregnancy levels. The Falicov study also found that women with a high interest in sexual activity before pregnancy tended to maintain higher levels during pregnancy. In addition, the Tolor and DiGrazia study showed evidence of a pregnant woman's increased need for closeness and touch.

Pattern 3 showed a steady decline in sexual desire throughout all three trimesters. This pattern is supported by Solberg, Butler, and Wagner (1973), who described an almost linear decline of coital frequency during pregnancy associated with a decrease in sexual interest. The frequency of coitus was higher in younger women and was inversely related to length of marriage except in the last 2 months of pregnancy. Variables such as race, religious preference, education of the woman or her partner, negative feelings about pregnancy, or whether or not the pregnancy was planned appeared to have no relation to coital frequency. A study by Perkins (1982) also supported a general trend toward a progressive decline in coital frequency toward the end of pregnancy. Fifty-eight percent of the study group indicated that pregnancy made them feel less attractive. Quality of coital sensations and frequency of sexual activity were directly correlated. Where there was a significant decrease in the quality of coital sensation, a significant increase in masturbation occurred. Perkins' data indicated that sexually experienced and satisfied women compensated better in the changed circumstances of pregnancy than inexperienced or sexually unfulfilled women. Positive sexual experiences may have retarded the rate of decline in interest or activity in late pregnancy but did not divert the eventual decline.

Pattern 4 shows no change in patterns of sexual interest in sex during pregnancy. Thus, for some women, pregnancy is a time of heightened sexual awareness and sensuality, whereas for others there is either no change or a decline in interest and frequency of coitus. Although not all the contributing variables have been studied, certainly the sexual interest of the partner of the pregnant woman and any sexual advice from health practitioners must be taken into account. In the 1966 Masters and Johnson study, the women thought the drop in frequency of intercourse in the last trimester was because they were less physically attractive. However, the husbands' primary explanation was fear of injuring the fetus or wife.

Primiparous women generally were more likely to experience a decline in sexual behavior whereas multiparous women often experienced an improvement, especially after the first 3 months. Approximately 77% of the women in this study were warned by their physicians not to engage in sexual intercourse until after the baby was born. The time period suggested for abstaining was from 1 to 3 months before the due date. Many of these women said they lost sexual interest in the last 3 months independently of the doctor's warnings. In the Solberg, Butler, and Wagner study (1973), the changes in patterns of sexual behavior were attributed to the following: physical discomfort (46%); fear of injury to the baby (27%); loss of interest (23%); awkwardness having intercourse (17%); recommendation of a physician (8%); reasons unrelated to pregnancy (6%); and the woman's imagined loss of attractiveness (4%). Women who did receive physician instruction to avoid intercourse were asked to refrain anywhere from 2 to 8 weeks before their due dates. The Falicov study (1973) participants mentioned the following factors as affecting decline in sexual desire, feelings of eroticism, and sexual satisfaction: nausea; vomiting; heartburn; vagina feeling smaller, making penetration painful; and vaginal numbness, making orgasm more difficult.

Finally, there may be women who do not enjoy sexual relations prior to pregnancy and use the pregnancy as an excuse to stop having sexual relations. This attitude is easily supported by a social and cultural concept of the pregnant woman as asexual, as if the two factors, pregnancy and sexual interest, were incompatible.

Arousal Phase Changes

During their original laboratory observation research, Masters and Johnson (1966) were able to record data on six pregnant women during arousal and orgasm. They learned that responses were much the same as in nonpregnant women, with a few exceptions. During arousal in primiparas, the combination of the breast engorgement of arousal and the breast swelling of pregnancy led some women to complain of severe breast pain, especially in the nipples and areolas, during advanced stages of arousal in the first trimester. Later in the pregnancy this tenderness did not recur during sexual arousal. The orgasmic platform was even more noticeable during pregnancy than before.

Orgasm Changes

Masters and Johnson's 1966 observations were that instead of the usual rhythmic series of contractions during orgasm, in late pregnancy the uterus sometimes engaged in a single tonic contraction lasting as long as a minute. During orgasm the fetal heartbeat sometimes slowed down a little, then quickly resumed its normal rate. Masters and Johnson (1966), Pugh and Fernandez (1953), and Solberg and colleagues (1973) all concluded that there were no deleterious effects on pregnancy outcome from sexual activity, including orgasm. However,

the role of orgasm as an independent variable was not assessed until a study by Goodlin, Keller, and Raffin in 1971. These authors concluded that the relative risk of premature labor or ruptured membranes is 15% in gravidas orgasmic after the 32nd week of pregnancy. Among gravidas with a history of premature births, the risk was 21% for premature labor from orgasm. Therefore, they recommended abstinence from orgasm after 31 weeks' gestation for women with a ripe cervix or with a history of premature deliveries. This study has been criticized on the grounds that the conclusions were based on unequal groups and that some of the subjects in the premature group already had a previous history of premature labor.

In a later study by Goodlin, Schmidt, and Creevy (1972), uterine contractions did occur with multiple orgasms and lasted up to 15 minutes after the last orgasm. Fetal heart rate showed some decelerations, which were considered innocuous and were not consistent with all contractions. Goodlin and associates interpreted these data as suggesting that premature labor might be initiated by these strong uterine contractions. These findings have not been supported by other studies.

A retrospective study by Perkins (1979) examined the association between coitus, orgasm, and other sexual experiences and the proximity to the onset of labor. No significant association between these variables could be made, and in contrast to the Goodlin studies, orgasmic patients appeared to have a consistently lower percentage of early deliveries. Masturbation was consistently associated with a lower risk of prematurity throughout various stages of gestation. This is interesting in light of the fact that masturbation has been shown to produce a more intense orgasmic response than coitus. In this study about one fifth of the women claimed at some time to have purposely prevented orgasm. The reasons given were fear of hurting the baby, fear of starting labor, instructions not to have sex or orgasm, or painful orgasm. Perkins' data also suggested that in the last 2 months of pregnancy, the uterus appears to be more intrinsically irritable to stimuli of all sorts and that coitus appeared to constitute a stronger stimulus to uterine contractions than orgasm. One criticism of this study was that the number of cases was too small and that the investigator should have asked about coitus during the preceding 7 days rather than just the last 24 hours before delivery.

In the 1973 Solberg study none of the 260 patients noted the immediate onset of labor after intercourse or orgasm. Frequency of coitus and rates of orgasm also showed no relation to gestational age at birth.

In a 1981 study by Mills, Harlap, and Hartley on 10,981 pregnancies, the data show no increase in risk of premature rupture of membranes, low birth weight, or perinatal death associated with coitus. Women abstaining from intercourse had more unfavorable outcomes in the 7th and 8th month. These differences, however, were almost eliminated by adjustment for maternal age. The abstainers tended to be older, of higher parity, less educated, and of lower social class. While this was a large study, it did not address whether the women had orgasms, or engaged in masturbation.

A study of 39,217 pregnancies was conducted by Klebanoff, Nugent, and Rhoads (1984), who found no association between third-trimester coitus and adverse outcome of pregnancy. In fact, the data show an almost protective effect of coitus, since increasing coital frequency was associated with increasing length of gestation in blacks, whites, and Puerto Ricans. These investigators suggest that coitus may not be a specifically protective factor itself, but rather simply a marker of good health. Women who went on to deliver prematurely may not have felt well in ways that were obscured from measurement and may have tended to become less sexually active. Data on orgasm were not collected in this large sample either.

Sexual Activity During Pregnancy

Safety Concerns

Intercourse, orgasm, or both seem to be safe for most pregnant women throughout pregnancy. Since sexual activity can cause uterine contraction, patients with prematurely dilated cervices, previous threatened premature labor, and multiple pregnancy should be considered for sexual restriction. Patients who have had more than one spontaneous abortion, who have threatened abortion, who have threatened abortion in the first trimester, or who are candidates for impending miscarriage in the second trimester should be considered for individual contraindications of sexual activity (coitus, orgasm, or both). Patients with ruptured membranes engaged fetal head or lightening, or the possibility of placenta previa should be considered for vaginal abstinence. Patients should be cautioned against blowing air into the vagina during cunnilingus in pregnancy because air embolisms have resulted in death (Guana–Trujillo and Grant–Higgins 1987). Some doctors have been concerned that prostaglandin found in male semen could trigger uterine contractions strong enough to begin labor or rupture membranes, but, in fact, normal semen does not contain enough prostaglandin to initiate these responses (Lavery and Miller 1981).

Situations in which the placenta may not function optimally, such as toxemia, diabetes, heart disease, and multiple gestation, should be considered for orgasm restriction. Doctors usually advise against coitus if a woman has any spotting of blood in the first 12 weeks or has miscarried in the previous pregnancy. A slight blood-stained discharge somewhere around the time of the first or second missed period is actually quite common.

The First Trimester

After the 6th or 7th week of pregnancy, it is not uncommon for nausea and possibly vomiting to get in the way of erotic feelings. Sexual activity, or the thought of it, can be enough to make the nauseated pregnant woman feel that she will lose control over her stomach. Often women find that their sense of smell is heightened during the first trimester, and any odor may become particularly nauseating or antierotic.

Breast tenderness is common in early pregnancy, and tenderness during arousal can be especially painful. Breast stimulation may have to be stopped altogether, or the couple may have to communicate about exactly what kind of touch is pleasurable, if any.

Tiredness and "overdoing things" play a part in curtailing sexual interest. The extent of this physical exhaustion due to hormonal changes can be surprising to some women, and they feel that they can barely wait to get to bed to fall asleep. Sex may only prolong the agony of exhaustion.

Fear of miscarriage creates anxiety that can cause couples to avoid any sexual expression at all, even cuddling. If the woman has previously lost a baby or has noticed any bleeding in the current pregnancy, she may naturally feel that sex is a threat to the fetus. Her partner may also feel this danger. If sexual activity does occur, there may be additional stress, guilt, and anxiety. Health professionals can help relieve this guilt by reassuring the couple when they are past any dangerous times. Very little is known about the effects of lovemaking on miscarriage in the first trimester (Kitzinger 1983).

The Second Trimester

The tissues around and inside the vagina "ripen" early in the 4th month. The tissues are engorged due to the increased vascularity and blood volume, which make them swollen and red to purple in color. The tissues remain this way throughout pregnancy, so the pregnant woman is in a constant state of early arousal. This arousal level also creates a constant state of extra lubrication, so the woman feels much more moist.

The pressure of the growing fetus and congested pelvic organs can make some women feel constantly in need of a sexual outlet. It is not uncommon for a woman to feel a persistent need to masturbate or have sex. Sometimes partners are too anxious about hurting the fetus to engage in sex fully at the level the pregnant woman is ready for. Some women reveal guilt over their heightened erotic needs and the use of masturbation as a solution. Both partners need reassurance that this is normal.

The resolution phase takes longer and is less complete, which adds to the feeling of congestion. Cramping and backache can occur after orgasm. As the second trimester progresses, the woman's body begins to look pregnant as her abdomen begins to enlarge. This is the time when the "missionary position" (man on top) can become uncomfortable because any weight on the breasts or abdomen feels painful. At this point couples may wish to try other positions that prevent any abdominal pressure or deep penetration. The following positions may be suggested:

- Side-lying with vaginal entry from behind
- Side-lying facing one another
- Woman sitting up supported by pillows with knees drawn up and resting over partner, who is on his side below her
- Woman superior (on top) facing partner's face
- Woman superior (on top) facing partner's feet
- Woman on hands and knees, entry from behind
- Woman standing bent over, entry from behind
- Man and woman both sitting facing one another with woman's legs over partner's legs

Finally, there may be problems of *dyspareunia,* painful intercourse, caused by vaginitis, pressure on the abdomen, or penile thrusting against the cervix, particularly after quickening as occurred. At times, fetal movement, if it is particularly active, may decrease interest in sex.

The Third Trimester

By the third trimester indigestion and heartburn are often of primary concern. If the woman lies down flat, these problems often worsen, so she may want to attempt coitus in a sitting position. Hemorrhoids can also have an inhibiting effect on sexual interest, especially if they are painful and inflamed.

The uterus may have one long sustained contraction after orgasm, lasting for a minute or more. For some women this is an interesting and pleasurable sensation, given the great size of the uterus. For others the sensation may be frightening because they fear the fetus will be deprived of oxygen or be injured during this contraction. As mentioned earlier, fetal heart tones may slow minimally, but there is no reported danger to the fetus. The resolution phase is still incomplete, so the sense of arousal is often constant. Some women complain that no matter how often they masturbate, have intercourse, or have orgasm, they cannot feel "satisfied."

As the pregnant woman becomes larger, she may feel her body is too awkward and enormous for sex, or she may feel like a beautiful, bountiful goddess. Her body image along with her physical state will direct her sexual interest. If she feels too ugly, she may be convinced that her partner finds her ugly too. Quite often men are awed and delighted by seeing a pregnant woman's body. Sometimes, however, they are turned off and cannot feel

aroused. The man may have his own fears of harming the baby, and this fear or the reaction to his partner's extremely womanly body may occasionally inhibit the ability to get an erection.

The medical focus on the pregnant woman as she nears her delivery may also reduce her feeling of self-confidence and her sense of her body as sexual. If she has had a particular special test or procedure, such as amniocentesis or ultrasound, she may begin to sense that the medical profession is more in charge of the pregnancy that she or her partner are (Kitzinger 1983). Frequent medical visits at the end of pregnancy reinforce this sense. Understanding and support from her obstetric care-givers may have an influence on the pregnant woman's sexuality and on her feelings of well-being.

The increased risks of preterm delivery, chorioamnionitis, and premature rupture of membranes (PROM) have been studied by Naeye and Flood (1984). They found an association between higher frequency of infection and increased mortality from infection when intercourse occurred more than once a week in the last month before delivery. Other variables strongly correlated with increased risks were race, advanced maternal age, parity, instrumentation of the cervix, smoking, incompetent cervix, and low weight gain during pregnancy. Naeye's theory is that infections weaken the membranes and render them more vulnerable to rupture.

Seven days from last intercourse was considered the critical time interval for clinical evidence of bacterial invasion to show up. It is known that sperm in seminal fluid can transport bacteria across ovulatory cervical mucus (Toth, O'Leary, and Ledger 1982). Naeye's studies have been criticized for not controlling for the loss of the mucous plug; narrowly defining rupture of membranes; collecting data between 1959 to 1966, when national perinatal mortality rates were higher than they are now; and assuming that neutrophilic infiltration of the placenta indicates amniotic fluid infection. Naeye (1984) does suggest fastidious perineal cleansing by the coital partners or the use of condoms to reduce infections.

There is often a return of fatigue during the third trimester owing to lack of sleep and the physical requirements of maneuvering an enlarged body around all day. Last-minute preparations for the baby may also be tiring, and fatigue is often an inhibitor of sexual interest.

Finally, there may be the problem of the male partner's sexual interest in persons other than his mate during pregnancy (Ellis 1980). In Masters and Johnson's (1966) study of the 79 men participating in the interview project, 71 were married to women whose doctors had forbidden intercourse for 2 to 6 months before delivery. Eighteen of those 71 husbands said they engaged in extramarital sexual activity during the pregnancy or in the postpartum period. Several continued the extramarital activity after the baby was born.

Labor and Delivery

If the mother is at term and the cervix is ripe, sexual activity, including orgasm, may even be encouraged. (If labor has already begun or the membranes have ruptured, then intercourse or manual stimulation could cause infection.) During sexual arousal, oxytocin is released into the pregnant woman's bloodstream. The uterus needs oxytocin for good tone during contractions, and the uterus becomes increasingly sensitive to oxytocin at the end of pregnancy. Breast stimulation in particular releases oxytocin, and this may play an important role in helping the cervix to ripen and dilate.

Labor is painful, and some women might find any connection between this process and sexual excitement impossible to see. Other women, on the other hand, describe the birth as a powerfully erotic experience of moving sexual energy. Yet even if a woman could envision herself having an intense sexual experience during birth, this would be difficult to express in an institutionalized labor and delivery setting (Kitzinger 1983). The freedom to fully experience spontaneous emotions is usually restricted unless the woman is at home or at an alternative birth center. In addition, if physical sensation is obliterated by the use of drugs or anesthesia, any possible sexual feelings will also be obliterated.

Thus, there is a great deal of variation in the extent to which women experience a connection between labor and delivery and their sexuality or self-concept as feminine and womanly.

Postpartum Sexual Activity

In the United States women are advised to wait 6 weeks before resuming sexual intercourse. This period allows resumption to be correlated with the 6-week medical checkup and makes it convenient for the physician to prescribe contraceptives at the same time. Despite medical advice, many couples resume sexual intercourse before the 6-week period, often between 3 and 4 weeks after the birth. Some couples feel guilty about having sex earlier than advised. The basic rule of thumb is that intercourse may be resumed once the vaginal bleeding has ceased, there is no perineal discomfort, and the couple is psychologically ready. Again, there is tremendous variation in when couples feel ready to resume sexual activity, especially intercourse (Guana–Trujillo and Grant–Higgins 1987). While some women have a tremendously heightened awareness of their bodies and feelings of sexiness in the first weeks after delivery, other women are just as intensely estranged from their bodies and find the idea of having sex unthinkable. It is not uncommon for women to require at least 6 months to recover adequately from the birth process before they feel interested in sex and physically ready to engage in it. Unless women are

informed that it may take a long time to comfortably resume sexual activity, they may feel inadequate and guilty when the traditional 6-week time period has come and gone and they still are not interested in sex.

In non-nursing mothers the resumption of ovulation and steroid production occurs some time after the 6th or 8th postpartum week. Mothers who nurse more than 60 or 70 minutes per day suppress ovulation and steroid production. However, nursing is not considered an effective birth control method because the pattern of hormonal change is unpredictable in each woman. Menstruation returns in 70% to 80% of mothers before lactation ends. The following effects of the decreased hormone

FAMILY CONSIDERATIONS

Men's Sexuality During the Childbearing Year

Current research suggests a complex relationship centering on a man's personality characteristics, his experience of his own sexuality during the childbearing year, and the quality of his relationships with his mate and his newborn child. Marital satisfaction is known to decrease upon the birth of the first child, and sexual satisfaction shows a parallel decline. Men are likely to be more distressed about this change, attributing it to childrearing, while women are less concerned about the change and are likely to attribute it to other life concerns.

However, it is clear that men's sexual functioning is closer to the core of their self-concept than appears to be true for women, so this decline in sexual satisfaction may impact more significantly on men. In one study, men who rated their own sexual satisfaction as high during the first trimester of pregnancy appeared to adapt more easily in the postpartum period. Mates of these men were psychologically healthier in the postpartum period themselves and established more positive relationships with their babies.

Thus, a man's sexuality during the childbearing year seems to be linked with the well-being of his mate and the family overall. Unfortunately, men often regard childbearing as the "kiss of death" for a satisfying sexual relationship, perhaps because they equate *change* with *decline*. The nurse working with childbearing couples should take every opportunity to discuss anticipated changes in the marital and sexual relationship, and help couples adapt creatively and maintain satisfying levels of intimacy through pregnancy and the first few months after childbirth.

May K: Men's sexuality during the childbearing year: Implications of research findings. Holistic Nursing Practice 1(4):60–66, 1987

(estrogen) production on sexual function are described by Masters and Johnson (1966). Orgasms are shorter and weaker, the vagina does not become as vasocongested or as lubricated, these responses take longer to develop, and the color of the labia minora and majora is not as deep a red. Responsiveness returned to normal in 3 months after delivery.

Vaginal bleeding generally lasts about a month, although it may start to diminish in as little as 2 weeks. Some women and some partners are bothered by the odor and feeling of the discharge, whereas others find it a natural or even exciting part of the postpartum experience. The placental site takes 6 weeks to heal completely, and the uterus takes 6 weeks to involute to prepregnant size. The release of oxytocin during breastfeeding helps the uterus involute more quickly. By the end of the first week, the cervix is healing, the external os remains open to varying degrees, and the internal os closes.

The vaginal walls, vulva, and other tissues gradually diminish in size but rarely return to their prepregnant condition. Tears in the vaginal vulvar system will cause a decrease in orgasmic reaction. A stretched or torn vaginal orifice may also decrease orgasmic reaction. If the pubic hair has been shaved, the vulva may be extremely tender and itchy where pubic hair is beginning to grow again.

The episiotomy is certainly a cause of sexual concern for many women. Although actual healing of the episiotomy takes about 2 weeks, it may be much longer before the scar feels elastic enough for penetration and there is no pain at the site. The scar may take as long as 4 months to reach a comfortable state. It helps a great deal for the woman to get up the courage to look at the scar, to watch it heal, and to check for problems such as infections or embedded stitches. The first resumption of intercourse should be preceded by lots of touching, some sexual encounters that do not involve intercourse, and careful exploration with fingers in the vagina to get an idea what penetration might be like and to check for any remaining painful areas. Penile entry needs to be slow and easy, using lots of added lubrication. If the woman is on top, she may have much more control over the angle and depth of penetration. Even women who have had a cesarean section experience pain during penetration for several months after delivery. This is probably due to lack of lubrication and changes in vaginal and pelvic tissues. Cesarean incisions heal in about 3 weeks, but special care should be taken to use positions for intercourse that do not put pressure on the incision.

Effects of Breast-feeding

Breast-feeding has many sexual aspects to it, and yet nursing mothers often feel so tired and drained that they are not interested in sex. Other women see breast-feeding as a wonderfully sensual experience, and some even have orgasms while nursing. Couples often feel relieved to know that the sexual aspects of nursing are normal. The breasts can leak or spurt large quantities of milk during arousal, which makes some couples avoid sex altogether, to avoid having to cope with the mess. Some couples are so impressed by the full size of the woman's breasts that they are more moved toward sexual expression. Partners may be exhilarated by watching their wives breast-feed or jealous that the baby has priority on the breast. The woman may view her breasts as having primarily a physiologic function now while her partner may continue to see her breasts as sexual. This can create different expectations and needs. Some male partners will not go near the lactating breasts because they seem so overwhelming. If there is any difficulty with breast-feeding, parents' emotional stress can cause them to feel exhausted from worry or lack of sleep. If the baby is constantly cranky or colicky, nerves become worn thin and sexual feelings are lost, since every ounce of energy is needed to cope with the baby.

Studies on whether breast-feeding women are more or less interested in sex have produced conflicting conclusions. One study showed that three quarters of breast-feeding women do not notice any difference in their sexual feelings after childbirth (Kenney 1971). A sizable minority said they were less interested in sex, although once they weaned the baby, desire was the same as it was before pregnancy. Masters and Johnson (1966) found nursing mothers had a more prompt return of sexual desire. Murray (1976) suggests that nursing mothers can feel overburdened, overtired, and resentful. Mothers are likely to maintain extra body fat as long as they nurse, which results in self-image problems and anxieties about desirability.

Emotional Adaptation and Sexuality

Fatigue from sleep deprivation, emotional stress, and physiologic changes reduces interest in sex. It takes approximately 1 month for the body to replace the lost blood supply, and resting is important to help this process. Postpartum depression will have a negative effect on sexual feelings, since a person with even mild depression has little interest in sex.

Many couples find that as soon as they start to make love, the baby seems to know and wants to be fed. Some people have speculated that the profound bond between the mother and baby seems broken as the mother involves herself with her partner, that the baby feels this, and that therefore it "seems to know" just when mother is beginning to make love. Another reason that a baby might start crying when parents are starting to make love is that the baby has been rushed through the feeding so that the scene can be set for the parents to enjoy themselves.

For parents who have lost their babies through either stillbirth or early neonatal death, the issue of resuming sexual relations may be very prominent. Some couples may feel that sexual expression is a loving expression shared between two grieving partners that brings a pleasurable relief from painful feelings. Others may feel so depressed that it will take quite a while to resume sexual interest. Finally, feelings of guilt that sexual activity during the pregnancy could have caused the death of the baby may have to be dealt with. The loss of the baby could be seen as punishment for sexual behavior that was laden with guilt feelings.

IMPLICATIONS FOR NURSING CARE

Quite often the aspect of human sexuality is left unconsidered throughout the patient's interaction with the health care system. Health care workers may believe patients do not have sexual concerns, may lack comfort with the subject of sex themselves, may believe discussing it takes too much time, may believe the patient will be offended if the subject is raised, or may believe someone else will do it. The practice of nursing emphasizes viewing the client as a whole human being, and if nursing care fails to include sexuality, then nursing also fails in its holistic goals.

Assessment

Prior to initiating any interaction with patients in regard to sexual well-being, the nurse should conduct a self-assessment, because personal attitudes and values in this area will have a major impact on the effectiveness of the care she renders.

Self-Assessment

Each nurse should ask herself whether or not she feels comfortable about including concern for sexual health in patient care, for not all nurses will be interested in doing so. Self-awareness begins by asking the following questions:

- How do I feel about providing sexual information, counseling, and support so that my clients can have a better sexual future?
- What is my own concept of *sexual adequacy* or of what is sexually *normal?* Do I want to impose that on my clients?
- Do I honestly want my clients to function better sexually?

- How ready am I for an honest discussion of sexuality with a client?
- How would I feel if I were this client, given the same set of circumstances?
- How do I feel about heterosexuality, homosexuality, masturbation, orgasm, unmarried mothers, lesbian mothers, surrogate mothers, and so forth?
- What verbal and nonverbal messages do I convey about my sexuality?

If the nurse wishes to explore the sexual concerns of clients, specialized knowledge and skills are necessary. If the nurse is not comfortable with sexuality, clients should be referred to others who are resource persons in sexual health.

Patient Assessment

Perinatal nurses need to include assessment of the sexual aspects of an individual's or couple's life, since sexual functioning is as much a part of health during the childbearing years as nutrition, exercise, sleep, and stress management (Guana – Trujillo and Grant – Higgins 1987).

Use of Language

Language is often a barrier to communication about sex. The cultural taboos surrounding the discussion of sexual topics have given rise to countless euphemistic terms, vague generalities, and oversimplifications. Both clients and health professionals assume meanings by implication. Many different levels of terminology can be used to discuss sex, including scientific language, religious language, common usage terminology, and street language or slang. Health professionals should familiarize themselves with all those levels and understand the definition of each term. From the client's choice of words, the nurse should gain an understanding of the terminology the client is most comfortable with. Nurses should use language that they feel comfortable with, keeping in mind that if the language is too scientific, the client may not understand it and that slang or common terms may offend certain clients.

Being Specific

The client should be encouraged to give specific details of a problem and to describe a typical situation in which the problem occurs. The nurse must continuously clarify each statement that could be misinterpreted. For example, a client might say, "I have so little desire for sex, and my partner wants to have sex so frequently." The nurse should first clarify what the term "so frequently" actually means. "So frequently" may actually mean anything from three times a day to once a month or so. The taboo in the culture that inhibits sexual discussions makes it difficult to remember to keep asking the client to be specific. For the pregnant family, a good way to bring up the topic might be something like, "Many couples have concerns about sexual activity during pregnancy. I'm wondering what concerns you may be having."

This line of questioning does several things. First, it is an open-ended question that prompts the client to answer with something other than "yes" or "no." Secondly, it lets the client know that she or he may not be the only one having a concern and that concerns about sexuality are considered normal. Thirdly, it brings up the subject so that the client knows that sexual functioning is a permissible topic to discuss in a health care setting. Often health professionals think that any concerns about sexuality will be initiated by the client. Surveys show, however, that the client wants the discussion to be initiated by the health professional.

If the client has no questions at the time, the nurse can offer some information by treating it as review. The nurse might begin by saying, "As you probably already know . . ." This allows the client to feel safer by not having to reveal a sexual concern and also imparts information. The nurse should keep in mind that even if the client has no immediate concerns, the door has been opened to the possibility of discussing sexual concerns in the future.

Clues to Patient Readiness or Interest

Because clients rarely ask direct questions, the nurse does not always know when a client is interested in having a discussion about sexual matters. Frequently clients drop hints in the form of jokes, a concern about someone else, or an afterthought to a conversation. Sometimes the clues are quite subtle, as when a client asks the nurse, for example, how long postpartum bleeding lasts or how long it will be before the baby sleeps through the night. The client's partner may also be the one dropping hints. As the nurse learns to listen for the clues and explore the underlying concern, more clients will be helped to get their sexual issues out in the open.

Clients and their partners believe health professionals should know about sex, that by virtue of having completed nursing or medical school training, the health professional has absorbed, synthesized, and made usable sexual knowledge. Most people have been deluged by a vast array of sex-related messages from magazines,

---

movies, television, books, and songs. They expect that health professionals will have answers to their sexual concerns, or they may avoid the issue to try to protect the health professional from embarrassment when they sense that the nurse or doctor is uncomfortable with the topic of sex.

Diagnosis

The nurse may encounter individuals who have concerns about their sexuality and who seek assistance with them in the course of routine health care. Based on information gained through a careful assessment, the following nursing diagnoses may be useful in guiding care:

- Disturbance in self-esteem or body image
- Potential for altered sexuality patterns
- Potential sexual dysfunction

Planning and Implementation

Even though she may not wish to become an expert on human sexuality, every nurse caring for childbearing families must be prepared to integrate aspects of sexual care into the overall plan. Nursing functions promoting sexual health are outlined by Woods (1984) as follows:

- Facilitation of a milieu conducive to discussion of sexual health
- Provision of anticipatory guidance
- Validation of normalcy
- Education
- Counsel for clients who must adapt to changes in their usual forms of sexual expression
- Provision of intensive therapy for clients with complex problems
- Consultation with other helpers

These functions are listed in order of increasing requirements for skill and knowledge.

A useful framework for integrating sexual health into the nursing process is the P-LI-SS-IT model proposed by Annon (1974). The letters represent four levels at which sexual concerns can be approached. Each level requires an increasing level of knowledge, skill, and comfort with the subject of human sexuality: *Permission, Limited Information, Specific Suggestions,* and *Intensive Therapy.*

At the first level, *permission,* the nurse initiates the discussion of sex, giving permission to talk about sexual subjects and legitimizing the existence of sexual feelings, thoughts, desires, or questions.

The P-LI-SS-IT Model

P	Permission	
LI	Limited Information	Brief
SS	Specific Suggestions	Therapy
IT	Intensive Therapy	

ASSESSMENT TOOL

Sexual Problem History

I. Description of the current problem (what the client sees as the problem)
- Ask about the effect on the patient:
  "How does this affect you?"
  "How do you feel about it?"
- Explore the effects on the partner:
  "How does this concern affect your partner?"
  "How has your partner dealt with the problem?"
- Explore the severity:
  "How often do you have this difficulty?"

II. Description of the onset and course of the problem
- Obtain a description of the onset (gradual or sudden, precipitating events) and consequences:
  "When did this start occurring?"
  "What was the situation the first time this occurred?"
- Obtain a description of the course (changes over time; increase, decrease, or fluctuation in severity, frequency, or intensity; relationship of problem to other variables).

III. Identification of the client's perception of the factors causing and maintaining the problem
- Ask about psychological, biologic, sociological, and environmental influences that the client thinks may be contributing factors

IV. Elucidation of previous interventions to deal with the problem and their results
- Ask about previous medical interventions (specialty, date, form of treatment, results, current medications of any kind).
- Ask about other professional or paraprofessional interventions (specialty, date, form of treatment, results). Include questioning that covers alternative treatments, such as biofeedback, special diets, polarity, movement, exercise, and so on.
- Ask about self-help (what, when, results).
  "How have you tried to solve the problem up until now?"
- Ask about communication with partner:
  "Have you discussed this with your partner?"
  "What were the results?"

V. Identification of current expectations and goals (specific and general)
- Explore how the client would like things changed:
  "How would you like the situation to be different?"

Often the permission alone is sufficient to reduce a client's anxiety or feelings of guilt. If the nurse has negative feelings about a patient's behavior, fantasies, or beliefs, she should acknowledge these feelings to herself and refer the patient to someone more comfortable with the situation. If the setting is not appropriate or if privacy, time, knowledge, or skills are lacking, the client should be referred to someone with expertise in human sexuality. Most important is that the nurse listen to what the client has to say.

At the second level, *limited information,* the nurse imparts information to the client that is relevant to the client's concern, particularly if the problem is one of altered sexuality patterns or disturbance in self-concept. If the client has a specific question, then the nurse gives whatever information is pertinent to the question. Even if the client indicates that there is no specific question or concern, the nurse can impart information on sexuality by treating it as review. For example, the nurse might say, "As you may already know, breast-feeding mothers often find that when they become aroused, their breasts leak milk." The nurse can then listen to the client's response to see if there is further need for discussion.

The third level of intervention, *specific suggestions,* requires the nurse to take a sexual problem history before formulating suggestions. This is a fairly detailed assessment of the client's problem. The accompanying sexual problem history format is adapted from Annon (1974).

If the suggestions are not perceived as helpful in a short period of time, or if a specific sexual dysfunction has been identified, the patient ought to be referred for intensive therapy.

The final level of intervention, *intensive therapy,* is provided by a sex therapist, sex counselor, or psychotherapist trained in human sexuality when the client needs more extensive intervention. As distinct from this last level, the levels of permission, limited information, and specific suggestion are considered *brief therapy.* Most nurses are not prepared to intervene beyond the level of giving limited information unless they have had a good deal of training in human sexuality. It is still appropriate, however, for nurses to make an assessment of the problem.

Evaluation

Evaluating the effectiveness of nursing care directed toward promoting sexual well-being is often difficult because the absence of stated patient concerns may either reflect well-being or the inability to seek help. Thus, expected outcomes may focus more generally on creating a supportive environment so that patients can voice concerns, providing appropriate information at the appropriate level (see Self-Care Teaching points), and providing appropriate care for specific patient problems, either through additional patient teaching or through referral.

SELF-CARE TEACHING

Sexual Activity During Pregnancy and Postpartum

First Trimester

- Don't have sex on an empty stomach.
- Breast tenderness and other changes are temporary.
- Decrease breast fondling.
- Wear a bra during sex if it seems to help.
- Use a coital position that does not put undue pressure on the breasts.
- Don't try to have sex when you're tired.
- If orgasm or sexual intercourse have been prohibited, you can use other means of loving expression, such as hugging, massage, together activities, and so on.

Second Trimester

- Increased lubrication may create a hygiene concern.
- Wash genitals with warm water and avoid deodorant soaps and all douches.
- A back rub after orgasm may ease discomfort.
- Become creative with new positions.
- Heightened or decreased interest in sex is normal.
- Masturbation and orgasm are not a threat in an uncomplicated pregnancy.

Third Trimester

- Sex may be better in the upright position.
- Alternatives to intercourse may become necessary.
- Remind your partner of increased need for cuddling and holding.
- Sustained tonic contraction has not been shown to hurt the fetus in an uncomplicated pregnancy.

Postpartum

- For both vaginal and cesarean deliveries, sexual intercourse may be resumed around 3 to 4 weeks postpartum.
- Do not resume sexual intercourse until vaginal bleeding has stopped, to prevent introduction of infection at the placental site.
- Check for healing of episiotomy and perineum by inserting a finger or tampon into the vagina.
- Sexual arousal may cause milk to leak from the breasts. Nursing the baby before sexual activity or wearing a bra with absorbent pads during lovemaking may help this problem.
- If additional lubrication is necessary, use contraceptive cream or a natural vegetable oil (safflower or soy, for example). K-Y jelly dries out rapidly and turns to little balls of dried lubricant.
- Have longer periods of foreplay to encourage lubrication.
- Communicate openly.
- You can use alternative forms of sexual expression (mutual masturbation, massage, oral or anal sex).
- Do not take baths for 2 or 3 weeks to avoid spreading bacteria from other parts of the body to the vaginal opening.
- Begin Kegel exercises immediately after birth and do them whenever you urinate and frequently during the day to strengthen pubococcygeal muscles and tighten the vaginal opening.
- Take sitz baths 3 times a day to help heal episiotomy scar.
- Examine the perineum with a good light and mirror within a few days of delivery and then again 3 weeks later to reassure yourself that it is healing.
- If something doesn't look right, contact a physician — it's easier to fix problems sooner rather than later.
- Intercourse and your body do return to "normal."
- Wear a bra 24 hours a day as soon as possible after delivery to help decrease engorgement.
- Encourage your partner not to put pressure on breasts while they're sensitive, especially during the night when the baby is sleeping for longer periods without feeding.
- Set priorities realistically. Arrange your schedule so that you nap when the baby does.
- Get a nap of at least 30 minutes every day or at least lie down and get off your feet.
- If you're depressed, get help from friends and family. Get further help if the depression lasts longer than 3 days.
- When the baby is weaned, your sex drive will return in full force.
- Don't rush feeding just before lovemaking.
- You can put the baby in another room or behind a screen during lovemaking.
- You can use music to soothe the baby during lovemaking.

CHAPTER SUMMARY

Nurses can promote sexual health for pregnant couples by anticipating information that these couples will need, by confirming the normalcy of changes in sexual patterns, and by facilitating communication about sexual issues between the partners. In particular, couples may need permission to continue what they were already doing or permission to stop doing something because it doesn't feel right. Often the most helpful thing the nurse can do is to listen supportively to the client's concerns after letting her know that concerns about sexuality are reasonable and just as valid as concerns about diet or exercise. It is important to keep in mind that each couple brings together a unique combination of sexual desires, concerns, behaviors, attitudes, and motivations. Also, each pregnancy is different and affects each couple differently. Therefore, the nurse who is interested in sexual health must investigate the factors that may have a bearing on sexual feelings, such as the couple's relationship or the pregnant woman's feelings about her body, in order to gain insight into potential areas of sexual concern.

Vaginal intercourse need not be prohibited during a normal pregnancy. Prohibition is necessary only if the cervix is ripe and there is a poor reproductive history. In such cases the nurses should make sure that the couple understands that the ban on intercourse is necessary and that orgasm either from intercourse or masturbation may be more powerful than intercourse alone in initiating labor. Finally, the pregnant couple can most benefit by being treated as humans with real strengths and vulnerabilities who are going through a transitional period in their lives. If the pregnant woman's body is respected and she feels in control of her pregnancy, she will be able to stay in touch with her body and feel it still belongs to her. In the long run, this will be very important for the return of good feelings about her sexual image, body image, and self-esteem.

STUDY QUESTIONS

1. Describe how vaginal lubrication occurs.
2. Discuss the controversies that exist about the nature of female orgasms.
3. List at least six factors that could affect the couple's sexual relationship during pregnancy.
4. Describe several ways that the woman's interest in sex may fluctuate throughout the pregnancy.
5. Discuss the circumstances under which sexual activity is contraindicated during pregnancy.
6. Identify the physiologic and anatomic changes that occur during pregnancy that may make intercourse more difficult.
7. Describe several positions for sexual intercourse that prevent abdominal pressure or deep penetration.
8. Discuss the ways that the changes in body image that occur later in pregnancy could affect a woman's sexual self-image.
9. When is resumption of coitus considered safe in the postpartum period and why?
10. Describe the effects that breast-feeding may have on a couple's sexual relations.

REFERENCES/BIBLIOGRAPHY

Annon J: Behavioral Treatment of Sexual Problems: Brief Therapy, Vol 1. New York, Harper & Row, 1974

Bing E, Coleman L: Making Love During Pregnancy. New York, Bantam Books, 1977

Calderone MS: Fetal erection and its message to us. Monthly report of Sex Information and Education Council of the United States (SIECUS) May–July, 1983

Comfort A: Refractory period after ejaculation. Lancet 1:1075, 1972

Covington TR: Sex Care. New York, Pocket Books, 1987

Crooks R, Bauer K: Our Sexuality, 2nd ed. Menlo Park, CA, Benjamin–Cummings, 1983

Ellis DJ: Sexual needs and concerns of expectant parents. J Obstet Gynecol Neonatal Nurs 9:306, 1980

Falicov CJ: Sexual adjustment during first pregnancy and postpartum. Am J Obstet Gynecol 117:991, 1973

Federation of Feminist Women's Health Centers: A New View of a Woman's Body. New York, Simon & Schuster, 1981

Francoeur RT: Becoming a Sexual Person, Chaps 3, 4. New York, John Wiley & Sons, 1982

Goodlin RC, Schmidt W, Creevy DC: Uterine tension and fetal heart rate during maternal orgasm. Obstet Gynecol 39:125, 1972

Goodlin RC, Keller DW, Raffin M: Orgasm during late pregnancy: Possible deleterious effects. Obstet Gynecol 38:916, 1971

Guana–Trujillo B, Grant–Higgins P: Sexual intercourse and pregnancy. Health Care for Women International 8:339, 1987

Hite S: The Hite Report. New York, Dell Pub, 1977

Kaplan HS: Disorders of Sexual Desire. New York, Brunner–Mazel, 1979

Kenney JA: Sexuality of pregnant and breast-feeding women. Arch Sex Beh 2(3):215, 1973

Kinsey AC, Pomeroy WB, Martin CE: Sexual Behavior in the Human Male. Philadelphia, WB Saunders, 1948

Kitzinger S: Women's Experience of Sex. New York, GP Putnam's Sons, 1983

Klebanoff MA, Nugent RP, Rhoads GG: Coitus during pregnancy: Is it safe? Lancet 10:914, 1984

Klein J: Scared sexless. American Health, p. 84. April, 1987

Langfeldt T: Aspects of sexual development, problems and therapy in children. In Samson JM (ed): Proceedings of the International Symposium on Childhood and Sexuality. Montreal, Editions Etudes Vivantes, 1980

Lavery JP, Miller CE: Effect of prostaglandin and seminal fluid on human chorionic membranes. JAMA 245:2425, 1981

Maddock J: Sexual health and health care. Postgrad Med 58(1):53, 1975

Masters WH, Johnson V: Human Sexual Response. Boston, Little, Brown & Co, 1966

Masters WH, Johnson V: Human Sexual Inadequacy. Boston, Little, Brown & Co, 1970

Masters WH, Johnson VE, Kolodny RC: Human Sexuality. Boston, Little, Brown & Co, 1982

Mills JS, Harlap S, Harley EE: Should coitus in late pregnancy be discouraged? Lancet 7:136, 1981

Moses AE, Hawkins RO: Counseling Lesbian Women and Gay Men. St. Louis, CV Mosby, 1982

Murray ME: Sexual problems in nursing mothers. Med Aspects Hum Sex 10:75, 1976

Muscari ME: Obtaining the adolescent sexual history. Pediatr Nurs 13(5):307, 1987

Naeye RL, Flood B: Factors that predispose to premature rupture of the fetal membranes. J Obstet Gynecol Neonatal Nurs 13(2):119, 1984

Perkins RP: Sexuality in pregnancy: What determines behavior? Obstet Gynecol 59:189, 1982

Perry JD, Whipple B: Pelvic muscle strength of female ejaculators: Evidence in support of a new theory of orgasm. J Sex Res 17:22, 1981

Proctor SE: A developmental approach to pregnancy prevention with early adolescent females. J Sch Health 56(8):313, 1986

Pugh WE, Fernandez FL: Coitus in late pregnancy. Obstet Gynecol 2:636, 1953

Rigg CA: Homosexuality in adolescence. Pediatr Ann 11(10):826, 1982

Solberg DA, Butler J, Wagner NN: Sexual behavior in pregnancy. N Engl J Med 288:1098, 1973

Tolor A, DiGrazia P: Sexual attitudes and behavior patterns during and following pregnancy. Arch Sex Behav 5:539, 1976

Toth A, O'Leary WM, Ledger W: Evidence for microbial transfer by spermatozoa. Obstet Gynecol 59:556, 1982

Woods NF: Human Sexuality in Health and Illness. St. Louis, CV Mosby, 1984

World Health Organization (WHO): Education and treatment in human sexuality: The training of health professionals. Report of WHO meeting (Technical Report Series No. 572), Geneva, WHO, 1975

Yoos L. Adolescent cognitive and contraceptive behaviors. Pediatr Nurs 13(4):247, 1987

7 fertility and infertility

Although science has begun to perfect some techniques that facilitate fertility, chance continues to play a large role in conception. Even under optimal conditions, only about 25% of couples who try to conceive will do so within 1 month. In the course of a year, approximately 85% of couples who attempt pregnancy will be successful (Menning 1988).

Involuntary childlessness, however, is on the rise, with the latest statistics indicating that approximately 15% to 20% of United States couples experience infertility (Glass 1982; Speroff 1983).

Infertility can be viewed as a major life crisis. Unwanted involuntary childlessness can harm self-esteem and contribute to stresses in a marital relationship. Infertility testing and treatments can be costly, time-consuming, painful, and, when results are unsuccessful, disappointing.

To understand the concept of human infertility, it helps to understand concepts related to human fertility. Therefore, this chapter begins with a brief look at reproductive potential and the normal process of conception. Infertility, as discussed in this chapter, is of three biologic kinds: female, male, and interactive. The second half of the chapter discusses the nursing process as a means of working with infertile couples. Both nursing assessment and diagnostic procedures are discussed. Specific treatment and nursing interventions are provided.

Nurses play a crucial role in helping couples who have concerns about their fertility potential. Persons experiencing infertility problems need emotional support, guidance, advocacy, education, and appropriate referrals for adequate care. Nurses contribute in all of these critical areas by providing skilled nursing care that encompasses both technical and psychosocial expertise. Nurses work not only with the infertile person but with the infertile couple and the larger family unit.

FERTILITY

Fertility patterns are dependent on many factors, including age, sex, and health. The nurse must understand the physiologic processes underlying male and female reproductive potential and conception in order to deliver effective care to those who want to control their own fertility either by avoiding pregnancy or by achieving it.

Male and Female Reproductive Potential

A major difference between male and female reproductive potential is that women have a finite reproductive life span, whereas men, after puberty, have the capacity to reproduce for the rest of their lives. Women are born with a set number of eggs, usually about 1 to 2 million. By the time a woman begins to menstruate, she has about

300,000 to 400,000 eggs left. It is believed that about 450 eggs are ovulated during a woman's lifetime, with the rest of the eggs regressing. Normally, a woman has a reproductive life span of about 35 years (Glass 1982).

In contrast, men constantly produce sperm. New sperm cells are generated approximately every 74 days. There are approximately 200 to 300 million sperm in each ejaculate, of which only about 200 reach the area around the egg. There is no known time in a man's life when he ceases to produce sperm (Glass 1982).

Normal Process of Conception

To understand the various causes of infertility, the nurse must be familiar with male and female anatomy and physiology and the normal process of conception. The following is a brief overview of the process that must take place for conception and implantation of a fertilized ovum to occur.

Sperm Production.   For conception to occur, mature, healthy spermatozoa must be produced and deposited into the vagina. Sperm production is induced by follicle-stimulating hormone (FSH) and luteinizing hormone (LH). These hormones are released from the pituitary gland under the influence of the hypothalamus and stimulate testosterone production by the testes. (Male reproductive organs were discussed in Chapter 5.)

Transport.   After deposition in the vagina, the sperm must be transported through the cervical mucus into the uterus and fallopian tubes. At the time of ovulation, the cervical mucus normally undergoes certain physiologic changes that aid it in protecting the sperm against the normal acidity of the vagina, which would be lethal to sperm. The semen's alkalinity also provides a measure of protection. Sperm remaining in the vagina for more than 2 hours become immobilized. Sperm rapidly migrate to the cervix and have been found in the cervical mucus within 90 seconds of ejaculation.

Capacitation.   After a short time in the cervical mucus, the sperm migrate up the uterus, aided by uterine contractions, and enter the fallopian tubes. (The fallopian tubes were discussed in Chapter 5.) Once within the fallopian tubes, the sperm undergo a process called *capacitation,* in which they change their surface characteristics and release enzymes, particularly hyaluronidase, that contribute to their ability to penetrate the ovum.

Ovulation.   During the transport and capacitation of the sperm, the ovum also undergoes essential changes. Before ovulation, estrogen secretion from the ovaries increases, under the influence of FSH and LH released by the pituitary gland in response to the hypothalamus. This increased estrogen production leads to the growth of many follicles in the ovary. Normally only one follicle reaches maturity and is released from the ovary at ovulation. This follicle, known as the graafian follicle, contains an ovum, which is released from the follicle ready to be fertilized. There is evidence that the fimbriae (or fingerlike projections at the ends of each fallopian tube) massage the ovaries to help extract the ovum. (Ovarian structure was discussed in Chapter 5.)

Fertilization.   The ovum can be fertilized only during the early stages of its journey in the fallopian tube. Fertilization normally occurs in the outer one-third of the fallopian tube. Cilia and muscle contractions in the tube are believed to facilitate transport of the ovum to meet the sperm. When one sperm has penetrated the ovum, the *zona pellucida,* a translucent coat surrounding the ovum, acts to block the entry of any others.

Implantation.   After fertilization, implantation of the conceptus must occur. Implantation is the process by which the fertilized ovum attaches to the uterine wall and penetrates both the uterine epithelium and the maternal circulatory system. This process can only occur if there has been developmental maturation on the surface of the conceptus to enable implantation. This developmental maturation occurs through the lysis (destruction) of the *zona pellucida.* At the time of implantation, the uterus is under the influence of progesterone. Adequate levels of progesterone are necessary for successful implantation and for maintenance of the conceptus in the uterine lining. When conception occurs, the woman begins to produce the hormone human chorionic gonadotropin (HCG), which is necessary to maintain the pregnancy. The *corpus luteum,* which is the yellow mass found in the graafian follicle after the ovum has been expelled, is essential to maintaining adequate levels of HCG until the placenta takes over this function. (Further information on fertilization, cleavage, and embryonic development are discussed in Chapter 14.)

INFERTILITY

Involuntary infertility is a serious problem for many people. There is much speculation about why the apparent incidence is increasing. Some possible reasons are the expansion of environmental hazards, the greater tendency on the part of women to delay childbearing until after the biologically optimal time, and the fact that more people are now seeking treatment for infertility rather than "hiding" it. Nurses play an important role in the management of infertility, both by being involved with the many diagnostic tests and treatments and by providing needed counseling and emotional support.

Infertility is defined as the inability to conceive and carry a pregnancy to viability after at least 1 year of regular sexual intercourse without contraception. *Primary infertility* is an inability to conceive and carry a pregnancy to viability with no previous history of pregnancy carried to a live birth. *Secondary infertility* is an inability to conceive and carry a pregnancy to a live birth following one or more successful pregnancies.

Although often used interchangeably, the terms *infertility* and *sterility* are not synonymous. *Infertility* implies that some potential may exist for conception under optimal circumstances, whereas *sterility* denotes a total and irreversible inability to conceive (Menning 1988). Broadly defined, infertility includes the inability to carry a pregnancy to viability. Thus, women who experience habitual abortion, defined as a history of three or more consecutive spontaneous abortions, can be described as infertile.

Causes of Infertility

In examining the causes of infertility, it is essential to consider not only the individual characteristics of the man

---

Causes of Infertility
Biological Causes
Female (40%)
- Vaginal: abnormalities, infections, highly acidic vaginal *p*H
- Cervical: hostile environment (insufficient estrogen or infection), incompetent cervix
- Uterine: abnormalities, hostile environment that does not allow implantation and survival of blastocyst
- Tubal: adhesions, scar tissue due to pelvic inflammatory disease (PID); endometriosis
- Ovarian: anovulation, irregular or infrequent ovulation, secretory dysfunction, inadequate luteal phase

Male (40%)
- Anatomical abnormalities/congenital factors
- Inadequate sperm production/maturation: maternal DES ingestion, varicocele, testicular inflammation, heat exposure, sexually transmitted disease, radiation exposure, stress, certain drugs
- Inadequate motility of sperm: same as above
- Blockage of sperm in male reproductive tract: same as above
- Inability to deposit sperm: problems with ejaculation

Interactive (20%)
- Sexual dysfunction
- Situational causes (lack of a partner; homosexuality)
- Unexplained causes (10%–15%)

and woman, but also their potential fertility as a couple. For example, a man with a low sperm count may be able to impregnate a partner who has no physiologic abnormalities but may be unable to impregnate a woman who ovulates very infrequently. In most instances, infertility can be traced to identifiable causes in the man, the woman, or the couple as a unit. However, in about 10% to 15% of cases, no specific cause for a couple's infertility can be identified. Until recent years, such couples were labeled as "psychogenically infertile," on the assumption that a psychological imbalance, usually in the woman, caused their infertility. This conclusion was based on poorly controlled research studies and conflicting findings and has been refuted by more recent well-controlled research. Such couples are now described as experiencing "unexplained" infertility, which acknowledges that medical technology does not yet have the means to diagnose and understand all forms of infertility. However, psychological factors cannot be completely discounted.

The other causes of infertility are more obvious, and stem from differences in customs and situation. The term *situational infertility* can apply to people, such as men or women without partners and homosexual men or women, whose life situation precludes the occurrence of conception. These people are not necessarily biologically infertile, but because of the absence of an opposite-sex partner, they are unable to conceive. This group is receiving more publicity lately because of the advent of sperm banks and *in vitro* fertilization as alternative means of achieving conception.

Since most causes of infertility are biologic, they are grouped as female causes, male causes, and interactive causes.

Female Infertility

Female causes account for about 40% of all cases of infertility. Figure 7–1 illustrates the anatomical areas where dysfunctions that interfere with fertility can occur.

Vaginal Causes

The vagina is the canal in which sperm are deposited. Certain conditions in the vaginal environment are hostile to sperm survival. Such conditions include vaginal infec-

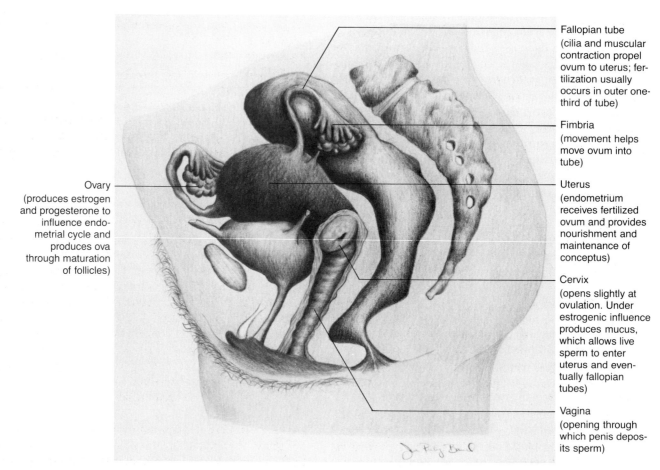

Figure 7–1. Female reproductive anatomy and function, indicating areas where dysfunction may occur. (Childbirth Graphics)

NURSING RESEARCH

Ambiguity and Infertility

An open-ended study of 26 private and 22 clinic infertility patients revealed the concept of ambiguity to be central to women's experiences with infertility. Ambiguity is linked to the concept of uncertainty as it exists in relation to the causes of infertility, the diagnosis of infertility itself, the treatments prescribed and their prognosis, the diagnosis of pregnancy and what the outcome of a pregnancy will be. In addition, ambiguity and uncertainty exist in relation to the life pursuits of infertile persons as well as to the control they perceive they have and their identity as infertile. The researcher raises many provocative and important questions from the results of this study, leading to interesting ideas for further research.

Sandelowski M: The color gray: Ambiguity and Infertility. Image: The Journal of Nursing Scholarship, 19(2):70, 1987

tions (vaginitis), anatomical abnormalities that may prevent access by the sperm to the cervix and uterus, and sexual dysfunction that prevents penetration by the penis. Vaginal infections may be lethal to sperm. Even under normal circumstances, the vaginal environment is acidic and is not conducive to sperm survival. However, if other factors are normal, enough sperm can survive the acidic environment and reach the cervix, which is alkaline under normal ovulatory conditions. A highly acidic vaginal environment decreases sperm survival markedly and contributes to infertility.

Cervical Causes

During the preovulatory period and ovulation itself, specific changes occur in the cervix that make the cervical environment conducive to sperm survival. The cervical os (the opening in the cervix) becomes slightly widened. The cervical mucus becomes more alkaline, more abundant, and watery. It acquires the consistency of egg whites and can be stretched 6 to 10 inches while remaining intact. It also displays a ferning pattern microscopically. These changes occur under the influence of the increased estrogen production and LH surge that occur around the time of ovulation.

A disruption in any of these physiologic changes can contribute to infertility by resulting in a cervical environment that is more hostile to sperm survival. Problems such as insufficient estrogen production or cervicitis (cervical infection) are examples of contributing factors. If estrogen production is deficient, an adequate amount of

healthy, ovulatory cervical mucus will not be produced, and the sperm will have a much more difficult time swimming up through the cervical os into the uterus and the fallopian tubes. The presence of cervicitis also renders the cervical mucus more hostile to sperm.

Cervical problems can also be more mechanical in nature. Occasionally, after conception a woman's cervix will dilate prematurely, leading to a spontaneous abortion. This condition is referred to as *cervical incompetence*. It has been found more frequently in women whose mothers were treated with diethylstilbestrol (DES) during pregnancy.

It is important to note that terms such as "hostile" cervical mucus, or "incompetent cervix," although widely used, are in disfavor because they convey some sense of blame and a negative image of women.

Uterine Causes

The uterus must provide a hospitable environment for sperm as they journey up the uterus into the fallopian tubes to fertilize the ovum. In addition, the uterus functions as the organ in which the fertilized ovum, or *blastocyst,* implants. Thus, the uterine lining, or *endometrium,* must be rich and healthy, with adequate secretory responses to increased progesterone to allow the blastocyst to implant and survive.

Difficulty with conception and implantation can be the result of uterine abnormalities. These may be structural, such as a bicornuate uterus, for example, or physiologic, such as uterine myomas or leiomyomas or Asherman's syndrome, in which the walls of the uterus remain closed. Contrary to common belief, retroversion or retroflexion of the uterus does not cause difficulties in achieving or maintaining a pregnancy.

Tubal Causes

Infertility related to problems with the fallopian tubes is becoming more common as a result of an increase in the incidence of pelvic inflammatory disease. Pelvic inflammatory disease can lead to adhesions (scarring) around the fallopian tubes, which creates obstructions in the tubes, preventing transport of the ovum and the sperm. The popularity of the intrauterine device has contributed to the rise in pelvic inflammatory disease, particularly since about 40% of pelvic inflammatory disease associated with intrauterine device use is asymptomatic. The absence of symptoms often means that treatment is not sought until after scar tissue and adhesions have formed.

Endometriosis, a condition in which endometrial tissue grows in areas outside the uterus, can also contribute to tubal problems. Excess endometrial tissue growing around the fallopian tubes leads to adhesions and decreased tubal mobility.

Ovarian Causes

The ovaries are endocrine organs and secrete estrogen and progesterone in addition to storing eggs and producing one mature egg each month at the time of ovulation. Ovarian dysfunction is a major cause of infertility. *Anovulation,* or lack of ovulation, is a common problem among women complaining of an inability to become pregnant. Clearly, if an egg is not produced, pregnancy cannot occur. Sometimes a woman ovulates very irregularly and infrequently, a condition known as *oligo-ovulation.* Stein–Leventhal syndrome, more commonly referred to as *polycystic ovary syndrome,* is a condition in which multiple cysts on the ovaries lead to anovulatory problems. Hirsutism and obesity are commonly associated with this syndrome.

Secretory malfunction of the ovaries may contribute to infertility as well. If progesterone secretion by the ovaries is inadequate, a woman may conceive and ovulate, but she will be unable to maintain the fertilized ovum and will experience a spontaneous abortion. An inadequate luteal phase, or second half of the menstrual cycle, that is related to inadequate progesterone secretion also contributes to infertility. LH is responsible for maintaining the corpus luteum, which in turn is necessary for the nourishment and support of the fertilized ovum. An inadequate luteal phase may be partially responsible for habitual abortions that are due to a uterine inability to support the fertilized ovum.

Male Infertility

Comparatively little is known about male infertility, even though about 40% of infertility problems are related to dysfunctions in the male, usually in sperm production. Figure 7–2 illustrates areas in which dysfunctions leading to infertility may occur.

Congenital factors may also result in infertility. Congenital absence of the vasa deferentia or of the testes, while rare, will obviously result in infertility. A maternal history of DES ingestion may be correlated with de-

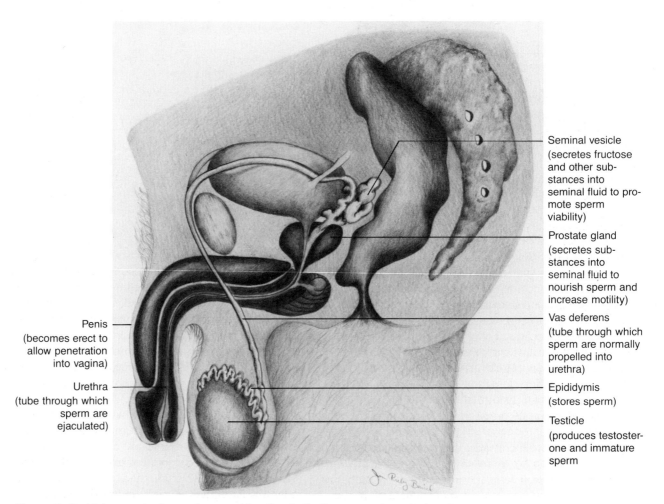

Penis
(becomes erect to allow penetration into vagina)

Urethra
(tube through which sperm are ejaculated)

Seminal vesicle
(secretes fructose and other substances into seminal fluid to promote sperm viability)

Prostate gland
(secretes substances into seminal fluid to nourish sperm and increase motility)

Vas deferens
(tube through which sperm are normally propelled into urethra)

Epididymis
(stores sperm)

Testicle
(produces testosterone and immature sperm

Figure 7–2. Male reproductive anatomy and function, indicating areas where dysfunction may occur. (Childbirth Graphics)

creased sperm count and with anatomical abnormalities of the testes. However, most problems in male fertility result from inadequate sperm production or maturation (spermatogenesis); inadequate motility of the sperm; blockage of sperm along the male reproductive tract; or inability to deposit sperm in the woman's vagina (Speroff 1983).

Problems in Sperm Production

Many cases of inadequate sperm production cannot be explained or treated. One of the few specific defects that can be treated with reasonable chance of success is a *varicocele,* or varicose vein in a spermatic cord, usually the left one. Researchers believe that the presence of a varicocele leads to a local increase in temperature, which has a detrimental effect on sperm production. Occasionally, sperm production may also be affected by the presence of a *hydrocele,* which is a small fluid-filled bag within the scrotum.

Any testicular inflammation, or *orchitis,* may lead to testicular impairment and atrophy. A major cause of testicular inflammation is an episode of mumps after puberty. Fortunately, such inflammation usually occurs unilaterally. If it is bilateral, sterility may result.

Another factor directly affecting the testes and sperm production is *cryptorchidism,* or undescended testicles. Normally, the testes are enclosed in the scrotal sac, an environment somewhat cooler than core body temperature. This cooler environment is optimal for producing sperm in adequate numbers and allowing them to mature and become motile. If the testes are not descended into the scrotal sac before puberty, they will be permanently damaged by the increased heat within the abdomen.

Other sources of heat may also be detrimental to sperm production. Men who wear tight underclothes or take frequent, long, hot baths or saunas may be at a higher risk for decreased sperm production and motility. Men with illnesses associated with a persistent high fever may temporarily experience a depressed sperm production.

Sperm production may also be affected by infections, specifically, infections of the reproductive organs, such as sexually transmitted diseases — particularly gonorrhea, T mycoplasmosis, and chlamydiosis. Tuberculosis is also a culprit, since it can spread to the reproductive organs. Exposure to radiation can adversely affect sperm production, as can traumatic injury to the testicles.

Stress and inadequate nutrition are also implicated in decreased sperm production, as is inadequate intake of vitamins A, B complex, and C. That stress can also be a factor is suggested by evidence from research done on men in concentration camps and by research that found that men living in urban areas had poorer sperm production than men living in rural areas (Menning 1988). Smoking, alcohol intake, and high-pressure work are often as-

sociated with stress, and each of these is believed to play a role in causing abnormal semen. The nicotine intake from smoking more than one pack of cigarettes a day is associated with impairments in the quantity and quality of spermatogenesis. Lowered testosterone levels are correlated with excessive alcohol intake, and impotence and decreased libido are associated with high-pressure work and alcohol intake (Speroff 1983).

Ingestion of certain drugs can have detrimental effects on the sperm. Methotrexate, a drug used to treat psoriasis and certain forms of cancer, has been found to have lasting effects on the sperm-forming germinal cells, leading to chromosomal abnormalities. Drugs used to treat urinary tract infections, such as nitrofurantoin can affect spermatogenesis, as can amebicides and sex hormones. Research on the effects of marijuana on sperm is inconclusive, but there is evidence that excessive use of the drug can result in suppression of gonadotropin-releasing hormone (GnRH), decreased testosterone production, and oligospermia.

The man may develop an antibody reaction to his own sperm after sperm cells have entered surrounding tissue as a result of trauma, vasectomy, or infection. Subsequently, otherwise healthy sperm will be destroyed.

Problems in Ejaculation

Occasionally, male infertility can be caused by ejaculatory problems that result in an inability to deposit sperm in the vagina. *Retrograde ejaculation* is a condition in which sperm are not ejaculated out of the penis, but rather are ejaculated backward into the bladder. The man will notice no fluid after orgasm, and his urine will appear milky-colored. Retrograde ejaculation may be caused by diabetes, nerve damage, certain medications, and surgical trauma (Menning 1988).

Interactive Causes of Infertility

Some cases of infertility result from problems specific to the couple in interaction with one another. The woman may develop antibodies to her partner's sperm, thus destroying otherwise healthy sperm and markedly decreasing the chances of conception. Sexual problems, such as very infrequent sexual intercourse or sexual technique not conducive to conception, can also lead to difficulty in achieving conception. It is often unclear whether sexual difficulties contribute to infertility or result from the stress of infertility. Although it must be stressed that there are no universal prescriptions for sexual satisfaction, certain sexual practices are more beneficial for achieving conception. Intercourse in positions where the woman lies on her back enhances the possibility that sperm will migrate up to the cervix due to gravity. Intercourse must also be timed with the woman's ovulation. Ovulation usually occurs approximately 14 days before the onset of the next menstrual cycle. Once an egg is ovulated, it has a life span of about 12 to 24 hours. Once sperm are ejaculated, they have a life span of about 24 to 48 hours. These factors are critical in timing intercourse to enhance the possibility of conception.

ASSESSMENT OF FERTILITY STATUS

Assessment of persons seeking evaluation and treatment of infertility begins with a detailed, comprehensive history. Included in this health history are activities of daily living, social habits, sexual practices, and more general health information that helps shed light on possible causes of infertility. Such a history may be followed by specific diagnostic procedures for infertility.

Assessment of Physiologic Aspects

As technological advances have been made in the treatment of infertility, the nurse's role has expanded. Nurses play an integral role in many assessment procedures — for example, nurses teach patients how to chart their basal body temperature and, in some cases, perform the postcoital tests. Some nurses take samples of cervical mucus and observe them under the microscope. Occasionally, nurses assess sperm count, motility, and morphology by observing the sperm microscopically.

Assessment of Psychosocial Responses

Nurses are responsible not only for helping to identify the possible reasons for infertility but also for assessing patients' responses to it. It is important to understand how infertility affects people's lives. If nurses understood more in this area, they could help to lessen the emotional impact of infertility. Assessing how well a person or couple is coping with infertility is an essential part of the domain of nursing, and helping people cope with the often overlooked emotional and psychosocial aspects of infertility is an integral part of the nurse's work.

Menning (1988) has identified several stages that people pass through as they resolve the emotional conflicts surrounding infertility. Wilson (1979) noted the following sequence of responses:

1. Disbelief and denial
2. Depression and anger
3. Optimism
4. Desperation
5. Depression
6. Acceptance

Infertile couples often have a sense of not being in control, which adds to their difficulties in resolving their feelings about their infertility. Involuntary infertility is often referred to as a "crisis." In terms of Erikson's developmental framework, it has been viewed as an impairment of the person's ability to resolve the conflict of "generativity versus stagnation" (Erikson 1963).

More recently, Unruh and McGrath (1985) have described infertility as "chronic sorrow." Current nursing research (Olshansky 1987; Sandelowski and Pollack 1986; Sandelowski 1987) sheds light on the emotional responses to infertility in general as well as responses to high technological procedures which are emerging in this field (Mahlstedt, MacDuff, and Bernstein 1987; Olshansky 1988; Seibel and Levin 1987).

Cultural beliefs also influence responses to infertility. In many cultures, childbearing is expected and childlessness is pitied. Infertility is often blamed on the woman, although in some cultures the man's virility is in question until he has fathered a child. In some Middle Eastern countries, a woman's infertility is sufficient reason for divorce. Beliefs about causes of infertility may suggest that the infertile person is somehow inadequate or is being punished for previous wrongdoing. These cultural beliefs may be held in part by people who see themselves as quite modern in other ways and may make the process of accepting and dealing with the diagnosis of infertility even more difficult.

Infertility can have profound effects on self-image, on sexuality, and on sexual relationships. Frequent sources of stress are the many procedures involved in an infertility workup, the need to engage in sexual intercourse "on schedule," and the repeated cycle of raised hopes followed by disappointment. Infertility can lead to feelings of loneliness and isolation and can create great strain on a marital relationship. Nurses need to understand these feelings and stresses so that they can better intervene in the care of their patients and help them to cope with their infertility.

Diagnostic Procedures for Infertility
History and Physical Examination

Before tests to determine the causes of infertility are made, a detailed medical, social, and family history must be obtained from both partners. Often the history will uncover important information. It can even reveal a need for education about the timing of sexual intercourse and about the woman's fertile period.

The history should elicit information about the duration of the infertility and whether it is primary or secondary; the frequency of sexual intercourse; the regularity, duration, and frequency of menstruation; and any premenstrual signs and symptoms. It should also include information on any history of vaginal discharge, cervicitis, pelvic infections, surgery, and accidents. General physical condition, illnesses, allergies, and drug intake should be noted, as should any significant family history. Prior use of contraceptives, including type, duration, and complications should be recorded. Information on maternal use of DES should be noted also.

Necessary information from the man includes any history of mumps, orchitis, diabetes mellitus, herniorrhaphy, or exposure to x-rays or toxic substances, such as lead, iron, zinc, or copper. He should also be questioned about exercise patterns, exposure to heat (from the environment or from wearing tight underclothes), duration of infertility, whether the infertility is primary or secondary, frequency of coitus, and history of maternal use of DES.

A complete physical examination of both partners is essential, particularly a thorough pelvic examination of the woman. Certain laboratory tests, such as a complete blood count, thyroid function tests, and urinary analysis are also included in an infertility assessment. If findings are negative, an infertility workup is begun. The workup consists of five basic tests: semen analysis, postcoital test, basal temperature recordings, serum progesterone test and/or endometrial biopsy, and hysterosalpingogram.

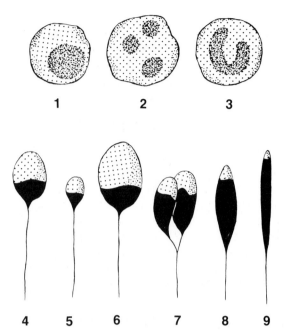

Figure 7–3. Morphologic variations of spermatozoa. *(1, 2)* Immature cells. *(3)* White blood cell (for comparison with immature cells). *(4)* Oval sperm (normal). *(5)* Small (microcytic) sperm. *(6)* Large (macrocytic) sperm. *(7)* Double-headed (bicephalic) sperm. *(8, 9)* Tapering forms. (Danforth DN [ed]: Obstetrics and Gynecology, 5th ed. Philadelphia, JB Lippincott, 1986)

Semen Analysis

The semen analysis should be done early in the infertility investigation because it is simple, noninvasive, and reveals very important information. For this test the man produces a masturbated specimen after 48 to 72 hours of abstinence. The specimen should be collected in a glass container, since plastic may affect the sperm. Condoms should not be used to collect the sperm because they contain spermicidal agents. Some men are uncomfortable with masturbation and can only produce a specimen by sexual intercourse while using a condom to collect the semen. Special sheaths can be provided for these men. The semen should be examined within 2 hours of ejaculation. Because a single semen analysis may not be indicative of the man's fertility potential, repeated semen analyses are often done, preferably at least 74 days apart to allow for maturation of new germ cells (Speroff 1983). The semen analysis provides information on sperm count, motility, and morphology (Fig. 7–3); volume of ejaculate (normal volume is 3–5 ml, with a range from 1–7 ml); presence of infection (evidenced by increased numbers of white blood cells); semen viscosity; and presence or absence of agglutination of sperm (agglutination may indicate the presence of an infection or immune reaction).

The normal values of a semen analysis include a count of greater than 20,000,000 cells, at least 50% motility 2 hours after ejaculation, and greater than 60% normal-appearing sperm. There is some debate about what should be considered a normal sperm count: some authorities believe that a count of 60,000,000 is the lower limit of normal. However, it has been found that men with counts of 20,000,000 are able to impregnate their partners (Glass 1981). Rarely, men with counts of 10,000,000 are able to impregnate a woman.

The Postcoital Test

The postcoital test, or Sims–Huhner test, provides information on the receptivity of the cervical mucus and the ability of the sperm to reach and survive in it. This test must be scheduled for the anticipated day of ovulation. The couple is instructed to have sexual intercourse at that time, after a 48-hour period of abstinence. The woman should then be examined within 8 hours. A sample of cervical mucus is observed microscopically for characteristics that enhance sperm survival and for indications of adequate estrogen production. Normal, healthy, ovulatory cervical mucus reveals a ferning pattern microscopically, is very watery and abundant (composed of 95% to 98% water), and demonstrates *spinnbarkeit,* or the ability to stretch as much as 6 to 10 inches without breaking (Fig. 7–4). The presence or absence of sperm is observed microscopically. Normally, some motile sperm should be seen. There is no agreement, however, as to what number of sperm constitutes a normal postcoital test.

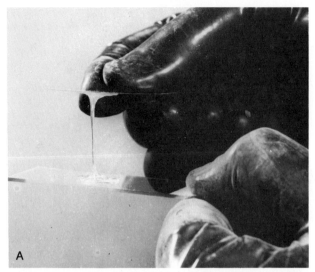

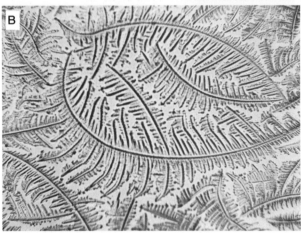

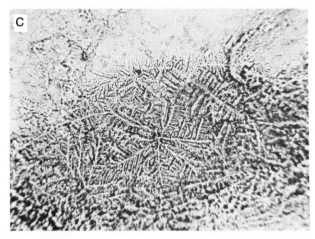

Figure 7–4. (*A*) Technique for determining spinnbarkheit (fibrosity) of cervical mucus. (*B*) Typical ferning of cervical mucus at midcycle. (*C*) Incomplete (atypical) ferning during early secretory phase of cycle. (Danforth DN (ed): Obstetrics and Gynecology, 5th ed. Philadelphia, JB Lippincott, 1986)

Basal Body Temperature Recordings

The basal body temperature (BBT) chart is an indirect method of determining whether ovulation has occurred. Basal body temperature in a normally ovulating woman shows a biphasic pattern, with temperatures below 98°F for the first half of the menstrual cycle and above 98°F for the second half of the cycle after ovulation. The woman is instructed to take her temperature before arising each morning with a special thermometer that is calibrated in tenths of degrees Fahrenheit and to record her temperature on a special graph. A BBT chart indicating normal ovulation, anovulation, and pregnancy is shown in Figure 7–5. Ovulation occurs under the influence of LH and progesterone. At midcycle, at the point of ovulation, there is a surge of LH, resulting in an abrupt rise in temperature to a peak. The second half of an ovulatory cycle is progesterone-dominant. This is referred to as the *luteal phase* of the menstrual cycle, since LH levels remain elevated to help support progesterone secretion and facilitate an optimal uterine environment for a fertilized ovum. Progesterone is thermogenic, leading to a temperature increase during the second half of the menstrual cycle. The BBT provides an indirect indication of whether the luteal phase is adequate for maintenance of the uterine lining should implantation occur. A temperature rise of less than 10 days' duration may be an indication that the luteal phase is inadequate and that insufficient amounts of progesterone are being produced.

Serum Progesterone Test and Endometrial Biopsy

The serum progesterone test is another indirect indication of ovulation. A blood sample is drawn during the presumed luteal phase of the menstrual cycle. At the midluteal phase, the normal serum level of progesterone is 10 ng/ml or higher, with a lower level of 3 ng/ml to 4 ng/ml at an earlier stage of the luteal phase. An adequate amount of progesterone suggests that ovulation has probably occurred. Additional information may be obtained from an endometrial biopsy, which is often done in addition to or instead of the serum progesterone test. Endometrial biopsy is a direct histologic examination of the endometrial tissue, which reveals whether there is adequate secretory tissue. If adequate secretory tissue is seen, secretion of progesterone and LH is normal, thus indicating the ovulation has occurred. This test also determines whether the endometrium is in harmony with the woman's phase of menstruation. If a lag time of more than 2 days is exhibited, progesterone levels may be inadequate. Specifically, if the endometrial lining does not show the amount of secretory tissue that would be expected for the day of the woman's menstrual cycle, the adequacy of the luteal phase and progesterone production is in doubt.

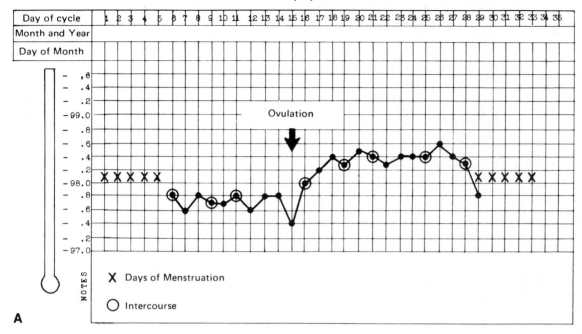

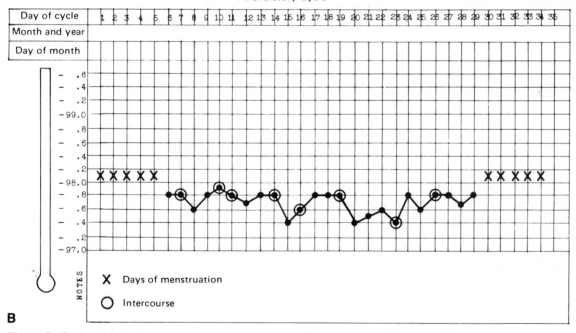

Figure 7–5. Basal body temperature records suggesting (*A*) ovulatory and (*B*) anovulatory cycles. As a rule, intercourse on day 16 (*A*) would be expected to be fruitful; but as is shown here, this is not always the case.

Hysterosalpingogram

The fifth basic test in an infertility workup is the hysterosalpingogram, in which radiopaque dye is injected through the cervix into the uterus. Fluoroscopy shows whether the fallopian tubes fill with dye. From this, the physician can determine whether they are patent (Fig. 7–6). An x-ray film is taken 24 hours later to determine if the dye has dispersed in the pelvic cavity, indicating patency of the tubes. This test must be scheduled during the

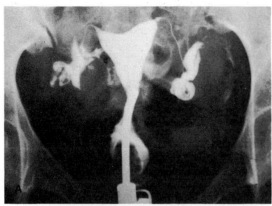

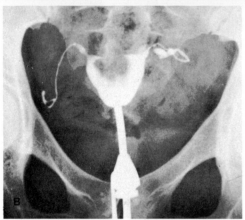

Figure 7–6. Hysterosalpingograms. (*A*) Normal uterus and fallopian tubes with peritoneal spill. Note outline of ovarian beds and leakage into proximal part of vagina. (*B*) Large filling defect in uterine cavity due to submucous fibroid. Note incomplete tubal filling and absence of peritoneal spill. (Danforth DN (ed): Obstetrics and Gynecology, 5th ed. Philadelphia, JB Lippincott, 1986)

first half of the menstrual cycle, after menstruation, to reduce the risk of infection and before ovulation to prevent inadvertent flushing of a fertilized egg out of the tubes. If an oil-based dye is used, this test is believed to have a possible therapeutic effect, enhancing the chances of conception up to 6 to 9 months after the procedure.

Occasionally, the tubal insufflation test, or Rubin's test, is used instead of the hysterosalpingogram. This test involves the injection of carbon dioxide into the uterus and tubes to determine tubal patency. If the tubes are patent, the carbon dioxide flows out of the ends of the tubes and into the abdomen, which produces abdominal sounds that can be heard on auscultation and causes referred shoulder pain. The Rubin's test is used less frequently than the hysterosalpingogram because it is more painful and has a high rate of false-positive results, which may be due to tubal spasm caused by carbon dioxide (Speroff 1983).

Laparoscopy and Culdoscopy

In addition to these five basic tests, several other procedures are performed if indicated. If all the previous tests are normal, a laparoscopy is often performed about 6 to 9 months after the hysterosalpingogram. The delay is to allow time for conception, since the hysterosalpingogram can exert a therapeutic effect by opening the tubes. *Laparoscopy* is direct visualization of pelvic structures through a lighted scope inserted through the woman's abdomen. It can reveal pelvic pathology, such as endometriosis, adhesions, and active infection. Tubal adhesions can sometimes be lysed during laparoscopy. *Culdoscopy* is also sometimes performed. This procedure involves visualizing the area behind the cul-de-sac, behind the posterior vaginal fornix.

Other Tests

Immunoassay Tests. If there is reason to believe that a woman may have antibodies to her partner's sperm or that a man may have antibodies to his own sperm, immunologic tests are done by taking a semen specimen and observing its interaction with the serum of the partner as well as with the serum of the man himself.

Sperm Penetration Assay. A test recently added to the repertoire of infertility tests is the *sperm penetration assay,* in which sperm are capacitated *in vitro* and observed for their ability to penetrate the zona pellucida of ova from superovulated hamsters (Speroff 1983). This test gives a possible indication of the ability of the sperm to penetrate and fertilize a human ovum.

Test Timing

The timing of infertility tests is critical. The postcoital test, for example, must be done at the presumed time of ovulation. The hysterosalpingogram must be done after menstruation has ceased in order to prevent the possibility of old menstrual blood being pushed into the tubes, where it might lead to infection. It must be done before ovulation, however, to prevent pushing a fertilized ovum out through the fimbrial end of the tubes. The accompanying display, Fertility Testing and Favorable Clinical Findings, summarizes the tests, the appropriate time for doing them, and favorable findings.

SPECIFIC TREATMENT FOR INFERTILITY

Once a diagnosis of the cause of the infertility has been made, treatment that involves the male partner, the female partner, or both may be initiated.

Fertility Tests and Favorable Clinical Findings

Male Factors

Evidence of Normal Ejaculation and Sperm Production

Semen Analysis:
Microscopic examination of semen sample is done early in workup, since it is a simple test that provides valuable information and may obviate more invasive procedures (done after 48 to 72 hours of abstinence from orgasm since less time may result in false low sperm count).

   Favorable clinical findings:
Normal amount of ejaculate (3–5 ml; range: 1–7 ml)

No agglutination of sperm (Agglutination suggests infection or autoimmunity.)

Normal seminal fluid; semen liquifies

Sperm count showing greater than 20,000,000 cells with at least 50% motility 2 hours after ejaculation and more than 60% normal-appearing cells

Female/Interactive Factors

Evidence of Normal Hormonal Cycle and Receptivity to Sperm

Basal Body Temperature (BBT) Measurement
Oral temperature taken daily before arising throughout several menstrual cycles provides overall assessment of cyclic hormonal changes.

   Favorable clinical findings:
Biphasic pattern with persistent temperature elevation for 12–14 days prior to menstruation

Postcoital Test
Vaginal examination within 8 hours after intercourse, during time of presumed ovulation, is done to determine whether normal ovulatory changes occur in cervical mucus and whether sperm survive in vaginal environment.

   Favorable clinical findings:
Cervical mucus suggestive of ovulation:

Microscopic ferning pattern is present.

Mucus is watery, slippery, abundant.

Spinnbarkeit is present.

Presence of normal live and motile sperm in cervical mucus

Serum Progesterone Measurement
Blood sample is taken to determine whether serum progesterone peaks during midportion of second half of menstrual period (days 22–24).

   Favorable clinical findings:
3–4 ng/ml in early luteal phase, 10 ng/ml at midluteal phase

Endometrial Biopsy
Endometrial tissue is collected during vaginal examination in second half of menstrual cycle (days 22–24) to determine presence and adequacy of secretory tissue. Secretory tissue is present if ovulation occurs and peaks at midphase of second half of menstrual cycle (luteal phase).

   Favorable clinical findings:
Biopsies at different points in menstrual cycle showing development of endometrium consistent with phase of cycle (lag time of more than 2 days suggests inadequate luteal phase/progesterone production)

Immunoassay tests
Immunologic tests are performed with semen and male/female serum.

   Favorable clinical findings:
Absence of antibody reaction

Evidence of normal pelvic anatomy and tubal functioning

Hysterosalpingogram
Dye is injected through cervix into uterus, with fluoroscopic visualization of spread of dye through fallopian tubes. This is usually done in first half of menstrual cycle, after menstruation has ceased, to lower risk of infection from pushing menstrual fluid into tubes, but before ovulation in order to avoid flushing out of tubes a fertilized ovum that might be present.

   Favorable clinical findings:
Patency of fallopian tubes, demonstrated by dispersal of dye from cervix and uterus up into peritoneal cavity

Absence of abnormalities in uterine cavities and fallopian tubes

Laparoscopy
Pelvic structures are visualized directly, using telescope and light source inserted through small abdominal incision.

   Favorable clinical findings:
Normal pelvic structures and absence of signs of infection, adhesions, endometriosis, or lesions

NURSING RESEARCH

Responses to High Technology Infertility Treatment

A recent article in *Image: The Journal of Nursing Scholarship* reported several findings that reflect infertile persons' responses to the new high technology treatments available to assist them in conception. Six themes were elicited in the research: (a) drivenness, that is, infertile persons feel compelled to try all the new technologies; (b) difficulty "getting on with life," because they waver between stopping infertility treatments and pursuing normal lives while involved in infertility treatments; (c) marital and sexual disruption; (d) uniqueness of personal responses, that is, members of a couple will probably respond differently to infertility and its treatment; (e) financial stresses; and (f) an exacerbated cyclical pattern of hope and despair.

Olshansky EF: Responses to high technology infertility treatment. Image: The Journal of Nursing Scholarship 20(3):128, 1988

Female Infertility

Vaginal, Cervical, and Uterine Treatment

For female infertility from vaginal causes, treatments include therapy for vaginitis, if indicated, sexual therapy for problems such as vaginismus, and surgical correction of structural or anatomical abnormalities, if possible.

Treating cervical causes of infertility involves many possibilities. If a cervicitis exists, it should be treated. Often the treatment of choice is with tetracycline, since this medication is effective against *Chlamydia,* an organism implicated in many cases of cervicitis. If the problem is poor cervical mucus, it can be treated in many ways. Sometimes douching with an alkaline solution (such as water with baking soda) half an hour before intercourse may improve the pH of the mucus, making it more alkaline and thus more conducive to sperm survival. Estrogen therapy often helps to increase the abundance of the cervical mucus and enhance spinnbarkeit and ferning. If the cervical mucus is resistant to treatment or if the cervicitis is not amenable to treatment, sometimes intrauterine artificial insemination with the partner's sperm may be used to bypass the hostile cervical mucus. If the problem stems from an incompetent cervix (which is often found in conjunction with a history of maternal use of DES), a cerclage can be performed at about 12 to 14 weeks of pregnancy, to be removed at term. This procedure involves placing an encircling suture in the cervix to prevent the cervix from dilating prematurely, thus helping to prevent a spontaneous abortion.

Treatment of uterine causes of infertility may include surgery for removal of uterine fibroids (myomas). If the uterine problem is a result of Asherman's syndrome, a condition in which the walls of the uterus (endometrium) adhere to one another, leading to amenorrhea, a dilatation and curettage is often done to break up the adhesions. Following this, a Foley catheter is inserted into the uterus and the balloon is filled with 3 ml of fluid. This catheter is left in place for 7 days. Sometimes an IUD is inserted and remains in place for about 3 to 6 months. A treatment regimen of high doses of estrogens for 2 months (for 3 out of 4 weeks each month) is then maintained (Speroff 1983).

Tubal Treatment

The rising incidence of tubal problems as contributing or major factors in infertility has resulted in an increase in research in this area. Consequently, more treatments are now available, although many are still somewhat experimental. Much effort is being expended on improving microsurgical techniques to reopen the tubes. Sometimes medications, such as danazol or oral contraceptives, are given to treat endometriosis (Speroff 1983). *In vitro* fertilization has been receiving widespread attention as a method of achieving conception and implantation while bypassing blocked fallopian tubes. This procedure involves removing ripe ova (often several ova that have been stimulated to mature by administration of human menopausal gonadotropin) and mixing them with fresh semen in a petri dish. After fertilization, several ova are implanted in the woman's uterus in the hopes that one will successfully grow into a healthy embryo and fetus.

Ovarian Treatment

Treatment of ovarian causes of infertility usually requires the induction of ovulation with medication. A summary of the ovulation-inducing medications used in infertility treatment is presented in Table 7–1. The major drugs used in such treatment are clomiphene citrate, human menopausal gonadotropin, HCG, and bromocriptine. Progesterone therapy is also used.

Clomiphene Citrate. Clomiphene citrate increases the secretion of FSH and LH. Ovulation occurs due to the influence of these gonadotropins on the growing follicle. It is unclear whether clomiphene works on the pituitary, directly on the hypothalamus, or on both. It produces an antiestrogenic effect that causes poor cervical mucus in about 15% of women taking this drug. For this reason, women taking clomiphene are sometimes simultaneously given estrogen. Clomiphene is administered orally and is begun on day 5 of the woman's menstrual cycle

Table 7–1   **Medications Used to Induce Ovulation**

Medication	Purpose and Method of Use	Disadvantages and Side-Effects
Clomiphene citrate	Increases secretion of FSH and LH, which stimulate follicle growth Administered orally, 50 mg/day to 250 mg/day, from day 5 to day 9 of menstrual cycle Ovulation should occur 5 to 10 days after the last dose	Antiestrogenic—may cause poor cervical mucus Other complications are vasomotor flushes, abdominal distention, bloating, pain, soreness, breast discomfort, nausea and vomiting, visual symptoms (spots, flashes), headaches, dryness or loss of hair, ovarian enlargement
Human menopausal gonadotropin and Human chorionic gonadotropin (HCG)	Stimulates follicle growth Administered IM daily for 7 to 10 days during first half of menstrual cycle After the ovaries have been stimulated, HCG is administered IM to induce ovulation	Ovarian hyperstimulation Multiple pregnancies Expensive Sometimes requires repeated ultrasounds to rule out ovarian enlargement
Bromocriptine	Inhibits pituitary secretion of prolactin, thus preventing suppression of pulsatile secretion of FSH and LH Administered orally, 25 mg/day, until pregnancy occurs (some practitioners do not administer it during luteal phase because of possible teratogenic effects)	Nausea Diarrhea Dizziness Headache Fatigue

and continued through day 9. If clomiphene is begun earlier than day 5, the risk of multiple gestation is increased if conception occurs. The initial dosage is 50 mg/day, and if no ovulation occurs, the dosage is increased in increments of 50 mg, up to a maximum of 250 mg/day. The ovulatory surge of gonadotropins occurs 5 to 10 days after the last day of clomiphene administration. The couple is advised to have sexual intercourse every other day for 1 week, beginning 5 days after the last day of medication. Results indicate that about 80% of women will ovulate and about 40% will become pregnant with clomiphene therapy (Speroff 1983). Complications and side effects of the drug include vasomotor flushes, abdominal distention, bloating, pain, soreness, breast discomfort, nausea and vomiting, visual symptoms (such as visual spots and flashes), headache, dryness or loss of hair, and ovarian enlargement. The ovaries should be checked for enlargement periodically by bimanual examination.

Human Menopausal Gonadotropin and Human Chorionic Gonadotropin (HCG).   Human menopausal gonadotropin is a purified preparation of gonadotropins extracted from the urine of postmenopausal women. It works by stimulating the growth of the follicles and is administered by daily intramuscular injection for 7 to 14 days. The patient's estrogen response is monitored by examining the quality and quantity of the cervical mucus, testing 24-hour urine samples to determine urinary excretion of estrogens, and obtaining plasma estradiol levels. Sometimes sonograms are taken periodically to

permit visualization of the ovaries under the influence of human menopausal gonadotropin so that undue ovarian enlargement can be prevented. HCG is administered to induce ovulation after the ovaries have been stimulated by human menopausal gonadotropin. Couples are advised to have intercourse on the day of the HCG administration and for the 2 days following.

Bromocriptine.   It is believed that high levels of prolactin interfere with normal function of the menstrual cycle by suppressing the pulsatile secretion of the gonadotropin-releasing hormones, follicle-stimulating releasing hormone and luteinizing releasing hormone. Bromocriptine, which inhibits the pituitary secretion of prolactin, is administered in a dosage of 2.5 mg/day until pregnancy occurs. Some practitioners, however, do not administer it during the luteal phase because of the possibility of teratogenic side effects should a pregnancy occur. The side effects include nausea, diarrhea, dizziness, headache, and fatigue.

New Types of Therapy.   Sometimes progesterone is administered to women with an inadequate luteal phase. Also, clomiphene citrate, which is used frequently for ovulation induction, is sometimes used for an inadequate luteal phase. A recent form of therapy involves the use of a portable intravenous pump that provides a pulsatile administration of 5 μ GnRH intravenously every 90 minutes through a device that allows the woman to go about her daily activities. At the beginning of the temperature rise that indicates ovulation, HCG is administered to support the corpus luteum, which produces progesterone.

Male Infertility

The goal of treatment in male infertility is to achieve an adequate sperm count, motility, and morphology and to have the sperm penetrate the egg to achieve fertilization. Often therapy for oligospermia consists of removing environmental hazards that are decreasing sperm production. These include heat sources — for example, tight underclothes, hot tubs, or saunas — certain drugs, chemicals, and toxins. Sometimes testosterone therapy is effective in increasing sperm production.

If the cause of infertility is found to be a varicocele, surgery to ligate the varicose vein is usually recommended. The success rate of such surgery is higher among men whose presurgery sperm count is greater than 10,000,000 (Glass 1981).

Retrograde ejaculation is sometimes treated by retrieving the sperm from the urine through catheterization and artificially inseminating the woman with it. Sometimes antidepressant drugs are given, since these drugs relax the bladder sphincter, helping to alleviate retrograde ejaculation.

If the sperm count continues to remain low, but the man is not *azoospermic* (zero sperm count), sometimes artificial insemination with his sperm is performed. This involves collecting a split ejaculate, where the first couple of drops of semen are collected in one container and the rest of the ejaculate is collected in another. After several specimens are collected, the first parts of each split ejaculate are combined to produce one larger-volume split ejaculate. In this combined ejaculate, the concentration of sperm is higher, since the first part of the split ejaculate is the richest in sperm. Another treatment is artificial intrauterine insemination with sperm from the partner that has been washed with a special solution to separate spermatozoa from seminal plasma. If the quality of the sperm cannot be improved by this method, the couple might consider the option of artificial insemination of the woman with donor sperm.

Interactive Causes of Infertility

If infertility is found to be due to the manufacture of antibodies by the woman to her partner's sperm, the treatment of choice is condom therapy for 6 months. This involves the use of condoms during sexual intercourse for 6 months to decrease the woman's sensitivity to her partner's sperm. After 6 months, the couple is advised to try to conceive in the hope that the antibody level has decreased.

If sexual problems are discovered in the infertility workup, sexual counseling or education is warranted. Sometimes marital counseling to deal with other aspects of the couple's relationship is also valuable.

When a specific cause of infertility is not found, a specific treatment cannot be determined. Various treatments may be considered and tried on the chance that they might be successful. Couples with unexplained infertility deserve to be given all available information about their condition and possible prognosis, as well as education about general aspects of infertility, possible causes, and solutions. Often such couples need emotional support as they decide when to stop their infertility workup and treatment and begin to consider other options available to them.

Discussing Alternatives to Childlessness

With recent advances in medical technology, many new and varied options are available to infertile couples in addition to the traditional choice between adoption and childlessness. The nurse should present these options to the patient and provide any additional information and referral requested by the patient.

Adoption. Adoption usually occurs through use of adoption agencies or through independent private attorneys. Adopting a child has provided many infertile couples with an excellent alternative to undesired childlessness. Some people adopt a newborn infant, while others may choose to adopt an older child. Couples who choose adoption must still resolve their feelings about the desire to experience pregnancy, as distinct from the desire to have a child.

Deciding to Be Childfree. Deciding to remain "childfree" (a term sometimes preferable to "childless," which may have more negative connotations), while becoming more acceptable, still has stigma associated with it. The decision is a difficult one for many people, particularly those who did not initially choose this state of affairs. Many infertile couples do eventually decide to remain childfree, which is quite different from merely accepting infertility. Some people seem to come to a point in their infertility workup at which they decide that being childfree is an acceptable and perhaps desirable life for them. In understanding this phenomenon, however, it is very important to differentiate between the motivations of infertile couples and the motivations of persons who assume they are fertile but choose to be childfree.

Artificial Insemination. The option of artificial insemination is not new, for it has existed for decades. Artificial insemination with the partner's sperm is sometimes employed in cases where the cervical mucus is not conducive to sperm survival; the insemination procedure can bypass the cervix and deposit the sperm directly into the uterus. Also, if the couple is having sexual difficulties, artificial insemination with the partner's sperm can be used, in this case to deposit the sperm at the cervical os. Artificial insemination with donor sperm is used in cases of male infertility where the female partner is able to conceive. Sperm from an anonymous donor is used for insemination, although sometimes the donor is known and, in fact, chosen by the couple. The option of artificial insemination has provided a viable alternative for many infertile persons. However, many issues surrounding artificial insemination with donor sperm have not, as yet, been well researched. Much secrecy is involved, and many parents are unsure about the ramifications of telling their children that they were conceived through artificial insemination by donor. Controversy continues about the most appropriate way to handle the issues of secrecy and confidentiality.

The procedure used for artificial insemination has been directly affected by the current Acquired Immune Deficiency Syndrome (AIDS) epidemic. Artificial insemination with fresh sperm is no longer used. All potential donors are tested for the human immunodeficiency virus (HIV), and then the sperm is frozen. Three to six months later the potential donor is again tested for HIV and, if negative, the frozen sperm is used. This procedure allows for more accurate testing for HIV, since the incubation time for development of HIV is taken into account when testing the donor. The use of frozen sperm, however, is believed to be less effective than fresh sperm.

In Vitro *Fertilization and Embryo Transplantation.* *In vitro* fertilization, the process leading to "test tube babies," has received much publicity in the last few years and has provided an alternative for couples whose infertility is due to fallopian tube problems. This procedure bypasses the fallopian tubes by retrieving mature ova from the ovary, fertilizing them in a test tube, and then implanting the fertilized ova in the woman's uterus.

Gamete Intrafallopian Transfer. In addition to *in vitro* fertilization, newer techniques have been developed. Gamete intrafallopian transfer (GIFT) is one of these techniques. It consists of surgically retrieving the ovum from the ovary and implanting it into the fallopian tube while separately implanting sperm into the fallopian tube, thus, it is hoped, allowing fertilization to occur naturally.

In vivo fertilization, or embryo transplantation, is an even newer technique, in which an embryo conceived in one woman is transplanted into the uterus of another woman who is unable to conceive naturally but can carry a fetus to maturity. The baby would genetically be the result of the union of the husband's sperm with the ovum of the woman from whom the embryo is transplanted.

Surrogate Mothering. Some women are not only unable to conceive but are also unable to carry a fetus, because of lack of a uterus or other problems. The use of a surrogate mother provides an alternative for such women. The male partner produces a semen specimen that is artificially inseminated into the host (or surrogate) mother. The fetus grows in the uterus of the surrogate mother and at birth is given to the infertile couple. Many legal and ethical issues surround this option, and cases have received much public attention. Some states are currently considering legislation aimed at regulating this practice.

Ethical Questions Concerning Options

Nurses must be acutely aware of the psychosocial and emotional aspects associated with the options open to infertile couples and of the painful process that persons must engage in to arrive at choices regarding those options. Many ethical questions surround options that appear to some to be tampering with nature and to others to be providing much-desired children who could not be produced by traditional means.

Much new medical research is focusing on perfecting the use of these options, with particular emphasis on *in vitro* fertilization and, more recently, on embryo transplants. It is also important to note that not all options are available to all people. *In vitro* fertilization, for example, assumes that the male partner has healthy, viable sperm (though donor insemination could also be used) and that the female has a healthy uterus that will provide a healthy environment for the embryo. Artificial insemination, whether with the partner's sperm or with a donor's sperm, assumes that the woman is able to conceive and to successfully carry a pregnancy to term.

LEGAL/ETHICAL CONSIDERATIONS

Ethical Dilemmas Posed By High Technology Infertility Treatments

Ethical dilemmas are created as a result of the newer infertility treatments. Because patients' decisions regarding treatment options may be influenced by them, nurses must be aware of these dilemmas:

- "Unnaturalness" of new technologies and the fact that they are not sanctioned by the Catholic church
- Acceleration of trend toward "genetic engineering"
- When life begins and the sanctity of life

In addition, many of these procedures are quite expensive, precluding their use for many couples. Even if a couple can afford the procedures, many issues are raised. The hope that is provided by these procedures is quite often negated by the low rates of conception and the emotional, physical, and financial stresses. Recent attention to the ethical and legal aspects of high technology infertility treatments is evident in the scientific literature (Andrews 1986; Donovan 1986; Grobstein and Flower 1985).

IMPLICATIONS FOR NURSING CARE

Although the diagnosis of infertility and the determination of the course of treatment are largely medical responsibilities, many problems related to infertility are clinical nursing problems.

The diagnosis and treatment of infertility usually extends over a period of years and involves many different steps. The standard course of diagnosis and treatment for an infertile couple is shown in Figure 7–7. At every step, those involved in this process are likely to need information, anticipatory guidance, and emotional support. These are primarily nursing responsibilities, and the effectiveness of the nursing care delivered depends on the nurse's knowledge of the causes and treatments for infertility and of its emotional and psychosocial consequences. The following section highlights nursing care for those being tested and treated for infertility.

Assessment

The assessment of a couple experiencing infertility involves eliciting a comprehensive history, with attention to reproductive and sexual factors in order to rule out any sexual dysfunction. In addition, an assessment must be made of the couple's perception of their stresses related to infertility as well as their ability to cope with the stresses. Understanding their responses to the infertility is essential in order to accurately diagnose the couple's ability to cope, the degree of grieving they may be experiencing, and their self-concept. Their level of knowledge regarding infertility diagnosis and treatment is also important information in arriving at an accurate assessment. A thorough physical examination and appropriate diagnostic and laboratory tests for both the man and woman provide essential information for a comprehensive assessment.

NURSING RESEARCH

Identity of Self as Infertile

A recent article reveals that persons experiencing infertility undergo a process of adopting and managing an identity of self as infertile. This process is described, as persons take on an informal identity of self as infertile with associated informal fertility work, and then take on a formal identity of self as infertile with associated formal fertility work. Managing this identity, which becomes all encompassing, can be accomplished in various ways: (a) overcoming it, by becoming pregnant after resolving the underlying cause; (b) circumventing it, by becoming pregnant without correcting the underlying cause; (c) reconciling oneself to it, by choosing such alternatives as adoption or being childfree; and (d) remaining in limbo, by failing to come to terms with infertility.

Olshansky EF: Identity of self as infertile: An example of theory-generating research. Advances in Nursing Science, 9(2):54, 1987

Diagnosis

The nursing diagnoses that are often related to the situation of a couple experiencing infertility include the following.

- Self-concept disturbance
- Ineffective individual coping
- Sexual dysfunction
- Ineffective family coping
- Knowledge deficit

Planning and Implementation

Planning for nursing care must include attention to the patient's needs for information about diagnostic tests, treatment alternatives, and options and for emotional support. Since individuals respond and adapt to this process over time, in repeated contacts with the patient or couple the nursing plan can be continually assessed and modified.

Nursing care of individuals and couples during evaluation and treatment of infertility spans a wide range of functions. Most nursing interventions are directed toward teaching — about effective self-care and about specific

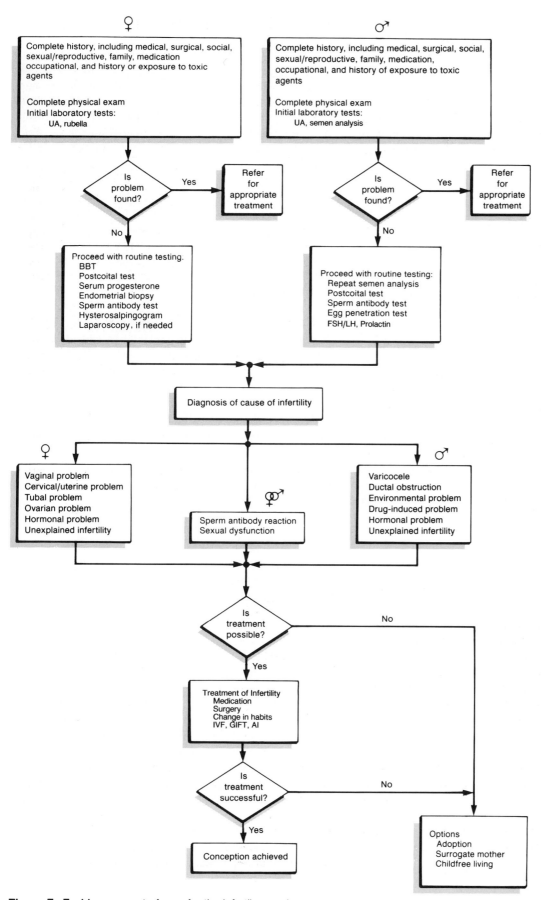

Figure 7-7. Management of care for the infertile couple.

SELF-CARE TEACHING

Guidelines in Reducing the All-Encompassing Nature of Infertility

Infertility can become all-encompassing and consequently can affect other important arenas of life. The following are suggestions the nurse can give couples to assist in reducing the all-encompassing nature of infertility:

- Cultivate other creative aspects of life (*e.g.*, hobbies, a career).
- Set aside time to discuss feelings related to infertility (with spouse, friends) and try to focus on other things at other times.
- Join an infertility support group (*e.g.*, RESOLVE) to help cope with the distressing feelings related to infertility.

diagnostic and treatment alternatives — and toward providing support for emotional and family concerns.

Teaching for Effective Self-Care

An important part of nursing care for infertile persons is emphasizing and teaching self-care. Infertility is often experienced as being "out of control." Identifying and using successful coping strategies helps the individual regain a sense of control. Stress-reduction techniques, such as exercise, relaxation techniques, and meditation may be especially useful both for those with general concerns about fertility and for those concerned about specific diagnostic or treatment procedures. The nurse should also encourage infertile individuals to maintain and improve their overall health.

Infertility can become an all-encompassing concern, resulting in alterations in health and recreation patterns and a loss of interest in other aspects of life. The nurse can emphasize that one can be creative, productive, and successful in other areas even if one is not able to produce children. Being involved with other interests and activities will result in a healthier lifestyle and a more balanced perspective on life.

Providing Support

The nurse working with infertile persons provides much-needed support and advocacy, as well as education and help in decision making. The nurse must be able to present options in a nonjudgmental way and facilitate the patient's own decision making. The emotional adjustment to the perceived loss of childbearing capacity is often difficult. Patients may have no one else with whom they feel they can discuss their sense of loss or anger; the nurse must be able to listen sensitively and acknowledge their feelings.

Providing referral to other sources of assistance is another way in which the nurse supports the infertile person or couple. One important source of information and support is Resolve, a national organization for infertile couples and individuals. This organization, composed of self-help groups that provide support and information about infertility, was started in 1973 by Barbara Eck Menning, a maternal-child nurse. Resolve conducts workshops, provides referral information for specialized services, and organizes support groups. It also provides preadoption meetings for individuals considering that option.

The nurse also acts as an advocate and resource person, making appropriate referrals to adoption agencies, to lawyers to help with adoption proceedings or surrogate mothers, and to specialists in certain areas of infertility treatment.

Providing Anticipatory Guidance

An important nursing responsibility is providing anticipatory guidance for the battery of tests to which patients are subjected during infertility evaluation. Explaining the procedures and any specific preparations needed is essential and helps relieve some of the anxiety and apprehension felt by patients. To fulfill this responsibility, the nurse must be familiar with the diagnostic and treatment protocols used in infertility evaluation in her particular setting. In addition to explaining procedures that couples will experience, the nurse must also discuss the range of human responses to the procedures, such as effects on sexual functioning and the marital relationship.

Dealing with Family Concerns

It is essential that the nurse consider the couple — and, if appropriate, the entire family — as a unit. Infertile couples often experience a great deal of anxiety about their inability to provide grandchildren for their own parents, and the potential grandparents may feel that their children are "letting them down," without understanding the anxiety that their children are experiencing. Perhaps treating the family in a holistic manner would help to improve communication and understanding among the various family members. The emotional problems surrounding infertility illustrate extremely well the need for a greater emphasis on family-centered care. Infertility is a highly charged emotional issue that has far-reaching implications for many family members. The nurse can play an integral role in helping family members to understand and deal with their reactions to infertility.

Providing Accurate Information

Nurses can help dispel the many myths that surround infertility. The myths that if couples would just relax, they would become pregnant or that if they adopt, they will

FAMILY CONSIDERATIONS

Viewing Infertility With a Family Focus

It is essential that the nurse adopt a family-centered care perspective and consider the entire family unit when assisting individuals and couples in coping with infertility. Family involvement is apparent in several ways:

Infertile couples often experience a great deal of anxiety about their inability to provide grandchildren for their own parents.

"Potential grandparents" may feel that their children are "letting them down." Or, they may be fearful of pressuring their children about conception.

Infertile couples may experience some marital disruption.

Socializing with family members during such "child-oriented" events as holidays may be quite difficult for infertile persons.

become pregnant are clearly shown to be unfounded in the literature. In helping to dispel such myths, nurses will promote better understanding among people in general of the stresses faced by infertile persons, and the stigma attached to infertility will be diminished.

As more and more people seek treatment for their infertility, nurses will have more visible and valuable roles in working with such people. In integral and important ways, the nurse can help infertile persons resolve their feelings about infertility.

Evaluation

Evaluation of the interventions discussed requires ongoing assessment of the couple over time. As the couple engages in the diagnostic and treatment procedures associated with attempting to overcome infertility, the nurse, through ongoing interaction with the couple, can assess the couple's responses to the interventions. Factors to be alert to are the couple's ability to "get on with their lives" despite the demands of diagnosis and treatment for infertility, their ability to put infertility in perspective in order to cultivate other areas of their lives, and their ability to maintain their marital relationship and relationships with significant others in the face of the stresses associated with infertility. The evaluation of the "success" of the interventions depends not on whether the couple actually conceives but rather on evidence of a

healthy emotional response to resolving the distressing feelings surrounding infertility.

CHAPTER SUMMARY

The field of fertility evaluation and infertility treatment is expanding rapidly, and much new and important knowledge is being developed. Along with this expansion of knowledge comes increasing nursing responsibility. Nurses must understand current methods of diagnosis and treatment and appreciate the important human issues related to infertility. Working with infertile individuals and their families is an exciting new field for clinical practice and research. Nursing practice focuses on coordinating the plan of care, and assessing and intervening on the basis of identified patient needs for support, anticipatory guidance, information, and referral.

STUDY QUESTIONS

1. List and describe the basic diagnostic tests that are included in an infertility workup and discuss the appropriate times for performing these tests.
2. Discuss the common causes of infertility for men and women and the treatment available for each.
3. Write a short summary of what is known about the emotional aspects of infertility, particularly how it affects the lives of those experiencing it.
4. Discuss the options for childbearing/childrearing that are available to infertile persons, including related emotional and ethical issues.

REFERENCES/BIBLIOGRAPHY

Andrews LB: Legal and ethical aspects of new reproductive technologies. Clin Obstet Gynecol 29(1):190, 1986

Donovan P: New reproductive technologies: Some legal dilemmas. Fam Plann Perspect 18(2):57, 1986

Erikson EH: Childhood and Society, 2nd ed. New York, WW Norton & Co, 1963

Glass RH: Infertility. In Glass RH (ed): Office Gynecology, 2nd ed. Baltimore, Williams & Wilkins, 1981

Glass RH, Ericsson RJ: Getting Pregnant in the 1980s. Berkeley, University of California Press, 1982

Grobstein C, Flower M: Current ethical issues in IVF. Clin Obstet and Gynecol 12(4):877, 1985

Mahlstedt PP, MacDuff S, Bernstein J: Emotional factors and the in vitro fertilization and embryo transfer process. J In Vitro Fert Embryo Transfer 4(4):232, 1987

Menning BE: Infertility: A Guide for the Childless Couple, 2nd ed. Englewood Cliffs NJ, Prentice-Hall, 1988

Olshansky EF: Identity of self as infertile: An example of theory-generating research. Adv in Nsg Sci 9(2):54, 1987

Olshansky EF: Infertility and its influence on women's career identities. Health & Care for Women International 8(2,3):185, 1987

Olshansky EF: Responses to high technology infertility treatment. Image: The J of Nsg Scholarship 20(3):128, 1988

Sandelowski M: The color gray: Ambiguity and infertility. Image: The J of Nsg Scholarship 19(2):70, 1987

Sandelowski M, Jones LC: Social exchanges of infertile women. Issues in Mental Health Nsg 8(3):173, 1986

Sandelowki M, Pollock C: Women's experiences of infertility. Image: The J of Nsg Scholarship 18(4):140, 1986

Seibel MM, Levin S: A new era in reproductive technologies: The emotional stages of *in vitro* fertilization. J In Vitro Fert Embryo Transfer 4(3):135, 1987

Speroff L, Glass RH, Kase NG: Clinical Gynecological Endocrinology and Infertility, 3rd ed. Baltimore, Williams & Wilkins, 1983

Unruh A, McGrath P: The psychology of female infertility: Toward a new perspective. Health Care for Women International 6:369, 1985

Wilson EA: Sequence of emotional responses induced by infertility. J KY Med Assoc 77:229, 1979

SUGGESTED READINGS

Borg S, Lasker JN: In Search of Parenthood. Boston, Beacon Press, 1987

Harkness C: The Infertility Book. San Francisco, Volcano Press, 1987

Salzer LP: Infertility: How Couples Can Cope. Boston, GK Hall and Co, 1986

Zion AB: Resourses for infertile couples. J Obstet Gynecol Neonatal Nurs 17(4):255–258, 1988

Zion AB: The process of developing patient educational materials for infertile couples. J Obstet Gynecol Neonatal Nurs 17(4):259–263, 1988

8 family planning and contraception

LEARNING OBJECTIVES

After studying the material in this chapter, the student should be able to

- Discuss the importance of family planning

- List the various methods of contraception

- Assess the efficacy of each contraceptive method

- Explain the mechanism of action for each method

- Discuss the side-effects and major contraindications of each method

- Assist in counseling couples seeking family planning information

- Prepare women for procedures necessary for IUD and diaphragm use and support them during those procedures

- Explain the use of barrier contraceptives to interested couples

- Describe the procedures for abortion and provide or ensure the provision of counseling and support to the woman

- Recognize the importance of fully informing couples regarding family planning alternatives

- Discuss male and female sterilization and its implications

KEY TERMS

Aerobes

Anaerobes

Androgen

Antiemetic

Azoospermia

Breakthrough bleeding

Cystocele

Ectopy/ectopic

High-density lipoproteins (HDL)

In situ

Leukorrhea

Low-density lipoproteins (LDL)

Macrophage

Mononucleated

Normotensive

Nullipara

Phagocyte

Rectocele

Spotting

Stenosis

Steroid

Steroidogenesis

Teratogenesis

Uterine prolapse

Withdrawal bleeding

Little was known about reproduction until fairly recently. In early times menstruation was not associated with conception because reproductive-aged women were continually gestating a pregnancy, and menstruation was an uncommon phenomenon. The discovery of spermatozoa in semen by the Dutch microbiologist Leeuwenhoek in 1677 was a major event in the history of natural science. It was not until 1843, however, that Baer observed the union of the sperm and ovum and conception was understood.

In the late 1800s and early 1900s women themselves became active in the birth control movement, but only in the late 1960s could birth control methods be openly discussed with women in health care settings. The timing was propitious, because it was in this period that concerns about the rapidly escalating world population inspired the slogan "Zero Population Growth."

This chapter discusses both the active planning of families and presently available methods of contraception. Actions, effectiveness, safety, and contraindications of the various methods are discussed. Nursing implications involve self-care teaching and counseling for decision making.

FAMILY PLANNING

In family planning, the couple decides the number of children they want and when to have them; that is, the birth of each child is planned and desired. Equally important to family planning is the spacing of children to protect the mother's health and to ensure the parents' ability to provide each child with individual care and attention.

Preconception Planning

It is important to prepare for the major event of pregnancy. This time interval allows for determining the health states of the parents and the existence in either partner of health problems that would complicate the pregnancy.

Couples contemplating pregnancy should seek advice prior to conception regarding their health status. Although an ideal expectation, it is one that would enhance the probability of a healthy baby.

The Prepregnant Appointment

A prepregnant appointment is scheduled with an obstetrician and/or nurse practitioner who will be the primary-care provider during the anticipated pregnancy. During this visit, the care provider collects health histories of both partners, performs a complete physical exam-

Objectives of Family Planning

- Avoid unwanted pregnancies
- Regulate intervals between pregnancies
- Decide the number of children in the family
- Control the time at which births occur in relation to the parents' age
- Facilitate wanted births for women with fertility problems
- Avoid pregnancy for women with serious disease whom an imposed pregnancy would place at additional risk
- Provide women who are carriers of genetic disease with the option of avoiding pregnancy

The overall goal of these objectives is to improve the health of the mother, the baby, and the family. Child spacing, limitation of family size, and timing of the first birth are recognized preventive health measures.

ination of the woman, refers the male partner to a urologist, obtains laboratory tests, and counsels the couple.

Couple: Health History

A health history collected from each partner should include all the information normally obtained in this process, but with special emphasis on the following information:

- Preexisting medical conditions and/or surgical procedures
- Menstrual history
- Contraceptive use
- Family history to determine risk for sickle cell disease or trait, diabetes, Rh factors, Tay–Sachs disease, trisomy 21, or other familial or genetic disease
- Immunization status of the woman (particularly rubella)
- History of herpes infection or other sexually transmitted disease; substance abuse

Woman

Physical Examination. A complete physical examination should be performed on the woman with special focus on the reproductive system. It should include the following assessments:

- *Abdomen:* to detect masses, lesions, scars, tenderness, muscle tone
- *Vagina:* to detect abnormal vaginal discharge due to infection, lesions, structural abnormalities, and/or DES (diethylstilbesterol) exposure, past surgery

- *Breasts:* to detect masses, nipple discharge or inversion, tenderness
- *Speculum examination:* to visualize the vagina for lesions, infection, deformities, inspect the cervix to describe its length, condition of the os, position, and color.
- *Bimanual examination of the uterus:* to provide information on uterine size, shape, consistency, presence of masses, fibroids, and position

Laboratory Data.   Blood tests include a CBC, rubella screen, blood type, serology, toxoplasmosis titer (if exposed to cats), hemoglobin electrophoresis if there is a family history of hemoglobinopathies, and glucose screening as appropriate. Other tests would include cervical cultures, Pap smears, gonorrhea smear, chlamydia culture, herpes smear if indicated, and urinalysis.

Man

Physical Examination.   The male urologic examination is performed by a urologist who would assess the male reproductive tract for lesions, infection, masses, cysts, hernia, undescended or small testicles.

Laboratory Data.   Blood tests would include a CBC, blood type, serology, hemoglobin electrophoresis (as appropriate), glucose screening, test of sperm for number, motility, and condition.

Health Teaching

Counseling is one of the most important functions the nurse can perform for couples seeking preconception advice. Examining and testing the couple is a necessity, but providing them with information that is vital for achieving their goal of producing a healthy baby is equally, or more, important. Health teaching is primarily focused on the female, but the male partner should also be involved in her activities. The information provided to them should not only give them the facts but the rationale for their compliance. (The accompanying display summarizes the information needed for preconception counseling.)

As well as being physically prepared for pregnancy, the couple should also be prepared psychologically and financially. For instance, the couple's disability insurance should be in place, and the adequacy of medical coverage for the mother and newborn confirmed.

The support system should be established. The emotional support and advice that can be offered the couple planning for pregnancy can have a significant impact on the quality of the pregnancy and its outcome.

Contraceptive Choices

Although the history of birth control goes back at least 5000 years, the search for a perfect contraceptive method continues. If sexually active fertile couples do not use

SELF-CARE TEACHING

Preconception Health Care

- Maintain an accurate menstrual calendar
- Discontinue use of birth control pills 3 months prior to conception
- Use condoms for contraception in the interim
- Have an IUD removed 1 month prior to conception
- Discontinue use of contraceptive foam or gel
- Avoid use of alcohol, recreational drugs, and cigarettes
- Optimize nutrition, and/or lose or gain weight as indicated
- Avoid X rays, or confine them to the first half of the menstrual cycle, using a lead apron
- Know the symptoms of pregnancy. After one missed period obtain a pregnancy test
- Know that cats may be infected with toxoplasmosis. Avoid emptying kitty litter boxes, do not eat raw meat, and wear gloves for working in the garden when cats are, or have been, in the area (see Chapter 18).

some form of birth control, they can expect to become pregnant in 6 months to 1 year. There are several good birth control methods; each has its advantages and disadvantages. There is no one perfect method.

Factors Influencing Contraceptive Choice

In considering available choices, there are additional forces that influence the choice of contraceptive.

Social and Cultural Beliefs.   The contraceptor may experience ambivalence because of individual religious beliefs, family tradition, cultural practices, or personal values. Many cultural groups place pressure on women to have children and may even encourage pregnancies until a male child is born. Lingering Victorian attitudes may classify sex as sinful, shameful, and engaged in only for purposes of procreation.

In some areas, information regarding contraception is restricted and access to birth control methods is lacking. Poor women may not have the money or the means of transportation to get to facilities where contraceptives are available, even if the contraceptives themselves are free.

Safety.   The hazards of contraception are meaningful only when compared with the alternative hazards of uncontrolled fertility. The fact is that all common methods of contraception present fewer risks than do pregnancy and childbirth. An exception is the use of the pill by women over 35 years of age, who smoke.

The safety of contraception has rightfully been an issue

RELATED RESEARCH

Subdermal Progestagen Implants

Studies of contraceptive systems that use the sustained release of a low-dose synthetic progestagen have been ongoing for 20 years. The most extensively studied is the Norplant* subdermal implant system. It is presently marketed in China, Finland, Sweden, Thailand, and the U.S.

The Norplant capsule is comprised of six silastic biodegradable rods that are inserted subdermally into the woman's upper arm; it remains in place and is effective for a period of 5 years. After this time, it must be replaced. Some of the advantages of the Norplant capsule are:

- It contains no estrogen
- It achieves contraceptive effects at a low dose
- It delivers the progestagen at a rate of 50–80 mcg/d over the first year and 30–35 mcg/d over the next five years
- It has a failure rate of 0.2% to 1% per year
- It offers a contraceptive method to women who cannot take combined oral contraceptives because of their age, or who are looking for an effective temporary or long-term contraception without opting for sterilization

A disadvantage of the system for some women is persistent spotting or irregular menstrual periods. Some studies also suggest Norplant may adversely affect lipid metabolism.

* Norplant is the registered trademark of the Population Council, New York, NY, for Contraceptive Subdermal Implants.

Darney P: Contraception: Are implants the answer? Contemp OB/GYN 28(1):29–37, 1986

for all women who use or contemplate using birth control. Each woman must weigh the risks and benefits when considering contraception. The primary issue in choosing a birth control method may be either safety or effectiveness. If a woman wants maximum security from pregnancy and considers safety a lower priority, then she may choose oral contraception even though she smokes. A woman wanting absolute safety from side-effects, who will risk the slight chance of pregnancy, may choose a diaphragm.

Women planning only to delay pregnancy may view safety — particularly in terms of preserving reproductive capability — as the highest priority.

The Ideal Contraceptive Method

The ideal contraceptive would have a variety of qualities, many of which are lacking in most contraceptives. These qualities include:

- Ease of use
- Independence from coitus
- Total safety
- Total effectiveness
- Low expense
- Complete freedom from side-effects
- Availability to everyone
- Instant reversibility
- Use with a minimum of advice and care from the health care provider

It is unlikely that such a contraceptive will be developed in the foreseeable future.

Implications for Nursing Care

In her role in the promotion of health and the prevention of disease, it is the nurse who can best provide women with the information that will enable them to make an informed choice about contraception.

It is the nurse's responsibility to be familiar with the various methods described here: hormonal methods, intrauterine devices, mechanical and chemical barriers, natural family planning, withdrawal, elective abortion,

NURSING RESEARCH

Clinical Use of a Fertility History Card

An author in the *Journal of Nurse-Midwifery* discusses the use and misuse of contraceptives and the approaches to improved contraceptive efficacy. Using a decision-making model as a theoretical base, she shifts from patient teaching to body awareness and self-care responsibility. With the use of a Fertility History Card, women learn about fertility and changes that occur during the normal menstrual cycle. The author predicts that the Fertility History Card will increase the correct use of contraceptives because it increases awareness of fertility risk, promotes self-care responsibility, and reinforces patient–patient teaching provided by other members of the health care team.

Riedmann GL: The fertility history card: Clinical use in improving contraceptive efficacy. J Nurse-Midwifery 33(1):15–24, 1988

Birth Control Methods

- Hormonal methods
- Intrauterine devices (IUDs)
- Mechanical barriers: diaphragm, cervical cap, vaginal sponge, condom
- Chemical barriers: foam, cream, jelly, suppository
- Natural family planning
- Withdrawal: coitus interruptus
- Elective abortion
- Surgical sterilization: male and female

and surgical sterilization. The nurse's knowledge of the actions, effectiveness, safety, and contraindications of each of these contraceptive methods will be invaluable in family counseling related to family planning. In the end, the best control method is one that makes the couple feel most natural and comfortable and that they will use correctly and consistently.

ORAL CONTRACEPTIVES

There are three types of oral contraceptives in use today: combination oral contraceptives, the mini-pill, and post-coital contraception.

Combination Oral Contraceptives

The *combination oral contraceptive pill* contains both estrogen and progesterone (the latter in the synthetic form called *progestin*). Oral contraceptives currently available in the United States are listed in Table 8–1.

Mechanism of Action

The estrogen and progestin in oral contraceptives are dissolved in the gastrointestinal tract, absorbed by the blood stream, and carried to the brain, where they exert their effect on the hypothalamus. Not only are the ovaries suppressed, but many functions of the reproductive tract meant to enhance fertility are altered in order to deter it.

Estrogen. There are two major forms of orally active estrogen: ethinyl estradiol (EE) and mestranol. The ethinyl estradiol is 50% more potent than is mestranol; doses of these estrogens range from 20 to 100 μg.

The hypothalamic–pituitary–ovarian axis becomes suppressed as a result of the intake of exogenous estro-

gen. In turn, the gonadotropic hormones LH and FSH are also suppressed, resulting in inhibition of ovulation.

Normal cyclical endometrial changes are disrupted, inhibiting implantation if, per chance, ovulation occurs.

Progestin. Progestin is a derivative of its parent compound 19-nortestosterone, and in the U.S. five of these compounds are currently used in birth control pills. These include norgestrel, ethynodiol diacetate, norethindrone acetate, norethynodrel, and norethindrone. These progestins have androgenic, estrogenic, and antiestrogenic properties, with the exception of norethynodrel, which has no antiestrogenic properties, and norgestrel, which has no estrogenic properties. Doses of these progestins range from 0.05 to 2.5 mg.

Progestin inhibits ovulation due to suppression of gonadotropin releasing hormone (GnRH) and pituitary release of follicle stimulating hormone (FSH). It causes cervical mucus to thicken, become cellular, and impervious to sperm penetration, and produces atrophic changes in the endometrium, inhibiting ovum implantation. Progestin also may decelerate ovum transport through the fallopian tube, disrupting the timing of implantation.

The contraceptive effect of estrogen results from its influence on ovulation, ovum transport, implantation, and maintenance of the corpus luteum. The contraceptive effect of progestin results from its influence on ovulation, cervical mucus, capacitation, ovum transport, and implantation.

Safety and Effectiveness

Other than surgical methods, the birth control pill is the most effective form of contraception. Women who are motivated to use the pill properly are at little risk for pregnancy and may achieve close to 100% effectiveness. The use effectiveness of the pill is difficult to determine, since only 30% to 50% of women who begin taking the pill will be using this method 1 year later. Low continuation rates are related to factors that cannot be controlled or that may be misunderstood. These include diverse medical reasons, such as nausea, missing pills, anxiety about side-effects, or bleeding that could be eliminated by adequate teaching and the availability of advice by telephone.

In nonsmoking women under 35 years of age, pregnancy presents greater risks than does oral contraceptive use. In oral contraceptive users over 30 who smoke, the risk of cardiovascular complications increases significantly. In women 40 to 44 who do not smoke, pregnancy and oral contraceptive use carry the same risk.

Contraindications

Even though oral contraception is safe for most women, contraindications to the pill should be evaluated

(text continued on page 165)

Table 8–1   Oral Contraceptives Available in the United States

Brand Names	Type	Number of Tablets	Estrogen (mg)		Progestin (mg)					Progestin Potency
			Mestranol	Ethinyl estradiol	Norgestrel	Norethindrone	Norethindrone acetate	Ethynodiol diacetate	Norethynodrel	
Brevicon (Syntex)	Comb.	21		0.035		0.5				Low
Norinyl 1 + 50, 21-Day 28-Day (Syntex)	Comb.	21/28	0.05			1.0				Low
Norlestrin 1/50 (Parke-Davis)	Comb.	21		0.050			1.0			Medium
Loestrin 1.5/30 (Parke-Davis)	Comb.	28		0.030			1.5			Medium
Lo/Ovral (Wyeth)	Comb.	21/28		0.030	0.3					Medium
Ovral (Wyeth)	Comb.	21		0.050	0.5					High
ModiCon 21 (Ortho)	Comb.	21/28		0.035		0.5				Low
Ortho-Novum 1/50 (Ortho)	Comb.	21/28	0.05			1.0				Low
Demulen 1/35 (Searle)	Comb.	28		0.035				1.0		High
Zorane 1/50 (Lederle)	Comb.	28		0.050			1.0			Medium
Zorane 1/20 (Lederle)	Comb.	28		0.020			1.0			Medium
Ovcon-35 (Mead Johnson)	Comb.	28		0.035		0.4				Low

		Days	Progestin	Estradiol	Androgenic Effect
Mini-Pill					
Micronor (Ortho)	Micro.	35	0.35		Low
Nor-Q.D. (Syntex)	Micro.	42	0.35		Low
Ovrette (Wyeth)	Micro.	28	0.075		Low
Biphasic					
Ortho-Novum 10/11 (Ortho)	Comb.	21	0.035	0.50 (1st 10 days)	Low
		28	0.035	1.00 (2nd 10 days)	Low
Triphasic					
Ortho-Novum 7/7/7 (Ortho)	Comb.	21	0.035	0.50 (1st 7 days)	Low
		28	0.035	0.75 (2nd 7 days)	Low
		Insert pills 28	0.035	1.00 (3rd 7 days) (last 7 days)	Low
Tri-Norinyl	Comb.	21	0.035 (all days)	0.5 (1st 7 days)	Low
				1.0 (8–16 days)	Low
				0.50 (17–21 days)	Low
Triphasil (Wyeth)	Comb.	21			Low
					High

Triphasil (Wyeth):

	Estradiol	Norgestril
(1–6 days)	0.30	0.50
(7–11 days)	0.40	0.75
(12–21 days)	0.30	0.125

Norethynodrel has no androgenic effect. Norethindrone, norethindrone acetate, and ethynodiol diacetate have a moderate androgenic effect. Norgestrel has a relatively strong androgenic effect.

SELF-CARE TEACHING

Oral Contraceptive Users

- Begin the first pack of pills in one of the following three ways:
  —Take the first pill from the pack on the first day of menstrual bleeding (day 1 of the cycle).
  —Start the first pack on the Sunday following your period, whether you are bleeding or not. This method ensures that you will have no menstrual periods on weekends.
  —Start the first pack of pills on the fifth day of your menstrual period.
- Use a back-up method of birth control, such as foam and condoms or a diaphragm, each time you have sex during the first month of pill-taking.
- Take the pill at approximately the same time each day to maintain the blood hormone level. Associate taking the pill with some routine activity, such as brushing teeth, getting ready for bed, or eating breakfast.
- If you miss a pill, take it as soon as you remember.
- If you miss a pill and don't remember until the next day, take two pills (yesterday's and today's). If this happens, use a back-up method of contraception until the pack of pills is finished.
- If you miss two pills in a row, take two pills as soon as you remember, and two the next day. *Be sure* to use your back-up method of birth control until the pack of pills is finished.
- If you miss three pills, it is possible to ovulate and get pregnant. Begin to use a second method of birth control immediately, and throw away the pills that are left in the pack. Begin a new pack on the Sunday after you missed three or more pills, even if you are bleeding. Continue to use your back-up method of birth control until you are two weeks into the new pack. If pills are frequently forgotten, especially for several days, it might be best to consider another birth control method.
  When a menstrual period is missed and the pills have been taken correctly, it is unlikely that pregnancy has occurred, and a new package of pills can be started at the regular time. Periods may occasionally be missed when you are using oral contraception. If you are concerned, call your health care provider for advice.
- If you have missed one or more pills and no menstrual cycle begins, stop taking the pill. Begin using another birth control method and obtain a pregnancy test.
- If you miss two periods after taking the pills correctly, a pregnancy test should be done.
- If pregnancy occurs while taking birth control pills,

there is a slight risk of having an infant with birth defects. A few providers may recommend abortion, although many would not.
- Use of the pill may initially cause minor side-effects, such as nausea, headache, breakthrough bleeding, breast tenderness, or bloating. These symptoms result from the hormones contained in the pill and usually disappear in 1 to 3 months. If they persist, a change of pill may be needed.
- If an illness causes several days of vomiting and diarrhea, use a back-up method of birth control until the next menstrual period.
- If you experience light bleeding (spotting) during two or more cycles, you may need a change of pill. Call your health care provider.
- If pregnancy is desired, the pill should be stopped. It is best to have several months of spontaneous menstrual cycles before becoming pregnant. This will ensure return of normal menses before pregnancy begins. An alternative method of birth control should be used during these 3 months.
- Never borrow pills or share yours with anyone. Women who have not been examined and taught pill use and danger signals may have contraindications to pill use unknown to the lender.
- If you are admitted to a hospital or see a physician for any reason, inform your health care providers that you are using oral contraceptives.
- Many physicians suggest to women taking birth control pills that they need a "rest period" from pill use. This practice has resulted in many unwanted pregnancies, and there is no evidence that this practice will decrease side-effects or complications.
- If you smoke more than 15 cigarettes a day, be aware of the danger signals that accompany smoking and pill use.
- Concurrent use with other medications may reduce the effectiveness of the pill or the other drugs. Such drugs include anticonvulsives, phenobarbital, rifampin, antibiotics, antacids, sedatives, hypnotics, phenothiazines, tranquilizers, insulin or oral hypogly-cemics, corticosteroids, and antihistamines.
- If *Candida* (yeast) vaginitis is a chronic problem, a pill with high progestin content may increase its incidence.

Danger Signals

If you experience the following symptoms (opposite page) contact your physician or clinic immediately:

SELF-CARE TEACHING *(continued)*

- *Severe abdominal pain* may indicate gallbladder disease, blood clot, hepatic adenoma, or pancreatitis.
- *Severe chest pain or shortness of breath* may indicate pulmonary embolism or myocardial infarction.
- *Severe headache* may indicate stroke, hypertension, or migraine headache
- *Eye problems — blurred vision, flashing lights, or blindness —* may indicate stroke, hypertension, or other vascular problems.
- *Severe pain in the calf or thigh* may indicate a blood clot in the leg.

early in any discussion of birth control methods. (See the display on Contraindications, page 166.)

Side-Effects and Complications

Minor side-effects occur in 40% of women and result from physiologic and metabolic changes caused by the hormonal action of the pill (Table 8–2). When the estrogen level of the pill is excessive, it may cause symptoms similar to those of pregnancy; when its level is low, menopausal symptoms may occur.

These effects may be temporary and appear only for the first few months of pill-taking. When the progestin level of the pill is excessive, symptoms arise from its androgenic properties. These effects, which may or may not worsen with time, primarily involve bleeding irregularities.

Delayed Return of Menstruation

In most cases, ovulatory function and menstruation return soon after oral contraception is discontinued. At 2 to 3 months, ovulation occurs in 50% of women; by 6 months, ovulation will have occurred in 80%. If the woman is anxious because menstruation has not returned by 6 months, she should be referred to a fertility specialist.

Increased Cardiovascular and Cancer Risk

In some women, use of oral contraceptives significantly increases their risk for serious complications.

Cardiovascular Complications. The most serious side-effect, thromboembolism, is primarily related to the estrogenic component. Some of the more catastrophic events that can result from deep thrombosis are myocardial infarction, stroke, and pulmonary embolism. Women on the pill at greatest risk of cardiovascular complications are those who smoke, are over 35 years of age, and have hypertension, diabetes, a history of vascular or heart disease, or a family history of diabetes or heart attack in a family member under age 50. Risk is compounded in the presence of multiple risk factors.

Oral contraceptives containing the more potent progestins have also been associated with coronary heart disease and death due to stroke, ischemic heart disease, and higher blood pressure levels. Blood changes also occur in women on the pill.

Symptoms of serious side-effects, which should be reported promptly, include pain and swelling of the legs, sudden severe headache, chest or abdominal pain, and unexplained visual disturbances.

Hepatocellular Adenoma. Hepatocellular adenoma, a rare benign liver tumor, occurs in about 3 of every 100,000 women who have been long-term users of oral contraceptives. Its primary symptom is abdominal pain, which may continue for months before it is diagnosed. When the tumor has been detected early, discontinuation of the pill may cause tumor regression. Risk of acquiring the tumor may be increased when the pill used has a high hormonal content and the woman is over 35.

Hypertension. Elevation of the systolic blood pressure has been linked to the progestin component of the pill.

Cancer. The possibility that the pill produces malignancies has been an issue for years and may be a major factor in the refusal or discontinuation of pills by some women. At this time, there are no valid data to support a cause-and-effect relationship between pill use and cancer.

Noncontraceptive Benefits

The noncontraceptive benefits of the pill have been ignored, and the rare, but more serious, problems have been given maximum attention by the media and some health professionals.

Numerous studies have documented the pill's effectiveness in reducing morbidity and mortality. Table 8–3 identifies the noncontraceptive benefits of oral contraceptives and their physiologic bases, when known.

Pill choice is less than scientific. There is no way to predict how the hormone levels in a specific pill will interact with an individual woman's metabolism. For this reason, many clinicians initially prescribe a low-dose preparation (35 μg or less of estrogen). Some general guidelines for pill selection are listed in the display, Factors in Pill Selection, page 169.

NURSING ALERT

Contraindications to Oral Contraceptive Use

Absolute Contraindications

- Thrombophlebitis, thromboembolic disorders, cerebral vascular disease, coronary occlusion; a history of these conditions; or conditions predisposing to these problems
- Markedly impaired liver function
- Known or suspected carcinoma of the breast
- Known or suspected estrogen-dependent neoplasia, especially carcinoma of the endometrium
- Undiagnosed abnormal genital bleeding
- Known or suspected pregnancy
- Obstructive jaundice in pregnancy (although not all patients with this history will develop jaundice on the pill)
- Congenital hyperlipidemia (because estrogen increases the risk of cardiovascular death in these patients)
- Obesity in women who smoke and are over 35 years old

- Heavy smoking (15 or more cigarettes a day) in women 30 years of age or older*
- Impaired liver function within the past year

Relative Contraindications

These require clinical judgment and informed consent.

- Migraine headaches
- Hypertension with resting diastolic blood pressure of 90 or greater, or a resting systolic blood pressure of 140 or greater on three or more visits, or an accurate measurement of 110 diastolic or more on a single visit*
- Uterine leiomyoma. (This condition does not seem to be a problem with the new low-dose formulations.)
- Elective surgery. (The pill should be discontinued, if possible, 1 month prior to elective surgery to avoid an increased risk for postoperative thrombosis.)
- Epilepsy. (The pill may increase the frequency of seizures.)
- Sickle cell disease or sickle C disease (but not sickle cell trait)
- Smoking in women over 35
- Undiagnosed, abnormal vaginal bleeding
- Diabetes mellitus
- Long-leg casts or major injury to lower leg
- Age: 45 years of age or older, or 40 years or older if there is a second risk factor for the development of cardiovascular disease*

Possible Contraindications

- Completion of term pregnancy within the past 14 to 20 days*
- Weight gain of 10 pounds or more while on the pill*
- Irregular menstrual cycles
- Profile suggestive of ovulation and infertility problems: late onset of menses or very irregular, painless menses
- Cardiac or renal disease (or history thereof)*
- Conditions likely to make patient unreliable in following instructions for pill use (mental retardation, major psychiatric problems, alcoholism or other drug abuse, pattern of taking oral medication incorrectly)
- Gallbladder disease or recent cholecystectomy
- Lactation*

Conditions Requiring Careful Observation

Pill use may be initiated by patients with the following problems with careful observation.

- Depression*
- Hypertension with resting diastolic blood pressure of 90 to 99 at a single visit*
- Chloasma or hair loss related to pregnancy (or history thereof)*
- Asthma*
- Epilepsy*
- Uterine leiomyomas*
- Acne
- Varicose veins*
- History of hepatitis, provided that liver function tests have been normal for at least 1 year

* This contraindication to combined birth control pills may not be a contraindication to progestin-only pills or may be less of a contraindication to them.

Table 8-2   **Side-Effects of Oral Contraception Due to Hormonal Imbalance**

Estrogen Excess	Estrogen Deficiency	Progestin Excess	Progestin Deficiency	Androgen Excess
Skin changes				
Chloasma Hyperpigmentation Telangiectasia	Insignificant	Oily scalp Acne Hair loss	Insignificant	Acne Oily skin Hirsutism Pruritus
GI Changes				
Nausea	Insignificant	Increased appetite Decreased carbohydrate intolerance	Insignificant	Increased appetite
Weight Changes				
Cyclic weight gain Increased fat deposition Edema	Insignificant	Noncyclic weight gain	Weight loss	Weight gain
Vascular Changes				
Headache Edema Leg cramps	Hot flushes	Headache between pill cycles Dilated leg veins Pelvic congestion	Insignificant	Insignificant
Psychological Effects				
Irritability	Irritability Nervousness Depression	Depression Fatigue Libido changes	Insignificant	Insignificant
Reproductive Tract Changes				
Menstruation				
Uterine cramps Heavy, frequent menses	Early and midcycle spotting Decreased menstrual flow No withdrawal bleeding	Shorter menstrual period	Late breakthrough bleeding and spotting Heavy menses with clotting Delayed onset of menses Dysmenorrhea	Insignificant
Uterus				
Growth of leiomyomas (fibroids) Cervical ectopy Leukorrhea	Pelvic relaxation Uterine prolapse	Insignificant	Insignificant	Insignificant
Vagina				
Insignificant	Dryness of mucosa Atrophic vaginitis	*Candida* infection (yeast)	Insignificant	Insignificant
Breasts				
Suppression of lactation Cystic changes Tenderness Increased size (ductal and tissue), fluid retention	Diminished size	Increased size (alveolar tissues) Tenderness	Insignificant	Insignificant

The Mini-Pill

The mini-pill contains only progestin and was developed for women who experience extreme estrogen-related side-effects and for women in whom estrogen is contraindicated. These pills are to be used daily and continuously.

The mini-pill's contraceptive action renders the endometrial and cervical mucus unfavorable to sperm motility and survival. Pregnancy rates for women using the mini-pill are two to three times greater than the rates for the combination pill. The advantages and disadvantages of mini-pill use, as well as the contraindications, are listed in the display on page 169.

Table 8–3   **Noncontraceptive Health Benefits of Oral Contraceptives**

Benefit	Cause
• Decreased iron deficiency anemia: 50% less than in nonusers of oral contraceptives	• Decreased endometrial proliferation during each menstrual cycle, resulting in increased iron stores
• Decreased menstrual flow: decreased menorrhagia decreased intramenstrual bleeding	
• Less pelvic inflammatory disease	• Decreased menstrual bleeding to act as culture medium
	• Less dilation of cervical canal during menstruation
	• Hostile cervical mucus, which deters pathogens from entering uterus
	• Weaker uterine contractions, which decrease spread of infection
• Reduced incidence of benign breast disease Incidence decreases with longevity of use Incidence decreases when progestin dose increases and estrogen dose stays the same	• Protection provided by progestin component; mechanism unknown
• Decreased incidence of benign ovarian cysts	• Suppression of cyclical ovarian activity
• Protection from ectopic pregnancy	• Decreased incidence of pelvic inflammatory disease, which would lead to blockage of fallopian tubes
	• Prevention of ovulation
• Decreased incidence of rheumatoid arthritis	• Cause unknown
• Decreased risk of endometrial cancer	• Regular endometrial sloughing, caused by progestin contained in combined oral contraceptive pills
In addition, oral contraceptive use • Decreases menstrual cramps • Decreases length of menstrual period • Regulates menstrual periods • Eliminates mittelschmerz • Diminishes fear of pregnancy • Can be helpful in the treatment of acne, ovarian cysts, endometriosis • May increase sexual enjoyment • Decreases premenstrual tension	

Postpartum Use of Oral Contraceptives. Breast-feeding provides little contraceptive effect and should not be depended upon as a reliable method of controlling pregnancy. However, lactation is well established by 6 weeks postpartum, and oral contraceptives are less likely to disrupt successful breast-feeding. When women are resistent to using barrier methods or an IUD, progestin-only oral contraception may be used. Combined pills that contain estrogen should not be used since the effect of estrogen on the infant is not well understood. The progestin-only mini-pill may be used for contraception, and does not appear to decrease lactation.

Women who are not breast-feeding should avoid pill use for 1 month after delivery. During this time the risk for thromboembolic disease is very high, and estrogen ingestion is contraindicated. Following abortion, there is little risk, and it is safe to begin oral contraception immediately.

Postcoital Oral Contraception

Postcoital contraception after unprotected mid-cycle sexual intercourse may be achieved with estrogen-only pills or with combination estrogen-progesterone therapy. Postcoital oral contraception is usually reserved for women who have been raped or for cases of barrier method failure (such as rupture of a condom). The mechanism of this method of pregnancy termination is not yet known, but clinical experience indicates that its failure rate ranges from 2% to 30%.

Factors in Pill Selection
Age

- Women under 35 years of age who have no contraindications are good candidates for pill use.
- Women over 35 years of age who smoke *should not* use oral contraceptives regardless of health status.

Pill Type

- Pills containing 35 μg or less of estrogen should be used initially.
- Adjustment of pill type can be made if minor side-effects become a problem.

Motivation

- For healthy women who desire the most effective contraceptive method, the pill is a good choice.
- Women with relative or possible contraindications who insist on pill use should be referred to a physician.
- Women must be able to remember to take a pill daily.
- Ambivalence about pill use may be caused by cultural or religious beliefs.
- Women who prefer spontaneous sexual activity would probably be more interested in the pill than in other methods of contraception.

Resources

- Resources should be readily available for follow-up appointments and care if problems should arise.
- The expense of this method may preclude its use by women with inadequate finances.

Implications for Nursing Care

The nurse has a crucial role in the evaluation of the woman prior to oral contraceptive use. The physician may prescribe the pill, but it is the nurse who usually assesses and manages the normal oral contraceptive user.

Assessment
Patient History

A complete health history is collected at the initial visit. In order to assess the woman's appropriateness for use of the pill, specific information is needed in addition to the usual data base.

Menstrual History. When the history reveals an erratic, irregular pattern of menses with bleeding problems, referral to a physician is indicated. If the woman's fertility has not been established, she may be anovulatory; if she is put on the birth control pill, it may be difficult to determine later if infertility was inherent or has been influenced by the use of the pill. If the woman insists on using the pill, however, it will stabilize her menstrual periods and decrease heavy bleeding. As long as she is fully informed, this could be an option for her.

Reproductive History. The record of past pregnancies, abortions, and complications of pregnancy and delivery not only documents the woman's fertility but shows the number of children, the spacing of births, and the woman's attitude toward future births. If she has several children and does not want more, she or her partner may be interested in surgical sterilization.

SELF-CARE TEACHING

Mini-Pill Users

- Begin taking the mini-pill on the first day of the next menstrual period.
- Take one pill a day continuously; never miss a pill or take a break from pill-taking.
- Take the pill at the same time each day to maintain hormonal level and prevent spotting.
- Be sure to use a second method of birth control for at least the first 3 months of pill-taking, and during midcycle after that.
- If a pill is missed, take it as soon as you remember, and take the next pill at the usual time. Use your back-up method of contraception until the next period.
- If two pills are missed, take one of the missed pills as well as the pill for that day as soon as you remember. Take the second missed pill the next day along with the regular pill for that day. Use a back-up method of contraception until the next period.
- If you have not had a period for 45 days, even though you have not missed a pill, get a pregnancy test.
- Menstrual cycles may change in length and amount of bleeding; spotting may occur; and missed cycles (without pregnancy) may be experienced.
- If severe abdominal pain occurs while you are on the pill, see your clinician immediately. Users of the mini-pill are at higher risk for ectopic pregnancy if a pregnancy should occur.
- Remember, it is important to perform breast self-examination monthly.
- Return for a check-up before the third package of pills is finished. At this time you will be given a 1-year supply, and yearly check-ups will be adequate. Return for care immediately if you experience any of the danger signals or feel that you are having problems with the pill.

Mini-Pill: Advantages, Disadvantages, and Contraindications

Advantages

- Can be used by women who have developed estrogen-related side-effects on the combination pill, such as chloasma, breast tenderness, nausea, and vomiting
- Is safer for women for whom estrogen use is contraindicated, such as those with obesity, hypertension or endocrine disorders or those with a history of thromboembolic or liver disease
- Can be used by women in the 35 to 40 age group who want oral contraception
- Decreases symptoms of dysmenorrhea
- May be used by postpartum lactating women. (The quantity of milk is not reduced, as it is with estrogen use, but the effect on the milk is unknown.)
- Are taken daily and therefore are less likely to be forgotten
- May reduce the risk of pelvic infection

Disadvantages

- Are less effective than combination pill
- Produce side-effects (primarily alterations in the bleeding pattern, such as breakthrough bleeding, heavy irregular bleeding, and amenorrhea)
- Require use of a back-up method of contraception for the first 3 months
- Are associated with an increased incidence of monilia (yeast) vaginitis

Contraindications

- All the absolute contraindications for the combination pill
- Undiagnosed abnormal genital bleeding
- Irregular menstruation
- History of ectopic pregnancy
- History of reproductive cancer

Especially important is information on the past use of contraception, including the method used, length of use, satisfaction, side-effects, and reasons for its discontinuation. A history of gynecologic surgery should also be obtained.

Sexual History. Included in the sexual history should be a record of sexually transmitted diseases, vaginal or pelvic infections, coital history, and attitudes toward sex.

Collection of the sexual history also provides data that may help to evaluate whether the contraceptive method desired is appropriate for the individual. For instance, if a teen-ager with no steady boyfriend has sexual intercourse once or twice a month, the pill would not be the best choice for her. If, on the other hand, she has a steady boyfriend with whom she has regular intercourse, use of the pill would be an ideal contraceptive method for her.

Health History. It is the health history that determines whether pill use is contraindicated. In some cases a history of an illness that is a contraindication for pill use does not mean that it absolutely cannot be used. An illness may fall into the category of relative contraindications, requiring clinical judgment by a physician and informed consent by the patient.

Family History. History of specific familial disease will provide genetic information that may have implications for a woman contemplating use of oral contraception. However, a young woman with a strong family history of disease, especially one under 30, may not be as concerned about pill use as would a woman over 35.

Social History. Collection of data on social history offers insights into the woman's daily activities, coping patterns, family life, aspirations for the future, reliability, judgment, and more. In conjunction with impressions already obtained, discussion of these areas will offer valuable information for an assessment of her probable reliability in taking the pill, in returning for follow-up visits, and in telephoning the health care provider if problems arise.

Nutritional History. A nutritional assessment is important for women on oral contraceptive pills. Even though we know that anemia occurs less often in such women because of decreased menstrual flow, there are certain dietary deficiencies, such as vitamin B_2, B_6, B_{12}, C, and folic acid deficits, that can occur if their diet is inadequate.

Review of Systems. The review of systems is one of the most important elements of the patient history. It is here that all data that have been overlooked or not provided by the woman up to this point are picked up. The process of reviewing each system with specific symptoms often prompts the memory of past of present events. Symptoms that may result from oral contraceptive use are outlined in the accompanying display.

Physical Examination

A complete physical examination of each family planning patient is the ideal. In reality, however, when the woman is young and healthy, as are most patients seeking birth control, a screening examination is adequate. When a health problem is found during this examination,

Information on Effects of Oral Contraceptives Obtainable from Systems Review
System and Possible Symptoms
Skin
Increased growth of body hair, hair loss

Development of acne

Chloasma, or darkening of the facial skin that may assume a butterflylike configuration over the face; also called "mask of pregnancy"

Telangiectasis, or spider nevi. Appear as tiny red dots with spiderylike capillaries extending outward from them; most commonly found on the upper chest and face

Eyes
Blurred vision, flashing lights, diplopia (double vision)

Improper fit of contact lenses due to swelling of the cornea

Ears
No apparent change

Nose and Sinuses
Increased symptoms of hay fever, rhinitis, nasal polyps

Mouth and Throat
Epulis, gingivitis, sweetish taste in mouth

Breasts
Increase in size, pain (mastalgia), fluid retention, tenderness, masses

Respiratory System
Increased nasal congestion

Chest pain, shortness of breath (may indicate pulmonary emboli or myocardial infarction—rate of both is increased in smokers)

Cardiovascular System
Generalized edema, varicosities, leg pain, increased blood pressure, pain in the chest, headache, migraine headache, color or temperature change in legs. Smokers are at increased risk.

Gastrointestinal System
Nausea, vomiting, loss of appetite, abdominal bloating or cramping, stomach pain, constipation, jaundice

Urinary Tract
Burning, pain, frequency, urgency of urination (symptoms of cystitis)

Frequency of intercourse

Musculoskeletal System
Unilateral leg pain, swelling, elevation and redness of leg

Genital Tract
Abnormal bleeding, spotting, amenorrhea, dysmenorrhea, vaginal itching, odor, increased discharge

Sexual activity

History of myoma

Insufficient vaginal lubrication

Nervous System
Headaches, flashing lights, tingling, numbness, change in affect, migraine, change in sex drive, depression

Hematopoietic System
Anemia, spontaneous or excessive bleeding, bruising

the system or systems identified with the problem are then examined in depth.

The purpose of this examination is to identify conditions that would contraindicate initiation of pill use. It also provides baseline data in the event that problems later arise from use of the pill. Special attention is needed in the following assessments:

- Measurement of blood pressure, weight, and height
- Eye examination
- Examination of head and neck for condition of hair and thyroid size
- Breast examination for detection of possible masses and teaching breast self-examination
- Abdominal examination for assessing liver size, tenderness, and nodes; gallbladder; kidney tenderness; and abdominal tenderness or masses
- Pelvic examination to assess the external genitalia: speculum examination to view the cervix, vagina, vaginal discharge; bimanual examination, including palpation of the uterus to determine its size and detect tenderness and the presence of leiomyomas; examination of the cervix and vagina; palpation of the ovaries for size and tenderness; and rectovaginal examination for rectocele and cystocele
- Examination of extremities to evaluate peripheral circulation, varicosities, edema, bruising

Laboratory Data

Baseline studies should include urinalysis, complete blood count, Pap smear, gonorrhea culture, Venereal Disease Research Laboratories (VDRL) test, and a wet mount when vaginal infection in suspected. Some settings also routinely do blood-clotting studies, a chest x-ray study, and liver function tests. If there is the least suspicion of pregnancy, a pregnancy test should be performed and its results reported as negative before any pills are taken.

Follow-up Visits

As a rule, a 3-month supply of oral contraceptives is prescribed at the first visit. This is done to ensure the woman's early return in the event that she experiences unreported side-effects and to permit her health care providers to check her physical and emotional parameters during the first few months of pill-taking.

The physical assessment includes measurement of blood pressure and weight, urine dipstick test, and palpation of the liver in long-term users. The history taking should identify abnormal symptoms that are warning signals of problems, such as severe headaches, eye problems (blurred vision, flashing), pain in calf or thigh, chest pain or shortness of breath, and, in long-term users, severe abdominal pain.

NURSING ALERT

Protection Against Sexually Transmitted Diseases

Every woman, regardless of age, who has multiple partners or is at risk for sexually transmitted disease, including HIV, should use a spermicidal preparation, in addition to her oral contraceptive, and have her partner wear a condom.

Reinforcement for positive pill-taking actions may encourage better compliance. Return visits should be scheduled for 6- to 12-month intervals, depending on the individual. It is advisable for women who have one or more risk factors to be examined more frequently.

Teaching for Effective Self-Care

Educating women in anticipation of contraceptive use is an important function of the nurse. Such education facilitates the optimum use of contraception and encourages its continuation. The amount of information to be covered is substantial. The creative use of visual aids that illustrate the female anatomy and the menstrual cycle will enhance understanding and expedite counseling. Sample packages of 21- and 28-day pills can be used to demonstrate pill-taking. Handouts that explain in simple language how to take the pill, what to do when pills are forgotten, common side-effects, danger signals, and phone numbers to call when problems occur will reinforce learning and provide a reference at home. Some settings provide classes for groups of women interested in oral contraception. These not only save time but allow a flow of information from group participation and interaction.

Informed Consent.   The birth-control pill is the most widely used drug in a population of healthy people. Since it involves some risk to health, it is important that pill users be fully informed about its use, side-effects, and possible association with complications. This is not only an ethical issue but a legal one as well. By law, clinicians are mandated to provide the information a woman needs to reach a reasonable and informed decision to use birth-control pills.

INTRAUTERINE DEVICES (IUDs)

The practice of inserting foreign devices into the uterus to prevent pregnancy dates back to antiquity. A variety of materials have been used by women in an attempt to prevent conception. It was not until the late 1950s, however, that efforts were made to mass produce intrauterine devices (IUDs).

The IUD became a popular method of contraception for approximately 2.2 million women because it is easy to use and its contraceptive effects are reliable. However, at the present time the Progestasert and the Copper T 380A are the only IUDs marketed in the United States and available to women who desire this method of contraception.

In 1974 one of the early IUDs, the Dalkon Shield, was removed from the market by the manufacturer. A number of women wearing this IUD were experiencing pelvic infections, some of which were so severe that major pelvic surgery was necessary for their survival, but rendered them infertile. The problem was identified as having been precipitated by the IUD's multifilimented tail, which facilitated passage of bacteria from the vagina into the uterine cavity. Numerous suits were brought against the manufacturer, the A.H. Robbins Company. As a result, the company recommended in 1980 that all remaining Dalkon Shields be removed from women still using them.

In 1985 the Ortho Pharmaceutical Company withdrew its IUDs from the U.S. market, and in 1986 the G.D. Searle Company followed suit. These decisions were made solely on the basis of economic and legal jeopardy and not because their IUDs were unsafe. Financial risk from increasing numbers of lawsuits for injuries allegedly related to their IUDs and difficulties in obtaining liability insurance prompted both companies to withdraw their IUDs from the market. However, IUDs manufactured by these companies are readily available to women in other countries.

Types of IUDs

There are two major types of IUDs currently in use: the Progestasert and the ParaGard (also known as the Copper T.)

Progestasert

The Progestasert, made of ethyl vinyl acetate, is T-shaped. Its vertical column contains 38 mg of progesterone in a silicon oil base that releases the hormone at a rate of 65 μg/day. Two threads extend from the base of the T into the vagina (Fig. 8–1). These threads serve two purposes: (1) their presence indicates that the IUD is in place and, (2) the threads expedite IUD removal.

The Progestasert system is the only intrauterine contraceptive that uses the hormone progesterone. The amounts of hormone released is slightly more than the body produces in one day, during the latter portion of the menstrual cycle. The progesterone in the system is delivered directly into the uterine lining and does not enter the general circulation.

Advantages of its use are: (1) reduced blood loss during menses; (2) lower incidence of anemia; and (3) decreased blood loss in women who experience heavy menses.

Its disadvantages are: (1) increased number of days of nonmenstrual bleeding and spotting, (2) the need for yearly replacement, and (3) higher cost. See the accompanying display for contraindications.

ParaGard (Copper T)

ParaGuard is an intrauterine copper contraceptive device, also known as the Copper T 380A IUD. It was devel-

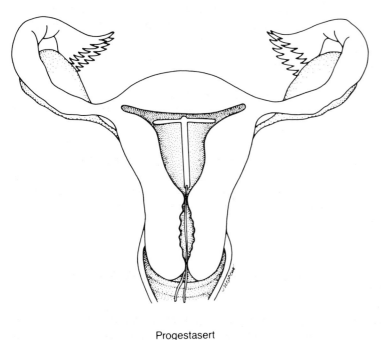

Progestasert

Figure 8–1. Placement of the Progestasert within the uterus with the strings extending from the cervical os. (Childbirth Graphics)

NURSING ALERT

Contraindications to Use of the Progestasert

- Abnormalities of the uterus
- Cancer of the uterus or cervix
- Corticosteroid therapy
- Current, suspected, or possible pregnancy
- Ectopic pregnancy
- Heart disease
- Heart murmur
- Uterine infection
- Leukemia
- Multiple sexual partners
- A sexual partner who has multiple sexual partners
- Pelvic or fallopian tube infection
- Recent abortion or miscarriage
- Recent pregnancy
- Sexually transmitted disease

Relative Contraindications

- Anemia or blood clotting problems
- Bleeding between periods
- Diabetes
- Fainting episodes
- Genital lesions
- Heavy menstrual flow
- IUD currently in place
- Prior IUD use
- Severe menstrual cramps
- Impairment in ability to check for IUD string or danger signals
- Concern for future fertility

oped by GynoMed Pharmaceutical, Inc., a New Jersey company interested in the needs of women's health. Although the device was approved by the United States Food and Drug Administration (FDA) in 1984, it was not available in the United States until 1988. It is now an available option to women who have not had previous access to a copper-bearing intrauterine device.

The ParaGard is a small, inert polyethylene "T"-shaped device that has copper wire wound around its stem and a copper sleeve fitted onto each half of the cross bar. The exposed surface area of the copper is 380 mm².

Prior to its release, clinical trials of the T 380A IUD, conducted in women over 25 by the Population Council, showed a failure rate of about 1%. The council contends that because of its low failure rate, the T 380A is one of the most effective contraceptives in the world.

Women who desire a reversible method that does not interfere with spontaneity or require daily maintenance are good candidates for the ParaGard device. Appropriate candidates for this IUD, according to the manufacturer, include women who:

- Are parous
- Are in a stable, mutually monogamous relationship, with a low risk of contracting sexually transmitted disease
- Have no history or suspicion of pelvic inflammatory disease.

Inappropriate candidates for the IUD, according to the manufacturer, are:

- Nulliparous women
- Those with more than one sexual partner or otherwise at risk for sexually transmitted disease
- Those with a history or suspicion of pelvic inflammatory disease, genital tract infections, or gynecologic malignancies.

Mechanisms of Action

The mechanism responsible for the effectiveness of the IUD is still unknown. The numerous cellular and biochemical changes that occur in the endometrium after IUD insertion may represent a sterile inflammatory response to the presence of a foreign body. The precise contraceptive effect of progesterone used in the Progestasert is not fully known.

Copper devices interfere with estrogen uptake by the endometrium. The chemical composition of the cervical mucus is altered by copper ions, which may also affect sperm motility, capacitation, and survival. IUDs may also increase secretion of prostaglandins, thus inhibiting implantation.

Safety and Effectiveness

The most serious health risks for IUD users are the potential for pelvic infection and the increased probability of an ectopic pregnancy. The risk of infection for IUD users may be four times higher than that for nonusers, and it may remain throughout the length of use, depending on the woman's parity and the number of her sexual partners.

In general, IUDs are highly effective. The incidence of unplanned pregnancy with the Progestasert is 2% to 3%, while the incidence of pregnancy with the Copper T 380A is 1%. The performance of these devices is influenced by their size; the woman's age, parity, and frequency of intercourse; and by the woman's diligence in checking for

SELF-CARE TEACHING

IUD Use

- You should not be aware that the IUD is in place, and your partner should not feel it during intercourse.
- Be sure to check the IUD strings frequently to ensure that the device has not been expelled. It should be checked before intercourse and after menstrual periods or bouts of uterine cramping. The strings can be checked in one of the following positions: (1) Lie down with your knees bent and separated. (2) Stand with one foot on a stool or chair. (3) Sit on the toilet and bear down. (4) Get into a squatting position.
- Insert your first finger into the vagina until you touch the strings or cervix. The cervix feels firm, like the tip of your nose, and the strings should be protruding from the os at its center.
- If you feel a hard object, the IUD may be in the process of being expelled. See your health care provider as soon as possible, and do not have sexual intercourse until you do.
- Whenever a period is missed or the string cannot be felt, seek care immediately.
- When cramping occurs during the first few menstrual periods, an analgesic may be taken.
- For added protection, use a back-up method of contraception such as foam, condoms and foam, and spermicides during the first 3 months of use. During subsequent periods use a back-up method during the midcycle fertile period. This practice will also help to reduce the risk of infection.
- When you are ready for pregnancy, the IUD should be removed by a medical professional. Never at any time try to remove the device yourself.
- It is best to wait 3 months after removal before attempting pregnancy. Be sure to use another method of contraception during that period.
- Side-effects may include heavy menstrual bleeding, lower back and abdominal pain, cramping, and midcycle spotting. If bleeding is consistently heavy, you may become anemic, and need iron supplementation or removal of the IUD.
- Be sure to learn what type of IUD you are wearing and the date of its insertion. The Cu 7 and Copper T must be replaced every 3 years. The Lippes Loop and Saf-T-Coil may remain in the uterus indefinitely unless problems arise. The Progestasert should be replaced each year.
- If the following symptoms occur, seek medical help immediately: abdominal pain, chills and fever, heavy vaginal discharge with or without odor, heavy bleeding, and pain during intercourse.

Danger Signals

If you experience any of the following symptoms, contact your physician or clinic immediately.

- Missed or late menstrual period
- Abdominal or pelvic pain
- Fever, chills
- Heavy bleeding, clots, spotting, heavy periods
- Strings absent or hard object felt in cervix
- Heavy, foul, or unusual vaginal discharge

its presence. The expertise of the person inserting the device, its ease of insertion, personal support through counseling, and prompt attention to problems or side-effects are the most important variables in successful IUD use, regardless of the type of device.

Side-Effects and Complications

Syncope. Syncope (fainting) at the time of IUD insertion results from vagal response to the pain of cervical dilatation and the distention of the uterine cavity by the device. This response may be anticipated in women who are overly anxious or have a narrow, tight cervix. Symptoms may include hypotension, bradycardia, pallor, weakness, and diaphoresis. When vagal response occurs, the IUD insertion procedure should be stopped immedi-

ately. To relieve the symptoms, the patient should be placed in a horizontal position and given spirits of ammonia to inhale. If the patient does not respond or symptoms are more severe, intravenous atropine may be ordered.

Pain and Bleeding on Insertion. Uterine cramps or low backache may occur at the time of insertion and may last for a few days. Mild pain medication usually relieves the pain of insertion. A small amount of bleeding may occur during insertion. The care provider may choose to insert the IUD during the end of the menstrual period for this reason. Also, this timing reduces the possibility of pregnancy at the time of insertion.

Perforation of the Uterus on Insertion. Partial or total perforation can occur during or after insertion. The disappearance of the tail may occur and should be checked. When the uterus is perforated, there is risk of abdominal adhesions, intestinal obstruction or penetration, infection, and loss of contractive protection. This complication requires surgery.

Changes in Menstrual Patterns. Spotting may occur during the first 2 or 3 months after insertion. Following insertion, the first few periods may be heavier and longer than usual. If bleeding continues after this time, the physician should be consulted.

When periods are missed, there is always the possibility of pregnancy. A pregnancy test should be done and, if positive, a physician should be consulted.

Expulsion of the IUD. Expulsion of the IUD may occur in 5% to 20% of users in the first year of use. The presence of threads assures that it remains within the uterus. When the threads cannot be felt, another contraceptive method should be used to protect against pregnancy, until the system can be checked. The use of contraceptive foam, cream, jellies, or condoms is advised to avoid a possible pregnancy.

Pregnancy With an IUD in Place. Pregnancies in women with an IUD in place are at risk for spontaneous abortion during the first or second trimester. When the IUD is removed in early pregnancy, the risk of spontaneous abortion is decreased by 50%. If the device is not removed, approximately 50% of women will abort.

Problems that can occur with an IUD *in situ* during pregnancy are premature delivery, stillbirth, and lower infant birth weight. No evidence of birth defects or complications in subsequent pregnancies has been reported.

Ectopic Pregnancy. An ectopic pregnancy is one in which the fertilized ovum implants outside the uterus; over 95% of these pregnancies occur in the fallopian tubes. The link between ectopic pregnancy and the IUD is well known but not well understood. For more complete information on ectopic pregnancy, see Chapter 19. Progestasert users are more apt to have an ectopic pregnancy than users of other types of IUDs. The World Health Organization conducted two studies, one on the risk of ectopic pregnancies in a progesterone-releasing IUD, similar to that of the Progestasert, and one study on the risk of ectopic pregnancies in women wearing copper-releasing IUDs. Results of these studies showed that the risk of ectopic pregnancy with the progesterone IUD was ten times higher than that with the copper-releasing IUDs.

Implications for Nursing Care

If a woman cannot use oral contraceptives or wants a method that does not intrude in her sexual activities, the IUD may be the method that best meets her needs. Experience has shown that women who are motivated and informed may have many years of uneventful and successful IUD use.

Assessment
Patient History

A complete health history is collected. The particular systems that may be affected by IUD use will be discussed.

Menstrual History. History of regular menstrual periods with a normal amount of blood loss and minimal or no cramping is ideal for women desiring IUD insertion. However, specific information regarding patient experiences with extended menstruation, dysmenorrhea, menorrhagia, metrorrhagia, or spotting must be obtained. If any of these symptoms have been experienced, it is important to identify when the pain or bleeding occurred, frequency of occurrence, length of symptoms, amount of blood loss, and whether anemia resulted. If these symptoms are no longer present and the patient has been experiencing normal menses over a long period of time, she may be given an IUD with the understanding that heavy bleeding or cramping might recur.

Young women with erratic menstrual patterns are not candidates for IUD insertion because of their small, underdeveloped uteri, increased incidence of expulsion, increased cramping, and risk for pelvic infection and possible infertility. However, young women who have given birth and live with a husband or steady partner may be considered for IUD use.

Reproductive History. The first information to obtain is a history of pregnancy and the possibility of a current undetected pregnancy. A history of pelvic inflammatory disease, gonorrhea, or ectopic pregnancy precludes IUD use. The incidence and etiology of past or present vaginal infections or cervicitis should be investigated.

Multiparous women are better candidates for IUD use than nulliparous women. A woman who intends to have more children should never be given an IUD.

The frequency of sexual intercourse, the number of partners, the personal hygiene, and willingness to use foam or condoms as back-up contraceptives are pertinent to the decision-making process.

Health History. A history that includes any of the following conditions would preclude IUD use: valvular heart disease (because of the potential for subacute bacterial endocarditis); diabetes, ongoing steroid treatment, or other condition that may impair the coagulation response; anemia; physical or mental impairment rendering the patient unable to check for the IUD strings or to recognize danger signals; previous episodes of vasovagal response; and allergy to copper.

Physical Examination

For the prospective IUD user with no contraindications, the pelvic examination is the most important portion of this examination.

During the speculum examination, the vagina and cervix can be inspected for inflammation, cervical or vaginal discharge, cervical stenosis or polyps, masses, cysts, ulcerations, structural abnormalities, and position of the cervix. Specimens from the cervix and vagina are also collected to detect possible infection.

The purpose of the bimanual examination is to detect a uterus that is too small or too large (the latter might indicate pregnancy); determine uterine position and mobility, which might influence the ease of IUD insertion; detect the lumpy presence of myomas within the uterine wall; identify structural abnormalities of reproductive organs; palpate and assess ovarian size and tenderness; establish the presence or absence of pain or tenderness in the pelvis; palpate the cervical os to determine patency; and assess the amount, consistency, color, and odor of the vaginal discharge.

Laboratory Data

Baseline laboratory studies should include urinalysis, complete blood count, Pap smear, gonorrhea culture, VDRL test, pregnancy test, and a wet mount when vaginal infection is suspected. Blood-clotting studies may also be ordered when appropriate.

Teaching for Effective Self-Care

The primary nursing intervention related to the IUD is to educate and support the user and assess her understanding of the device's use. Emphasis on the urgent need to seek care when problems arise is equally important.

The use of visual aids and plastic models that show the position of the IUD in relation to the female anatomy will effect understanding better than an extended explanation. Support for the woman during insertion will help make the process more acceptable to her and confirm your interest in her well-being. If possible, remain in the room for a short time after insertion to reassure her that the procedure went well and that cramping will soon decrease. Obtain an order from the physician for analgesic when the pain is severe.

BARRIER METHODS OF CONTRACEPTION

Barrier methods are popular with women who dislike or are unable to use the pill or IUD. Barrier methods are generally easy to use and available to almost anyone. They include the diaphragm, the cervical cap, the vaginal con-

---

Users and Nonusers of Barrier Method Contraception

Women most inclined to use barrier methods are those who

- Are postpartum or lactating
- Have infrequent intercourse
- Forget to take pills
- Are awaiting sterilization
- Are unable to get medical care
- Have many sexual partners, increasing their risk of sexually transmitted disease
- Want to increase IUD effectiveness
- Want an interim method before attempting pregnancy
- Have male partners with recent vasectomies
- Are over 35
- Are premenopausal

Women who dislike barrier methods are those who

- Want more effective contraception
- Do not want to insert a device just prior to intercourse
- Find them greasy or messy, or dislike the sensation of burning or itching experienced with some products
- Do not want to wait for or interrupt intercourse
- Have a male partner who does not like the method
- Need a contraceptive that can be used without the partner's knowledge
- Are uncomfortable about touching themselves or inserting devices or spermicidal preparations into the vagina

---

traceptive sponge, and vaginal spermicides in the form of creams, jellies, foams, and suppositories.

Barrier methods of contraception have assumed an important new dimension in women's health. Now viewed as an equal and, perhaps, a more important barrier to HIV and other sexually transmitted diseases, barrier methods are no longer seen as just contraceptive in nature. Chlamydia, herpes, gonorrhea, syphilis, genital warts, and HIV are becoming endemic.

Barrier methods such as diaphragms, condoms, and contraceptive sponges, are now being looked at as preventive measures against disease. When used in conjunction with a spermicide, barrier devices offer sexually active women (especially those with multiple partners) an additional degree of protection from infection.

While the pill remains the most popular birth control method, users need to be informed on an individual basis as to risk of infection and the need for a barrier method to provide a fail-safe combination equally effective as a contraceptive and in disease prevention.

Diaphragm

The diaphragm is a soft, thin, dome-shaped latex cup rimmed with a firm, flexible coiled spring or metal band. The diaphragm is placed with its posterior rim fitting firmly within the posterior fornix and the anterior rim placed securely under the pubic bone (Fig. 8 – 2). It is used in conjunction with spermicidal cream or jelly and inserted into the vagina before intercourse. It is used by women who are knowledgeable about their bodies and the various contraceptive methods, who are willing to think ahead and prepare for sexual activity, and who desire a method that does not produce systemic or other invasive effects in their bodies.

Types of Diaphragms

The *arching spring* diaphragm is probably the most commonly used, since the average woman can use it comfortably. The rim of this diaphragm is strong and firm. When bent, its spring arches, facilitating insertion by slipping naturally behind the cervix into the posterior fornix (Fig. 8 – 3). These features make it a good choice for women who have weak vaginal musculature, a cystocele or rectocele, a shallow pubic arch, a retroverted uterus, or a firm nulliparous uterus.

The *flat spring rim* diaphragm has a flat, thin, compressible but gentle spring within its rim (see Fig. 8-3). When it is folded, insertion past the cervix into the posterior fornix is easy to achieve. It is used primarily in nulliparous women with firm vaginal tone, or in women with a shallow notch posterior to the pubic bone.

The rim of the *coil spring* diaphragm contains a firm, spiral wire, making it flexible at any portion. When compressed, the rim is flat. It is more flexible than the flat

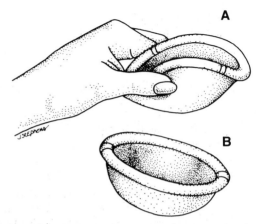

Figure 8 – 3. Two commonly used diaphragms. *(A)* The arching spring rim type has a sturdy rim with a firm spring. *(B)* The flat spring rim type folds at two points only for easy insertion. (Childbirth Graphics)

spring and causes less pressure on the tissues. This diaphragm is used in women with average vaginal muscle tone and average pubic arch.

The choice of diaphragm for an individual woman depends on physiologic parameters rather than the patient's wishes. Only when a woman's body build is such that she could use either of two types of diaphragms equally well does she have a choice in the selection.

Safety and Effectiveness

When used properly, the diaphragm is a safe method of contraception. Risks associated with the diaphragm may result from the user's resentment of the device's inconvenience; her need for a method of contraception that can be used without the partner's knowledge; lack of privacy for insertion, removal, cleaning, and storage; and dislike of the diaphragm by the partner.

Contraindications

There are many medical and social contraindications to diaphragm use. These include:

- Allergies to rubber or spermicide
- History of recurrent urinary tract infection
- Genital tract abnormalities resulting from weak musculature, such as uterine prolapse, cystocele, rectocele, and decreased vaginal tone, most of which occur in multiparous women (Some women with these problems can use an arching spring diaphragm.)
- Fixed retroflexed or retroverted uterus
- Lack of time or trained personnel to fit the diaphragm and instruct the patient in its use
- Past history of toxic shock syndrome
- Inability of the woman to learn to insert and remove the diaphragm

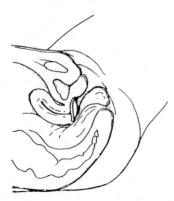

Figure 8 – 2. Lateral view of a correctly fitted diaphragm.

- Lack of facilities and privacy for insertion, hygiene, or storage
- Tight vaginal musculature that impedes diaphragm insertion
- A notch behind the pubic bone too shallow to support the diaphragm rim

Diaphragm effectiveness rates vary from 88% to 98%. Use effectiveness depends on four variables: (1) the diaphragm's ability to act as a barrier against sperm entering the cervical canal; (2) its ability to contain spermicidal jelly or cream and to hold it against the cervix; (3) the motivation of its user; and (4) the quality of teaching that accompanies the initial prescription. The diaphragm's effectiveness is greatly reduced when women do not adhere strictly to the rules for its use.

Side-Effects and Complications

No serious side-effects are likely from use of a well-fitted diaphragm as recommended. Side-effects that might occur include:

- Itching, burning, or swelling of the vaginal or penile tissue as a result of exposure to latex, rubber, or spermicidal jelly or cream
- Recurrent urinary tract infection related to rim pressure on the urethra.
- Interference with bowel movements or size of stool and hemorrhoids may occur when posterior pressure is exerted on the descending colon through the vaginal wall.
- Vaginal trauma from rim pressure or prolonged wear.
- Toxic shock syndrome, which has been reported to occur after diaphragm use. Its signs are temperature elevation of 101°F or more, diarrhea, vomiting, muscle aches, and a sunburnlike rash.

The advantages of diaphragm use include the following:

- No interference with breast-feeding
- Ability to insert the device 2 to 6 hours prior to intercourse
- Avoidance of daily pill taking
- Avoidance of interference in the metabolic and physiologic processes of the body
- Some protection against sexually transmitted diseases and the development of cervical dysplasia

Implications for Nursing Care
Assessment

The nurse plays an important role in contributing to successful diaphragm use. Not only does she have ade-

quate time to spend teaching patients its proper use, but the family planning nurse also understands women's motivations in attempting to avoid unwanted pregnancy.

Patient History.   The purpose of the patient history is to assess the appropriateness of the diaphragm for the woman, to discover possible contraindications to its use, and to assess whether the woman is likely to use it properly.

The menstrual history is not as crucial for women anticipating diaphragm use as for women planning to use the pill or IUD. It does, however, help diaphragm users to determine the approximate days of fertility, thus enabling them to avoid positions during intercourse that might displace the diaphragm or to abstain from sex altogether during those days.

Knowledge of the number of pregnancies and deliveries will probably dictate the size and type of diaphragm used. A diaphragm cannot be fitted too soon after delivery, since the wrong size may be prescribed if the woman is measured before full uterine and vaginal involution has occurred.

Information gained from the sexual history is important. For instance, a woman who has infrequent intercourse and is comfortable about touching her body may find the diaphragm a good choice. On the other hand, a woman who has frequent and active sex may not be a good candidate for diaphragm use, since the device may be displaced by deep penile thrusting or by intercourse in the female superior position.

The most serious problem to rule out in the health history is a past episode of toxic shock syndrome. A positive history contraindicates use of the diaphragm. Other, less serious problems that would preclude diaphragm use are recurrent urinary tract infections and physical abnormalities of the vagina or cervix.

Physical Examination.   A screening examination is performed with particular attention to the pelvic examination, since this is the only system affected by diaphragm use.

Speculum inspection of the vagina and cervix to exclude local problems is particularly important. These might include vaginitis, which may prevent diaphragm fitting if the tissues are tender, reddened, and edematous; masses or fluid-filled cysts; and structural abnormalities.

Bimanual findings that are essential for proper use of the diaphragm are: (1) an adequate notch behind the symphysis pubis, necessary to hold the anterior rim of the diaphragm in place; (2) adequate space in the posterior fornix to accommodate the posterior rim of the diaphragm; (3) adequate muscle tone to maintain the device in place; and (4) lack of structural abnormalities that would interfere with the use of the diaphragm. (See Figure 8–3).

Laboratory Data

Laboratory studies should include urinalysis, complete blood count, Pap smear, gonorrhea culture, VDRL test, and a wet mount when vaginal infection is suspected.

When health assessment has been completed, contraindications have been excluded, and the woman has chosen the diaphragm as her contraceptive method, the nurse should assess the woman's understanding of its use. This is accomplished by the woman's ability to demonstrate its correct insertion and removal, her comfort in handling the diaphragm and touching her body, and her ability to verbilize instructions for diaphragm use.

Cervical Cap

The cervical cap was approved by the FDA in 1988. It is eventually to be marketed as a prescription contraceptive device.

The cervical cap is a soft, thimble-shaped rubber device that fits tightly over the cervix and blocks the passage of sperm (Fig. 8–4). It is deeper and smaller in diameter than the diaphragm and is held in place by the action of suction. The cap must be half filled with spermicidal jelly to improve its effectiveness.

Like the diaphragm, the cervical cap must be fitted by specially trained personnel. Its rim must fit securely around the base of the cervix but not touch the os. Placement and removal of the cervical cap may be more difficult than placement and removal of the diaphragm.

Safety and Effectiveness

There has been too little experience with long-term use of the cervical cap to determine its safety. Clinicians providing the cap and studying its use express concern about the possible risk of infection from the prolonged exposure of the cervix to secretions or bacteria trapped in the cap and trauma or chronic irritation of cervical and vaginal tissue. The ultimate safety concern is the possible role of the cap in pelvic infection.

Contraindications to the use of the cervical cap are the following:

- Lack of trained personnel to fit and teach its use
- Allergy to rubber or spermicide
- Anatomic abnormalities of the cervix or vagina
- Inability of the woman to learn the technique of insertion
- Cervical or vaginal infections
- Delivery of a full-term infant within the past 6 weeks
- Abnormal Pap smear
- History of toxic shock syndrome

Few studies have been conducted to determine the effectiveness of the cervical cap, but it is thought to be about as effective as the diaphragm.

Side-Effects and Complications

Side-effects and complications of cervical cap use include the following:

- Discomfort caused by the device to either partner
- Vaginal lacerations or abrasions
- Acute cervicitis
- Pelvic infection
- Development of abnormal Pap smear

The last three conditions have been observed in cap users, but their association with its use has not been documented.

Advantages of the Cervical Cap

- Insertion of the cap is unrelated to the time of intercourse.
- It can be used by women with poor pelvic muscle tone.
- It does not put pressure on the bladder or rectum.
- It can remain in place for 3 days or longer.

Implications for Nursing Care

See this section under Diaphragm Use.

Vaginal Contraceptive Sponge

Natural collagen and synthetic sponges incorporating spermicide were approved by the FDA in 1983 for use in the United States. The Today Vaginal Contraceptive Sponge is available in one size only and may be purchased

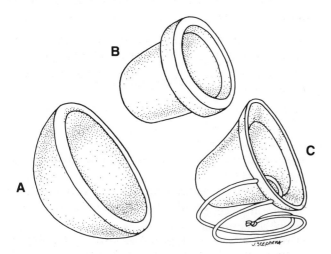

Figure 8–4. Three types of cervical caps. *(A)* Dumas Cap. *(B)* Prentif cavity rim cervical cap. *(C)* Vimule cap. (Childbirth Graphics)

over the counter without prescription. The sponge is small and pillow-shaped and is made of polyurethane that contains 1 g of spermicide. In addition to its spermicidal properties, the sponge acts as a cervical barrier and traps sperm within it. On one side, the sponge has a concave depression into which the cervix fits; on the reverse, a loop is attached to expedite its removal.

The sponge provides protection for 24 hours. Prior to insertion it is moistened with water. Repeated intercourse may occur during this period without further precautions. After 24 hours, the sponge is removed and discarded.

Safety and Effectiveness

The safety of the vaginal sponge is not clearly known; however, risks appear to be small.

Contraindications to the use of the vaginal sponge include:

- Allergy to spermicide or polyurethane
- Abnormalities of pelvic structures that would interfere with its placement, retention, or removal
- Inability of the woman to insert or remove the device

SELF-CARE TEACHING

Foam Use

- The foam must be used every time you have sex.
- Read the instructions on the can of foam.
- The foam may be inserted 30 minutes before intercourse but will be more effective if used just before it. If after 30 minutes intercourse has not occurred, insert another applicator of foam.
- Shake the can of foam vigorously to ensure complete mixing and foaming action before use.
- Place the applicator on the can and fill it by applying pressure to the top of the can. Use one or two applicators as indicated on the label.
- Lie on your back with your knees bent and spread apart. With your fingers, spread the lips of the vagina and carefully insert the applicator into the vagina as far back as possible.
- Push the plunger to insert the foam and then remove the applicator from the vagina. Repeat this process if two applications are specified. Wash the applicator with soap and water.
- If douching is desired, wait at least 8 hours after the last intercourse for optimum spermicidal effect.
- To avoid running out of foam, have a spare can available.

- Inability to remember to use the sponge
- History of toxic shock syndrome
- Vaginal colonization by *Staphylococcus aureus*

Side-effects and complications of sponge use include:

- Redness, irritation, and itching of the vulva, resulting from allergy to spermicide
- Tearing of the device during insertion, removal, or intercourse
- Dryness of the vagina, resulting from absorption of vaginal secretions by the sponge

The effectiveness of the vaginal sponge is thought to be similar to, but probably lower than, that of the diaphragm.

Vaginal Spermicides

Vaginal spermicides are currently available in a variety of forms, including creams, jellies, suppositories, foam, and foaming tablets. These preparations all contain an inert vehicle that works in two ways: (1) by physically blocking the passage of the sperm into the cervix and (2) by releasing spermicides that kill the sperm.

They are being viewed more favorably as a contraceptive method partly because of their safety and their availability without a prescription.

Types of Spermicide
Contraceptive Foam

Spermicidal foam is sold in pressurized cans and can be bought in drugstores without a prescription. It is a thick, white foam that not only blocks the entrance of sperm into the uterus, but kills sperm from the chemical action of its spermicide. The use of foam has no known serious side-effects. It is a good method to use in the following instances:

- As an interim method for women who have stopped taking the pill to prepare themselves for pregnancy
- As a contraceptive method used in conjunction with the condom
- As a protective measure against sexually transmitted infection or disease
- As a back-up method:
  When pills run out or pill use has been stopped for some reason
  When increased effectiveness is desired at midcycle by users of IUDs, condoms, or the fertility awareness method
  When a woman is waiting to begin the initial pill cycle and during the first month of pill use
  For the first few months after the insertion of an IUD
  After an IUD has been expelled

When a condom breaks (foam can be quickly inserted into the vagina; it may or may not be effective, as sperm enter the cervix within seconds)

Spermicidal Creams, Jellies, and Suppositories

In many family planning settings foam is recommended over creams, jellies, or suppositories, since its effectiveness rates are generally higher.

Spermicidal creams and jellies are packaged in tubes and can be purchased over the counter at drugstores. Caution in the choice of these products is advised. Spermicidal creams and jellies meant to be used alone may be confused with products meant for use with the diaphragm or hygienic products that contain no spermicide. Labels should be read carefully.

Spermicidal creams and jellies are inserted with an applicator similar to the one used for foam. The cream or jelly is squeezed into the applicator that screws into the top of the tube. The waiting time for their dispersal is specified in the directions on each tube.

Safety and Effectiveness

The safety of the vaginal spermicides is one of the major reasons for their increased popularity. Spermicidal chemicals are active against many bacteria and provide a measure of defense against sexually transmitted disease. However, because vaginal mucosa is capable of absorbing a range of substances, questions have arisen about the possibility of systemic effects in spermicide users. To date, no evidence of teratogenic effects has been reported when used during an undetected pregnancy. Nevertheless, vaginal spermicides should be avoided if there is the least suspicion of pregnancy.

The effectiveness of vaginal spermicides depends on the quality of their use. The effectiveness rate has been estimated to be between 80% and 95%.

Spermicidal suppository effectiveness rates are difficult to obtain but are known to be less than those for foam. The suppositories are inserted by hand and must be placed deep in the vagina in order to protect the cervical os from the entrance of sperm and provide optimal spermicidal effect.

Noncontraceptive Benefits

Vaginal spermicides have some important noncontraceptive benefits. They kill many organisms responsible for sexually transmitted disease, and they decrease the incidence of pelvic inflammatory disease by as much as 50%.

Condom

The major form of male barrier contraceptive is the condom (rubber). Condoms rank in popularity second

SELF-CARE TEACHING

Condom Use

- Use the condom each time you have sex.
- Carry a condom for "emergency" situations.
- Handle the condom carefully to avoid tearing.
- Apply the condom to the erect penis (either partner may do this) before the penis is put into the vagina.
- Unroll the condom to its full length over the penis, leaving a half-inch empty space at the bottom, or purchase condoms with nipple tips.
- Use a lubricant, such as contraceptive cream, when the vagina is dry to prevent friction, pain, or tearing of the condom.
- When withdrawing the penis, hold the rim of the condom to avoid spilling sperm in or near the vagina.
- Withdraw the penis before erection is lost in order to prevent the condom from slipping off in the vagina.
- Store condoms in a cool, dry place.

only to the pill as a contraceptive method in the United States and worldwide may be used by as many as 40 million couples.

The majority of condoms are made of latex or processed collagenous sheaths. The latter are superior in preserving sensitivity and are reusable. The FDA has stringent standards of quality for condom manufacture. A variety of condoms are now on the market. Newer types are thinner and may be prelubricated. They are also available in bright colors, and some contain erotic ribbings.

Safety and Effectiveness

Rare sensitivity reactions can occur as a result of the material from which the condom is made, the spermicide, or the lubricant. Otherwise the condom does not cause adverse side-effects. Allergies and the man's inability to maintain an erection while using a condom are the only contraindications to condom use.

Condom effectiveness is reported to be between 97.0% and 98.5%. If used in conjunction with a vaginal barrier method, the combined effectiveness approaches that of the pill.

Noncontraceptive Benefits

The condom offers many benefits in addition to pregnancy prevention. These include:

- Prevention of vaginal infections, the spreading of sexually transmitted disease, and possibly pelvic inflammatory disease

- An increase in comfort and sexual satisfaction when lubricated condoms are used
- Inclusion of the condom in the sexual foreplay when the woman puts it on
- Reduction of antibody titers in couples where the woman is producing antibodies against her partner's sperm

Implications for Nursing Care

Vaginal sponges, spermicides, and condoms are non-prescription contraceptives and are often purchased by patients over the counter without recommendation from a health care provider. If the patient has concerns or questions about these methods, the nurse should instruct the patient on their correct use, including review of manufacturers' instructions, if available. (See Self-Care Teaching: Foam Use and Condoms.)

FERTILITY AWARENESS METHODS

Increasing numbers of couples are turning to less intrusive and more personal methods of contraception known collectively as natural family planning or fertility awareness methods. This group is motivated, often for religious reasons, to spend time and effort learning to assess and maintain control of their own fertility. All fertility awareness methods require regular abstinence from sexual intercourse for a specific number of days. They do not depend on regular menstrual cycles but rely on signs and symptoms of fertility.

Types of Fertility Awareness Methods

There are currently four methods of fertility awareness (referred to as periodic abstinence by some).

- Calendar rhythm method
- Temperature, thermal, or basal body temperature method
- Cervical mucus or ovulation method
- Sympto-thermal method

These terms are used to describe specific techniques for identifying or predicting the fertile period. Rules for the days when abstinence is maintained depend on the method being practiced. Advantages of fertility awareness methods include the following:

- They are free or inexpensive.
- Once learned, they are helpful in achieving as well as avoiding pregnancy.

- Such methods are not controversial and may be taught in sex education programs.
- They encourage couple communication concerning family planning and sexuality.

Calendar Rhythm

Before the calendar rhythm method can be used and fertile days approximated, 12 months of recorded menstrual cycles are needed to determine the longest and shortest cycles experienced by the woman in order to predict the possible fertile days of future cycles. The process of counting days of the menstrual cycle begins at day 1 of menstrual bleeding and ends when the next period begins. The beginning of the fertile period is estimated by subtracting 18 days from the shortest of the woman's previous 6 to 8 cycles. The end of the fertile period, taking into account sperm and ovum survival at 2 to 3 days and 24 hours respectively, is estimated by subtracting 11 days from the longest of those 6- to 8-month cycles. For example, if a woman's cycle lasts 23 to 32 days, abstinence would be required from day 10 to day 21, a total of 11 days. A woman whose cycle varies from 23 to 31 days would abstain from intercourse from day 5 to day 20 of her cycle, or a total of 16 days. Charts are available that show how to calculate the fertile period, and these may be provided by the health-care setting.

The calendar rhythm method has several disadvantages:

- Incorrect calculations can result in pregnancy.
- Variations in normal menstrual patterns and changes in menstrual cycles over time can lead to incorrect calculations.
- Irregular bleeding confused with a menstrual period can result in incorrect calculations.
- Consistent recording of menstrual cycles is necessary.
- Long periods of abstinence from sexual intercourse are necessary.

Temperature Method

The temperature method of birth control uses the single physical sign of a rise in basal body temperature (BBT) to predict ovulation. A temperature rise at midcycle, called the *thermal shift,* normally occurs in all fertile cycles. A temperature elevation of approximately 0.5°F occurs after ovulation and continues for the rest of the cycle, as shown in Figure 8-5. (See Chapter 7.) This slight elevation occurs in response to the production of progesterone from the corpus luteum and verifies ovulation as well as fertility.

The daily BBT is recorded each day of the cycle, but since the temperature elevation occurs after ovulation, this event can never be anticipated. For this reason, absti-

SELF-CARE TEACHING

Natural Family Planning

How to Determine Your Fertile Period

Follow these steps to determine exactly when the fertile, or unsafe, days occur in your monthly cycle.

1. Keep a written record of your monthly cycle for 12 consecutive months. Count the first day of menstruation as day 1 of the cycle and the day before the next menstruation as the last day of the cycle. At the end of 12 months, determine how many days were in the longest cycle and how many were in the shortest one.
2. To establish the first fertile, or unsafe, day of your period, subtract 18 from the number of days in the shortest cycle.
3. To establish the last fertile day of your period, subtract 11 from the number of days in the longest cycle.

Example

Suppose that for the previous year your cycles varied from 26 to 29 days in length. Your fertile, or unsafe, period would be from day 8 (26 days minus 18) to day 18 (29 days minus 11). Counting from the first day of menstruation (day 1), you could have intercourse safely up to day 8 and after day 18. Intercourse would not be safe during the 11 days in between. Similarly, if your cycles varied from 30 to 34 days over a 12-month period, you could not have intercourse safely on the 12 days between day 12 and day 23 of your cycle.

Tables to Determine Your Fertile Period

If your shortest cycle has been:	Your first fertile (unsafe) day is:	If your longest cycle has been:	Your last fertile (unsafe) day is:
21 days	day 3	21 days	day 10
22 days	day 4	22 days	day 11
23 days	day 5	23 days	day 12
24 days	day 6	24 days	day 13
25 days	day 7	25 days	day 14
26 days	day 8	26 days	day 15
27 days	day 9	27 days	day 16
28 days	day 10	28 days	day 17
29 days	day 11	29 days	day 18
30 days	day 12	30 days	day 19
31 days	day 13	31 days	day 20
32 days	day 14	32 days	day 21
33 days	day 15	33 days	day 22
34 days	day 16	34 days	day 23
35 days	day 17	35 days	day 24

nence from intercourse begins the first day of menses and continues until the third day of temperature elevation. Coitus is confined to the postovulatory period, which lasts for approximately 10 days.

Some disadvantages of the temperature method are:

- BBT does not predict ovulation.
- Long periods of abstinence are required.
- Daily temperature must be carefully taken before arising in the morning.
- BBT is inaccurate when illness or fever occurs.
- Some women may not be able to recognize the temperature elevation.
- Temperature charts are sometimes uninterpretable.

Cervical Mucus Method

Women who use the cervical mucus method of birth control must become familiar with their daily cervical mucus discharge. They must be taught by trained and skillful professionals to recognize and interpret cervical mucus changes that respond to varying estrogen levels.

To learn this method, women must be able to differentiate feelings of dryness, moistness, and wetness at the vaginal opening that occur during various phases of the menstrual cycle. In addition, different types of mucus must be distinguished. During the pre- and postovulatory phases, the mucus is yellowish and viscous (the viscosity discourages the movement and maintenance of sperm). At ovulation, the mucus becomes clear and slippery

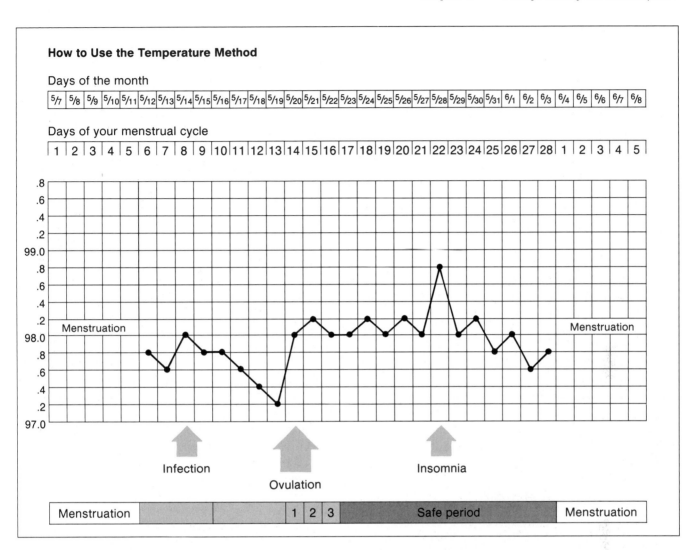

How to Use the Temperature Method

Days of the month

| 5/7 | 5/8 | 5/9 | 5/10 | 5/11 | 5/12 | 5/13 | 5/14 | 5/15 | 5/16 | 5/17 | 5/18 | 5/19 | 5/20 | 5/21 | 5/22 | 5/23 | 5/24 | 5/25 | 5/26 | 5/27 | 5/28 | 5/29 | 5/30 | 5/31 | 6/1 | 6/2 | 6/3 | 6/4 | 6/5 | 6/6 | 6/7 | 6/8 |

Days of your menstrual cycle

| 1 | 2 | 3 | 4 | 5 | 6 | 7 | 8 | 9 | 10 | 11 | 12 | 13 | 14 | 15 | 16 | 17 | 18 | 19 | 20 | 21 | 22 | 23 | 24 | 25 | 26 | 27 | 28 | 1 | 2 | 3 | 4 | 5 |

The basal body thermometer, also known as an ovulation thermometer, only measures temperatures between 96°F and 100°F and can be used orally or rectally. You will want to keep one of these special thermometers at your bedside. You also should have handy graph paper for your temperature chart, and a pencil to record your temperature before getting up.

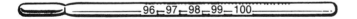

• In the morning, just after waking and before any activity, take your temperature and record it as a dot on the chart like the one shown.
• Note on the chart any event other than ovulation that might make your temperature rise. Insomnia, infections, tension, even using an electric blanket may cause a daily rise in temperature.
• Note your menstruation period on the chart.
• Keep this chart for 6 months. Your safe days for intercourse will be from 3 days after the sudden drop in temperature until 3 or 4 days after your period is over. For some women, it is difficult to attend to the temperature-taking procedure first thing in the morning. It has been shown that if the temperature is taken regularly at 5:00 p.m., or at bedtime, these temperatures can be charted in the same way as the basal body temperature. Whenever you choose to measure your temperature, accuracy and consistency are of great importance.

Figure 8-5. Using the temperature method.

(much like egg white) in response to high estrogen levels. It becomes stretchable (a quality referred to as *spinnbarkeit*) and produces a ferning pattern when dried on a slide and viewed with a microscope. (See Figures 7–4 and 7–5.)

Time and motivation are required by this method. Daily assessment of the mucus pattern and interpretation of its quality and quantity demand not only a knowledge of reproductive physiology but dedication to the use of the method as well.

To prevent pregnancy, abstinence begins on the first day after menses on which mucus is observed and continues until the fourth day after the peak of symptoms.

Disadvantages of the cervical mucus method are:

- Menstrual flow may disguise the onset of cervical mucus secretions.
- During the dry "safe" days without mucus, intercourse is not permitted on consecutive days, since seminal fluid might be confused with cervical mucus.
- Abstinence is recommended if at any time during the cycle there has been confusion about the quality of the mucus.
- Douching will change the quality and quantity of the cervical mucus.
- Vaginal infections may mask mucus changes.
- Lubricants used for intercourse will change or mask the mucus.

Sympto-Thermal Method

The sympto-thermal method combines techniques for determining the fertile period. The calendar and mucus changes are used to estimate the onset of fertility; the BBT and mucus changes are used to estimate the end of fertility. For example, abstinence begins when indicated by calendar calculations or when mucus is first noted—whichever comes first. In the calendar method, the start of the fertile period is calculated by subtracting 20 days from the length of the shortest period noted of the six preceding cycles. The end of the fertile period is determined to begin on the fourth day after the peak of cervical mucus, or on the evening of the third day of consecutive high temperatures. Other indicators that can be used are midcycle spotting or pain (*mittelschmerz*), observation of the position and dilation of the cervix, breast tenderness, mood changes, and edema.

This method provides the couple with more information to use in assessing cyclical changes. Advocates of the method strongly recommend the partner's inclusion in fertility regulation. They suggest that the woman make the observations while the partner records the information.

The sympto-thermal method is more difficult to learn than other natural family planning methods because of the number of indicators that must be monitored. Six months of guidance and careful supervision by a trained person may be needed before the method can be used with confidence.

Disadvantages of the sympto-thermal method include:

- All the disadvantages of the temperature, calendar, and mucus methods
- The need for lengthy and concentrated instruction
- The impossibility of spontaneous sex

Effectiveness

Although all of these techniques identify the fertile period, not one of them is precise, and therefore prolonged periods of abstinence may be required. It may be necessary for the couple to abstain from sex for one quarter to one half of the normal menstrual cycle. Depending as they do on the motivation of the user, these methods are generally less effective in preventing pregnancy than some of the other contraceptive methods.

Implications for Nursing Care

With additional training and experience with these methods, the nurse then may be responsible for instructing the patient in the correct use of the selected method of natural birth control. (See Fig 8–5 and Self-Care Teaching: Natural Family Planning.)

MALE CONTRACEPTION

Only about 6% of the world's population uses some method of birth control. The primary method used by men is the condom since one in three couples rely on male contraception.

In a 1987 survey 46 million couples were believed to use condoms, while 75 million men worldwide had vasectomies. Unknown millions were believed to rely on the withdrawal method (coitus interruptus). The search for an acceptable antifertility drug for men has proven to be formidable. To be effective, such a drug would have to assure 100% absence of spermatozoa in the semen (azoospermia) over an extended period of time.

A safe antifertility pill for men may be in the offing. The pill will need to fulfill certain criteria: (1) be capable of suppressing sperm production or maturation; (2) be reversible; (3) not interfere with libido; and (4) not compromise the health status of the male.

Researchers have thus far focused their attention either on hormonal interventions to suppress spermatogenesis or chemical approaches that would interfere with sperm maturation.

The use of Glossypol, a polyphenolic substance found in the seed and root bark of certain cotton plant species in China, offers promise. An antifertility effect is seen in users of the cooking oil made from the seeds. The anti-spermatic effect on men is being investigated and is currently undergoing animal studies.

Coitus Interruptus

Coitus interruptus (withdrawal) is one of the oldest methods of fertility control. In some parts of the world it is still used more often than either the condom or the pill. The practice of coitus interruptus requires the male to withdraw his penis from the vagina just before ejaculation occurs. He must be careful not to spill semen in the vagina or at the introitus as he withdraws. Pregnancy has been known to occur from ejaculate remaining at the introitus even when penetration has not occurred. Moreover, pre-ejaculatory fluid may leak from the penis without either partner's awareness. One of the major disadvantages of this method is its high failure rate.

There are no medical side-effects from use of coitus interruptus. However, the sex act itself may cause anxiety if the woman or man fears that he may not be able to control ejaculation. Thus, sexual experience is less than optimal for both the man and the woman.

Coitus interruptus has several advantages:

- The method is medically safe.
- No preparation for sex is needed.
- No expense is entailed.
- Its use is better than no contraception at all.
- It is a good back-up method of contraception.
- It permits sexual spontaneity.

The disadvantages of coitus interruptus are as follows:

- High incidence of pregnancy
- Interruption of sexual excitement or plateau
- Diminished pleasure for the couple
- Anxiety about the man's ability to withdraw before ejaculation

ELECTIVE ABORTION (THERAPEUTIC ABORTION)

In January 1973 the U.S. Supreme Court issued a landmark decision legalizing abortion in the United States. Since that time numerous controversies have arisen concerning funding, state regulation of abortion, where, when, and how abortions can be performed, and restriction of services. Recently, there has been controversy over

Common Reasons for Unwanted Pregnancies

- Lack of access to birth control
- Lack of knowledge of where to seek care, or fear of doing so
- Failure of the contraceptive method
- Failure to use a back-up method during early use of a new method or after missing pills
- Use of less effective contraceptive methods, such as douching, withdrawal, rhythm method
- Late or no return visits to the health care setting to obtain more pills or have IUD replaced or diaphragm refitted
- Lack of funds to pay for a contraceptive method
- Psychosocial conflicts:
  Denial that pregnancy can occur (most common among teen-agers)
  Belief that sex must be completely spontaneous
  Ambivalence regarding pregnancy
  Desire for independence (among teen-agers)
  Attempt to involve partner in marriage or relationship through pregnancy
  Prior pregnancy that was aborted because of peer or family pressure
  Desire to confirm femininity
  Thrill of risk taking
  Identity conflicts

policies requiring parental notification when pregnant minors seek abortions.

Since 1982 the federal government has provided funding for abortion only when there is a threat to the pregnant woman's life or the pregnancy was a result of rape or incest. This does not mean that abortions are illegal, but simply that funding for them is restricted.

Factors contributing to pregnancies that are neither wanted nor planned are multiple and complex. They include physical, social, and emotional stressors that women may not be able to recognize or control. Some common reasons for unwanted pregnancies are listed in the accompanying display.

Elective abortion (often called therapeutic abortion) is a voluntary method of terminating an unplanned, unwanted pregnancy. When unplanned pregnancy occurs, there are several options for the woman to consider. The woman or couple may choose to continue the pregnancy and keep the baby, continue the pregnancy and relinquish the baby for adoption, or request a therapeutic abortion. Since back-up abortion after contraceptive failure is a family planning issue, it is discussed here.

Methods of Abortion

Menstrual Extraction

Vacuum extraction of the uterine contents 5 to 7 weeks after the last menstrual period is rarely performed today, since detection of pregnancy within 6 days of conception is now possible with the radioimmunoassay pregnancy test. Before the development of this test, pregnancy could not be diagnosed until 42 days after the last menstrual period. Thus, menstrual extraction was performed before it was known whether pregnancy had actually occurred. Early vacuum abortion has now taken the place of this procedure.

Early Vacuum Abortion (Suction Curettage)

Early vacuum abortion now accounts for 80% of abortions performed in the United States. Uterine contents are removed by suction under local or general anesthesia. When general anesthesia is used, the procedure must be performed in a hospital, and cost to the patient is high. When local anesthesia is used, the abortion can be safely done in an office as long as medical facilities are available nearby if serious problems or side-effects are encountered.

The cervix is dilated with metal dilators or with laminaria that have been set in place 6 to 24 hours prior to the procedure. Laminaria are short, rounded pieces of a Japanese seaweed that is hygroscopic (i.e., that absorbs water). When one or more of these small sticks of compressed seaweed are inserted into the cervix, they draw fluid from the cervical canal and expand, causing the canal to dilate. Cervical dilation occurs slowly, and this method is preferred by many physicians over the use of metal dilators, since it is less traumatic to the cervix.

A suction tube is inserted into the uterus and the uterine lining is aspirated within 3 to 5 minutes (Fig. 8–6). A uterine curette is then used to scrape any remaining tissue from the uterine wall. Cramping may last up to 20 minutes after the procedure is completed. The physician examines the uterine tissue carefully to identify the placental villi that signal successful abortion. The specimen can also be sent to the pathology lab if villi are not seen or the tissue appears abnormal.

Dilatation and Evacuation

Dilatation and evacuation may be performed at 13 to 24 weeks and vacuum curettage and curette scraping used as in early vacuum abortion. However, it requires greater dilatation of the uterus, since the products of conception are larger. The use of crushing instruments and a large-bore vacuum curette may be necessary in pregnancies approaching 24 weeks.

The cervix is dilated with laminaria. After the administration of local or general anesthesia, the laminaria are removed and the cervix is dilated with metal dilators. The uterine contents are evacuated with suction and other instruments as necessary. This method is safer than amniocentesis but may be more stressful to the physician performing the abortion and to the nurse assisting him or her.

Amniocentesis

Amniocentesis, performed at 15 to 24 weeks, involves inserting a hollow needle into the amniotic sac surrounding the fetus. Amniocentesis can only be performed after 15 weeks of pregnancy when the amount of fluid in the amniotic sac is adequate to permit the removal of a small amount.

A local anesthetic is used to numb the skin over the site where the needle is injected. An 18-gauge needle is inserted through the abdomen into the amniotic sac, and a small amount of fluid is removed. Over a 10-minute period, a dose of prostaglandin is infused into the sac to initiate uterine contractions. The patient is awake, and an intravenous infusion of saline maintains her hydration. Uterine contractions begin in 12 to 48 hours, and the patient experiences contractions until the fetus is born (usually dead but occasionally alive).

Side-Effects and Complications

Infection.   Postabortion infection may occur 24 to 36 hours after the abortion and may cause fever, vaginal discharge, cramping, and general fatigue. When the infection is mild and in its early stages, it can be treated on an outpatient basis. If the problem involves products of conception retained in the uterus, dilatation and curettage (D&C) is required after sufficient intravenous antibiotic levels are obtained. When infection spreads further into the pelvis or abdominal cavity, hospitalization is required. Nursing care of pelvic infections is discussed in Chapter 30.

Continuation of Pregnancy.   In rare cases abortion is unsuccessful and pregnancy continues, evidenced by symptoms of pregnancy and a growing uterus. Such cases are the result of inadequate curettage of the uterine lining.

Bleeding.   Excessive bleeding can occur after any abortion procedure, but it is less common when local anesthesia is used. General anesthesia relaxes the uterine musculature, rendering it unable to contract and clamp down on bleeding vessels. Bleeding is more common after late prostaglandin amniocentesis.

Uterine or Cervical Trauma.   Injury can occur to the cervix during dilatation but is less likely when laminaria

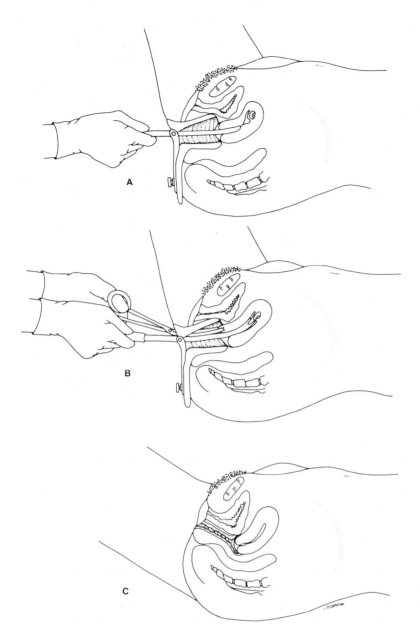

Figure 8–6. First trimester abortion: vacuum aspiration. *(A)* A speculum is inserted into the vagina, and the cervix is anesthetized. The cervix is gradually dilated with increasingly larger dilators. *(B)* A ring forceps holds the cervix steady while the suction tube is passed through the cervix. Suction is applied until all the products of conception (fetus, placenta, membranes) have been aspirated. *(C)* The suction tube, clamp, and speculum are removed. The vagina, cervix, and uterus will quickly return to their nonpregnant state. (Childbirth Graphics)

are used. Perforation of the uterus may occur during suction or D&C abortions. In many cases the perforations heal spontaneously and without symptoms. If cervical injuries are extensive, incompetence of the cervical os may result and present problems with maintaining subsequent pregnancies.

Implications for Nursing Care

The nurse's role in caring for women desiring therapeutic abortion is one of physical and emotional support. Collection of historical, physical, and laboratory data will depend on the routine of the health care setting in which the nurse is functioning. Counseling and support of the patient are uniquely nursing functions, unless a designated abortion counselor performs these services.

Assessment

Patient History

Health History.   Previous conditions that could affect the well-being of a woman seeking a therapeutic abortion include a history of heart disease (such as rheumatic fever in childhood), blood-clotting disorders, drug allergies and usage, seizure disorders, urinary tract infections, metabolic disorders (*i.e.,* diabetes), and hereditary diseases such as sickle cell anemia. Her blood type (including Rh factor) and that of her partner should be supplied if known. Episodes of sexually transmitted diseases or vaginal infections should be documented.

SELF-CARE TEACHING

Following an Abortion

- Normal activities may be resumed, but avoid strenuous work or exercise for a few days.
- Resume normal eating and drinking habits.
- Bleeding and cramping may occur for a week or two. If either becomes severe, seek medical advice. Light bleeding and spotting are normal for about a month.
- Menstruation should resume in 4 to 6 weeks.
- Use a method of birth control if you have sex before menstruation resumes. It is possible to get pregnant during this period.
- Do not use tampons for the first week after the abortion to avoid possible infection. Use sanitary pads instead.
- Refrain from intercourse for 1 week after abortion. You are vulnerable to infection until the uterine lining heals.
- Refrain from douching for 1 week to prevent infection.
- Take your temperature twice a day to detect possible infection. If it goes up to 100°F or more, seek medical help.
- Keep your follow-up appointment in 2 weeks. It is important to ensure your full recovery.

Reproductive History. The patient's menstrual history should include the date of the last menstrual period (LMP) in order to determine the length of the pregnancy; the accuracy of this date is important, and it should be obtained carefully. The regularity of past menstrual periods, their length, the amount of bleeding, and presence of pain or premenstrual symptoms should also be documented.

The history of previous pregnancies should include the dates and outcomes. Previous abortions (spontaneous or therapeutic) and past major or minor surgery, such as tubal ligation, cesarean sections, cervical cryosurgery or conization, or myomectomy (removal of fibroids), should be noted.

The contraceptive history should include all past use of contraception, methods, length of use, effect on menstrual cycles, side-effects or other problems, and reasons for discontinuing their use. Plans for future contraceptive use should be noted.

Physical Examination

A physical assessment may be performed by the nurse or physician. If it is done by the nurse, the physician performing the abortion will repeat the pelvic examination to verify the size of the uterus in weeks (necessary for determining the type of abortion procedure), to examine the vagina and cervix for abnormalities and tenderness, and to collect Pap smear and gonorrhea and chlamydia cultures if they were not previously done. The position of the uterus must be assessed to determine the placement of instruments during the abortion procedure. The adnexal area is palpated for tenderness or ovarian enlargement.

Laboratory Data

Laboratory data to be collected include a serum or urine pregnancy test, complete blood count to check for anemia and evidence of possible hereditary blood disorders, blood type, and Rh factor; VDRL test, urinalysis, and maternal antibody screen for the Rh-negative woman, who would be given RhoGam after the abortion to prevent isoimmunization.

Part of the responsibility of the family planning nurse is to counsel the pregnant woman about her alternatives. When a definite decision has been made to proceed with the abortion, the nurse arranges for the procedure with the woman or couple, including an early appointment and assurance that a support person will take her home after the procedure. The procedure and possible complications are discussed before the informed consent form is signed. The nurse should plan to discuss postabortion complications, their signs, and the need for immediate care (see Chapter 19); make an appointment for a follow-up visit; and discuss the use of postabortion birth control, guided by her earlier assessment.

PERMANENT CONTRACEPTION: SURGICAL STERILIZATION

Sterilization is a permanent method of contraception available to both men and women, who choose it for the following reasons:

- They are unsatisfied with reversible contraceptive methods
- They have completed their families
- They need 10 to 20 years of pregnancy protection.

More than 60 million women have chosen sterilization to control their fertility, making it the world's leading family planning method.

Informed Consent

Because sterilization must be considered an irreversible procedure, a couple's decision must be based on complete and clear information. Many couples do not realize that once the procedure is performed, fertility is permanently ended. Moreover, increasing numbers of young women under 25 are seeking permanent sterilization. Some have no children and want to remain childless, while others feel that they have completed their families. These women need time and careful counseling prior to their decision making. Their life situation may change, and along with that change may come a desire for children.

When procedures are funded by the Department of Health and Human Services, federal regulations apply. Approximately 10% of sterilizations performed are funded by the U.S. government. Regulations for these procedures require that the woman be at least 21 years old and receive counseling before signing consent forms. After signing, there is a mandatory 30-day wait to give her time to reconsider. The consent form is then valid for 180 days only. In emergency situations there are exceptions to this rule.

The regulations require that the following information be supplied before surgery is performed:

- Complete explanation of the procedure
- Discussion of minor and life-threatening risks and possible side-effects
- Discussion of alternative birth control methods and the irreversibility of the sterilization procedure
- Description of possible benefits
- Reassurance that a change of mind will not jeopardize future health care or monetary benefits

The woman must also be given an opportunity to ask questions, and an informed consent form must be signed.

Female Sterilization

Tubal ligation blocks the fallopian tubes and prevents the ovum from migrating into the uterus. A variety of methods are used, including ligation, coagulation, and the application of clips, rings, or bands. All of these are accomplished by entering the pelvis through the abdominal wall or the posterior vaginal cul-de-sac.

Abdominal Tubal Ligations

Minilaparotomy. Minilaparotomy can be performed during the postpartum period or at any other time for women wanting an outpatient procedure with local anesthesia. It is an easy procedure for the physician to perform, requires only simple instruments, and has a short recovery period.

A small horizontal incision is made 1 inch above the pubic bone, and the fallopian tubes are occluded one at a time. The Pomeroy technique is commonly used. The two ends of the tube will heal, and scar tissue will close the lumen. Recovery from this procedure is swift, and the woman can return home within a few hours.

The procedure can only be performed on women who are slim and have freely movable tubes and uterus. The many women who prefer general to local anesthesia would not be suitable candidates for this procedure. Reversibility is unpredictable.

Laparoscopic Tubal Ligation. Another tubal ligation procedure is performed with a laparoscope under general anesthesia. Patient recovery is rapid, and there is a low rate of complications.

The laparoscope is an endoscopic instrument that, when inserted into the abdomen or pelvis, permits visualization of the organs. The tubes are occluded by coagulation, excised by the Pomeroy technique, or clamped with bands or clips. The procedure cannot be used in women during the early postpartum period. Laparoscopy requires experience and skill and is costly. Reversibility is unpredictable.

Vaginal Tubal Ligations

Colpotomy. Colpotomy involves making a surgical incision through the posterior vaginal fornix to provide access to the pelvic cavity. It is used primarily in women of high parity and may be performed under general or local anesthesia in an outpatient or inpatient setting. The whole procedure is concluded within one half hour. Little postoperative pain is experienced by the patient.

Colpotomy cannot be used in the early postpartum period and has a higher rate of complications from infection and hemorrhage than other forms of tubal ligation. Reversibility is unpredictable.

Culdoscopy. In *culdoscopy* the physician gains access to the fallopian tubes and uterus through the posterior cul-de-sac by means of an endoscope. This procedure is seldom used. It cannot be performed in the early postpartum period, and the skill of the physician has to be great. Reversibility is unpredictable. The use of colpotomy and culdoscopy has been largely replaced by the minilaparotomy procedure.

Reversibility of Tubal Ligations

As the volume of voluntary tubal ligations escalates, so does the number of women seeking reversal procedures. Presently, the odds for sterilization reversal are not good. Sterilization methods now used cause such damage to the tubes that reanastomosis is difficult at best. Risk of ectopic pregnancy is ten times greater than normal after tubal reversal.

Some sterilization methods are easier to reverse than others. Electrocautery destroys about 4 cm or more of the tube and is the most difficult method to reverse. The popular Pomeroy technique removes 3 cm of the tube,

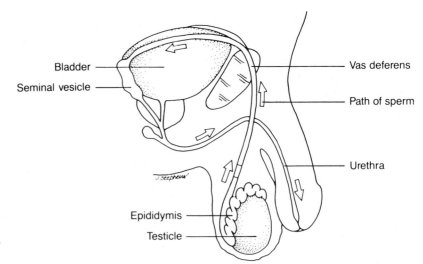

Figure 8–7. Pathway of sperm in ejaculation. (Childbirth Graphics)

making it less difficult to rejoin. Tubal ligation using the newer rings and clips may be more easily reversed, since less of the tube is involved.

Hysterectomy

The risk of serious complications, including death, is 10 to 100 times higher for women having hysterectomies than for those having tubal sterilization. Hysterectomy is major abdominal surgery, and the cost, recovery time, and psychological trauma are such that this procedure should be considered only when pathologic problems dictate its use. It should never be used for voluntary sterilization alone.

Male Sterilization: Vasectomy

Bilateral partial vasectomy is an uncomplicated operative procedure and the simplest and safest method of surgical sterilization. It produces sterility by interrupting the vas deferens and preventing sperm from being ejaculated in the semen (Fig. 8–7).

Local anesthesia is used, and the procedure takes less than 30 minutes in a doctor's office or clinic. A small incision is made in each of the scrotal sacs. The vas deferens is pulled through the incision, cut, and tied as shown in Figure 8–8. The stumps of the vas are often coagulated for greater safety (but less reversibility). The man is able to walk almost immediately following surgery. Some discomfort, such as soreness and swelling of the scrotum, and some minor bleeding under the skin might be experienced for a day or two. Use of a jockstrap, ice packs, rest, and aspirin usually relieves the symptoms.

The patient must be informed that he will not become immediately sterile, since the vas contains sperm for 1 to 3 months. Pregnancy can occur during this time, so contraception will have to be used. After 3 months, a specimen of semen is examined, and if it is free of sperm, sterilization is complete. Reversibility depends to a large extent on the type of procedure that was done.

CHAPTER SUMMARY

The nurse plays a variety of important roles in the family planning setting: teacher, counselor, supporter, and re-

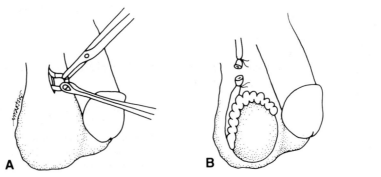

Figure 8–8. Vasectomy. *(A)* Local anesthetic is injected, a small incision is made in both scrotal sacs. The vas deferens is pulled through the incision in each. *(B)* The vas deferens is cut and tied or coagulated. *(C)* The incisions are closed. (Childbirth Graphics)

source person. Most of all, she brings a special understanding and empathy to patient care. She understands the couple's need to control the number and spacing of children. In today's world, control of fertility is basic to the couple's relationship, their ability to provide for their offspring, the health of the mother, and their plans for the future.

The nurse can give the couple the information they need to make an appropriate and informed decision about birth control. By urging the couple to seek ongoing care from the family planning setting when problems or questions arise, the nurse encourages proper use of their birth control method, and therefore greater success with it.

STUDY QUESTIONS

1. Why is family planning important to our world and to the quality of human life?
2. What physiologic mechanisms are responsible for the effectiveness of oral contraception?
3. Name some health benefits that result from oral contraceptive use. Name some of the most common side-effects and contraindications to oral contraception.
4. How can the nurse help to increase compliance in oral contraceptive users?
5. Discuss the patient population most favorably disposed to the use of a diaphragm and the reasons for their choice.
6. What makes the nurse's role in diaphragm use so important?
7. Name the currently used IUDs. What are the most common reasons why women discontinue IUD use?
8. What problems may arise when pregnancy occurs in a woman wearing an IUD? How is this situation resolved?
9. Discuss the concept and the various methods of natural family planning. Why do couples choose these methods?
10. What are the advantages and disadvantages of surgical sterilization for men and women? What methods of sterilization are used?
11. How can the nurse prevent personal bias from intruding into the teaching of birth control methods?

REFERENCES/BIBLIOGRAPHY

A fresh look at barrier contraceptives. Contemp OB/GYN 31(3):132, 1988

Alza Corporation, Projestasert Intrauterine Progesterone Contraceptive System. Informational package insert, 1986

Connel EB: Moderator: What's new in contraceptive methods? ACOG/AMA/CME Forum. Female Patient 10:(11):24, 1985

Cramer DW, Schiff I, Schoenbaum JB, et al: Tubal infertility and the intrauterine device. N Engl J Med 321(15):941–947, 1986

Darney P: Contraception: Are implants the answer? Contemp OB/GYN 28(1):29–37, 1986

Dickey RP: Managing Contraceptive Pill Patients, 5th ed. Durant, Creative Informatics, 1987

Elliot J, Anderson L, Bernstein S: Progress report on a study of the cervical cap. Center for Population Planning, University of Michigan, Ann Arbor, 1984

Forrest JD: The end of IUD marketing in the United States: What does it mean for American women? Fam Plann Perspec 18(2):52–55, 1986

Greydanus DE: Contraception. In Lavery JP, Sanfilippi JS (eds): Pediatric and Adolescent Obstetrics and Gynecology, p 234. New York, Springer–Verlag, 1985

Henshaw SK, Binkin NJ, Blaine E, Smith JC: A portrait of American women who obtain abortions. Fam Plann Perspec 17(2):90–96, 1985

Herceg–Baron, Furstenburg FF, Shea J, et al: Supporting teenager's use of contraceptives: A comparison of clinic services. Fam Plann Perspec 18(2):61, 1986

Kugel C, Verson H: Relationship between weight change and diaphragm size change. J Obstet Gynecol Neonatal Nurs 15(2):123–129, 1986

Oral-contraceptive Use and the Risk of Breast Cancer: The Cancer and Steroid Hormone Study of the Centers for Disease Control and the National Institute of Child Health and Human Development, 1986

Population Reports Family Planning Programs, Series J #32, Sept/Oct 1986. Baltimore, Population Information Program, The Johns Hopkins University

Rosenfield A: Contraception: Where are we in 1985? Contemp OB/GYN 25(2):79–97, 1985

Speroff L: Which birth control pill should be prescribed today? Contemp OB/GYN 29(3):102, 1987

Waites GN: Male fertility regulation recent advances. Bull WHO 64(2):151–158, 1986

Whitley N: Contraceptive Sterilization: A Manual of Clinical Obstetrics, pp 727–765. Philadelphia, JB Lippincott, 1985

Willson JR, Carrington ER, Laros RK et al: Obstetrics and Gynecology, 8th ed, pp 205–209. St. Louis, CV Mosby, 1987

SUGGESTED READINGS

Copper-bearing IUD introduced in United States. NAACOG Newslet 15(1):9, 1988

Dirubbo NE, The condom barrier. Am J Nurs 87(10):52, 1987

Forrest JD: The end of IUD marketing in the United States: What does it mean for American women? Fam Plann Perspec 18(2):52, 1986

Johnson MA: The cervical cap as a contraceptive alternative. Nurse Prac 10(1):37, 1985

Kellinger KG: Factors in adolescent contraceptive use. Nurse Pract 10(8):55, 1985

Matis N: Natural family planning: A birth control alternative. J Nurse-Midwifery 28(1):7, 1983

Neidhardt A: Why me: Second trimester abortion. Am J Nurs 86(10):1133, 1986

Speroff L: Which birth control pill should be prescribed today? Contemp OB/GYN, 29(3):102, 1987

Schneider TR: Voluntary termination of pregnancy. J Obset Gynecol Neonatal Nurs (Suppl): 1984

Vansintejan GA, Purdy PJ: International family-planning training for Nurse Practitioners. J Obstet Gynecol Neonatal Nurs 15(6):42, 1986

Youngkin EQ, Miller LG: The triphasics: Insights for effective clinical use. Nurse Pract 12(2):17, 1987

9 genetics and genetic counseling

LEARNING OBJECTIVES

After studying the material in this chapter, the student should be able to

- Identify those patients who should be referred for genetic counseling, genetic screening, and prenatal diagnostic testing

- Discuss how genes are transmitted in families

- Describe common genetic disorders

- Explain genetic screening methods and prenatal diagnostic techniques

- Describe the process of genetic counseling

- Discuss psychological and social problems encountered in genetic counseling

- Explain the goals of nursing care for women and families who have a history of genetic disease or who are in need of genetic counseling

KEY TERMS

Alleles

Autosome

Amniocentesis

Carrier

Chromosomes

Chromosome disorder

Deoxyribonucleic acid (DNA)

Dominant trait

Gene

Heterozygote

Homologous chromosomes

Homozygote

Karyotype

Locus

Meiosis

Mitosis

Monosomy

Mosaicism

Multifactorial

Mutation

Proband

Recessive

Recurrence risk

Sex chromosome

Trisomy

Genetics is the science of heredity, and genes are the coded sequences of information by which cellular organisms regulate their embryologic development, metabolic functioning, growth, and reproduction. The study of human genetics is becoming increasingly important to the childbearing process because genetic factors play a role in the etiology of many birth defects and a variety of human diseases. Several studies of newborns indicate that approximately 1 in 50 newborns (2%) has a major congenital abnormality. Although environmental factors, such as infection and nutritional deficiencies, are thought to be the underlying cause in about 60% of these congenital abnormalities, about 40% are thought to have a hereditary origin. An even more dramatic example of the importance of genetic factors in the causation of medical events is the finding that in over 60% of first-trimester spontaneous abortions, the conceptus has a chromosomal abnormality.

Most prospective parents are not aware of these facts. Therefore, there is an ongoing need to identify those at increased risk of having a child with a serious genetic disorder so that they can be offered genetic counseling and appropriate genetic testing. There is a need for nurses to play an active role in helping to identify and refer high-risk patients and their families for genetic services and in meeting the special psychosocial needs of those dealing with genetic disorders and congenital anomalies. The most supportive nursing care can be given only when the nurse has a thorough understanding of the principles of medical genetics and the process of genetic counseling.

This chapter provides a basic understanding of human genetics, an appreciation of the medical aspects of genetic services as they relate to obstetric care, and an overview of the variety of genetic diseases and of the services developed to meet the health care needs of those at risk for hereditary disorders.

THE GENETIC CODE

Genetic information is organized in small cellular structures known as chromosomes. Chromosomes are primarily composed of DNA (deoxyribonucleic acid), histone proteins, and nonhistone proteins. DNA is a macromolecule composed of three types of chemical units: (a) a five-carbon sugar (deoxyribose); (b) a phosphate group (PO_4); and (c) a nitrogen-containing base subunit of which there are two types, purines and pyrimidines. In DNA, there are two purines, adenine (A) and guanine (G), and two pyrimidines, thymine (T) and cytosine (C).

In humans, DNA occurs as a double-stranded helix, or spiral. Two long chemical chains of DNA molecules are wound around one another and are linked by chemical bonds so that the whole forms a shape like a spiral stair-

case (Fig. 9–1). The adenine (A) in one strand is bonded to thymine (T) in the other strand, and cytosine (C) in one strand is bonded to guanine (G) in the other strand. All the information needed for the development of an individual human being is carried in the sequence of these four nitrogen base subunits. The genetic code is a series of triplet sequences of the A, G, T, and C nitrogen bases. Three nitrogen bases, in a particular order, code for each of the 21 amino acids that are the building blocks of proteins.

A gene, or unit of hereditary information, is that region on a chromosome that codes for one particular cellular product or outcome. It is composed of coding sequences interrupted by noncoding sequences that are initially transcribed but are not represented in the mature messenger RNA. Messenger RNA (mRNA) molecules carry information originating in DNA that is subsequently used in the production of proteins. Each chromosome is thought to contain thousands of genes, lined up in a specific sequence. Therefore, each gene has a specific location on a particular chromosome. There are thought to be two types of genes: structural genes, which control the manufacture of proteins, and regulatory genes, which control the activity of structural genes.

Genetic mutations occur when there are changes in the sequence of nitrogen bases in a gene. These changes can occur in one of three ways:

One or more bases may be changed.

During chromosome replication or as a result of breakage, a part of a gene or the whole gene may be lost.

During replication or as a result of translocation, additional nitrogen bases may be added to a gene sequence.

The consequence of these changes is a misreading of the genetic code, leading to one of the following:

Absence of production of the product

Underproduction of the product

Overproduction of the product

Production of a structurally abnormal product that may be biochemically inactive or inefficient

HOW GENES ARE TRANSMITTED IN FAMILIES

Hereditary disorders are classified into three main etiologic categories. Diseases in which there is a demonstrable change in the number or structure of an individual's chromosome complement are called *chromosome disorders*. Diseases caused by a mutation at the gene level are called *single gene disorders*. Abnormalities that are

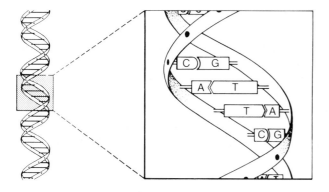

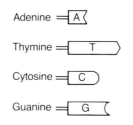

Figure 9–1. Structure of DNA.

due to the interaction of many genetic factors (polygenic inheritance) or to an interaction of environmental factors and genetic factors are termed *multifactorial disorders.*

Most hereditary diseases can be neatly placed into one of these three categories, but some appear to be caused by combinations of these etiologies. This chapter focuses on the three main categories.

Chromosomal Inheritance in Families

Classification and Replication of Human Chromosomes

With the exception of mature red blood cells, which have no nucleus, chromosomes are present in every cell in the body. Genes are arranged in specific sequences on each chromosome and serve as vehicles for the transmission of genetic information. The movement of chromosomes during cellular division and sexual reproduction closely follows the basic laws of inheritance first described by Gregor Mendel in the 19th century.

The number, sizes, and shapes of chromosomes within a cell are fixed properties for all normal members of any species. With the exception of ova and sperm, all somatic cells in the normal human have 46 chromosomes. These include 22 pairs of chromosomes called *autosomes.* Each autosome is structurally identical to its partner, but different from all other autosomes. In addition to autosomes, there are two sex-determining chromosomes in each cell. These are labeled X and Y. Normal males have one X and one Y chromosome, and normal females have two X chromosomes (Fig. 9–2). Sperm and egg cells, or *gametes,* each have 23 chromosomes, one autosome from each pair, and one sex chromosome.

At conception, an ovum and sperm, each containing 23 chromosomes, fuse to form the *zygote,* or fertilized ovum. The first cell of a new individual now has 46 chromosomes. Each parent has contributed equally to the offspring's genetic makeup. The mechanism by which the single-celled zygote and each resulting somatic cell reproduces its chromosomes and divides into two genetically identical daughter cells is termed *mitosis.* Mitosis usually leads to the exact duplication of genetic information, which is necessary for the differentiation, growth, and biologic maintenance of a new individual (Fig. 9–3).

Meiosis is the term applied to the division process that occurs during the production of ovum and sperm. Exchange of genetic material, which enhances genetic variability among individuals, may occur between homologous chromosomes during this division process. Meiosis allows each of these germ cells to contain half the individual's genetic information (Fig. 9–4). The fusion of gametes from two individuals promotes genetic variability, since new and potentially advantageous gene combinations can emerge at conception.

Chromosome Structure and Identification

Chromosomes are visible as compact, well-defined structures only during cell division; therefore, the tissues used to study chromosomes under the microscope must have many viable and rapidly dividing cells. Specially developed tissue culture techniques are used to obtain cells that have high rates of mitotic or meiotic divisions so that the chromosomes can be studied under the microscope and photographed. After applying one of several different chemical stains, the underlying structural features of the chromosomes, called *bands,* are revealed (Fig. 9–5).

The most common tissues used for chromosome analysis are lymphocytes, skin fibroblasts, and amniotic fluid cells. Other tissues occasionally used to study chromosomes are testicular or ovarian biopsy tissues, bone marrow, and fibroblasts from other organ tissues. The morphology of chromosomes is most easily distinguished during the early parts (metaphase and prophase — see Fig. 9-3) of the cell division cycle. In metaphase, chromosomes observed under the microscope look like *Xs* and are made up of two identical DNA double helical strands. These strands are attached to each other by a structure called the centromere (see Fig. 9–5). Each identical DNA strand is called a *sister chromatid.* The centromere divides the chromosome into a short arm region and a long arm region.

(text continued on page 201)

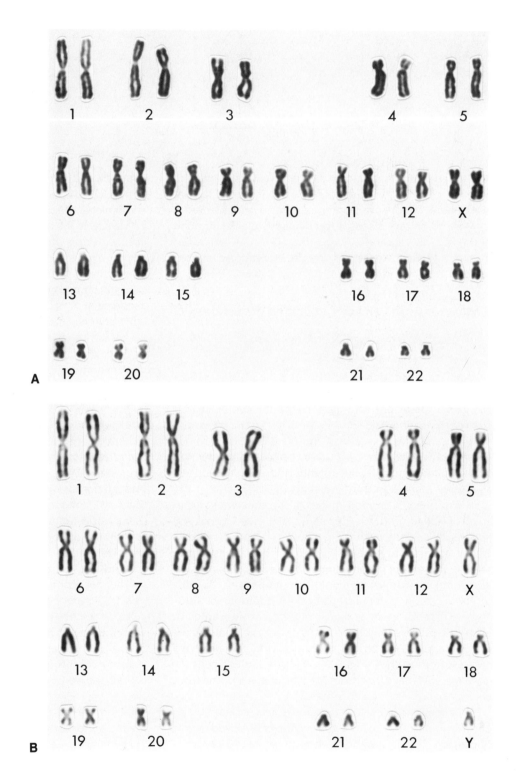

Figure 9-2. Chromosomes. (*A*) Normal female. (*B*) Normal male.

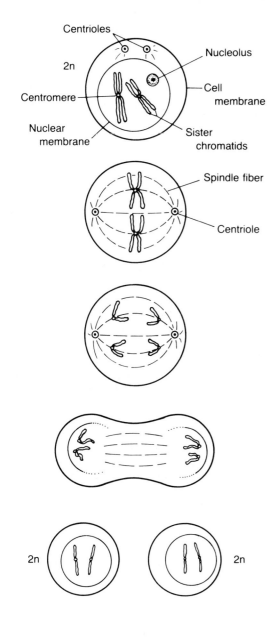

Prophase

Chromosomes are doubled, each consisting of two sister chromatids as they enter prophase. They are joined at the centromere. In late prophase/prometaphase, the nuclear membrane begins to disintegrate; centrioles separate and spindle fiber formation is seen.

Metaphase

Chromosomes line up on metaphase plate and are attached to spindle fibers at their centromere.

Anaphase

Centromeres divide, single-stranded sister chromatids (now chromosomes) are pulled to opposite poles.

Telophase

Chromosomes reach poles and begin to uncoil and elongate; division furrow is seen at cell membrane; nucleolus and nuclear membrane reform at end.

Cell divides and new daughter cells enter interphase

Figure 9–3. Mitosis (shown with one autosomal pair).

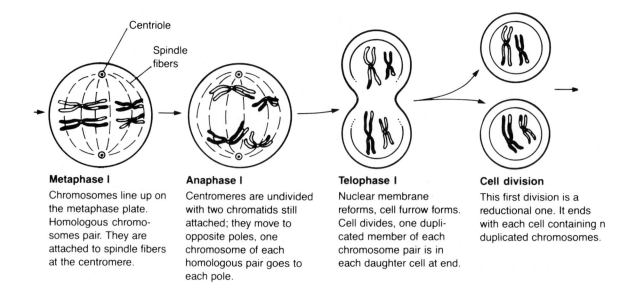

Metaphase I

Chromosomes line up on the metaphase plate. Homologous chromosomes pair. They are attached to spindle fibers at the centromere.

Anaphase I

Centromeres are undivided with two chromatids still attached; they move to opposite poles, one chromosome of each homologous pair goes to each pole.

Telophase I

Nuclear membrane reforms, cell furrow forms. Cell divides, one duplicated member of each chromosome pair is in each daughter cell at end.

Cell division

This first division is a reductional one. It ends with each cell containing n duplicated chromosomes.

As cells enter the second part of meiosis, chromosomes elongate and the nuclear membrane disintegrates. No DNA replication occurs. Each cell contains 1 set (n) of duplicated chromosomes.

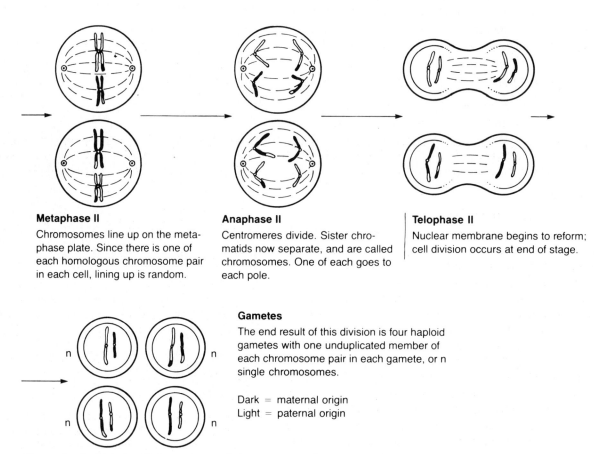

Metaphase II

Chromosomes line up on the metaphase plate. Since there is one of each homologous chromosome pair in each cell, lining up is random.

Anaphase II

Centromeres divide. Sister chromatids now separate, and are called chromosomes. One of each goes to each pole.

Telophase II

Nuclear membrane begins to reform; cell division occurs at end of stage.

Gametes

The end result of this division is four haploid gametes with one unduplicated member of each chromosome pair in each gamete, or n single chromosomes.

Dark = maternal origin
Light = paternal origin

Figure 9–4. Meiosis with two autosomal chromosome pairs.

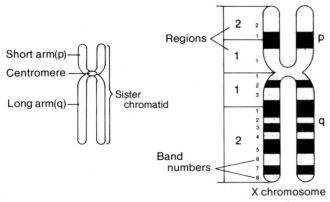

Figure 9–5. Diagrammatic representation of chromosome structure at mitotic metaphase.

The most efficient and accurate way to examine an individual's chromosomal makeup is to make a photographic *karyotype* (Fig. 9–6). A karyotype shows all the chromosomes of a single cell arranged by matching pairs from the largest to the smallest. Chromosome analysis involves the microscopic examination of 20 to 30 properly prepared cells. The number of chromosomes in each cell is counted. About five cells are also photographed so that the sequence of bands can be examined and numerical changes and structural rearrangements can be identified.

Clinical Aspects of Chromosome Disorders

Changes in chromosome number or chromosome structure are a significant cause of fetal wastage in pregnancy and, in newborns, lead to congenital abnormalities and usually severe mental retardation. The incidences of some chromosomal abnormalities are shown in Table 9–1.

Numerical Abnormalities

A change in the amount of chromosome material usually has detrimental effects during prenatal and postnatal development. The absence of a single chromosome is called *monosomy* and is almost always lethal to the embryo. The presence of an extra chromosome, called *trisomy,* is also usually incompatible with life. However, trisomies involving the smaller chromosomes are found in liveborn infants with congenital defects and mental retardation (Fig. 9–7, page 203).

Monosomies and trisomies are usually caused by mechanical accidents during meiosis. *Meiotic nondisjunction* is the term applied to the faulty mechanism whereby both members of a chromosome pair migrate together into the same cell during the first meiotic division rather than separating and each going into one of the two newly created cells. The result of this failure to separate is that two of the newly formed gametes will have 24 chromosomes and two will have 22 chromosomes, rather than each

having the normal 23. If such an abnormal ovum or sperm is fertilized, the resulting embryo will have either 47 chromosomes (trisomy) or 45 chromosomes (monosomy) in each somatic cell. The numerical chromosomal disorders are summarized in Table 9–2, page 204.

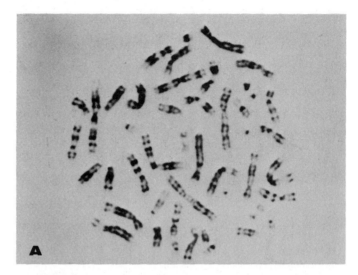

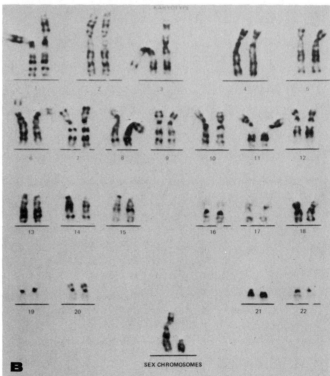

Figure 9–6. (*A*) A chromosome preparation showing a metaphase spread. (*B*) The chromosomes from this spread arranged in a karyotype, showing a normal 46, XY male. (Bannerman RM: Basic human genetics. In Iffy L, Kaminetsky HA [eds]: Principles and Practice of Obstetrics and Perinatology, Vol 1, p 26. New York, John Wiley & Sons, 1981. Courtesy of Dr. Richard L. Neu)

Table 9–1   **Incidence of Chromosomal Abnormalities in Liveborn Infants**

Abnormality	Incidence
Numerical Aberrations	
Sex Chromosomes	
47,XYY	1/1,000 MB*
47,XXY	1/1,000 MB
Other (males)	1/1,350 MB
45,X	1/10,000 FB
47,XXX	1/1,000 FB
Other (females)	1/2,700 FB
Autosomes	
Trisomies	
13–15 (D Group)	1/20,000 LB
16–18 (E Group)	1/8,000 LB
21–22 (G Group)	1/800 LB
Other	1/50,000 LB
Structural Aberrations	
Balanced Robertsonian	
t(Dq;Dq)	1/1,500 LB
t(Dq;Gq)	1/5,000 LB
Reciprocal translocations and insertional inversions	1/7,000 LB
Unbalanced	
Robertsonian	1/14,000 LB
Reciprocal translocations and insertional inversions	1/8,000 LB
Inversions	1/50,000 LB
Deletions	1/10,000 LB
Supernumeraries	1/5,000 LB
Other	1/8,000 LB
Total	1/160 LB

* LB, livebirths; MB, male births; FB, female births.
(Simpson JE: Pregnancies in women with chromosomal abnormalities. In Schulman JD, Simpson JE [eds]: Genetic Diseases in Pregnancy: Maternal Effects and Fetal Outcome. New York, Academic Press, 1981)

Autosomal Disorders

Down syndrome is the most common clinically recognized chromosome disorder. It has an incidence of 1 in every 800 births and occurs whenever an individual is born with an extra number 21 chromosome. In 95% of all cases of Down syndrome, the affected person has three structurally normal number 21 chromosomes instead of two (trisomy 21). Down syndrome (DS) refers to the clinical features mentioned below, while trisomy 21 refers to the cytogenic finding of three number 21 chromosomes. It is thought that this configuration is the result of a meiotic nondisjunction occurring in one of the parents (see Fig. 9–7). Clinical diagnosis is usually made at birth and is confirmed by karyotype analysis. The most common physical stigmata present at birth are a round face that has a flat profile; palpebral fissures characteristically slanted upward; epicanthal folds; speckling on the irises, called *Brushfield's spots;* short, flat nasal bridge; small mouth with large protruding tongue; high-arched palate; excessive loosening of skin at the nape of the neck; and simian palm creases. None of these clinical features is pathognomonic for Down syndrome.

Congenital heart defects are present in 40% to 60% of persons with trisomy 21 and often cause death in early childhood. Gastrointestinal defects are also often present, the most frequent being congenital duodenal obstruction. Mental retardation ranges from mild to severe. The incidence of leukemia in persons with Down syndrome is 20 times higher than that in the population as a whole.

Two other types of Down syndrome are known. Four percent of cases have a chromosome *translocation* in which a third number 21 chromosome is present in the cell but is attached to another chromosome (see discussion of structural abnormalities, which follows). The clinical findings are virtually identical to those in trisomy 21 Down syndrome. One percent of Down syndrome cases are the result of *mosaicism.* In this situation the affected person has two different populations of cells, one with the normal chromosome number and one with 47 chromosomes in each cell because of the presence of an extra number 21 chromosome (see discussion of structural abnormalities, which follows). The severity of clinical findings is variable and may be related to the percentage of abnormal cells and the tissues affected.

Trisomy 13 (Patau's syndrome) is a severe disorder characterized by microphthalmia, cleft lip, and postaxial polydactyly. Other clinical features include microcephaly with sloping forehead, malformed ears, congenital heart defects, urogenital defects and polycystic kidneys, and severe mental retardation. Fifty percent of children with trisomy 13 die within the first year of life.

Trisomy 18 (Edwards' syndrome) is characterized by growth retardation; micrognathia; clenched fists with the second and fifth fingers overlapping the third and fourth; rocker-bottom feet; low-set, malformed ears; prominent occiput; and congenital heart defects. Trisomy 18 infants invariably suffer severe mental retardation, and most die in early childhood.

Sex Chromosome Abnormalities

Triple X (XXX) syndrome, XXY syndrome (Klinefelter's syndrome), and *XYY syndrome* are the most common sex chromosome trisomies in newborns (see Fig. 9–7). The only monosomy compatible with life is known as *Turner's syndrome* (XO) and is caused by the loss of one sex chromosome. The effects of alterations in the sex chromosomes are less severe than those of alterations in the autosomes.

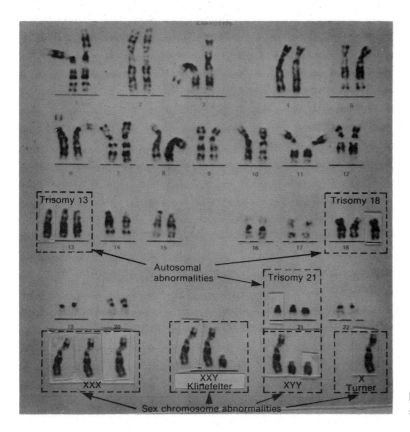

Figure 9–7. Karyotype illustrating the major chromosome abnormalities in a composite.

Klinefelter's syndrome (XXY) occurs in approximately 1 of every 1000 men. Sterility due to abnormal testicular development is the primary clinical feature. Clinical signs, such as gynecomastia, tall stature, thin build, and small genitalia, usually do not appear until after adolescence, making diagnosis difficult in childhood. Most men with Klinefelter's syndrome have normal intelligence or mild mental retardation.

Most people with 47, XYY or 47, XXX karyotypes have normal physical and intellectual development. However, the incidence of mental retardation in these people is higher than that in the population as a whole. Most men with a 47, XYY karyotype have normal gonadal development, and they usually father chromosomally normal offspring. Many adult 47, XXX women lead a normal sexual life and have children, most of whom are chromosomally normal.

Women with Turner's syndrome, 45, XO, frequently show the following clinical features: short stature, webbing of the neck, cubitus valgus (abnormal lateral deviation of the forearm from the elbow), low hairline at the nape of the neck, and lack of sexual development. Their ovaries are usually only a streak of connective tissue, and thus, they present with primary amenorrhea. Approximately 5% to 10% of 45, XO women have normal menses and are fertile. Pregnant 45, XO women should be offered prenatal counseling because they have an increased risk of having children with chromosome abnormalities.

Other clinical problems found at increased rates in women with Turner's syndrome are coarctation of the aorta, malformation of the nails, renal abnormalities, and pigmented nevi of the skin. Although they have normal intelligence, most have difficulty with spatial perception.

Structural Abnormalities

Minor structural variations in regions of the chromosome containing no hereditary information are known to exist in the normal human population and are thought to be benign. On the other hand, structural alterations of chromosomes may lead to birth defects or fetal wastage if a loss or duplication of genes accompanies the rearrangement.

Simple duplications or deficiencies arise either by chromosome breakage or by errors in the chromosomal reproductive process. Chromosomal *translocations* arise when chromosomal breakage is followed by an exchange of material either between parts of a single chromosome or among different chromosomes. If no genetic information is lost, the individual is clinically normal and is said to be a *balanced translocation carrier*. If genetic information is lost during a chromosome translocation, a partial monosomy results. When genetic information is duplicated, a partial trisomy results. The clinical features caused by such an *unbalanced chromosome translocation* depend on the size and the chromosome location of the rearrangement.

Table 9-2 **Summary of Numerical Chromosomal Abnormalities**

Type	Synonym	Incidence	Diagnostic Features at Birth	Prognosis	Detection
Autosomal Monosomy					
		Rare Usually incompatible with fetal survival			
Sex Chromosome Monosomy					
XO	Turner's syndrome*	1/10,000 live female births Most common chromosomal abnormality in spontaneous abortions (18%)	Edema of hands and feet Increased incidence of coarctation of the aorta Somatic abnormalities may be few, and condition often is not recognized at birth.	Normal intelligence Sterile	Buccal smear for X chromatin bodies may be negative. Endocrine levels are abnormal. Abnormality usually revealed in adolescence by presence of short stature, ovarian streaks, and amenorrhea. Estrogen at puberty may aid development of secondary sex characteristics.
Autosomal Trisomy					
		Usually incompatible with fetal survival			"Older" mother is at higher risk for offspring with these syndromes.
Trisomy 13	Patau's syndrome	1/20,000 live births	Microphthalmia (very small eyeballs) Cleft lip Postaxial polydactyly (extra digits) Microcephaly Malformed ears Congenital heart defects Urogenital defects Polycystic kidneys	Severe mental retardation 50% die within first year of life	Karyotype analysis confirms diagnosis.
Trisomy 18	Edwards' syndrome	1/8,000 live births	Micrognathia (small jaw) Clenched fist with 2nd and 5th fingers overlapping the 3rd and 4th Rocker-bottom feet Low-set, malformed ears Congenital heart defects	Severe mental retardation in all cases Death usual in first few months	Karyotype analysis confirms diagnosis.
Trisomy 21	Down syndrome	1/800 live births Most common chromosome disorder	Typical round face with flat profile Protruding tongue Epicanthal folds	Mild to severe retardation Increased incidence of leukemia	Karyotype analysis confirms diagnosis; "older" mother is at higher risk for offspring with this syndrome.

* Turner's syndrome can also be the result of other chromosomal abnormalities, but these are extremely rare.

(continued)

Table 9–2   **Summary of Numerical Chromosomal Abnormalities** (continued)

Type	Synonym	Incidence	Diagnostic Features at Birth	Prognosis	Detection
Sex Chromosome Trisomy					
XXX	Triple X syndrome	1/1,000 female births	None	Usually normal intelligence, but slightly increased incidence of mental retardation Fertile, with normal offspring	"Older" mother is at higher risk for offspring with this syndrome. Buccal smears may reveal triple-X karyotype.
XXY	Klinefelter's syndrome	1/1,000 live male births	None	Usually normal intelligence Mild mental retardation does occur Sterile	Feminine characteristics appear in puberty, including gynecomastia. Typically, sufferer is tall and gangly with small testes and underdeveloped facial and body hair. Breast reduction may be advised for psychological and cosmetic reasons.
XYY		1/1,000 live births	None	Rarely, may be associated with some intellectual impairment Fertile	Abnormality may remain undetected until revealed on karyotyping. In persons with XYY syndrome, sperm count may be reduced and plasma testosterone levels may be high.

Deletions of genetic material from an autosomal chromosome usually lead to severe mental retardation and physical abnormalities. For example, *cri du chat syndrome* arises when an individual is born with a deletion of genetic material from the short arm of the number 5 chromosome. Affected infants have a characteristic catlike cry; microcephaly; round face with the appearance of widely spaced eyes, which have a downward slant; epicanthal folds; flat nasal bridge; and micrognathia. Severe mental retardation, failure to thrive, and hypotonia are characteristic of this disorder.

Translocations may arise *de novo,* for the first time, in an individual, or they may be inherited. Normal balanced translocation carriers have an increased risk of passing an unbalanced amount of chromosome material to their offspring. Therefore, when a deformed fetus or infant is found to have an unbalanced translocation, the parents should be offered karyotype analysis and genetic counseling to determine whether one of them is a balanced translocation carrier. This will allow both parents to be informed of the possibility of increased risks in future pregnancies.

Mosaicism is another cytogenetic abnormality. As mentioned previously, a mosaic individual is born with two populations of cells, each with a different chromosomal constitution. Such a situation arises after fertilization, during embryonic growth, and is caused by an accident in cell division in a single cell line during mitosis. The range of clinical symptoms varies a great deal in mosaic individuals and is thought to be related to the percentage of abnormal cells and to the particular tissues of the body that are affected.

Causes of Chromosomal Abnormalities

The internal and environmental events that lead to the formation of chromosome abnormalities are not clearly understood. Radiation, drugs, viruses, toxins, and chemicals are all known to induce chromosome damage. However, it is extremely difficult to determine the cause in individual cases. Women exposed to these environmental hazards during their first trimester should be referred for genetic counseling to explore the possibility of increased risks to their fetus. The most significant factor predisposing the chromosomal abnormalities (most commonly Down syndrome) is increased *maternal* age. As Table 9–3 shows, the risk of having a child with Down syndrome rises substantially with the age of the mother. Common medical practice dictates that all women who will be 35 or older at the time of delivery be counseled and offered

Table 9-3   **Risk of Down Syndrome by Maternal Age**

Maternal Age	Frequency of Down Syndrome	
	Fetuses	*Live Births*
–19	—	1/1550
20–24	—	1/1550
25–29	—	1/1050
30–34	—	1/700
35	1/350	1/350
36	1/260	1/300
37	1/200	1/225
38	1/160	1/175
39	1/125	1/150
40	1/70	1/100
41	1/35	1/85
42	1/30	1/65
43	1/20	1/50
44	1/13	1/40
45–	1/25	1/25

(Thompson JS, Thompson MW: Genetics in Medicine. Philadelphia, WB Saunders, 1980)

prenatal testing to determine the karyotype of their fetus. The reason for the connection between age and incidence is not known. The age of the father has not been found to have a pronounced effect on the incidence of chromosome abnormalities.

Single Gene Inheritance in Families

The term *single gene traits* refers to those genetic diseases that are caused by a mutation of a gene at a single locus (site) on a chromosome. They are sometimes called *Mendelian traits* because the mutant phenotypes occur in the fixed proportions described by Gregor Mendel, indicating that the genes are segregating and reassorting according to Mendel's genetic principles.

There are four basic patterns of single gene inheritance:

- Autosomal dominant
- Autosomal recessive
- X-linked dominant
- X-linked recessive

A knowledge of the patterns of inheritance is essential to genetic counseling, since the risks vary with each inheritance pattern. Patterns of inheritance may be pictorially represented on a diagram called a *pedigree*. The pedigree is developed during assessment and history-taking. It helps provide a quick reference source for other members of the genetic team and helps determine which members of the family need further examination and

testing. Common symbols used in pedigree charting are shown in Figure 9-8.

Since chromosomes come in pairs (called homologous chromosomes), genes also come in pairs. Genes that are located at the same locus on a pair of homologous chromosomes are *alleles*. When the genes in a pair are identical, the person is called a *homozygote* for that locus. When the genes in a pair are different, the person is a *heterozygote*.

The terms *dominant* and *recessive* refer to the clinical expression of a trait or genetic mutation in a heterozygous individual. If the presence of a mutant gene is clinically expressed in the heterozygous individual and masks the presence of the normal allele, the mutant gene is called *dominant*. If the presence of the mutant gene is not clinically expressed and does not mask the presence of the normal allele, the mutant gene is called *recessive*. There are examples, such as the ABO blood group alleles, where both allelic genes are expressed equally as *codominants*.

Autosomal Dominant Inheritance

Autosomal dominant disorders are disorders that are clinically expressed when *either* allelic gene at a given autosomal chromosome locus is mutant. Most people affected with dominant disorders are heterozygotes because the mutant homozygous state is usually lethal or severely debilitating.

Figure 9-9 illustrates the classic characteristics of autosomal dominant inheritance. We can see that the trait appears in every generation, with no skipping. Male and female offspring are equally likely to be affected. Male-to-male transmission of the disorder is an important clue. Unaffected persons do not transmit the trait to their children.

Dominant traits have several characteristics that may modify the pedigree in a particular family and may even lead to a misinterpretation of the data. In working with a family affected by a chronic genetic condition, nurses might note variations in the degree to which family members are affected. The interaction of a gene with its biologic environment may modify the expression of a dominant trait and may account for the variation within a family. The variation of clinical manifestations from person to person even within a given family is referred to as variable expressivity.

A trait is said to be *penetrant* if a mutant gene is clinically expressed, and *incompletely penetrant* if the heterozygous state cannot be clinically distinguished from the normal homozygous state. A gene that occasionally is incompletely penetrant in a family may appear to skip a generation; that is, a heterozygote for a dominant disorder may be asymptomatic.

When a family seeks genetic counseling for a dominant disorder, the pedigree is examined to see whether an

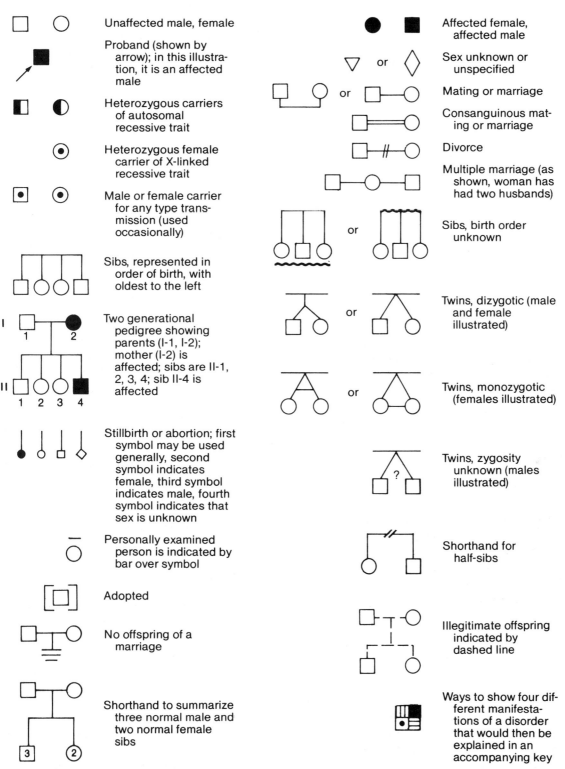

Figure 9–8. Commonly used pedigree symbols.

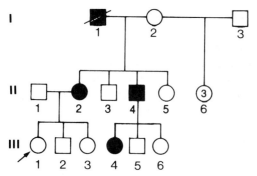

Figure 9–9. Pedigree illustrating autosomal dominant inheritance in Huntington disease; the age of III-1 must be taken into account when risk is determined.

affected parent transmitted the mutant gene or whether the mutant gene arose as a new mutation in a germ cell of a genetically normal parent. If both parents are unaffected and the patient has a new mutation, the recurrence risk for the normal parents is no greater than the risk for the general population because it is unlikely that the mutation will occur again in that family. However, the patient has a 50% risk in each pregnancy of transmitting the mutant gene.

A parent who carries a mutant gene for a dominant disease can transmit either the normal gene or the mutant gene of that gene pair to children (Fig. 9–10). The gene is selected randomly through the natural process of meiosis. Parents have no control over which genes their children inherit. Therefore, in each pregnancy, the child

Affected   Normal
Father   Mother

One affected parent has a single faulty gene (*D*) that *dominates* its normal counterpart (*n*).

Dn   nn

Dn   nn   Dn   nn

Affected   Normal   Affected   Normal

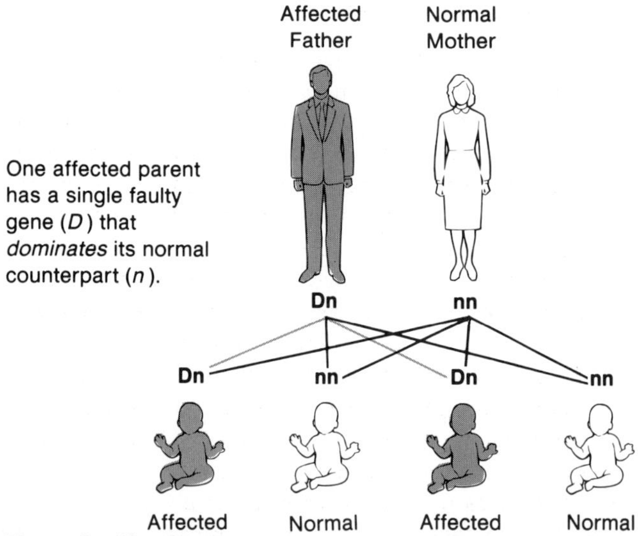

Figure 9–10. Dominant inheritance. (Paris Conference 1971): Standardization in Human Cytogenetics. Birth Defects: Original Article Series, VIII:7, 1972. The National Foundation, New York. (From Wisniewski LP, Hirschhorn K [eds]: A Guide to Human Chromosome Defects. White Plains, New York, the March of Dimes Birth Defects Foundation, BD:OAS XVI[6], 1980.)

has a 50% (1 in 2) chance of inheriting the mutant gene and manifesting the disease. Each child also has a 50% (1 in 2) chance of inheriting the normal gene and being free of the disease.

Achondroplasia, a dominantly inherited skeletal disorder consisting of short-limbed dwarfism, large head size, and bulging forehead, is an example of an autosomal dominant disorder. True achondroplasia is distinguished from other types of dwarfism by radiologic examination. Most persons with achondroplasia have normal intelligence and can lead normal lives.

It is not unusual for two people of very short stature to marry. Before their risk of producing a child with a similar skeletal disorder can be accurately assessed, an exact clinical diagnosis must be obtained in order to distinguish among the many forms of short stature. When two true achondroplastic dwarfs mate, they have a 25% chance that their offspring will inherit a mutant gene from each parent (homozygous achondroplasia) and have a lethal skeletal disorder; a 50% chance that their offspring will be a heterozygous achondroplast; and a 25% chance that their offspring will inherit a normal gene from each parent (normal homozygote) and grow to normal height. Interestingly, some parents with short stature perceive the possibility of having a child of normal height as a problem. This underscores the necessity of communicating with parents without imposing one's personal biases.

Autosomal Recessive Inheritance

Autosomal recessive disorders are disorders that are clinically expressed only when *both* allelic genes at a given chromosome locus are mutant (homozygous). In recessive inheritance, both parents are usually clinically normal carriers (heterozygotes) of the same mutant gene (Fig. 9–11). Pedigree analysis reveals that male and fe-

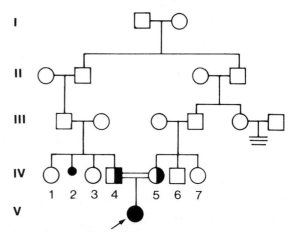

Figure 9–11. Autosomal recessive pedigree illustrating consanguinity. The diagnosis indicates that the parents, IV-4 and IV-5, are heterozygotes.

male offspring are equally likely to be affected. If partners are consanguineous, the likelihood that they carry the *same* mutant gene is increased. The offspring of an affected individual are usually normal unless the affected person is married to a heterozygote for the same gene.

People who are heterozygous for a mutant gene produce two types of gametes: gametes containing the normal gene and gametes containing the mutant gene. When both parents are carriers of the same mutant gene, each of their offspring has a 25% (1 in 4) risk of inheriting *both* mutant genes and developing the disease; a 50% (2 in 4) chance of inheriting one normal and one mutant gene and being a clinically normal carrier; and a 25% (1 in 4) chance of inheriting the two normal genes and being free of the disease (Fig. 9–12). Unaffected siblings have a 67% (2 in 3) chance of being heterozygotes.

Although everyone is believed to carry a few mutant recessive genes in the heterozygous state, the genes responsible for most autosomal recessive disorders are rare. Unless the partners in a couple are blood relatives, the likelihood that both are carriers of a mutant gene at the same locus depends on the incidence of the mutant gene in the population.

Some examples of autosomal recessive disorders are

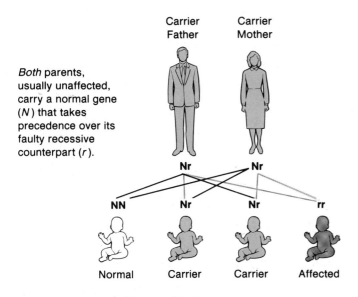

Both parents, usually unaffected, carry a normal gene (*N*) that takes precedence over its faulty recessive counterpart (*r*).

The odds for each child are:

1. a 25% risk of inheriting a "double dose" of *r* genes which may cause a serious birth defect
2. a 25% chance of inheriting two *N*s, thus being unaffected
3. a 50% chance of being a carrier as both parents are

Figure 9–12. Recessive inheritance. (Paris Conference 1971): Standardization in Human Cytogenetics. Birth Defects: Original Article Series, VIII:7, 1972. The National Foundation, New York. (From Wisniewski LP, Hirschhorn K [eds]: A Guide to Human Chromosome Defects. White Plains, New York, the March of Dimes Birth Defects Foundation, BD:OAS XVI[6], 1980.)

cystic fibrosis, phenylketonuria (PKU), Tay–Sachs disease, oculocutaneous albinism, infantile polycystic kidney disease, and sickle cell anemia.

Cystic fibrosis may be the most common hereditary disorder in the Caucasian population. Approximately 1 in 20 Caucasians carries the cystic fibrosis gene. Therefore, approximately 1 in 400 white couples (1/20 × 1/20) is at risk to have a child born with the disorder. Since the risk of the offspring inheriting a defective allele from each parent is 25% (see Fig. 9–12), the actual incidence of cystic fibrosis among Caucasian infants is approximately 1 in 1600. The carrier rate among blacks is about 1 in 50, and it is even lower among other racial groups. Cystic fibrosis is usually manifested between birth and early childhood. It is primarily a disorder of the exocrine glands of the skin, gastrointestinal tract, pancreas, respiratory tract, and male reproductive tract. Clinical problems include meconium ileus, malabsorption, pancreatic insufficiency, respiratory distress, and frequent respiratory infections due to defective, increasingly viscous secretions that obstruct the airway. A suspected diagnosis is confirmed by a sweat test that reveals elevated concentrations of sodium, potassium, and chloride. The prognosis is variable, but death in adolescence or early adulthood is common as a result of severe chronic lower respiratory tract infection. In some cases, indirect DNA analysis is available for prenatal diagnosis and carrier detection of cystic fibrosis in a particular family. It is important to refer such individuals for genetic counseling, since this information may play an important role in their childbearing decisions.

X-Linked Inheritance

Traits that are determined by genes located on the X-chromosome are referred to as *X-linked*. In relation to X-linked traits, the terms *dominant* and *recessive* apply only to females. Females have two X chromosomes and will be symptomatic if they are heterozygous for an X-linked dominant trait but asymptomatic if they are heterozygous for an X-linked recessive trait. Females who are homozygous for an X-linked recessive disorder will, of course, manifest the symptoms of the disease. Males, on the other hand, having only one X chromosome and a Y chromosome, will *always* be affected if they inherit an X-linked mutant gene. Males are said to be *hemizygous* (carrying only one allele) for each X-linked gene locus.

The X-linked recessive pedigree illustrates several important features of this inheritance pattern (Fig. 9–13). Carrier (heterozygous) females have a 50% (1 in 2) chance of transmitting the mutant X-linked gene and of having affected sons. The daughters of heterozygous females have a 50% (1 in 2) chance of being heterozygotes like their mothers. An affected (hemizygous) father transmits his X chromosome to all of his daughters, who therefore *must* be carriers. An affected father cannot have affected daughters unless he mates with a carrier female. Affected fathers will have only disease-free sons because there is no male-to-male transmission of X-linked genes. Fathers pass on their Y chromosomes to their sons.

When a male affected with an X-linked disorder is born into a family with a negative family history, the possibility that he may be a new mutation must be considered. This creates a counseling problem because it may not be possible to determine with certainty whether or not his mother and sisters are carriers. Carrier detection tests are available for only some of the X-linked disorders.

An interesting genetic principle called *lyonization* may be seen in carrier females who manifest symptoms of X-linked recessive disorders. It has been noted that in most somatic cells, one X chromosome becomes inactivated and remains genetically inactive (turned off) for the life of that cell. Chance determines which of the two X chromosomes becomes inactivated in any given cell. It is postulated that mildly affected carriers have a higher percentage of cells with an active mutant X chromosome and inactive normal X chromosome. Although the X chromosome is involved in sex determination, most of the genes on the X chromosome have functions unrelated to sex. Some examples of X-linked recessive disorders are color blindness, hemophilia A and B, Duchenne muscular dystrophy, Lesch–Nyhan syndrome, and glucose-6-phosphate dehydrogenase deficiency.

X-linked dominant disorders are rare. They can appear in every generation of the family. The ratio of affected females to affected males will be on average 2 to 1, because affected males can have only normal sons and only affected daughters, and affected females can have affected sons and daughters, as well as unaffected sons and daughters.

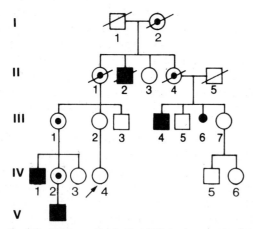

Figure 9–13. Pedigree illustrating X-linked recessive inheritance; the status of III-2 and IV-4 are not yet known and cannot be determined from the pedigree, although IV-2 must be a carrier because both her brother and son are affected, and, retrospectively, this marks III-1 and II-1 as carriers.

Hemophilia A (Factor VIII$_c$ deficiency) is an X-linked recessive disorder of blood coagulation that may become manifest any time after birth. The underlying metabolic defect is the complete absence of the Factor VIII coagulation component. The main life-threatening symptoms are severe, uncontrollable bleeding from wounds; deep tissue bleeding; and bleeding into joints. The recent availability of therapeutic Factor VIII concentrate has led to a longer life expectancy in hemophilic patients. The overall incidence of hemophilia in the general population is likely to increase in the future because, with treatment, affected males can survive to adulthood and can reproduce. Heterozygous females require special management during pregnancy. The potential for coagulation-related problems should be evaluated when amniocentesis or surgery (*e.g.,* cesarean section) is considered.

Carrier detection testing is available for hemophilia A. However, the test has a reliability of only 72% to 94%. Prenatal diagnosis until recently consisted primarily of amniocentesis for sex determination to provide the option of avoiding the birth of males. Now, indirect DNA analysis employing chorionic villus sampling or amniocentesis has permitted the accurate prediction of the pregnancy outcome in several cases.

Duchenne muscular dystrophy is an X-linked recessive disorder characterized by the onset of muscle weakness by the age of 3 to 5 years, progressive loss of strength, confinement to a wheelchair, and death in the late teens or early adulthood due to respiratory infection or cardiac failure. Almost all affected boys have pseudohypertrophy of the calf muscles; diagnosis is confirmed by extremely elevated serum muscle enzyme levels (especially creatine phosphokinase) and typical pathologic findings on muscle biopsy. However, only 60% to 70% of heterozygous females can be identified by increased levels of creatine phosphokinase, since there are many variables that confound the findings and only 5% have been reported to have some muscular weakness. Carrier screening and prenatal diagnosis by means of indirect DNA analysis is available to some families with Duchenne muscular dystrophy.

Cystic fibrosis and Duchenne muscular dystrophy place an extremely heavy physical, emotional, and economic burden on affected individuals and their families. Health professionals need to approach these families with sensitivity, support, and with knowledge about recent scientific advances in order to create an atmosphere in which the medical, genetic, and psychosocial ramifications of these disorders can be discussed.

Multifactorial Inheritance in Families

Multifactorial inheritance refers to the third major etiologic category of genetic disorders, defined as those traits

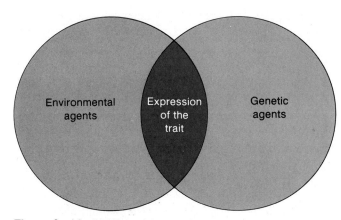

Figure 9–14. Multifactorial causation.

and disorders that arise as a result of the interaction of many genetic factors (polygenic inheritance) or the interaction of genetic and environmental factors (Fig. 9–14). The multifactorial model was created to explain the observation that some disorders cluster in families but have a lower incidence than would be expected if they had a Mendelian single gene model.

Families affected by multifactorial disorders, unlike families with chromosomal abnormalities and single gene disorders, cannot usually be provided with precise counseling about genetic probabilities. Information about recurrence risks for multifactorial disorders is arrived at empirically, on the basis of population and family studies. The nature and number of contributing genes is unknown, and although environmental factors are thought to be significant, a causative role for them has not been clearly documented. Nor have specific environmental agents been identified in the majority of multifactorial diseases. It is postulated that some multifactorial disorders result when a critical threshold is reached. The threshold levels necessary to trigger the disease process can be achieved in one of two ways: (a) a person may inherit at least the requisite number of deleterious genes to achieve the threshold for a particular disorder; or (b) a person may inherit less than the threshold level of deleterious genes but have the abnormal developmental process initiated by exposure to unknown environmental factors.

A particular multifactorial disorder is often found to occur more frequently in one sex than the other. One's risk of a multifactorial disorder within a family is in direct proportion to the degree of one's relationship to the affected individual(s). The closer the relationship, the greater the number of genes shared in common. Some of the more common multifactorial disorders, such as congenital heart defects, club foot, neural tube defects, pyloric stenosis, cleft lip and cleft palate, and congenital hip dysplasia, have a 2% to 5% recurrence risk for first-degree relatives of the affected individual if no other family mem-

bers are affected. The risk of recurrence increases (1) when more than one family member is affected, (2) in proportion to the severity of the disorder in the proband, and (3) if an affected individual is a member of the less susceptible sex.

Neural tube defects are midline abnormalities of the spine or brain caused by failure of the neural tube to close properly during the fourth week of development. The incidence of neural tube defects in the United States is approximately 1 in 700 births. The incidence varies throughout the world. Isolated anencephaly, encephaloceles, meningoceles, myelomeningoceles (spina bifida cystica), and some forms of spina bifida occulta are attributed to multifactorial inheritance. In spina bifida, unknown factors early in embryonic life trigger the abnormal development of the neural tube, precursor of the brain and the spinal cord, causing an opening in the vertebrae where the normally protected nerves can push through into a membranous sac. The nerves in the exposed part of the spinal cord are stretched and damaged, often to the extent that nerve impulses are not transmitted beyond the lesion. This can cause lower limb paralysis and loss of bowel and bladder control. Severity varies among affected individuals.

Anencephaly results when the closure defect occurs at the cranial end of the neural tube. This is a lethal condition and often results in a delayed stillbirth in which the cranium is absent and the brain is exposed and malformed.

Neural tube defects can be diagnosed prenatally by amniocentesis for alpha-fetoprotein in amniotic fluid and by high-resolution ultrasound examination. General population screening by measuring maternal serum alpha-fetoprotein levels is available in some locations. These techniques are discussed later in this chapter. Medical and surgical techniques have been developed to reduce the risk of life-threatening spinal infection and hydrocephaly in newborns with spina bifida. The variability of the defect in kind and severity, the availability of prenatal diagnosis and postnatal medical and surgical intervention, and the burden that the disorder places on the affected individual and family raise many issues that need to be discussed and clarified during visits with the family physician and nurse as well as at genetic counseling sessions.

In order to provide accurate recurrence risk estimates and accurate clinical information, it is important to inquire of anyone reporting the occurrence of a neural tube defect in his or her family whether other malformations were also present in the affected person. Neural tube defects occur along with some chromosome abnormalities and are also found as part of Meckel's syndrome (polycystic kidneys, occipital encephalocele, polydactyly, cleft lip and palate, congenital heart defects). Meckel's syndrome has an autosomal recessive mode of inheritance, and, therefore, parents of an affected child have a

25% risk of recurrence rather than the 2% recurrence risk that is associated with an isolated neural tube defect.

SCREENING POPULATIONS FOR GENETIC TRAITS AND DISEASES

Genetic screening involves testing a specific population to identify those who are affected by a genetic disease, those who may be predisposed to a genetic disease, and those who are clinically normal carriers of a mutant gene and are at risk of having abnormal offspring.

For any screening program to be efficacious, the disorder and mutant gene must be fairly frequent in the test population; the test must be easy and cost-effective to administer and be sensitive, accurate, and reliable in identifying carriers of affected and normal genes; and the test must cause little inconvenience, discomfort, or health risk to the person being tested.

Newborn Genetic Screening

Newborn genetic screening programs aim to identify those presymptomatic newborns affected with a genetic metabolic disease so that preventive treatment can be initiated before permanent damage is done.

Nearly 3000 genetic diseases have been catalogued. Of these, the basic biochemical defect is known in fewer than 200 inborn errors of metabolism. Preventive therapy is available for only a handful of these disorders.

The number of disorders for which a newborn is screened varies from state to state and is usually mandated by state law. Nevertheless, tests should be administered with the informed consent of the mother.

The classic newborn screening programs involve obtaining a specimen of cord blood, newborn blood, or newborn urine. A few drops of blood are collected on a small piece of filter paper after a heel stick in order to perform the microbiologic assays to screen for phenylketonuria (PKU), maple syrup urine disease, galactosemia, homocystinuria, and tyrosinemia. It is essential that these tests be performed at least 3 to 5 days after birth so that the infant has begun protein ingestion, since inability to metabolize certain ingested amino acids is what allows the metabolic disorder to be detected.

It must be emphasized that these are screening tests and not diagnostic tests. An abnormal screening test must be confirmed by more sensitive, often more complex tests that can distinguish a transient abnormality, or artifact, from a true abnormality and also identify the specific etiology in a particular case.

Couples are often not aware that their newborn is being routinely tested for these genetic diseases. Abnormal screening test results usually cause confusion and great anxiety. Prior to discharge, nurses should help to educate parents about newborn screening tests in order to reduce the likelihood that their significance will be misunderstood and to facilitate the confirmatory testing stage. Genetic counseling is an essential component of any genetic screening program and should be offered to couples whose infant is found to have a genetic disease through newborn screening.

In addition to the tests mentioned above, newborn screening programs may include tests for some or all of the following genetic disorders: congenital hypothyroidism, hemoglobinopathies, alpha$_1$-antitrypsin deficiency, cystic fibrosis, Duchenne muscular dystrophy, hyperlipidemia, adenosine deaminase deficiency, and congenital adrenal hyperplasia.

Maternal Serum Alpha-fetoprotein Screening

Approximately 90% of infants with neural tube defects are born in families with no previous history of neural tube defects. Most of these pregnancies are not monitored by prenatal diagnostic tests because the increased risk of the couple has not been previously established. However, a screening test developed in the United Kingdom in the early 1970s and utilized extensively there and in some areas of the United States permits the identification of previously unrecognized high-risk pregnancies.

Elevated levels of alpha-fetoprotein in the maternal serum (MSAFP) are associated with the presence of an open neural tube defect in the developing fetus. The optimal time to obtain the maternal serum specimen is at 16 to 18 weeks of gestation. If an elevated alpha-fetoprotein level is detected, a second sample is obtained. If the second level is elevated, ultrasonography is performed. Ultrasound findings may indicate the necessity of an amniocentesis to confirm diagnosis.

It is essential that nurses note and convey to couples being screened that maternal serum alpha-fetoprotein testing is a screening procedure and not a diagnostic test. An elevated level of alpha-fetoprotein in the maternal serum indicates a 5% to 10% risk that an open neural tube defect is present. Low levels of maternal serum alpha-fetoprotein are correlated with an increased risk of a trisomic fetus (*i.e.,* trisomy 13, 18, or 21). Since approximately 80% of infants with trisomy 21 are born to women under the age of 35 years, this screening test has wide applicability, especially since it also serves to screen for neural tube defects. However, a woman with a low MSAFP level may have a fetus with normal chromosomes and a woman with a normal MSAFP level may have a fetus with a chromosome abnormality. Since MSAFP levels may be low due to overestimation of gestational age, an ultrasound should be performed in order to confirm the gestational age. If the gestational age based on the last menstrual period agrees with that determined by ultrasound, then the only way to rule out a chromosome abnormality is amniocentesis.

Genetic counseling must be available as part of maternal serum alpha-fetoprotein screening programs so that, when necessary, the psychosocial and medical issues can be dealt with in depth. However, to ensure proper understanding of the benefits and limitations of this screening procedure, and to reduce parental anxiety when an abnormal level is detected, parent education must begin and continue with the obstetric nurse and obstetrician.

Heterozygote Screening

The objective of heterozygote screening programs is to detect clinically normal carriers of a disease-causing mutant gene so that couples at increased risk for affected offspring can be identified and counseled. Each available test is offered to members of ethnic groups known to have a high frequency of the mutant gene under investigation.

Three autosomal recessive conditions (Tay–Sachs disease, sickle cell anemia, and thalassemia) are common enough in their ethnic subpopulations that heterozygote screening is considered medically appropriate and should be offered. Most couples undergoing screening tests for these three disorders have no prior family history of these genetic diseases and are unaware of their potential increased risk. In these disorders *both* prospective parents must be carriers before they are at risk (25% risk in each pregnancy) of having affected offspring. Once a high-risk couple is identified, genetic counseling is essential so that all reproductive options, such as prenatal diagnosis, artificial insemination, or possible medical therapy can be discussed.

Tay–Sachs Disease

Tay–Sachs disease is much more common among Jews of Eastern European (Ashkenazi) descent than among other ethnic groups. Approximately 1 in 25 Ashkenazi Jews is a clinically normal carrier of the mutant Tay–Sachs gene. And 1 in 625 Ashkenazi Jewish couples has a risk of producing a Tay–Sachs child.

Tay–Sachs disease is a fatal degenerative disease of the central nervous system. Newborns affected with the disease appear normal at birth. However, development after the sixth month slows, and neurologic impairment progresses until the child becomes blind, with progressive muscle weakness and hypotonia and uncontrollable seizures. By the end of the second year of life, the child deteriorates to a vegetative state. The child usually dies between the ages of 3 and 5 years.

Tay–Sachs disease is caused by the absence of a vital enzyme called hexosaminidase A. Without this enzyme the body cannot metabolize a naturally occurring lipid called GM_2 ganglioside. This lipid accumulates primarily in nerve cells, which accounts for the progressive neurologic manifestations.

Tay–Sachs disease has no cure or treatment. Like all autosomal recessive disorders, it frequently strikes families with no previous history of the disease. Prevention of Tay–Sachs disease is possible only through prenatal diagnosis and genetic screening programs that identify carriers of the mutant hexosaminidase A gene. The screening test measures the level of hexosaminidase A enzyme in leukocyte, plasma, and tear specimens. Carriers have intermediate levels of the enzyme because they have only one active hexosaminidase A gene. Both parents must be carriers of the recessive hexosaminidase A gene in order to produce a Tay–Sachs baby. Recent data indicate that as a result of extensive voluntary screening and the availability of prenatal diagnosis, over the past 14 years there has been a 60% to 85% decrease in the incidence of this disorder in Jewish infants in North America.

Sickle-Cell Disease

Sickle-cell disease is a common disorder among people of black African descent. About one in ten American blacks carries the sickle gene, which is a clinically normal condition, and is said to have sickle-cell trait, which is clinically normal. One in a hundred black couples has a risk of having offspring affected with sickle-cell disease, a hemoglobin disorder. The adult hemoglobin molecule is composed of two alpha globin chains (coded for by the alpha globin gene) and two beta globin chains (coded for by the beta globin gene). Individuals with sickle-cell trait have a mutation in one of the two beta globin genes, while those with sickle-cell disease have mutations in both beta globin genes. The mutations for sickle cell disease lead to the formation of sickle hemoglobin (hemoglobin S). During certain clinical conditions, such as hypoxia, sepsis, acidosis, high fever, dehydration, and emotional and physical stress, the hemoglobin S molecule forms rodlike structures that cause erythrocytes to assume a sickle shape. Sickle-shaped erythrocytes become occluded in capillaries and arterioles, leading to a lack of oxygen in affected areas of the body. The clinical manifestations of sickle-cell disease are variable. Some of those affected are symptom free, and others suffer life-threatening complications. Symptoms may include chronic hemolytic anemia; shortness of breath; lethargy; bouts of pain in arms, legs, back, and abdomen; loss of appetite; jaundice; swelling at joints; and susceptibility to infections.

At present, there is no cure for sickle-cell disease. A number of antisickling drugs that may prevent the occurrence of clinical symptoms are undergoing clinical trials. Treatment at present is symptomatic and supportive: antibiotics for infections, transfusions for severe anemic crises, and daily folic acid supplementation to prevent folate deficiency.

Carriers of the sickle-cell gene, who are said to have *sickle-cell trait,* do not have anemia and do not suffer illness as a result of their carrier state. In rare instances, under extreme conditions of exercise or high altitude, erythrocytes may sickle in the bloodstream of people with sickle-cell trait. The heterozygote screening method for sickle-cell trait involves analyzing a small blood specimen by electrophoresis to separate the globin chains of the hemoglobin molecule. Because over 180 mutant hemoglobins are known, and more than one mutant hemoglobin may migrate to the same position, additional laboratory tests must be performed after a positive first test in order to arrive at a precise genetic diagnosis. Prenatal diagnosis and genetic counseling are now available to identified carrier couples.

Beta Thalassemia

Beta thalassemia (Cooley's anemia) is an autosomal recessive hemoglobin disorder caused by defective synthesis of the beta globin chain. The syndrome is associated with marked pallor that begins in infancy, varying degrees of jaundice, hepato-splenomegaly, retarded physical growth and development, and a characteristic facial appearance. Repeated blood transfusions are necessary to maintain life, a treatment that eventually leads to the clinical problems associated with chronic iron overload. Death often occurs by 15 to 20 years of age. Treatment to prevent the clinical symptoms from developing is not available.

A high incidence of β-thalassemia is found among people of Mediterranean descent (from Italy, Sicily, Sardinia, Greece, Cyprus, and Turkey). It is also found with increased frequency in the Middle East and Far East. Among those of Greek and Italian ancestry, about 1 in 25 is a carrier of the mutant beta globin gene, and 1 in 2500 has the disease. Heterozygotes for beta thalassemia (who are said to have beta thalassemia trait) are usually asymptomatic, although they may have mild anemia and moderate splenomegaly.

The beta thalassemia gene has a wide racial distribution. Therefore, the target population for screening is not clearly defined. Certain ethnic groups that have a high frequency of the gene, such as those of Italian, Greek, Southeast Asian, Sephardic Jewish, and Arab descent, should be offered the option of heterozygote screening. Carrier couples identified through screening programs

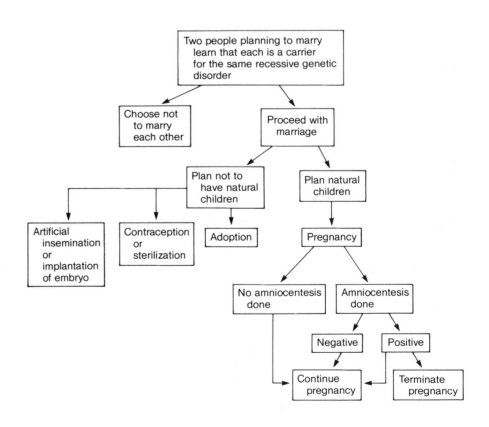

Figure 9–15. Flowchart for decision-making in premarital carrier screening.

and through family history have the option of prenatal diagnosis in future pregnancies.

Summary

Heterozygote (carrier) testing for most other disorders is usually available on a case-by-case basis and depends on a previous family history of the disease under investigation.

The continued success of heterozygote screening programs in preventing tragic genetic diseases and offering various reproductive options to at-risk couples depends on the identification of the patient's ethnic origin, and on education and advocacy by the physicians and nurses caring for those of reproductive age.

The purpose of heterozygote screening is to prevent further occurrence of a genetic disorder. Prevention may occur at three points (Fig. 9–15):

- If premarital screening reveals that both prospective partners are carriers, plans to marry can be abandoned.

- If both partners are carriers, the couple can decide not to have children.

- If the couple decides to have children, pregnancies in which amniocentesis reveals that the fetus has the disorder may be terminated.

Couples may decide to have children even though they are carriers. Health professionals must support the family in any decisions it makes.

PRENATAL DIAGNOSIS

One of the most significant advances in human genetics has been the development of prenatal diagnostic tests that allow physicians to diagnose accurately nearly 200 different genetic diseases in the developing fetus. Obtaining knowledge about the genetic health of a fetus gives a pregnant woman several options that would otherwise not be available during routine prenatal care. A small but growing number of birth defects appear to be treatable *in utero*. For example, a fetus diagnosed as having the metabolic disorder galactosemia, if treated prenatally by restriction of maternal galactose intake and postnatally by dietary control of lactose intake, appears not to develop the clinical manifestations of this disease. In one case, a fetus diagnosed as inheriting a vitamin-responsive form of methylmalonic acidemia received prenatal therapy through a maternal vitamin B_{12} dietary supplement and postnatally was placed on a low-protein diet. These treatments appear to have had favorable effects on the child's development.

NURSING ALERT

Who Should Be Offered Prenatal Diagnosis

Prenatal diagnosis should be offered to

- Gravidas who will be 35 or older at time of delivery
- Clients who have previously had a child with any kind of chromosome abnormality
- Couples in which either parent is a known balanced translocation chromosome carrier
- Couples in which *both* partners are carriers for a diagnosable metabolic or structural autosomal recessive disorder
- Couples in which *either* partner or a *previous child* is affected with a diagnosable metabolic or structural dominant disorder
- Gravidas who are known or presumed carriers for a serious X-linked recessive disorder
- Couples for whom there is a personal or family history (*i.e.*, first-degree or second-degree relative) of a neural tube defect
- Clients who exhibit extreme anxiety or concern

Intrauterine surgery to correct an anatomical defect is a very recent experimental procedure offered in cases where the prognosis is otherwise extremely poor. In one such case, a woman undergoing amniocentesis because of advanced maternal age was found to have a twin pregnancy during ultrasound examinations. One twin appeared normal and the other twin was noted to have ascites at 17 weeks of gestation. Over the next 13 weeks, periodic ultrasound examinations revealed that an obstructive urethral malformation in the ascitic twin had led to a dilated and hypertrophied bladder, hydroureters, and hydronephrosis. At 30 and 33 weeks of gestation, a catheter was introduced through the maternal and fetal abdominal walls into the fetal bladder. Placement of the catheter allowed urine to drain from the fetal bladder and permitted fetal development to continue. The infant was born at 34 weeks of gestation with prune-belly syndrome (abdominal muscle deficiency syndrome) but with normal pulmonary and renal function. The infant responded well to postnatal surgery. Children born with untreated high-grade prenatal urinary obstruction often have advanced hydronephrosis that is incompatible with life.

Some parents whose affected offspring may not be amenable to treatment *in utero* may choose to be spared the birth of a child with a tragic genetic disease and opt for a midtrimester abortion. Those parents who choose to maintain a pregnancy when a fetal defect has been detected can benefit from their foreknowledge by preparing emotionally and medically for the birth of a child with special needs. It must be emphasized, however, that in the great majority of cases (95%–98%), prenatal tests indicate that the fetus will be born *free* of a detectable disorder. The alleviation of anxiety produced by this knowledge is immeasurable.

In genetic counseling, timing is critical. Most prenatal tests are performed between the 16th and 20th week of pregnancy. The genetic counseling process should ideally begin several weeks before the optimal test date. Not only does the family medical history have to be genetically evaluated, but often the expectant parents or other family members have to undergo genetic screening tests to maximize the benefits to be gained from prenatal testing. Although some expectant parents obtain genetic counseling prior to pregnancy, most of those needing referral are identified after conception has taken place. Therefore, it is imperative that high-risk patients be identified and referred for genetic counseling at their *first* prenatal visit, if not before.

Counseling Process

The genetic counseling process begins when a pregnancy is identified as being more likely than usual to lead to the birth of an infant with a defect. Advanced maternal age is the most common indication for prenatal diagnosis. Table 9–3 illustrates the significant increase in the incidence of Down syndrome in women over 35 years of age. The incidence increases each year. Women over 40 years of age have a greater than 1% chance of giving birth to a child with Down syndrome.

Genetic screening tests can identify other high-risk pregnancies. To identify couples who are at increased risk for children with birth defects, family medical and pregnancy history and ethnic heritage must be determined.

It is important to note, however, that most *rare* disorders occur for the first time in families with no previous history of the problem and with no other indications that they are at increased risk. Every couple expecting a child has a small chance (approximately 2%) that their child will be born with a birth defect or hereditary disorder. No one can guarantee that any child will be perfectly normal.

Once it is established that a couple is potentially at high risk, they should be referred to the genetic counseling team, who will thoroughly review their medical histories with a pedigree. The efficacy of any family genetic screening tests and appropriate prenatal tests will then be discussed. It is extremely important that the couple understand the benefits, the risks, and the limitations of the recommended procedures before they decide whether or not to have the tests. The final decision always rests with the patient.

The results of most cytogenetic tests and biochemical tests are available within 4 weeks. When a fetal abnormality is detected, the referring obstetrician is also notified so that the couple may discuss their pregnancy options. Ideally, the couple should also meet again with the genetic counseling team so that any questions they have about the diagnosis, the developmental potential of their fetus, and their feelings can be discussed. This is always a tumultuous time for the couple. They will have strong feelings — of disbelief, anger, and sadness at the loss of a normal child — that need to be ventilated. They must make decisions that may have lifelong consequences in a very short period of time, usually 1 or 2 weeks. This is hardly enough time for them to assimilate their feelings or to understand the medical details so that they can make a decision about whether to terminate the pregnancy. Therefore, the couple often need from health care professionals repetition of the information on several occasions, so they can understand the diagnosis, and empathic listening to their feelings during this crisis. It is important for the nurse to support the couple's decision, regardless of one's personal feelings; one must realize that such a circumstance makes enormous physical, emotional, and psychological demands on them. Whether the couple decide to terminate or continue with the pregnancy, they must be informed of the mourning process so that they realize that anger, denial, and guilt are normal feelings. The loss of a fetus, whether it be through a therapeutic termination, miscarriage, or stillbirth, represents the loss of a real child to the couple. The birth of a child with a defect represents the loss of the hoped-for perfect child. The couple needs to mourn and should be allowed to express their feelings. Genetic counselors can provide bereavement counseling in conjunction with the maternity nurse's empathic support.

Techniques Used in Prenatal Diagnosis

Several diagnostic techniques have been developed that can reliably monitor the development of the fetus *in utero*.

Amniocentesis

Transabdominal amniocentesis in combination with ultrasonography is the most widely used prenatal diagnostic technique. The technique was developed in 1962 to treat fetuses suffering from fetal/maternal Rh incompatibility. In the 1970s it was applied to the diagnosis of genetic disease.

Before amniocentesis is done, ultrasonography is used to (a) verify fetal viability, (b) determine the gestational age of the fetus by measurement of the biparietal diameter, (c) determine placental and fetal positions, (d) diagnose multiple gestations, and (e) detect gross fetal malformations. Amniocentesis should be performed by an obstetrician trained and experienced in the technique. Under strict aseptic conditions, a 3.5-inch 20- or 22-gauge spinal needle is inserted through the abdominal wall into the amniotic fluid. The stylet is removed and 20 to 30 ml of fluid is gently aspirated into a syringe, transferred to sterile tubes, and transported at room temperature to the laboratory as quickly as possible (Fig. 9–16). After the procedure, the woman may return to her normal activities and is instructed to report any cramping, leaking of amniotic fluid, or vaginal bleeding. Techniques have also been developed to allow successful amniocentesis on twin and triplet pregnancies.

Cells from the developing fetus are present in the amniotic fluid. The cells are separated from the fluid by centrifugation and placed in tissue culture medium so that they can be grown and harvested for subsequent karyotyping to identify chromosome disorders. The cell-free fluid is used to analyze the level of the fetal protein alpha-fetoprotein. Findings of higher than normal levels of alpha-fetoprotein are diagnostic for the presence of neural tube defects: anencephaly or spina bifida. Other, less common disorders may also be associated with elevated levels of alpha-fetoprotein in the amniotic fluid: missed abortion, congenital nephrosis of the Finnish type, severe Rh immunization, esophageal atresia, duodenal atresia, omphalocele, Turner's syndrome with cystic hygromas, and several chromosome abnormalities. Therefore, the diagnosis of the cause of the elevated alpha-fetoprotein level must then be confirmed by a high-resolution ultrasound examination. On the basis of family history, biochemical studies are performed on the cultured cells to test for the presence of some of the over 100 detectable metabolic disorders. Among these are Tay–Sachs disease, Lesch–Nyhan syndrome, Hunter's syndrome, Hurler syndrome, and various hemoglobinopathies.

Hereditary metabolic disorders are caused by the absence of an enzyme due to a gene deletion, the alteration of an enzyme structure due to a gene mutation, or a mutation of the gene that regulates the synthesis of the enzyme. If the enzyme in question is expressed in amniotic fluid cells, it can potentially be used for prenatal diagnosis. An unaffected fetus would have normal levels of the enzyme, a clinically normal "carrier" of the mutant gene defect would have approximately half the enzyme level, and an *affected* fetus would have very low enzyme levels or none at all. For disorders in which an abnormal protein is not expressed in amniotic fluid cells, other test procedures utilizing DNA for genetic diagnosis are available.

Amniocentesis has been carefully studied in several countries (the United States, Canada, and the United Kingdom) and has been found to be a safe and reliable procedure if performed by an experienced physician under ultrasonic guidance. Fetal loss, the major risk of amniocentesis, occurs in less than 0.5% of those pregnancies having amniocentesis. Repeat amniocentesis is necessary in 0.1% of the cases. The possibility of injury from fetal puncture at the time of amniocentesis has been found to be minimal. Amniotic fluid leakage and vaginal bleeding occur in less than 1% of women and usually have no clinical significance.

Amniocentesis has several limitations. In rare instances, more than one needle insertion is necessary in order to obtain the amniotic fluid. Occasionally, the amniotic fluid cells cannot be successfully cultured in the laboratory and a second amniocentesis is necessary to obtain a viable culture. In addition, although the level of accuracy of most diagnostic tests is extremely high (99.8% accuracy for cytogenetic analysis), the couple must be informed of the unlikely chance of a missed diagnosis.

Fetoscopy

Fetoscopy involves the transabdominal insertion of a cannula into the womb. A fetoscope, which consists of a fiberoptic light source and a self-focusing lens, can then be inserted through the cannula opening. The initial procedure is similar to amniocentesis. Ultrasound is an essential accompaniment in order to identify placentation and fetal position. Fetoscopy permits direct visualization of the fetus (in 2–4-cm segments) so that developmental deformities can be identified. In addition, a fetal blood sample can be obtained through a 27-gauge flexible needle, permitting the diagnosis of such disorders as hemophilia A and B, which are not presently detectable by other means. A fetal biopsy may also be obtained if needed for diagnostic purposes.

Fetoscopy carries an increased risk of spontaneous abortion (5%–10%) or premature delivery (10%) and is therefore offered only to those women who have a significant risk of producing a child with a birth defect that is detectable only by this method.

Ultrasonography

Ultrasonography uses high-frequency sound waves to create echoes that are generated by the reflection of the ultrasound off maternal organs and fetal internal and external organs. During the second trimester ultrasound can be useful in estimating fetal size and in determining the volume of amniotic fluid to identify cases of oligohydramnios and polyhydramnios. Neural tube defects, limb anomalies, fetal ascites, and hydrops fetalis may also be diagnosed by routine ultrasound. The use of ultrasonography for the prenatal diagnosis of congenital heart defects is currently under study. It is believed that, at the levels used in obstetric ultrasonography, high-frequency sound waves present no risks to the mother or the devel-

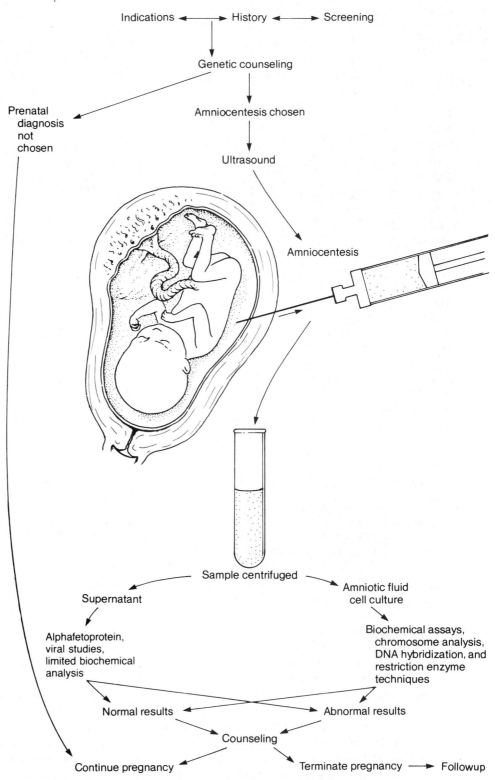

Figure 9-16. Amniocentesis: options and disposition of sample.

oping fetus. Questions about the risks of ultrasonography have recently been raised and are under investigation.

Chorionic Villi Sampling

Chorionic villi sampling is a recent development in prenatal diagnosis. It permits first-trimester testing for chromosomal and biochemical disorders. The procedure is done at 8 to 10 weeks after the last menstrual period and involves the passage of a plastic catheter with a metal obturator vaginally into the uterus. Under ultrasonic guidance the catheter is positioned in the chorion frondosum, where a small sample of chorionic villi is aspirated under negative pressure. Chorionic villi are rapidly dividing cells; consequently, test results can be obtained within 10 days and often as quickly as 1 to 2 days.

The advantages of chorionic villi sampling are that the procedure is performed in the first trimester and that results are obtained relatively quickly so that a first-trimester pregnancy termination is an option if an abnormality is detected.

Another advantage is that chorionic villi sampling utilizes living fetal tissue directly (as opposed to the shed epithelial cells in amniotic fluid used in amniocentesis), and, therefore, the number of potential disorders that can be detected is somewhat greater than that in amniotic fluid studies.

The risks involved with chorionic villi sampling, that is, miscarriage, infection and septic shock, damage to placental membranes, and incorrect interpretation of results, are estimated to be less than 1%, and the risk of complication declines as the experience of the practitioner increases. Since the procedure is relatively new and the full range or significance of findings is not fully understood, an abnormal result requires careful counseling and possibly referral for second-trimester amniotic fluid studies.

GENETIC COUNSELING

Genetic counseling attempts to address questions about hereditary disease and reproductive risks. This process has an educational component and should be offered at a level appropriate to the patient's ability to comprehend. Since questions of this nature involve one's basic identity as a sexual being — am I capable of producing a normal, healthy child? — health professionals must approach the area of genetics in a humane, sensitive fashion. They need to be alert to the patient's fear of being "different" or "flawed" as a person or in the ability to produce normal children.

The process of genetic counseling involves taking a

NURSING ALERT

Who Should Be Offered Genetic Counseling

Genetic counseling should be offered to patients and families whose medical history reveals one of the following conditions:

Congenital abnormalities
  mental retardation
  congenital malformations
  ambiguous genitalia
Parental exposure to environmental agents (drugs, irradiation, certain infections)
Known inherited disorders
Identified carriers of metabolic, biochemical, or chromosomal disorders
Multiple miscarriages or stillbirths
Infertility
Consanguinity
Advanced maternal age (35 and over)
Anxiety about potential offspring

detailed family medical history, extending as far back as two generations for each side of the family. The information gained from this effort is assembled by a genetic counselor in the form of a pedigree or family tree (see Figs. 9–8, 9–9, 9–11, and 9–13). The pedigree, in association with various diagnostic tests, forms the basis on which a genetic diagnosis is made. When a child with a birth defect or a genetic disease has already been born, counseling is important to explore the family's handling of and adjustment to this trauma. Some families are able to accept the birth of such a child without being devastated, but many are unable to overcome the trauma and throughout their lives experience what has been termed "chronic sorrow."

When a genetic diagnosis is made, the counselor educates the parents about the genetic mechanisms that led to the abnormality, explains the natural history and prognosis of the defect, and encourages the couple to ventilate their feelings about their child's condition. The genetic counselor should inform the parents about community facilities that assist in the care of the affected infant, such as infant stimulation and physical therapy programs and parent support groups. Parents should also be encouraged to have an ongoing relationship with a genetics center so that they will have access to the most up-to-date therapies and diagnostic procedures.

Team Setting

Genetic counseling is best offered in a team setting that enables patients to receive sophisticated care from health professionals who specialize in caring for patients at risk for genetic diseases. The technology applied to diagnosing genetic conditions is advancing so rapidly that only those at the cutting edge of genetics research are able to provide the latest methods of diagnosis and care. The medical genetics team can include a physician geneticist, a genetic counselor, a cytogeneticist, a neurologist, a psychiatrist, a pediatrician, an obstetrician, a nurse, and a social worker. Other medical specialists are consulted as needed.

Because so many specialists may be involved in diagnosing a genetic condition, patients should be told that they will be seen by several people and that their genetic workup will be a group effort. Patients often feel that their condition is so rare that they are freaks. They can be relieved to learn that the team is experienced in dealing with similar problems and that their condition is not so rare that it cannot be diagnosed or managed.

Differences Between Genetic Counseling and General Medical Practice

Patients generally expect the medical system to provide a definitive diagnosis and a prescribed form of treatment that only occasionally allows for decision making by the patient. Genetic counseling differs from traditional medical care from the start in that the patient must actively participate in arriving at the diagnosis by providing a detailed family medical history or pedigree. When the diagnosis is determined, the patient hears that he or she has a certain estimated risk of producing an affected child and that this risk will be present with each pregnancy. The counselor must not interpret these risks as "high" or "low" on the basis of her own perspective, for this is the patient's task. Since interpretation of statistical probability is highly subjective, a genetic-risk figure may have different meanings for the counselor and the patient. A patient may have a preconceived idea of the recurrence risk that may serve as an anchor or starting point, which may be adjusted upward or downward as a result of counseling. Therefore, it is important to review all possible options so the patient can make an informed decision. Individuals beyond the reproductive years may learn that they have transmitted a genetic disease or defective genes to their offspring. This is very different from hearing, for example, that one has a condition that can be treated with surgery. Learning about the uncertainty of genetic risk is often disturbing to patients, but some who are carriers of a genetic defect value the possibility of having an unaffected child so highly that it overshadows the risk.

Once risk figures have been determined, genetic counseling patients seen for reproductive reasons are expected to make their own decisions about the course of action they will follow. The options include selective reproduction (prenatal diagnosis in each pregnancy with abortion when results are unfavorable); adoption; artificial insemination by donor (where appropriate); medical intervention following an affected birth, for rare conditions; or "taking one's chances." The burden of making these kinds of decisions can be painful to patients who wish and expect to be told the best course of action.

Psychosocial and Ethical Aspects of Genetic Counseling

Cultural and Religious Considerations

As the treatment and prevention of genetic disease have become increasingly important components of health care, the ethical and social issues raised by this proliferating medical service have become rather complicated. Serious public policy issues that cannot easily be ignored arise in the daily delivery of genetic services. Nursing personnel need to be aware of these ethical issues and sensitive to their implications.

Cultural and religious values play an important role in an individual's approach to genetic counseling, and nurses should make every effort to view patients within the social framework of their particular family. If a person comes from a large extended family, for example, and is expected to bear children as soon as he or she is married, any inability to reproduce healthy children can be particularly traumatic. In initiating an informational session about genetic issues, the nurse should attempt to provide a supportive, nonjudgmental environment that will encourage patients to share their questions and concerns freely.

Religious attitudes permeate considerations of reproductive plans. The nurse needs to determine what a couple's religious values and practices are and to organize the information offered accordingly. In working with a Catholic or an Orthodox Jewish couple, the use of the term *abortion* may be counterproductive; the word *termination* might have less emotional overtones. The nurse should guard against allowing her own personal and religious values to unduly influence the way she presents genetic information. Although all health professionals risk presenting information in a biased manner, imposing one's values to another person's family planning is, to say the least, unprofessional.

Cultural differences between nurses and patients are even more difficult to deal with, particularly in view of the number of refugee and foreign-speaking populations who have settled in most large American cities. Although it is impossible to be knowledgeable about all population groups, a nurse involved in providing genetic information to a couple whose cultural background is unfamiliar to her would be wise to make an effort to get the couple to discuss their expectations about family size and constitution early in her contact with them. Such discussions reveal much about reproductive attitudes as well as about the interpersonal relationship of the couple.

Economic Considerations

Economic factors strongly affect a family's attitude toward their reproductive potential. When the birth of a chronically ill child is a possibility, parents need to be made aware of the financial responsibilities the child's condition will involve and to have an open discussion of the natural history of the disease as well as its potential impact on the family structure. Few medical conditions threaten the fabric of the marital relationship as much as a defect that is transmitted by parents to their offspring. Historically, women have been considered responsible for their children's abnormalities, and even when presented with evidence to the contrary, couples often cannot accept the truth. The presence of an imperfect gene in a family implicates members of the extended family as well, especially the grandparents. Sides are quickly drawn and harsh words often exchanged about "the other side of the family."

Effects on Family Functioning

A diagnosis of genetic disease usually has a major impact on family functioning. The associated distress is expressed in a different way by each family, but a variety of coping mechanisms will be developed by each member of the nuclear family in an attempt to manage this distress. The birth of an affected child may bring about a tremendous change in the parents' self-image, which renders the marital relationship particularly vulnerable. Caring for an affected child provides a daily reminder that the marital partnership is responsible for the affected child and his or her future. Divorce and sexual dysfunction are common sequelae when poor communication between parents and inadequate social supports produce an environment in which the parents are unable to maintain their sense of personal worth.

When a dominant condition is diagnosed or a chromosomal problem is known to be transmitted from one parent only, the sense of guilt experienced by the responsible parent can be intense. The partner's anger or frustration can be equally damaging. These feelings are often suffered in silence, and a nurse working with such a couple must explore these possible reactions sensitively and attempt to help both partners ventilate their feelings as they learn to cope with this new image of themselves. Not everyone will feel comfortable discussing such emotionally charged areas. The nurse who does not feel confident of her ability to engage in discussions at this level would

do well to suggest a referral to another health professional, preferably a genetic counselor experienced in dealing with families at risk for transmitting a genetic condition.

Confidentiality

Although confidentiality should be provided for patients in all areas of medical service, it is particularly important to families seeking genetic counseling. Because flaws in one's genetic makeup arouse powerful feelings of vulnerability, patients seeking genetic counseling need to be openly assured that the information they provide about themselves and their family will be kept in the strictest confidence. Patients need reassurance that no information will be shared with employers, since genetic screening in the workplace is a matter of company policy in some instances and therefore of increasing concern to the employee.

A genetic diagnosis requires complete documentation of a family's medical history; when patients first come for genetic counseling, the counselor must raise the issue of assembling information from the extended family and help the clients to appreciate the value of sharing the diagnosis with family members. Providing relatives with information they would not otherwise have can prevent serious medical complications. For example, when cystic fibrosis is diagnosed in a family, other members of the family need to be alerted to the fact that the cystic fibrosis gene is carried in the family. The diagnosis of polyposis of the colon, a precursor to cancer, should also be shared with family members because early detection and treatment of this condition greatly improve the prognosis. Genetic counselors face an ethical dilemma when individuals refuse to share information about genetic susceptibility with members of their extended family. There is a fine line between the patient's right to privacy and the counselor's responsibility to family members who have not sought his or her help. In general, patients who refuse to share a genetic diagnosis with their family do so because of fear that this information will result in their being labeled or stigmatized by the family.

Informed Consent

The concept of informed consent permeates most areas of medical care today. In the context of genetic counseling and screening, it is particularly important that, at the center of the shared process of decision making about issues of reproductive life, there should be a truly informed patient — one who understands not only the genetic information on which a diagnosis was based but also the implications of that diagnosis for the family and the potentially affected child.

The question of informed consent raises another important issue in genetic care that is somewhat unusual in the medical service field, namely, patient autonomy. Genetic decision making is a uniquely personal affair. Reproductive choices that result in the birth of a child who will be cared for by an individual couple are viewed by society as the unique responsibility of that couple, even though their decision may eventually involve public responsibility for the medical care of that child. The prevailing concepts of medical care also dictate the right of individuals to make these choices independently, unburdened by the overt influence of health professionals. Genetic counselors generally support the concept of nondirective counseling and are conscientious in their effort to make clear to patients that they have the right to refuse any genetic screening or diagnostic procedure. The educational responsibilities of genetic counselors include explaining these patient rights. Clearly, informed consent can only be exercised when adequate medical information has been provided.

IMPLICATIONS FOR NURSING CARE

Probably every nurse practicing today has had contact with a client or family affected by a genetic disorder. The amount of involvement depends on the nurse's education, understanding of genetics, job description, and the type of genetic disorder the client has. Some nurses may specialize in genetics and become genetic counselors. But most nurses are in a liaison position with more specialized personnel. Although nurses in any type of practice may be involved to some degree in some aspect of genetic care, this section relates specifically to care by nurses specializing in maternal care fields.

Nurses specializing in maternal health care play a key role in the prevention of genetic disease. By accruing knowledge of genetic disorders and using their powers of observation, nurses may be the first to discover "clues" and identify a genetic problem. Knowledge of available facilities will help the nurse to refer clients to the proper professionals. Nurses should be alert to the heritability of many disease entities, such as cystic fibrosis, hemophilia and sickle-cell disease, and should take responsibility for helping patients to obtain a genetic referral. They should inform all women aged 35 or older of their increased risk of giving birth to a child with a chromosomal abnormality, such as Down syndrome, and of the availability of prenatal diagnosis.

Assessment

Women of childbearing age and their partners should always be screened for a genetic history. The nurse should be able to make a referral to an obstetric or genetic service where prenatal diagnosis and amniocentesis are available. A federal program providing genetic services throughout the United States has been in effect since 1978. The program is organized on a statewide basis, and genetic counseling facilities are now available in nearly every state in the nation.

A high degree of nursing skill and training combined with the public's perception of nurses as knowledgeable, sympathetic, and caring people may encourage some patients to communicate more easily with nurses than they might with other medical professionals. Open communication between patients and nurses is essential so that as many high-risk individuals and families as possible can be identified.

Interviewing skills are extremely important in obtaining the relevant preliminary genetic history. The experienced nurse may also chart the family's pedigree in preparation for genetic counseling. In many cases, family medical records will be needed for further research into the occurrence or potentiality of a disorder in a family. Sometimes clients do not want others in the family to know that they are concerned about familial defects, or

Services Provided by the Nurse

In working with clients the nurse can be called on to

- Provide referral for genetic counseling
- Plan, implement, administer, or evaluate screening programs
- Provide health teaching
- Monitor and evaluate clients
- Work with families under stress engendered by problems related to a genetic disorder
- Coordinate care and services
- Manage home care and therapy
- Follow up on positive newborn screening tests
- Interview clients, assess needs, take family histories, and draw family pedigrees
- Reinforce genetic counseling information
- Support families when they are receiving counseling and making decisions
- Recognize the possibility of a genetic component in a disorder and take appropriate referral action

(Adapted from Cohen FL: Clinical Genetics in Nursing Practice. Philadelphia, JB Lippincott, 1984)

older members of the family may have kept "secrets" within the family for so long that they hesitate to disclose them now to strangers. The matter of obtaining permission to see family records must be handled with the utmost delicacy and in a nonthreatening way.

The nurse may help the pregnant woman prepare for diagnostic tests both by discussing the tests, the procedure, the possible outcomes, and the length of time needed for the test and for the results and by assisting with procedures in the physician's office, the clinic, or the hospital.

The initial appraisal of family dynamics may also be made by the primary-care nurse. The family should be encouraged to verbalize feelings. For instance, how will the family accept the test results? If the client is considering the possibility of terminating the pregnancy, has she indicated that this is a planned pregnancy or does she feel ambivalent about it? Does she have coping mechanisms or support persons to help her after she reaches a decision? The nurse must be sensitive to marital stress or potential stress on a family. Any information of this type that the nurse can supply along with the family history and pedigree chart will be helpful to the genetic counselor.

When finishing the history taking and preparing the client for the referral sessions, the nurse should caution the client or family against expecting immediate results. The genetic counselor may not be able to give immediate answers. Counseling may take several sessions, and time is needed for testing and for obtaining results from those tests. And then the team must work together to formalize their findings. The nurse can be very helpful in preparing the family for this period of waiting.

Diagnosis

The nurse may assist in preparing family members for specific genetic diagnostic tests, but she is also responsible for diagnosing responses to the process of genetic testing and counseling. Although it is likely that a family undergoing evaluation will have ready access to a genetic counselor, the nurse may still be in a position to identify specific nursing or collaborative problems requiring additional attention. The following are some diagnoses that may be particularly useful in the care of families with genetic problems:

- Decisional conflict
- Grieving
- Knowledge deficit
- Disturbance in self-concept

Planning and Implementation

Planning and implementing follow-up is probably the most important care the nurse can give a couple undergoing genetic counseling.

Interpretation and Reinforcement.   The nurse is needed to interpret and reinforce information given by the geneticist. Sometimes, because of the stress involved, couples do not understand clearly what they have been told. The nurse should be able to answer further questions and clarify the information given. The nurse may discuss treatment, facilities, community agencies for support, and alternatives.

Guidance for Decision Making.   The couple needs to be assured that they do not need to rush into a decision — unless the client is well into her pregnancy and there is a question of terminating a pregnancy (and even then, the couple must not feel that they are being pressured into making a decision). Support should be given both in making a decision and after the decision has been made. A nurse assuming responsibility for this kind of genetic support should maintain a close association with the patient's medical genetics team in order to avoid providing conflicting information.

Decisions will be emotionally painful. They may involve the birth of a defective baby or such things as termination of a pregnancy, sterilization, adoption, or artificial insemination. The nurse should give support and make arrangements to facilitate decisions.

Resources.   The nurse as a resource person should be familiar with community resources: where the family can go for financial aid, where equipment for a child is available, what agencies will give further support, where local support groups for a particular disorder are located.

Supporting.   The family must be encouraged to verbalize their feelings while they are arriving at a decision and after the final decision has been reached. Denial, sorrow, guilt, fears, and anger may all be near the surface, needing to be expressed. The nurse may find that further referral is necessary. The nurse is important in helping individuals establish feelings of self-worth.

Providing support during difficult decisions or during grieving subsequent to decisionmaking is another key element of nursing care. Families dealing with the birth, or potential birth, of a newborn who has congenital abnormalities often stress the need for — and sometimes the lack of — sympathetic discussions with knowledgeable professionals who appreciate the grief they are experiencing. Parents who have given birth to an abnormal infant or who have terminated a pregnancy for genetic reasons are outspoken in their criticism of medical professionals who deny them the opportunity to ventilate their feelings. Special consideration must be given to parents selectively terminating a pregnancy so that the personal biases of the medical and nursing staff do not interfere with supportive care.

Providing Information. Providing needed information for family members at critical points in the life cycle may also be a nursing responsibility. Chronic genetic conditions stress family members in different ways at different times in the life cycle; the nurse must be sensitive to the family's changing needs for information and support. Adolescents may have a crucial need for information about their reproductive risks. Affected parents may have misinformed adult children about the transmission of the disease with which they are affected. They may also, because it is something they cannot deal with emotionally, have failed altogether to discuss the genetic implications of their illness with their children. Nurses should be vigorous in their exploration of these areas of concern and be knowledgeable about the resources available to patients who need referral for genetic counseling.

Evaluation

The nurse may have contact with couples of childbearing age in a variety of settings; as part of her care, she must ensure that couples are appropriately screened for genetic problems and given appropriate referral. Further, once genetic care is indicated, the nurse should evaluate the adequacy of patient teaching and supportive care on an ongoing basis. Finally, when families are faced with difficult decisions with respect to genetic outcomes, the nurse is responsible for ongoing follow-up to ensure that adequate information and anticipatory guidance is available. The effectiveness of nursing care may be reflected in the psychological adaptation of family members to grief and loss and in their ability to cope with stresses related to genetic problems.

CHAPTER SUMMARY

Obstetric nurses can play a key role in the prevention of genetic disease by learning the indications for patient referral for prenatal testing. It is extremely important that the nurse use her interviewing skills to obtain a relevant preliminary genetic history so that pertinent family and medical history can be evaluated and appropriate referrals made. These efforts will help to ensure that all patients, regardless of socioeconomic status, have access to genetic services. Additional efforts should be made to educate colleagues about the psychological needs of patients with genetic disease in order to protect them from insensitive care.

STUDY QUESTIONS

1. What are the three main categories of hereditary diseases?
2. What is a karyotype?
3. What is a pedigree?
4. Who should be referred for genetic counseling?
5. What is the difference between amniocentesis and chorionic villi sampling?
6. What is heterozygote screening?
7. What is the risk of Down syndrome in a 35-year-old woman?
8. What do genetic counselors do?
9. How does genetic counseling differ from traditional medical care?
10. As a nurse, how can you help women avoid transmitting a genetic disease to their offspring?
11. For which genetic disorders is prenatal diagnosis and carrier detection available even though the nature of the gene defect has not yet been determined?
12. What issues affect the mourning process when a woman gives birth to a child with a hereditary disease?

REFERENCES/BIBLIOGRAPHY

Dillon LS: The Gene: Its Structure, Function, and Evolution. New York, Plenum, 1987

Hawkins JD: Gene Structure and Expression. Cambridge University Press, London, 1985

Levin B: Genes, 2nd ed. New York, John Wiley & Sons, 1985

Reznikoff W, Gold L: Maximizing Gene Expression. Stoneham, MA, Butterworths, 1986

Setlow JK: Genetic Engineering Principles and Methods, Vol. 10. New York, Plenum, 1988

Thompson E: Pedigree Analysis in Human Genetics. Baltimore, Johns Hopkins University Press, 1986

Vogel F, Motulsky AG: Human Genetics: Problems and Approaches, 2nd ed. New York, Springer–Verlag, 1986

10 adolescent sexuality and childbearing

LEARNING OBJECTIVES

After studying the material in this chapter, the student should be able to

- Outline historical trends in the emergence of adolescent health care as a subspecialty area

- Obtain an adolescent health history

- Perform Tanner staging as it relates to pubertal assessment of sexual maturity

- Describe the psychosocial development of the adolescent

- Explain the negative impact of onset of sexual activity during adolescence

- Understand issues of consent and confidentiality as it relates to the provision of adolescent health care

- Discuss ways in which the nurse can support and promote health maintenance for the pregnant adolescent

- Name and discuss three possible pregnancy complications in the adolescent

KEY TERMS

Acquired immunodeficiency syndrome (AIDS)

AIDS-related complex (ARC)

Amenorrhea

Chlamydia

Confidentiality

Consent

Contraception

Gonorrhea

Gynecologic examination

Herpes

Human immunodeficiency viral (HIV) infection

Human papillomavirus (HPV)

Mature minor doctrine

Menarche

Menstruation

Oligomenorrhea

Pelvic inflammatory disease

Pregnancy-induced hypertension

Preterm labor

Puberty

Pubescence

Sexually transmitted disease (STD)

Sexuality

Syndrome of failure

Syphilis

Tanner staging

The fact that adolescents have special health care needs based on their unique developmental status has not always been appreciated. In 1938 the American Academy of Pediatrics issued a policy statement that included adolescence as a unique population requiring specialized health care. However, this remained a neglected area of care until J. Roswell Gallagher established the first adolescent clinic in 1952 at Boston Children's Hospital. In 1968 the Society for Adolescent Medicine, an interdisciplinary professional organization that has as its purpose the development and dissemination of scholarly and scientific information regarding the unique developmental and health care needs of adolescents, was founded. Nurses involved in the delivery of health care to adolescents are active participants in the Society. However, formalized and professional education of nurses in the area of adolescent health care has lagged. Colleges of nursing are only now beginning to provide formalized graduate education in adolescent health, some based on an interdisciplinary approach with medicine.

This chapter reviews the interaction of the physiologic changes in puberty and psychosocial developmental changes in the female adolescent. Specific attention will be given to the need for gynecologic services, health teaching regarding changing body habitus, the negative outcomes of early sexual activity, and adolescent pregnancy. A discussion surrounding the issues of consent and confidentiality, as they relate to the provision of services to the adolescent client, is also included.

ADOLESCENT HEALTH

Adolescence is a period of dramatic changes in physiologic growth and psychologic development, with a maturation of the emotional self and a transition in social roles to those of adult status. The rapidity of overlapping changes in each of these areas makes provision of nursing care complex and challenging.

Clinicians must be prepared to make assessments of adolescents based not only on their physical development but also on their growth in the areas of psychologic and social maturity. Therefore, it is important to understand the distinction and the overlap between the physiologic and psychosocial aspects of adolescence, and the need for individualized care based on these aspects.

Physiologic Development

The word *puberty* is derived from the Latin word *pubescere,* which, literally translated, means "to grow hair." It typically refers to the pervasive growth that affects all bodily tissues: peak growth velocity for the reproductive,

RELATED RESEARCH

Priorities for Adolescent Health

In 1986 a conference sponsored by the Division of Maternal and Child Health of the US Department of Health and Human Services brought together experts in adolescent health research and health services to develop priorities in adolescent health through the year 2000. The recommendations proposed by this group are as follows:

1. In order to promote adolescent health, it is critically important that we expand our knowledge of adolescence as a developmental stage within the context of the entire life span, distinct from the stages of childhood and adulthood.

    Research must continue to focus on the influence of positive relationships with adults and peers in order to determine what kinds of psychological environments foster optimum psychosocial development.

2. We must explore strategies for improving the health of adolescents within the social contexts that are critical for this age group.

    Socioeconomic conditions strongly influence adolescent health. Health promotion and disease prevention programs must be tailored to reflect social factors. Further, schools must provide unified programs, including school nursing, counseling, and social service work in high-risk areas.

3. We need to expand the kind and number of indicators used to evaluate the health status of adolescents at both national and local levels in order to plan health care and evaluate present services.

    Lack of uniform and accessible data prevents accurate assessment of adolescent health and health care. Each state is encouraged to assemble data on adolescent health in order to monitor programs and make recommendations for policies and services. Nurses with specialized backgrounds in policy and program development and in clinical services can contribute to this effort.

4. In order to effectively serve adolescents, health services must respond to their unique needs and to changes in the organization and financing of our health care system.

5. Health professionals who plan to work with youth must receive an education organized around an interdisciplinary core curriculum and supplemented by formal training in their specialty as well as by continuing education courses in adolescent health.

Bearinger L, Gephart J: Priorities for adolescent health: Recommendations of a national conference. MCN 12:161–163, 1987

cardiovascular, and musculoskeletal systems occurs during adolescence.

The onset of puberty in girls is controlled by the central nervous system in the areas of the hypothalamic/pituitary regions of the brain. The specific mechanisms responsible for initiating puberty are not clearly understood; however, genetic factors, along with improved nutrition and general health status, have been implicated (Tanner 1987). The neuroendocrine regulation of the brain through the stimulation of releasing factors of gonadotropin-releasing hormone (Gn-RH) stimulates the production of follicle-stimulating hormone (FSH) and luteinizing hormone (LH) in a positive feedback mechanism. The most obvious outcome is the stimulation of the reproductive organs, the ovaries; this results in the development of such secondary sex characteristics as breast development and axillary and pubic hair (Moscicki and Shafer 1986; Tanner 1987).

Sexual Maturity Rating

Chronologic age (actual age) correlates very poorly with physiologic maturity. While the sequence of pubertal events is predictable, the rate at which it occurs varies for each individual. For female adolescents the length of puberty can range from 1.5 to 8 years, with an average of 4 years. The progression of sexual development can be assessed by clinical measurements of height, weight, and sexual maturity. Height and weight measurements are easily obtained and are cost-effective; good longitudinal data have been collected and have established norms that can be used to monitor growth.

The level of sexual development is described by Tanner staging. This method of assessment is based on the progression of secondary sex characteristics and assigns numbers for stages of maturation of pubic hair, breasts, and genitalia. The scale measures from prepuberty (Tanner I) to achievement of adult status (Tanner V). Adolescent health care specialists commonly employ this method to summarize growth, to ascertain whether development is progressing normally, and to predict future developmental events (see Assessment Tool and Figs. 10–1 and 10–2).

With the onset of puberty, an adolescent's body image may be disrupted, and concerns over the normalcy of rapid body changes become paramount. Comparison with same-sex peers is common during early adolescence.

The typical progression of body changes associated with puberty is reviewed in Table 10–1. Nurses may find Tanner staging a helpful adjunct in providing health teaching and reviewing physical development with the young female adolescent. Table 10–1, Figures 10–1 and 10–2, and the Assessment Tool may be used as educational pieces for the adolescent.

ASSESSMENT TOOL

Stages of Sexual Development for the Female (Tanner Stages)

Stage I (Prepubertal)

- There is no breast or pubic hair development.
- Vaginal mucosa is thin, red, and dry.

Stage II (Ages 10–11)

- Breast buds appear and diameter of the areola increases.
- Labia majora is more vascular and wrinkled and develops hair follicles.
- Vaginal mucosa becomes moist, pink, and thick.
- Uterine fundus begins to enlarge.
- Body fat is redistributed and hips widen.
- Height spurt begins.

Stage III (Ages 11–12)

- Breast enlargement continues.
- Pubic hair becomes coarser and curly, its texture more adultlike.
- Labia minora enlarges and becomes more pendulous.
- Vaginal mucosa thickens, the vagina lengthens, and a white vaginal discharge may appear.
- Fallopian tubes increase in diameter.
- Uterine fundus size increases.
- Axillary sweat glands begin functioning and axillary hair begins to appear.
- Facial sebaceous glands activate and acne may appear.
- Rapid growth and peak height velocity occur.

Stage IV (Ages 12–13)

- Breasts enlarge and areola form a separate mound from the surrounding breast tissue.
- Pubic hair covers the perineum and mons but does not reach the thighs.
- Uterus and vagina continue to enlarge.
- Menarche occurs.
- Linear growth decelerates.

Stage V (Ages 13.5–15)

- Breasts and genitalia are adult.
- Pubic hair spreads to thighs.
- Ovulation begins and becomes regular.
- Linear growth ceases.

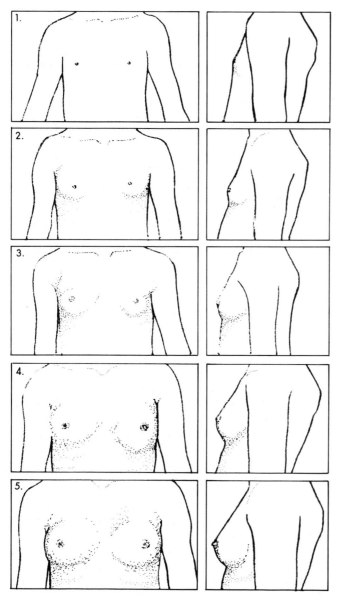

Figure 10–1. Sexual maturity rating in adolescent women, based on breast development.

NURSING RESEARCH

Preparation of Adolescents for Menstruation

A study of 74 female students in the 8th and 10th grades focused on their perceptions of menstruation and how they were prepared for it. Questionnaires were administered in a health education class. Eighty percent had already started menstruating; the majority had been prepared by their mothers, although many stated that this teaching had occurred at the time they had started menstruating. Common initial reactions were surprise, fear, and embarrassment; the most common perception expressed was the inconvenience of menstruation because it interfered with activities.

The majority of girls thought that boys should also be taught about menstruation, but only a third wanted that teaching to occur in coed groups. Nearly 40% wanted parents to inform other family members about the onset of menstruation but often indicated specific conditions they wanted parents to consider. The majority thought that fifth and sixth grades were the best times to introduce information about menstruation.

Nurses involved in education of pre-adolescent and adolescent girls should consider the adolescent's need for control of the learning experience and for the selective sharing of the event with others. Assisting girls to plan for and cope with the inconvenience of menstruation should be incorporated with other teaching: by including nurses, teachers, and mothers in this planned teaching, the development of positive female identification may be enhanced.

Havens B, Swenson I: Menstrual perceptions and preparation among female adolescents. J Obstet Gynecol Neonatal Nurs 15(5):406–408, 1986

Table 10–1   **Progression of Adolescent Female Growth Parameters**

Physical Characteristic	Average Age	Range	Tanner Staging
Breast development (thelarche)	10 years	8–13 years	Tanner 2–5
Pubic hair (adrenarche)	11 years	11–14 years	Tanner 2–5
Height spurt (25% adult height achieved)	11.5 years	24–36 months duration, one year prior to onset of menarche	Tanner 2–3
Menarche	12.8 years	10–16.5 years	Tanner 3–4

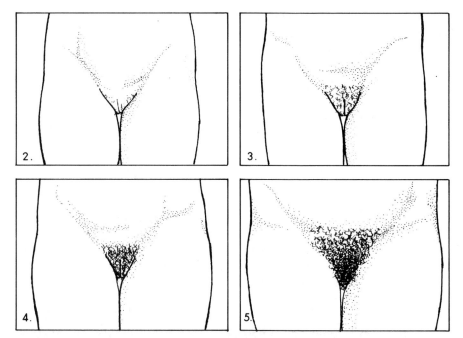

Stage 1: Preadolescent — no pubic hair except for the fine body hair (vellus hair) similar to that on the abdomen

Stage 2: Sparse growth of long, slightly pigmented, downy hair, straight or only slightly curled, chiefly along the labia

Stage 3: Darker, coarser, curlier hair, spreading sparsely over the pubic symphysis

Stage 4: Coarse and curly hair as in adults; area covered greater than in stage 3 but not as great as in the adult and not yet including the thighs

Stage 5: Hair adult in quantity and quality, spread on the medial surfaces of the thighs but not up over the abdomen

Figure 10–2. Sexual maturity rating in adolescent women, based on pubic hair development.

Menarche

A major landmark in female adolescent development is menarche, or the onset of menstruation. The physiologic processes involved in the onset and maintenance of menstruation are discussed in Chapter 5, Normal Reproductive Anatomy and Physiology.

Exercise: Effects on the Menstrual Cycle

Physical exertion is a healthy and beneficial activity; regular exercise is known for its physiologic and psychologic advantages. However, female adolescents who participate routinely in strenuous physical activities may experience menstrual irregularities. While regular activity is an excellent way of maintaining a healthy body, it may also cause delayed menarche and oligomenorrhea (scanty flow) in the adolescent. These menstrual irregularities are believed to be mediated at the hypothalamic level. In response to acute physical exertion, β-endorphins are released from the anterior pituitary gland along with adrenocorticotropic hormone (ACTH), the "stress syndrome."

The central nervous system–hypothalamic–pituitary regulatory system is sensitive to changes in its environment. Research suggests that attainment and maintenance of a normal menstrual cycle and reproductive function in the adolescent may be dependent upon a certain body weight and height ratio. Generally menstruation does not occur in girls who are more than 15% below the ideal weight for their height.

It has also been established that vigorous physical training, such as running, gymnastics, swimming, and ballet dancing, causes delay in breast development as well

as menarche. The causes of exercise-induced amenorrhea and delays in menarche are still unclear. In most instances these changes are reversible when strenuous exercise is discontinued (Moscicki and Shafer 1986).

Psychosocial Development

According to Muuss (1988), there are three major developmental tasks of adolescence. These are listed in the accompanying display. Accomplishing these tasks requires much energy and time during adolescence; roadblocks to accomplishing them may cause problems.

Adolescent development has been conceptualized as three distinct time periods: early, middle, and late adoles-

---

Developmental Tasks of Adolescence

Developmental tasks of adolescence include

- Establishment of sexual and reproductive maturity
- Attainment of a vocational or life work plan that is consistent with one's actual competencies
- Establishment of autonomy from the family system while maintaining an interdependent link with family and friends and allowing for true intimacy and mutual sharing

Muuss RE: Theories of Adolescence, 5th ed. New York, Random House, 1988

cence. Although overlap between these periods is expected, they do provide a framework that assists the nurse in assessing the adolescent's developmental status.

Early Adolescence. In girls early adolescence usually occurs between 11 and 13 years of age. During this time rapid growth occurs, as evidenced by the attainment of secondary sex characteristics and peak height. Preoccupation with the rapid body changes and a reworking of body image are common themes. Timing of changes appears critical: comparisons with same-age peers, in an attempt to define what is normal, are to be expected. Cognitively, the adolescent is in a period of concrete operational thinking, which is egocentric, focused on the "here and now," and unable to take into account cause and effect or the probability of outcomes or future implications of one's behavior. A movement away from the family begins during this period so that independence–dependence struggles are common. Sexuality concerns usually occur within same-sex peer groups; talking on the phone about crushes on significant adult role models is common. Exploration of sexual self-concept begins before actual dating or sexual activity occur.

Middle Adolescence. Middle adolescence begins around age 14 to 15 and blends into late adolescence at age 17. Physiologic growth is usually completed during this period, and body image and size stabilize. Family issues over emancipation continue. Use of the peer group to establish behavioral norms is common during this emancipation phase. Cognition shifts to formal operations, with emergence of abstract thought and the generation of multiple options to solve problems. During stressful events regression to earlier modes of problem solving is common. Emergence of sexual self-concept is evidenced by dating behavior in group situations or as a couple. Progression of sexual activity from kissing, petting, and genital touching to sexual intercourse can occur. Since heterosexual behavior is the culturally accepted norm, it is the most commonly observed. Gay or lesbian youth may actually engage in a heterosexual rehearsal phase or may delay their "coming out" until late adolescence or young adulthood (Troiden 1988). Exploration, experimentation, and the absence of true psychological intimacy in this period is normal. The lack of a mature sexual self-concept, in addition to societal and environmental factors, may result in adolescents engaging in sexual activity without adequate protection against pregnancy or sexually transmitted infections.

Late Adolescence. Late adolescence occurs at approximately age 17 to young adulthood. Physical growth is now complete. In most late adolescents cognition is abstract and future-oriented. The importance of the peer group recedes, and relationships assume a new quality of mutuality and reciprocity, as evidenced by a caring for another person instead of a narcissistic orientation (Sarrel and Sarrel 1981). Relationships with the family assume an adult-to-adult quality.

Adolescent Sexuality

Whether adults accept it, whether adolescents themselves accept it, whether there are restrictive laws, and whether there is sex education in the schools or not, adolescent sexual activity is a normal part of the maturation process. Over half of adolescents between the ages of 15 and 19 years have had sexual intercourse. One in five has had sexual intercourse by age 15, yet the majority of adolescents have fewer than three partners in their teenaged years (Marsiglio and Mott 1986).

There are some who believe that the way to slow down or discourage adolescent sexual activity is to withhold sexual information and contraceptive services. This supposition is based on the belief that sexual knowledge stimulates sexual experimentation. Conversely, there are those who believe that today's adolescent is already well informed about sexual knowledge, has access to contraceptives, has the motivation to use them, and has the knowledge to use them correctly. Neither argument is true, and both arguments limit access to education and services that are needed for adolescents to become responsible, well-educated sexual beings (Dawson 1986).

Many adolescents say they will not seek services from health professionals because they anticipate judgmental attitudes about their previous sexual activity or their contemplation of future sexual activity. It is important for health professionals to listen carefully to adolescents and ask questions that demonstrate a genuine interest. The use of moralizing attitudes that merely say "don't" often makes little sense to young people (Burke 1987). Health professionals need to consider whether they are unwittingly encouraging sexual rebellion by setting forth rigid guidelines that the adolescent is likely to reject altogether.

Adolescents want some sensible adult guidance in making decisions. Discussions about not exploiting or hurting others or themselves by bringing an unwanted child into the world can make a great deal of sense to many adolescents. Adolescents must feel they can make their own sexual decisions, and to do this they must have specific facts and knowledge about their options and the consequences of their decisions (Burke 1987).

COMMON HEALTH CONCERNS

Adolescents of the 1990s usually experience advanced pubertal development before psychosocial development, as evidenced by the decreasing age at menarche or first period of 12.5 years. Since the early 1970s the age of sexual debut has declined. The absence of a future orientation and the inability to see consequences of behavior put sexually active adolescents at considerable risk, because they may lack the ability to plan ahead for health care appointments or to engage in responsible health practices. During this time of evolving identity and emerging sexuality, many adolescents with reproductive capabilities are without sufficient social maturity to engage in responsible sexual behavior.

Access to Reproductive Health Care

Since the early 1970s there has been a demonstrable trend toward unmarried female adolescents engaging in sexual activity at a younger age. Survey data documented that 50% of 15- to 19-year-old females in the United States are sexually active. This change in behavior pattern over the last 20 years has resulted in one million pregnancies in adolescents, with nearly half of these resulting in live births and one third resulting in abortion (Hofferth, Kahn, and Baldwin 1987). National physician survey data indicate a shift in health care needs for adolescent females in the area of gynecologic and obstetrical care.

The use of obstetrical and gynecologic care emerges as one of the 20 most common reasons for visits to physician offices during late adolescence. Nearly 11% of all visits made to physician offices in the United States are for prenatal care (9.1%), contraceptive management (1%), and disorders of menstruation (0.9%) (Cypress 1984). Since available data only represent physician office visits, the true incidence of health care delivered to youth, such as that rendered by hospital and public health department clinics, Planned Parenthood, and other such agencies, is even greater. Thus, demands are being placed on the nursing profession to provide care to this population in a variety of health care settings from inpatient facilities to primary care settings.

Consent and Confidentiality

Adolescents have not always possessed the right to make decisions regarding their own health care. Prior to the twentieth century, two doctrines or approaches to the legal status of minors prevailed. The ''parental sovereignty'' doctrine assumed exclusive ''ownership'' by the parent of the youth. With the emergence of child labor laws and mandatory education, the ''child welfare'' approach restricted parental rights in circumstances in which parental ownership was determined to be injurious or dangerous to the child. In both cases, either parent rights or state rights defined the best interests of the child. In the past two decades the concept of the ''mature minor doctrine'' has emerged; this permits a care-giver to assess the adolescent's psychosocial maturity before consenting to provide care, instead of requiring a reliance on an arbitrary assumption that the adolescent is incompetent to make decisions. Reliance on the parent or state occurs only when the adolescent is deemed immature. The implication of the mature minor doctrine is that assessment of competency is based on a case-by-case review of maturity by the care provider. Members of the health care team, such as physician, nurse, and social worker, are involved either as individuals or as a team in assessing competency. The role of the nurse involves providing assessment and documentation of cognitive competency within the clinical interview.

Consent is defined as the process or ability whereby the client agrees to participate in a specific treatment regimen. Consent implies that the client has received adequate information to understand the risk–benefit ratio, alternatives to treatment (including no treatment), and expected outcomes.

Confidentiality involves a private and personal relationship between the provider and the client. In most states adolescents have the right to give consent for their own care in a private and confidential manner for health services related to sexuality, and, to a limited extent, mental health and substance abuse. Adolescents should also be judged on their own ability or inability to pay for these services, irrespective of their parents' health insurance or economic status. Reliance on parental health care benefits for payment may adversely affect confidentiality, since bills generated for the diagnosis and treatment of pregnancy or sexually transmitted disease (STD) may violate the adolescent's right to privacy.

Concerns about confidentiality and fear of disclosure of services to parents clearly contribute to an adolescent's reluctance to seek essential services. Although adolescents may want parental involvement in nonsensitive health care issues, they may delay seeking services in such sensitive areas as emotional problems, sexuality, and substance abuse. As a result, even when adolescents have ready access to primary health care, they may have unmet needs in areas that they perceive as sensitive. Considering the complexities of all these variables, the rise of pregnancy and sexually transmitted diseases among adolescents is not surprising.

Laws that protect confidentiality are not intended to exclude parents in the delivery of health care to their child. Since adolescents may delay seeking services because of fear of disclosure to parents, the law allows them to access care so that they do not experience the negative outcomes of inadequate health care. These include poorer pregnancy outcomes when prenatal care is delayed or absent and such negative sequelae as pelvic inflammatory disease resulting from untreated sexually transmitted disease. Inclusion of the parent can occur, if indicated, after the adolescent is in the health care system and a plan has been negotiated between the adolescent and the provider regarding parental involvement.

Implications for Nursing Care

Adolescents often are concerned about the normalcy of their body; added reassurance regarding these concerns is necessary throughout the health visit. The use of sophisticated medical terminology is confusing and often perceived as indicating pathology. The nurse should use accepted slang along with appropriate medical terminology. This will enable the nurse to obtain a reliable health history while providing health education. The use of three-dimensional models or pictures is helpful in teaching about the adolescent's changing body.

The Health History

The setting of the health interview should occur where adequate privacy can be ensured, thereby reducing client embarrassment. The interviewer should be perceived as nonjudgmental regarding the adolescent's beliefs, values, and behaviors. Ensuring the privacy of health information disclosed by the adolescent is of paramount importance. From the start the nurse should inform the youth that all information shared between provider and client is confidential except in the following situations: an acutely suicidal adolescent, for whom direct adult intervention would provide a safe environment; the disclosure of unreported physical or sexual abuse; and particular areas in which state regulations include mandatory reporting laws. The emphasis is on providing a safe environment for the youth and disclosure is not to be construed as a punitive measure.

The health history, as it relates to the provision of gynecologic or reproductive health, is usually very focused and problem oriented; the progression of questioning is from the least sensitive to the most sensitive. The nurse must recognize the importance of the female adolescent's perception of her sexuality so that psychosexual maturity can be fostered (Woods 1987). The exclusion of concerned persons, such as boyfriends or parents, during the initial interview sends a clear message to the adolescent that the interviewer is concerned about maintaining confidentiality. Inclusion of male partners and parents may occur after the adolescent has consented to this and may be beneficial by providing health education that dispels myths and enhances compliance by those in the adolescent's social support network. An example of the types of questions asked on the reproductive health history are given in the accompanying Assessment Tool.

Initial Gynecologic Examination

The optimal experience of an initial pelvic examination is an examination performed as a result of the adolescent's request for gynecologic health care. The initial examination is aimed at evaluating the possibility of existing health problems. Indications for a pelvic examination are listed in the accompanying display.

Frequently the first pelvic examination triggers concerns about the discovery of pathology, fear of pain, and embarrassment about nudity, all of which enhance the adolescent's anxiety about her own sexuality.

The role of the nurse emerges in several areas: obtaining an adequate health history, preparing the adolescent for her pelvic examination by providing knowledge about the procedure and skills which enhance relaxation and decrease anxiety, and providing essential health information following the examination.

Preparation for the first pelvic examination is important. Millstein and associates (1988) have documented that adolescents can experience heightened levels of anxiety prior to the pelvic examination. Preparation for the pelvic examination should include not only an explanation of the order in which the examination will proceed but also a description of anticipated feelings or sensations. For example: "You may feel a stretching and tugging sensation while I slip the speculum into place." Al-

ASSESSMENT TOOL

Content Areas of Reproductive Health History for an Adolescent Female

Menarche	Age of onset	"How many days do your periods usually last?"
	Duration of flow	"How often do your periods come? Do you keep track of them by using a calendar?"
	Frequency	
	Date of last normal menstrual period (LNMP)	"When was the date of your last menstrual period? Was it normal?"
	Dysmenorrhea	"With your periods do you ever have cramps? Does this affect your activities or school attendance? Do you use any remedies/medications?" (Be specific to include name of drug, dosage, and frequency of ingestion.)

(continued)

ASSESSMENT TOOL   (continued)

Sexual activity	Age of sexual debut	"Has anyone ever touched you on any part of your body where you didn't want to be touched?" (Issues of past sexual abuse or date rape by an acquaintance may be important areas of discussion.)
	Sexual orientation	"Whom do you find yourself most attracted to, men or women?" (Question allows youth to admit feelings of attraction and does not imply a behavior, such as actually having intercourse with a same-sex individual.) "Have you ever had sexual contact with a person of your gender?"
	Frequency of coitus	"When you have sex, how often might that be? Once a month, once a week, or twice a week . . . ?" (Allow the adolescent to have a range of choices.)
	Number of sexual partners	"How many partners have you had in the past two months? How many in the past year? How many since you first started having sex?"
	Sexual practices	(Include questions that ask about the full range of sexual expression, including kissing, touching, and masturbation (solo or mutual) as well as oral, vaginal and anal intercourse. To counsel youth regarding safer sex practices, the clinician must be aware of the adolescent's entire repertoire of behaviors.)
	Sexual pleasure	"Is having intercourse/sex pleasurable for you? Are you satisfied with your sexual life the way it is now? Do you think your partner is satisfied?"
Contraceptive history	Current method of birth control used	(It may be helpful to list the choice of specific methods: i.e., foam, sponge, condoms, withdrawal, birth control pills, etc. Ask about the frequency with which a method is used, i.e., "never," "sometimes," or "always" and about any perceived or real side-effects from using a specific method.
Ob/gyn history	Number of pregnancies	(List exact number, including number of live births and spontaneous and therapeutic abortions.)
	Recent gynecologic procedures	(List dilatation and curettage [D&C], recent abortion, and any subsequent complications.)
	Prior history of pelvic inflammatory disease	(Ask when and where treatment was obtained and if management was on an inpatient or outpatient basis.)
STD history	History of previous sexually transmitted disease (STD)	(Determine the type of STD, its treatment and if the partner was treated.)
Drug history	Onset, duration, and frequency	(It is important to ask about the use of cigarettes, alcohol, and other illicit drugs. Ask about intravenous drug use. Inclusion of this is essential in the assessment of behaviors at risk for HIV infection.)
Partner	Male partner involvement	Is the female adolescent's partner involved in the visit today? (Have there been any prior discussions regarding contraception?)
	Male partner STD assessment	"Does your boyfriend have any symptoms of infection?" (Include symptoms of urethritis [discharge or dysuria] and any open sores or warts in the genital region.)
Support system	Parents and friends	(Ask who is aware of the client's sexual activity and if she anticipates any negative effects from disclosing her behavior to her parents or friends. Ascertain what support is available and/or needed.)

Indications for an Adolescent Pelvic Exam

Menstrual disorders, including the following:

- Amenorrhea
- Irregular uterine/vaginal bleeding
- Dysmenorrhea unresponsive to therapy

Undiagnosed abdominal pain

Rape

Request for prescription method of birth control

Suspected pelvic mass

Any sexual activity

Request by the patient

lowing the adolescent to see and feel the sensation of the speculum opening in her hand will approximate this feeling. Telling the patient, "I'm going to touch you now," prior to touching the vulva or inserting a gloved finger into the vagina, may decrease the likelihood of startling her. Talking to the adolescent throughout the examination, use of such relaxation techniques as controlled deep breathing or visual imagery, or the strategic placement of a poster over the examination table may foster a more relaxed environment (Kohen 1980). Inclusion of a significant person (friend or family member) who can be supportive during the examination can be helpful but should be done only if the adolescent consents. If the examiner is male, an adult female should be present during the examination.

A mirror may be included in the examination if the patient is interested. In addition to viewing the cervix and vagina, the adolescent can be allowed to view her external genitals and learn the relationship between them and internal structures that are not usually visible. A common criticism of menstrual education materials has been that they provide drawings that make the internal genitals appear disembodied from their external anatomy, particularly the clitoris and labia. Use of the mirror should help to facilitate an integrated approach to the gynecologic examination.

Promoting Health Maintenance Through Teaching

Menarche is the most observable phenomenon signifying the transition from girl to woman. Preparation prior to the event will decrease negative perceptions of it. Premenarcheal and menarcheal girls need to receive accurate and developmentally appropriate information regarding not only the physiologic and hygienic aspects of menstruation but also the associated emotional changes.

Given the adolescent's lack of life experience and her need to interpret new body changes, sensations, and feelings, health education becomes increasingly important. The nurse can provide health teaching so that the adolescent may incorporate health-promoting behaviors into her life-style. The display shown below lists areas of health teaching that should be included in the health visit. Assessment of cognitive status may influence the amount and complexity of instruction given to the adolescent, and the teaching itself may be integrated with the questions for the health history and with the pelvic examination.

Patients, at best, retain five to six major ideas from a health visit. Thus, timing patient teaching carefully in

Anticipatory Guidance with the Adolescent Client

Breast Development	Discuss level of comfort regarding rapid body changes. Reassure regarding size, shape, and appearance of breast asymmetry. Teach breast self-exam.
Vaginal Development	Educate regarding the appearance of physiologic leukorrhea. Teach about changing vaginal secretion throughout ovulatory cycle.
Menstruation	Instruct on the use of a menstrual calendar to record last menses and document frequency, duration, and character of menses. Discuss concerns about menstrual cramps. Instruct on appropriate use of medications, when indicated.
Sexuality	Discuss sexual orientation. Issues regarding romantic attraction to same sex or opposite sex individual need to be discussed in a nonstigmatizing approach.
Sexual Activity	Discover if sexual debut has been initiated or is contemplated. If so, include contraceptive counseling for prevention of pregnancy and sexually transmitted disease. Teach health care regarding safer sex practices to reduce acquisition of sexually transmitted diseases.

relation to anxiety-provoking procedures may be advisable. Repetition of important concepts, such as instruction about the correct use of a contraceptive device or method, may be necessary to facilitate internalization of new information. Educational materials should use simple language and incorporate the use of visual aids whenever possible (Streiff 1986).

Understanding the psychologic development of the female adolescent helps the nurse comprehend the discrepancies between an adolescent's motivation to comply with health-promoting activities and her actual behavior. An example of this is the adolescent who states that she does not want children until early adulthood but who initiates sexual activity without contraception at age 15 and experiences an unplanned pregnancy. The motivations for pregnancy are complex and not easily elucidated; however, some health care workers support the concept that assessment of cognitive function is essential in providing health education. Decisions to engage in a certain behavior, such as avoiding sexual activity or using a reliable method of contraception, may occur if options are known.

Categorizing a female adolescent's cognitive ability into either concrete or formal/abstract thinking should guide the nurse in providing different educational strategies (Sachs 1987). Adolescents who are concrete thinkers would benefit from teaching methods that enhance problem solving, such as cognitive rehearsal used in role playing and the use of the pronoun "you" in any scenario so that answers generated can be personalized for their own situation. Abstract thinkers are better equipped to apply information learned in a counseling session to future situations.

SEXUALLY ACTIVE ADOLESCENTS

Two significant threats to well-being among sexually active adolescents are the acquisition of sexually transmitted diseases and the occurrence of unintended pregnancy.

Sexually Transmitted Diseases

Venereal disease was first identified in Europe in 1530 when a Verona physician described the signs and symptoms of the so-called "French disease" and gave it the name "syphilis." Syphilis quickly became the most recognizable and debilitating of the venereal diseases. Not until Fleming's discovery of penicillin and its development was syphilis effectively treated.

Prior to the 1970s five diseases were recognized to be transmitted through sexual contact: gonorrhea, syphilis,

chancroid, lymphogranuloma venereum, and granuloma inguinale. Since then, the term "venereal disease" (named for the goddess of love Venus) has been supplanted by the term "sexually transmitted disease" (STD). The number of causative agents of STDs has grown to more than 20: technological advancement and sophistication in identifying the causative agents of STDs has added a substantial number to the list. Alterations in sexual behavior have increased the spread of STDs, and microbial resistance to antibiotics has made management of these diseases increasingly difficult.

The expanding incidence of STDs since the 1960s and the emergence of the first untreatable and fatal sexually transmitted disease, AIDS, has made the public aware of the implications and importance of STDs. Widespread education about prevention of these diseases may yet emerge as one of the more effective control measures. In the meantime, *continence, condoms,* and *caution* are the major weapons against the spread of STDs.

This section discusses currently common STDs and their description, clinical features, symptoms and diagnosis, complications, and teaching and management. The nurse can play a major role in helping to prevent the spread of STDs. Appendix D reviews critical information about the most common treatable STDs.

Common STDs
Chlamydia Trachomatis

The most common bacterial STD and the least publicized is *Chlamydia trachomatis*. The incidence among all age groups is estimated to be 4.5 million new cases annually. This exceeds gonorrhea by a ratio of 2 : 1. Sexually active adolescents, especially girls, represent the highest risk age group with a chlamydial prevalence rate of 15% to 20%, compared to 10% in women age 20 to 24 and less than 4% in women over 30 years old. Approximately 1 in 6 sexually active adolescents will have *C. trachomatis*. Unfortunately, one half of females are asymptomatic, thus emphasizing the need for routine screening within this population. Another risk factor for *C. trachomatis* infections, besides age, is the presence of *Neisseria gonorrhea* infection. Approximately 40% to 50% of persons with *N. gonorrhea* have concomitant *C. trachomatis* infections. Thus, testing and treating of dual infections is essential (Schachter, Stoner, and Moncada 1983).

Gonorrhea

Among sexually active females prevalence rates for *Neisseria gonorrhoeae* have been reported to range from 3% to 18%. The increased rate of gonorrheal infections in black adolescents may be due to the epidemic use of crack cocaine and other drugs in urban areas, which diminishes the likelihood of their engaging in safer sexual practices (Bell and Hein 1984).

Human Papillomavirus

New attention has recently been drawn to one of the oldest STDs, human papillomavirus (HPV). HPV was once regarded as a self-limiting nuisance. Rates of HPV infections have been difficult to obtain because of this earlier lack of interest and reporting. Recent evidence, however, has established a correlation between HPV and the development of cervical cancer. Current studies reveal that referrals for genital warts have risen 460% from 1966 to 1981, the major increase occurring in females. More than 65% of these patients were in the 15- to 19-year-old group (Becker, Stone, and Alexander 1987). HPV is now thought to be the second most common STD, exceeding *N. gonorrhoeae*.

Cervical HPV infections are not readily discernible to the naked eye. HPV infection of the cervix is usually diagnosed by pathologic changes seen in Papanicolaou smears or by new DNA viral typing. Colposcopic evaluation of the cervix, vagina, and vulva may reveal suspicious areas of white epithelium after the application of 3% acetic acid. Definitive diagnosis is achieved through tissue biopsy. Treatment involves a variety of options and is based on the type of lesion and its distribution. There is no medication at present that eradicates the virus.

Complication: Pelvic Inflammatory Disease

Pelvic Inflammatory Disease (PID) is the most serious common complication of STD. It is estimated to cost over $1 billion in health care each year. Approximately 1 million women are affected each year, and 20% to 36% are less than 19 years old. Major morbidities as a result of this disease are tubo-ovarian abscess; ectopic pregnancy which occurs once in every 125–150 pregnancies in women without PID but once in every 20–25 women after PID because of tubal scarring; chronic pelvic pain; and infertility (which will occur in 20% of those women with first infections). The long-range economic and emotional impact on these women is immeasurable. It has been estimated that 1 out of 8 sexually active adolescents will develop PID, compared to 1 out of 80 sexually active 24-year-olds (Washington, Sweet, and Shafer 1985).

The etiology and pathogenesis of PID remain obscure. Both *Chlamydia trachomatis* (CT) and *Neisseria gonorrhoeae* (NG) have been implicated in the etiology of 50% to 80% of PID. However, over 90% of PID cases are associated with multibacteriologic isolates. Thus, the direct role of CT and NG are not understood. It has been estimated that 11% of women with cervical *Chlamydia trachomatis* and 10% to 20% of women with cervical *Neisseria gonorrhoeae* will develop PID.

HIV Infection and AIDS

A new and more frightening threat emerged in the 1980s: human immunodeficiency virus (HIV) infection and the resulting disease, acquired immunodeficiency syndrome (AIDS). This infection, transmitted through sexual activity or blood contact, is not treatable and is regarded by many as the major public health problem of the 1990s. The following section discusses HIV/AIDS as a threat in the general population. See Chapter 20 for a discussion of AIDS during pregnancy and Chapter 34 for nursing care of the high-risk neonate.

HIV infection causes a collapse of the body's immune system and eventual death from opportunistic infections. AIDS was first identified in the United States in 1981 when several cases of *Pneumocystis carinii* pneumonia and Kaposi's sarcoma were seen in male homosexuals. AIDS is endemic in Haiti and central Africa and has spread to the heterosexual community worldwide.

The human immunodeficiency virus (HIV) is a member of a recently described class of virus called a retrovirus. The HIV selectively infects human T lymphocytes, most often the subset of helper T_4 lymphocytes known as the T_4 cell. After HIV enters a T_4 lymphocyte host cell, it may become inactive for a period of time or may rapidly replicate. This rapid replication first interferes with the function of the T cell (which is central to the immune response) and then kills the cell. As a result, severe immunodeficiency develops, presenting clinically in recurrent Kaposi's sarcoma, *Pneumocystis carinii* pneumonia and other opportunistic infections, and/or severe neurological deterioration. It was the presence of the two aforementioned diseases that unmasked the presence of AIDS in the United States (Williams 1986). Persons infected with HIV fall into four categories:

- Those who have a negative HIV antibody test because they are in an incubation stage, which may last from 6 months to 5 years
- Those who are HIV positive but are asymptomatic
- Those who have AIDS Related Complex (ARC) and who have developed a cluster of chronic, severe physical symptoms, such as night sweats, fever, and nonspecific diarrhea; extreme weight loss; persistent generalized lymphadenopathy; fatigue; and yeast infections (usually of the mouth)
- Those who actually have AIDS, as demonstrated by severe immunodeficiency, presence of Kaposi's sarcoma, pneumocystic pneumonia, or characteristic neurological symptoms (Carr and Gee 1986)

Incidence

Since its identification in 1981, the incidence of AIDS has risen to pandemic proportions worldwide. As of March 14, 1988, a total of 56,212 cases of AIDS had been reported in the United States, with more than 31,400 cases ending in death. In the year from March 1987 to March 1988, a total of 23,000 cases was reported, representing an increase of 58% over the previous year. The

Centers for Disease Control (CDC) have projected that by the end of 1991 there will be 270,000 diagnosed cases of AIDS in the United States (Centers for Disease Control 1988). Since the beginning of the epidemic in the United States, the majority of AIDS cases have occurred in the following subgroups:

- Homosexual or bisexual men
- Intravenous drug users
- Hemophiliacs
- Prostitutes
- Recipients of blood products by transfusion
- Children born to a woman infected with the virus

Heterosexual partners of members of these groups and children born of women of high-risk groups now constitute a significant new portion of cases.

Transmission of HIV

The modes of HIV transmission are parenteral, sexual, and perinatal. The most frequent mode of HIV transmission to *women,* who represent about 7% of the infected population, has been through sharing needles with IV drug users or sexual contact with a male partner who is himself likely to have been infected through needle sharing.

Parenteral Transmission. Parenteral transmission involves person-to-person contact with infected blood, such as with contaminated needles or blood products. The greatest danger for parenteral infection (other than among IV drug users who share needles) has occurred from blood products transfused between 1979, when the virus seems to have first appeared, and the spring of 1985, when the antibody test came into use for screening donated blood.

The absolute risk for HIV infection among health care workers is very low, less than 0.5% for an HIV needle stick and much lower for exposure to the nonintact skin or mucus membrane of an HIV-infected patient. Estimated risk for a surgeon operating on an HIV-infected patient is 1 : 4,500 to 1 : 130,000 (Hagen, Meyer, and Pauker 1988). Although the risk of HIV infection through a needle stick or puncture wound is low, such infections have occurred; thus, health care workers should follow standard blood and body fluid precautions with all patients (see Nursing Alert: Universal Precautions in Chapter 23).

Sexual Transmission. Sexual transmission occurs from the passage of contaminated semen or vaginal fluids to another person.

It is presumed that multiple exposures to the body fluids of an infected person will increase the probability of transmission of the virus. A factor that seems to influence the acquisition and transmission of HIV is the presence of a concomitant sexually transmitted disease, especially one that causes genital ulcers. Studies in the United States have shown that syphilis and genital herpes have been specifically associated with HIV infection (Cates and Schultz 1988). The loss of the epithelial integrity associated with these diseases may provide a portal of entry or exit that may be needed for HIV to cause infection. Studies confirm that HIV is not transmitted through casual contact, that is, touching, working next to, or sharing living space with individuals who have HIV. Those who have nonsexual or nonblood household contact with a person with HIV/AIDS are not at risk for infection (Mead 1988). Currently there is no epidemiologic evidence of transmission of HIV through casual contact, even though the virus is found in semen, blood, urine, saliva, amniotic fluid, and tears. Transmission occurs almost totally through intimate sexual contact or needles (Centers for Disease Control 1988).

Most women experiencing HIV infections are heterosexual. The means by which the chain of transmission is established in the heterosexual population is illustrated in Figure 10-3.

Perinatal Transmission. Perinatal transmission involves passage of the virus from the mother to infant transplacentally during gestation, delivery, or through breast milk. The number of infants thus infected with HIV is expected to rise as the number of heterosexual carriers rises.

Diagnosis

Following exposure to and infection from the HIV virus, most individuals develop specific antibodies (or seroconvert) within 2 to 3 months of infection. The onset of *symptoms* is thought to occur anywhere from 6 months to 6 to 10 years following HIV infection. This means that there are a significant number of infected individuals who have not yet developed symptoms, have therefore not been tested, and who may unknowingly transmit the virus to others (Carr and Gee 1986).

AIDS is most often diagnosed by the presence of a set of complex infectious processes, with or without the presence of HIV antibodies in the blood. The HIV antibody test is not diagnostic although most patients with AIDS are seropositive. The number of seropositive individuals who will eventually develop AIDS after 5 years is estimated at 5% to 25%. The Centers for Disease Control (1988) estimate that 1 to 1.5 million individuals are seropositive. The HIV antibody test involves the analysis of a blood sample for the presence of antibodies that are produced by the immune system after the virus enters the bloodstream. When the initial test is positive by Enzyme-Linked ImmunoSorbent Assay (ELISA), an additional confirmatory test (Western Blot) is performed to reduce the risk of a false-positive result.

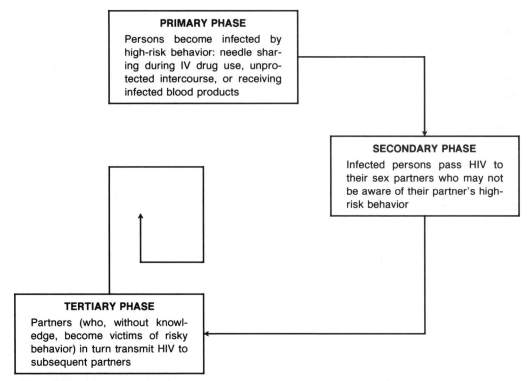

Figure 10–3. Manner in which chain of transmission of human immunodeficiency virus (HIV) is established within the heterosexual population. Transmission probably occurs in three stages in the United States.

Treatment

Presently there is no known treatment for HIV. Some compounds, such as azido-deoxythymidine (AZT), have been shown to be effective in slowing the disease process. Many compounds are still in various trial phases of research, and the FDA has permitted accelerated clinical trials of new drugs. Treatment is palliative, and therapy is aimed at combating opportunistic infection (Fischl et al 1987). Prevention is essential because of the severity and extremely poor prognosis of the disease.

Implications for Nursing Care

A significant number of women worldwide are infected with HIV. Approximately one half of women in Central Africa are infected, while in Haiti more than one quarter of women are infected. In 1988 in the United States, women accounted for 6.7% (about 100,000) of all AIDS cases. Of these, 50% were black, 29% Hispanic; 52% were drug users and 21% became infected after sexual contact with infected men. Of these men 67% were IV drug users and 16% were bisexual. Of all women with AIDS 79% are between the ages of 13 and 39 years, the childbearing years. These figures have startling implications; 80% of pediatric AIDS cases have been traced to infected mothers (Mead et al 1988). When women have been in a strictly monogamous relationship with a partner who is not infected, measures to avoid infection are not necessary. However, women in relationships with men who are bisexual, who have sexual contact with multiple partners, or who share needles during IV drug use, or women who themselves engage in the latter two practices must protect themselves from HIV infection. Women should be counseled to use the precautions shown in the display on the opposite page.

Sexually Transmitted Diseases in Adolescents

Sexually transmitted diseases represent one of the major morbidities occurring during adolescence and young adulthood, afflicting approximately 10 million persons under the age of 25 annually. Adolescents represent one of the highest risk groups affected, considering that not all adolescents have initiated sexual activity.

A growing concern for adolescents is exposure to HIV. Many adolescents know (or think they know) about HIV but lack the specific information they need not only to prevent the spread of a deadly disease but also to calm unwarranted fears. Adolescents may be avoiding discussing these fears with health professionals because they do not want to appear ignorant or because they are terrified that a rash or fever means the diagnosis of HIV. However, HIV is not the only sexually transmitted disease for adolescents to worry about (Selvin and Marvin 1987). It is estimated that there were 2.5 million adolescents in 1987 who contracted chlamydia, gonorrhea, genital warts, or herpes.

Several unique biological, behavioral, and developmental phenomena make these diseases of particular concern in the adolescent population. The immature adolescent cervix undergoes major physiologic transitions in the endocervical transformation zone. Infectious agents, such as *Chlamydia trachomatis, Neisseria gonorrhoeae,* and human papillomavirus (wart virus), may invade immature cervical columnar cells and account for a higher prevalence of these infections in adolescent females. Also, the unchallenged immune system does not afford female adolescents the localized antibody response when exposed repeatedly to infectious agents. Another factor yet to be well understood is the contribution of cervical mucus in anovulatory menstrual cycles to pelvic infection. The predominance of estrogen in the menstrual cycle of the physiologically immature adolescent provides for a cervical mucus that is clear and watery and facilitates the transport of pathogens to the upper genital tract (Bell and Hein 1984).

Implications for Nursing Care

STDs play a significant role in impairing the adolescent's future fertility and leading to the possible development of cervical cancer. Two thirds of sexually active adolescents report using an effective method of contraception at their last occurrence of intercourse, but less than 20% report using a barrier method (15% use condoms and 3% use a diaphragm) which would afford some protection against the acquisition of STD. The role of the nurse in health education is apparent. Adolescents not only need information regarding the correct use of contraceptive methods but also information regarding STD risk reduction strategies, including abstinence, condom use, avoidance of high-risk practices such as anal sex and IV drug use, use of spermicides, and the reduction of the number of sexual partners. In addition to knowledge, adolescents require skills that enhance values clarification and decision making regarding their sexuality (Tauer 1983).

When advising women about preventing HIV infection, the nurse should

- Instruct patients about basic female and male anatomy and physiology.
- Explain how HIV is transmitted. Oral, anal, or vaginal intercourse with multiple partners, prostitutes, or strangers and needle or syringe sharing with an infected person are very high-risk practices. Needle and puncture wounds have also been shown to transmit the virus. Breast-feeding by an infected mother and using blood that has not been screened for the presence of HIV antibodies are not safe practices.
- Explain that HIV is not spread by casual contact.

SELF-CARE TEACHING

Preventing HIV Infection

- *Absolutely* safe sex involves only abstinence, massage, or mutual masturbation.
- Avoid sex with multiple partners, anonymous partners, prostitutes, and partners with multiple partners.
- Avoid sexual activities that could create cuts in the skin through which the virus could enter the body.
- Avoid sexual contact with persons who have genital discharge, genital warts, genital herpes lesions, or other suspicious genital lesions.
- Avoid oral–anal sex.
- Avoid genital contact with oral "cold sores."
- Use latex condoms in combination with spermicides with any new partner.
- Avoid sex with people who have AIDS or its symptoms and with those who are known as HIV carriers or who have a positive antibody test or evidence of hepatitis B.
- Never share needles or syringes with anyone.
- If you use IV drugs, enter a treatment program as soon as possible.
- Have periodic examinations for sexually transmitted agents and syndromes if you are at high risk for a sexually transmitted disease.

Adolescent Pregnancy Risk

Adolescent pregnancy occurs in a girl under 18 years of age and is typically an unplanned and often an unwanted event.

Incidence

The United States has the highest rate of adolescent pregnancy in the developed world. Forty percent of sexually active adolescents are under 18 years of age, almost one third of the 15- to 17-year-old group are sexually active, while 70% of females have intercourse before age 20 (Dash 1989). Thus, the majority of American adolescents are at some level of risk for adolescent pregnancy (Fig. 10-4).

Etiology

The risk of pregnancy in adolescents is increased by

- Lack of knowledge about where and how to obtain contraceptive preparations or devices
- Lack of concern by the male partner about contraception

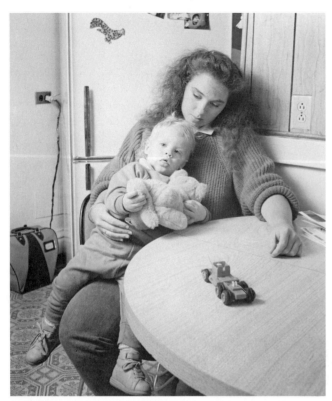

Figure 10 – 4. As a single mother the adolescent may find it difficult to continue her education when family and/or financial support is lacking. (Photo: Nancy M. Stuart. Copyright 1988)

for adolescents is abstinence. Since this is not a realistic option for many, it is important for the nurse counseling the adolescent to put the risks of early sexual activity in perspective. The obstetric and social risks of early childbearing for the mother and baby and the possibility of contracting sexually transmitted diseases, with the associated problems of infertility, cervical neoplasia, and acquired immune deficiency syndrome, present strong arguments for delaying sexual activity. The adolescent may reject the idea that these problems could happen to her, but she must be informed.

The role of the nurse in promoting use of contraception by adolescents is a challenging one, since they do not easily identify with health care providers and do not often seek out health care assistance on their own.

Nurses who practice in such settings as neighborhood family planning clinics and school-based clinics have the greatest access to this group of young women. When an adolescent voluntarily attends one of these clinics, she has made the first step in preventing pregnancy.

In these types of settings, it is possible for the nurse to schedule groups of adolescents to assess and increase their knowledge or use of contraception. Issues presented should include the importance of avoiding unwanted

When contraceptives are not used, pregnancy risk is highest in the first 6 months of a sexual relationship. This risk increases from 36% in the first three months to 45% at six months; thus, overall risk of conception is about 50/50. Among adolescents who do seek contraceptive services, the probability of becoming sexually active is high. Even though the nation's adolescent pregnancy rate has stabilized during the 1980s, rates for girls under 15 years continue to rise, thus reflecting an increase in sexual activity for this age group. Between 1970 and 1980 the number of sexually active adolescents increased nearly 60%. Adolescents risk pregnancy by continuing unprotected intercourse for months or years prior to seeking contraception.

Implications for Nursing Care

Many sexually active adolescents are uninformed about the various methods of birth control and are reluctant to seek help within the health care system. Therefore, it should be a priority of the nurse working with sexually active adolescent females to encourage adoption of a safe method of birth control. A full discussion of contraception is contained in Chapter 8. Elements particular to the care of adolescents are addressed in this chapter.

The safest and most beneficial method of birth control

Psychological and Socioeconomic Factors Affecting Adolescent Failure to Use Contraception

- Denial of the ability to get pregnant (especially under age 18)
- Feeling that contraception is "unromantic"
- Low self-esteem and lack of concern for personal health
- Fear of acknowledging sexual activity by requesting contraceptive services
- Feeling of embarrassment, ambivalence, or fear of public exposure
- Exaggerated fears of the effects and safety of contraception
- Delay of the partners in discussing contraception
- Disapproval of parents or peers
- Lack of or inaccurate knowledge regarding the risk of pregnancy
- Lack of knowledge about where or how to obtain contraceptive services
- Misunderstanding of the legal aspect of services to minors
- Inability to afford services and/or fear that a bill will be sent to parents, revealing her sex life
- An unsupportive partner who has a negative attitude toward conception.

pregnancy and infection, and the different ways in which these situations can be accomplished through the use of a contraceptive method. The group process provides the adolescent comfort, safety, and openness to such discussions without singling out individuals. The nurse should also encourage ongoing self-care through regular gynecologic follow-up, especially for screening for STDs or when problems arise with a contraceptive method.

The adolescent should be instructed regarding the various methods of contraception, their use, advantages, and disadvantages. Once explained, the choice of contraceptive method must be the adolescent's.

The latest information on adolescent contraception suggests that the low dose (<50 μg) oral contraceptive pills are the safest and most effective birth control method for adolescents, regardless of their smoking habits (Hatcher et al 1988). While the use of condoms in conjunction with an oral contraceptive would not only increase efficacy but protect from infection and add an element of shared responsibility for contraception, adolescents are usually not motivated or effective users of the barrier methods. The use of IUDs has not been widespread with adolescents because of the increased risk of pelvic inflammatory disease with multiple sexual partners.

Adolescent Pregnancy

Incidence

The adolescent pregnancy rate climbed during the 1980s, with at least one girl in ten becoming pregnant; nearly one third of adolescent girls risk pregnancy. Concern about adolescent childbearing and parenting has existed for decades. It is estimated that 1.2 million adolescents in the United States become pregnant each year, accounting for as many as 20% of births. Of today's 14-year-olds, one in four will become pregnant while still an adolescent; one in seven will choose abortion (Marsiglio and Mott 1986).

The rate of first births to women 15 to 19 years of age fell from about 54 per 1000 in 1970 to about 40 per 1000 in 1986, as shown in Figure 10-5. Although fewer adolescents were bearing children, proportionally more were becoming pregnant and having abortions, and the proportion of adolescent births out of wedlock increased from 43% in 1970 to 67% in 1986. In addition, the birth rate for unmarried adolescents age 15 to 17 years increased from 17 per 1000 in 1970 to 26 per 1000 in 1986. Adolescent pregnancy has become a major health concern; although the overall birth rate is stable, the birth rate among the youngest unmarried adolescents is rising.

Pregnant adolescents have been described (Waters 1969) as being caught in a "syndrome of failure," a term used to describe the effect that pregnancy can have on the life of the adolescent girl. Rarely will she finish her school year or graduate from high school. Thus, her chances for attaining her full educational potential are limited. She may marry as a result of her pregnancy, but the marriage frequently ends in divorce. As a single parent, she will have difficulty supporting herself and her child financially and may require governmental assistance in the form of welfare (Fig. 10-6). In addition, society may doubt her ability to parent, since infants of adolescent mothers frequently experience developmental lag, neglect, or abuse, thus adding to the problems of an already compromised family unit.

Etiology

Research aimed at identifying the causes of adolescent pregnancy has met with limited success. Distinguishing between an adolescent's desire for intercourse and a desire for pregnancy remains a problem (Fogel 1981). Numerous interrelated factors contribute to adolescent childbearing.

Socioeconomic factors may play a most important

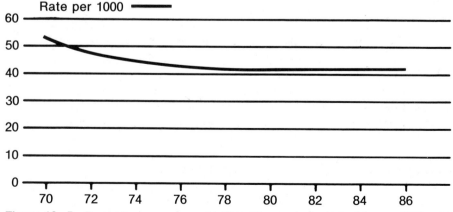

Figure 10-5. First births in women aged 15 to 19 years in the United States, 1970-1986

part. Adolescents of minority groups, especially blacks, who are overrepresented among lower socioeconomic levels, have an increased risk of teen pregnancy, have their first occurrence of intercourse at an earlier age, and are much more likely to have an out-of-wedlock birth than whites. The educational level of the adolescent's parents is correlated with the adolescent's effective use of birth control: as parental level of education increases, the adolescent's risk of pregnancy decreases. Age at first sexual experience is also a factor. When intercourse is postponed until an older age, the likelihood that contraception will be used increases. In 1979 approximately 50% of girls age 15 to 19 and 70% of boys aged 17 to 21 were engaging in sexual intercourse. The mean age at first intercourse was 16.2 years for girls and 15.7 years for boys (Zelnik, 1983).

The emphasis on sexual content in the media has been implicated in adolescent pregnancy. Adolescents receive conflicting messages when explicit sexual content is used to sell products aimed at their age group while, at the same time, readily available sex education is limited. This encourages adolescents to explore sex with little knowledge of the means to prevent conception (Panzarine and Gould 1988). Further, since physical maturation occurs much earlier than does cognitive maturation, it is no wonder that the adolescent has an unrealistically optimistic view of her chances of avoiding pregnancy.

Sexual intercourse for most adolescents is a spur-of-the-moment decision. The primary impetus for first inter-

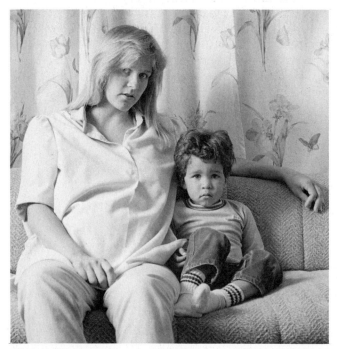

Figure 10-6. Recurrence of adolescent pregnancy within 24 months of an initial pregnancy occurs in 40%–50% of adolescents. (Photo: Nancy M. Stuart. Copyright 1988)

course among boys is peer pressure. Contraceptive knowledge and use among boys is erratic at best, since they tend to assume that girls are more informed and responsible. Girls more often are eager to be seen as grown-up and feminine. Adolescent girls with low self-esteem and low achievement may use sexual activity as a way to gain affection and a secure relationship.

Maternal/Fetal Implications

Reporting of risk factors associated with adolescent pregnancy is complicated by varying definitions of "adolescent" (*i.e.,* under 20, under 18, or under 16 years of age). Mercer (1984) notes that younger adolescents (14 years old and younger) are at greater perinatal risk. Middle (15–17 years old) and older adolescents (18 and older) have more positive perinatal outcomes when other risk factors are controlled for. Mercer further states that there is little evidence to suggest that youth or physiologic immaturity by themselves are related to poor maternal and neonatal outcomes: other factors, such as inadequate prenatal care, nutritional deficiencies, noncompliance with health regimens, and adverse social conditions, are more critical.

Adolescents are more likely to have preterm and small-for-gestational-age births, in part because of their lower socioeconomic status, poor nutritional habits, and lower prepregnancy weight, and because of delays in receiving prenatal care (Mercer 1984). Adolescent pregnancy has also been found to be associated with preeclampsia, eclampsia, and spontaneous abortion in the 15 year old and younger mother and with increased perinatal mortality and slow cognitive development for the infant (McAnarney and Thiede 1981).

Pregnant adolescents are at high risk for infections and sexually transmitted diseases, including chlamydia and trichomoniasis, which may play a part in premature birth and infant morbidity. Adolescents between 15 and 19 years of age have the second highest rate of gonorrhea in the United States (Carey, McCann-Sanford, and Davidson 1983). Infections that persist late in pregnancy and are present when membranes rupture may contribute to chorioamnionitis, postpartum endometritis, and neonatal septicemia. Pregnant adolescents are also particularly at risk for anemia. The fetal period and adolescence are the two most rapid periods of human growth and are associated with the highest iron requirements. This, compounded by the tendency of adolescents to eat irregularly, presents an even greater risk of iron-deficiency anemia. (Nutritional status among pregnant adolescents is discussed in more detail in Chapter 15.)

Family Implications

Adolescent childbearing is also associated with other long-term psychosocial factors that may have lasting effects on the health and later development of both mother and infant. The high rate of single motherhood may be associated with later marital instability. The limitations early childbearing puts on educational attainment usually result in less-skilled, lower-paying jobs. Stress caused by these two factors may result in higher rates of child abuse and neglect among mothers whose first children were born in adolescence (McAnarney and Thiede 1981).

Adolescent fathers also experience considerable stress from their premature parenthood. Although adolescent fathers are typically 3 to 4 years older than their partners, they tend to experience the same types of psychosocial risks: lower educational achievement, an earlier entry into the work force and lower-paying jobs, and increased family stress, as evidenced by a divorce rate two to four times higher than the rate for men who delay marriage and childbearing (McAnarney and Thiede 1981).

The adolescent father is often regarded as the "guilty" party and may encounter extremely negative reactions from others. He may feel tremendous responsibility for the situation but be left without supportive services. He may actually be denied contact with his partner and eventually with his child (Card and Wise 1978). However, most adolescent fathers want to maintain a relationship with their partner and want to be a positive presence in the child's life (Hendricks 1980). In major cities in recent years supportive services have been developed and specially tailored for the adolescent father, but many needs are still unmet (*Nurturing News* 1984).

Recurrent Adolescent Pregnancy

Another significant problem associated with adolescent pregnancy is recurrence. Within 24 months of an initial pregnancy, 40% to 50% of adolescent mothers are pregnant again (Fig. 10–7). Such short intervals between pregnancies are associated with

- Early termination of maternal education
- Increased dependence on public assistance

Factors that appear to increase the likelihood of recurrent adolescent pregnancy include

NURSING RESEARCH

Contraceptive Knowledge and Conception Among Adolescent Mothers

While lack of knowledge about contraceptives and conception is one of many factors placing sexually active adolescents at risk for pregnancy, little is known about the knowledge levels of adolescent women who have already borne children. This descriptive study was conducted to determine the knowledge that urban, black adolescent mothers had regarding contraceptive use and conception. A sample of 57 adolescents receiving prenatal care in a specialized adolescent maternity program was asked to complete a structured interview related to sex knowledge. While subjects gave accurate responses related to the risk of conception even on first intercourse and to oral contraceptive use, results suggest that they were inadequately informed about other methods of birth control, and a majority thought that douching and rhythm method were highly effective contraceptive methods.

This study suggests that even when receiving specialized prenatal care, the knowledge level of sexually active adolescent mothers may be inadequate to ensure appropriate use of contraception. While adolescent mothers may appear to understand how to use oral contraceptives effectively, care must also be taken to explain alternative methods of birth control and to eliminate misinformation.

Panzarine S, Gould C: Knowledge about contraceptive use and conception among a group of urban, black adolescent mothers. J Obstet Gynecol Neonatal Nurs 17(4):279–282, 1988

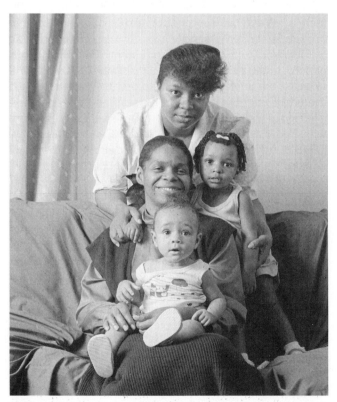

Figure 10–7. The adolescent mother with more than one child may need assistance from the nurse for ongoing planning and counseling to meet family needs. Help may also come from an older family member (the grandmother, for instance). (Photo: Nancy M. Stuart. Copyright 1988)

- Dropping out of school
- Lack of perceived life options
- Continued unprotected intercourse

Thus, interventions targeting these factors may be effective in decreasing pregnancy recurrence. Such interventions might include

- Flexible return-to-school policies
- Available and affordable child care
- Incentives to continue education
- Cultivation of and education about job opportunities for adolescent mothers
- Available and affordable contraceptive care in the context of comprehensive family care (Moore 1989).

Socioeconomic Implications

The socioeconomic implications of adolescent childbearing are alarming. Many adolescent mothers are unable to complete their education, resulting in lower work status and earning capacity than their peers who do not become pregnant. Edward Pitt, the director of a male adolescent responsibility program for the National Urban League, notes that "the poorest people in America today are children living in homes of adolescent mothers, their families living on an income of less than $4000 per year. Untimely parenting adversely affects the education, employment, and income prospects for both male and female adolescents."

A variety of services and programs on national, state, and local levels have been targeted to meet this need. These groups include Healthy Mothers, Healthy Babies Coalition, The Girls Club of America, the Children's Defense Fund, and Planned Parenthood Federation of America. Many high schools have also established comprehensive health clinics for adolescents, which provide family planning care, counseling, and medical care.

Implications for Nursing Care

When a sexually active adolescent becomes pregnant, she is thrust into a role for which she is often inadequately prepared. Support from the nurse becomes especially crucial when the pregnant adolescent lacks family support.

The adolescent mother has long been seen to be at increased psychological and obstetric risk. The normal developmental tasks of adolescence are challenging enough (described earlier in this chapter). The pregnant adolescent must complete these tasks in addition to the developmental tasks of adapting to pregnancy.

The extent of the psychosocial risk can be seen in the outcomes of adolescent childbearing. In the 1970s most adolescent mothers did not finish high school (Furstenberg, 1976). In recent years, specialized programs have been established to allow adolescent mothers to complete their education while receiving prenatal care and learning to care for their infants. However, additional support is needed to prevent long-term social disadvantage. Most adolescent mothers lack the skills to secure a well-paying job; many end up relying on welfare to support their families. Even if the adolescent mother marries the father of the baby, their economic future is not bright, since his opportunities for employment are as bleak as hers, and the cycle of poverty is continued with their children.

The goal of prenatal care for the adolescent is to promote the health of the mother and her infant. The actual care of the adolescent is much the same as that for women in their twenties, as discussed in Chapters 16–18. The process of pregnancy management is similar to that of the more mature woman, but planning for care must consider the individual adolescent's understanding and psychological needs.

Because of the adolescent's multiple needs, perinatal care is most effective if done from a multidisciplinary team approach. The health care team caring for the pregnant adolescent may include a nurse, physician, social worker, nutritionist, and psychologist. Each member of the team must not only be knowledgeable about the prenatal care of the adolescent but also sensitive to both her physical and psychological needs. The care and nurturing of the adolescent must be assumed by the nurse who is patient, understanding, and interested and who will work to assist the adolescent with the process required to aid the growth and well-being of herself and her baby.

Prenatal providers must be aware that the adolescent who becomes pregnant may become angry and rebellious, is typically concerned about other people's reactions to her pregnancy, and is often in personal turmoil. She may be economically disadvantaged, less future-oriented, and less cooperative with health care providers than other adolescents in planning her own care. She may resist nutritional advice and the use of such supplemental medications as iron and vitamins and have difficulty describing symptoms, past illnesses and their treatment. She is also more inclined to be late for or miss prenatal appointments. As a consequence, adolescents who behave in these ways are at increased psychosocial and perinatal risk because of incomplete care.

The pregnant adolescent is often characterized as being a high-risk obstetrical patient. In part this is due to the high probability for a number of problems that may occur from life-style and age-related factors: low socioeconomic status, smoking, substance abuse, and venereal disease. Risk is multiplied when the adolescent receives delayed prenatal care or when, receiving it, she neglects to follow the advice of the care provider.

Complications in Adolescent Pregnancy

Complications are much more likely to occur in this group, and every effort must be made by the nurse to convince the adolescent of the importance of consistent prenatal care. (For a complete discussion of nursing assessment and management of the following pregnancy risks, see Chapter 19; aspects specific to the adolescent are highlighted here.) Complications common in pregnant adolescents include low birth weight (LBW), pregnancy-induced hypertension (PIH), intrauterine growth retardation (IUGR), and preterm labor (PTL).

Low Birth Weight. The nutritional status of the pregnant adolescent is one of the vital influences in the overall quality of pregnancy and its outcome. (See Chapter 15 for nutrition in pregnancy.) Foods eaten during pregnancy have a profound effect upon fetal growth and development. Poor nutrition is common in pregnant adolescents and increases their risk of complications, such as stillbirth and birth defects (Picchnik and Corbett 1985). When the diet is improved, the adolescent experiences fewer problems before delivery and her baby will have fewer difficulties after birth.

Inadequate weight gain can negatively influence the birth weight of the infant. Weight gain of less than two pounds per month after the first trimester is considered inadequate. When the pregnant adolescent is underweight, she should try to gain a total of 30 pounds to assure that the baby's nutritional needs are met. Obesity in the adolescent mother also reflects a probable dietary problem, which may result in inadequate nutrition during pregnancy. (See Chapter 34 for full discussion of low-birth-weight-infants.)

Pregnancy-Induced Hypertension. The incidence of pregnancy-induced hypertension (PIH) in the general population is 5% while in the pregnant adolescent population it has been estimated to range from 7% to 34%. Specialized multidisciplinary prenatal programs that provide intensive support for pregnant adolescents can significantly reduce the incidence of pregnancy-induced hypertension, in some cases reducing it to the same level as for 20- to 25-year-old women. (See Chapter 19 for full discussion of PIH.)

Preterm Labor. Preterm birth is defined as a delivery that occurs before 37 completed weeks of gestation, as calculated from the first day of the last menstrual period. Because preterm infants are born before they have sufficient time to achieve optimal intrauterine development, they are at risk for a number of perinatal problems. Labor that begins prior to term is one of the greatest problems in obstetrics today because of the dangers to the infant. Risks of prematurity and perinatal death are higher in mothers 15 years of age and younger, and their infants, compared to those of women in their twenties,

NURSING RESEARCH

Specialized Prenatal Programs for Adolescents

A study was conducted to test the effects of a specialized multidisciplinary prenatal education program on perinatal outcomes in an urban adolescent population. Fifty pregnant adolescents attended the program and were compared with 50 nonattender controls. Those who attended the program had fewer perinatal complications than those who did not; this was true for the younger (13–15 years old) as well as the older (16–18 years old) adolescents. Significant differences were noted in incidence of anemia (4% of attenders vs. 28% of nonattenders), urinary or vaginal infections (6% of attenders vs. 72% of nonattenders) and use of drugs during pregnancy (8% of attenders vs. 64% of nonattenders).

These results are consistent with other studies documenting that it is the presence or absence of excellent prenatal care, and not maternal age, that best explains perinatal outcomes in pregnant adolescents. This program was directed by a clinical nurse specialist and corroborates other studies that found that nurses in advanced practice can significantly improve maternal and infant outcomes in populations of pregnant adolescents.

Slager–Earnest S, Hoffman S, Anderson–Beckman C: Effects of a specialized prenatal adolescent program on maternal and infant outcomes. J Obstet Gynecol Neonatal Nurs 16(6):422–429, 1987

are two to three times more likely to die during their first year of life. Adolescents who have subsequent pregnancies are also at risk for delivery of a premature infant or one who will die during the perinatal period.

Obstetrical problems, as mentioned above, occur more often in the adolescent than they do in postadolescent women. Rather than being an inherent trait within the adolescent, the increased numbers of problems experienced are directly related to the obstetric care received. This means that complications can be expected when prenatal care is delayed or is inadequate in quality. Conversely, when early comprehensive care is received, the adolescent should experience a normal, uncomplicated course of pregnancy and a healthy, thriving infant.

Psychosocial Risk

The extent of psychosocial risk to the pregnant adolescent depends on such factors as availability of care, family support, and socioeconomic status as well as the adolescent's own developmental status.

The young adolescent (14 years and younger) is often incapable of consistent conceptual or abstract thinking, so she has difficulty in anticipating the consequences of actions and in problem solving. She is not prepared for the responsibility or the decision making associated with pregnancy and parenthood, gives little thought to the future, and focuses primarily on the present. Thus, she has trouble understanding the need for preparation for the baby, since that time is so far off. The younger adolescent has had little time to adjust to the normal physical maturation that occurs at her age and now must also adjust to the dramatic physical changes associated with pregnancy. She has a very tentative sense of her own feminine identity and is not prepared to internalize the adult role of mother in any real way. She is far more likely to rely on her own mother to assume responsibility for the coming child. She cannot provide for herself or her own baby, because in many ways she is herself still a child. Even with intensive supportive services, pregnancy is likely to retard the social, educational, and emotional development of the young adolescent mother.

The middle adolescent (ages 15 and 16) has more resources for coping with pregnancy. She is more likely to use logic and abstract thinking, and can prepare for future events more effectively. She is more independent in her behavior. The middle adolescent is more comfortable with her feminine identity and with her maturing body. She may be ready to internalize aspects of the mother role, and her own mother may more readily accept her as a mother, instead of assuming responsibility for the coming child. The middle adolescent is likely to complete more of her schooling and is more likely to be in a stable relationship with the father of the baby. Often the father can be a significant source of emotional support for her, although physical and financial support still is likely to come from her own parents.

The older adolescent (17 years and older) is much more like an adult in her response to pregnancy. Her relationship with the father is often a stable one, and he is often able to provide some financial support. The older adolescent is close to establishing her own independence. Although her position is much better than that of younger adolescents, pregnancy is still likely to prevent her from obtaining additional schooling. Her future employment opportunities will be extremely limited, and she will have to rely on support from her mate or her own family (Fig. 10–8).

The Adolescent Father

The adolescent father is typically 2 or 3 years older than his partner. Prenatal services have been largely unavailable for adolescent fathers until recently. In the past, teenage fathers were often regarded as troublemakers. They often were actively excluded from services available to mothers and kept from having contact with their

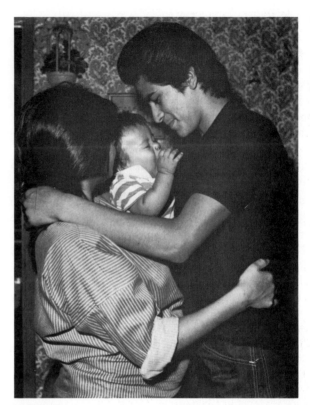

Figure 10–8. The adolescent couple can make a positive adaptation to parenthood with specialized care and adequate social support. (Courtesy of Morning Glory Press. Photo: Joyce Young)

partners and their infants. However, in recent years, this has changed; many communities now have specialized social and health care services for adolescent fathers.

The adolescent father must struggle with the same developmental tasks as his partner, as well as adapting to the specific demands of his partner's pregnancy. The adolescent father experiences a range of emotional responses: anger, fear, shame, pride, a sense of responsibility to the mother and baby, a wish to escape altogether from the situation, and sometimes hopelessness, when he feels he cannot cope with the various demands being made on him.

The adolescent father's adaptation to pregnancy is further complicated by several factors:

- He is often not living with his partner; thus, although he may have ongoing contact with her, he is not directly involved in many aspects of the pregnancy.

- He may regard the pregnancy as a source of pride and proof of his masculinity or as a source of intense shame, depending on his social and cultural background.

- The typical role of father-as-provider is usually not available to him because of his age and lack of job opportunities.

NURSING RESEARCH

Prenatal Education with Unwed Adolescent Fathers

This study examined the impact of a prenatal education program on knowledge about sexuality, pregnancy and birth and child care in a volunteer sample of 28 urban black adolescent fathers, aged 15–18 years. Subjects were randomly assigned to either of two groups, one of which received four prenatal classes of 2 hours in length.

Findings suggest that the adolescent father who received prenatal education demonstrated significantly more knowledge about pregnancy and prenatal care and infant care and development than fathers who received no instruction. There were no differences in knowledge related to sexuality or labor and birth. However, regardless of whether or not the father received prenatal education, the higher his knowledge of maternal and infant development and care, the more supportive behaviors he reported toward the mother and the expected infant.

Although the sample is small and further study is needed, this study suggests the importance of providing as much information as possible to the prospective adolescent father about maternal and infant needs since increased knowledge levels may contribute to increased support for the mother during pregnancy and in the early months of parenthood.

Westney O, Cole O, Munford T: The effects of prenatal education interview on unwed prospective adolescent fathers. J Adoles Health Care 9:214–218, 1988

However, programs that have been specifically developed to assist adolescent fathers can help tremendously. Counseling and support can be tailored to the teenage father's special needs, among which are the following:

- Deciding how to manage the changes pregnancy makes in his relationship with his partner
- Finding a job or some other means to make a tangible contribution to her support
- Learning about pregnancy and how he can be involved in childbirth
- Learning about child care in preparation for an ongoing relationship with his child

Health professionals are finding that when these services are available, adolescent fathers want to maintain a relationship with their partner (although not necessarily a mate relationship) and their child and want to be an influence in the child's life. Adolescent fathers can be helped to achieve this goal if they receive support as they adapt to the demands of the partner's pregnancy (Westney et al 1988).

Adolescent Parenting

Much of the existing research on adolescent parenting suggests that parenting by adolescent mothers is less than optimal. Problems identified in adolescent mothering include

- Insensitivity to infant cues
- Proneness to physical punishment
- Tendency to provide less than the needed stimulation, including verbal interaction, play, and cuddling

These characteristics are of concern because it is clear that maternal behavior affects the infant's development and well-being. Recent research (Ruff 1987) suggests that while adolescent mothers may not initially be as responsive to their newborns, their responsiveness increases over the first two months and they tend to interact more actively with their infants. The extent to which the mother's behavior adapts to the infant's needs may depend to some degree on the mother's self-esteem, her level of understanding of infant development, and her own level of education and developmental status (Ruff 1987; Mercer 1986). Thus, maternal–newborn behavior as well as maternal developmental status are factors that are important to assess in the early postnatal period. By assessing whether the adolescent mother's understanding of newborn behaviors and needs is sufficient to allow a good start in the parenting role, the nurse is able to identify mother–baby couples most in need of supportive nursing care to help establish a positive relationship in the early weeks and months of life.

CHAPTER SUMMARY

Adolescence is a period of dramatic changes; clinicians must be prepared to assess adolescents on physical and psychological development and social maturity. Sexual development has been described by Tanner, and his stages are helpful in assessing sexual maturity.

Many adolescents with reproductive capacity have neither the emotional maturity nor the social support to engage in responsible sexual behavior. Because adolescent girls are engaged in sexual activity at a younger age, greater demand is placed on the nursing profession to provide care and education.

Unintended pregnancy and sexually transmitted disease (STD) are two significant threats to the well-being of sexually active adolescents. STDs represent one of the major morbidities occurring during adolescence and young adulthood. The threat of AIDS has become especially significant to this age group. Birth to single mothers and recurrent pregnancy are of concern as socioeconomic factors as well as physical factors for the mother and newborn. The nurse is challenged to provide information concerning sexuality, pregnancy, and contraceptives to adolescent girls and their partners.

STUDY QUESTIONS

1. What is the purpose of Tanner staging? What two parameters are used to assess adolescent sexual development?
2. Describe the characteristics of young, middle, and late adolescence. What implications do these developmental phases have for sexuality? For childbearing?
3. Why are adolescents at particular risk for STDs? What are the most common STDs today? What are the risks associated with them?
4. Explain how HIV is transmitted. What precautions are recommended for sexually active individuals? For health care workers?
5. What risks are associated with adolescent childbearing? What interventions have been shown to be effective in reducing these risks?

REFERENCES/BIBLIOGRAPHY

Becker TM, Stone KM, Alexander ER: Genital human papillomavirus infection: A growing concern. Obstet Gynecol Clin North Am 14(2):389–397, 1987

Bell TA, Hein K: Adolescents and sexually transmitted diseases. In Holmes KK, Mardh PA, Sparling PF, Wiesner PJ (eds): Sexually Transmitted Diseases. New York, McGraw-Hill, 1984

Burke PJ: Adolescents' motivation for sexual activity and pregnancy prevention. Issues Compr Pediatr Nurs 10:161, 1987

Card J, Wise J: Teenage mothers and teenage fathers: The impact of early childrearing on the parents' personal and professional lives. Fam Plann Perspect 10(4):199, 1978

Carey W, McCann–Sanford T, Davidson E: Adolescent age and obstetric risk. In McAnarney E (ed): Premature Adolescent Pregnancy and Parenthood. New York, Grune & Stratton, 1983

Carr GS, Gee G: AIDS and AIDS-related conditions; Screening for populations at risk. Nurse Pract 11:25, 1986

Cates W, Schultz SL: Edidemiology of HIV in women. Contemp OB/GYN 32(3):94, 1988

Centers for Disease Control Update: Acquired immunodeficiency syndrome an HIV infection among health care workers. MMWR 37:229, 1988

Cypress BK: Health care of adolescents by office-based physicians: National ambulatory medical care survey, 1980–81. NCHS Advance Data 99: Sept. 1–8, 1984

Dash L: When Children Want Children: The Urban Crisis of Teenage Childbearing. New York, William Morrow, 1989

Dawson DA: The effects of sex education on adolescent behavior. Fam Plann Perspect 18(4):163, 1986

Fischl MA, Richman DD, Greico MH et al: The efficacy of Azidothymidine (AZT) in the treatment of patients with AIDS and AIDS-related complex. N Engl J Med 317:185, 1987

Fogel C: Adolescent pregnancy. In Fogel C, Woods N (eds): Health Care of Women. St. Louis, CV Mosby, 1981

Furstenberg F: The social consequences of teenage parenthood. Fam Plann Perspect 8:148–156, 1976

Hafner DW: Safe sex and teens. SIECUS Report 17(1):2–9, 1988

Hagen MD, Meyer BK, Pauker SG: Routine preoperative screening for HIV. JAMA 259:1357, 1988

Hatcher RA, Guest F, Stewart GK, Trussell J et al: Contraceptive Technology, 1988–1989, 14th rev. ed., pp 65–94. New York, Irvington Publishers, 1988

Hendricks L: Unwed adolescent fathers: Problems they face and their sources of social support. Adolescence 15:861, 1980

Hofferth SL, Kahn JR, Baldwin W: Premarital sexual activity among U.S. teenage women over the past three decades. Fam Plann Perspect 19(2):46–53, 1987

Kohen DP: Relaxation/mental imagery (self-hypnosis) and pelvic examinations in adolescents. J Dev Behav Pediatr 1(4):180–186, 1980

Marsiglio W, Mott FL: The impact of sex education on sexual activity, contraceptive use and premarital pregnancy among American teenagers. Fam Plann Perspect 18(4):151, 1986

McAnarney R, Thiede H: Adolescent pregnancy and childbearing: What we have learned in a decade and what remains to be learned. Semin Perinatol 5:91, 1981

Mead PB: Infection control in the era of AIDS. Contemp OB/GYN 32(3):116, Sept. 1988

Mead PB, Galask RP, Minkoff HL, Sever JL: AIDS looking ahead. Contemp OB/GYN 32:106, 1988

Mercer R: Adolescent pregnancy. In Kowalski K, Sonstegard L, Jennings B (eds): Women's Health: Crisis and Illness in Childbearing. New York, Grune & Stratton, 1984

Mercer R: Relationship of developmental variables to maternal behavior. Res Nurs Health 9:25–34, 1986

Millstein SG, Adler NE, Irwin CE: Sources of anxiety about pelvic examinations among adolescent females. Sexually Active Teenagers 2(2):66–72, 1988

Moore M: Recurrent teen pregnancy: Making it less desirable. MCN 14:104–108, 1989

Moscicki AB, Shafer MA: Normal reproductive development in the adolescent female. J Adoles Health Care 7(6S):41S–63S, 1986

Muuss RE: Theories of Adolescence, 5th ed. New York, Random House, 1988

Nurturing News: A Quarterly Forum for Nurturing Men 6(4): Special issue on teenage fathers, 1984

Panzarine S, Gould CL: Knowledge about contraception use and conception among a group of urban, black adolescent mothers. J Obstet Gynecol Neonatal Nurs 17(4):279, 1988

Picchnik S, Corbett M: Reducing low birth weight among socioeconomically high-risk adolescent pregnancies. J Nurse Mid-wife 30(2):88–89, 1985

Poole L: Human immunodeficiency virus infection in women — Nursing Prespective. In Schinazi RF, Nahmias AJ (eds): AIDS in Children, Adolescents, and Heterosexual Adults. New York, Elsevier–North Holland, 1988

Ruff C: How well do adolescents mother? MCN 12:249–253, 1987

Sachs B: Cognitive screening for adolescent health education. J Pediatr Nurs 2(2):113–119, 1987

Sarrel LJ, Sarrel PM: Sexual unfolding. J Adolesc Health Care 2(2):93–99, 1981

Schlachter J, Stoner E, Moncada J: Screening for chlamydial infections in women attending family planning clinics: Evaluation of presumptive indicators for therapy. West J Med 138(3):375–379, 1983

Selvin AP, Marvin CL: Safe sex and pregnancy prevention: A guide for health practitioners working with adolescents. J Commun Health Nurs 4(4):235, 1987

Streiff LD: Can client's understand our instructions? Image 18(2):48–52, 1986

Tanner JM: Issues and advances in adolescent growth and development. J Adolesc Health Care 8(6):470–478, 1987

Tauer K: Promoting effective decision making in sexually active adolescents. Nurs Clin North Am 18(2):275–292, 1983

Troiden RR: Homosexual identity formation. J Adolesc Health Care 9(2):105–113, 1988

Washington AE, Sweet RL, Shafer MA: Pelvic inflammatory disease and its sequelae in adolescents. J Adolesc Health Care 6(4):298–310, 1985

Waters J: Pregnancy in young adolescents: A syndrome of failure. South Med J 62:655, 1969

Wattleton F: American Teens: Sexually active, sexually illiterate. J Sch Health 57(9):379–380, 1987

Westney O, Cole O, Munford T: The effects of prenatal education interview on unwed prospective adolescent fathers. J Adoles Health Care 9:214–218, 1988

Williams AB: Public health implications of HIV infection. Nurse Pract 11:8, 1986

Woods NF: Toward a holistic perspective of human sexuality: Alterations in sexual health and nursing diagnoses. Holistic Nursing Practice 1(4):1–11, 1987

Zelnik M, Shah F: First intercourse among young Americans. Fam Plann Perspect 15:64, 1983

SUGGESTED READINGS

Bearinger L, Gephart J: Priorities for adolescent health: Recommendations of a national conference. MCN 12(3):161–164, 1987

Davidson J, Grant C: Growing up is hard to do in the AIDS era. MCN 13(5):352–357, 1988

Fullar S: Care of the postpartum adolescent. MCN 11(6):398–403, 1986

Sachs B: Reproductive decisions in adolescence. Image 18(2):69–72, 1986

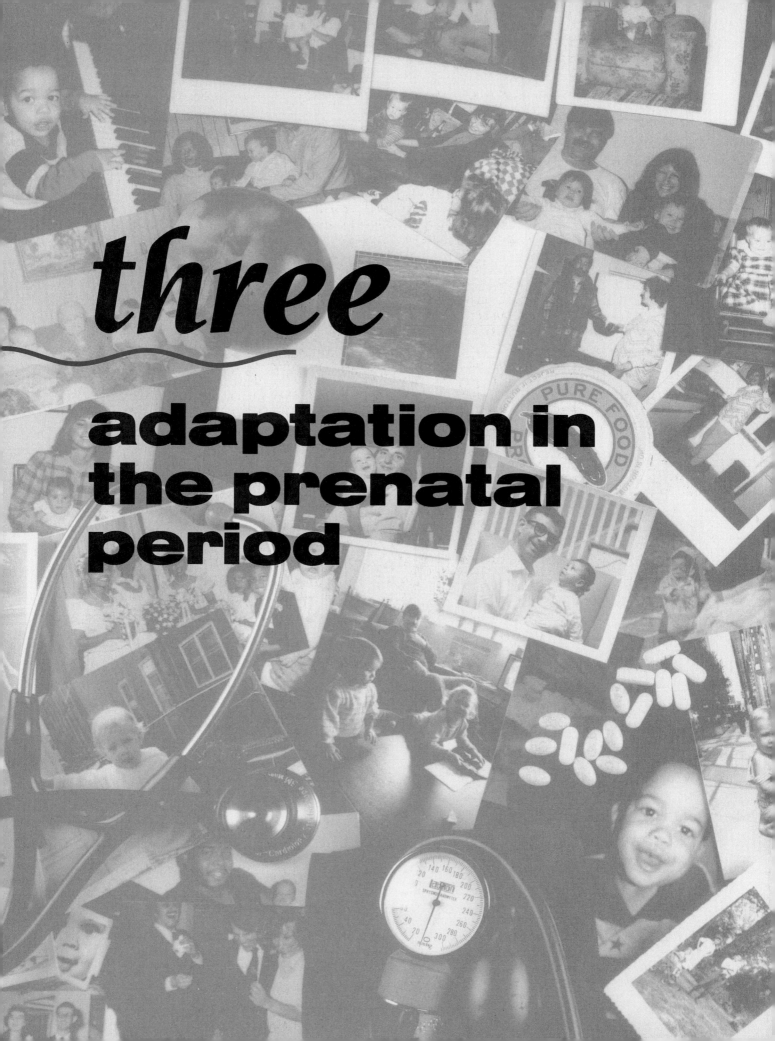

three

adaptation in the prenatal period

11 psychosocial aspects of childbearing

LEARNING OBJECTIVES

After studying the material in this chapter, the student should be able to

- Describe some major social factors that influence decisions about childbearing

- List characteristics that reflect a person's psychosocial readiness for childbearing

- Discuss the psychosocial conse- quences and perinatal risk factors associated with early and delayed childbearing

- Describe major areas in which birth practices may vary across cultures

- Discuss nursing strategies for assessing cultural variations in birth practices

- Explain the importance of culturally appropriate nursing care for the health of childbearing women and their families

KEY TERMS

Acculturation

Adolescence

Cognitive processes

Cultural relativism

Development

Ethnocentrism

Psychosocial responses

Puberty

Role

The nurse has a unique responsibility and challenge in maternity care. Because of its holistic view of human health, and especially because of its concern with emotional health, nursing must concern itself with a broad range of factors that affect how women and their families adapt to pregnancy and childbirth.

Pregnancy and childbirth are events that touch nearly every aspect of the human experience: biologic, psychological, social, and cultural. Individual adaptations to childbearing on each of these levels may be quite different, depending on the age, health, socioeconomic status, and cultural background of the woman and her family. These differences result in a wide range of individual and family needs for information and assistance during the childbearing year.

Despite this tremendous natural variation, however, there are also recurring themes or patterns that can guide the nurse in providing sensitive and effective care for childbearing families. This chapter discusses some major social, cultural, and psychological patterns in how people adapt to the childbearing experience. The study of these patterns spans several disciplines, including sociology, anthropology, and psychology. An in-depth discussion of every psychosocial aspect of pregnancy and birth that has implications for nursing is beyond the scope of this book. The purpose of this chapter is to discuss how some of the more important psychological, social, and cultural aspects of childbearing affect women and their families and how they guide the provision of maternity nursing care.

Childbearing has strong psychological and social meanings in human culture, and these meanings affect human *health*. The current strong consumer movement for family-centered maternity care, as discussed in Chapter 2, arose in part because these important issues were ignored in traditional obstetric care for too long (Puls 1987). There is also some evidence that the improved obstetric outcomes noted even among high-risk women cared for by nurse midwives and nurse practitioners might result in part from the delivery of more sensitive and culturally appropriate care (Schuster and Ashburn 1980).

SOCIAL ASPECTS OF CHILDBEARING

One's conceptions of health and illness and the decisions one makes about reproductive behavior are, in large part, products of the larger society and the social class and cultural group to which one belongs. Pregnancy and childbearing have specific social significance, and decisions about childbearing may be regarded as of major importance or of little consequence depending on that significance. To function most effectively with childbearing families, the nurse must understand the larger social context in which maternity care is delivered and must recognize the social factors that influence reproductive behavior and decisions about pregnancy and birth (Burst 1987).

Social Factors Influencing Childbearing Decisions

In most Western countries, the decision about whether or not to risk pregnancy is a most significant one, ultimately affecting many lives. Pregnancy usually marks a person's entry to the parental role and, as such, has life-long implications. However, people do not always make a clear, conscious decision for pregnancy or parenthood. The pros and cons of parenting, with its expectations and life changes and the necessity of taking on a permanent new life role, are not always considered in the conscious or unconscious decision to risk pregnancy. Often the decision to risk pregnancy is based more on emotional responses in a particular situation than on rational thought and a life plan. One example of such a decision can be seen when a person who does not want to become pregnant or cause a pregnancy participates in unprotected intercourse.

Many factors determine whether a person behaves in ways that risk pregnancy, consciously chooses to have a child, or chooses to remain childfree. Among these factors are knowledge about human sexuality; the availability of contraceptive options; the nature of socially acceptable sex roles; influences from peers, partners, and family; and larger social and cultural influences.

Knowledge of Human Sexuality

Whether or not to bear children initially requires a sound knowledge base for decision making. In the not-too-distant past the topic of sexuality was considered a forbidden topic in polite company. The mid-1800s, known as the Victorian era, were characterized by sexual repression and a strong sense of modesty, required because of the presumed purity and innocence of women and children. Women were believed to have little or no capacity for sexual response and were viewed as inferior to men both physically and intellectually. Thus the need for sex education was considered useless and inappropriate for females and superfluous for the more sophisticated male. This attitude prevailed until the 1920s. Influenced by new social and economic freedom for women, sexual attitudes during the Jazz Age became increasingly less inhibited. Information on birth control and marriage manuals with detailed descriptions of sexual techniques were widely published. The work of Sigmund Freud stressed the psychological importance of sexuality in motivating human behavior in both health and disease. Following World War II Alfred C. Kinsey, a zoologist from Indiana University, began his revolutionary inquiry into human sexual behavior, opening a floodgate of research on this once taboo topic. Kinsey's work was modified and advanced by such leading sex researchers as William Masters and Virginia Johnson. The belief that to understand the complexities of human sexuality a person must understand sexual anatomy and physiology as well as psychological and sociological factors became widely held (Masters, Johnson, and Kolodny 1983).

Today the majority of young people now receive some kind of formal sex education (Editorial, *Family Planning Perspective,* 1986). The nature of this instruction, however, varies widely from a simple description of the biological aspects of reproduction covered in a single class period to a comprehensive program of study that includes accurate information about sexuality, including contraception, exercises to improve decision making and communication skills, and guidance in developing satisfying interpersonal relations integrated throughout the 12 years of elementary and secondary schooling (Muraskin 1986).

In spite of these efforts to increase young people's knowledge of human sexuality, controversy still exists as to whether or not formal sex education should be mandated for all school-age children. Proponents of mandatory sex education claim that a sound knowledge base would decrease teen-age pregnancies and virtually halt the spread of sexually transmitted disease in the adolescent population. Opponents, on the other hand, believe that making such instruction mandatory usurps the role of the parents as sex educators of their children and decreases the authority of local school officials to determine curricular content (Muraskin 1986). While many agree that sex education should be taught in schools (Lester and Cox 1986) and several studies have demonstrated that formal sex education programs have not led to an increased risk of premarital pregnancy (Dawson 1986; Marsiglio and Mott 1986), most research thus far has sug-

RELATED RESEARCH

The Impact of Sex Education on Sexual Activity, Contraceptive Use, and Premarital Pregnancy Among American Teenagers

A longitudinal study conducted by sociologists Marsiglio and Mott examined the impact of sex education on adolescent behavior. Data from the National Longitudinal Survey of Work Experience of Youth were used for the study. In the survey yearly personal interviews were conducted with a nationally representative sample of 6015 women and 6054 men from 1979 to 1984. The primary objective of Marsiglio and Mott's analysis was to determine whether teen-agers who take a sex education course are any more likely than other adolescents to later become sexually active, use effective contraception, or have a premarital pregnancy.

Results indicated a number of interesting findings. Sixty percent of the women and 52% of the men had taken a course in sex education by the time they reached 19. Instruction about contraception was far less common than instruction about the menstrual cycle and sexually transmitted diseases. Somewhat surprisingly, the researchers found that most participants had a relatively low current knowledge level about the menstrual cycle. Young white women were the most knowledgeable about the likelihood of pregnancy of any of the study subgroups. A large portion of the teen-agers, particularly males, were having sex before they had the opportunity to take a course.

Exposure to a course was associated with a slight increased probability of subsequent sexual activity. This tendency was counterbalanced by the increased use of effective contraception by those who reported having a sex education course. As a net result, no significant association was found between taking a sex education course and subsequently becoming premaritally pregnant before age 20.

Several limitations of the study existed. First, the study did not take into consideration the quantity and quality of the sex education received. Second, the reliability of the data depended solely on the openness and recall ability of the participants. Finally, benefits of sex education other than prevention of unplanned adolescent pregnancies were not explored. The researchers concluded that until the public resolves its ambivalence over what sex education should and should not do, it is unlikely that sex education courses will substantially alter teen-age sexual behavior.

Nursing is in a prime position to help promote the adaptation of the school-age child by sensitizing the public to the sociosexual needs of students. Conducting nursing research in this area can help clarify the type and timing of sex education needed in school curricula. Based on these findings, professional nurses can influence the development of consistent comprehensive sex education curricula by being visible leaders and enlisting the support of parents and school officials.

Marsiglio W, Mott FL: The impact of sex education on sexual activity, contraceptive use, and premarital pregnancy among American teenagers. Fam Plann Perspect 18(4):151, 1986

gested that sex education, as it is currently taught, has little if any effect on the decision of young people to initiate sexual activity. It is clear that further research is needed to identify the necessary components of a successful formal sex education program and to develop satisfactory methods of presenting this important information.

Availability of Contraceptive Options

The dramatic development in contraceptive options since the 1960s has directly affected the way people make decisions about childbearing; in fact, contraceptives have to a large extent *created* the opportunity for decision making in this area. In realistic terms, throughout most of human history, parenthood (more particularly, motherhood) could not be chosen; childbearing was simply a predictable consequence of intercourse. Although techniques for contraception have been recorded throughout history, only in the last half-century has contraception been reliable enough to allow people to choose the timing of pregnancy.

Some continuous-action methods of contraception (oral contraceptives and intrauterine devices) not only greatly reduce the incidence of unwanted pregnancy but eliminate the need for intentional contraceptive behavior to be closely associated with sexual behavior. Other methods, such as diaphragms, condoms, and spermicides, require the contraceptive behavior to occur in conjunction with sexual activity, but even these intermittent-action methods greatly reduce the incidence of accidental pregnancy. Increased protection against sexually transmitted diseases, especially HIV, has contributed to the increased use of condoms. Permanent contraception or sterilization can be provided through surgical intervention, such as tubal ligation or vasectomy, with minimal risk. Even when an unwanted conception occurs, birth can be prevented through therapeutic abortion. Despite strong opposition in some segments of the population, abortion is still generally available in the United States and is a widely used contraceptive option in many countries around the world.

Contemporary Male and Female Roles

The nature of socially acceptable sex roles plays a large part in decisions about childbearing. Male and female adult sex roles in Western culture are still defined predominantly in terms of parenthood. Although some progress has been made in breaking down barriers between acceptable sex roles for men and women, boys and girls are still socialized differently to conform to their expected future roles as mothers and fathers. Furthermore, most young adults in the United States still hold childbearing as a positive value and intend to become parents at some time. This orientation toward parenthood may be more in evidence in women than in men, since women tend to be socialized throughout life in nurturing functions and with the expectation of motherhood. Men are socialized primarily toward a productive occupational career and only secondarily toward future fatherhood (Tiedje and Collins 1989).

Even though sex roles still reflect an orientation toward parenthood, there are now competing social roles, especially for women. The costs and benefits of parenthood, especially motherhood, may be evaluated in terms of occupational roles. The modern family in America relies heavily on the earnings of the female partner employed outside the home. More than 50% of women in families with children under 5 years of age were employed outside the home in the early 1980s, and this income contributes substantially to the total household income. Childbearing, however, typically interrupts a woman's earning power, at least temporarily, and lost financial income and career development usually cannot be recovered (Campbell, Townes, and Beach 1982).

Women tend to be primarily responsible for management of the home and for providing or arranging for child care, even when they are also employed outside the home (Kratz, 1987). This may be changing in some segments of the population; some middle-class couples are now exploring more equal participation by the father in child care. In other cases fathers, sometimes called "house-husbands," assume the primary responsibility for taking care of small infants. These arrangements usually result in some financial sacrifice and loss of occupational advancement for the father. However, these changes still affect only a small minority of adults of childbearing age.

Peer, Partner, and Family Influences

Pressures from a partner or peers can persuade a person to risk pregnancy even when that person is not ready to do so. In adolescence, peer pressure often influences a teenager to initiate sexual activity that may lead to a pregnancy. In couple relationships, pressure to become pregnant may be used as a way to test or force a partner into commitment.

Family pressures also influence childbearing practices. The family continues to be the basic societal unit serving to perpetuate the species and socialize the young. Although childless-by-choice marriages are increasingly common and accepted, pressures on adults to bear children are still strong. Parents expect to be provided with grandchildren, and friends and siblings who have children often try to persuade others to follow their example. Finally, with the increasing life expectancy in Western countries, the fear of growing old and being alone may be an influential factor in the decision to bear children.

Sociocultural Influences

Social, economic, and cultural factors also influence childbearing decisions. Socioeconomic status, usually described in terms of occupation, education, and income, reflects values and lifestyles that directly affect decisions about procreation. This can be seen in part in the differential birth rate among socioeconomic groups in the United States. The birth rate reached an all-time low in 1974 and has increased only slightly since that time. Middle-class Americans are restricting their family size to two children more consistently than are lower-class or upper-class groups, although the differences in contraceptive use and family size between social classes are becoming smaller. More couples are deferring marriage until their middle or late twenties and delaying the first birth for several years after marriage (Fogel 1981). Concerns about overpopulation, environmental pollution, or global warfare may lead some couples to delay, limit, or avoid childbearing, while motivating others to start families sooner. Some will delay pregnancy until adequate financial resources are available, while others feel that if they waited to be financially secure before starting a family, they would never start one.

Cultural influences play a large part in childbearing decisions. In cultures that view children as valuable assets, a large family may be desirable to demonstrate status or success. In some parts of the world, children are still regarded as necessary to assist with family work. If male children are perceived as more valuable, a couple may have more children in an attempt to bear a son. Cultural values also dictate the age at which sexual activity may begin, whether or not marriage is a prerequisite for sexual activity and childbearing, and whether contraception is an acceptable practice.

Another important recent development which has only begun to impact society is the lethal epidemic of human immunodeficiency virus (HIV) infection and acquired immunodeficiency syndrome (AIDS), first identified in 1981. Since that time more than 70,000 cases of the retroviral infection have been reported to the Centers for Disease Control, with underreporting estimated to be around 20% in the United States (Miramontes 1988). Currently the majority of people with HIV have been males, particularly blacks and Hispanics, who are homosexual or bisexual or who are intravenous drug users. A review of recent studies on HIV indicates that high-risk groups have shown initial rapid and profound changes in behavior to avoid infection (Becker and Joseph 1988). This risk reduction behavior most frequently involves modification rather than elimination of sexual behavior (such as decreasing the number of sexual partners, avoiding anal intercourse, and using condoms during sexual intercourse) or drug-use behavior (such as sterilizing needles before reuse). However, longitudinal studies tend to reveal a high degree of reverting back to unsafe practices after a period of time (Jones et al 1987; McKusick, Conant, and Coates 1985). Much less common are behavior changes in members of potentially high-risk heterosexual adolescent and young

LEGAL/ETHICAL CONSIDERATIONS

Needed: Effective National Policy on AIDS/HIV Infection

According to experts, such as Miramontes, a critical care nurse, HIV infection is not only the most significant health problem of the twentieth century but is also one of the most significant social issues of our times. The social, political, and economic issues raised by this disease are numerous and complex.

Since 1981 the number of persons with AIDS has grown tremendously. Currently no national policy has been established to control the AIDS epidemic. Miramontes identifies several reasons for this situation. Fear, fueled by misinformation and ignorance, has affected the reaction to the epidemic. Early connection with such stigmatized risk groups as homosexual and bisexual males and IV drug users has contributed to the belief of many that the disease is self-inflicted and the result of deviant behavior. The fatal nature of the disease has led to an avoidance response by those who have difficulty in dealing with death and dying. The lack of a national policy has resulted in a failure to appropriate sufficient funds to stem the disease's spread.

Miramontes points out three major areas of controversy surrounding the AIDS crisis that deserve careful consideration: testing, education, and funding. Thought-provoking questions arise in each of these areas.

Routine Testing: Should testing be voluntary or mandatory? Should test results be disclosed to others? Under what circumstances?

Education: Is education an effective way to change high-risk behavior? What should be included in such education programs? At what age should these programs be introduced?

Health Service Funding: Who should bear the cost of AIDS treatment? Is health care a right for all individuals or open only to those who can afford to pay for it?

One thing is clear. As the numbers of those infected increase, everyone will be affected in some way by this epidemic.

Miramontes H: Needed: Effective national policy on AIDS/HIV infection. Nurs Outlook 36(6):262, 1988

adult populations, who tend to be present-oriented and believe that they are invulnerable (Becker and Joseph 1988; Davidson and Grant 1988). New infections among women are occurring mainly in intravenous drug users and sexual partners of intravenous drug users. Because most of the women at risk for HIV infection are of childbearing age, the number of children with AIDS is expected to increase. The implications of HIV infections for the childbearing family and for society in general are complex and profound. An organized and vigorous national effort will be needed to bring this threatening epidemic under control.

Motivations for Childbearing

With so many influences on contraceptive and childbearing decisions, it is rare for persons to be fully aware of their own motivations to bear a child. Some motivations can be classified as healthy ones and persons may be aware of them. For example, there is the simple desire of a couple in an emotionally satisfying relationship to have a family. Some people may be aware of a desire to share a part of themselves with the world or to leave a legacy for the future. Some may feel childbearing is part of the adventure or challenge of life, a pathway toward achieving their own potential. For others, parenthood is a desirable status, one that permits them to share experiences with parents, peers, and siblings. Some may feel incomplete as adult members of society without children.

Other motivations for childbearing are less healthy and reflect unresolved problems. Often the people concerned are unaware of these motivations or refuse to acknowledge them. These motivations are more common among adolescents and reflect their psychosocial immaturity (Poole 1987). Such motivations may include having a child to save a faltering relationship, to provide a source of affection and security, or to replace a loss (such as a miscarriage, death of a significant other, or some personal failure). Others may choose childbearing as a means to prove sexual ability or fertility or as a means to escape an unhappy home life or work situation.

PSYCHOLOGICAL ASPECTS OF CHILDBEARING

We can have ex-spouses and ex-jobs but not ex-children (Rossi 1980).

This comment points to the irrevocable nature of the psychological change that results from childbearing. Even when an infant is placed for adoption and there is no further contact between the infant and the natural parents, the parents may feel a lifelong pull toward their unknown child. The following section highlights some important psychological aspects of childbearing; the reader is referred to Chapters 12 and 36 for in-depth discussion of the psychological adjustments required during pregnancy and the transition to parenthood.

Individual Development and Parenthood

Parenthood is a major transition point in the lives of adult men and women, and particularly for adolescents who become parents. The timing of parenthood affects the timing of other life events, such as marriage, the completion of basic education, job or career changes, and even retirement. Parenthood also affects one's self-concept and values, and changes one's interests and one's ability to pursue some directions in life. Becoming a parent changes the nature and direction of further psychological development and sets the stage for many future life changes. Finally, parenthood profoundly alters relationships with other family members and especially the relationship with the mate (Miller and Newman 1978). A major factor influencing the psychological impact of parenthood is the individual's own maturity and readiness for childbearing.

Psychosocial Readiness for Childbearing

Psychosocial readiness for childbearing is defined as the ability to adapt to the demands and complete the tasks of pregnancy, childbirth, and parenthood. Psychosocial readiness and physiological readiness for childbearing are not the same thing, as evidenced by the many social problems encountered by adolescents who bear children. A person might be said to have achieved psychosocial readiness for childbearing if he or she has the following characteristics:

- The capacity to establish and maintain intimate relationships
- The ability to give to and care for another human being
- The ability to learn and to adjust patterns of daily life
- The ability to communicate effectively with others
- An established sexual identification

However, individuals themselves often have additional benchmarks that they see as important factors in psychosocial readiness for childbearing. Adults in social groups where contraception and planning of first pregnancies are common may consciously focus on and think about these benchmarks much more than adults in social groups where conception is not usually controlled or planned. For example, a middle-class, well-educated couple may think of establishing careers and a comfortable household and of having time as a couple before feeling ready for the first child. A couple from a lower-class minority group may see those goals as out of reach and may perceive pregnancy and childbirth more as an inevitable consequence of life as a couple.

However, some benchmarks for readiness are generally recognized by most adults. Since in our culture most children are born to women in relatively stable monogamous relationships with male partners, both men and women often cite the existence of a stable couple relationship as a major factor in readiness for childbearing. Financial security also tends to be an important factor—one that may be mentioned more often by men than women. This probably reflects the fact that the "breadwinner" function is a large part of the traditional male sex role in Western society (Kay 1982). The attainment of personal goals may also be an important benchmark; these goals will vary and may range from finishing high school and getting a job to successfully taking over the family business.

Impact of Childbearing on Adult Roles

Pregnancy and childbirth signal the acquisition of a new role for the man and woman involved—that is, the role of father or mother of a particular child. The term *role* refers to a set of behaviors that reflect the goals, values, and sentiments of a particular social position. Roles are developed through meaningful interactions with others. The acquisition of the parent role affects other roles the person may play, such as the role of worker, spouse, friend, sibling, and child. People also learn and develop roles in relation to others in similar or complementary roles. Thus, a young mother learns about the mother role both from her own mother and from her mate as he develops his father role. The paired or complementary roles are patterned to mesh so that interactions between the *role partners* are satisfying and meaningful.

Roles are learned through formal and informal means, and the socialization to function in major roles begins in childhood. For example, girls are encouraged to learn to care for younger children and to meet and anticipate the emotional needs of others and are socialized in preparation for their future roles as mothers. Boys are less often socialized as future fathers, but that may be changing as sex roles change in Western countries. Much learning about the parent roles is indirect. The child observes his mother and father and the examples provided by other family members and, as a new parent, may mimic behaviors seen as a child.

Taking on new roles is both a cognitive and emotional process. Emotional ties with others influence the way we enact important roles. This is especially true of the parent role, because it is enacted within the intimate and important context of the spousal couple and the family unit and because the transition involves both emotional and physical change.

Childbearing and Women's Roles

Pregnancy and childbirth have significant psychological and physical effects on women. These changes are irreversible. Rossi's point about "ex-children" is particularly pertinent to women. They carry children in their bodies and have a relationship with the developing fetus through pregnancy and childbirth that changes them physically and emotionally (Fogel 1981). A woman can never "not know that she is a mother," even if she relinquishes her infant. Childbearing has been described as a major psychological and social influence in a woman's life (Grossman, Eichler, and Winickoff 1980). The changes brought about by childbearing are discussed in the next chapter.

Childbearing has major social implications for women as well. The changes in women's roles in the last two decades have been dramatic. The role of wife and mother in the home was considered the norm in the 1950s among the middle class, and pregnancy often signaled a departure from other roles and a focusing of attention on childrearing and home management. Women in lower socioeconomic classes did not have the luxury of giving up paid employment but continued to be employed in traditional semiskilled or unskilled women's jobs while rearing their children. However, as more women moved into the job force and into nontraditional work roles, childbearing gradually became a function that was *added on* to other responsibilities rather than substituted for them.

Several recent nursing studies have examined the relationship between employment and maternal role conflict (Brown 1987; Majewski 1986). Tiedje and Collins (1989) point out that nurses are in a key position to assist the new generation of employed mothers.

Childbearing creates profound changes in women's roles within the home. Women are likely to report more overall change and more change in their personal lives after the first birth than do their partners (Harriman 1983). Even if she is employed outside the home, major responsibility for childrearing and home management decisions typically fall to the woman. Thus, raising children constitutes a second or even a third "full-time job" for many women when added to outside employment and home management. The women's movement has focused on this issue, referring to the "superwoman syndrome"—the problem of the woman who is compelled to fill all these roles and who lives at a frantic pace to meet their demands.

Even though this state of affairs is clearly not healthy for women or families over the long term, sex roles are slow to change in some areas. The man's share of household management and childrearing responsibilities still tends to be less than half, even among men who say they believe in sexual equality and want to participate more in home life. Thus, pregnancy and the first birth often mean a shift to a more traditional division of labor than may have existed in a couple relationship before.

There are several reasons why this shift occurs. First,

men tend to be socialized to expect that they do not know enough to care for an infant, and so they do not expect to do so. Women, while they may not know any more than their male partners, are socialized to expect that they should know how to care for an infant; this pattern persists throughout childrearing. Second, breastfeeding, which is gaining in popularity once again, requires the woman to be engaged in most direct infant caretaking. Third, while maternity leave is a common option for women, paternity leave is still quite rare in the United States. Thus, from a financial standpoint, women are encouraged to stay home for some period of time after birth whereas men are not. Although it is true that women need this time for physical restoration and to establish the mother–infant relationship, this period of primary child care responsibility sometimes delays the man's skill development in this area and further contributes to the pattern in which women assume major child care and home management responsibilities after the first birth.

Childbearing and Men's Roles

Childbearing also causes changes in men's roles, although the changes are usually not as apparent as those experienced by their partners. Men may father children and never know that they have done so. They experience childbearing as if they were "one step removed," at least in the biological sense. However, fatherhood has always introduced important changes in men's lives, and more attention is now being paid to the experience of fatherhood than ever before.

Men are not socialized to delve into the emotional aspects of their lives and their relationships. The typical male sex role in Western countries is to deny, or at least avoid, emotional responses except in certain acceptable "male" arenas, such as competition, sports, protection of family, and occupational strivings. The primary role for adult men is their occupational role, and for many men that role changes little with the birth of a child, although often men will report that they feel "more responsible" and compelled to be a better provider after they have a child. It is only recently that men have been expected to take a more active role in pregnancy, birth, and early parenting, and as yet we know little about the long-term consequences of this role change on fathering behavior. Some speculate that this type of nurturing activity during the childbearing year might contribute to more nurturant fathering and less rigid sex-role behaviors among men, but this remains to be seen. (Expectant fatherhood is discussed in more detail in Chapter 12).

Husbands tend to report less overall change in their lives and less personal change with parenthood than do their wives (Harriman 1983). This perhaps is to be expected given the fact that pregnancy is a biologic event for women whereas men can only observe this biologic shift.

Several studies have found that husbands tend to express more negative response to any change in sexuality in the marital relationship than do their wives (Grossman, Eichler, and Winickoff 1980; Harriman 1983; May 1987). This may suggest that the sexual relationship is of more significance to men in the couple relationship, and so even fairly predictable changes in sexuality caused by childbearing may cause more stress for the father. This might in part be explained by the fact that the primary source of support and nurturance for most men is their spouse, and the sexual relationship may be the main way in which they feel cared for and loved.

One important aspect of childbearing that touches men's views of themselves is the notion of having responsibility for a child. Men often see the father role as a great responsibility — their tie to the future and their link to the past. Having a child to "carry on" may be important, even if it isn't a male child to carry the "family name." The notion of having a child to carry on the family traditions or to provide a future for an aging grandparent is often important to men as they anticipate and experience fatherhood.

Childbearing and the Couple Relationship

Childbearing also has a profound effect on the couple as a unit. Depending on how the pregnancy is viewed, it can signal the initiation into full family status for the couple or the beginning of hard times, stress, and unmet emotional needs. A research project in which couples were followed throughout pregnancy and into the first year of parenthood found that how couples fared in the transition to parenthood depended in part on their typical style of interaction and the amount of time they spent together (Cowan et al 1978; Lewis J 1988; Lewis W 1988). Partners who showed a greater tendency toward mutuality (or "coupleness") in their relationship coped with the transition to parenthood better if their lifestyle and the division of labor supported that mutuality. For example, a flexible work schedule that allowed the man to spend more time with his partner and their baby contributed to the sense of "coupleness" and made the transition easier. A rigid work schedule, on the other hand, could make it more difficult to maintain the couple relationship after birth. However, couples who tended toward more separateness in their relationship during the pregnancy were more satisfied after the birth if their situation reinforced this separateness while still allowing some tasks to be shared.

This research has also shown that shifts occur in three primary areas of the couple relationship: in the sense of self, in role behavior, and in communication patterns. Changes in the sense of self within the couple relationship were reflected in the growing importance of viewing oneself and one's partner as parents and in widening gaps between the ideal self and the actual self. Men and women took on higher, more idealized standards for themselves but often experienced some difficulty in meeting them.

Shifts in role behavior, or in "who does what," also produce some disequilibrium in the couple relationship. Again, Cowan and colleagues found that couples tended to adopt more traditional divisions of labor. Even in couples who had intended to share infant care responsibilities, within 8 weeks after birth the woman had taken over most or all of the responsibility, regardless of whether she was breast-feeding or employed (Cowan et al 1978).

Communication patterns were affected by these shifts in role behaviors and by each partner's sense of self, as well as by such practical issues as the mother's and infant's physical status and fatigue level. It is interesting to note that the partners tended to perceive the same event or milestone differently. A period of worry for one might be a period of happiness for the other. This difference in perception not only reflects a shift in how the couple communicates about their experience but also indicates that the process of becoming a family is different for each member, even if they live and experience the process together.

Early and Delayed Childbearing

Childbearing usually occurs in Western countries in late adolescence (18 years and up) and into the 20s. Early childbearing (*i.e.*, among adolescents younger than 18) and delayed childbearing (usually defined as postponement of the first birth until age 30 or later) have unique psychological and developmental consequences for both mother and father. Both types of childbearing are also sometimes associated with adverse health outcomes for mother and child. Adolescent childbearing is discussed in detail in Chapter 10.

Delayed Childbearing

The number of American women becoming pregnant for the first time after age 30 has increased dramatically in the 1980s. The rate of first births to women aged 30 to 34 years increased significantly between 1970 and 1986, climbing from 7.3 per 1000 women to 17.5, as shown in Figure 11–1. Among white women the proportion still childless at 30 years of age increased from 17% in 1976 to 25% in 1986.

Causes of Delayed Childbearing. Any discussion of the causes of delayed childbearing should acknowledge the occurrence of unplanned pregnancies, especially in the over-40 age group. Such pregnancies may result from ineffective contraception and irregular menstrual cycles in premenopausal women. Often this occurs in a multipara whose last pregnancy was 6 to 8 years earlier. In contrast, planned pregnancies usually occur in the 30- to 35-year-old age group. Often this is a first pregnancy, delayed consciously. However, in this age group, once the decision for pregnancy is made, there is often a further delay before conception actually occurs. Within 1 year of trying to conceive, 86% of 20- to 24-year-olds will do so. In contrast, only 52% of 35- to 39-year-olds will succeed. (Devore 1983). Two causes for this difficulty in conceiving are the increased incidence of reproductive tract disorders in women over 30 years of age and irregularity of ovulation following years of oral contraceptive use.

In a recent study conducted by Meisenhelder and Meservey (1987), 68 white, married, middle-class, primiparous, career women were surveyed concerning their reasons for delaying parenting. The main reasons given by this group of women were development of the marriage relationship, career development, and financial need.

A common motivation for pregnancy after age 30 is the

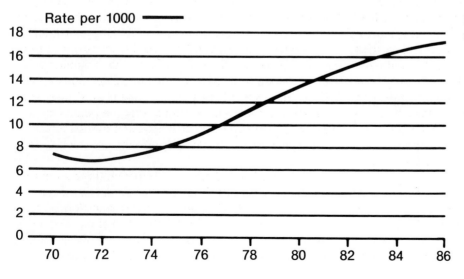

Figure 11–1. First births to women aged 30 to 34 years in the United States, 1970–1986.

feeling that time is running out. These women may be engaged in careers but feel that it is "now or never" for a successful pregnancy. Women may also choose pregnancy at this point in life to experience a revitalization. In a society that places great emphasis on youth, the older woman may feel that a pregnancy will "keep her going" and youthful. Women may also *postpone* pregnancy into their 30s for psychological reasons. They may have had time to experience life and a career and to solidify their own identity. They may feel quite secure in their relationship with their mate. Financial status also tends to improve with increased age.

Far less is known about the man who becomes a father later than is typical. There is some evidence that men in their 30s may feel more secure in their identity and in their relationship with their mate, and these factors may help make being an "older" father a positive experience. For these reasons and because many men go through developmental changes in their 30s, "older" fathers may be more nurturant and tolerant and may engage in less authoritarian and sex-stereotypical behavior with their children than men who become fathers in their early 20s (Nydegger 1973).

Perinatal Risk Factors for Delayed Childbearing. The relationship between maternal age and infant mortality is well recognized. Women who become pregnant over age 35 are routinely designated as "elderly gravidas" and may be considered to be at high risk. Delayed childbearing has been associated with second-tri-

mester spontaneous abortions; chromosomal abnormalities; twinning; low birth weight, particularly among primiparous women; and labor abnormalities (Cohen, Newman, and Friedman 1980; Ventura and Hendershot 1984).

Fetal and neonatal deaths increase in frequency with increasing maternal age, especially after age 35. This increased perinatal mortality is often associated with chronic maternal hypertension, placenta previa, and uterine inertia and with the increased rate of breech deliveries in this population. Decreased uteroplacental blood flow may be responsible for placental and uterine problems. Changes in fetal growth rate may also be observed in pregnancies in older mothers. As maternal age increases, infant birth weight decreases, especially in underweight women or those who have low weight gains during pregnancy (Naeye 1983).

Risks to the health of mother and infant increase when childbearing is delayed until after age 30, but the increases do not become marked until ages 35 to 40. The risks are more likely to be the result of underlying medical problems that are likely to increase with age than the result of maternal age alone. In one study healthy gravidas ages 35 and older receiving care in a nurse-midwifery service did not experience higher than normal perinatal morbidity or mortality (Stein 1983).

Psychosocial Risk Factors. Relatively little is known about the psychosocial consequences of delayed childbearing for parents, since the phenomenon has not

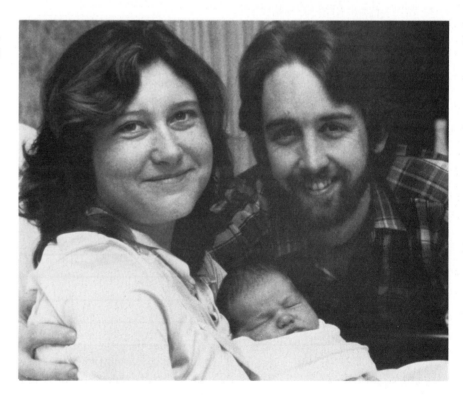

Figure 11–2. Many couples are waiting until the woman is in her mid-thirties before having their first child. (Photo: BABES, Inc.)

attracted much scientific interest until recently (Fig. 11 – 2). A study following mothers in their teens, 20s, and 30s through the first 8 months of motherhood found that older mothers made a slower physical recovery from childbirth, experienced more fatigue, and expected more of themselves in the maternal role than did mothers in their 20s (Mercer 1986). These mothers also experienced a significant decrease in self-concept at 8 months after birth. This may reflect the high standards these women set for themselves in their mothering as well as loss of the satisfaction they might have derived from their occupational role. The same study also found that older women experience greater emotional change with motherhood, reflecting the higher "cost" of the intense involvement of self required by early mothering.

Childbearing has profound social and psychological effects on women, on men, and on their relationships with each other. The nurse who understands the complex factors affecting the psychosocial experience of childbearing is equipped to give more appropriate, sensitive, and effective care. The nurse is also then able to anticipate potential risk factors for women, such as those posed by early and delayed childbearing, and intervene before the woman's health is compromised.

CULTURAL INFLUENCES ON CHILDBEARING

Culture exerts a major influence on childbearing practices. The following section provides an overview of cultural variations in childbearing practices and highlights ways in which those variations can affect adaptation to childbearing and the delivery of nursing care to childbearing women and their families.

Culture is defined as a system of goals, beliefs, attitudes, and roles that change but tend toward stability, that are shared by a distinct human group, and that are transmitted by that group and learned by succeeding generations. The culture of any particular group consists of its technology, its social structure and norms, and its belief systems. Culture develops in response to the unique psychological and physical environmental conditions experienced by a given group (Griffith 1982). Thus, cultural norms both shape human behavior and are shaped by it in a continuous process of social interaction.

The more central an event is to human existence, the more highly developed cultural practices are likely to be around that event. Events that mark changes in status, such as puberty, marriage, or the death of a spouse tend to be particularly important, as are events that involve many unknowns and physical risk. Pregnancy and childbirth, as human events of individual and social importance, are reflected in the practices of the wider culture, and practices related to these events tend to be highly developed and associated with strong and persistent beliefs (Kay 1982).

As people of different cultural backgrounds come together, there is a process of *acculturation,* in which some beliefs and practices are modified or dropped in favor of practices of the dominant culture while other practices or beliefs are retained or change more slowly. How quickly individuals or groups become acculturated depends on many factors, such as the opportunities for learning in the new setting, the extent to which the dominant culture discriminates against minorities, and the amount of physical and cultural differences between the two groups.

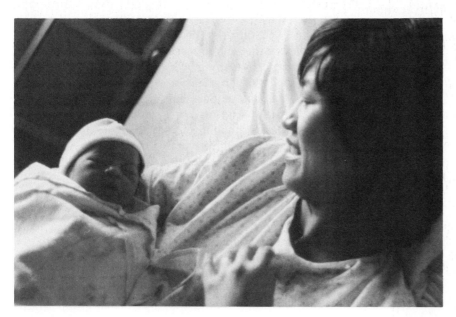

Figure 11 – 3. Cultural beliefs dictate how women and their families view childbearing and care for their newborns. (Photo: BABES, Inc.)

Individuals also vary tremendously in their traditionalism or modernism, even within the same cultural group (Fig. 11–3). An example of this can be seen in the changing role of the American woman. An outside observer of a metropolitan area might state with confidence that most American women believe that a woman should have roles outside the traditional ones of wife and mother. The same observer might find, however, that most American women in some other area do not hold that belief. Even generalizations that are true on a global level may not be very useful in explaining behavior for a given individual. Generalizations about cultural groups are often oversimplifications and, as a result, may not apply to many individuals within a particular group.

Cultural Differences and Socioeconomic Differences

There is a strong tendency for *socioeconomic patterns* to be mistaken for cultural patterns. For example, writings in sociology in the 1960s described a pattern of female-headed households among blacks as a cultural tendency toward matriarchy. However, more careful examination showed that this was true only among blacks in the lowest socioeconomic levels. In fact, this pattern appears to be related much more to economic issues than to cultural ones. That is, female-headed households are no more common among blacks than among whites of equivalent socioeconomic status (TenHouten 1970).

This type of misconception arises in large part because ethnic minorities are poorer than whites overall and are overrepresented among the very poor. Thus, people from these cultural groups have less opportunity for education and upward mobility. The economic gap accentuates differences from the dominant white middle-class culture, and soon the assumption is made that observed differences are cultural in origin.

Ethnocentrism and Cultural Sensitivity in Health Care

Since most nurses and other health care providers in the United States are white, middle-class, and well educated, they have been socialized to the dominant cultural practices surrounding pregnancy and birth and take for granted that these practices are desirable. They may regard other sets of beliefs and practices as deviant or, at best, questionable.

Ethnocentrism, or the practice of judging cultural beliefs or practices by standards from another culture, is a common human behavior. Culture is by its very nature taken for granted and rarely examined by those within it, and people of every culture tend to assume that their ways are the only reasonable ones. Health professionals must avoid this kind of "tunnel vision," since it can complicate interactions with patients and undermine the effectiveness of health care.

Cultural relativism is the practice of judging the customs of a particular culture by standards that are consistent with the values of that culture. Culturally sensitive health care does not require the professional to become an expert in cultural differences in health practices. However, it does require the professional to acknowledge belief and value systems different from her own and to take them into account when delivering care to childbearing women and their families.

Cultural Patterns in Pregnancy and Birth

Most cultures view pregnancy and birth not as an illness per se but as a period of increased vulnerability and risk. Many birth practices appear to be aimed at decreasing this risk by protecting the mother and unborn baby from harmful influences. Cultural beliefs about the relative risks of pregnancy, the intrapartal period, and the postpartum period also differ. For instance, the traditional Chinese custom of "doing the month" — in which the mother stays in the house, rests, and avoids activities other than caring for the baby — reflects the underlying belief that the postnatal period constitutes a time of vulnerability. In contrast, the dominant American view is that the birth is the period of highest risk, and the postpartum period is of much less concern.

Balance as a Cultural Value in Childbearing

A recurring theme in many cultures is the notion of maintaining a balance in the woman's physical, emotional, and spiritual nature during pregnancy. Anthropologists refer to *humoral pathology,* or the belief that a balance between intrinsic body qualities, such as heat and cold or moisture and dryness is essential for good health during the childbearing year. If one of these qualities is diminished through childbirth, practices are aimed at restoring the balance. Balance is also a value in emotional and spiritual matters in many cultures. Strong emotions are sometimes thought to "mark" or threaten the fetus, and a pregnant woman may attempt to avoid certain kinds of thoughts, emotions, or interactions for this reason.

Cultural variations tend to cluster around such activities as self-care practices during pregnancy and the postpartum period — for example, diet, activity and rest, maternal emotions, preparation for birth and for parenthood. It is beyond the scope of this chapter to discuss these variations in detail, even as they relate to the most prevalent cultural groups in the United States. Furthermore, a listing of cultural practices for a particular group is basically a generalization that may or may not be useful in clinical care. However, a brief discussion of cultural variations in pregnancy and birth practices does help to sensitize the reader to areas in which the dominant and subcultural beliefs differ. In these areas careful and thoughtful nursing assessment before planning and implementing care is most important.

Self-Care Activities During Pregnancy and Postpartum

Prenatal care as practiced in Western countries is quite unique, reflecting the view that pregnancy is a condition that requires medical observation to ensure health. Many cultures regard pregnancy as a normal state, and women only seek the help of a healer if problems arise. Women from other cultures often present themselves for prenatal care late in pregnancy because they regard their condition as one that requires only self-care.

Diet During Pregnancy and Postpartum. Most cultures encourage the pregnant woman to maintain a diet that is generally considered a normal one for that culture. Food taboos are common, usually reflecting a cultural belief that certain foods are unclean or fears that ingesting certain foods will produce undesirable physical characteristics in the newborn. Food cravings are considered normal among pregnant women in many cultures, and satisfaction of the woman's craving may be seen as vital to the well-being of the fetus.

Foods may also be considered important in maintaining a physical balance in the pregnant or newly delivered woman. Asian and Mexican practices emphasize the importance of "hot" foods after childbirth as a way to restore health and prevent complications arising from the loss of body heat through birth.

Activity and Rest. Most cultures encourage a pregnant woman to maintain normal activities, excluding strenuous work, although some encourage more rest during pregnancy. Norms for sexual activity during pregnancy are more variable, ranging from no change to strict prohibitions of sexual intercourse through the second half of pregnancy.

Usually the postpartum period is characterized by more restrictions on maternal activity. Most cultures encourage a period of rest, some as long as 40 days, during which time the mother is confined to her home, often to her bed. Some cultures regard the postpartum woman as unclean and prohibit her participation in religious activities. When this is the case, there is usually provision for a ritual cleansing for both mother and infant at the end of the confinement period.

Preparation for Birth

Preparations for the actual birth may include intensive preparation of the house and actual physical preparation

of the mother through specific exercises, religious practices, or diet. However, some cultures, notably of Arab peoples, view preparation in advance of the event as potentially dangerous. Advance preparation, or even referring to the fetus by name, may be seen as tempting fate and making the mother and fetus vulnerable to evil influences.

Birth Practices

Birth practices vary primarily according to norms about who may attend the birth, what positions and activities are healthy and acceptable for the laboring woman, and practices involving the placenta and umbilical cord. Most cultures provide for female members of the family to be present at birth. A few traditional cultures include the father or other men (Heggenhougen 1980). Many groups encourage use of tonics, teas, or certain foods during or just before labor to prevent a state of imbalance in the woman. In American culture the custom of prohibiting food and drink in labor started in the middle of the 20th century with the use of general anesthesia. Today, although methods of anesthesia have improved, food and drink are still prohibited (Broach and Newton 1988). Expression of pain during labor varies considerably from culture to culture. Some cultures, notably Arab and some Hispanic groups, consider crying, moaning, and other verbal expressions of pain as normal. Others, including many Asian groups, have a tradition of stoicism, and responses to pain are quite subtle.

Cultural practices surrounding the umbilical cord and placenta are also quite varied. Some groups follow specific practices in cutting the cord and caring for the umbilical stump. The umbilical stump is often seen to be a vulnerable area, and folk practices of binding the umbilicus with "belly bands" or binders are common among southern blacks and Mexican Americans. Some cultures view the cord as spiritually related to the infant. For example, traditional Japanese practices include preserving the cord and keeping it in the family home (Perry 1982).

Preparation for Parenthood

Culture dictates the nature of preparation for the parental role. Women are usually socialized clearly to expect to become mothers. Only in the most industrialized countries are there many acceptable roles for women outside the family unit. Many cultures begin preparation for parenthood through sibling caretaking of younger children, usually by the older daughters. Lifelong preparation for motherhood may be reinforced by religious beliefs or traditions emphasizing the importance of motherhood. A dramatic example of this influence may be seen among those of the Mormon faith, who believe that marriage and many children assure parents of a high place in heaven. Mormon families with six children or more are not unusual, even though the prevailing practice among Americans in general is to limit births to two or three.

Preparation for fatherhood tends to be less distinct in many cultures, including most Western countries. However, so-called primitive cultures usually have some male rituals related to birth and fatherhood. These rituals are called "ritual couvade" and often involve dietary restrictions or a set of behaviors mimicking the woman in labor and birth (Fishbein 1981). Anthropologists described these rituals in great detail in the early part of this century, believing them to be a form of sympathetic magic aimed at warding off evil influences from the vulnerable woman and unborn child. The father-as-labor-coach role, which has become quite common in the United States, has some similarities to this practice (Heggenhougen 1980).

Common Cultural Variations in the United States

As individuals and families leave their countries of origin and come to the United States, their traditional practices and the practices of the larger American culture may blend, conflict, or coexist. The following is a brief discussion of practices related to pregnancy and birth among common ethnic groups in the United States. Again, some variations that may appear to be cultural in fact reflect the socioeconomic conditions in which many people from minority groups live.

The nurse must not assume that these generalizations will apply to any individual patient she may encounter in clinical practice. They are presented here only to increase the reader's awareness of ways in which approaches to pregnancy and birth may differ. In clinical practice, the soundest approach is to *ask* what the woman considers normal practice during pregnancy, birth, and the postpartum period (see the Implications for Nursing Care section later in this chapter for some useful questions), to observe family behavior carefully, and to base nursing care on this assessment.

African Americans. Black women tend to view pregnancy as a normal healthy state, and their experience of a pregnancy may be strongly influenced by social factors, such as the couple relationship, economic pressures, and whether or not the pregnancy was intended. Although single motherhood is not a desirable situation, children born to single mothers are cherished and are not stigmatized. Children of adolescents are often raised by the grandmother as her own. In a descriptive study of 19 black grandmothers, Flaherty, Facteau, and Garver (1987) found that the adolescent mothers were clearly expected to and did make the daily care decisions concerning the infant. Decisions about medical care, however, were most frequently made by the grandmother.

The extended family, especially her own mother, is a source of significant support for the pregnant woman. Many women prefer the maternal grandmother, rather than the baby's father, to be the labor support person (Carrington 1978).

Southern black women may engage in a practice called *pica,* or the eating of clay, laundry starch, or other substances generally considered nonnutritive. This is probably a learned behavior characteristic of lower socioeconomic groups, in which blacks are overrepresented. (See Chapter 15 for further discussion of pica.) Other dietary practices may include avoidance of "acid" or "strong" foods during pregnancy to prevent having a hard-to-manage baby. The mother's behavior during labor may be subdued and stoic so as not to draw undue attention to herself, or her response to pain may be verbal and pronounced. Rarely, a black woman may express a wish or preference for lighter-skinned children, possibly a reflection of more overt discrimination against blacks with distinct Negroid features.

Southeast Asian Americans. Since 1975 the United States has resettled approximately 500,000 Southeast Asian refugees, three quarters of whom are Vietnamese. Those who immigrated in the early 1970s tended to be middle-class and well-educated. Later immigrants, however, were more likely to be poor, to be less educated, to have little experience of Western culture, and to have spent time in refugee camps before arriving in this country. Among these are Cambodian, Laotian, and Hmong people. Most of these immigrants are young and of childbearing age. If families have lost many relatives in fighting or in refugee camps, there may be a strong desire to have a large family, and birth control information may be refused.

Southeast Asians may hold Catholic, Buddhist, Confucian, or spiritualist beliefs that influence childbirth practices. In general, there is a commitment to stoicism. Women may consider crying out or complaining to be shameful, especially in the presence of a man. This may result in unexpectedly imminent births unless the nurse is alerted to the possibility that the woman may be in active labor even though she may show no distress during contractions (Nelson and Hewitt 1983).

There is a strong cultural tradition of politeness and deference to authority. This may be reflected in a tendency to avoid eye contact and social physical contact (shaking hands, touching shoulders) and to answer questions affirmatively regardless of true feelings.

Squatting may be the preferred position for birth. The woman is taught to conserve body heat during childbirth and in the postpartum period. The nurse can provide warmed extra blankets and drinking water without ice. Bathing after childbirth may be considered risky. Women may take only "hot" traditional foods from home during the early postpartum period. The woman's activities may be restricted for 40 to 60 days after birth, with other female relatives assuming household and infant care responsibilities (Wadd 1983).

Mexican Americans. Mexican Americans are the second largest minority group in the United States. The majority of Mexican Americans and Mexican immigrants are of childbearing age, and the fertility rate of this group is 50% higher than that of any other ethnic group in the United States (Tamez 1981). Women of Mexican descent may view pregnancy as a natural condition requiring no medical care under usual circumstances. However, the woman and fetus are considered vulnerable to outside bad influences. The woman may wear a *cinta* (a belt with keys attached) or a *muñeco* (a knotted cord around the abdomen) to prevent complications. Women may avoid drinking milk and may stay physically active to help prevent a large baby and a difficult delivery. An interesting study by Cummins, Scrimshaw, and Engle (1988) found that a majority of low-income Mexican American women in the study group looked on cesarean birth in a positive light rather than the negative view held by some other cultures.

Female family members are often present during labor and birth. Among more traditional couples, the father rarely participates.

Attitudes about breast-feeding may vary in this population. Some may believe colostrum to be unclean and so will not breast-feed until the second day after birth. There is some evidence that the incidence and duration of breast-feeding among Mexican American women is decreasing (Huffman et al 1982). Mexican American women may observe a 40-day resting period after birth called *la cuarentina*, during which dietary and activity restrictions apply, including a prohibition on sexual intercourse. Mothers may bind the infant's umbilicus to prevent *mal aire* (bad air) from entering. Consequently, mothers may resist allowing the umbilicus to air-dry. The nurse should be alert to this possibility and provide information about cleanliness, frequent changing of binding, and appropriate fit to prevent infection (Zepeda 1982).

Filipino Americans. Because of the long-standing relationship between the United States and the Philippines, Filipino Americans may demonstrate a range of traditional and Western practices. Western medicine is generally well accepted, but traditional practices may be maintained in such areas as the mother's activity level and diet patterns during pregnancy and postpartum. Hot, spicy, or salty foods may be avoided during pregnancy, and satisfying food cravings may be seen as important in preventing premature birth. Women are encouraged to decrease their activity during pregnancy and especially during the postpartum period. This may be misinterpreted as laziness or non-compliance by hospital staff.

Politeness, ease in social interaction, and deference to family authority, particularly the mother's mother, may create misunderstandings between staff and the family: the mother may smile pleasantly and indicate that she understands certain instructions, but later will not follow staff recommendations, instead adhering to traditional ways as encouraged by her mother. This reflects an effort to avoid contradicting the nurse directly (Stern, Tilden, and Maxwell 1980). Women are socialized toward motherhood at an early age, and the extended family is seen as having an important role in child care.

Asian Americans. Large populations of Japanese Americans and Chinese Americans can be found in most metropolitan areas on each coast. Practices among Asian Americans range from fairly traditional Oriental practices to near-total adoption of American patterns. Japanese Americans are more concentrated on the west coast and have attained the highest median income and educational level of any minority group in the United States. Cultural norms place a high value on deference and politeness, emotional reserve, conformity, and allegiance to family. More traditional families may show strong male dominance, and the extended family may be important in daily life. The birth of a male child may confer high status on the mother. Western medicine tends to be well accepted, and pregnancy is viewed as a state of health requiring little change in normal activities. Child rearing habits in Japan greatly encourage dependence on the mother, who is expected to satisfy infant needs immediately and to maintain very close contact with the infant. The patterns may be seen to a lesser extent among Japanese American women (Chung 1977).

Chinese American customs related to childbearing vary according to the length of time the parents' families have been in this country and their educational level. Beliefs in the value of maintaining physical and spiritual balance during pregnancy and the postpartum period may be present. Herbal teas may be used as tonics during pregnancy, and certain foods may be avoided. A prime example of the importance of balance in maintaining health is the custom of "doing the month," a period of 40 days after birth during which the woman is advised to stay in the house, rest, and avoid unnecessary activity. The woman may avoid contact with water during this period, reflecting a belief that she has an excess of cold in the body and is vulnerable to arthritis and other body aches later in life if she becomes chilled during the postpartum period.

Arab Americans. Arab immigrants are estimated to number 2 to 3 million in the United States. Arab Americans may adhere to either Christianity or Islam but have common cultural practices. Meleis and Sorrell (1981) present a comprehensive perspective of childbearing practices among Arab Americans. Childbearing is a major role for women, whose domain is primarily the home and family. Infertility in a married woman is grounds for divorce in some Arab countries. Male children are highly valued; the sex of the infant may appear to be more important to parents than its health. The husband is involved in all aspects of his wife's care, and often the woman will defer to him in decisions about her own care. Arab women are expected to be modest and deferential. It is considered normal for Arab women to moan and cry during labor, yet few request anesthesia.

Advance preparation for the birth and the infant is avoided for fear of attracting the "evil eye." Compliments about the infant are avoided for the same reason.

A traditional mistrust of written agreements may present difficulties when informed consent for medical procedures is being obtained. Trust is more readily placed in verbal agreements, especially with others of similar background. Arab families thrive on a high level of interaction and cohesiveness. Visiting by the extended family during the postpartum period is considered an obligation. Children are included in all aspects of family life, and women may have a strong desire to have older children greet the newborn in the hospital.

Pregnancy and Childbirth in American Culture

McBride (1982) points out that "just as there is no 'the American family,' there is no 'the American way of childbirth.' " There is at least as much variation among Americans as a group as there is among other cultural groups and probably more, because of the diversity of backgrounds represented. However, McBride points out that there are two opposing trends that characterize childbirth in America: the trend toward increasing medical and technological intervention in childbirth and the consumer movement toward family-centered childbirth. These trends are discussed in detail in Chapter 2. From a cultural perspective, these opposing trends do characterize a typically American approach to childbirth: an emphasis on technological intervention to ensure a good outcome and an emphasis on a family-centered approach and participation by members, especially fathers.

High standards of living, widespread access to health care, and the high value placed on educational and occupational advancement also contribute to a pattern sometimes called "the premium birth/baby syndrome." Middle-class couples expect to have only two or three children, perhaps only one. Thus, they do everything in their power to ensure a good outcome: getting into good physical shape before trying to conceive, getting early prenatal care, taking every available class and every possible precaution. This pattern may also include disdain for those who fail to take advantage of current technology and to eliminate unhealthy practices, such as smoking, during pregnancy. Unfortunately, this perspective can

also lead to intense self-doubt and guilt if expectations for a good birth and a healthy baby are not met, even if the outcome was not preventable.

One recent development that cannot be considered uniquely American but that does seem to illustrate the American orientation toward use of technology to achieve desired ends is the practice of *surrogate childbearing.* Individuals or couples unable to bear children may contract with a healthy young woman to be artificially inseminated and bear a child, whom they will subsequently adopt.

Such arrangements are legal in many states as "private adoptions," and usually include a payment to the surrogate mother, as well as payment of medical costs and living expenses during the childbearing year. Often the prospective adopting father's sperm is used. In some cases, the adoptive parents establish and maintain a close relationship with the surrogate mother; they may be her labor support people, and in some cases, they take the mother into their home for her postpartum recovery so that the infant can be breast-fed.

Surrogate childbearing seems to challenge many of our assumptions and beliefs about the nature of maternal feelings during pregnancy and birth. One experienced labor nurse expressed unease in caring for a surrogate mother in labor when the adoptive parents were her labor "coaches." The nurse's concern was that there appeared to be no opportunity for the surrogate mother to reconsider her decision after seeing her newborn, and the nurse described her own confusion in the delivery room—to whom should she hand the newborn, to the natural mother or the adoptive mother?

The American way of birth seems as foreign to people outside the United States as non-American ways do to health professionals here. As health professionals we face a challenge: to provide care without letting our own ethnocentrism blind us to the actual needs and concerns of patients. Whether or not a particular birth practice is "rational or "normal" is not the issue. The issues for the professional must always be: is it safe? is it feasible? is it important to the patient? The nurse must evaluate cultural practices in the light of these questions. If they can be answered affirmatively, there usually is no reason not to support the wishes of the woman and her family even if they do not fit with the nurse's own belief system. On the other hand, there may be some very important reasons why they should be supported.

IMPLICATIONS FOR NURSING CARE

Cultural practices related to birth are important because women and their families believe they are important. If a woman believes she is in danger of becoming ill because she took a shower during her postpartum hospitalization, she may be at risk because of that very belief. Thus, cultural practices have important implications for the provision of nursing care.

A nurse cannot reasonably hope to become an expert on every cultural group and on its birth practices. Even if she could, this level of knowledge might not be helpful in many individual cases because of the uneven rate of acculturation and because of the natural variability even among people of the same cultural group. However, the nurse can be open and interested in learning about her patient's concerns and needs in relation to traditional practices, and she can treat these practices with respect. By doing so, she demonstrates respect for her patient and facilitates the woman's transition to motherhood.

The nurse cannot expect to *change* her patient's developmental status or socioeconomic level to reduce risk, but care can be planned to meet the woman's individual needs. In this way, the nurse can work toward the major goal of assisting women and their families to attain and maintain optimal health even in the presence of significant risk factors.

The material in this chapter provides only the basis for a deeper exploration of the psychological and emotional tasks for mothers, fathers, and their families as they move through pregnancy, birth, and early parenthood. Units III through V discuss in detail the nursing care required to support families through the childbearing year. However, some points in this chapter have particular importance for the delivery of clinical nursing care.

The psychosocial aspects of maternity care can be just as important as the physical ones in producing positive obstetric outcomes. A simple example can be provided by a comparison of two pregnant women, of whom one is pleased to be pregnant and one is distressed.

From a purely obstetric standpoint, there may be no reason to expect that one woman's health would be any different from the other's. However, if the nurse assesses the woman's psychosocial status carefully and is aware of the woman's reaction to the pregnancy, she may anticipate that this might affect her overall health. The nurse may recognize that, in fact, the second woman is likely to be experiencing considerable stress and may not be caring for herself in a way that will sustain good health throughout her pregnancy. If this stress continues, her physical health may suffer, and her psychological state may eventually lead to physiologic risk. Comprehensive assessment and sensitive psychosocial care by the nurse could make the difference between successful adaptation to an unexpected pregnancy and complications induced by acute unresolved stress.

Unfortunately, it is far too easy to make assumptions about psychosocial aspects of childbearing and thus about the care that is needed. A care provider would never *assume* that a pregnant woman's blood pressure was nor-

mal, even if the woman was at low risk. Even though most pregnant women remain healthy and experience no complications, blood pressure would be measured and recorded. Psychosocial aspects of maternity care, however, are often relegated to routines that *assume* that there are no differences in the psychosocial responses of women and their families to childbearing. A practical example is the "routine" shower for the mother after childbirth. Most nurses might assume that the mother would like to be "cool, clean, and fresh" after the hard work of childbirth. Most new mothers might agree. However, as discussed earlier in this chapter, some ethnic groups believe that loss of body heat is dangerous to the new mother, and their cultural practices are designed to prevent heat loss, not encourage it. Women with these cultural beliefs would regard the "nice shower" as an unnecessary risk. Another example might be the nurse who assumes that a father should be at the birth of his child. Again, many men want to be present and need relatively little encouragement. However, some men, because of their traditional beliefs or because of their own fear and discomfort, may not wish to be present, and their spouses may not expect or want them to be present.

One might argue that these concerns are relatively unimportant when compared to more life-sustaining types of care that nurses must also give. However, a large part of nursing care for most childbearing women is not of the *life-sustaining* variety. Childbearing women by and large are a healthy population seeking assistance and support through a fairly predictable course of events. Nursing care for healthy childbearing families should be aimed at promoting health *and* maximizing the family's satisfaction with their experience.

The nursing process provides the framework for effective psychosocial care. Before the nurse can plan and implement care, she must view health in relation to childbearing in its broadest sense and carefully assess the needs and strengths of each woman and her family. Assessment in this area requires an openness to the woman's point of view and that of her family and a willingness to ask questions and to listen. The nurse can then individualize care on the basis of a systematic physical and psychosocial assessment of the woman and her family.

Making nursing diagnoses, formulating a plan, and implementing interventions for aspects of psychosocial care proceed from this base. Nursing diagnoses help to focus attention on the aspects of health that may be most adaptable during the childbearing year. Evaluating the effectiveness of psychosocial aspects of care may be more difficult, because psychosocial outcomes are not as measurable as other outcomes, such as infant birth weight, for example, or success at breast-feeding. However, results of sensitive nursing care will be reflected in the woman's satisfaction, comfort, and self-confidence and in the family's positive response to the childbirth experience.

Assessment

An assessment of the psychosocial and cultural characteristics of the childbearing woman and her family is the first step in effective maternity care. However, before the nurse can perform an accurate assessment of her patient, it is essential that she do an assessment of herself.

Self-Assessment

Everybody has biases and preconceptions about other groups of people and other ways of life. It is human nature to make assumptions about others, at times on the basis of relatively little information. However, this human tendency can be a problem in nursing assessment. The nurse who is unaware of her own biases and blind spots may make inappropriate judgments about a patient because the patient's behavior or attitudes do not fit the nurse's own view of the world.

The maternity nurse is especially at risk in this regard because of the emotional nature of such issues as abortion, teen pregnancy, women's rights, and alternative birth practices. For instance, an Arab American father is *expected* to oversee all decisions about his wife's care and may be seen as an inadequate husband if he does not do so. The nurse who is unaware of this cultural difference may view his behavior as overbearing and chauvinistic and may respond with anger, especially if she highly values sexual equality and the idea that women should take responsibility for their own care.

The nurse should note her own response and assess whether or not she can provide care to this family without imposing her own value judgments. She should also examine her own biases and acknowledge that the belief systems she and her patients hold are different. Once that is done, the important issue for the nurse is to validate the patient's desires in this situation and support them through her own nursing care.

Differences may also arise in terms of specific birth practices. A nurse who highly values a scientific approach to care may react with frustration when an Indochinese woman refuses to drink ice water after her delivery. The nurse "knows" that there is no scientific basis for the mother's fear that drinking ice water during the postpartum period will cause her to develop arthritis later in life. The nurse may even try to explain to the mother that her fears are unfounded and may be surprised to discover that the mother holds to her belief and refuses to take cold fluids. This is an ethnocentric approach to care. In contrast, a culturally sensitive approach would be to ac-

---

Assessment of Cultural Practices in Childbearing

What is the meaning and value of reproduction in this culture?

How is pregnancy viewed? Is it a state of illness, vulnerability, or health?

What responsibilities do the parents have as a result of pregnancy?

Is birth seen as a normal process or as being related to illness and danger?

Is birth considered a public or private event? Who should be present?

What practices govern diet and food preparation before birth?

What practices govern the mother's activity level and the types of activities acceptable during pregnancy and labor?

What precautions are important for the mother and infant after birth?

When is the infant accepted into the family?

What type of help is acceptable after birth and from whom?

What kinds of behaviors are expected of the mother, father, and other family members in relation to the infant?

Affonso D: Assessing cultural perspectives. In Clark A, Affonso D (eds): Childbearing: A Nursing Perspective. Philadelphia, FA Davis, 1979

---

knowledge that beliefs are different and to help the mother to get access to warm fluids. Again, this approach requires the nurse to examine how her own beliefs are intruding into her plan of care and to recognize that in most situations, there is no single "right" way of behaving. Again, when confronted with a difference in birth practices, the nurse should approach the issue systematically by evaluating the *safety* of the practice, the *feasibility* of incorporating it into the plan of care, and the *importance* of the practice to the patient.

Patient and Family Assessment

Some basic information about psychosocial factors is usually reflected in the routine patient assessment forms used in clinical practice: age, sex, marital status, race, socioeconomic status, educational level, and language barriers are usually noted. However, there are some important variables that are often ignored. *Readiness for pregnancy* is often overlooked in early prenatal care. Whether the pregnancy was planned and wanted should be noted, as well as the *partner's* response to the timing of the pregnancy and the responses of any other important family members. If a mother's significant others are not happy about a pregnancy, the nurse should be aware that the woman may be at increased emotional risk and may need additional support. However, if that information is never gathered or documented, the nurse cannot anticipate problems and help the patient to cope with them. This underscores the importance of a *family assessment* in maternity care. The family assessment is discussed in detail in Chapter 16.

Cultural assessment is also an area often neglected in prenatal nursing assessment. This type of assessment may be difficult because of language barriers or differences in customary patterns of interpersonal interaction. Communication barriers that may result from cultural differences and that may themselves signal a need for a more complete assessment, as well as strategies the nurse can use to avoid communication barriers and some useful questions she can employ in obtaining a cultural assessment for maternity care, are listed in the accompanying displays.

Diagnosis

The data on the psychosocial and cultural factors in a particular patient's case are analyzed with the other data gathered in the nursing assessment. Psychosocial and cultural variables are often important contributing factors in a nursing diagnosis. The following two nursing diagnoses may be significant when planning care using information on psychosocial and cultural variables.

* Impaired communication related to language barrier
* Altered health maintenance related to self-care in pregnancy

Planning and Implementation

The planning of appropriate psychosocial and cultural approaches to care must include the patient and members of her family and usually involves other health professionals as well. Often patients have a variety of psychosocial needs that complicate their health care. Thus, the nurse will need to plan referral to and coordination with social workers, nutritionists, and community agencies to ensure that the resources available to the patient's family are effectively utilized.

Planning of nursing care can also be directed toward a group of maternity patients when a pattern of needs is identified frequently in a practice setting. Nurses in facilities that regularly care for pregnant adolescents will need to make special plans to meet the adolescents' specialized social, emotional, and nutritional needs during pregnancy. Nurses in settings in which cultural diversity is common will need to plan for availability of interpreter services and bilingual/foreign language materials for patient teaching.

Nursing interventions are planned and implemented after adequate information has been gathered and are directed at the patient needs set forth in nursing diagnoses. Many interventions related to psychosocial and cultural aspects of pregnancy fall into two general categories: communication and teaching for effective self-care.

Strategies for Avoiding Barriers in Communication

Approach

* Consider whether a direct approach is acceptable or whether direct questions are embarrassing or offensive.
* Take time to engage in some social interaction to show respect and gain confidence and knowledge.
* Safeguard the patient's sense of modesty; avoid discussing matters related to her care when outsiders are present.

Customs

* Recognize that all human behavior is influenced by cultural patterns. Never assume that a practice is unimportant. Learn the significance of practices and facilitate them whenever possible.
* Learn the rationale for unusual practices and incorporate them whenever possible into your plan of care. When they cannot be incorporated, for reasons of safety or practicality, find out whether there are alternatives that would be acceptable to the patient.

Language

* Never assume that the patient is understanding you if English is her second language. Arrange for translation when possible and obtain written patient information sheets in other languages that you encounter frequently.
* Avoid using American slang and medical jargon. Speak slowly and quietly.

Stern P, Tilden V, Maxwell E: Culturally induced stress during childbearing: The Filipino American experience. Issues Health Care Women 2:67, 1980

Practicing Effective Communication

The nurse is in a unique position to close any communication gaps between physicians and patients of different social and ethnic groups. Often such patients are in awe of physicians and may hesitate to ask questions or make requests. In addition, physicians are trained to focus on illness aspects of care and may not recognize potentially important cultural variations in birth practices. Nurses, on the other hand, are usually regarded as approachable and knowledgeable, and patients, if given the opportunity, may share their concerns first with a nurse.

The nurse should be alert to communication gaps between providers and patients in the practice setting and should be prepared to evaluate the problem and propose solutions. For example, to decrease communication gaps in maternity practice settings, the nurse could provide specially prepared patient information sheets in languages, and at reading levels, suitable for bilingual families and those with limited education. The nurse may also be able to assist colleagues to provide culturally sensitive care by identifying and helping to change policies that prevent families from maintaining their own traditions related to pregnancy and birth.

Promoting Health Maintenance Through Teaching

A major type of nursing intervention when psychosocial or cultural factors are of concern is teaching for effective self-care. The term *self-care* in nursing has gained popularity since the late 1950s, in large part because of the work of Dorothy Orem. Orem developed a theory of nursing in which the concept of self-care was central. The self-care model places great emphasis on helping the patient to identify her own health-related needs and goals.

Although the needs identified by the nurse and patient may be different, the nurse assists with what the *patient* sees as high priorities and also gives information about other health needs she has identified herself. Once a relationship of trust and a pattern of success has been established, the patient will generally recognize the importance of the latter needs and will choose to concentrate on them as well. As the patient sets her own priorities for self-care, the nurse provides supportive intervention by, for example, giving necessary information and encouragement and by helping her to implement her self-care plan. The nurse may also intervene more directly by anticipating major unmet needs and planning intervention, reducing the negative effects of stressors, and augmenting the resources available to the patient.

Childbearing women and their families are often especially open to teaching that will assist them in their self-care. Since many women want to improve their diet,

activity level, and stress reduction routines during pregnancy, they are receptive to information, provided it is understandable and useful. Another area where self-care teaching is important in maternity nursing is in teaching new parents about infant care. Infant care is usually a high priority for parents, and a nurse who provides them with the information they need *when* they need it has intervened effectively. The nurse's ultimate goal in teaching for effective self-care is to reduce the family's future need for nursing or medical care.

Evaluation

The effectiveness of nursing care is determined by the extent to which results match expectations. This evaluation process should be continuous so that the plan of care can be modified as the patient progresses or fails to progress toward specified goals.

Evaluation of maternity care on a large scale often uses reductions in maternal care and infant morbidity and mortality rates (discussed in Chapter 1) as indicators of success. This approach is often used in populations designated as "high-risk," such as the poor or refugee populations. These rates do reflect the effectiveness of nursing care, although in a rather indirect way.

For instance, a specialized plan of care for a young pregnant adolescent that emphasizes increasing the girl's self-esteem and building her confidence in dealing with the world may directly affect the girl's ability to obtain the social support she needs during her pregnancy. That ultimately may help to improve her overall obstetric course. If a similar plan of care is implemented for most adolescents in that practice setting, a reduction in maternal morbidity among that population might eventually be seen. Effective nursing care in these settings may also be reflected in improved self-care routines that persist after pregnancy and in family satisfaction with the birth experience.

This rather indirect effect is often characteristic of the contribution nurses make to maternity care. The improved outcomes among high-risk pregnant women receiving care from nurse midwives and nurse practitioners provide another example (Neeson et al 1982; Stein 1983). Improvements in maternal and neonatal health are achieved by the maternity nurse's holistic approach to care, which takes into account psychosocial and cultural variations as major factors affecting human health.

CHAPTER SUMMARY

Psychosocial and cultural aspects of childbearing are sometimes regarded as less important than other aspects that seem more "clinical" in nature. However, a good understanding of a particular woman's response to pregnancy or her behavior in labor is impossible without some knowledge about what the pregnancy means to her, what she believes is normal and healthy behavior, and what she believes can be harmful to her. More important, the nurse cannot plan an effective course of care for a woman without such knowledge.

Many factors influence how people make decisions about reproductive behavior and how childbearing affects their lives. The individual's readiness for parenthood, motivations for childbearing, and view of what is acceptable male and female behavior often influence his or her reproductive decisions. The availability and acceptability of contraception and the amount of peer and family pressure toward parenthood also help determine whether an individual risks pregnancy, avoids it, or works to achieve it. Once pregnancy occurs, the ease or difficulty of the adjustment to it are determined in large part by the individual's sex, age, and developmental status and the extent to which cultural norms can guide his or her behavior.

The nurse cannot hope to change psychosocial or cultural aspects of a patient's life experience. Nor can the nurse expect to eliminate all of her own biases about what is "right" for childbearing families. However, if she is knowledgeable and careful in her assessment and willing to examine her own beliefs, the nurse can avoid imposing her own value system on the women and families with whom she works. By including psychosocial and cultural assessment as part of her knowledge base, the nurse may be able to anticipate family problems and strengths within the context of maternity care. Assessment of psychosocial and cultural aspects of the patient's life experience is the foundation for comprehensive maternity nursing. The adequacy of the information derived from that assessment can determine whether the subsequent nursing care is appropriate and effective in promoting the health of childbearing women and their families.

STUDY QUESTIONS

1. List some social factors that might influence a person's decision about whether or not to risk pregnancy.
2. What characteristics might be considered important in determining a person's psychosocial readiness for pregnancy?
3. Keeping in mind the characteristics you identified in Question 2, explain why adolescent pregnancy is associated with high psychosocial risk.
4. Discuss the perinatal risk factors associated with early and delayed childbearing.
5. List some cultural variations in birth practices that

you have seen or heard about in your clinical setting. Outline how you could assess those patients' cultural beliefs and practices and how you would adjust your care to maintain safety and deliver culturally sensitive nursing care.

REFERENCES/BIBLIOGRAPHY

Affonso D: Assessing cultural perspectives. In Clark A, Affonso D (eds): Childbearing: A Nursing Perspective. Philadelphia, FA Davis, 1979
Alan Guttmacher Institute: Teenage Pregnancy: The Problem That Hasn't Gone Away. New York, Alan Guttmacher Institute, 1981
Becker MH, Joseph JG: AIDS and behavioral change to reduce risk: A review. Am J Public Health 78(4):394, 1988
Broach J, Newton N: Food and beverages in labor. Part I: Cross-cultural and historical practices. Birth 15(2):81, 1988
Brown MA: Employment during pregnancy: Influences on women's health and social support. Health Care of Women International 3(2/3):151, 1987
Burst HV: Women's health: Pregnancy and childbirth—issues and concerns of healthy pregnant women. Public Health Reports Supplement 52(4):57, 1987
Campbell F, Townes B, Beach L: Motivational bases for childbearing decisions. In Fox G (ed): The Childbearing Decision. Beverly Hills, Sage Publications, 1982
Card J, Wise J: Teenage mothers and teenage fathers: The impact of early childrearing on the parents' personal and professional lives. Fam Plann Perspect 10(4):199, 1978
Carey W, McCann–Sanford T, Davidson E: Adolescent age and obstetric risk. In McAnarney E (ed): Premature Adolescent Pregnancy and Parenthood. New York, Grune & Stratton, 1983
Carrington B: The Afro American. In Clark A (ed): Culture/Childbearing/Health Professionals. Philadelphia, FA Davis, 1978
Chung J: Understanding the Oriental maternity patient. Nurs Clin North Am 12:67, 1977
Cohen W, Newman I, Friedman E: Risk of labor abnormalities with advancing age. Obstet Gynecol 55:414, 1980
Cowan C, Cowan P, Coie L et al: Becoming a family: The impact of the first child's birth on the couple relationship. In Miller W, Newman L (eds): First Child and Family Formation. Chapel Hill, Carolina Population Center, 1978
Cummins LH, Scrimshaw SCM, Engle PL: Views of cesarean birth among primiparous women of Mexican origin in Los Angeles. Birth 15(3):164, 1988
Davidson J, Grant C: Growing up is hard to do—in the AIDS era. MCN 13(5):352, 1988
Dawson DA: The effects of sex education on adolescent behavior. Fam Plann Perspect 18(4):162, 1986
Editorial: Sex education and sex-related behavior. Fam Plann Perspect 18(4):150, 1986
Fishbein E: The couvade: A review. J Obstet Gynecol Neonatal Nurs 10(5):362, 1981

Flaherty MJ, Facteau L, Garver P: Grandmother functions in multigenerational families: An exploratory study of black adolescent mothers and their infants. Matern Child Nurs J 16:61, 1987

Fogel C: Adolescent pregnancy. In Fogel C, Woods N (eds): Health Care of Women. St. Louis, CV Mosby, 1981

Fox G (ed): The Childbearing Decision. Beverly Hills, Sage Publications, 1982

Gaffney KF: Maternal–fetal attachment in relation to self-concept and anxiety. Matern Child Nurs J 15:91, 1986

Griffith S: Childbearing and the concept of culture. J Obstet Gynecol Neonatal Nurs 11(May–June):181, 1982

Grossman F, Eichler L, Winickoff S: Pregnancy, Birth and Parenthood. San Francisco, Jossey–Bass, 1980

Harriman L: Personal and marital changes accompanying parenthood. Fam Relat 32:387, 1983

Heggenhougen H: Father and childbirth: An anthropological perspective. J Nurse Midwife 25(6):21, 1980

Hendricks L: Unwed adolescent fathers: Problems they face and their sources of social support. Adolescence 15:861, 1980

Huffman S, Mhango C, Rockert R et al: Trends in the incidence of breast-feeding for Hispanics of Mexican origin and Anglos on the U.S. Mexican border. Am J Public Health 72:59, 1982

Jones CC, Waskin H, Gerety B, Skipper BJ et al: Persistence of high-risk sexual activity among homosexual men in an area of low incidence of the acquired immunodeficiency syndrome. Sex Transm Dis 14(2):79, 1987

Kay M (ed): Anthropology of Human Birth. Philadelphia, FA Davis, 1982

Kratz CR: Matters for concern: Still left holding the baby. Community Outlook 4:11, 1987

Lester B, Cox JL: Involving nurses in public school sex education. J Sch Health 58(3):108, 1988

Lewis JM: The transition to parenthood: 1. The rating of prenatal marital competence. Family Process 27:149, 1988

Lewis WM: The transition to parenthood: 2. Stability and change in marital structure. Fam Process 27:273, 1988

Majewski JL: Conflicts, satisfactions and attitudes during transition to the maternal role. Nurs Res 35(1):10, 1986

Marsiglio W, Mott FL: The impact of sex education on sexual activity, contraceptive use, and premarital pregnancy among American teenagers. Fam Plann Perspect 18(4):151, 1986

Masters WH, Johnson VE, Kolodny RC: Human Sexuality. Boston, Little, Brown & Co, 1983

May K: Factors contributing to readiness for fatherhood: An exploratory study. Fam Relat 31:353, 1982

May KA: Men's sexuality during the childbearing year: Implications of recent research findings. Holistic Nurs Pract 1(4):60, 1987

McAnarney R, Thiede H: Adolescent pregnancy and childbearing: What we have learned in a decade and what remains to be learned. Semin Perinatol 5:91, 1981

McBride A: The American way of birth. In Kay M (ed): Anthropology of Human Birth. Philadelphia, FA Davis, 1982

McKusick L, Conant M, Coates TJ: The AIDS epidemic: A model for developing intervention strategies for reducing high-risk behavior in gay men. Sex Transm Dis 12(4):229, 1985

Meisenhelder JB, Meservey PM: Childbearing over thirty: Description and satisfaction with mothering. West J Nurs Res 9(4):527, 1987

Meleis A, Sorrell L: Arab American women and their birth experiences. MCN 6:171, 1981

Mercer R: Adolescent pregnancy. In Kowalski K, Sonstegard L, Jennings B (eds): Women's Health: Crisis and Illness in Childbearing. New York, Grune & Stratton, 1984

Mercer R: Relationship of developmental variables to maternal behavior. Res Nurs Health 9:25, 1986

Miller W, Newman L (eds): First Child and Family Formation. Chapel Hill, Carolina Population Center, 1978

Miramontes H: Needed: Effective national policy on AIDS/HIV infection. Nurs Outlook 36(6):262, 1988

Muraskin LD: Sex education mandates: Are they the answer? Fam Plann Perspect 18(4):171, 1986

Naeye R: Maternal age, obstetric complications and outcome of pregnancy. Obstet Gynecol 61:210, 1983

Neeson J, Patterson K, Mercer R et al: Pregnancy outcomes for adolescents receiving prenatal care by maternity nurses practicing in extended roles. J Adolesc Health Care 4:94, 1982

Nelson C, Hewitt M: An Indochinese refugee population in a nurse–midwife service. J Nurse Midwife 28:9, 1983

Nurturing News: A Quarterly Forum for Nurturing Men 6(4): Special issue on teen-age fathers, 1984

Nydegger C: Timing of fatherhood: Role perception and socialization. Unpublished paper, University of California, San Francisco, 1973

Panzarine S, Gould CL: Knowledge about contraception use and conception among a group of urban, black adolescent mothers. J Obstet Gynecol Neonatal Nurs 17(4):279, 1988

Perry D: The umbilical cord: Transcultural care and customs. J Nurse Midwife 27:25, 1982

Poole C: Adolescent pregnancy and unfinished developmental tasks of childhood. J Sch Health 57(7):271, 1987

Puls KS: Birth alternatives for consumers. Chart 84(5):3, 1987

Rossi A: Transition to parenthood. J Marr Fam 30:26, 1968

Schuster C, Ashburn S: The Process of Human Development. Boston, Little, Brown & Co, 1980

Slager–Ernest SE, Hoffman SJ, Beckmann CJA: Adolescent program on maternal and infant outcomes. J Obstet Gynecol Neonatal Nurs 16(6):422, 1987

Speraw S: Adolescents' perceptions of pregnancy: A cross-cultural perspective. West J Nurs Res 9(2):180, 1987

Stein A: Pregnancy in gravidas over 35 years. J Nurse Midwife 28:17, 1983

Stern P, Tilden V, Maxwell E: Culturally induced stress during childbearing: The Filipino American experience. Issues Health Care Women 2:67, 1980

Tamez M: Familism, machismo, and childrearing practices among Mexican Americans. J Psychiatr Nurs 19:21, 1981

TenHouten W: The black family: Myth and reality Psychiatry 33:145, 1970

Tiedje LB, Collins C: Combining employment and motherhood. MCN 14(1):29, 1989

Troll L: Early and Middle Adulthood. Monterey, CA, Brooks/Cole, 1975

Tyler L, Duarte J: Guiding adolescents' choice of a contraceptive. Contemp OB/GYN 23:172, 1982

Ventura S, Hendershot G: Infant health consequences of childbearing by teenagers and other mothers. Public Health Rep 99:138, 1984

Wadd L: Vietnamese postpartum practices: Implications for nursing in the hospital setting. J Obstet Gynecol Neonatal Nurs 12:252, 1983

Waters J: Pregnancy in young adolescents: A syndrome of failure. South Med J 62:655, 1969

Zelnik M, Shah F: First intercourse among young Americans. Fam Plann Perspect 15:64, 1983

Zepeda M: Selected maternal–infant care practices of Spanish-speaking women. J Obstet Gynecol Neonatal Nurs 11(6):371, 1982

SUGGESTED READINGS

Cummins L, Scrimshaw S, Engle P: Views of cesarean birth among primiparous women of Mexican origin in Los Angeles. Birth 15(3):164, 1988

Meisenhelder J, Meservey P: Childbearing over thirty: Description and satisfaction with mothering. West J Nurs Res 9(4):527, 1987

Tiedje L, Collins B: Combining employment and motherhood. MCN 14(1):29, 1989

12 individual and family adaptation to pregnancy

LEARNING OBJECTIVES

After studying the material in this chapter, the student should be able to

- Discuss basic functions and developmental tasks of the child-bearing family

- Discuss the crisis potential of pregnancy and explain why family crises may occur during pregnancy and how they can be prevented

- List parental tasks during pregnancy and discuss their significance for healthy individual and family adaptation

- Identify common maternal and paternal responses to pregnancy and suggest nursing interventions

- Identify situational and developmental factors that influence parental adaptation to pregnancy and suggest nursing interventions

KEY TERMS

Attachment

Bonding

Development

Developmental task

Family life cycle

Grief process

Growth

Loss

Transition

"Conception is the beginning not only of a growing fetus, but also of the family in a new form, with an additional member and with changed relationships. For couples having their first child, this is especially true; for already established families new demands and needs arise that must be dealt with in order to insure the successful incorporation of the new offspring into a changed family system" (Grossman et al 1980).

Pregnancy demands that parents make adjustments on all levels in preparation for the birth of a child. The adjustments are far more apparent in the woman, but evidence is growing that paternal adjustments during pregnancy have important consequences not only for the father's own emotional well-being, but also for the physical and emotional well-being of the woman and the overall health of the family unit.

Much research continues to be directed at understanding how individuals and families accommodate a pregnancy and eventually a newborn in their lives, and what difference the quality of their adaptation to pregnancy makes in later family adjustments. Two major concerns face clinicians providing care during pregnancy: first, the fact that the quality of a woman's psychosocial adaptation to pregnancy is related to her physical health during the childbearing year, and second, the fact that problems in the family unit during pregnancy may contribute to later family problems: marital discord and separation, failure to provide optimal infant caretaking, and deterioration in other family relationships.

A major goal of maternity nursing care is to help families make the healthiest adjustment to the normal stresses of the childbearing year. This chapter presents an indepth discussion of the psychosocial adaptation to pregnancy of family members and the family as a whole.

Knowledge that can help the nurse to understand how a woman and her family adapt to the changing demands of pregnancy comes from current research and from clinical practice. The following areas are emphasized in this chapter:

- Basic structures and functions of the family unit
- Why the demands of pregnancy may increase the potential for crisis in a family
- How attachments are formed and losses are experienced by family members during pregnancy
- How expectant mothers, fathers, and other family members typically adapt to the changing demands of pregnancy

An understanding of these areas is essential if the nurse is to be able to assess individual and family needs and establish accurate nursing diagnoses as well as a realistic

plan of care. Nursing interventions based on this knowledge provide a structure for promoting optimal individual and family health.

THE CHILDBEARING FAMILY

The family is the fundamental unit of all human societies, all of which are organized with the family as the unit responsible for reproduction and socialization of their young. Although all families share some common functions, such as the ones just mentioned, family structure — that is, who is considered a member of the family, and what each member's roles and responsibilities are — varies widely among, and even within cultures. How the term *family* is defined reflects this variability in structure. The following are some currently accepted definitions of family as used by social scientists:

- A social system made up of two or more interdependent persons that remain united over time and mediate individual needs with demands of the larger society
- A group of interacting and interdependent personalities
- A group of individuals related by blood, marriage, or adoption, residing in the same household, sharing a common history, and interacting with each other on the basis of their roles in the group

All of these definitions center on the idea that a family is composed of at least two interacting individuals bound together by emotional or social ties. However, an unmarried pair of adults sharing a household may be considered a family under the first two definitions, but not the third.

One problem in defining the word is that each individual's view of "family" tends to be based on his or her own experience. For instance, some people may consider neighbors, housemates, or even household pets as "members of the family" and interact with them on that basis. Some may believe that a living unit not bound by blood or marriage cannot be defined as a family. Others may believe that the presence of children is what distinguishes a family from other groups.

For the purposes of scientific writing, it is important to select a definition of "family" and use it consistently. However, in providing care or services to individuals and their family members, identifying the patient's definition of family and then providing care on that basis is essential. Pregnancy and childbirth are usually considered major family events. A woman's "family," whatever that means to her, is most often her primary support during the childbearing year. Her family environment will have a direct influence on her emotional and physical health and is likely to be the environment in which the infant will be nurtured and raised. For these reasons, the nurse must have some understanding of the common variations in family structure and function in contemporary society.

Family Structure

One way scientists and clinicians examine families is by analyzing family structure and function. *Family structure* refers to the arrangement of members and their roles. If asked to describe the typical American family structure, many would probably describe a family with a husband, a wife, and two children. This "typical" family was portrayed prominently in television and fiction during the 1950s, usually as white and middle-class, with a father who worked to support the family, a mother who was a homemaker and cared for the children, and children who behaved well and got into little trouble.

This tranquil view of the family probably reflected the nation's need to return to stability and traditional values after the disruption of World War II. So many young people established families of this type that, in the 1950s, there was a dramatic increase in the birth rate, called the "baby boom." However, political, social, and economic changes during the 1960s focused attention on long-ignored aspects of American society, such as racism, sexism, and political dissent, which seemed to be in direct conflict with this complacent view of the family. Many people, especially the young middle-class people who at-

tended college in record numbers in the 1960s, began to explore and debate sensitive issues related to the family, such as women's roles, abortion, birth control, overpopulation, divorce, and social justice.

This reexamination of the American family led to the recognition that family structures in the United States were far more diverse than the predominant view of the 1950s had suggested. Not only was the two-parent household, with father as breadwinner and mother as homemaker, not universal, it was, in fact, becoming less common as new family structures emerged. New structures continued to emerge into the 1980s. The following are family structures the maternity nurse is likely to encounter in her practice.

Nuclear Families

The term *nuclear family* is used to describe families in which parents and their dependent children live in a single family residence away from either parent's family of origin. The nuclear family is still the most common family unit in the United States. In recent years, however, the total number of people represented by that type of family has decreased.

When the term was first used in the 1950s, it usually referred to a family in which the father was the sole breadwinner. In recent years, the two-income family has become the norm in the United States. In 1980 nearly half of American families were dual-earner families; by the 1990s, this number is expected to increase to 80% (Benokraitis 1985). The economic climate of the 1970s forced more families to depend on two incomes and to limit their total family size.

The nuclear family is often characterized by increased mobility as employed parents relocate for economic reasons. One result of this increased mobility can be isolation from the support of the extended family and community. However, closer examination of family interaction patterns often shows that nuclear families maintain ties with both families of origin through frequent telephone calls and visits. Childbirth is an event that typically brings grandparents and siblings into the home; the nurse will often hear an expectant mother report that her mother will be coming to help around the time of the birth. Nuclear families in groups where frequent relocation is the norm — such as the military or large corporations in which transfers are common — often establish a support network that may substitute in some ways for the support of the extended family.

Kin Networks or Extended Families

The terms *kin network* and *extended family* refer to two or more households of any type, which look to each other for support and frequent interaction and which may exchange goods, services, and information. Often, a newly established nuclear family is in fact part of a kin network,

---

Family Structures Encountered by the Maternity Nurse

- Nuclear family: Group made up of parents and dependent children living in a single family residence, separate from family of origin. The nuclear family is the most common family unit in the United States.
- Kin network or extended family: Group made up of two or more nuclear family units that provide mutual support.
- Single-parent family: An adult head-of-household with one or more dependent children. This structure is becoming more common in the USA.
- Nuclear dyad: Male–female couple living without children in single family residence.
- Reconstituted or blended family: Arrangement in which remarried adults are raising children from previous marriage and/or from current marriage.
- Three-generation family: Arrangement in which one or more grandparents and adult children and grandchildren live together. This arrangement is especially common among immigrants from Asia and Central and South America and other minority groups.

if relatives by blood or marriage are nearby and are part of the family's social group.

Single-Parent Families

The single-parent family unit is characterized by an adult head of household with one or more dependent children. Single-parent families are becoming increasingly common in the United States, largely as a result of rising divorce rates, rising birth rates among unmarried women, and the growing practice of adoption by unpartnered adults.

The circumstances leading to the information of the single-parent family dramatically affect the quality of family life. In situations where a spouse has died and the remaining spouse has income-earning capacity, the combination of insurance benefits and earned income may result in only a small decline in financial resources. The same can often be said of families experiencing divorce, although failure to meet child-support obligations is becoming more common. Although the mother is still most often awarded custody of children, the number of single custodial fathers is increasing (Hansen 1985, Hansen and Bozett 1985). When a single adult chooses to adopt a child, economic resources are carefully considered and must be judged adequate to support the family before custody is awarded. However, unmarried women who keep and raise their children are frequently at high social and economic risk. Most often they have little or no earning power and are forced to apply for welfare support. If the mother does have paid employment, wages are usually low and may not even provide sufficient income for necessities and child care costs during work hours. In a study conducted by Hogan, Buehler and Robinson (1983), the researchers concluded that the increased stress in single parents in the study led to survival-type decision making in which long-term goals were sacrificed to get through just one day at a time.

These problems result from the lack of effective social and economic supports for single-parent families, rather than from a deficit in the family structure itself. When adequate supports exist, family life can be rewarding, and children often receive high-quality time and attention from parents and other adults in the social network.

Nuclear Dyads

The term *nuclear dyad* is used to describe male-female couples living without children in a single family residence. In contemporary Western countries, both partners are usually employed outside the home until the birth of their first child. Young married couples may delay the first pregnancy for several years as they attempt to establish their couple relationship and their own economic base. The term can also apply to older adults whose children no longer live with them.

LEGAL/ETHICAL CONSIDERATIONS

The Father and the Law

The court system in the United States has traditionally held that the state should not interfere with the way parents rear their children. Beginning in the early 1900s, however, a gradual change occurred, resulting in a tendency to favor individual rights over the preservation of the family unit. This shift resulted in the slow loss of the father's advantaged position in the eyes of the law.

By the twentieth century, court rulings showed a clear preference for awarding custody to mothers involved in divorce proceedings. While today greater attention is being given to the nurturing capabilities of fathers, the vast majority of custody cases are still decided in favor of the mother; it is virtually impossible for a homosexual father to receive custody of his children. Yet to be determined is who will be responsible for the children when neither parent wants them.

Child support has recently become a second major social issue. The increased economic burden of child support to society, along with the women's movement, has led to (1) "desexing" the legal obligation to support children and (2) increased government involvement in enforcing child-support payments.

Finally, the legal system has gradually begun to extend protection to less traditional families, specifically unwed fathers. Recent court decisions have made it clear that a state cannot ignore the claim of an unwed father to his child, although such claim will not necessarily result in the father's receiving custody of that child.

With a focus on holistic health care, nurses are in an advantageous position to help fathers. Divorcing fathers who want custody should be advised that they must be able to present objective evidence of (1) their ability to provide an adequate income and (2) their ability to be nurturant. In addition, fathers will need to avoid all appearance of sexual promiscuity. Unwed fathers who wish to share custody and/or control of their children should be counseled to take the steps required in their state to establish paternity.

Walters LH, Elam AW: The father and the law. Am Beha Sci 29(1):78, 1985

Reconstituted or Blended Families

The terms *reconstituted family* and *blended family* are used to refer to families in which adults have remarried and are raising children from the previous marriage and/or children from the current marriage. This type of family is becoming increasingly common as divorce and remarriage rates remain high.

Three-Generation Families

The term *three-generation family* refers to families in which one or more dependent grandparents live with adult children and grandchildren. Three-generation families also include grandparents who share their homes with dependent children, primarily adolescent women and grandchildren (Flaherty et al 1987). In the United States this pattern is more common among minority groups, especially immigrants from Asia and Central and South America. Caring for grandparents in the home is often considered the obligation of the oldest grown child. Such arrangements also conserve financial and human resources; three-generation families can benefit from the wisdom and experience of grandparents. The grandmother's role may also include responsibility for child care, as in many Asian and Southeast Asian families, thus freeing the mother to seek paid employment.

Family Function

The family carries out certain functions or tasks essential to the survival of the individual as well as the larger society. Family functions center around meeting individual human needs while maintaining some sense of order and predictability in social interaction. In general, families work as cooperative groups to achieve the goals listed in the accompanying display, Basic Social Functions of the Family.

Maslow's hierarchy of needs, shown in Figure 12–1, suggests that basic physiologic needs must be met before the individual can reach his or her fullest potential. A comparison might be drawn with family functions. A family unable to meet its members' basic needs for food, shelter, safety, and security is unlikely to be able to meet other, "higher" needs, such as providing affiliation and affection, socializing the young, or meeting recreational or religious needs. On the other hand, a family in which basic needs are readily met is likely to have more resources to devote to those higher needs.

Basic Social Functions of the Family

- Providing basic needs for food, shelter, safety, and security
- Providing stable sexual relationships for the adult
- Providing affiliation, affection, and love
- Facilitating reproduction
- Conferring roles and status
- Socialization of the young
- Meeting recreational needs
- Meeting religious and spiritual needs

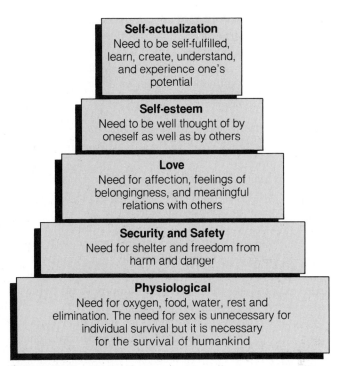

Figure 12–1. Maslow's hierarchy of needs.

Since family structures vary, not every family unit will engage in all of these higher functions. However, societies are structured so that those human needs are most often met within the family. Other social institutions, such as churches, schools, and government agencies, are created to augment family resources in certain areas, but the primary responsibility for these functions still lies with the family unit. Some functions that are of particular significance to the childbearing family are discussed in greater depth.

Providing for Affiliation, Love, and Affection

The family must be able to fulfill individual needs for affectionate relationships and a sense of belonging to a group. Often these needs are fulfilled by having a spouse or lover, children, friends, and a place to call "home." Individuals in families in which these needs are not adequately met may develop a sense of helplessness, hopelessness, and diminished self-esteem. The family unit is likely to disintegrate, with adults and older children escaping the family situation and younger children depending on the parents' ability to reestablish a secure home.

The importance of a secure, loving base can be seen in recent research on the influence of psychosocial stress on maternal adaptation to pregnancy, birth, and motherhood. Several researchers have found that pregnant women in troubled marital and family relationships experienced significantly higher levels of stress and increased rates of perinatal complications (Brown 1986; Mercer et al

1988a, Richardson 1987). Further, there was a correlation between the mother's evaluation of her relationship with her mate during pregnancy and her responsiveness to the child and to the child's intelligence at 4 years of age. This illustrates how individual needs for affiliation and love must be met in order for the family to thrive.

Conferring Social Roles and Status

To confer social roles and status is a particularly important function of the family in today's society. Role theory, a major theoretical framework used in social psychology and sociology, is often applied to family study. A *role* is a set of behaviors that reflect the goals and values associated with a particular position or status in a social group. Roles are learned through interaction with others and are first learned within the family unit. Members of a particular group have a shared understanding of the nature of particular roles, and expectations about behavior are usually fairly clear within the group.

However, there is also room for individual variation and interpersonal negotiation about a person's enactment of a role, within certain limits. For example, an expectant mother may plan to return to work shortly after the birth of her child. She has learned what is expected of her as a mother as she begins to take on the maternal role but has not learned as clearly what is expected of the working mother. She will need to negotiate this variation of the maternal role with her significant others, such as her spouse, and, perhaps, her own parents and siblings. This negotiation reflects the fact that roles are learned in complementary pairs. Complementary roles, such as husband and wife, mother and father, mother and child, mesh with each other. By learning about the complementary role and how another will enact that role, one can learn about one's own role and what is acceptable and expected behavior.

Roles are not static. They are constantly being renegotiated in response to changes either in the family unit or in the individual. Some role changes are gradual and highly predictable, such as those involved in growing from an adolescent to an independent adult. Other changes are more abrupt, such as the transition to the parent role. Although people are prepared in general terms for parenthood throughout life as part of their socialization into male or female sex roles, preparation for the specific behaviors required in the parent role is vague and highly variable. The transition from expectant parent to new parent is fairly abrupt and dramatic.

The importance of the family as a social unit that confers roles and status is apparent when we consider how many major life roles, such as parental, spousal, and child roles and male and female sex roles, are learned within the family of origin. This also explains why some attitudes and behaviors related to family life seem so slow to change.

Family Development

Families can be analyzed according to how family structures and functions change over time. Researchers in the fields of sociology, psychology, and home economics in the post–World War II years observed that families appeared to grow and mature just as individuals do. This observation was the basis for work by Evelyn Duvall, who proposed a theory that described changes in structure and function over the usual lifespan of the family.

The Family Life Cycle

Duvall (1977) proposed that family development occurred in a predictable sequence of stages throughout the life cycle. As shown in the accompanying display, Stages in the Family Life Cycle, the sequence begins with a married couple and progresses through childbearing and child-rearing into middle age, old age, and eventual dissolution of the family with the death of both spouses.

This theory of family development has many similarities to other developmental theories that apply to individuals, such as Erik Erikson's "Eight Ages of Man." The following principles underlie Duvall's theory of family development:

- The needs of individual members may determine how long a family spends in a particular stage; generally, movements to a new stage are linked to the age of the first-born child.
- When certain developmental tasks are completed, they provide the basis for the emergence and eventual

---

Stages in the Family Life Cycle

- Married couple/beginning family
- Childbearing family (from birth of first child through age 30 months)
- Child-rearing family
    With preschool children (oldest child 30 months through 6 years)
    With school age children (oldest child 6 through 13 years)
    With teen-age children (oldest child 13 through 20 years)
- Launching family (from departure of oldest child until departure of youngest child)
- Middle-aged family (from departure of youngest child to retirement of oldest spouse)
- Aging family (from retirement until death of both spouses)

Adapted from Duvall E: Marriage and Family Development. Philadelphia, JB Lippincott, 1985

completion of future tasks. When developmental tasks are not completed, subsequent tasks are more difficult and may not be accomplished.

Duvall's theory of family development was developed during the 1950s and 1960s and has been refined by other family scientists. The framework has some limitations: it describes only families with children, and it does not seem to account for family development when unexpected or unusual events occur, such as adolescent pregnancy, single parenthood, divorce, and remarriage. However, it does serve as a useful framework to examine the tasks that face families as they enter the childbearing and child-rearing period.

Tasks of the Childbearing Family

As it adapts to pregnancy, the family must accomplish certain developmental tasks in preparation for birth and child-bearing. The accompanying display, Developmental Tasks of the Childbearing Family, lists these tasks. Accomplishing these tasks during pregnancy lays the groundwork for the later, more complex adaptations required when the newborn is added to the family unit.

The nurse can observe families as they work to accommodate these tasks during pregnancy. Each of the tasks requires some reorganization in current patterns of activity and interaction. The adjustments required of families during pregnancy are major ones and take considerable amounts of time and energy to accomplish. If a family is unable to reorganize itself to meet these developmental requirements, unmet needs will begin to mount up and may overwhelm the family's coping mechanisms. The nurse must be able to identify individuals and families who are beginning to experience problems in adapting to pregnancy and intervene early to promote optimal individual and family health. The following sections discuss in more detail the nature of individual and family adaptations to pregnancy.

Pregnancy as Crisis

Because some degree of change is unavoidable during pregnancy, and because change is often required over a fairly short period of time, a number of social scientists and clinicians have described pregnancy as a type of crisis — that is, an unsettling event that leads to a state of disequilibrium.

Crisis Theory Applied to Expectant Families

Crisis theory has been widely used to examine the impact of pregnancy on individuals and the family. A pregnancy, especially a first pregnancy, is quite unlike other previous life experiences and brings with it stressors to which the couple involved must adapt. Some stressors can be described as *frequent stressors,* meaning that they happen with enough regularity that they might be expected to affect most families. Other stressors may be *unanticipated,* such as complications of pregnancy or unexpected personal and family losses. The combination of frequent and unanticipated stressors experienced by each family is unique. Whether or not these stressors produce a crisis in the family depends in large part on factors present to balance those stressors.

Balancing factors include the individual's or the family's ability to perceive the stress in their situation realistically and their coping mechanisms to reduce and adapt to that stress. The expectant mother and father first respond to stress by using coping patterns that have been successful in the past. If these are successful, then a crisis does not result. However, quite often, previously successful coping patterns are not adequate for the demands of pregnancy, and a crisis can result (Lewis 1988). Aguilera and Messick (1986) point out that the degree to which a crisis is successfully resolved depends on:

- How realistically the situation is perceived
- The individual's and family's precrisis level of functioning
- The range of coping patterns available
- Past success or failure in dealing with crisis, anxiety, and stress
- The resources available to the individual and family
- The ability to mobilize and use those resources

Developmental Tasks of the Childbearing Family

Acquiring knowledge and plans for the specific needs of pregnancy, childbirth, and early parenthood

Preparing to provide for the physical care of the expected baby

Adapting financial patterns to meet increasing needs

Defining evolving role patterns

Adjusting patterns of sexual expression to accommodate pregnancy

Expanding communication to meet present and future emotional needs

Reorienting relationships with relatives

Adapting relationships with friends and community to take account of the realities of pregnancy and the anticipated child

Maintaining a healthy morale and philosophy of life

Adapted from Duvall E: Marriage and Family Development. Philadelphia, JB Lippincott, 1985

Crises are by their nature time-limited; individuals and families cannot continue with anxiety and stress at high levels and will adapt in whatever way possible to reduce the distress to tolerable levels. Gerald Caplan, one of the early writers in the field of crisis theory, emphasizes that the acute phase of a crisis lasts only 4 to 6 weeks (Caplan 1964).

The crisis potential in the process of family adaptation to pregnancy is shown in Figure 12–2; the following clinical example shows how well crisis theory can apply to this aspect of maternity care.

A couple, Mary and Ted, find themselves expecting a baby long before they had planned for one. Financially, things have not gone as hoped, and the loss of Mary's income after the baby is born will be difficult to manage. Ted avoids discussing his fears and financial concerns with Mary, and instead focuses his attention on his work. For minor problems in the past, this has worked well for him. Mary experiences a lot of nausea and other physical discomforts in the first trimester and is worried that labor and birth will be difficult for her.

Mary confides in friends at work about her fears, again a coping pattern that has been satisfactory in the past. This time, however, instead of receiving support, she hears several "horror stories" about friends' pregnancies that further increase her own anxiety. (Combination of frequent and unanticipated stressors and use of past coping mechanisms.)

Mary believes that Ted is concerned only about their financial situation and feels he is being insensitive to her needs. Ted is angry that he can't provide any more financial security for his family

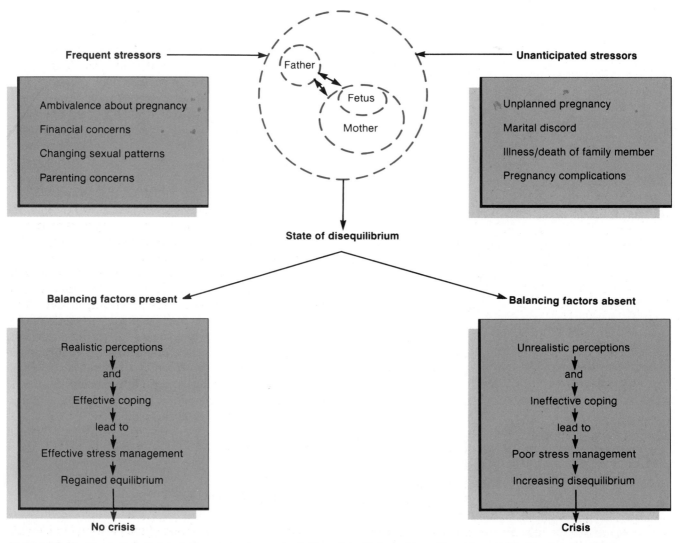

Figure 12–2. Family adaptation during pregnancy: potential for crisis. (Adapted from Donaldson N: The postpartum follow-up clinician. J Obstet Gynecol Neonatal Nurs 10(4):249, 1981)

and worries that Mary thinks he has let her down. (Unrealistic perception of situation.)

Mary's and Ted's fears and concerns grow and soon create considerable tension in their relationship. Ted begins working even longer hours to avoid his own fears and his partner's worry. Mary stops discussing her worries with friends, but when she tries to talk things over with Ted, he acts as frightened as she does. Mary feels compelled to reassure him, and while neither is comfortable in the situation, neither knows how to alleviate the tension. They soon find themselves alternately arguing and avoiding each other. (Ineffective coping and increasing stress leading as crisis.)

Characteristics of a Crisis

The pregnancy has precipitated a crisis for this couple, requiring them to adapt in ways different from coping patterns that have worked in the past. The resulting disequilibrium produces discomfort and anxiety and motivates the individual to find other ways of reestablishing balance. Crisis can be seen as a turning point or, as the word translates in Chinese, a "dangerous opportunity." A crisis is dangerous because if adaptation is not successful, there is potential for further deterioration in the individual's status and psychological regression. A crisis is an opportunity, because if adaptation is successful, there is potential for considerable psychologic growth and maturation.

Crises can be categorized as either *situational,* arising from a change in events or life circumstances, or *maturational* (or normative), arising from internal changes, in the individual or family, associated with normal growth and development. Most often pregnancy is regarded as a maturational crisis. Childbearing is a predictable event in most people's lives and is regarded in society as an important part of the transition to adulthood. However, pregnancy can also be a situational crisis: for Mary and Ted, this is certainly true. Other unexpected problems, such as maternal complications or a financial setback, can result in a situational crisis for an expectant family.

One feature of childbearing that complicates the process of adaptation and increases the potential for crisis is the fact that mother and father have qualitatively different experiences of pregnancy and birth. Most adults in couple relationships regard their partners as their primary support person and rely on that support in periods of stress. Pregnancy and birth, because of their profound biologic effects on the woman, create an experience gap between the woman and her mate. This gap may make it difficult to continue previous patterns of communication and interaction in the relationship, especially if the pregnancy is a first pregnancy occurring early in the couple's relationship. This "experience gap" will be discussed in

more detail later in this chapter when the impact of the pregnancy on the couple's relationship is examined.

The crisis potential of pregnancy may be heightened because one partner may feel that the other cannot understand and meet his or her needs adequately and because pregnancy is changing something that partners usually take for granted and consider very stable: their characteristic ways of relating to each other. The process of reorganizing relationships—forming new attachments, loosening old ones—is basic in human interaction, but it takes on new significance during the childbearing year. The following section explores the concepts of attachment and loss as they relate to the experience of pregnancy.

ATTACHMENT AND LOSS IN THE PRENATAL PERIOD

In each person's life, much of the joy and sorrow revolves around attachments or affectional relationships—making them, breaking them, preparing for them and adjusting to their loss (Klaus and Kennell 1982).

Attachment and loss are an intrinsic part of the childbearing experience. The process of parent-infant attachment has received much scientific and clinical attention. Much of this work has focused on the discovery of steps in the process of attachment, the identification of factors that enhance or inhibit the formation of parent-infant attachment, and the investigation of how clinicians can influence the process. These important aspects of maternity nursing care are presented in depth in Unit V, in the context of postpartum and neonatal care.

Attachment usually refers to a strong affiliative tie with another, based on a long period of mutual stimulation and response, more like the process of "staying in love." The earliest use of the term typically referred to the infant's tie to the parent or caretaker. However, current use also includes the parent's emotional tie to the infant (Klaus and Kennell 1982).

The beginnings of attachment and the potential for loss can be seen during pregnancy as parents prepare to enter into a new relationship with the soon-to-be-born child. The following section discusses the process of attachment and adaptation to loss as they occur in the expectant family.

Prenatal Attachment

Mothers are usually aware of the growing fetus for 20 weeks or more before birth and know that the fetus is there for an even longer period. Mothers usually demonstrate some investment in a relationship with the fetus by the middle trimester. This is true even in high-risk situations in which the mother is herself at physical risk because of the pregnancy (Kemp 1987). Mothers may interact with the fetus either by talking or by interpreting movements and may try to stimulate or stop fetal movement by changing positions and activities.

How the mother views the fetus varies considerably across cultures. Some groups in Southeast Asia believe that the fetus should receive tender, loving care and be taught about life almost from the moment of conception, whereas other groups, including many in Western countries, do not consider the fetus fully human until after quickening. Cultural beliefs will probably influence how prenatal attachment develops.

Maternal attachment during pregnancy is probably influenced to some extent by the biologic and hormonal changes caused by the pregnancy itself. An example is the nesting behavior of mammals; whether an animal recognizes it is carrying young is questionable, but hormonal influences do trigger behaviors like nestbuilding shortly before labor begins. Prenatal attachment in humans cannot be explained entirely on that basis, because fathers also appear to demonstrate attachment to the unborn child during pregnancy (Mercer et al 1988c).

Although research on paternal prenatal attachment has begun only recently, findings appear to be similar in many ways to those among mothers. However, fathers may express their attachment to the fetus more through their involvement in activities related to the pregnancy than in interaction with the fetus. Partly, this is because they have to "go through" the mother to interact with the fetus; the father's experience of fetal life is always "one step removed." This may explain in part why fathers are often so thrilled to hear the fetal heart tones or see the fetus on sonography. These experiences are, in a way, much more direct for them.

The mother and father together may engage in attachment behavior. Parents may use pet names for the fetus, and may "play games" with the fetus in three-way interaction. The mother may try to stimulate fetal movement so the father can feel it. Often parents will talk about the personality of the fetus and draw conclusions about sex and temperament from these early interactions.

The Significance of Parent – Fetal Attachment

Nurse researchers have begun to explore how to assess prenatal attachment more systematically and to consider what significance, if any, prenatal attachment has for the quality of later parent – infant interaction. Tools have been developed to measure prenatal attachment, and some studies suggest that high levels of prenatal attachment may be associated with more positive perceptions of the infant after birth among mothers (Cranley 1981).

Some researchers also have wondered about the effects of antenatal diagnostic techniques such as amniocentesis and sonography on prenatal attachment. Findings have been inconsistent. Grace (1984) found that knowing the baby's sex after amniocentesis did not appear to affect maternal – infant attachment. Likewise, Davis and Akridge (1987) found that nursing interventions designed to promote intrauterine attachment appeared to have no effect on attachment. A study by Carter – Jessop (1981), on the other hand, suggested that asking mothers to keep track of fetal movement during pregnancy led to higher maternal attachment. Much more work is needed before clinical practice can be based on these research findings, but nursing care could potentially be dramatically improved if the quality of parent – infant relationships could be affected by supportive intervention during pregnancy.

Prenatal attachment is also an important aspect for the nurse to consider in working with expectant couples when pregnancy is threatened or lost. The following section will examine the concept of loss during pregnancy and the significance that loss may have for individual and family adaptation to pregnancy.

Loss During Pregnancy

Since pregnancy holds the potential for new attachment, it also must hold the potential for loss. *Loss* is defined as the deprivation of a desired or valued object or wished-for outcome. Loss is resolved through the grieving process, or grief work, in which a person painfully reexamines memories of the lost object. As the memories are relived, the emotional tie is reexperienced, each time with less pain. Gradually the emotional pain is reduced to a level that permits the person to set new goals or make new attachments.

Any type of loss may cause a grief response, even changes that appear to be minor shifts in self-image or in significant relationships. Pregnancy, particularly for women, signals an irrevocable change in self-image. The woman will never again be only a young woman, someone's daughter and mate; even if the pregnancy is terminated intentionally, her self-concept will be adjusted to take into account that life experience. This new view of the self will be created in part by grieving for what must be given up.

Taking on the parental role often means relinquishing parts of other roles. Grief work is seen as an important part of taking on the maternal role. For example, becoming a mother may force a woman to give up her view of herself as a carefree gadabout or her cherished fantasy of becoming a company president before her 35th birthday. A pregnancy will cause reorganization in her relationship with her spouse. She may grieve over the loss of her trim, attractive body and what she perceives to be the loss of her husband's passionate interest.

Pregnancy forces similar, although less dramatic shifts in the father's self-concept and will require grief work to resolve some losses. Many men feel the loss of their partner's undivided attention acutely with the first pregnancy, and some have difficulty resolving this loss. One father told a nurse, "The pregnancy is an absolute gain for her; she gets to have me *and* the baby. I feel like I've lost her and gained a stranger." A father may require some time to adjust to the increasing responsibility he feels and resolve in his own mind some loss of mobility and freedom. He may also need to resolve goals and expectations he will likely not accomplish because of his new expectant father status.

Losses caused by changes in self-image and in relationships with important others are usually subtle, and the man or woman may not even recognize the emotional adjustments he or she is making. However, more obvious loss — loss of a pregnancy through miscarriage or fetal demise — also occurs.

The Impact of Pregnancy Loss

Pregnancy loss always seems unexpected. Pregnancy and birth are regarded as happy events, and the emotional impact of pregnancy loss can be a significant threat to individual and family mental health. Pregnancy loss is not uncommon, however; approximately one pregnant woman in five will experience a loss through miscarriage or fetal demise (Borg et al 1981).

Loss of a pregnancy is experienced on several levels. First, the woman must acknowledge her body has failed to complete the physiologic function of childbearing. This can be a threat to her self-esteem and to her sense of her own femininity. Second, to the extent that attachment to the fetus has begun, the bond must be broken. Finally, during pregnancy, the unborn child is regarded as part of the mother. With a pregnancy loss, the mother loses a part of herself as well as her fantasy of herself as a mother (Friedman et al 1982). Parents, especially mothers, are in a state of psychologic and physical readiness for a baby, but instead must cope with the fact that there will be no baby.

Loss of a pregnancy is often associated with feelings of guilt. Most women and their partners feel some ambivalence about pregnancy. If a loss occurs before that ambivalence is resolved, the parents may feel they deserved to lose the pregnancy. Parents may review their recent lives in great detail, searching for something they may have done or did not do that caused the loss. For example, both

partners may experience guilt and assume they caused the miscarriage, if the loss occurs after sexual intercourse. In the majority of cases, the actual cause is never known, but parents may persist in their search for an explanation until their grief work is completed.

Health professionals sometimes assume that a first-trimester miscarriage is easier to accept than a later pregnancy loss. They may consider the woman "hardly pregnant" and give cues that grief over a miscarriage is somehow inappropriate. Comments such as "you're young — you can always try again" and "it was for the best" or "be thankful you have other children," while well-intentioned, fail to acknowledge the pain associated with a pregnancy loss. Such comments may also communicate the health professional's lack of understanding of the patient's situation. Women and their partners do sometimes grieve over the early loss of pregnancy, if they wanted the pregnancy very much and if they had begun to establish an attachment to the unborn child (Borget et al 1981).

The nurse should also recognize that grief may not be limited to just the parents themselves. Siblings, grandparents, and other relatives interested in the pregnancy will experience pain and grief. These other family members may need some guidance in ways they can assist the parents in adjusting to the loss.

Steps in the Grieving Process

Scientists and clinicians have observed that the grief process consists of several phases. These are summarized by Mercer (1977) as:

Numbness and shock

Protest

Anger and yearning

Disorganization

Reorganization

The first phase usually lasts only days. The later phases may become progressively longer and may overlap, so that the grieving person vacillates between two phases for a period of time. The acute mourning period may last from 6 months to 2 years, depending on the nature of the loss (Estok et al 1983). Steps in the grief process are shown in Figure 12–3.

Parents may find that friends and relatives expect them to bounce back quickly from a pregnancy loss and are unwilling or unable to understand their grief. A variety of self-help groups have been formed, for example, SHARE (Source of Help in Airing and Resolving Experiences), AMEND (Aiding a Mother Experiencing Neonatal Death), and HAND (Helping After Neonatal Death), to serve as networks for grieving parents. Most health care

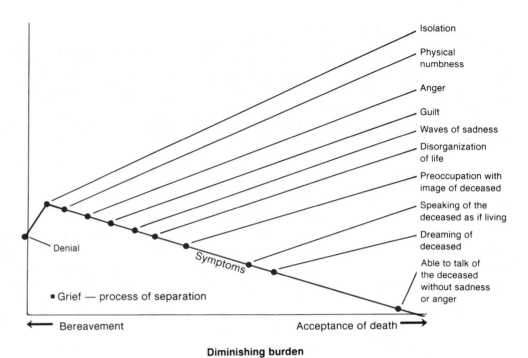

Figure 12–3. Steps in the grief process. (Hallett E: Birth and grief. Birth and the Family Journal 1(4):21, 1974)

facilities can provide referral information to local groups. Many institutions also have special follow-up services for parents experiencing miscarriage or perinatal loss.

Effect of Pregnancy Loss on Subsequent Pregnancies

Most pregnancy losses are of unknown cause. Many couples who experience a pregnancy loss go on to conceive within 2 years, and some may attempt to conceive immediately. Experts generally agree that the couple should mourn the loss before conceiving again. Pregnancy will not diminish the parents' grief and will likely prolong it, at the same time interfering with their ability to attach to the new unborn child.

A pregnancy loss can have definite effects on an individual's adaptation to a subsequent pregnancy. A woman who lost an earlier pregnancy at 20 weeks may not be able to invest herself emotionally in the pregnancy until after she passes that benchmark and realizes that the event will not recur. Both partners may make changes in their daily life as if the woman were extremely vulnerable. Patterns such as restricting physical activity and avoiding sexual intercourse may not be medically indicated, but parents will impose such restrictions on themselves out of fear and protectiveness. Other couples may delay a subsequent pregnancy, not wanting to expose themselves to the potential for loss and grief again. Although the fact is of little comfort to parents who experience a pregnancy loss, most pregnancies proceed quite normally and result in the birth of a healthy newborn.

MATERNAL ADAPTATION TO PREGNANCY

Pregnancy is a time when women quite literally begin to share themselves and their bodies with another being, a relationship that will continue for the many years of motherhood. This event naturally produces profound changes in the ways a woman views herself, her body, her relationship with the child's father, and her future with her as yet unknown offspring (Grossman et al 1980).

The maternity nurse must be knowledgeable about the processes involved in maternal adaptation to pregnancy so that she can provide appropriate emotional support, supply needed information, and help expectant women to anticipate events and their future needs. The following section highlights some aspects of expectant motherhood, and then discusses maternal tasks of pregnancy.

The Expectant Mother

The miracle of a woman's ability to conceive and bear children has been a major theme in art and literature throughout human history. The theme of the pregnant woman as being unusually powerful and in harmony with the forces of nature is repeated in ancient mythology and in nearly all cultures.

Western culture has devoted much scientific attention to the physical and psychologic process of pregnancy.

Early psychoanalytic thought, emerging during the restrictive Victorian era, reflected both the fascination with and the fear of the woman's ability to create life. This conflict was clear in the societal view of expectant motherhood during that era. The word "pregnant" was not used in polite company. Instead, women were said to be "indisposed" and "in a period of confinement." Expectant mothers were rarely if ever seen in public in the latter half of pregnancy. They were considered to be unusually frail and vulnerable during this time.

However, as women's roles changed in the years before and after World War II, pregnancy gradually came to be regarded as a more natural part of a woman's life. The baby boom of the 1950s reinforced this as women in record numbers were conceiving and bearing children. Maternity clothes, once limited to one or two outfits made to last throughout a pregnancy, became a booming business. The prepared childbirth movement, with its strong grassroots origins, brought pregnancy even more into public view. Women began keeping paid positions later into pregnancy, and pregnant women in public places were no longer regarded as unusual.

The women's movement of the 1960s and 1970s continued this trend, as pregnancy began to be viewed as a state of health that should not interfere with a woman's activities. Conventional prenatal and birth-care practices began to be challenged, and decisions about maternity care were increasingly seen as matters over which the woman should have control (Burst 1987, Puls 1987).

Contemporary clinicians now recognize that a woman's psychologic adaptation to pregnancy is as important as her physiologic health in determining whether obstetric outcomes are good. Major tasks have been identified in this process of maternal adaptation. The following section discusses these in detail.

Maternal Tasks of Pregnancy

Several developmental tasks that reflect healthy maternal adaptation to pregnancy and provide a basis for the acceptance of the maternal role have been identified. These tasks are often discussed within a framework of trimesters of pregnancy, since some concerns are more pressing at one point in pregnancy than another, and because the biologic nature of pregnancy provides some predictable sequences of events.

However, the nurse should recognize that tasks overlap and may emerge in different ways at various points in pregnancy and that distinctions between completion of one task and the beginning of another are not clear-cut. Furthermore, these developmental tasks, which are listed in the accompanying display, are perhaps better described as parental tasks of pregnancy, since many of them apply as well to the expectant father.

Developmental Tasks of Pregnancy

Accepting the pregnancy
Establishing a relationship with the unborn child
Adjusting to changes in self
Adjusting to changes in the couple relationship
Preparing for birth and early parenthood

Accepting the Pregnancy

Women often are surprised to realize that they may be pregnant, even if they have been actively trying to conceive. Some women may ignore or not even notice early symptoms and not seek confirmation of pregnancy until after several missed menses. Others may delay confirmation because they are unwilling to hear definite news one way or the other. However, recent advances in home pregnancy testing now make it possible for women to confirm their own pregnancy with high levels of accuracy before a second missed period, and this may change how women respond to suspicion and early symptoms of pregnancy.

A woman's initial response to the news that she is pregnant may be shock, joy, delight, anger, or a combination of all of these feelings. Typically, if her response is a happy one, she will announce the news to her partner fairly soon. If her initial response is more negative, or if she anticipates that his response will be negative, she may wait for several days or weeks before disclosing the news.

In most cases, regardless of whether or not she planned the pregnancy, the woman experiences some early ambivalence about the pregnancy. She may feel the timing is not right and can find many reasons why she should not be pregnant. An early nurse researcher in maternity nursing, Reva Rubin, described this as the "someday, but not now" phenomenon (1970).

Accepting the pregnancy first requires the woman accept the reality of her pregnancy and the fact that her body will become the vehicle for supporting another life. The woman may first view the fetus as an intruder; this reflects a normal egocentric reaction to this remarkable experience. The woman's behavior is typically self-centered, attending to her own needs and concerns first. The fetus is not a separate being, yet it is not part of her. Although accepting the *fact of pregnancy* on an intellectual level is a first step, the woman must then acknowledge it on an emotional level as *her* pregnancy.

Another important part of this maternal task is securing the acceptance of her pregnancy by other important people. Usually, acceptance of the pregnancy by her mate is of the utmost importance to the mother. The father is usually told first, and a woman's own emotional response to the confirmation of pregnancy often reflects whether or not she believes her mate will be pleased. The responses of other important people in her life, such as parents, friends, or co-workers, are also of concern to the pregnant woman. A woman who believes that her significant others are not supportive of the pregnancy is at risk for difficulties in later adaptation (Cranley 1981). This can cause special problems for the single mother, whose family members and friends may not welcome the pregnancy and may even respond very negatively to the news (Tilden 1983).

Establishing a Relationship With the Fetus

For the woman to establish a relationship with the fetus, she must come to see it as a being separate from herself. However, a risk in this process is that the woman will see the fetus as separate and *intrusive*. If the fetus remains an alien presence and a threat to her selfhood, the woman will not nurture and protect it. Psychologically, this risk is avoided by the process of incorporation.

Incorporating the Fetus. As the woman accepts the pregnancy and begins to adjust to the physiologic and emotional changes it produces, she gradually comes to see the pregnancy and the fetus as part of herself. She begins to see herself as pregnant and, as such, deserving of special attention. She may begin wearing maternity clothes far earlier than is actually necessary, an announcement to the world that she is pregnant. This self-absorption enables the woman to incorporate the fetus and the pregnancy as part of herself, and to accommodate the changes pregnancy causes without experiencing a significant threat to her self-concept. Once this is accomplished, the woman can allow herself to view the fetus as a separate being with whom she is beginning to establish a relationship.

Separating Fetus from Self. The process of identifying the fetus as a separate being usually begins with the increased uterine growth and sensations of fetal life in the middle trimester, although some women may begin this process sooner. Separation begins as the mother identifies the fetus as a separate being with its own boundaries and selfhood, but still a valued part of her and dependent on her. The woman comes to think of the fetus as a fantasized baby; she may begin to daydream about her baby, and engage in conversations and interactions with the fetus. This signals the beginning of maternal–fetal attachment, as the mother invests herself emotionally in a relationship with the unborn child.

This process of separating fetus from self while forming a growing attachment to the unborn child continues throughout pregnancy. In the last weeks, the physical discomforts of the pregnancy and the feelings of "being tired of being pregnant" signal a tipping of the scale: she is now ready to give up the pregnancy, separate physically from the fetus through childbirth, and welcome her newborn.

Adjusting to Changes in Self

Another set of maternal tasks of pregnancy is related to the changes the woman experiences in her emotions and attitudes, and in her body.

Adjusting to Physical Changes. The pregnant woman must adjust to changes in her perceived body size, in mobility, in body function, and in her emotional investment in her physical appearance. These adjustments begin almost immediately after conception. The rapid physiologic alterations of early pregnancy are felt more than seen, but hormonal fluctuations, the subtle abdominal growth, and breast swelling may combine to produce a negative response to her own body. Women often are concerned that others understand they are pregnant and "not just getting fat." Later, when more pronounced physical changes are noticeable, the woman must also adapt to the limitations of a larger, heavier body. She probably will experience a sense of increased vulnerability and physical awkwardness.

Some women welcome these changes as part of being pregnant, whereas others dislike them intensely. Many women will avoid cameras and mirrors, while others appear to be fascinated with their changing bodies and have more pictures of themselves pregnant than at any other time. Most women accept their pregnant bodies with some regret and some pleasure. Although women who have a large investment in their physical appearance and their trim bodies may have more difficulty accepting these changes, in most cases acceptance is not stressful enough to disrupt maternal adaptation to the pregnancy overall. However, concerns about body image persist through pregnancy and into the postbirth period and have been identified as a major concern.

Adjusting to Emotional Changes. Emotional changes have come to be associated with pregnancy just as closely as unusual food cravings and maternity clothes. Expectant mothers exhibit a degree of *emotional lability* that in the nonpregnant woman would be regarded as pathologic. Rapid and dramatic mood swings may be a result of hormonal fluctuations, or may simply reflect elevated anxiety levels. Mood swings usually occur in response to some environmental cue; the mother may respond with great happiness to a kind word and later be reduced to tears by a stranger's stare. Such mood swings can be confusing to the woman herself and to family members.

Another characteristic emotional change of pregnancy is *increasing anxiety*. Fears about her own physical vulnerability and that of the fetus, worries about the anticipated pain and work of childbirth, and changes in her relationship with her partner all produce increased anxiety. Another source of increasing anxiety is the fact that pregnancy signals a transition to motherhood with its responsibility and long-term commitment. The pregnant woman must, in a sense, rediscover who she is. The woman's status with friends, relatives, even her own mother, changes with pregnancy, and she must renegotiate these relationships in terms of her future motherhood.

One outlet for this increased anxiety during pregnancy may be through fantasies and dreams. Women often report having strange, sometimes bizarre fantasies and dreams about the baby, and birth process, or highly erotic encounters. These may reflect processing of unconscious fears and conflicts, and are regarded as a normal side-effect of the mother's emotional adaptation to pregnancy.

Adjusting to the Changing Couple Relationship

Another maternal task of pregnancy is to adjust to the changes pregnancy causes in her relationship with her mate. The couple's relationship changes because both partners are changing and their anticipated future together is changing. Research has found that both positive and negative changes occurred in the marriage relationship as a result of pregnancy (Saunders et al 1987, Tomlinson 1987). The woman experiences shifts in her usual emotional responses to her partner. Two areas are particularly important: increases in her dependence on her mate and shifts in her sexual relationship.

Increases in Dependence.   The pregnant woman becomes more dependent on others, particularly her mate, for physical and emotional support (Fig. 12–4). Signs of this may be seen in extreme worry about her partner when away from home; in increased impatience with activities and interests that do not include her; and in more practical matters, such as relying on him for physical help at home.

Experienced maternity nurses have observed that to adapt to pregnancy and motherhood successfully, a woman must herself "be mothered." In a sense, the woman's needs for affection, attention, and support must be met before she can give to her infant. Reassurance of support from partner and friends becomes extremely important, even to a woman who, at other times in her life, is independent and self-reliant. The single mother with little economic security and without the support of a family will experience extremely high levels of stress because her needs for support are not being met.

Changes in the Sexual Relationship.   Another area in which the woman must adapt is in her sexual relationship with her mate. Although most women feel an increased need for love and affection during pregnancy, the desire for sexual activity during pregnancy varies among women, and even in the same woman at various times during pregnancy. These changes, which are both physio-

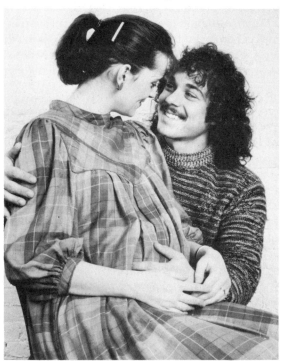

Figure 12–4. Warm, loving support from her mate is an important factor in healthy maternal adaptation to pregnancy. (Photo: Erika Stone)

logically and psychologically based, are discussed in detail in Chapter 6. Changes in the woman's desire for sexual activity tend to have a "ripple effect" in the relationship. Her decreased interest may cause the mate's interest to decline, which in turn causes her to worry about her attractiveness, making her even more uncomfortable and concerned. The woman may also worry that sexual activity will have a harmful effect on the pregnancy or the fetus and may discourage her partner's interest for that reason. Women in relationships in which open communication about sexuality has been established are likely to have less difficulty in this area than women who are unaccustomed to discussing sexual matters with their partners.

Preparing for Birth and Early Motherhood

The process of maternal adaptation to pregnancy is completed as the mother prepares herself to experience labor, to give birth, and to take on the maternal role. Although this process occurs to some extent throughout pregnancy, the woman begins this preparation in earnest in the last trimester (Bliss–Holtz 1988). This preparation is institutionalized to some extent through prepared childbirth classes, baby showers, and physical preparation of the nursery for the baby. The women may also engage in a flurry of activity in the last weeks of pregnancy, sometimes called "nesting behavior." She will hurry to finish preparing the baby's layette or clean the entire house in preparation for the baby. Folk wisdom suggests that nesting behavior signals that labor will begin soon. Although there is no scientific proof that this is true, experienced labor and delivery nurses have observed that women often come into labor tired, having had a burst of energy and activity a day or two before they went into labor.

Resolving Fears About Childbirth.   A woman typically has fears and worries about the process of labor and birth. These fears are understandable; while the primigravida has not experienced the process and so fears the unknown, the multigravida may know what can go wrong and exactly what to anticipate. A woman often has fears about how she will respond to the pain and work of labor, about losing control emotionally and physically, and about whether she and her baby will survive. Some of these fears can be resolved with information and reassurance from care providers. Support from her partner can also help, but ultimately the woman must cope with fear in her own way (Fig. 12–5).

Prepared childbirth classes can assist in resolving some worries and give the woman some additional coping mechanisms that may be useful in labor and birth. One

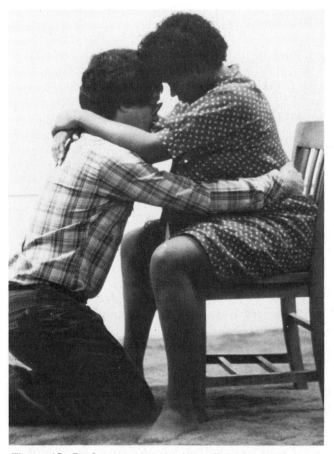

Figure 12–5. Couple rehearsing labor. Rehearsing with her mate how she will cope with labor helps the pregnant woman prepare for childbirth. (Photo: BABES, Inc.)

way women sometimes cope with fear is by making elaborate plans for their birth, by reading and asking many questions, and by talking with other women about their experiences. Some may cope by not wanting to know, and by leaving matters in the hands of their care providers. Although the nurse may value information-seeking behavior on the part of the pregnant woman, the nurse must also realize that avoiding information may be an effective coping mechanism for some women and should not be discounted.

Accepting the Maternal Role.   Accepting the maternal role is a process in which the mother internalizes the maternal role in preparation for actually enacting the role with her newborn. The processes that take place during the attainment of the maternal role are discussed in greater depth in Unit V. However, the nurse should recognize that the woman begins the process of learning the maternal role during pregnancy at the same time as she begins to attach to her unborn child, and each process affects and is affected by the other. Anticipatory socialization into the mother role occurs as the mother fantasizes about herself and her baby, observes other mothers and chooses behaviors to mimic or avoid, and engages in role play as she cares for other children. With the birth of the infant, the mother continues the process of maternal role attainment, with the end point being the establishment of a sense of comfort and competence in the role.

Situational Factors Affecting Maternal Adaptation

Certain situational factors are known to affect the woman's adaptation to pregnancy. Some of these are of particular importance to the maternity nurse, since they also may have a significant impact on the woman's health during the childbearing year.

Partnered Versus Unpartnered Status

There is still little known about the experience of the single mother. Women who have less social support and perceive a troubled relationship with the father of the baby are known to experience higher rates of perinatal complications and higher stress than other women, but the differences may have more to do with socioeconomic or psychological distinctions than with an unmarried or unpartnered status itself. Tilden (1983), a nurse researcher, did identify some areas of concern during pregnancy which are uniquely different for single mothers. Single mothers have a more difficult time making a decision to keep a pregnancy, because they were choosing to be a solo parent and could not count on partner support. Single mothers experienced some stress and uncertainty in deciding how to disclose the news of their pregnancy to friends and family, and whom to tell. The single mother also had to take legal issues into consideration: who would care for the infant if something happened to her; whom to list as father of the baby on birth records; what arrangements, if any, should be made to allow the father contact with the baby. Single mothers also had to enlist social support to substitute for the support of a partner and to replace family support, which was sometimes withdrawn after the pregnancy was announced.

This research suggested that the first and second trimesters were particularly stressful for single mothers, because of the unique issues they faced, and pointed to the need for specialized supportive care for women who choose to become single mothers.

First and Subsequent Pregnancies

Recent research has begun to underscore some important differences between women's experiences of first and subsequent pregnancies. The multigravida experiences all of the changes pregnancy brings but, in addition, must cope with the demands of older children and concerns about how the coming baby will affect her relationships with them (Walker 1986). She is also older, may have less energy and require a longer time to recover from physical stress, and may have specific fears about labor and birth based on previous experiences. The multigravida may also complain that her partner is not as excited about this pregnancy and does not treat her as special; she may perceive this as a lack of support. Health care providers may also tend to assume that she knows what to expect and will not have as many questions. Sometimes a multigravida is given less time in prenatal visits because of this assumption. However, even an experienced mother will have many questions. Each pregnancy is unique; past experiences may be very different from those in the present pregnancy. The multigravida also needs special assistance in planning how to prepare her older children for the arrival of the baby and in arranging for help to permit her adequate rest and time to be with the new baby after it arrives (Fig. 12–6).

High-Risk Pregnancy

Although about 20% of all pregnancies in the United States come to be labeled "high risk," to date relatively little attention has been given to the woman's experience of high-risk pregnancy. One team of nurse researchers has done extensive work in developing several models, which attempt to explain the effect of antepartum stress on how the family functions during pregnancy (Mercer et al 1986, 1988b).

The woman whose pregnancy comes to be labeled "high-risk" must accomplish the same tasks of pregnancy but faces additional challenges: a physical threat to her own well-being and that of her fetus, treatment regimens designed to reduce physiologic risk but may in-

crease her psychologic stress, and uncertainty about outcomes even in the best of circumstances.

The woman and her partner may have much difficulty in resolving ambivalence and in establishing a relationship with a fetus who may not be healthy and may not survive. Concerns about the welfare of the mother and fetus predominate. The couple may curtail their sexual relationship completely and find that they talk about nothing but the latest lab reports or the status of the baby. New developments in antenatal assessment may give parents more information but not necessarily more certainty about the outcome of the pregnancy.

An at-risk pregnancy may also have widespread effects on the family as a whole. The mother may be on bed rest for weeks, without reliable household help. Her family not only loses her work in the home but her income as well, if she was employed outside the home. If there are older children, they may not understand why family routines are so disrupted and may themselves become more difficult for the mother to care for. Additionally, one study indicated that during the first postpartal week, mothers of preterm infants were more anxious and depressed than mothers of term infants (Gennaro 1988). All of these factors further complicate the process of maternal adapta-

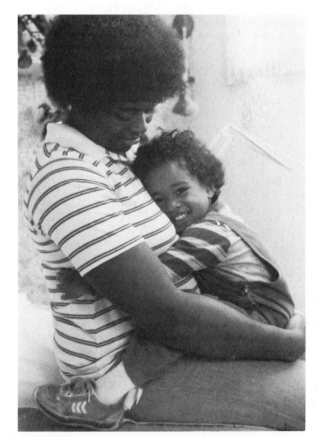

Figure 12–6. The secundigravida must prepare herself to care for and love two children. (Photo: BABES, Inc.)

NURSING RESEARCH

Effect of Stress on Family Functioning During Pregnancy

A recent study reported in *Nursing Research* examined the effects of stress on family functioning in a group of 593 subjects experiencing low-risk and high-risk pregnancies. Anxiety and depression levels were compared between men and women in the study population as well as between high-risk and low-risk pregnancy experiences. The research team of Mercer, Ferketich, DeJoseph, May and Sollid found that partners in the high-risk group reported similar levels of family functioning, whereas in low-risk pregnancies, men reported significantly more positive family functioning than their partners.

A sense of mastery was a significant predictor of family functioning for high-risk women. Unexpectedly, the extent of pregnancy risk was not a major stressor for these women.

For low-risk women, depression and perceived, rather than actual, social support received were directly linked to family functioning.

Perceived support was found to be particularly critical for men. The researchers suggest that this may be because of man's major source of support, his wife, is less available to him because of her preoccupation with the pregnancy.

The study underscores the complex effects of antepartal stress on family functioning and points to the particular need to examine the stress of hospitalization itself on high-risk pregnancies. Additional studies should also help nurses identify the most appropriate interventions for childbearing families experiencing both high-risk and low-risk pregnancies.

Mercer RT, Ferketich SL, DeJoseph J et al: Effect of stress on family functioning during pregnancy. Nurs Res 37(5):268, 1988

tion in a high-risk pregnancy, and may create a situation with high crisis potential.

Developmental Variations in Maternal Adaptation

The mother's own developmental status also affects how she adapts to pregnancy. Most first pregnancies occur among women in their early to middle twenties. However, both adolescent mothers and first-time mothers over 30 years of age are increasing in number. Maternal adaptation to pregnancy during adolescence is discussed in Chapter 10.

Older Mothers

The older first-time expectant mother also has some unique characteristics that affect how she adapts to pregnancy. Recent research has indicated that multiple demographic factors rather than maternal age alone are important predictors of reproductive outcomes (Mansfield 1987, Woods 1987).

These characteristics are related to her occupational status, her self-image, and the status of her marital relationship. Although the older woman seems to have more definite assets to assist her in her adaptation to pregnancy, she also has some characteristics that may make adjustment more difficult.

First, since women in their thirties have worked longer, they are much more likely than younger women to have made a significant personal commitment to their work. Women of this generation are also more career-oriented than women of earlier generations. In fact, one study found that the second reason for delaying childbearing was career development, exceeded only by development of the marriage relationship (Meisenhelder et al 1987). Thus, the older expectant mother may worry about leaving her position, even for a short time. She may also feel self-conscious about her pregnant body in the workplace, especially if she is in a workplace where men predominate or her job requires a certain amount of physical activity.

Second, the older mother is more likely to have a clearly defined sense of self than a younger woman. She is probably more self-confident and able to handle change, but she may also value her self-reliance and ability to control matters in her own life. Pregnancy may disrupt much of this; the changes may feel unpredictable and out of control, and the woman may have difficulty accepting the increase in dependence that may occur. In addition, the fact that she is at slightly increased risk for some complications, such as Down syndrome or cesarean delivery, may also threaten her self-image. She may be aware that her body does not function quite as it did when she was 21 years old. She may have less tolerance for fatigue, may gain weight more easily, and may worry about her body's ability to "bounce back" from pregnancy. These feelings may be intensified if she knows no other women her age who are pregnant and can only compare herself to women 10 years younger.

Finally, the older woman usually has been in a couple relationship longer. Although this is a definite asset in some ways, it may also be a source of concern. The woman may worry more about how her relationship with her mate will change with pregnancy than will a younger woman whose relationship with her mate is still being established when she conceives. She and her partner have had longer to establish habits that will change with a new baby, such as much uninterrupted quiet time, mobility, and a household routine suitable for adults.

PATERNAL ADAPTATION TO PREGNANCY

Relatively little is known about the process of paternal adaptation to pregnancy, since expectant fatherhood has only recently become a topic of interest in social science and health research. The following section reviews current knowledge about expectant fatherhood, highlighting some areas of particular importance to the maternity nurse. In this chapter, as throughout the book, the term "father" refers to the male who participates in the pregnancy in a biologic and psychological sense. Virtually no research has been conducted on the experiences of men who are "social" fathers — that is, men who participate in pregnancies for which they are not biologically responsible or who know that they have fathered a child but abandon their partner and psychologically cut themselves off from the pregnancy.

The Expectant Father

Prior to the 1960s, there was no clearly defined role for expectant fathers in Western society, other than providing emotional and financial support for the pregnant woman. Published research before 1960 tended to focus on abnormal psychological reactions among expectant fathers, such as clinical depression and unusual sexual behavior. However, the focus changed with the advent of the prepared-childbirth movement.

The prepared-childbirth movement of the 1960s most often involved well-educated, middle-class couples who saw participation by the father an important aspect of the childbearing experience. These consumers pressured hospitals and health professionals to change policies that prevented fathers from participating in normal childbirth. Gradually, research about expectant and new fatherhood began to appear in scientific journals. Most research focused on the effects of participation by the father on the course of labor and on later parent-infant interaction. However, attention was later directed toward exploration of the experience of expectant fatherhood itself, and nurse researchers played an important part in generating knowledge in this area.

There are still large gaps in our knowledge about expectant fatherhood. To date, little attention has been paid to the experience of men from ethnic and lower socioeconomic groups. Most recent research has been done with middle-class, well-educated, Caucasian fathers; their experience of expectant fatherhood is likely to be different from those of minority and lower-class fathers in important ways. Other aspects of expectant fatherhood that need further exploration are differences between the responses to pregnancy of first-time and experienced fa-

thers as well as single expectant fathers, and the responses of expectant fathers to high-risk pregnancy.

Paternal Tasks of Pregnancy

Paternal tasks of pregnancy are similar in many ways to those described for mothers. Like mothers, fathers experience psychologic and sometimes physical changes as pregnancy progresses. However, the father's response to pregnancy is primarily *psychological*, without the biologically induced changes women experience. Although it is convenient to examine paternal adaptation by trimesters of pregnancy, the nurse should realize that the timeframe of trimesters may not fit as well for fathers as it does for mothers.

For instance, fathers experience fewer benchmarks of pregnancy than do their partners, and probably will feel them later. The woman feels her body changing dramatically in the first trimester; all the father can see is that she is gaining a little weight and may be sleeping more. The mother typically feels fetal movement long before the father can feel it. Furthermore, not all events of pregnancy will have the same meaning for fathers. Feeling fetal movement or participating in prenatal classes may be mildly positive experiences for some fathers but may be absolutely thrilling "peak experiences" for others, depending on their overall outlook on the pregnancy. Therefore, the nurse should recognize there may be more variation in men's experiences of pregnancy, both in the nature and in the pace of change over time, and should take care not to assume that expectant fathers are all alike.

Accepting the Pregnancy

The process by which an expectant father accepts the pregnancy as a fact and incorporates it into his own life is an interesting one to observe. Most men are proud and happy when a pregnancy is announced. Most will communicate pleasure and happiness about the pregnancy to their partner. Often this is an important reassurance for the woman, since she is also likely to be experiencing some reservations about the pregnancy.

A pregnancy typically does not feel real for the father until the physical changes in his partner are apparent, and sometimes not until he can feel or hear fetal life. Intellectually, he may know his partner is pregnant, but he can forget that fact because the pregnancy is not yet a central part of his life. He may feel increasing anxiety about the long-term future commitment and financial demands of parenthood, but this reflects acceptance on a cognitive level; he may not feel an emotional investment in the pregnancy until much later. How readily the father accepts the pregnancy on an emotional level depends in large part on how ready he feels for it.

Men experience ambivalence about a pregnancy just as women do, perhaps more so, because men are not socialized to anticipate parenthood to the extent that women are in our society. Men are at a further disadvantage in that they do not feel profound physical and physiologic changes as do their partners. These changes do reinforce the reality of the pregnancy for the woman and help her to resolve her own ambivalence.

Furthermore, men often will not discuss their reservations about a pregnancy with their partners, in part to spare their partner additional emotional pain. In addition, complaining about a pregnancy they helped create is also regarded as "unmanly" by many men.

Unfortunately, expectant fathers often have no one else with whom they can discuss such matters, so they are left to resolve their feelings as best they can. During the process of resolving his doubts about a pregnancy, an expectant father will usually maintain some emotional distance from the pregnancy and resist efforts of others to involve him more, until he can overcome his ambivalence. A father who feels relatively ready for pregnancy may need only a few days for this process, whereas a father faced with a pregnancy for which he was totally unprepared may spend much of the pregnancy attempting to adjust (May 1982a).

In this age of highly reliable contraceptives, pregnancies do seem to catch more fathers by surprise than one might expect. In one study of 20 expectant couples, over half of the men reported that a pregnancy was unplanned, while their partners reported the opposite (May 1982b). Despite the effect unreadiness for pregnancy might have on the amount of emotional support an expectant father may be able to give his partner, prenatal records often fail to include any information about the father's readiness for pregnancy. Any information recorded usually is collected from the woman rather than first-hand from the father.

Establishing a Relationship With the Unborn Child

Establishing a relationship with the unborn child appears to be a somewhat different process for the expectant father than for the mother. The mother's relationship with the fetus is direct and personal, reinforced by physical sensations. The father's relationship is more indirect until late in pregnancy, and there are no physical reminders of the growing relationship.

One of the major indicators of the father's growing relationship with the unborn child is his involvement in pregnancy and preparation for birth. To some extent, this has been institutionalized by the current widespread acceptance of participation by the father in childbirth.

One of the consequences of the prepared childbirth movement was the evolution of the expectant father's

role as "labor coach." The United States is unique among Western countries in its acceptance of and emphasis on active participation by the father in childbirth. This trend was welcomed by many men and their partners, because it made possible a level of participation in pregnancy and birth for the father, unheard of in the 1950s and early 1960s.

However, one slightly less positive consequence has been a tendency to treat all expectant fathers as if they desired and were prepared to assume the same type of involvement in pregnancy and birth. By the 1970s, over 90% of expectant fathers were attending prenatal classes and childbirth in some areas of the country. Fathers who chose *not* to be actively involved in those ways were sometimes regarded with concern and suspicion by health professionals; some assumed that there must be some serious underlying problem in the father or in the marital relationship, if the father chose not to attend the birth.

Styles of Paternal Involvement in Pregnancy.   Recent research clearly shows many variations in the type of involvement in pregnancy that men find most comfortable for themselves and their spouses (May 1982a). Some men are quite comfortable being highly emotionally invested in the pregnancy and exploring the changing emotional impact the pregnancy has on them. Often these men see themselves as "full partners" in the experience and welcome participation in prenatal classes and childbirth because it allows them to share the experience with their spouses.

Other men may see their role in pregnancy as more task-oriented; they may take responsibility for some aspects of the pregnancy, such as keeping the partner on her prenatal diet plan, making purchases for the baby, or remodeling their living quarters. Men who are more comfortable in this style of involvement may prefer the more traditional sex role expectations of the husband and father. Men who see themselves as "managers" may also be comfortable with prenatal classes and involvement in childbirth as the "coach."

Others are not comfortable with much emotional or active participation in the pregnancy, and adopt a quiet "observer" stance. Sometimes men who prefer to watch from the sidelines are those who may still be resolving their own ambivalence about a pregnancy. Some are quiet and less participatory by nature and are uncomfortable in a more active role. Often their partners know they are pleased to be expectant fathers and feel well supported, but may think they have to "explain" the father's apparent uninvolvement since it does not seem to fit the typical pattern (May 1982b). The type of involvement the father chooses and the extent of his involvement in the pregnancy experience appear to depend on a number of factors.

Sociocultural Factors. The prepared childbirth movement and its emphasis on the father's role as labor coach has generally been well accepted by middle-class American families. Most middle-class fathers fully expect to be actively involved in pregnancy and preparation for childbirth. However, the male sex role among minority and lower socioeconomic groups tends to be more traditional, and men in these groups have been slower to adopt this type of participation. This is especially true among lower-class Hispanic and Asian American men. The division of labor between the sexes is particularly distinct in these groups. Since pregnancy is regarded as a woman's concern, expectant fathers from these cultures may be more hesitant about becoming involved. Men from these groups may tend to adopt a more task-oriented involvement because it is consistent with their view of the husband and father role.

Personality Factors. The man's personality type also influences his level of involvement in pregnancy. Men with highly masculine personalities (a strong need for dominance, high assertiveness, and a strong orientation toward activity rather than toward interpersonal interaction) may feel uncomfortable with close involvement in pregnancy. Pregnancy is inherently a feminine arena; men with traditionally masculine self-concepts may feel out of place. Such men may tend to be more distant from the pregnancy or may concentrate on concrete physical preparations for the baby.

On the other hand, some men have personalities more balanced between masculine and feminine traits (a strong need for affiliation, high empathy with others, and a strong orientation toward interpersonal interaction). Personalities of this kind are called *androgynous* personalities. Recent research suggests that such men are more comfortable with emotional involvement in pregnancy as full partners, may be more sensitive and effective labor support people, and can be more nurturant caregivers with infants and small children (May and Perrin 1985).

The Woman's Preferences About Paternal Involvement. The expectant woman may determine to a large extent how involved her partner may become in the pregnancy. In a sense, the woman may function as a gatekeeper: if she wants her partner to be highly involved in pregnancy and childcare, he is likely to be involved. However, if the woman wants to keep those experiences more for herself, the father is much less likely to be actively involved.

Adjusting to Changes in Self

Pregnancy typically triggers a range of emotional responses among expectant fathers. The man's self-concept begins to shift to take on the new father role. He begins to rediscover himself as an adult and must decide what it means to him to become a father. He may become bored and dissatisfied with aspects of his life that seemed acceptable only months before, such as his job, the size of the living quarters, or his educational status. Certain themes are common as the expectant father adjusts to changes in himself.

Feelings of Increased Responsibility. Men frequently report that their mate's pregnancy heightens their own sense of responsibility. Often this is expressed in concern about financial security. Men may take on additional work to provide more income for their family. Men from minority or lower socioeconomic groups may feel this increased responsibility most acutely, since their traditional view of their role of husband and father is strongly oriented toward providing for their family. If they are unable to do so, they may experience much self-doubt and shame.

Men may also become increasingly concerned about their own and their wife's personal safety. Expectant fathers report being hesitant to take ordinary chances because there is now "someone else" to think about. Often men will also be more protective of their partners and their homes at this time.

Concerns About Fathering Ability. Most men express some worry about their own ability to be a good father. In part, this reflects the fact that in Western countries men are poorly prepared to take on the parent role. Boys are subtly discouraged from learning about childcare and grow up believing that women "naturally" know how to care for children. Thus, many men face pregnancy feeling insecure about their own parenting ability.

This concern may also stem from their own experiences of being fathered. If they had a nurturant, available father, men are able to pattern their own behavior on their father's. But many men had fathers who were somewhat emotionally distant and were not very involved in childrearing. This pattern was the norm throughout most of the years after World War II. Thus, many men now are starting their own families with no positive role model on which to pattern their behavior; they only know they do not want to be the type of father they had.

Pregnancy Symptoms in the Male. Men also can experience a physical response to their mate's pregnancy. The *couvade syndrome* (after the French verb *couver,* meaning "to hatch or brood") is a constellation of symptoms much like those that women experience: weight gain or weight loss, digestive disturbances, particularly morning nausea, fatigue, headache, and backaches. Couvade symptoms are more likely to occur in early pregnancy and tend to diminish as pregnancy progresses. They may also be fairly common; from 25% to 65% of expectant fathers may experience some physical symp-

NURSING RESEARCH

Physical and Emotional Responses of Expectant Fathers Throughout Pregnancy and the Early Postpartum Period

A comparative, repeated measures survey design was used to study the physical and emotional health of 81 expectant fathers and 66 nonexpectant men at monthly intervals over the course of a year. The aim of the study was to examine the incidence, duration, and perceived seriousness of couvade symptoms. Compared to nonexpectant men, expectant fathers experienced more colds that lasted longer during the first trimester, and a greater unintentional weight gain perceived as more serious during the third trimester. Expectant fathers differed most from nonexpectant fathers in terms of emotional health, particularly during the immediate postpartum period. The symptoms found most frequently included excessive fatigue, nervousness, difficulty concentrating, insomnia, headaches, restlessness, and irritability. Dr. Clinton particularly points out that all symptoms found to be a problem for these expectant fathers can be highly influenced by nursing care. She recommends that nurses and other health care providers include anticipatory health counseling for fathers as well as mothers throughout pregnancy and the postpartum period.

Clinton JF: Physical and emotional responses of expectant fathers throughout pregnancy and the early postpartum period. Int J Nurs Stud 24(1):59, 1987

toms associated with their mate's pregnancy (Clinton 1986, Strickland 1987).

Despite the fact that couvade symptoms appear to be fairly common, they often go unrecognized. Lipkin, a nurse researcher interested in couvade syndrome, conducted a retrospective review of over 200 expectant fathers' medical records and compared them with records of men whose mates were not pregnant. Not only did the expectant fathers present with a higher number of physical complaints for which they sought treatment, but most of the complaints were ones that might well be pregnancy-related. However, in less than 15% of cases was there any notation on the medical record that the man was an expectant father. Furthermore, medical treatment for these symptoms included procedures such as upper and lower GI radiography, proctoscopy, and a range of prescription medications. This raises the possibility that at least some of these symptoms were psychosomatic couvade symptoms. If so, they likely would have resolved

on their own, but in fact may have been overtreated because they were misdiagnosed (Lipkin and Lamb 1982).

A classic example of couvade symptoms can be seen in the following case.

> Rob is a professional athlete whose wife is expecting their first baby. About 6 weeks after the pregnancy was confirmed, he developed a craving for ice cream and began making trips to a local soda fountain several times a week. He proceeded to gain weight, almost pound for pound with his wife, until the last trimester. His craving for ice cream is particularly interesting because, as an athlete, he was usually careful about his diet. In addition, Rob had mild lactose intolerance and generally avoided dairy products. His craving and weight gain stopped in the last trimester since he compared symptoms with other fathers in a prenatal class and realized that his behaviors were probably related to his wife's pregnancy.

Couvade symptoms may be caused by a combination of stress, anxiety, and empathy for the pregnant spouse. They are usually quite harmless or, at most, annoying. In rare cases, a father experiences physical symptoms that become disabling; this signifies a more serious emotional disturbance, and intensive psychological evaluation is indicated. Occasionally, an expectant father exhibits the delusion that he is, in fact, pregnant. This extremely rare condition, known as *pseudocyesis,* requires psychiatric care.

Adjusting to Changes in the Couple Relationship

Pregnancy profoundly influences the man's relationship with his mate because both are changing, often in seemingly very different ways. The man often is surprised at the emotional changes in his mate and may experience her increasing introspection and self-centeredness in a negative way. Some men find their mate's growing preoccupation with pregnancy fascinating, while others see it as annoying and a little boring. A major step in the father's adaptation to pregnancy is learning how to adjust to his changing mate to meet her needs while at the same time keeping his own satisfaction and security in the relationship (Fig. 12-7).

Learning to Share the Mate's Attention. Pregnancy may be the first time the man has ever felt that he had to share his mate's attention in a real way. He may have to resolve feelings of rivalry with the baby and learn to put some of his own emotional needs "on hold" for a time. This process is directly related to his own maturation as an adult. If he is insecure about his importance in his mate's life, this adjustment may be very threatening and can sometimes lead to marital discord. Failure to

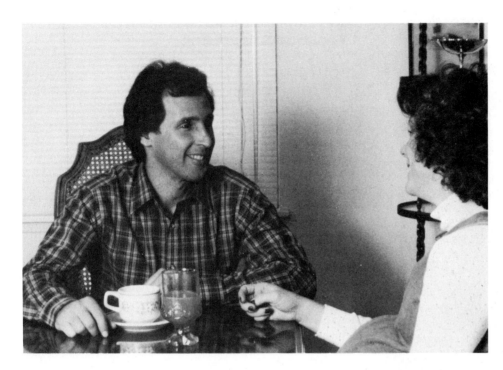

Figure 12-7. The expectant father must adjust to physical and emotional changes in his mate. (Photo: BABES, Inc.)

make this adjustment can signal future problems in his adjustment to parenthood, since caring for a child requires the parent to sacrifice some of his own needs and to take some satisfaction from doing so. However, the process can also contribute to his own development, as he learns to put other priorities above his personal needs, and prepare him for the future demands of parenthood.

Changes in the Sexual Relationship. Changes in the couple's sexual relationship are almost inevitable during pregnancy. These changes occur because of the physical, physiologic, and emotional impact of pregnancy on the woman and because the man then must adjust to a changing intimate partner. (See Chapter 6 for an indepth discussion of sexuality during pregnancy.) Men appear to be more sensitive to and more bothered by these changes than are their mates. Sexual satisfaction appears to be more central to a man's satisfaction with his marital relationship than to a woman's. Thus, if the pregnancy has had a distinctly negative effect on a couple's sexual life, the man will probably feel the loss more acutely, and his satisfaction with life overall will suffer more (May 1987).

Preparing for Labor, Birth, and Early Parenthood

Preparation for birth is most apparent late in pregnancy. Prenatal classes in almost every community prepare fathers for their role as support people in labor and birth. Sometimes men may come to regard the birth as a testing ground and worry that they may not measure up to their partner's or their own expectations as a labor coach. Men have many fears about their partner's well-

being through the labor process; they worry about how they will react to their partner's pain, and whether she and the baby will survive.

Some fathers will prepare for birth on their own, by reading or seeking out fathers' classes. Others who see themselves as less involved in the process may prepare little for birth but concentrate instead on making physical preparations for the baby. Preparation may also focus on certain concerns that reflect the father's fears; he may rehearse driving to the hospital or may read about emergency delivery in case they do not get to the hospital in time.

Fathers also recognize that they need to prepare to take care of their infants; most men have little or no experience in caring for small children and realize that there is much to learn. However, this important aspect may be neglected, in part because of the overemphasis on preparation for labor and birth. If infant care classes are available and designed to accommodate fathers easily, many men will attend and see them as very valuable. Again, this depends on how involved the father expects to be in child care. Some men quite realistically see themselves as rather uninvolved until their children are older and so will prepare less during pregnancy.

Situational Factors Affecting Paternal Adaptation

Some situational factors seem to influence paternal adaptation to pregnancy; however, very little research has been done to date in these areas. The nurse must keep in mind that her nursing diagnosis and interventions with fathers in these situations will be based solely on assessment of the father's individual situation and that the current literature may not be of much assistance.

The Expectant Father and the High-Risk Pregnancy

The expectant father whose mate is experiencing a high-risk pregnancy is often coping with a crisis that is both situational and developmental in nature. Men normally worry about their partner's well-being and the well-being of the fetus during pregnancy. When complications of pregnancy develop, these fears are greatly intensified. Again, the expectant father may have no one with whom he can discuss these concerns except his mate, and most men are unwilling to burden their mates in this way.

If the mother's condition requires hospitalization or strict bedrest, the father must then manage the household affairs, his job, and his worry about his wife and baby. He may experience shock and fear, and worry that his mate and baby are going to die, even if that risk is remote. He may feel torn between staying with his partner, staying with older children, and fulfilling work responsibilities. The father may not think to ask for help that might be available, or may underestimate the problems of finding childcare and household help.

An exploratory study of the effect of antenatal stress on families suggests that some fathers whose mates are hospitalized feel as if no one is concerned about their own stress levels. Several fathers whose mates had been hospitalized reported that the first time anyone had asked about their own experience was in the research interview itself, which usually took place 3 or 4 days after admission (May 1985).

First and Subsequent Pregnancies

Little is known about the differences between paternal adaptation to first pregnancies and adaptation to later ones. Some fathers may have an easier adjustment in subsequent pregnancies because they know what to expect, whereas others may be more fearful because of problems during the first pregnancy. A subsequent pregnancy is more complicated because relationships with the older child must be renegotiated. Often fathers take over more responsibility for caretaking of the older child during pregnancy, in preparation for the mother's involvement with the newborn. There may be a tendency for some fathers to become less involved with a subsequent pregnancy because the novelty and thrill may be lessened and because they believe their partner needs their support less. However, this is often not the case and, as mentioned before, multigravidas often complain they are not being treated as special during pregnancy and miss their partner's active and obvious support.

Developmental Variations in Paternal Adaptation

The father's own developmental status has a profound influence on his adaptation to pregnancy. Paternal adaptation to pregnancy in adolescence is discussed in Chapter 10.

Older Fathers

Men usually marry women 2 or 3 years younger than themselves and become fathers in their middle to late twenties. However, as the trend toward delaying first pregnancies into the thirties continues, more men are becoming expectant fathers for the first time in their late thirties and early forties. There is little research on the older father, and the differences his age makes on his adaptation to pregnancy are not well understood. One might reasonably assume that the couple's relationship will be more mature and better established if pregnancy has been delayed, and that the man will be more confident of his identity and his relationship with his spouse. If so, his own adaptation to pregnancy may be easier. However, the same factors may have the opposite effect: the older father may be unwilling or unready to adjust to changes in the well-established couple relationship, and his self-concept as a successful, competent adult may suffer more with the lack of control he may feel as he anticipates labor and birth.

SIBLING ADAPTATION TO PREGNANCY

Sibling adaptation to pregnancy will vary according to the developmental level of the older child. The areas in which the sibling is likely to experience the most change during pregnancy are maternal appearance; parental behavior; and home environment, particularly sleeping arrangements.

Children under 2 years of age are usually unaware of pregnancy and do not understand explanations about the future arrival of a new brother or sister. They may, however, pick up and respond to the emotional atmosphere in the household, particularly around the time of birth and shortly after. Children from 2 to 4 years of age may only respond to obvious changes in the mother's body and behavior and may not remember from month to month why the changes are occurring. However, changes in the physical environment may be disruptive for them. For this reason, if their sleeping arrangements must be changed to accommodate the new baby, these changes should be made well before the mother leaves home for birth and the arrival of the newborn.

Children aged 4 and 5 often enjoy listening to the baby's heartbeat and learning about the baby's development at a level appropriate to their age (Fig. 12–8). They understand that the new baby will be a brother or sister, but usually have unrealistic expectations about having a "playmate" when the baby arrives. Children at this age may sense a shift in the mother's attention, and may resent her physical limitations, such as her inability to lift and hold them or to engage in roughhousing late in pregnancy.

Schoolage children take a keen interest in the "hows" and "whys" of pregnancy and birth. They have many questions and may welcome age-appropriate books and pictures about birth. Often they plan elaborate welcomes for the baby and want to be able to help when the baby comes. Children of this age may express interest in being present at the birth and enjoy preparing for participation in the event.

The responses of adolescents to pregnancy also depend in large part on their developmental status. Younger adolescents may be uncomfortable with the obvious evidence of their parents' sexuality and may be quite negative and embarrassed about the changes in their mother's appearance. They may be fascinated and repelled by the process of birth; girls may not want to be present at birth because of their own fears, while boys may be more interested.

Middle and older adolescents, in the process of loosening their ties to their parents and families, may be somewhat indifferent to the changes associated with pregnancy, unless these interfere with their own activities and independence. They may also respond in a more adult fashion by imagining themselves in the parent role and offering support and help.

Preparing the sibling for birth and the arrival of the new baby can make for a smoother adjustment. Research to date has not shown that preparing the sibling during pregnancy eliminates sibling rivalry and adjustment problems after the birth. However, most parents choose to prepare children in some way during pregnancy in an effort to ease the child's adjustment to changes in the household. Preparation must be carried out at the child's level of understanding and in response to readiness to learn. (See Chapter 21 for discussion of sibling preparation for birth.)

Changes in Other Relationships

Pregnancy not only causes shifts in the relationship between the mother and father but also creates changes in other relationships. Many relationships are affected by a pregnancy. Often expectant parents find themselves spending more time with friends who have children and see their single or childless friends less as pregnancy progresses. Expectant couples often adjust their leisure activities to include "family" types of entertainment, such as visits to amusement parks and zoos; this anticipatory work seems to be important in helping the couple to establish a sense of their future together as a family and to reorient their adult friendships to fit their future status. Pregnancy also affects other family relationships. Ties with other siblings may become closer, since the burdens and rewards of parenthood can now be shared.

Grandparents

One especially important area that changes in response to pregnancy is the relationship with parents, who are soon to become grandparents. Expectant parents often find that their relationship with their own parents, particularly the mother's parents, whether actual or only remembered, seems to become more important and positive during pregnancy (Cronenwett 1985). For women, and perhaps for men, the first pregnancy signals true adult status and the beginning of a new, more equal kind of relationship with parents. Grandparents are often the first people told about a pregnancy; there is a recognition that the tie to the future represented by the unborn child is of special significance to the grandparent.

Women may seek their own mothers out for advice and reassurance about concerns of pregnancy; often, the older woman's experiences of pregnancy and birth will be discussed in great detail. If the pregnant woman's mother is unavailable to her, she may seek out another older woman to act as substitute. Many men also find themselves thinking about and talking with their own fathers more, seeking out advice and reassurance.

The adjustment grandparents themselves must make is a complicated one. The coming child may be a painful reminder of their own advancing age, or it may rekindle

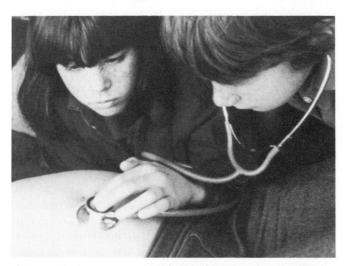

Figure 12–8. Schoolage children are fascinated by hearing fetal heart tones and feeling fetal movement. (Photo: BABES, Inc.)

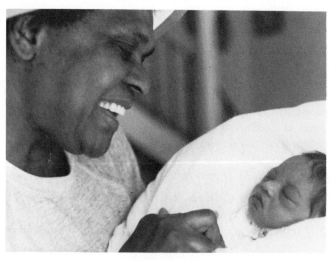

Figure 12-9. The birth of a child is an important event for grandparents. (Photo: BABES, Inc.)

their own energy for life and create a sense of hopeful expectation (Fig. 12-9). Grandparents are often unsure how much they should be involved in preparing for and caring for a new baby. Most grandparents are aware that childbearing and child-rearing practices have changed dramatically since they were young. Thus, they may think they have nothing to offer the new family. Others may interfere in the family's affairs and may create more strain in the young couple's life than they realize. To assist with this problem, many institutions and community groups are establishing classes designed to help grandparents adjust to their new roles and to give them current information about birth and child-rearing so they can be more effective sources of support for young families.

IMPLICATIONS FOR NURSING CARE

The nurse assumes a variety of roles in providing the psychosocial aspects of care during pregnancy. She may function as a teacher, role model, counselor or resource person, as well as a clinician. Much of her care is aimed at promoting healthy adaptation and preventing and reducing stress caused by the many individual and family adjustments required by pregnancy. In many instances, the nurse is the only health professional to have repeated and extended contact with the pregnant woman and her family throughout pregnancy.

Often mothers and their mates adjust well to pregnancy; they have functional support systems, communicate their love and concern about each other, and need only encouragement, anticipatory guidance, and factual information from the nurse in order to maintain equilib-

rium during the prenatal period. However, other mothers and their families are known to be at psychosocial risk. In those cases, the nurse is in an excellent position to identify psychosocial problems early and intervene before individual and family functioning begins to deteriorate.

The following section emphasizes the steps of assessment, diagnosis, planning and implementation of psychosocial prenatal care. Nursing interventions to assist in resolving psychosocial concerns in pregnancy are discussed briefly. These interventions are also important in the provision of overall nursing care and are discussed in Chapters 16-20 within the context of comprehensive nursing care of the pregnant woman and her family.

Assessment

The nurse's psychosocial assessment begins at the initial prenatal visit. As noted in Chapter 18, the nurse collects a health history that includes the following preliminary psychosocial data:

- Woman's developmental status/emotional state
- Status of pregnancy (planned or unplanned)
- Woman's response to confirmation of pregnancy
- Status of relationship with partner
- Partner's response to pregnancy
- Status of other support systems
- Living situation and financial status

Often the nurse cannot complete a comprehensive psychosocial assessment during the initial prenatal visit because of time constraints and the woman's need for specific information. The nurse continues to collect information about the woman's response to pregnancy in subsequent contacts. The nurse should make every effort to include the expectant father in early prenatal visits. This provides an opportunity to assess his adaptation to the pregnancy and his capacity to support his partner emotionally. Ongoing nursing assessment then focuses on maternal and paternal adaptation to the pregnancy and on the individual's and her family's ability to adjust to unexpected stressors.

A sample tool designed to assist the nurse in assessing parental adaptation to pregnancy is shown in the display, Assessment/Intervention for Parental Adaptation to Pregnancy, later in this chapter. Maternal and paternal tasks are discussed as they change with pregnancy, expected parental responses are noted, and nursing interventions are suggested. If the nurse detects slow progress or difficulties in adaptation in a particular area, that area should be assessed in greater detail.

Factors Signaling Increased Risk in Maternal Adaptation to Pregnancy

- Prior negative experiences in childbearing or child-rearing
    Loss of own mother without adequate substitute
    Previous birth that resulted in stillbirth or defective child
    Previous child emotionally or behaviorally disturbed or physically ill
- Conflicts or defects in support systems
    Chronic marital discord
    Family violence
    Partner opposition to pregnancy
    Chronic conflict with female relatives
- Inadequate preparation for childbearing or child-rearing
    Unplanned earlier pregnancies
    Previous children cared for by others
- Significant health concerns
    Presence of condition that mother believes will worsen with pregnancy
- Negative responses to current pregnancy
    Pregnancy rejection
        Denial or ignorance of pregnancy
        Overreaction to bodily changes
        Preoccupation with vague emotional and physical complaints
        Dress and behavior that suggest nonpregnancy
    Failure to develop emotional tie to fetus
    Lack of preparation for newborn

Adapted from Cohen R: Maladaption to pregnancy. Semin Perinatol 3(1):15, 1979

Difficulties in adapting to pregnancy often center on five major categories of risk factors (Cohen 1979).

- Prior negative experiences in childbearing or child-rearing
- Conflicts or defects in support systems
- Inadequate preparation for childbearing or child-rearing
- Significant health concerns
- Negative responses to current pregnancy

Specific examples of factors signaling an increased risk in adaptation to pregnancy are listed in the accompanying display. These factors were originally seen as signaling psychosocial risks for the childbearing woman, but they could also be problematic for expectant fathers and create high levels of stress in the family system. The nurse should pay particular attention to a mother who describes

problems or concerns in any of these areas and immediately conduct a more comprehensive and detailed assessment of the woman's status.

A more detailed assessment may require more time than is usually allotted for a "routine" prenatal visit, and in such cases the woman should return within days to complete the assessment. Since mothers are often seen only every 3 to 4 weeks early in pregnancy, it is not advisable to wait for the next routine prenatal visit to complete this assessment. The assessment tool on page 307 is an example of an interview guide designed to identify women who may be at risk and to collect additional information about the nature of that risk.

Diagnosis

The nurse establishes nursing diagnoses from the data collected in her assessment. Since most families are likely to be coping well with adaptation to pregnancy, nursing diagnoses may often be stated as potential problems, rather than actual ones. The nurse should also recognize that, as work proceeds in the field of nursing diagnosis, more categories with specific application to the childbearing family will be developed. Many nursing experts in the field of maternity care believe that current lists of nursing diagnoses do not always include categories that fit well with individual and family problems related to childbearing, and tend to focus on problems rather than on normal developmental challenges.

The following examples illustrate nursing diagnoses that may be useful in psychosocial aspects of prenatal nursing care.

- Fear of childbirth related to lack of previous experience and lack of knowledge about birth process
- Altered family process related to illness of mother during pregnancy
- Anxiety related to pregnancy
- Disturbance in self-concept related to changes in body image
- Knowledge deficit regarding normal psychosexual changes of pregnancy related to expectant fatherhood

Planning and Implementation

Since psychosocial support should be provided to the mother and her family throughout pregnancy, the nurse should plan opportunities at various points in pregnancy to spend extra time answering questions and assessing the woman's psychosocial status. The nurse might plan to have individual visits or to have groups of women at similar stages of pregnancy. The nurse should also plan for involvement by the partner whenever possible.

Successful prenatal care relies on communication about the expectant woman's needs among the various care providers who may be providing care. Essential laboratory data and physical findings always have a prominent place in the medical record, but important psychosocial findings may be lost in the midst of routine written communication. The nurse should formulate a plan of care based on clearly specified nursing diagnoses and make sure that other team members know about and understand the plan of care.

An expected outcome of nursing care, then, would be that all family members make a healthy adjustment to the demands of pregnancy. In many cases, necessary nursing intervention to foster this care is limited to providing sensitive listening and support along with information and suggestions about effective self-care.

Teaching for Effective Self-Care

Education is a major part of assisting parents and their families to adjust to the demands of pregnancy. Reassuring a woman that her emotional responses, while confusing and strange to her, are actually expected changes of pregnancy, and suggesting some ways she can keep these changes from intruding too much into her daily life is an example of this type of teaching. Women also may welcome information about their family members' adaptation to pregnancy; women tend to know very little about what is "normal" behavior for expectant fathers and siblings.

As noted before, most nursing intervention in the area of psychosocial care can be called "watchful waiting": observing how women and their families are adjusting and filling in with needed information, some encouragement, and some anticipatory guidance. However, this "watchful waiting" is also designed to alert the nurse to situations in which more intervention is necessary. As shown in the accompanying display, the nurse can take steps to reduce rising stress levels in a family in which adjustments are becoming more difficult. The goal of these more focused interventions is to prevent individual and family crises.

Reducing Stress and Crisis Potential

A single stressful event may not by itself lead to a crisis, but a combination of stress factors can suddenly overwhelm an individual's coping mechanisms. Part of comprehensive nursing care is the systematic assessment of stress factors in the pregnant woman's life; this assessment should be done early in pregnancy and should be updated as the pregnancy progresses or as the woman's life situation changes.

Typically, the nurse can gain important information simply by asking the woman about any concerns she may have, reassuring her that concerns and worries are a normal part of pregnancy. The nurse will be most effective in collecting this type of information if she communicates a willingness to listen and a caring attitude.

If a pregnant woman or her family is experiencing high levels of stress that may precipitate a crisis, four specific nursing interventions may be useful:

- Encouraging positive coping behavior
- Providing support
- Manipulating environmental stressors
- Providing anticipatory guidance

Encouraging Positive Coping Behaviors. The nurse can help the woman clarify sources of stress and review the coping patterns that have worked for her in the past. The nurse may also suggest new ways of coping with pregnancy: attending prenatal classes or support groups, seeking out an experienced friend for support, or acquiring needed information about specific concerns.

Providing Support. The nurse can also help by communicating her availability and concern. This can be done by a phone call to the mother between prenatal visits to see how she is getting along, or an unhurried and receptive attitude during a prenatal visit. Appropriate and caring reassurance from a professional is a powerful, though sometimes underused, way in which stress can be reduced.

SELF-CARE TEACHING

Reducing Stress Levels

The nurse may recommend the following to parents to reduce stress:

- Walk for exercise; it is an excellent way to avoid excessive fatigue and may help to even out mood swings
- Spend time with other parents of small children, and talk with them about what you like and don't like about parenthood
- Take a little more time than you ordinarily would with your appearance early in pregnancy; this may keep your self-confidence up and prevent you from getting discouraged about physical changes
- Seek out experienced parents and talk about concerns you may have
- Take time to have fun alone with your partner early in pregnancy; this will help you talk things out and support each other better

Manipulating Environmental Stressors. The nurse may also be able to identify environmental stressors that can easily be reduced or eliminated. Arranging for a more convenient prenatal visit schedule that allows for child care at home and involvement by the father in the visit, helping the mother to plan travel so that long car rides or crowded conditions on public transportation are avoided, and helping the family to plan for assistance after the birth are concrete interventions designed to reduce environmental stress for the expectant family.

Providing Anticipatory Guidance. The nurse may also help reduce stress levels by anticipating learning needs and providing information about what events can reasonably be expected. Examples of anticipatory guidance for the expectant family might be reassuring a pregnant woman that morning nausea usually decreases after the first trimester, or explaining to a father that many men do not feel involved in pregnancy until the last weeks and that he still will likely feel a strong bond with the fetus/newborn later. Even if the parents seem to have a considerable amount of information already, often they will still welcome discussion with a knowledgeable nurse about what they might expect.

If these steps do not seem to meet the woman's need for support, the nurse should consider consultation with the physician and other members of the health care team and, if appropriate, referral to more specialized counseling and psychiatric services.

Evaluation

Evaluation of the quality of psychosocial interventions is a challenging process. Psychosocial health may not be as easily measured as physical health, and results of interventions may not be seen immediately, or even within the time the nurse has contact with the woman. However, some immediate evaluations can be made about the relative success of interventions, in terms of the mother's expressed comfort level, satisfaction with increased knowledge, resolution of conflicts, and progress toward healthy adaptation to pregnancy. The nurse will need to rely on her interpersonal skills to assess the effects of her interventions with clients in this arena and to recognize that the effectiveness of her care may be reflected only in long-term outcomes: healthy parent and family adaptation to the childbearing process.

CHAPTER SUMMARY

Psychosocial adaptation to pregnancy is a complex process that requires extensive psychological, physical, and social adjustments over a fairly brief period of time. This adaptation lays the groundwork for the later transition to the parental role. Thus, adaptation to pregnancy is important to the long-range health of childbearing women and their families, and early assessment and intervention may prevent or greatly reduce later family problems.

Pregnancy is a time of increased vulnerability to crisis, if the demands facing an individual overwhelm usual coping patterns. However, maternal and paternal responses to pregnancy tend to show fairly predictable patterns that assist the nurse in the assessment and diagnosis of actual or potential difficulties in adaptation. Because of her repeated contact with expectant women and their partners, the nurse can play a central role in assessing individual and family adaptation to pregnancy and in intervening in ways appropriate to the identified level of need. Providing psychosocial support to individuals and families during pregnancy is a major nursing responsibility, one that contributes directly to the psychologic and physical well-being of expectant parents and their families.

STUDY QUESTIONS

1. List some basic functions of families, and identify ways in which some functions may be fulfilled outside the family unit.
2. Explain why pregnancy can be a crisis for some individuals and families. List the factors that determine whether or not change in a family unit becomes a crisis.
3. List parental tasks of pregnancy for mothers and fathers. Explain why these tasks are important in the healthy adaptation to pregnancy.
4. Discuss common parental concerns for each trimester of pregnancy, and outline appropriate nursing interventions.
5. List factors that predispose a woman to increased risk in adapting to pregnancy. Explain how the nurse can assess those factors while providing prenatal care.

REFERENCES/BIBLIOGRAPHY

Aguilera D, Messick J: Crisis Intervention: Theory and Methodology, 2nd ed. St Louis, CV Mosby, 1986
Benokraitis N: Fathers in the dual-earner family. In Hansen S, Bozett F (eds): Dimensions of Fatherhood. Beverly Hills, CA, Sage Publications, 1985
Bliss–Holtz V: Primiparas' prenatal concern for learning infant care. Nurs Res 37(1):20, 1988
Borg S, Lasker J: When Pregnancy Fails: Families Coping With

Miscarriage, Stillbirth and Infant Death. Boston, Beacon Press, 1981

Brown MA: Social support, stress, and health: A comparison of expectant mothers and fathers. Nurs Res 35(2):72, 1986

Burst H: Women's health: Pregnancy and childbirth—Issues and concerns of healthy pregnant women. Public Health Rep Suppl 52(4):57, 1987

Carter–Jessop L: Promoting maternal attachment through prenatal intervention. MCN 6:107, 1981

Clinton J: Expectant fathers at risk for couvade. Nurs Res 35(5):290, 1986

Cranley M: Roots of attachment: The relationship of parents with their unborn. Birth Defects: Original Article Series 17(6):59, 1981

Cronenwett L: Network structure, social support, and psychological outcomes of pregnancy. Nurse Res 34(2):93, 1985

Cronenwett L: Parental network structure and perceived support after birth of first child. Nurs Res 34(6):347, 1985

Davis M, Akridge K: The effect of promoting intrauterine attachment in primiparas on postdelivery attachment. J Obstet Gynecol Neonatal Nurs 16(6):430, 1987

Duvall E: Marriage and Family Development. Philadelphia, JB Lippincott, 1977

Estok P, Lehman A: Perinatal death: Grief support for families. Birth Fam 10(1):17, 1983

Fawcett J, York R: Spouses' physical and psychological symptoms during pregnancy and the postpartum. Nurs Res 35(3):144, 1986

Flaherty M, Facteau L, Garver P: Grandmother functions in multigenerational families: An exploratory study of black adolescent mothers and their infants. Matern Child Nurs J 16:61, 1987

Friedman R, Gradstein B: Surviving Pregnancy Loss. Boston, Little, Brown, & Co, 1982

Gennaro S: Postpartal anxiety and depression in mothers of term and preterm infants. Nurs Res 37(2):82, 1988

Grace J: Does a mother's knowledge of fetal gender affect attachment? MCN 9:42, 1984

Grossman F, Eichler L, Winickoff S et al: Pregnancy, Birth and Parenthood. San Francisco, Jossey–Bass, 1980

Hansen S: Parent–child relationships in single-father families. In Lewis R, Salt R (eds): Men in Families. Beverly Hills, CA, Sage Publications, 1985

Hansen S, Bozett F: Dimensions of Fatherhood. Beverly Hills, CA, Sage Publications, 1985

Hogan M, Buehler C, Robinson R: Single parenting: Transitioning alone. In McCubbin H, Figley C (eds): Stress And The Family I: Coping With Normative Transitions. New York, Brunner/Mazel Publishing, 1983

Kemp V, Page C: Maternal self-esteem and prenatal attachment in high-risk pregnancy. Matern Child Nurs J 16:195, 1987

Klaus M, Kennell J: Parent–Infant Bonding. St Louis, CV Mosby, 1982

Lewis J: The transition to parenthood: II. Stability and change in marital structure. Fam Proc 27:273, 1988

Lipkin M, Lamb G: The couvade syndrome: An epidemiological study. Ann Intern Med 96:609, 1982

Mansfield P: Teenage and midlife childbearing update: Implications for health educators. Health Educ 18(4):18, 1987

May K: Three phases in the development of father involvement in pregnancy. Nurs Res 31(6):377, 1982a

May K: The father as observer. MCN 7:319, 1982b

May K: An exploratory study of fathers' responses to their mates' antenatal hospitalization. Unpublished paper, 1985

May K: Men's sexuality during the childbearing year: Implications of recent research findings. Holis Nurs Pract 1(4):60, 1987

May K, Perrin S: The father in pregnancy and birth. In Hansen S, Bozett F (eds): Dimensions of Fatherhood. Beverly Hills, CA, Sage Publications, 1985

Meisenhelder J, Meservey P: Childbearing over thirty: Description and satisfaction with mothering. West J Nurs Res 9(4):527, 1987

Mercer R: Nursing Care For Parents At Risk. Thorofare, NJ, Charles B. Slack, 1977

Mercer R, May K, Ferketich S et al: Theoretical models for studying the effect of antepartum stress on the family. Nurs Res 35(6):339, 1986

Mercer R, Ferketich S: Stress and social support as predictors of anxiety and depression during pregnancy. Adv Nurs Sci 10(2):26, 1988a

Mercer R, Ferketich S, DeJoseph J et al: Effect of stress on family functioning during pregnancy. Nurs Res 37(5):268, 1988b

Mercer R, Ferketich S, May K et al: Further exploration of maternal and paternal fetal attachment. Res Nurs Health 11:83, 1988c

Puls K: Birth alternatives for consumers. Chart 84(5):3, 1987

Richardson R: Women's important relationships during pregnancy and the preterm labor event. West J Nurs Res 9(2):203, 1987

Rubin R: Cognitive style in pregnancy. Am J Nurs 70:502, 1970

Saunders R, Robins E: Changes in the marital relationship during the first pregnancy. Health Care Women Int 8(5/6):361, 1987

Strickland O: The occurrence of symptoms in expectant fathers. Nurs Res 36(3):184, 1987

Tilden V: Perceptions of single vs partnered adult gravidas in the midtrimester. J Obstet Gynecol Neonatal Nurs 12:40, 1983

Tomlinson P: Spousal differences in marital satisfaction during transition to parenthood. Nurs Res 36(4):239, 1987

Walker L, Crain H, Thompson E: Mothering behavior and maternal role attainment during the postpartum period. Nurs Res 35(6):352, 1986

Woods S: Myths and realities of the biological time clock: The childbearing years. Health Val 11(5):21, 1987

ASSESSMENT TOOL

Interview Guide for Assessing Parental Adaptation to Pregnancy

(This guide should be used at the first prenatal visit and updated throughout the perinatal period.)

Mother's Name _____ Age _____

Father's Name _____ Age _____

Married: Yes _____ No _____ **Length of Time Married** _____ **Number of Children** _____

Pregnancy Planned: Yes _____ No _____ **Gravida** _____ **Para** _____ **Abortion:** Elective _____ Spontaneous _____

Stillbirths _____

History of birth defects, prematurity, or illness in infants or family: _____
_____

Current health status: Mother _____
                       Father _____
                       Other children _____
Have they any close friends, relatives, or organizations that they can talk with or turn to for support? Yes _____
No _____ Name two: _____

Interview Questions

1. How does the woman feel about being pregnant? _____
   _____

2. Has anything happened in the past or is there a current condition that is causing the client concern?
   _____

3. What effect does the client believe this pregnancy will have on her future lifestyle?
   _____

4. What has been the expectant father's reaction to the pregnancy?
   _____

(continued)

ASSESSMENT TOOL (continued)

5. What child-rearing practices were used by the woman's parents when she was a child? _____
    _____
    a. Which of these child-rearing practices will the couple use with their child? _____
    _____
    b. Which practices will they avoid? _____
    _____

6. What does the couple do when faced with a serious problem? _____
    _____

7. Do they plan to attend childbirth education classes? Yes _____ No _____
    Why? _____

8. Does the expectant father plan to be with the woman during labor and delivery? Yes _____ No _____

9. Does the woman plan to have rooming-in? Yes _____ No _____

10. How much physical help do they expect
    a. During pregnancy: _____
    b. After pregnancy: _____
    c. Who supplies this help? _____

11. To what extent will this pregnancy and the infant alter the couple's plans for:
    a. Career and employment: _____
    b. Education: _____
    c. Lifestyle: _____

Additional Comments _____   **Note**

_____   Risk for crisis should be considered to be increased if:

_____   1. The mother experiences any pregnancy complications

_____   2. There is a probability of multiple birth

_____   3. Mother or infant requires transfer to a high-risk center

_____   4. There is continued stress that has not been alleviated

_____   5. The client or family has no support systems

ASSESSMENT TOOL

Assessment/Intervention for Parental Adaptation to Pregnancy

Tasks	Expected Behavior	Nursing Intervention	Possible Signs of Maladaptation
First Trimester: Maternal Adaptation			
Incorporation of intruding fetus	Ambivalence: "Not me, not now" response. May forget about pregnancy for short periods	Stress normalcy of ambivalence, encourage discussion of feelings. If pregnancy is unplanned and ambivalence strong, assess whether patient should consider terminating pregnancy.	Strong, intense resistance to pregnancy.
Acceptance of pregnancy by self, partner	Informs partner of pregnancy; anticipates partner's response. Negative or ambivalent response usually stressful and worrying.	Give anticipatory guidance about partner response to and needs in early pregnancy. Encourage participation by partner in early prenatal vist.	
Adjustment to changes in self:			
Emotional changes	Increasing introversion, narcissism, dependence, mood swings; changes in sexual patterns.	Discuss time-limited, hormonal nature of changes; emphasize meeting woman's own needs. Identify and suggest appropriate reading materials.	
Physical changes	Concern about signs and symptoms (weight gain, breast tenderness, nausea, fatigue)	Give anticipatory guidance about kind and duration of expected symptoms and practical comfort measures.	Disabling physical symptoms
Sexual changes	May report decreased interest in sexual activity and fears about intercourse during pregnancy.	Teach about physiologic causes of shifts in sexual patterns; give guidelines for intercourse during pregnancy.	
First Trimester: Paternal Adaptation			
Adjustment to news of pregnancy	Surprise, joy, or anger, depending on whether or not pregnancy was planned and intended	Stress normalcy of response. Encourage discussion of feelings.	Anger, suggestions for therapeutic abortion, "it's *her* problem"
Acceptance of pregnancy	Ambivalence. May forget pregnancy for long periods.	Stress normalcy of response; point out that many men get more interested later in pregnancy.	

(continued)

ASSESSMENT TOOL (continued)

Assessment/Intervention for Parental Adaptation to Pregnancy

Tasks	Expected Behavior	Nursing Intervention	Possible Signs of Maladaptation
Adjustment to changes in partner			
Emotional changes	Recognition of emotional changes and increasing needs.	Reinforce importance of giving partner extra support; give anticipatory guidance about changes and duration. Give specific examples of ways to help: helping her eat well, helping with heavy work, giving extra affection.	Anger at partner's emotional needs
Physical/sexual changes	Acceptance of changes in sexual relationship	Explain physiologic causes of changes. Encourage expression of feelings. Counsel about alternative methods of sexual expression.	Unwillingness to accept temporary sexual changes.
	Fears about partner's physical vulnerability	Counsel about pregnancy as state of health; give guidelines for intercourse in pregnancy.	
Adjustment to changes in self:			
Emotional changes	Increasing sense of responsibility; fears about ability to be good father.	Encourage discussion of feelings and concerns, especially with other men.	
Physical changes	May exhibit physical symptoms: weight gain or loss, nausea, fatigue	Explain nature of physical changes in positive light as sign of involvement; give practical suggestions for comfort.	Disabling physical symptoms
Second Trimester: Maternal Adaptation			
Separation of fetus from self; beginning attachment to fetus	Wonder, joy in response to quickening; pet naming of fetus, interactions with fetus.	Encourage "tuning in" to fetal movements; discuss fetal capacities for hearing, responding to interaction and maternal activity.	Quickening experienced as unpleasant; avoidance of maternity clothes.
Acceptance of fetus by others	Increasing need for contact with mother or maternal figure; dreams/fantasies about others' response to child.	Encourage discussion of changing relationships with family and friends.	
Adjustment to changes in self:			
Emotional changes	Tendency to focus on fetus and "leave out" partner;	Emphasize partner's need for nurturance, reassurance.	Denial of any need for change in couple relationship.

(continued)

ASSESSMENT TOOL (continued)

Assessment/Intervention for Parental Adaptation to Pregnancy

Tasks	Expected Behavior	Nursing Intervention	Possible Signs of Maladaptation
Physical changes	increasing dependence and demands on partner. Increasing feelings of well-being; more energy. Wearing maternity clothes; grief work about loss of figure. Avoidance of some activities for self-protection; concerns about sexual relationship.	Encourage open communication with partner. Discuss symptoms and causes; give anticipatory guidance about future changes. Encourage discussion of concerns.	Total avoidance of sexual contact with partner. Avoidance of weight gain; strong distress about pregnant figure.
Preparation for maternal role	Mimicry and role playing in maternal role; observing other women; accepting and rejecting behaviors as suitable for themselves. Grief work for roles being relinquished.	Discuss preparations for birth; parenthood. Encourage making early plans. Identify and suggest appropriate reading on parenthood.	

Second Trimester: Paternal Adaptation

Establishment of relationship with fetus	Excitement at feeling/hearing fetal life; "getting into" pregnancy.	Facilitate partner hearing/ feeling fetal life; discuss fetal capabilities (hearing, responding to activity, stimulation).	Continued strong ambivalence and emotional distancing. Uneasiness; anger about fetal movements.
Adjustment to changes in self: Preparation for paternal role	Increasing sense of self as father; increasing introspection, reflection on own father.	Encourage discussion of future role as father, plans for involvement in birth and care-taking. Encourage discussion of plans, expectations with partner.	Strong resistance to participation in preparations; continued inability to think about self as father.
Adjustment to changes in partner: Emotional changes	Accepting her increasing dependence; protectiveness of her increasing vulnerability. Learning to share her attention with fetus.	Discuss changes in couple relationship during pregnancy and early parenthood. Emphasize need for expression of affection and open communication.	Continued anger at partner's emotional changes.
Physical/sexual changes	Surprise, uneasiness, or enjoyment of partner's pregnant figure; gradual acceptance of changes. Concern over sexual changes in relationship.	Encourage discussion of sexual concerns. Encourage affectionate holding, reassurance of partner. Reinforce guidelines for safe, comfortable sexual activity during pregnancy.	Strong expressions of displeasure with partner's body, sexual relationship.

(continued)

ASSESSMENT TOOL (continued)

Assessment/Intervention for Parental Adaptation to Pregnancy

Tasks	Expected Behavior	Nursing Intervention	Possible Signs of Maladaptation
Third Trimester: Maternal Adaptation			
Preparation for birth and separation from fetus.	Eagerness for pregnancy to end; fears about labor and birth; disturbing birth dreams.	Stress normalcy of fatigue and fears. Focus teaching on preparation for labor and birth, expectations and worries. Give anticipatory guidance about hospital policies. Review signs and symptoms of labor and "danger signs." Assess plans for labor support; encourage presence of second support person if appropriate.	Denial of fears about childbirth. Unrealistic expectations about birth.
Preparation for early motherhood: acceptance of maternal role	Nesting behavior (preparing home and self for infant); fantasies about motherhood and child; concerns about ability to be good mother.	Discuss preparations for baby; advise against overdoing physical preparations causing excessive fatigue. Encourage attendance at infant care classes. Focus teaching on infant care, feeding methods. Identify and suggest appropriate reading. Discuss expectations and plans for father involvement in care-taking; plans for teaching father infant care skills.	Lack of preparation for infant.
Adjusting to changes in self:			
Emotional changes	Increasing sensitivity and anxiety	Provide reassurance and encouragement.	
Physical changes	Impatience with physical discomforts and awkwardness. Increasing feeling of physical vulnerability.	Give practical suggestions for easing discomforts. Reassure that discomforts are temporary.	
Adjustment to changes in couple relationship	Acceptance of increasing dependence on partner, increasing need for reassurance. Decreasing sexual activity.	Encourage joint activities; stress normalcy and temporary nature of changes. Encourage alternative forms of affection: holding, massage, and so on.	

(continued)

ASSESSMENT TOOL (continued)

Assessment/Intervention for Parental Adaptation to Pregnancy

Tasks	Expected Behavior	Nursing Intervention	Possible Signs of Maladaptation
Third Trimester: Paternal Adaptation			
Preparation for birth	Fears about labor and birth; worries about well-being of partner and child, about ability to support partner.	Stress normalcy of worries. Review signs and symptoms of labor and "danger signs," hospital admission procedures. Assess comfort with labor coach role and reassure as needed. Stress that help in labor will be available. Encourage presence of second support person if appropriate.	Denial of fears or unrealistic expectations about birth.
Preparation for early fatherhood.	Nesting behavior, purchasing items for baby. Questions about infants; concerns about ability to be good father.	Encourage attendance at infant care classes. Focus teaching on infant care, feeding methods, anticipated changes in household routine. Identify and suggest appropriate reading.	Absence of involvement in preparations.
Adjustment to changes in couple relationship: Sexual changes	Concerns about decreasing sexual activity; worries about future sexual relationship.	Stress normalcy; suggest alternative means of sexual expression. Give anticipatory guidance about slow return to normalcy after infant comes.	Continued anger and unwillingness to accept changes in sexual patterns.

13 physiologic adaptations in pregnancy

LEARNING OBJECTIVES

After studying the material in this chapter, the student should be able to

- Describe the major physiologic adaptations that occur during pregnancy and recognize their causes
- Describe the altered physiology of pregnancy to the woman as appropriate
- Demonstrate an understanding of these adaptations and their effects on the pregnant woman

KEY TERMS

Collagenous

Diaphoretic

Essential hypertension

Focal

Glomerular filtration rate (GFR)

Glucocorticoids

Glucogenesis

Homeostasis

Hyperemic

Hyperplasia

Hypertrophy

Hyperventilation

Hypervolemia

Hypocalcemia

Hygroscopic

Interstitial

Ketones

Neurohumoral substances

Metabolite

Nocturia

Precursor

Shunt

Sinusoids

Stasis

Synctiotrophoblasts

The period from conception to delivery is about 40 weeks long. During these weeks the mother's body undergoes complex physiologic changes of such magnitude that many are still not well understood. In just 24 days, an orderly conglomerate of growing human cells that already has a beating heart is constructed in the human uterus. The swiftness with which the fetus grows and develops into a recognizable human being is one of nature's wonders. The mother, whose body nourishes and sustains the new life, experiences nearly total immersion in its growth and well-being. The growth of the uterus, which makes the woman's pregnancy obvious, is only one of the multitude of transformations that have occurred or are occurring in every system of her body. These changes are so dramatic they would be considered pathologic in the nonpregnant woman. They are the body's adaptive response to the growing fetus's requirements for nutrients, removal of wastes, protection from harm, and space in which to grow.

This chapter discusses the changes produced by pregnancy in the structure and function of the various systems and organs of the body. Because of the dynamic endocrinologic influences that orchestrate these changes, hormonal functions are included as each system is addressed. Teaching and counseling of patients experiencing symptoms of pregnancy is covered in Chapter 18.

ADAPTATIONS OF BODY SYSTEMS

Adaptations in Reproductive Organs

Changes in body systems are most apparent in the reproductive organs (Table 13-1).

Uterus

The uterus is designed for childbearing, and the changes that occur in its structure, position, and function support the all-important physiologic process of replication of human life.

Growth

The expansion of the uterus is essential to accommodate the growing products of conception. To achieve this goal, the uterine muscle (myometrium) grows spectacularly, becomes more compliant, and its spiraling muscle bundles uncoil. Its weight increases 20-fold, from 70 g in the nonpregnant state to 900 to 1200 g at term (or from 2 ounces to 2 pounds). The volume of its cavity increases from 10 ml to 2 to 10 liters (or 1 to 2 gallons) at term, representing a 1000-fold increase (Fig. 13-1).

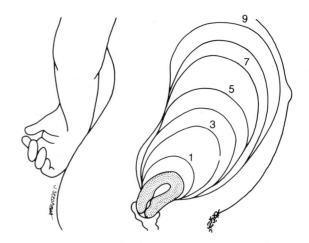

Figure 13-1. Uterine growth during successive months of pregnancy. (Childbirth Graphics)

Growth of the uterus in the first trimester is more rapid than that of the conceptual mass. Growth of the myometrium is due partly to hyperplasia in early pregnancy, but is more directly related to hypertrophy of the muscle cells (myofibrils). In conjunction with muscle growth, fibrous tissue is accumulated into the outer muscle layer of the uterus, and an increase in the amount of elastic tissue occurs. These events substantially increase the strength of the uterine wall.

The population and density of the myofibrils is highest in the corpus and least in the isthmus, an arrangement that is structured for uterine function during normal labor. During labor, contractile forces are strongest in the corpus and are known as *fundal dominance,* while contractions in the miduterus are much less forceful.

Muscle fibers in the upper corpus pull toward the top of the uterus and exert an upward and outward traction on the horizontal and circular muscle bundles of the lower segment during labor. At this time, total uterine length decreases, the upper uterine segment thickens, and the lower segment becomes thinned.

Hormonal stimulus to the growth and compliance of the pregnant uterus results from the release of estrogen and progesterone initially supplied by the corpus luteum and later by the placenta. Estrogen affects myometrial growth through the synthesis of proteins of the contractile mechanism. Progesterone is necessary for the preparation of the endometrium for ovum implantation in early pregnancy. Later in pregnancy, it renders the smooth muscle quiescent by inhibiting the contractile activity of the myometrium, thereby maintaining the pregnancy.

Late in pregnancy, the uterine wall begins to thin and soften, becoming saclike and pliable. The movement of the fetus can be observed and its body palpated for position and size.

Table 13-1   **Summary of Reproductive Tract Adaptations in Pregnancy**

Physiologic Changes	Clinical Significance
Uterine Endometrium	
Endometrium, or the uterine lining, proliferates in preparation for ovum implantation.	Estrogen stimulates this process and when inadequate, the uterine lining is not primed for implantation and early abortion may result.
Glycogen is stored within the endometrium to nourish the blastocyst should conception occur.	Implantation occurs when levels of estrogen and progesterone are adequate to maintain the endometrium.
Ovaries	
The ovaries are responsible for the formation of the corpus luteum	Implantation of the blastocyst and development of the placenta is secured by progesterone secretion.
	Human Chorionic Gonadotropin (HCG), by the eighth gestational day, has begun to provide nutrition and hormones to sustain the corpus luteum for 7–10 weeks until the placenta attains full function.
	HCG may remain in postpartum circulation for 3 days.
Fallopian Tubes	
The fallopian tubes facilitate fertilization of the ovum by the sperm	With stimulation from estrogen and progesterone, fluid in the oviduct conveys signals that condition the events of sperm capacitation and cleavage in the gametes.
Control timing of egg transport into the uterus.	Provides adequate preparation of the endometrium for implantation of the egg.
Uterine Cervix	
There is increased vascularity, edema, softness, and hypertrophy of the cervical glands.	Estrogen is responsible for cervical changes, and these signs are known as Chadwick's or Goodell's signs.
	A mucus plug forms in the cervical canal that becomes a barrier to protect the fetus from mechanical or bacterial invasion.
	In early labor this plug separates and as its blood vessels are severed, it is expelled as "bloody show"
Breasts	
Increase in size, nodularity, and sensitivity.	Under the stimulation of estrogen and progesterone, the breasts enlarge in size, the nipples enlarge, become dark, erect, and the gland of Montgomery enlarges.
The breast ductal system has intense growth during the first 3 months of pregnancy	Preparation for lactation
As pregnancy progresses, the alveolar cells become secretory.	Production of colostrum occurs late in pregnancy, and the breasts continue to enlarge.
Vagina	
The vagina becomes congested and vascularized.	Under the influence of estrogen there is proliferation of vaginal cells that causes the vaginal walls to become thickened, pliable, and distensible in preparation for the passage of the fetal head.
There are increased secretions that are white, thickened, and acidic.	Acidity of the vagina is maintained by lactic acid produced by lactobacilli that favor sperm survival. It also controls growth of pathogens in the vagina (pH 3.5–5.0).
Uterine Growth	
Uterine weight: increased from 70 g to 900–1200 g at term.	Estrogen and progesterone stimulate uterine growth and compliance. Progesterone prepares implantation site and inhibits myometrial contractility.

Uterine volume: increases from 10 ml to 2–10 liter at term (1000 times increase in size).	Uterus becomes palpable:
	    3 months at symphysis
	    5 months at umbilicus
	    9 months at xyphoid process.

Uterine position: lifts into the pelvis at 12 weeks and dextrorotates to the right as it enlarges	Fetal movement observed. Causes pressure on the right ureter. Weight of the 3rd trimester uterus on the vena cava and aorta may cause supine hypotensive syndrome.
Uterus maintains longitudinal position in line with the pelvic axis.	Palpation of fetal growth. Loss of center of gravity as uterus enlarges.
Anterior support is provided by the abdominal wall.	Diastasis recti may occur.

(continued)

Table 13–1   **Summary of Reproductive Tract Adaptations in Pregnancy** (continued)

Physiologic Changes	Clinical Significance
Uterus is less sensitive to contractility until midpregnancy when it becomes more sensitive due to oxytocin stimulation.	Oxytocin causes the myometrium to contract.
	Contractions early in pregnancy may cause abortion.
	Preterm birth may be a risk when contractions occur in the second trimester.
In the latter half of gestation, the uterus is more susceptible to contractions.	Initiates labor at term.
	Causes ripening, dilatation, and effacement of the cervix at term.
Braxton Hicks contractions are irregular, sporadic, and nonrhythmic contractions that continue throughout pregnancy.	Estrogen causes stretching and distention of the myometrium.
	The pregnant woman feels a sensation of painless uterine tightening and pressure.
	Contractions can be palpated by the examiner.
	Contractions may be mistaken for labor in the third trimester.

Position

As the uterus grows, its position changes. Early in pregnancy it maintains its pear shape, but it becomes more globular (spherical) by 3 months and, as it continues to grow, becomes more ovoid in shape. By 12 weeks of pregnancy, the uterus has risen into the pelvis, and its fundus can be palpated just above the symphysis pubis.

At first the uterus is more anteflexed than the non-pregnant uterus, but as it lifts from the pelvis it becomes dextrorotated, or turned to the right, as a result of pressure from the rectosigmoid located in the posterior pelvis.

As the uterus increases in size, it comes in contact with the abdominal wall and displaces the intestine laterally and superiorly (sideways and up). It maintains a longitudinal position in line with the pelvic axis, as shown in Figure 13–2, and the abdominal wall supports it anteri-

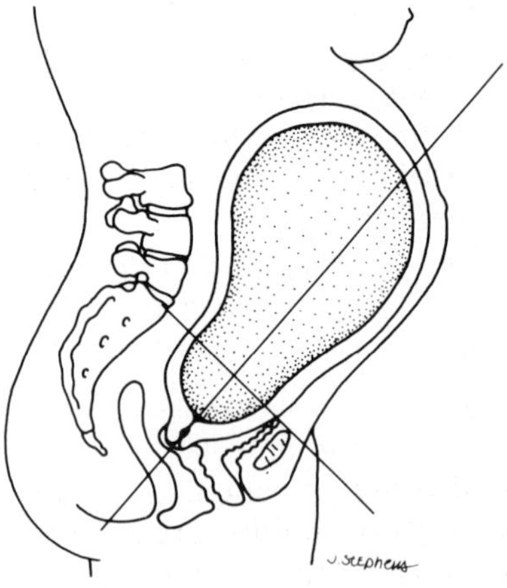

Figure 13–2. Relationship of the axis of the pregnant uterus to the pelvic axis, showing anterior support of the uterus by the abdominal wall. (Childbirth Graphics)

orly. In late pregnancy, when the pregnant woman lies on her back, the uterus rests posteriorly on the vertebral column, the vena cava, and the aorta. These major blood vessels become compressed between the uterus and the vertebral column, decreasing the blood flow to the brain and uterus. *Supine hypotensive syndrome* may occur, and the woman becomes faint and diaphoretic. She should be immediately turned to her side to relieve pressure on the vessels and restore adequate circulation.

Contractility

Uterine contractions begin to occur in early pregnancy and continue until delivery. These contractions are painless and usually occur every 5 to 10 minutes, but usually go unnoticed. These are known as *Braxton Hicks contractions,* named after the obstetrician who described them. (See Chapter 18.) These contractions are nonrhythmic, irregular, sporadic, and begin about the sixth week of gestation. They are thought to arise from the stretching of the uterine muscle as it grows, and the patient may comment on the sensation of painless uterine tightening and pressure. In late pregnancy, uterine contractions can also be felt by the examiner during abdominal palpation. Many women mistake strong, painful Braxton Hicks contractions for true labor. When no cervical dilatation results from these contractions, the patient is asked to walk or exercise; their disappearance is a sign that true labor has not yet begun.

Oxytocin is a pituitary hormone that stimulates uterine muscle to contract. Until midpregnancy, the uterus is relatively insensitive to the effect of oxytocin, but during the latter half of pregnancy, in preparation for labor and delivery, the uterus becomes increasingly susceptible to contractions. Positive stimulation from oxytocin correlates with the ripening and increasing dilatation and effacement (thinning) of the cervix. This means that oxytocin will effectively induce labor only in late pregnancy, when cervical ripeness has occurred. For the greatest effectiveness, the dose given to initiate or accelerate labor must be titrated for each woman individually.

Endometrium

The endometrium, or lining of the uterine cavity, is the primary target organ of the estrogen produced by the ovarian follicle and the progesterone produced by the corpus luteum. During the normal follicular phase of the menstrual cycle, estrogen acts on the tissue and glands of the endometrium, producing a typical proliferative pattern. After ovulation, in anticipation of conception, progesterone from the corpus luteum stimulates two important changes in the endometrium: storage of glycogen for the nourishment of a blastocyst and modification of endometrial microvilli to ensure contact between the blastocyst and the sustaining endometrial lining. By day 22 of the menstrual cycle, preparation of the endometrial site for implantation of the blastocyst is complete. When progesterone stimulation of the endometrium is insufficient to prime it for receiving the blastocyst, either implantation will not occur or an early first-trimester spontaneous abortion will result. Progesterone output that consistently remains low, a condition known as an inadequate luteal phase disorder, is a common cause of infertility and early repeated spontaneous abortion.

Cervix

During pregnancy the cervix has a dual role: to retain the uterine contents during the prenatal period, and to soften, dilate, and efface to permit parturition.

Primarily consisting of collagenous tissue, the cervix is structurally quite different from the main body of the uterus. The collagenous tissue is responsible for the rigidity of the cervix and controls the extent to which it will dilate.

Some of the earliest signs of pregnancy are changes in the appearance of the cervix. As early as 1 month after conception, estrogen stimulation has increased its vascularity, causing it to have a bluish cast known as *Chadwick's sign*. Edema resulting from the increased blood flow gives the cervix the characteristic appearance of cyanosis and the palpable softness that are presumptive signs of early pregnancy.

Hypertrophy of the cervical glands occurs to such an extent that they fill about one-half of the cervical structure and exude enough thick mucus to block the cervical canal. This barrier protects the fetus against mechanical or bacterial invasion from the outside. Called the "mucus plug," it is expelled from the vagina in early labor. As the mucus plug separates from the cervical canal, capillaries are severed and traces of blood are mixed with the mucus, giving it a pinkish color. The "bloody show," as it is known, is an early sign of labor.

Fallopian Tubes and Fertilization

When ovulation is complete, the ovum surrounded by the *corona radiata* is expelled directly into the peritoneal cavity. To become fertilized, it must find its way into one of the fallopian tubes. Passage into the tube is assisted by the fimbriated ends of the tube that fall naturally around the ovaries. Cilia lining the tubes beat toward the tube opening, assisting passage of the ovum into its lumen.

Meeting of ovum and sperm within the fallopian tube is essential for fertilization. This event is orchestrated in the tube by its muscular contractions, the ciliary movements that transport the ovum, and the composition of the ductal fluid. The function of the oviductal fluid was previously assumed to be strictly nutritional, but it is now believed that its major function is to convey biochemical signals that condition the events of sperm capacitation and cleavage in the gametes.

Events that take place in the tube are critical for successful pregnancy. The tube temporarily halts the movement of the sperm and ovum while penetration of the egg takes place.

After ejaculation, sperm are transported through the vagina, cervix, and into the uterus where they are transported to the ovarian end of the fallopian tube. This achievement takes but 5 to 10 minutes and may be aided by contractions of the uterus and fallopian tubes initiated by the female orgasm. Approximately one-half million sperm are ejaculated; only 1000 to 3000 successfully reach the ovum. If fertility is realized, it usually occurs shortly after entrance of the sperm into the fallopian tube.

However, prior to this event the sperm must open a pathway to the ovum through the many layers of its corona radiata. It is unusual for more than one sperm to enter the ovum, because the lattice-type structure of the corona radiata becomes defused and impermeable to other sperm once it is penetrated by a single sperm.

When fertilization is achieved, the ovum contains 23 male chromosomes and 23 female chromosomes, forming a complete complement of 46 chromosomes, or 23 pair in the ovum.

From this time on, the passage of the fertilized ovum into the uterine cavity is rigidly controlled. If the egg reaches the uterine cavity too early, preparation of the endometrium to receive the fertilized egg (blastocyst stage) may not have been completed; if too late, a breakdown of the uterine lining may have already begun.

Vagina

Increased estrogen stimulation during pregnancy causes many changes in the vagina. It becomes increasingly vascularized and congested and, like the cervix, takes on the dark red or violet sheen characteristic of pregnancy (Chadwick's sign). The proliferation of cells and hyperemia of the vaginal connective tissue and its supports cause the vaginal walls to become thickened, pliable, and distensible in preparation for the passage of the fetal head.

Cervical and vaginal secretions become thickened, white, and acidic as a result of the increased glycogen content of the vaginal epithelium. Glycogen is a normal constituent of the vaginal environment, and it increases as estrogen levels rise. Bacteria normally residing in the vagina (lactobacilli or Döderlein's bacilli) produce lactic acid as a by-product. Maintenance of the normal acidic *p*H of the vagina and its secretions depends upon lactic acid production. During pregnancy, high levels of estrogen help to maintain increased vaginal acidity (ranging from a *p*H of 3.5 to 5.0) and control the growth of the many pathologic bacteria that may inhabit the vagina.

Breasts

Remarkable changes occur in the breasts during pregnancy. As early as the first trimester, the breasts become enlarged and sensitive. The nipples also become larger, darker, and more erectile, and the primary areola darkens while a secondary, less pigmented areola develops around its outer border. The sebaceous glands within the primary areola (Montgomery's tubercles) become hypertrophied.

Growth of breast tissue by cellular proliferation occurs as early as the third or fourth week of gestation. Ductal sprouting is intense for the first 3 months, after which the lobulo-alveolar formation becomes dominant (see Chapter 5, Fig. 5–24). During the second half of pregnancy, the alveolar cells begin to become secretory with a thick, yellowish fluid called colostrum. As they mature during the third trimester, their blood vessels dilate and the breasts become increasingly enlarged. This enlargement in late pregnancy contributes to the change in the pregnant woman's center of gravity.

Hormonal Preparation for Lactation

The ovarian hormones estrogen and progesterone are necessary for breast development. Ductal development depends on the presence of estrogen, growth hormone, and glucocorticoids (adrenal hormones). Development of the lobulo-alveolar system requires progesterone, prolactin, and adrenal steroids.

Lactogenesis, the initiation of milk flow, requires fully developed mammary glands. The hormones necessary for milk production include prolactin growth hormone, glucocorticoids, insulin, and parathyroid hormone. These hormones supply the necessary amino acids, fatty acids, glucose, and calcium required for milk formation. Some hormones are discussed here as they relate to preparation for lactation. They are discussed more fully in relationship to let-down and milk-ejection reflex and suckling in Chapter 37.

Estrogen and Progesterone. Although estrogen and progesterone are responsible for the growth of the ductal and lobulo-alveolar systems, they inhibit milk production during pregnancy and the postpartum period and must be withdrawn for lactation to occur. This is accomplished by the loss of the placenta, which is the main source of estrogen and progesterone secretion during pregnancy.

Prolactin. An essential requirement for lactation, prolactin is secreted by the mother's pituitary gland. The concentration of her blood prolactin level rises from the fifth week of pregnancy until the birth of the infant, when its level becomes ten times that of the normal prepregnant amount.

Prolactin secretion is regulated by hypothalamic control of prolactin inhibitory factor (PIF) and thyrotropin releasing factor. The suckling of the infant at the breast inhibits the PIF, and prolactin is released. When the concentration of prolactin in the blood is high, the hypothalamus responds by secreting PIF.

Glucocorticoids. The glucocorticoids, the adrenal steroid hormones, regulate water transport across the cell membranes in pregnancy and during lactation.

Parathyroid Hormone. The parathyroid hormone limits the calcium content of the mother's milk and adjusts the iron content to the needs of the infant. It also protects the mother against hypocalcemia and excessive calcium depletion.

Thyroid Hormones. Thyroid hormones have no direct influence on the breasts, but are limited to generalized regulation of metabolic processes. Their effects on the mother include stimulation of appetite, enhanced absorption of nutrients, and maintenance of glucose and prolactin concentrations in maternal plasma.

Adaptations of the Cardiovascular System

During pregnancy, after the reproductive system, the cardiovascular system exhibits the most profound adaptations of all body systems. The mother's circulatory system has the steadily increasing burden of delivering nutrients to the fetus as well as excreting its wastes. As pregnancy progresses, the work of maintaining the fetus adds to the metabolic burden of the mother's body. Physiologic changes and their clinical significance are discussed in Table 13–2.

Heart

The position of the heart changes in pregnancy as the growth of the fetus elevates the diaphragm. It appears larger; it is pushed upward and to the left; and its apex is moved laterally from the nonpregnant position. This displacement may make the heart appear to be enlarged in

Table 13-2 **Summary of Cardiovascular Adaptations in Pregnancy**

Physiologic Changes	Clinical Significance
Mechanical Adaptations	
Cardiac volume increases by 10% (to 75 ml).	Size of the heart on x-ray films increases.
Elevation of the diaphragm from pressure of the uterus displaces the heart to the left and upward.	Changes (murmurs) in cardiac sounds that would be considered abnormal in the nonpregnant state occur: Pulmonic systolic murmurs are common. Apical systolic murmurs are heard in 60% of pregnant women.
Blood viscosity is lowered and torsion of the great vessels occurs because of displacement by the enlarged uterus.	Exaggerated splitting of first heart sound and loud third sound may be heard. Diastolic murmurs are abnormal (18% of women have soft, transient murmurs).
Blood Volume Adaptations	
Plasma volume increases by 50% (to 1250 ml), peaking at 30 to 40 weeks.	There is significant hydration of maternal tissues. Physiologic anemia from hemodilution occurs.
Total plasma albumin decreases from a nonpregnant value between 4.0 and 4.5 g/dl to pregnant value between 3.0 and 3.5 g/dl.	Colloidal pressure of vessels decreases. Vessel walls are more permeable.
Cardiac Output Adaptations	
Heart rate increases.	Pulse increases 10 to 15 beats/min, reaching maximum in third trimester. Kidney filtration increases. Oxygen transport increases.
Cardiac output increases. The nonpregnant heart pumps 5.0 to 5.5 liter/min. This rate is increased 30% to 50% by the end of the first trimester. It increases a further 10% during the last two trimesters when the patient is in the lateral recumbent position.	
The distribution of cardiac output changes.	Maternal–placental circulation in late pregnancy receives blood at a rate of 1,000 ml/min. This is 10% of cardiac output. The following factors decrease uterine blood flow: Uterine contractions Hypertonus, hypertension, hypotension Strenuous exercise Smoking Pathologic states: anemia, placental problems, infarcts, abrupt, preeclampsia The following factors increase uterine blood flow: Bed rest Lateral recumbent position
The increase in red cell volume (erythrocytes) is less than one-third of the increase in plasma volume.	Packed cell volume (hematocrit) and hemoglobin values fall.
The production of red cells accelerates.	The reticulocyte count increases. With a regular diet (no iron supplementation), red cell volume increases 18%, to 250 ml. With therapeutic iron supplementation, it increases 30%, to 400 to 450 ml. Oral supplementation of 60 to 80 mg/day of elemental iron from early pregnancy allows near maximum red cell volume expansion but does not maintain or restore iron stores. Therefore, women with iron stores should receive 30 to 60 mg/day of elemental iron, and those without stores should receive therapeutic amount of 120 to 240 mg/day.
Of the red cells added to the maternal circulation, 50% (about 600 ml) are lost during delivery and postpartum.	A total of 800 mg of iron is needed during pregnancy to meet maternal and fetal demands (200 mg is excreted during the pregnancy).
Peripheral Circulatory Adaptations	
Total peripheral resistance decreases.	Venous return to the heart increases.
Uteroplacental circulation is a low-resistance system that works as an arteriovenous shunt, decreasing total body vascular resistance by bypassing systemic circulation.	
The uterus presses on pelvic veins and inferior vena cava.	Stagnation of blood in lower extremities may occur.

(continued)

Table 13-2   **Summary of Cardiovascular Adaptations in Pregnancy** (continued)

Physiologic Changes	Clinical Significance
Blood flow to the skin increases.	Dissipation of fetal heat produces feelings of warmth in the mother. Vascular dilation of nasal mucous membranes may cause nose bleeds. Increased blood flow to the skin of the hands may cause erythema.

Blood Pressure Adaptations
Systolic and diastolic pressure is decreased during the first half of pregnancy (5–10 mm Hg), and then rises to nonpregnant level.
	Any rise of 30 mm Hg systolic or 15 mm Hg diastolic pressure above the norm is an abnormal finding.
	Brachial artery blood pressure varies with the patient's position:
	    Highest: sitting
	    Intermediate: supine
	    Lowest: lateral recumbent

Compression of the inferior vena cava and aorta in third-trimester pregnant women who lie on their backs may cause a decrease in cardiac output.	Supine hypotensive syndrome may occur. Faintness may result from an 8% to 30% decrease in systolic blood pressure. Bradycardia may ensue, and the cardiac output may be decreased by 50%. This can cause a decrease in uterine arterial pressure, which may be deleterious to the fetus if it occurs with hemorrhage or conduction anesthesia during delivery.

its transverse diameter. There may be an actual increase in heart size resulting from the increased workload of the heart and cardiac output.

Changes in the position and the circulatory dynamics of the heart may cause systolic murmurs as pregnancy proceeds. Apical systolic murmur can be heard in about 90% of pregnant women. Diastolic murmurs are heard in about 20% of women during gestation and pulmonic murmurs may be heard at some point in the pregnancy. These physiologic murmurs must be differentiated from organic murmurs, which are audible in both sitting and supine positions and during inspiration and expiration, and become louder as the heart rate increases.

Blood Volume

Blood volume increases dramatically as the pregnancy progresses. During the first trimester, a slight rise occurs, and by the end of the second trimester blood volume has increased by 50%. This hypervolemia of pregnancy is induced to meet the demands of an enlarged uterus and its growing vascular system and to protect the mother and fetus against circulatory insults, including impaired venous return of blood to the mother's heart, and against an anticipated blood loss of approximately 500 ml at parturition.

The increase in the plasma content of the blood during pregnancy occurs earlier and is greater than the increase in red cell mass. The result of the increased ratio of plasma to red cell mass is a decreased hemoglobin or hematocrit. By late pregnancy, the hematocrit may drop from the average nonpregnant norm of 41% to 37% and the hemoglobin from between 12 and 14 g/dl to 11 g/dl. This is known as physiologic dilutional anemia of pregnancy. However, the woman's nutritional state in terms of iron

and folate levels also has to be considered when anemia exists in pregnancy. After the 13th week of pregnancy, plasma volume ceases to expand while the red blood cell mass continues to rise. As a result, hemoglobin concentration increases to more normal levels.

Cardiac Output

The increase in the output of blood from the heart is the most profound change that occurs in the cardiovascular system during pregnancy. The output begins to increase early in the first trimester and rises rapidly to 30% to 50% above normal during the first 13 weeks of pregnancy. From 30 weeks to term, the cardiac output remains elevated 30% above normal baseline levels.

The physiologic rationale for increased cardiac output is not well understood. Two possible causes are the increased amount of circulating estrogen, which stimulates increased cardiac output, and decreased peripheral resistance, which itself may be caused by the large placental vascular bed, which acts as a shunt for the blood flowing through it.

The pregnant woman's position has a strong influence on cardiac output, especially during the third trimester when the uterus is greatly enlarged. When the pregnant woman lies on her back (supine), venous return from the lower extremities via the inferior vena cava is obstructed by pressure from the enlarged uterus. Blood becomes trapped in the extremities, and venous return to the heart is decreased. Cardiac output is compromised, and the blood pressure drops precipitously (Fig. 13–3). An episode of supine hypotensive syndrome is experienced by about 10% of pregnant women near term. When it occurs, the woman appears anxious, becomes light-headed, is diaphoretic, and will faint if the situation is not reversed.

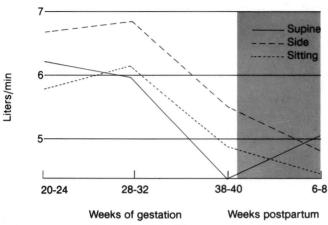

Figure 13-3. Cardiac output at different stages of pregnancy and puerperium according to patient's position.

Reversal is accomplished by her turning to the lateral (side-lying) position, which quickly removes pressure from the vena cava, allowing cardiac output to increase almost immediately.

Increased venous pressure in the lower extremities may also aggravate existing varicose veins or initiate their appearance. As pregnancy progresses, varicosities may become increasingly symptomatic and require specially constructed support hosiery that will prevent venous pooling in the lower legs.

Heart Rate

Increased cardiac output is accompanied by an increase in pulse rate. The resting heart rate, or the number of beats per minute, is elevated from the 70 beats per minute seen in the healthy nonpregnant woman to about 78 beats per minute during the first trimester, and to 85 beats per minute at term. The heart rate returns to normal within 6 weeks of delivery.

Stroke Volume

The stroke volume (amount of blood ejected by the heart per minute) is increased between 13 and 23 weeks of gestation to a maximum of 30% over the normal rate. This may continue unchanged, or it may gradually decrease to prepregnant levels by term. This parameter is difficult to determine, since the woman's position (supine, lateral, or standing) influences its measurement.

Blood Pressure

Changes in blood pressure during pregnancy are minimal in women who were previously normotensive. In fact, a slight decrease in blood pressure — the systolic pressure decreasing approximately 2 to 3 mmHg and the diastolic pressure decreasing about 5 to 10 mmHg — is considered normal. As term approaches, these levels tend to rise to their prepregnant norms.

Blood pressure is also affected by position. It is highest when the pregnant woman is sitting, intermediate when she is supine, and lowest when she lies on her side.

Hypertension associated with pregnancy is defined as an increased systolic blood pressure of at least 30 mmHg or an increased diastolic pressure of at least 15 mmHg above normal nonpregnant levels. If the baseline blood pressure is unknown, a systolic pressure of 140 mmHg or a diastolic pressure of 90 mmHg is diagnostic of hypertension. Pregnant women demonstrating these levels of blood pressure need further medical attention.

Pregnant women with essential hypertension may experience a significant decrease in their blood pressure levels during the first and second trimesters, but the hypertensive state returns during the third trimester. When a woman has been unaware of a prepregnant hypertensive condition, the problem of distinguishing preeclampsia from essential hypertension must be resolved by the health care provider.

Uterine Blood Flow

Blood flow to the uterus increases dramatically during pregnancy in order to supply the placenta, myometrium, and endometrium. Blood flow to the nonpregnant uterus is less than 35 ml/min. In early gestation, when the uterus and placenta are still relatively small, most of the blood flow is to the myometrium and endometrium. At 10 weeks, uterine blood flow is about 50 ml/min, and at 28 weeks it is 125 ml/min; this amount gradually increases to between 500 and 1000 ml/min at term.

Perfusion of the placental intervillous space by the mother's blood is necessary to provide nutrients and oxygen to the fetus and placenta and to remove metabolic wastes. As the fetus grows, the amount of placental blood flow required for its maintenance increases exponentially.

Blood Flow to the Skin

As pregnancy advances, blood flow to the skin increases proportionately. Capillary blood flow increases, and the veins become more dilated. Resting blood flow to the hand is increased seven times, and flow to the feet increases two to three times. Blood flow to the skin may increase to 400 to 500 ml and accounts in a large measure for the total increase in cardiac output. This increase promotes the loss of heat from the skin, which offsets the heat generated by the increased metabolic rate imposed by the pregnancy.

Adaptations of the Respiratory System

The major anatomic change in the respiratory system of pregnant women is flaring of the lower ribs. As a result, the subcostal angle widens, and the transverse diameter

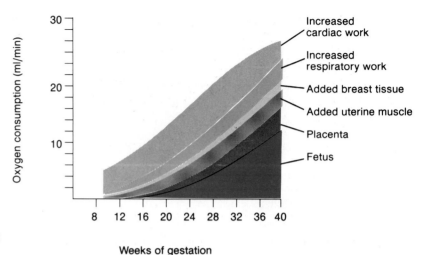

Figure 13–4. Components of increased oxygen consumption in pregnancy.

of the thoracic cage increases about 2 cm. The level of the diaphragm rises about 4 cm because of the increasing upward growth of the gravid uterus. Despite these changes, diaphragmatic excursion with breathing is slightly increased in pregnancy.

Women appear to breathe more deeply during pregnancy. The tidal volume, or the amount of air breathed out during quiet expiration, is 500 ml in nonpregnant women; this amount increases to 700 ml in pregnancy. The respiratory rate remains about 16 breaths per minute and may drop slightly at term. Minute volume, the volume of gas expired from the lungs per minute, increases

about 37% during pregnancy. Oxygen consumption increases about 14%, half of which is used by the products of conception and the rest by the growing uterus, breast tissue, and increased respiratory and cardiac work (Fig. 13–4).

When the increase in ventilation exceeds the increase in oxygen consumption, hyperventilation results, with consequent respiratory alkalosis. In pregnancy, the mother's body adapts to this change while the lowered serum CO_2 levels expedite passage of fetal plasma CO_2 to the mother for excretion. (Physiologic changes and their clinical significance are discussed in Table 13–3.)

Table 13–3   **Summary of Respiratory Adaptations in Pregnancy**

Physiologic Changes	Clinical Significance
Anatomical Changes	
Changes that improve gaseous exchange occur.	The movement of tidal air (the volume of air with each breath) increases.
The lower ribs flare to increase space long before mechanical pressure occurs. They may not return to original position after delivery.	More complete expiration is possible.
The level of the diaphragm rises 4 cm, and the transverse diameter of the chest increases 2 cm.	
Hormonal Influences	
Estrogen levels increase.	Estrogen causes decreased pulmonary resistance by increasing the pliability of connective tissue.
Progesterone levels increase.	Progesterone causes decreased pulmonary resistance by relaxing smooth muscle.
	Minute ventilation increases 37%.
	Hyperventilation and respiratory alkalosis may occur.
Respiratory center in the brain is sensitive to progesterone, which maintains low serum CO_2 levels. Fetal plasma CO_2 level exceeds that of maternal plasma by 4 to 8 mm Hg.	This permits easy passage of CO_2 from fetal to maternal circulation.
	Dyspnea may occur as a consequence of low CO_2 levels. Its immediate cause is not necessarily related to exercise.
Vocal cords increase in size because of increased circulation due to the influence of progesterone.	The voice becomes deeper.

Adaptations of the Urinary Tract

Renal function changes dramatically during pregnancy. (These changes and their clinical significance are discussed in Table 13–4.) The kidneys handle increased maternal blood volume and metabolic products and also act as the primary excretory organ for fetal waste products.

The kidneys become heavier and larger as a result of the increased blood volume and enlargement of their interstitial spaces. The length of the kidney increases about 1 cm and returns to its normal size after delivery.

Table 13–4   Summary of Urinary Tract Adaptations in Pregnancy

Physiologic Changes	Clinical Significance
Mechanical Adaptations	
The uterus enlarges, causing compression of the bladder against the pelvis.	Bladder capacity is reduced, causing more frequent urination.
Enlarged, dextrorotated uterus compresses the ureters as they pass over the pelvic brim, especially on the right side. (The sigmoid colon cushions the left ureter.)	Dilatation of the ureters and renal pelves occurs. These may contain as much as 200 ml of urine, causing stagnation and increased susceptibility to urinary tract infection (2% of pregnant women suffer from pyelonephritis).
Vesicoureteral reflux may occur.	This may cause changes in 24-hour urine collections (for HCG or estriol testing).
Dilatation of the ovarian vein complex over the right ureter occurs.	Blood drainage decreases.
Base of the bladder is pushed forward and upward from the engaged presenting part of the fetus.	Increased edema and possible trauma may occur.
	The possibility of infection is increased.
Circulatory Adaptations	
Renal blood flow increases up to third trimester.	Glomerular filtration rate increases 50% (greater in lateral recumbent position and less when standing or sitting).
	Renal threshold for glucose is lowered (tubules reach maximum of readsorption); glucose is spilled in the urine.
Hormonal Influences	
Under the influence of estrogen, total water retention is 6 to 8 liters in late pregnancy, distributed among the mother, fetus, placenta, and amniotic fluid.	Physiologic edema may occur.
Progesterone increases the size of the kidneys.	Sodium and electrolyte loss in the urine (natriuresis) may occur.
Aldosterone secretion from the adrenals and estrogen secretion from the placenta balance progesterone, causing:	Readsorption of sodium chloride and water by renal tubules occurs.
Dilatation of ureters and renal pelvises	Volume of urine for secretion does not increase.
Relaxation of bladder and trigone	Urine secretion in late pregnancy decreases; fluid retention increases.
	Bladder becomes edematous and easily traumatized.
Postural Effects	
Posture affects blood flow and renal function.	When the patient sits or stands there is a:
	decrease in renal blood flow and glomerular filtration rate from pooling of blood in pelvis and legs
	decrease in urine volume and secretion
	decrease in cardiac output, causing compensatory renal vasoconstriction.
	Water accumulates in the body during the day, causing dependent edema.
	When the patient is in the lateral position at night, the effect of gravity is removed, distributing fluid throughout the body, with the following effects:
	increased kidney filtration, causing nocturia
	increased secretion of water and salt
Changes in Nutrient Value of Urine	
The proportion of nutrients in pregnant urine is high	There is increased excretion of folates, glucose, lactose, amino acids, vitamin B_{12}, and ascorbic acid.
	Higher nutrient content of urine favors rapid growth of urinary bacteria, with greater risk of urinary tract infection.

Dynamic changes occur in the collecting system of the kidney. Dilatation of the renal calyces, renal pelvis, and ureters occurs during the first trimester and persists for 3 to 4 months postpartum. Decreased peristaltic activity of the system is observed as early as the third month of pregnancy. The maximum expansion of the organs is reached at term, when 90% of women exhibit ureteral dilatation.

Hypertrophy of the smooth muscle of the ureter and hyperplasia (increased growth) of connective tissue also occur. One of the functions of progesterone is to decrease smooth muscle tone, and its production may contribute to ureteral dilatation. These overall changes contribute to urinary stasis and a risk of increased infection.

Hydroureter (retention of water and swelling of the tissue) is common to all pregnancies and is more marked on the right side, where the ureter lies over the bony brim of the pelvis. Dextrorotation of the uterus, causing pressure on the right side, may also be implicated in the swelling of the ureter on that side. Again, these developments predispose the pregnant woman to urinary tract infection.

The growing uterus displaces the bladder forward and upward, making it more of an abdominal than a pelvic organ. As pregnancy progresses, the bladder mucosa becomes congested with blood (hyperemic). Its walls become hypertrophied as a result of stimulation from estrogen and pressure from the fetus. Decreased drainage of blood from the base of the bladder results in edema of its tissue and renders the bladder more susceptible to trauma and infection during labor and delivery. The effect of progesterone in relaxing the smooth muscle of the bladder wall also increases the bladder's capacity to hold urine. General dilatation of the urinary tract during pregnancy not only increases the risk of infection, but makes collection of specimens and evaluation of kidney function tests difficult.

Kidney Function

Changes in the glomerular filtration rate and renal plasma flow begin early in gestation and become fully functional by the second trimester. At this time the glomerular filtration rate has increased by 30% to 50% and remains at this level until term.

Because of increased filtration, laboratory values that measure kidney function are altered. Although the glomerular filtration rate increases, there are no changes in the production of serum creatinine or urea nitrogen. This means that the levels of these solutes are decreased from their nonpregnant level of 0.7 and 12.0 mg/dl respectively to 0.5 and 9.0 mg/dl. When nonpregnant levels of these solutes are found in pregnancy, impaired renal function may be present.

Other solutes are excreted in greater quantities because of the kidneys' increased workload. These include glucose, B_{12}, folic acid, amino acids, uric acid, and some water-soluble vitamins. Excretion of these nutrients may explain the rapid growth of bacteria in the urine. Excretion of protein is also increased, but until its level is greater than 300 to 500 mg/day, it may be considered normal.

Glucose in the urine (glucosuria) may not be an abnormal finding in pregnancy. The increased glomerular filtration rate, in conjunction with the decreased capacity of the tubules to reabsorb glucose, may cause one-sixth of pregnant women to spill glucose in the urine. However, if glucose is spilled consistently or there is a family history of diabetes mellitus, further diabetes testing is necessary.

Fluid Retention

Women should gain a minimum of 24 pounds during pregnancy. Ten pounds should be gained by 20 weeks of gestation, the remaining weight accumulating during the following 20 weeks. The added weight is shared by the fetus, breast growth, blood volume, and increased formation of tissue and fat. To supply the demands of the various tissues for water and electrolytes, 6 to 8 liters of water are retained in the body during pregnancy. Approximately 4 to 6 liters of this fluid passes into the extracellular spaces, causing a physiologic blood volume increase (hypervolemia). The body's volume receptors adapt to the increased fluid load, and the excretion of sodium in the normal pregnant woman is similar to that in nonpregnant women. Sodium retention is proportional to the amount of water accumulated during pregnancy. When sodium intake is severely limited in normal pregnancy, decreased kidney function and urine volume may result. Pregnancy outcome may be adversely affected by this practice.

Physiologic edema is normal in pregnancy and usually occurs during the third trimester. Swelling of the ankles and "stiffness" of the fingers signal water accumulation. Ankle edema results from the dependent position of the legs, which favors gravitation of fluid. Because of venous obstruction from the weight of the gravid uterus, blood flow back to the heart is decreased when the woman is supine, stands, or sits. As a result, fluid pools in the lower extremities. When the side-lying position is assumed, three important processes occur: the weight of the gravid uterus is removed from the vessels; venous flow to the heart increases; and kidney function improves. The excessive fluid is mobilized and excreted by the kidneys. Pregnant women who are retaining fluid are strongly advised to assume the side-lying position several times a day to help relieve this problem. When edema occurs in conjunction with increased blood pressure, proteinuria, or excessive weight gain, preeclampsia must be suspected, and further assessment and treatment are needed.

Adaptation of the Gastrointestinal System

The general performance of the gastrointestinal tract in pregnancy seems sluggish and somewhat impaired. Women commonly have symptoms of nausea, vomiting, heartburn, and constipation, the effects of hormones and a slowed-down digestive tract. The discomforts many women experience cloud the purpose behind these distressing symptoms — to provide for greater absorption of nutrients and enhance their utilization. (Changes and their clinical significance are discussed in Table 13–5.)

Appetite and Food Consumption

There are both quantitative and qualitative changes in the pregnant woman's appetite. Early in the pregnancy, women usually experience a surge in appetite, but this tends to decrease as pregnancy progresses. Some women experience aversions to certain foods, find their senses of taste and smell dulled or enhanced, or crave particular foods or other substances.

Craving for and ingestion of substances that are not necessarily food is called *pica*. Women may ingest coal, clay, laundry starch, toothpaste, or any number of other inappropriate substances. The cause of these taste changes and cravings is unknown but is generally attributed to estrogen and progesterone. Iron deficiency anemia or malnutrition may occur because of a reduction in the intake of necessary nutrients as a result of faulty eating habits.

Mouth

There are few physiologic changes in the mouth during pregnancy, but hyperemia is present there, as it is in many areas of the body. Pregnancy gingivitis may result from proliferation of local blood vessels and softening of

Table 13–5   **Summary of Gastrointestinal Adaptations in Pregnancy**

Physiologic Changes	Clinical Significance
Mechanical Adaptations	
Enlarging uterus puts increasing pressure on the stomach and intestines.	Hiatal hernia from partial rupture of the stomach through the diaphragm may occur.
Stomach and intestines are displaced; the appendix is moved upward and laterally.	Constipation and heartburn (pyrosis) are common.
Venous pressure increases below the enlarged uterus.	Hemorrhoids and varicosities may occur.
Hormonal Influences	
Tone and mobility of the smooth muscle of the gastrointestinal tract are lowered. Gastric emptying time increases.	Reflux esophagitis, constipation, and nausea may occur.
Water absorption from the colon increases.	Constipation may occur.
Cholestasis (suppression of bile flow) may occur.	Pruritus (generalized itching of the skin) results from increased retention of bile salts.
	Jaundice may occur.
Gastric secretion of hydrochloric acid and pepsin decreases (usually after the first trimester).	Indigestion may occur.
	Peptic ulcers improve because of decreased secretory response to histamines.
Estrogen affects adhesiveness of fibers in collagenous tissue.	Epulis may occur. Swollen, spongy gums bleed easily; condition regresses spontaneously after delivery.
Eating disorders of unknown etiology occur.	Pica is a craving for substances that may or may not be foods, such as clay, laundry starch, soap, toothpaste, plaster.
Saliva production increases (etiology unknown).	Ptyalism is a problem for some women. However, some feel that nauseated women find it difficult to swallow saliva, making it appear excessive.
Dental caries do not increase during pregnancy.	Routine dental care is needed during pregnancy.
Metabolic Adaptations	
Pregnancy has a profound effect on carbohydrate metabolism. Carbohydrates in the form of glucose are the primary energy source for the brain and fetoplacental unit.	Fasting plasma glucose levels drop during pregnancy.
	Plasma insulin levels show little change until the third trimester, when they rise about 30%.
Lipid metabolism in pregnancy causes fat stores to accumulate for periods of fetal growth and lactation.	About 3.5 kg of extra fat is stored by 30 weeks of gestation.
Protein is used by the fetus for growth.	Protein is probably not stored during pregnancy. If inadequate protein is ingested, the pregnant woman's muscle mass may be enlisted as a protein reserve.

the gums. A focal vascular hypertrophy of the gums is called *epulis*. The gums appear reddened and swollen and partially cover the upper portion of the teeth. These lesions may bleed excessively if traumatized by a toothbrush or the chewing of hard objects. The teeth are not affected, and the lesions regress spontaneously during the postpartum period. Their cause is unknown but is probably related to the high levels of estrogen.

Ptyalism is the seemingly excessive production of saliva, particularly in women experiencing nausea. Normally, 1 to 2 liters of saliva are produced each day, and this amount does not appear to be exceeded in women who experience ptyalism. Women who are suffering from severe nausea may find it difficult to swallow saliva, so that it accumulates and appears unusually copious.

Digestive Tract

As the uterus grows, the stomach and intestines are displaced upward. The motility of the entire alimentary tract is decreased as a result of the action of progesterone on its smooth musculature. The tone of the esophagus is also decreased, and with increased intragastric pressure, small amounts of stomach contents may reach the lower esophagus and cause heartburn (a condition known as *reflux esophagitis*).

Gastric motility is decreased, as is the production of hydrochloric acid and pepsin. The intestinal transit time of digested food is increased to facilitate the maximum absorption of nutrients from the *chyme,* a mixture of digested food, digestive secretions, and water found in the stomach and small intestines during digestion of food. Iron is absorbed during this digestive process, and in women with iron deficiency anemia or low iron stores, more iron will be absorbed. Another element absorbed readily from the intestinal contents is water. Since the transit time of the chyme in the gut is increased, excessive water is absorbed from it. The feces become hard and dry, and constipation results. Straining at stool causes increased venous pressure to the rectal vessels, and hemorrhoids may develop or become exacerbated.

Liver and Gallbladder

Significant liver changes are rare in pregnancy. The position of the liver changes during the third trimester, when it is pushed upward and backward toward the right. Its blood flow and metabolic activity are increased, but its volume remains unchanged. The increased metabolic processes of the liver are reflected in increased levels of cholesterol, lipoproteins, and triglycerides.

Spider nevi and palmar erythema, usually found in patients with liver disease, are common in pregnancy. They result from increased circulating estrogens rather than altered liver function, and disappear shortly after delivery.

The gallbladder becomes sluggish during pregnancy, and its bile becomes viscous from prolonged retention. Its incomplete emptying may cause formation of cholesterol crystals and increase the risk of developing gallstones.

Carbohydrate, Lipid, and Protein Metabolism
Carbohydrates

During pregnancy, carbohydrate metabolism is controlled by glucose levels in the plasma and the metabolism of glucose in the cells. A major source of quick energy for the body, glucose is also the primary energy source for the brain and the fetoplacental unit.

The liver receives nutrients from the mother's digestive process and also controls her plasma glucose level. The liver not only stores glucose as glycogen, but converts it back to glucose when blood sugar is low. Glycogen is also stored in other organs, such as the muscles, but can be used only as a local source of energy within these organs because they lack the liver enzyme necessary to convert glycogen back to free glucose.

Carbohydrates, which provide 50% of the total energy from the diet, are obtained from starch, sugars, and some animal glycogen. As the carbohydrates are absorbed from the digestive tract, they pass through the portal venous blood into the liver, where they are converted to glucose or stored as glycogen. After a high carbohydrate meal, plasma glucose rises and stimulates the release of insulin from the beta cells of the pancreas. The blood sugar is reduced when, in response to the effect of insulin, glucose is converted back to glycogen in the liver and muscles. When plasma glucose falls too low, the pancreatic hormone glucagon is released and converts liver glycogen back to free glucose for release into the plasma.

In nonpregnant women, fasting plasma glucose is about 80 mg/100 ml. In pregnant women, it drops to 75 mg/100 ml by 12 weeks of gestation and drops further, to 70 mg/100 ml, as pregnancy progresses. Plasma insulin levels change little until the third trimester, when they rise about 30%.

The effect of pregnancy on intracellular carbohydrate metabolism is not yet known, but pregnancy appears to have little effect on the body's carbohydrate homeostasis.

Lipids

Lipid metabolism during pregnancy causes considerable accumulation of fat stores. The plasma lipids most commonly involved during pregnancy are cholesterol, phospholipids, and triglycerides. These lipids promote high levels of fat storage in the mother but appear to have negligible influence on the fetoplacental unit.

It has been calculated that 310 g of extra fat is stored in the mother by the tenth week of gestation, 2.0 kg by 20 weeks, and 3.5 kg by 30 weeks. After 30 weeks, no further fat storage takes place. The stored fat is useful as a source of energy during periods of rapid fetal growth and during lactation.

Protein

Adequate protein intake to permit tissue growth of the fetus and placenta is essential during pregnancy. Plasma proteins generally decline during pregnancy but may also exhibit a hemodilutional effect. Protein gain during pregnancy is estimated at 925 g. Of this amount, about 440 g are used by the fetus, 100 g by the placenta, 166 g by the uterus, 135 g by the expanded blood volume, and 81 g by the breasts.

There is controversy over whether protein is stored during pregnancy, but it is generally considered unlikely. During the third trimester, however, 1.2 g of nitrogen is retained in the body daily, and this is equivalent to 7 g of protein. If maternal stores are lacking and inadequate protein is ingested, fetal growth can continue only if protein from the mother's body is used. The pregnant woman's muscle mass can be mobilized by the fetus as a protein reserve when adequate amounts are not otherwise available.

Adaptation of the Musculoskeletal System

The principal musculoskeletal changes of pregnancy are the hormonal relaxation of the joints and the adjustments in posture caused by the growth of the uterus (see Table 13–6).

As pregnancy advances and the uterus enlarges, the woman's center of gravity is displaced. The upper spine is thrown backward to compensate for the heavy anterior weight of the uterus. Lordosis results and gives the pregnant woman her characteristic stance and gait (Fig. 13–5). Some women also experience aching, numbness, and weakness of the upper extremities. These symptoms are due to the compensatory position of the back, which causes the woman to flex her neck and slump her shoulders anteriorly. This position places stress and traction on the peripheral nerves, causing pain and discomfort. Exaggeration of this position may also lead to paresthesia over the ulnar and median nerve, causing motor weakness and tenderness of the muscles of the thumb (carpal tunnel syndrome).

Relaxin, a hormone of pregnancy, is thought to be responsible for the softening and increased mobility of the sacroiliac, sacrococcygeal, and pubic joints. During delivery these joints may give just enough to allow passage of a fetal head that might otherwise have been unable to negotiate the passage.

The muscles of the abdomen are placed under great stress during the latter half of pregnancy. The vertical muscle located just beneath the skin of the abdomen is called the rectus abdominis. As the uterus grows, a midline lateral separation of the two halves of this muscle may occur, creating a vertical space between them. The width of this space can be palpated when the woman assumes a supine position and places her chin on her chest. A fairly common occurrence in pregnancy, the diastasis is not painful, and unless it is extreme, the muscle will return to its normal position some time after delivery. If the diastasis is extreme, the gravid uterus may herniate through the muscle opening.

Adaptation of the Skin

Many skin changes occur during pregnancy. Most are benign, and some are reversible. Estrogen affects the skin, as shown in Table 13–7.

Table 13–6 Summary of Musculoskeletal Adaptations in Pregnancy

Physiologic Changes	Clinical Significance
Hormonal and Mechanical Influences	
Joints relax under the influence of relaxin.	Mobility and pliability of sacroiliac, sacrococcygeal, and pubic joints increases in preparation for delivery.
Weight of the enlarging uterus increases.	Round ligament pain may occur.
Postural changes occur.	Center of gravity shifts, and some women experience backache. Leaning backward to compensate may cause lordosis and back strain.
	Spasm of the uterosacral ligaments may occur.
	Women may experience aching or numbness of upper extremities as a result of anterior slumping of the shoulders and chest.
Diastasis recti may occur.	Uterus may partially herniate.
Carpal tunnel syndrome.	Paresthesia, motor weakness and muscle tenderness may be experienced in the wrist and thumb.

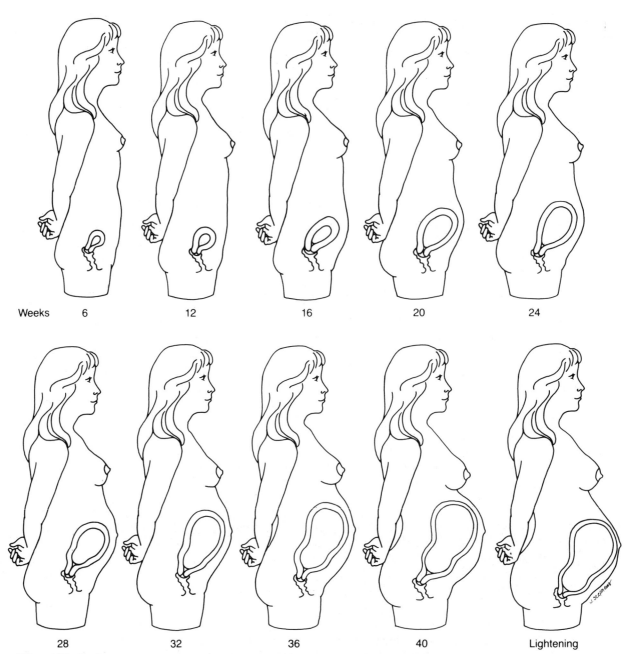

Weeks   6   12   16   20   24

28   32   36   40   Lightening

Figure 13–5. Development of postural changes during pregnancy. Significant postural changes occur as pregnancy progresses, causing accentuated curvature of the lumbar spine. Low back pain, one of the most common complaints of pregnancy, results from the pregnant woman's attempting to maintain her balance by leaning backward. (Childbirth Graphics)

Pigmentation

The increased skin pigmentation specific to pregnancy may be striking in some women. Face and body pigmentation resulting from the action of melanocyte-stimulating hormone may occur as early as 8 to 16 weeks of pregnancy. Chloasma gravidarum (the mask of pregnancy) is the brownish pigmentation that appears on the face in a butterfly pattern in 50% to 70% of women. It is usually symmetrical and is distributed on the forehead, cheeks, and nose. More common in dark-haired, brown-eyed women, it is progressive during the pregnancy. The pigmentation regresses after delivery and usually completely disappears. Women using oral contraception may also experience some increased facial pigmentation.

The nipples, areola, vulva, and thighs may become darker in color, and the linea nigra, a dark vertical line, may appear on the abdomen between the sternum and

Table 13–7   **Summary of Skin Adaptations in Pregnancy**

Physiologic Changes	Clinical Significance
Hormonal Influence	
Estrogen has decided effects on the skin.	In many women the influence of estrogen produces:
	Increased pigmentation (chloasma, linea nigra)
	Stretch marks
	Spider angiomas (vascular telangiectases)
	Palmar erythema

the symphysis pubis. Chloasma may persist for some time after delivery, but the other skin changes usually regress after the postpartum period.

Striae

Striae, also known as "stretch marks," are common in pregnancy, especially in areas such as the abdomen, breasts, buttocks, and thighs, where weight gain tends to stretch the skin. Their appearance is believed to be hormone-related, but it is not known why some women experience numerous striae while others may have very few or none. They appear in about 90% of women during the second trimester. They appear as reddish or purplish linear marks (Fig. 13–6) and may cause itching in some women. After delivery, they recede to silverish marks but never fully regress. Women have applied all manner of creams and lotions to prevent or reduce their appearance; rarely do they succeed.

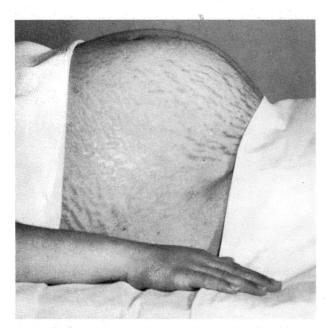

Figure 13–6. Abdomen of patient at term, showing striae gravidarum and prominent linea nigra. (Bookmiller MM, Gowen GL: Textbook of Obstetrics and Obstetric Nursing. Philadelphia, WB Saunders, 1963)

Spider Angiomas

Spider angiomas, also known as vascular spiders, or vascular telangiectases, are small clusters of thin-walled, dilated capillaries that resemble spiders in shape. They generally appear on the pregnant woman's chest, are thought to be estrogen-related, and usually disappear after delivery.

Palmar erythema, or redness of the palms of the hands, frequently occurs in conjunction with vascular spiders. About two-thirds of white women and one-third of black women experience these conditions. Neither is of any clinical significance.

ENDOCRINE FUNCTION DURING PREGNANCY

When the blastocyst enters the uterine cavity, its presence initiates events that transform the corpus luteum of the menstrual cycle (from which the ovum was derived) into the corpus luteum of pregnancy. Pituitary inhibition of the formation or maturation of new ovarian follicles prolongs the lifespan of the corpus luteum. The progesterone it secretes secures the implantation of the blastocyst, the development of the placenta, and the maintenance of pregnancy until the placenta has developed sufficiently to assume control. By the eighth day of gestation, concurrent secretion of human chorionic gonadotropin (HCG) has begun to provide nutrition and essential hormones to sustain the corpus luteum for 7 to 10 weeks. Production of HCG declines at this point as the placenta takes over, but low levels of HCG remain in circulation until approximately 3 days postpartum.

The human fetus sustained within the maternal uterus is well protected as it develops from a single zygote into a complex organism consisting of millions of cells. All the needs of the growing fetus—nutrition, removal of wastes, temperature control, and safety—are supplied by the mother. To achieve this ideal situation for fetal maintenance and growth, the mother's support system must double its normal capacity while maintaining the homeostasis necessary to supply her own needs. This amazing feat is accomplished through the alteration of maternal endocrine function.

An efficient communication system enables the fetus to relay information to the mother's body. In this way its requirements for nutrients and metabolic products that are essential for its growth and development are signaled to the mother, whose body promptly responds to supply fetal needs. This endocrine function, activated at the moment of conception, assures the fetus of a mechanism to control its environment. A summary of hormonal influences is given in Table 13–8.

Steroid Hormones

In nonpregnant women, the steroid hormones, estrogen and progesterone, are produced by the ovaries. In pregnancy, this mechanism is shut down, and instead these hormones are synthesized in the maternal–fetal–placental unit, and not solely by the placenta as previously believed.

Estrogen

During pregnancy, the function of estrogen production is assumed by the placenta, with precursors from the fetal liver and adrenals, in conjunction with androgens (male hormones) from the mother's circulatory system. By 20 weeks of gestation, the majority of estrogen excreted in the maternal urine is derived from fetal androgens.

During normal human pregnancy, a hyperestrogenic state of continually increasing proportions exists, which terminates abruptly after expulsion of the products of conception. The amount of estrogens produced by the normal pregnant woman near term in one day may exceed the total amount of estrogens produced by a nonpregnant, ovulatory woman in 3 years. Moreover, during the course of a normal pregnancy, the gravid woman produces more estrogen than an ovulatory woman produces in 150 years (Pritchard 1985).

Over 25 different estrogens have been found in the urine of pregnant women. The majority are maternal and fetal metabolites of hormones secreted by the placenta. The three classic estrogens of pregnancy — estrone, estradiol, and estriol — all secreted by the placenta, are the best-known and studied. These placental hormones produce estrogens by conversion of circulating androgens. It has become clear that the production of estrogen by the placenta depends upon androgen precursors from the mother and fetus. These organs are all responsible for the production of estrogen and androgens, but the role of the placenta is paramount.

Over 90% of the estrogen excreted in maternal urine is estriol. The concentration of estriol is 1000 times greater in pregnant than in nonpregnant women. It is thought that estriol may function to increase uteroplacental blood flow. Synthesis of normal amounts of estriol depends on an intact fetus and an intact placenta. Estriol secreted by the placenta enters the maternal circulation, is transferred into the amniotic fluid, and is excreted in the urine. When the mother or fetus is compromised, decreased estriol levels may reflect the problem.

Estriol measurements to assess fetoplacental function can be performed on urine, plasma, and amniotic fluid. Since urinalysis is an easy and accurate method of determining estriol levels, it has been used most commonly. When estriol levels fall more than 30% to 40% below their normal level, maternal or fetal problems can be suspected.

Currently, maternal estriol determination is less commonly used as a primary method of determining fetal well-being in high-risk pregnancies. It has been largely replaced by the simpler, less expensive, and more accurate method of nonstress testing.

Functions of estrogens during pregnancy are to assure:

- Uterine growth and enlargement
- Maintenance of uterine elasticity and contractility
- Maintenance of breast growth and its ductal structures
- Enlargement of the external genitalia

Progesterone

Progesterone production by the placenta does not depend on precursors, perfusion of the uteroplacental unit, or even the presence of a live fetus, since the fetus contributes no precursor.

After implantation, progesterone is produced by the corpus luteum until 10 weeks of gestation. The function of its secretion is transferred from the corpus luteum to the placenta between the 7th and 11th weeks of gestation, when it becomes the major source of progesterone. It produces about 250 mg/day, and its levels at term range from 100 to 200 ng/ml/day. Placental progesterone depends on the availability of maternal cholesterol. Cholesterol used for progesterone synthesis enters the trophoblast as a low density lipoprotein. The protein component of the low density lipoprotein may supply essential fatty acids for use by the fetus.

Progesterone may have a role in suppressing the maternal immunologic response to the fetus and in preventing rejection of the trophoblasts. The question of why the maternal organism does not reject the fetus as a foreign body has been studied for years. Its resolution may eventually change the face of the growing practice of organ transplantation.

Other, better-documented functions of progesterone include:

- Development of endometrial decidual cells containing glycogen to meet the embryo's nutritional needs

(text continued on page 335)

Table 13-8 **Summary of Hormonal Influences in Pregnancy**

Site of Production	Actions	Clinical Implications

Estrogen (Primarily estriol E₃) (Increases 1000-fold during pregnancy) Ovary
 	
Adrenal cortex
 	
Fetoplacental unit (after the seventh week of gestation, a 50% increase in secretion is ascribed to the placenta). Fetal liver and adrenals (secreted with precursors)
	Growth and function of the uterus
	   Hypertrophy of the uterine musculature
	   Proliferation of the endometrium
	   Increased blood supply to the uteroplacental unit
		Index of fetal wellbeing provided by measurement of estriol in urine or amniotic fluid:
		   Decreased level indicates: anencephaly; Addison's disease in mother; fetal demise; use of drugs, such as ampicillin, stilbestrol, meprobamate, or glucose in urine
		   Increased level indicates: twins, erythroblastosis

	Development of ducts, alveoli, nipples of the breasts	Increased breast size and tenderness
	Enlargement of external genitalia.	

	Increased pliability of connective tissue (tissues become hygroscopic and softer)
	   Relaxation of pelvic joints and ligaments
	   Stretching capacity of the cervix(?)
		Lordosis, backache
		
		Tenderness of the symphysis pubis
		Cervical dilatation

	Decreased gastric secretion of hydrochloric acid and pepsin	Indigestion, nausea, heartburn, decreased absorption of fat
	Increased pigmentation of skin (increased melanocyte-stimulating hormone to pituitary)	Hyperpigmentation: chloasma, darkened genitalia and areola, linea nigra
	Sodium and water retention	Edema, increased plasma volume (physiologic anemia)
	50% increase in clotting potential of blood fibrinogen (factor I)	Increased sedimentation rate Palmar erythema, vascular spiders (angiomas)
	Increased production of estriol in the late third trimester (may stimulate prostaglandin production)	Enhancement of rhythmic uterine contractions; increased vascularity and responsiveness to oxytocin stimulation
	Psychologic changes	Emotional lability, possibly changes in libido
Progesterone (Increases tenfold in pregnancy) Corpus luteum of the ovary for the first 7 weeks of pregnancy; then maternal-fetal unit	Development of decidual cells in the endometrium	Meets early nutritional needs of the embryo by deposition of glycogen
	Possible role in suppression of the maternal immunologic response to the fetus	
	Decrease in contractility of gravid uterus	Prevention of premature labor
	Development of lobulo-alveolar system of the breasts (secretory character)	Breast tenderness

	Apparent resetting of three hypothalamic centers, causing:
	   Extensive fat storage to protect mother and fetus during starvation or strenuous physical exertion
		Changes in fat storage, respiration and sensation:
		   Average storage of 3.5 kg of body fat (7.7 lb)

	Stimulation of the respiratory center; decrease in pCO_2 to facilitate transfer of CO_2 from fetal to maternal blood	Decreased alveolar and arterial pCO_2 in mother; hyperventilation
	Increase of 0.5°F in basal body temperature until midpregnancy; then return to normal	Sensation of being overly warm; increased perspiration
	Stimulation of natriuresis	Secretion of aldosterone (sodium saver) to maintain water and electrolyte balance
	Relaxation of smooth muscle	Nausea, reflux esophagitis, indigestion
	Decrease in stomach motility, colonic activity	Delayed emptying with readsorption of water from the bowel, resulting in constipation and hemorrhoids
	Decrease in tone of bladder and ureter; dilatation throughout the system	Stasis of urine, urinary tract infections

(continued)

Table 13–8   **Summary of Hormonal Influences in Pregnancy** (continued)

Site of Production	Actions	Clinical Implications
Human Chorionic Gonadotropin (HCG)		
Placenta, secreted by the syncytiotrophoblasts (appears as early as 8 days after conception; peaks at 60 to 90 days, when corpus luteum function is no longer needed to maintain the pregnancy). Peak secretion is 50,000–100,000 mIU/ml/day; (it drops to 25,000 to 50,000 mIU/ml after 4 months of gestation).	Maintenance of the function of the corpus luteum in early pregnancy Possible use in regulating steroid production in the fetus	Possible relationship with nausea Use in pregnancy testing (negative test after 16 to 20 weeks) Use in testing for multiple pregnancies (amount increases) Indication of threatened abortion (amount decreases) Use in diagnosis of trophoblastic disease and ectopic pregnancy (measured by the subunit HCG radioimmunoassay; no cross reaction with luteinizing hormone)
Human Placental Lactogen (HPL)		
Placenta, syncytiotrophoblasts (detected in the serum of pregnant women at 6 weeks of gestation; reaches 6,000 ng/ml at term)	Action similar to that of growth hormones Anti-insulin effect; sparing of maternal glucose Maintenance of adequate supply of nutrients for the fetus when the mother is fasting (amount of HPL secreted correlates with fetal and placental weight) Possible effect of the increased incorporation of iron into erythrocytes (currently under study) Stimulation of breast development, casein synthesis, and milk production	Increased availability of glucose for fetal use Increased protein synthesis Increased circulating fatty acids to meet increased metabolic needs; conservation of glucose and amino acids for use by the fetus Avoidance of ketosis that might be caused by inadequate maternal glucose intake and that might impair fetal brain development Association between high levels of HPL and multiple pregnancies
Prostaglandin		
Maternal-placental-fetal unit (widely distributed in all cells of the body)	Uncertain role in pregnancy: prostaglandin F_2 found in amniotic fluid, decidua, and maternal venous blood before labor Synthesis inhibited by anti-inflammatory drugs such as aspirin and indomethacin	Possible oxytocic effect on the uterine muscle Prostaglandin E used vaginally or in amniocentesis for second-trimester abortions and in labor induction Possible function in increasing length of gestation Use of indomethacin to halt premature labor
Prolactin		
Fetal pituitary, maternal pituitary, uterus (elevated blood levels at 8 weeks of gestation, reaching a peak of 200 ng/ml at term)	Sustaining milk protein, casein, fatty acids, lactose, and volume of milk secretion during lactation	Necessity of suckling response for release of prolactin
Thyroxine		
Thyroid gland, with stimulation from adenohypophysis (T_3 decreases until the end of the first trimester, then stabilizes; returns to normal 12 to 13 weeks postpartum; T_4 increases during pregnancy)	Thyroid enlargement with a 20% increase in function from tissue hyperplasia and increased vascularity	Increase of 25% in basal metabolic rate resulting from metabolic activity of the feto-placental unit. Increase of protein-bound iodine from 3.6–8.8 to 10–12 units/dl during pregnancy Palpitations, tachycardia, emotional lability, heat intolerance, fatigue, perspiration
Oxytocin		
Hypothalamus to pituitary for release	Stimulates uterine contractions (is not responsible for initial labor, but increases the intensity of contractions) Ferguson's reflex—release of oxytocin by cervical and vaginal distention during labor Stimulates milk let-down and ejection	Uterine involution Role in onset of labor unknown Lactation

- Decreasing uterine motility
- Stimulation of the respiratory system
- Relaxation of smooth muscle
- Maintenance of the early corpus luteum

Protein Hormones of the Placenta

Human Chorionic Gonadotropin

Human chorionic gonadotropin (HCG) is secreted by the syncytiotrophoblasts of the implanting placenta and reaches a maximum level of 50,000 to 100,000 mIU/ml at 10 weeks of gestation. Continued survival of the corpus luteum depends upon the presence of HCG. This hormone doubles the growth of the corpus luteum to assure continued adequate secretion of estrogen and progesterone. It also maintains the decidual layer of the endometrium to ensure early placental and fetal tissue development.

Survival of the pregnancy depends upon the hormones secreted by the corpus luteum until the 7th weeks of pregnancy. After this point, the corpus luteum is gradually replaced by the placenta, which sustains the pregnancy until term.

By 20 weeks of gestation, the HCG levels decrease to 10,000 to 20,000 mIU/ml and remain at this level until term. It has been shown that HCG levels near term are higher in women carrying female fetuses. The reason for this higher level is unknown.

Sophisticated immunologic and receptor tests are available to detect the presence of HCG in blood or urine. These tests are now standard for the determination of pregnancy. Determinations of HCG are extremely useful, and probably life-saving, for patients with ectopic and molar (trophoblastic disease) pregnancies. Levels of serum HCG can be measured in these patients to help guide the assessment and management of these conditions.

Another possible function of HCG, currently under investigation, is its role in stimulating the production of androgenic steroids in the early fetal testes to ensure masculine differentiation.

Human Placental Lactogen

Human placental lactogen (HPL) is also known as human chorionic somatomammotropin. It is secreted by the syncytiotrophoblasts and is very similar to human growth hormone and can be detected in maternal serum as early as week 6 of gestation. The hormone can be measured by radioimmunoassay, and in late pregnancy its levels are higher than that of any other known protein hormone.

Levels of HPL in the maternal circulation is directly correlated with fetal and placental weight. Since HPL is primarily found in the maternal circulation (minute amounts enter the fetal circulation), it is believed that it is metabolized in the maternal rather than the fetal tissues. High levels of maternal HPL are associated with multiple pregnancies, and levels up to 40 μg/ml have been found. By the end of pregnancy, levels lower than 4 μg/ml are considered abnormal. Serum HPL levels have been used in the past as a test for fetal wellbeing. Their use is presently limited, since tests that provide more accurate assessment are now available.

HPL is important to a number of essential metabolic processes of pregnancy. It facilitates the breakdown of fats to elevate the amount of circulating free fatty acids, which are an important energy source for maternal metabolism and fetal nutrition. It also inhibits the use of maternal glucose and the formation of glucose from noncarbohydrate sources such as protein, glucogenesis, and the formation of glycogen from amino and fatty acids in the mother. This is called "sparing," and its purpose is to save these products for use by the fetus.

HPL is also responsible for increased levels of insulin in the maternal circulation, causing protein synthesis and providing a source of amino acids for use by the fetus.

All these mechanisms help to supply the fetus with the nutrients it needs when the mother is fasting (between meals). If the mother does not eat sufficient carbohydrates for sustained periods, ketosis develops from the metabolism of fat as an energy source. Fetal development may be impaired by constant exposure to ketones; thus, caloric intake should not be severely restricted during pregnancy.

Other Hormones

Prostaglandins

Prostaglandins are a complex group of fatty acids that require an essential fatty acid (linoleic) as a precursor for production. They contain two double bonds of arachidonic acid and are metabolized in the lungs, liver, and kidneys. Since they are not stored in the tissues, prostaglandins E and F are metabolized in the lungs and in most instances exert their action at the site of their synthesis.

Levels of prostaglandin F in maternal blood vary widely, ranging from 35 pg/ml to 500 pg/ml, and no differences have been seen in these levels over the three trimesters. Thus, prostaglandin F levels cannot be used to predict or interpret reproductive events, including pregnancy. However, actions of prostaglandins in the body are numerous, and although these are not fully understood, they contribute to pregnancy and parturition. (See the box on page 336 for clinical applications.)

Prolactin

Secretion of prolactin during pregnancy is limited to the fetal pituitary, maternal pituitary, and the uterus, specifically the myometrium and endometrium. The

Clinical Applications of Prostaglandins and Prostaglandin Inhibitors

Prostaglandins

Established applications:

- Termination of first- and second-trimester pregnancies
- Termination of molar pregnancy in case of fetal death or missed abortion
- Menstrual induction
- Preoperative cervical dilatation in the first and second trimesters of pregnancy
- Termination of third-trimester pregnancy with fetal anomaly
- Management of third-stage labor and prevention of postpartum hemorrhage
- Induction and acceleration of labor at term
- Preinduction cervical softening and dilatation at term
- Maintenance of patency in ductus arteriosus in neonatal congenital heart disease

Potential applications:

- Treatment of toxemia of pregnancy
- Treatment of disseminated intravascular coagulation
- Treatment of male infertility

Prostaglandin Inhibitors

Established applications:

- Prevention of premature labor
- Treatment of dysmenorrhea
- Closure of ductus arteriosus

Potential applications:

- Prevention of spontaneous abortion
- Ovulation block
- Male contraception

(From Schulman H: Prostaglandins. In Fuchs F, Klopper A (eds): Endocrinology of Pregnancy, p. 242. Philadelphia, Harper & Row, 1983)

RELATED RESEARCH

Prostaglandins

In 1930 gynecologists Kurzok and Lieb observed that human semen, or a substance contained within it, caused the uterus to contract. Subsequent experimental research performed by Von Euler using sheep seminal vesicles purified this unknown substance. He called his discovery "prostaglandin."

By 1971 prostaglandins were being purified from a particular species of Caribbean coral and became widely available for research purposes. As a result, continued research determined that prostaglandins were mediators of pain and inflammation, and that most nonsteroidal antiinflammatory drugs were inhibitors of prostaglandin synthesis.

In 1982, the Nobel prize in medicine was awarded to Bergstrom, Samuelsson, and Vane for their work in the biochemistry, pharmacology, and physiology of prostaglandins and related substances.

Obstetrical uses of prostaglandins and their inhibitors are shown in Clinical Applications of Prostaglandins and Prostaglandin Inhibitors

Schulman H: Prostaglandins. In Fuchs F, Klopper A (eds): Endocrinology of Pregnancy, p 242. Philadelphia, Harper & Row, 1983

Prolactin levels in maternal and fetal blood have not been found to be significant in testing for abnormal pregnancies. However, in hypertensive pregnancies and in the presence of hydramnios during pregnancy, decidual and amniotic fluid prolactin levels are low.

IMPLICATIONS FOR NURSING CARE

Nursing practice is predicated upon a strong physiologic knowledge base. This knowledge is especially important for nurses caring for pregnant women in both the inpatient and outpatient setting. The body's physiologic adaptations to pregnancy and the major alterations that occur in the pregnant woman's body during the prenatal period stretch the imagination. At no time in a woman's life is her body subjected to such abrupt body changes and symptoms. The majority of these adjustments are normal manifestations of the pregnant state and may be easily explained. However, more troubling symptoms, such as bleeding, uterine cramping, or pain, require immediate attention.

presence of progesterone in the endometrium is necessary for prolactin secretion, whereas progesterone in the myometrium suppresses prolactin release.

The prolactin-inhibiting factor in the hypothalamus passes to the pituitary to control prolactin release into the maternal system. The function of prolactin during lactation is paramount, as discussed earlier. It is essential for maintaining the mother's milk supply via the suckling response.

Thorough understanding of the underlying physiologic adaptations during pregnancy allows the nurse to assess and diagnose potential or actual problems accurately and to implement an optimal plan of care for the pregnant woman.

CHAPTER SUMMARY

The events involved in the development of a new human are complex and astounding. The fact that the majority of pregnancies result in a healthy infant seems an unparalleled accomplishment in view of the fact that fetal deformity or death could result from displacement or malformation of a few cells during early pregnancy.

Thus, the responsibility of the nurse caring for pregnant women is challenging and rewarding. Not only must she help the mother maintain her health and emotional wellbeing, but the development and growth of the fetus must always be taken into account when any action or decision regarding care of the mother is made.

STUDY QUESTIONS

1. Why is it important for the nurse to know and understand the physiologic changes that occur in pregnancy?
2. Briefly describe the major physiologic changes that occur in the body systems.
3. Describe the symptoms of pregnancy that arise from these changes.
4. What body system is most affected by pregnancy, and why?
5. Describe the mechanism and treatment of supine hypotensive syndrome.
6. Explain the possible implications of the decreased motility of the tissues of the urinary tract during pregnancy.
7. Name the major hormones of pregnancy and describe their functions.
8. Describe some of the major physiologic adaptations of the reproductive tract in pregnancy.
9. Explain why women are concerned about the skin and body changes that occur during pregnancy.
10. How would you care for a pregnant woman in an outpatient setting who complains of backache, constipation, and nocturia?

REFERENCES/BIBLIOGRAPHY

Artal R, Wiswell KA: Physiological and Endocrine Adjustment to Pregnancy. Exercise in Pregnancy, pp 59–74. Baltimore, Williams & Wilkins, 1986
Catanzarite VA, Aisenbrey G: Prostaglandins: Mundane and visionary applications, Contemp OB/GYN 30(4):21–41, 1987
Guyton AC: Textbook of Medical Physiology, 7th ed. Philadelphia, WB Saunders, 1986
Hacker NF, Moore JG: Essentials of Obstetrics and Gynecology. Philadelphia, WB Saunders, 1986
Pauerstein CJ: Clinical Obstetrics, pp 65–80. New York, John Wiley & Sons, 1987
Pritchard JA, MacDonald PC, Gant NF: Williams Obstetrics, 17 ed. New York, Appleton-Century-Crofts, 1985
Schulman H: Prostaglandins. In Fuchs F, Klopper A (eds): Endocrinology of Pregnancy, p 229. Philadelphia, Harper & Row, 1983
Speroff L, Glass RH, Kase NG: Clinical Gynecologic Endocrinology and infertility, 3rd ed. Baltimore, Williams & Wilkins, 1984
Willson JR, Carrington ER (eds.): Obstetrics and Gynecology, 8th ed. St Louis, CV Mosby, 1987
Yen SS, Jaffe RB: Reproductive Endocrinology: Physiology Pathophysiology and Clinical Management, 2nd ed. Philadelphia, WB Saunders, 1985

SUGGESTED READINGS

Alexander LL: The pregnant smoker: Nursing implications, JOGGN 16:167–173, 1987
Corbett M, Meyer J: The Adolescent and Pregnancy, Chap 2. Boston, Blackwell Scientific Publications, 1987, pp 11–23
Cumming DC: The reproductive effects of exercise and training. Curr Prob Obstet Gynecol Fertil 10:231–285, 1987
DeFlorio IA, Duncan PA: Design for successful patient teaching. MCN J 11:246, 1986
Lee PA: Neuroendocrine maturation. In Lavery JP, Sanfilippo JS (eds): Pediatric and Adolescent Obstetrics and Gynecology. New York, Springer-Verlag, 1985
Pritchard JA, MacDonald PC, Gant NF: Williams Obstetrics, 17 ed. New York, Appleton-Century-Crofts, 1985, pp 31–59

14 fetal development

By the time the woman has missed her second menstrual period, all major organs and external structures of her baby are present in rudimentary form. To ensure the continuing healthy growth and development of the fetus, early diagnosis of pregnancy and regular assessment of fetal well-being throughout the prenatal period are essential. Teratogens and maternal medications that affect the embryo or fetus are listed in Appendix C.

Nurses interact with childbearing families in the prenatal period to observe and assess the well-being of the mother and the growth and well-being of her fetus. Nursing interventions will be directed by the information gained through assessment of maternal–fetal well-being and identification of the needs of the expectant parents. Evaluation of the growth and development of the fetus can be shared with the parents to promote prenatal parent–infant attachment and reassure them of their baby's normal growth.

Development from fertilization to birth includes three periods:

- Preembryonic Period (weeks 1–3) involving fertilization of the ovum, development of the conceptus, and formation of the three layers of the embryonic disc.

- Embryonic Period (weeks 4–8) involving rapid growth, tissue differentiation, and formation of all major organs

- Fetal Period (weeks 9–40) involving growth and development of major body organs and differentiation of organ systems

These periods can be further broken down initially into daily development. A visual timetable of the first 10 weeks is presented in Figure 14–1. Fetal heart and circulation are discussed at the end of the chapter.

PREEMBRYONIC PERIOD (FIRST TO THIRD WEEKS OF LIFE)

First Week of Life

Day 1: Fertilization

A new and unique individual cell arises at the moment of conception, the meeting of sperm and ovum, each containing one-half the number of chromosomes (*i.e.*, 23, the haploid number) and half the amount of DNA nor-

(text continued on page 344)

Major Events of First Week

Normal Events

- Fertilization and formation of the zygote (30 hours).
- Cleavage of the zygote into 12 to 16 blastomeres — the morula (days 2 and 3)
- Formation of the blastocyst (day 4)
- Attachment of the blastocyst (days 5–8)

Possible Abnormal Events

- Attachment of the blastocyst in the lower uterine segment rather than in the fundal area may restrict its growth and cause early abortion.
- Attachment of the blastocyst to an abnormal growth within the uterus can result in the death of the embryo.
- Abnormal implantation may occur. The blastocyst may contain defective blastomeres, or the trophoblastic cells may develop abnormally. Either may cause spontaneous abortion.
- Maternal infection or a genetic defect may interfere with the development of the zygote.
- Hydatidiform mole results from excessive invasion of the syncytiotrophoblastic cells in the uterine cavity. The fetus dies but the trophoblastic cells continue to proliferate and fill the uterine cavity with grapelike clusters. The pregnant woman experiences exaggerated pregnancy symptoms, such as nausea and vomiting, increased blood pressure, a uterus large for dates, and dark spotting before 20 weeks of pregnancy. Sonography of the uterus shows a typical snowflake pattern that is diagnostic of hydatidiform mole. Treatment of the disorder takes months of continual attention, and there is continued potential of malignancy.

- Abortions that occur spontaneously before 3 weeks of pregnancy are primarily due to severe chromosomal abnormalities. They usually occur before the woman knows she is pregnant. Estimates are that from 50% to 60% of early spontaneous abortions are of this type. Other causes may include underdevelopment of the endometrium, implantation problems, exposure to noxious substances, blighted ovum, uterine myomas, and hydatidiform mole.

- Ectopic implantation may occur. The blastocyst may implant at sites other than the endometrium, leading to an ectopic pregnancy. The most common ectopic sites of implantation are the fallopian tubes, accounting for 90% of these pregnancies. The fertilized egg may also stray from the tube and implant itself in the pelvis or abdomen. All of these sites present serious and possible fatal problems for the pregnant woman, and swift action is needed for their early resolution. A rare abdominal pregnancy may proceed normally, and in such cases a cesarean section is performed at term.

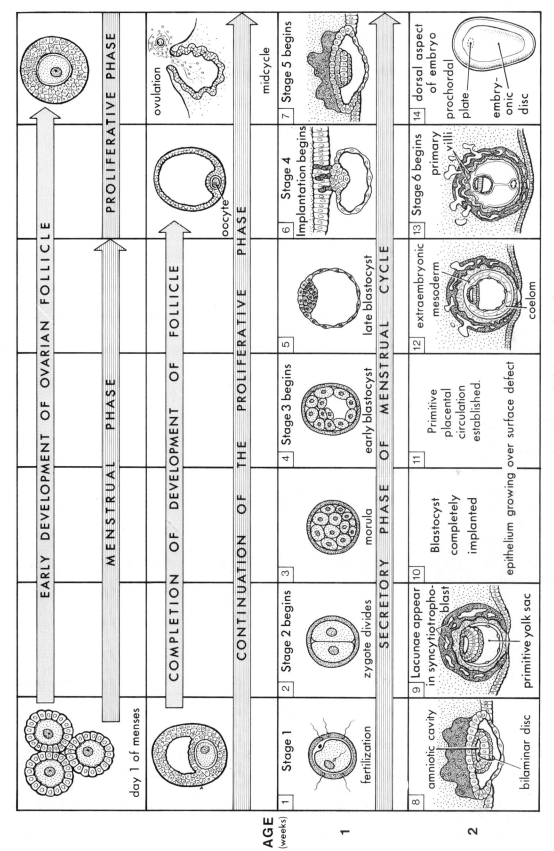

Figure 14–1. Timetable of human prenatal development, 1 to 2 weeks. See pages 342 and 343 for a continuation of this timetable. (Moore KL: The Developing Human. Philadelphia, WB Saunders, 1982)

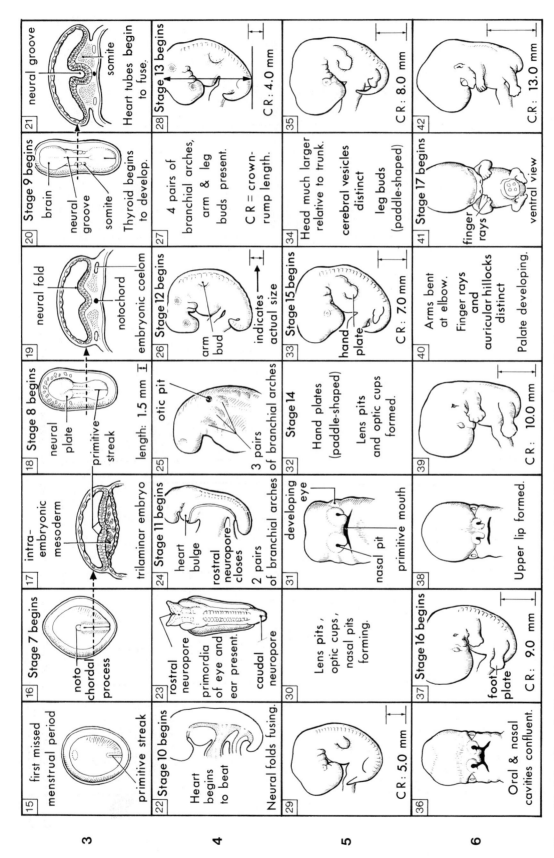

Figure 14–1 *(continued).* Timetable of human prenatal development, 3 to 6 weeks. (Moore KL: The Developing Human. Philadelphia, WB Saunders, 1982)

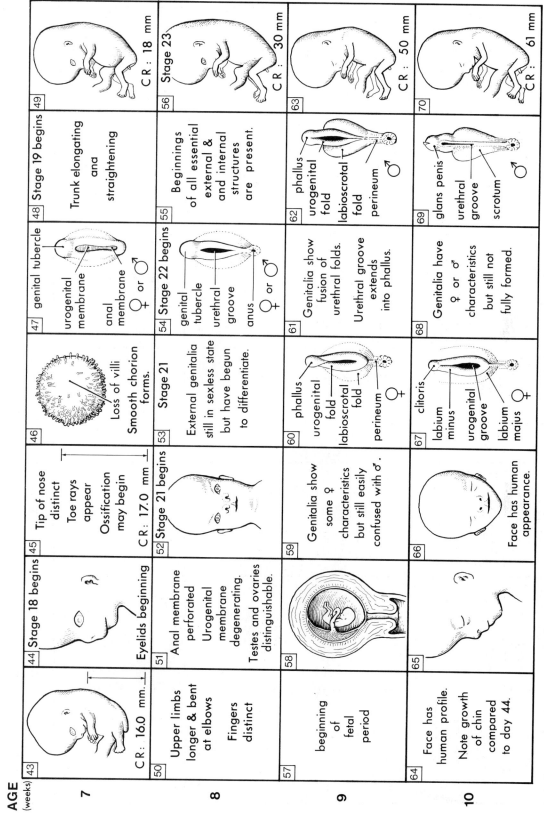

Figure 14–1 (*continued*). Timetable of human prenatal development, 7 to 10 weeks. (Moore KL: The Developing Human. Philadelphia, WB Saunders, 1982)

mally found in body cells. When fertilization occurs, the sperm contributes 23 chromosomes and provides the ovum with the diploid number, 23 pairs, as well as DNA to equal the amount contained in the ovum. The full complement of genetic information supplied by both parents provides the zygote with the building blocks necessary to form a new human being.

The sex of the individual arising from the new cell is also determined at this time. If the sperm fertilizing the egg contains an X chromosome, the new individual will be female (XX). If the sperm contains a Y chromosome, the new individual will be male (XY).

Days 2 and 3: Cleavage

As it passes through the fallopian tube, the original zygote divides about 30 hours after conception into two daughter cells called blastomeres. As the zygote traverses the tube, continued subdivisions of the original cell result in increasing numbers of blastomeres. Interestingly, during cell division the dividing cells decrease in size. This type of cell division is called *cleavage*. By the time the zygote is ready to enter the uterus, it contains a solid ball of 12 to 16 blastomeres called the *morula* (from the Latin word for mulberry), as shown in Figure 14–2.

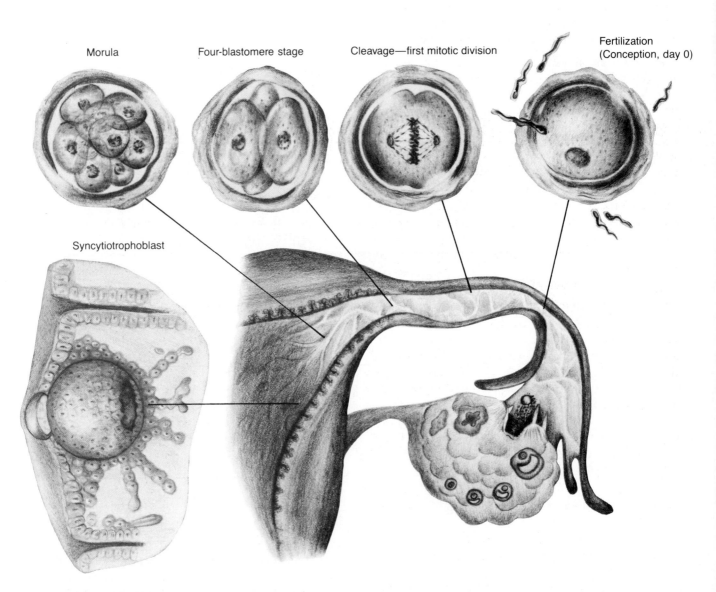

Morula   Four-blastomere stage   Cleavage—first mitotic division   Fertilization (Conception, day 0)

Syncytiotrophoblast

Implantation of the blastocyst

Figure 14–2. In the first week of life, the ovum is fertilized, goes through cleavage, becomes a blastocyst, and is implanted in the endometrium of the uterus. (Childbirth Graphics)

Day 4: Formation of the Blastocyst

Fluid within the intercellular spaces of the morula gradually increases, and spaces on one side of the inner cell mass come together, forming a single cavity, the *blastocele.* The cells separate into two layers. The outer layer organizes into the trophoblasts, which give rise to the placenta, and the inner layer of cells congregate to form the embryoblast, from which the embryo will form. The cavity of the blastocele fills with fluid, and the conceptus is now called the *blastocyst.*

The blastocyst floats freely in the uterus, receiving its nourishment and oxygen from secretions of the endometrial glands. Cells of the inner cell mass continue to proliferate and undergo differentiation in preparation for the formation of a new individual. At this point, the new life consists of a double layer of cells called the *embryonic disc.*

Preparation of the Endometrium. In its usual monthly fashion, the endometrium prepares itself for the implantation of the blastocyst. This initial preparation occurs during the proliferative phase of the menstrual cycle, when the endometrium becomes thicker and more vascular and its glands become elongated and dilated. After ovulation, the corpus luteum is formed and produces high levels of progesterone and estrogen in anticipation of pregnancy. Secretory changes also cause additional endometrial thickening, elongation, and tortuosity of its glands. The glands are rich in nutrients such as glycogen, lipids, and mucopolysaccharides.

When conception occurs, the corpus luteum continues to support the growing conceptus until the fourth month of pregnancy, when the placenta takes over production of estrogen, progesterone, and HCG.

Attachment of the Blastocyst. The blastocyst attaches to the uterine lining in the V-shaped portion of the anterior part of the uterine wall. When the trophoblast (the outer cell layer) attaches to the endometrium, it proliferates and separates into an inner cytotrophoblastic layer (fetal side) and an outer syncytiotrophoblastic layer (placental side). The outer layer develops fingerlike projections that proliferate and superficially attach the blastocyst to the endometrium within 6 days after conception, as shown in Figure 14–2.

Second Week of Life

Shortly after implantation, changes occur in the inner cell mass, the embryo portion of the blastocyst. A slitlike amniotic cavity appears about day 8, and the yolk sac appears as a second cavity on day 12. Two of the three layers that will form the embryo lie between these two cavities, and the pair is called the *bilaminar embryonic disc.* These two layers consist of a single cell layer of columnar embryonic ectoderm, which lies next to the amniotic cavity, and a flattened layer of cells making up the endoderm, which lies next to the cavity of the yolk sac. This endodermal disc becomes thicker at its cephalad end, forming the prochordal plate, which consists of an area of columnar cells attached to the overlying bilaminar disc. During early development of the nervous system, the function of the prochordal plate is to indicate the site of the mouth and to form the membranes of the mouth and throat.

The formation of the decidua, fetal membranes, and placenta extends beyond the second week, but their development begins at this point.

Development of Decidua

On approximately the ninth day after conception, spaces, or lacunae, appear in the invading syncytiotrophoblasts. Erosion of the maternal blood vessels by these cells fills the lacunae with blood and endometrial secre-

---

Major Events of Second Week
Normal Events

- Formation of the inner cytotrophoblast and outer syncytiotrophoblastic layers (days 7 and 8)
- Trophoblasts invade maternal endometrium and sinusoids (day 8)
- Appearance of the amniotic cavity (day 8)
- Formation of lacunar networks (day 9)
- Establishment of primitive uteroplacental circulation (day 11)
- Formation of primitive chorionic villi (day 13)
- Decidualization of the uterine lining (day 14)
- Development of prochordal plate (day 14)

Possible Abnormal Events

- Presence of a blighted ovum or genetic pathology may cause early spontaneous abortion
- The usual implantation site of the blastocyst is in the posterior wall of the uterus. However, ectopic implantations can occur in the cervix, ovary, intestines, fallopian tubes, or abdominal mesentery of the mother. Over 90% of ectopic implantations occur in the fallopian tubes and may result from a delay in the zygote's passage along the tube. The mother is always at risk for a massive bleeding episode when an unknown ectopic pregnancy has implanted and begins to grow. For this reason, the care provider must document the presence of an in-utero pregnancy.

tions, a highly nutritive solution that diffuses to the embryonic disc. Uteroplacental circulation begins with the flowing of maternal venous and arterial blood into the trophoblastic lacunae. Oxygenated blood from the spiral arteries of the endometrium enters the lacunae, and the deoxygenated blood from the embryo is removed by the uterine vessels. Early uteroplacental circulation develops from the fusing of lacunae and sinusoids formed from capillaries around the embryo and from the erosion of the syncytiotrophoblasts.

About day 14 the endometrium is in its secretory phase and has begun to change at the implantation site. It is now called the *decidua.* The decidua is the endometrium of pregnancy and is shed following pregnancy. The decidua responds to progesterone secretion after ovulation that prepares the endometrium for the implantation and nourishment of the blastocyst. During the development of the embryo, the cells of the endometrium enlarge and form decidual cells that extend over the entire endometrial surface. As pregnancy progresses, the decidua becomes thickened and extremely vascular. The portion of the decidua beneath the implantation site forms the *decidua basalis;* the portion that lies over the developing embryo is the *decidua capsularis;* and the remainder of the uterus is lined with *decidua vera,* as shown in Figure 14–3.

Development of Fetal Membranes

The *fetal membranes* do not in fact form part of the embryo. They include the yolk sac, allantois, amnion, and chorion. Their function is to protect the embryo, provide it with nourishment, and aid in its respiration and excretion in the intrauterine environment. The placenta is also considered one of these structures.

Yolk Sac and Allantois.   Part of the *yolk sac* is taken into the embryo and forms its foregut, midgut, and hindgut. As pregnancy progresses, the remainder of the yolk sac shrinks. Although it has no role in the storage of nutrients, it is believed to play an important role in the transfer of nutrients to the embryo.

The *allantois* arises from the hindgut of the yolk sac. As it grows, it becomes part of the body stalk and is later incorporated into the umbilical cord as the umbilical vessels.

Amnion.   The *amnion* forms the wall of the amniotic cavity. Amniotic fluid is produced by the cells that line it. Later, with the beginning of kidney function, urine is added and may eventually contribute the bulk of the fluid produced.

By term, the volume of amniotic fluid reaches 1 liter. It is 99% water and contains, in addition, small amounts of

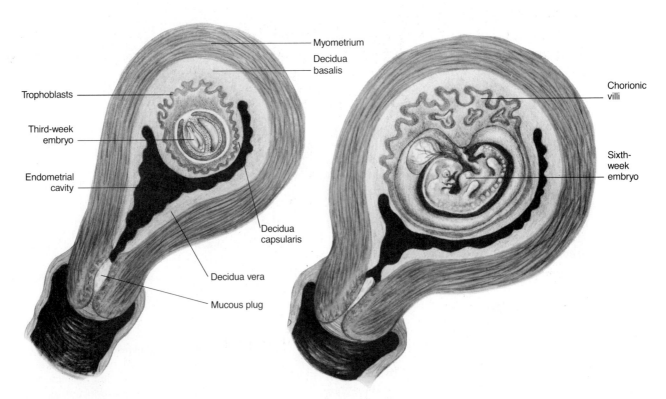

Figure 14–3.   Uterine decidua. *Decidua* is the name given to the endometrium that envelops the developing ovum. The *decidua basalis* unites with the chorion to form the placenta. The *decidua capsularis* surrounds the chorionic sac. The *decidua vera* is the endometrium of pregnancy that covers all but the blastocyst. (Childbirth Graphics)

protein, glucose, and inorganic salts. It provides fluid for the conceptus to drink and keeps it moist and warm. Amniotic fluid circulates continuously and has been estimated to flush one-third of its volume per hour during the last weeks of pregnancy.

Continuing growth of the embryo causes it to bulge into the amniotic cavity, where it is protected and allowed full movement. As the amniotic cavity expands, the amnion and chorion become fused, and the body stalk and yolk sac come together to form the umbilical cord. In this way the umbilical cord acquires the amnion as its outer cover.

Chorion.   The *chorion* consists of the lining of the extraembryonic mesoderm, with a layer of cytotropho-

blasts. Between days 9 and 20, the chorion becomes differentiated and grows rapidly. Groups of cytotrophoblasts (fetal side or inner core) migrate to the syncytiotrophoblastic layer (maternal or outer side) to form primary villi. Intervillous spaces filled with blood lie between the primary villi. The core of each villus is invaded by the extraembryonic mesoderm and the cytotrophoblastic layer to form the secondary villi (see Figure 14–6). These villi grow until they reach the basalic layer of the uterine decidua, where some project into the bloodfilled spaces.

Small blood vessels begin to form in each secondary villus and in the embryo, and the umbilical veins soon convey blood from the chorion into the primitive heart of the embryo. Blood is returned from the embryo by the developed umbilical arteries.

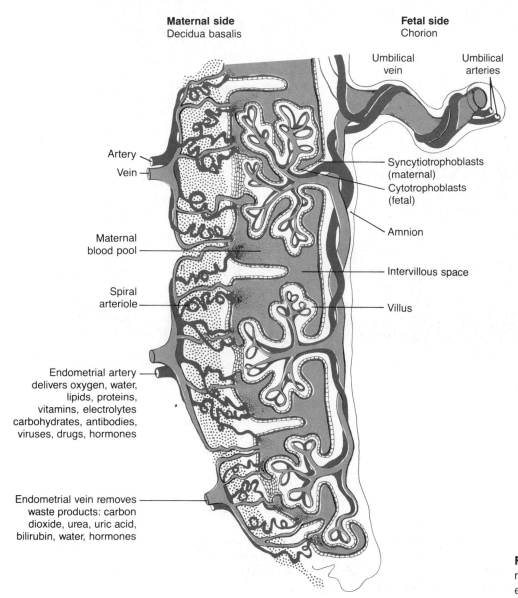

Maternal side
Decidua basalis

Fetal side
Chorion

Umbilical vein

Umbilical arteries

Artery

Vein

Syncytiotrophoblasts (maternal)

Cytotrophoblasts (fetal)

Amnion

Maternal blood pool

Intervillous space

Spiral arteriole

Villus

Endometrial artery delivers oxygen, water, lipids, proteins, vitamins, electrolytes carbohydrates, antibodies, viruses, drugs, hormones

Endometrial vein removes waste products: carbon dioxide, urea, uric acid, bilirubin, water, hormones

Figure 14–4. Placental membrane and fetal–maternal exchange. (Childbirth Graphics)

Development of Placenta

The *placenta* is a temporary organ, shared by the mother and fetus, that allows exchange across the maternal and fetal circulation, as shown in Figure 14–4. Maternal and fetal blood do not mix; nutrients, oxygen, and fetal waste products diffuse across fetal and maternal membranes. The placenta produces some hormones independently, such as HCG and human placental lactogen (HPL), and produces estrogen in conjunction with fetal precursors. The circulation of the fetus, which links it with the placenta, depends on the generation of blood flow by the fetal heart (60 ml/min at term). The maternal circulation surrounds the fetal villi, and its blood flow (600 ml/min at term) enters and exits the intervillous space by way of the uterine blood vessels.

The placenta has the following functions:

- *Respiratory:* By the process of diffusion, oxygen from the mother passes into the placenta and then into the fetal blood.
- *Nutritional:* The mother's blood supplies the fetus with nutrients such as carbohydrates, water, inorganic salts, fats, proteins, and minerals.
- *Excretory:* End products of fetal metabolism cross the placenta into the maternal circulation, from which they will be excreted.
- *Protective:* The placental barrier protects the fetus from many harmful substances. However, more and more teratogenic substances are being discovered that may pass the placental barrier.
- *Endocrine:* Estrogen, progesterone, HCG, and HPL are produced in large quantities.
- *Passive immunity:* Immunity to smallpox, diphtheria, and measles is passed to the fetus from maternal antibodies.

Third Week of Life

During the third week of life, the conceptus develops rapidly. This period also coincides with the first missed menstrual cycle of the mother.

The primitive streak (see Fig. 14–2) is formed during the third week, and three germ layers develop. This period, from approximately day 15 to day 21, is called the "period of threes"; not only do the three germ layers develop, but the primitive streak, the notochord, and the neural tube are formed.

Gastrulation

Gastrulation is the process by which the bilaminar embryo becomes a trilaminar embryo. On about day 15, the cytotrophoblast cells proliferate into the blastocyst to form the extraembryonic mesoderm, which later co-

---

Major Events of Third Week
Normal Events

- Formation of blood vessels within the chorionic villi (day 13)
- Gastrulation or conversion of the bilaminar embryonic disc into the three-layered trilaminar disc (day 14)
- Continued development of the chorion with formation of tertiary chorionic villi (day 15–20)
- Development of the neural tube (day 18)
- Formation of somites (day 21)
- Beginning of blood circulation (day 24)

Possible Abnormal Events

- If one fertilized ovum splits to form two identical embryos, monozygous twins result. Rarely, splitting of the inner cell mass may be incomplete, resulting in incomplete splitting of the primitive streak and embryonic disc. As a result, conjoined twins are formed. The amount of deformity may range from a small skin fusion to a double monster with shared trunk, organ, and limbs.
- The heart is most susceptible to teratogens between the 19th and the 41st days.

---

alesces to become the extraembryonic coelom. The mesoderm lies between the ectoderm and the endoderm, completing the trilaminar disc of the *primitive streak*. All tissues and organs of the embryo are developed from these three layers, as shown in Figure 14–5.

Ectoderm. The *ectoderm* forms the outermost tissues of the body, such as the skin, hair, and nails. The entire nervous system develops from the ectoderm, including the brain, spinal cord, and motor neurons. The full complement of nerve cells, numbering 100 billion or more, is present from the time of birth. No new cells will be added during the lifetime of the individual, but those that are present enlarge to keep pace with body growth.

Mesoderm. The cells of the *mesoderm* develop to form the skeleton, bone marrow, cartilage, and connective tissue; the smooth, voluntary, and cardiac muscles; the heart, blood vessels, and corpuscles; the inner skin layer; the lymphoid tissue; and the kidneys and gonads.

Endoderm. The *endoderm* gives rise to the epithelial linings of most of the body's internal organs, such as the alimentary canal, thyroid, parathyroid, thymus, liver, pancreas, respiratory tract, pharyngotympanic tube and middle ear, urinary bladder, parts of the female and male urethras, greater vestibular glands, prostate gland, bulbourethral glands, and the lining of the uterus.

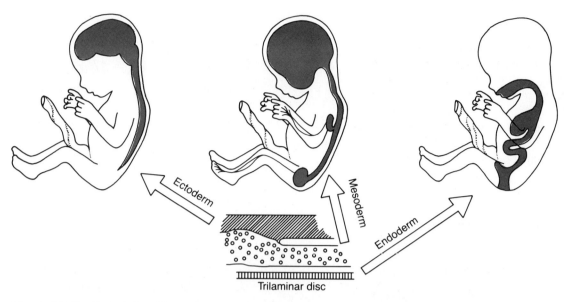

Figure 14–5. Gastrulation. *Gastrulation* is the process of converting the bilaminar disc into a trilaminar embryonic disc. The cells of the three germ layers divide and migrate to form the tissues and organs as depicted. (Childbirth Graphics)

Neurulation

A midline groove appears in the ectoderm over the primitive streak. As the ectoderm continues to elongate and expand, the underlying mesoderm moves cephalad and laterally. A column of cells, the notochord process, forms and in conjunction with the ectoderm joins to develop a notochord plate about day 16. The notochord plate then folds inward to form the *notochord,* the structure around which the vertebral column develops. As the notochord becomes surrounded by vertebral bodies, it disappears from under these structures. However, it persists between the vertebral bodies as the nucleus pulposus of the intervertebral discs.

The neural tube is developed from the closure of the neural plate and the neural fold—a process called *neurulation*—at about 21 to 26 days.

Growth of Chorionic Villi

Continued growth of the chorionic villi has increased their size (Fig. 14–6). They cover the entire surface of the chorion by day 15 and are now called *secondary chorionic villi*. When the cells within the villi begin to differentiate into capillaries, the villi are called *tertiary chorionic villi*. By day 22 these blood vessels have connected with the fetal heart, and blood begins to circulate within the chorionic villi. The function of the villi is to absorb nutrients from the maternal blood and excrete wastes from the embryo into the blood.

Division into Somites

About day 20, the mesoderm divides into paired bodies called *somites*. Located on either side of the developing neural tube, these paired bodies give rise to the skeleton and muscle tissue. During the somite period, days 20 to 30, 38 pairs of somites develop. Their total number eventually reaches 42 to 44 pairs, of which 4 are occipital, 8 cervical, 12 thoracic, 5 lumbar, 5 sacral, and 8 to 10 coccygeal. Some of the somites—the first occipital and the fifth to seventh coccygeal—disappear, while the rest form the axial skeleton. One criterion for determining the age of the embryo is the number of developed somites.

By the end of the third week of life, the conceptus is about 1.0 mm in length.

EMBRYONIC PERIOD (FOURTH TO EIGHTH WEEKS OF LIFE)

During this short, 4-week period, embryonic development is extremely rapid (see Fig. 14–1). All major internal and external organs and organ systems are formed, a process known as *organogenesis*. The embryo changes in shape, and major features of the external body are recognizable by eight weeks *(morphogenesis)*. This stage of growth and development holds the potential for major congenital malformations if the embryo is exposed to

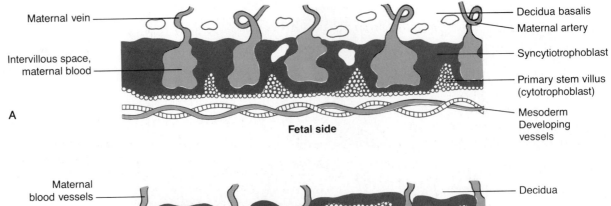

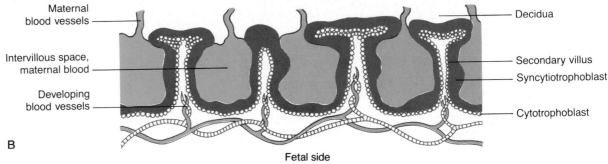

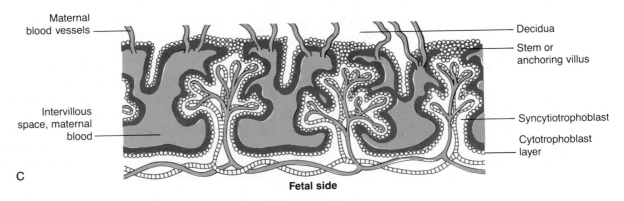

Figure 14–6. Development of the chorionic villi. (*A*) By the beginning of the third week, the primary stem villi consist of a primary stem core made up of cytotrophoblasts, covered by syncytiotrophoblasts. (*B*) The mesoderm of the chorion invades the core of each primary villus, which then becomes known as a secondary villus. (*C*) By the end of the third week, the tertiary villi are formed, and by the end of four weeks, tertiary villi cover the entire surface of the chorion. (Childbirth Graphics)

teratogens, such as drugs, chemicals, viruses, and other substances.

Fourth Week of Life

The embryo grows dramatically during the fourth week. It more than triples its length to 3.5 mm, and its weight approximates 5 mg. Elongation of the embryo has occurred, and it has become curved upon itself with the formation of a head and tail fold. Lateral body folds develop, making the embryo tubular rather than flat and disc-shaped.

Closure of the neural tube begins in the area of the occiput and proceeds upward and downward from that point. Somites, formed in a craniocaudal sequence as the neural tube closes, can be observed through the ectoderm.

The pericardial sac around the heart enlarges, causing the head region to elevate. The laryngotracheal groove and lung buds, which will become the respiratory system, are present. The mandible and maxilla of the jaw become distinct, and rudimentary forms of the eyes, ears, and nose are present. The intestinal system is formed from the yolk sac, and differentiation of the buds, which will become the esophagus, stomach, liver, and pancreas, is

Major Events of Embryonic Period (4–8 Weeks)

Normal Events

- Conversion of the flat trilaminar embryonic disc into a C-shaped cylindrical embryo
- Formation of the head, tail, and lateral folds
- Formation of the primitive gut by incorporation of the yolk sac into the embryo
- Formation of the lateral and ventral body walls
- Acquisition of an epithelial covering by the umbilicus through the expansion of the amnion
- Establishment of ventral position of the heart and development of the brain in the cranial region of the embryo
- Differentiation of the three germ layers into various tissues and layers that will become established as the major organ systems
- Appearance of the brain, limbs, ears, eyes, and nose
- Development of a human appearance by the embryo

Possible Abnormal Events

- Critical development of organ systems between 4 and 8 weeks of life renders the embryo vulnerable to developmental or environmental influences that may cause malformation:

  Abnormalities of the genes and chromosomes

  Alterations of maternal health, such as infection from rubella or herpes

  Ingestion of teratogenic substances
- During the embryonic period, the risk of mortality is greater than at any other time of life.

progressing. The thyroid and thymus glands are also developing. The primitive circulatory system is established, and the heart is beating. The placenta is also forming, while the chorionic villi are steadily growing and developing. The budlike projections on the surface of the embryo are the beginning of the limbs.

Fifth Week of Life

As the embryo and then the fetus grows during the first half of pregnancy, it is measured by its crown-rump length (CRL). The fetus is measured during the last half of pregnancy by its crown-heel length (CHL), or standing height, as shown in Figure 14–7. The CRL grows from 4 to 8 mm in this week, and the weight from 5 to 50 mg.

The growth of the head is rapid and exceeds the growth of the body during this week. The embryo lengthens and bends into a *C* shape, while an additional 42 to 44 pairs of somites are added to its caudal end.

The umbilical cord is formed from the union of the amnion, the yolk, and the connecting stalk. It now contains two umbilical arteries and one umbilical vein.

The doubling of the size of the heart makes it prominent, and its atria and ventricles are visible through the

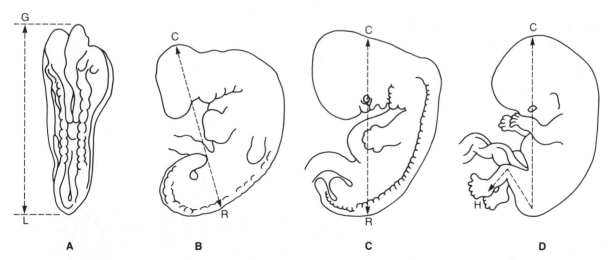

A   B   C   D

Figure 14–7. The embryonic period: Carnegie embryonic staging system. (*A*) From the third to the fourth week, embryos are straight and measured by their greatest length (*GL*). (*B*) Sitting height, or crown-rump length (*CRL*) is used for older embryos. (*C*) In embryos with flexed heads, the *CRL* actually measures the distance from the neck to the rump. (*D*) Standing height, or crown–heel length (*CHL*), is used for 8-week embryos. (Childbirth Graphics)

ectoderm. The embryo's four limb buds are most vulnerable to teratogens at this time.

Sixth Week of Life

The head has become larger than the trunk and is bent over the heart prominence. Elevations in the facial ectoderm are evident, and the position of the eyes, nose, mouth, and the groove that is to become the external acoustic meatus is established. In the upper limbs, the elbows and wrists are identifiable, and the hand plates develop ridges called finger rays. The lower limbs are not developed to the same degree. Changes are beginning to

occur in the genital region. (The CRL is 8 to 14 mm; the weight, 50 to 400 mg.)

Seventh Week of Life

Cerebral hemispheres appear as the head enlarges rapidly. The eyes move from a lateral to a more frontal position as the face elongates. Prominences appear over the ventral body wall from the large heart and liver, two organs that form early because their function is vital to the maintenance and survival of the embryo.

As the embryo continues to grow, the umbilical cord shrinks. The arm and hand of the upper limbs and the

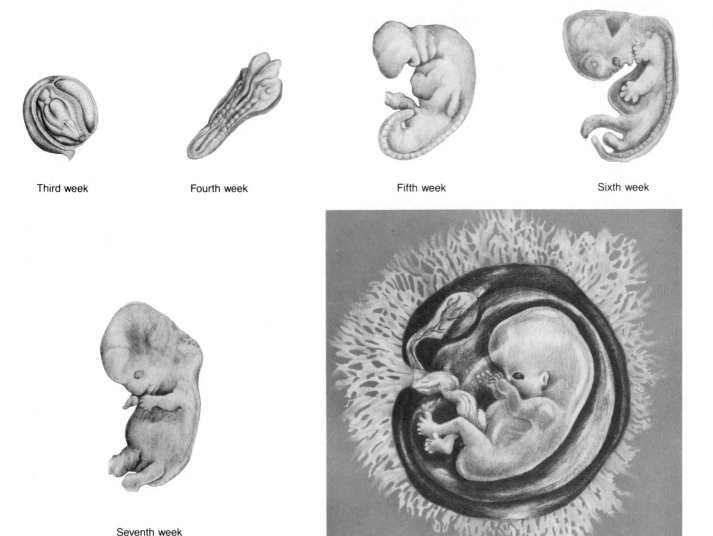

Third week   Fourth week   Fifth week   Sixth week

Seventh week

Eighth week

Figure 14–8. The relative growth of the human embryo is rapid from the third through the seventh week, while it undergoes a spectacular transformation from a conglomerate of specialized parts to a recognizable early human form. (Childbirth Graphics)

thigh, leg, and foot segments of the lower limbs become apparent. The fingers develop, and their growth is critical at this point (40 to 50 days). (The CRL is 14 to 20 mm; the weight, 400 to 1000 mg.)

Eighth Week of Life

During this final week of the embryonic period, the embryo exhibits definite human characteristics. The cerebral hemispheres have grown so rapidly that the head now makes up 50% of the mass of the embryo. The face occupies the lower half of the head, and the eyes continue to move to a more frontal plane. Eyelid folds develop. These will become fused during the ninth week and remain so until the seventh month. The fingers lengthen, and the toes are distinct by the end of the eighth week. The external ears are set low and are taking on their final shape. Sexual differences in the external genitalia can now be seen by the trained eye (Fig. 14 – 8). (The CRL is 21 to 30 mm; the weight, 1000 to 3000 mg.)

FETAL PERIOD (9TH TO 40TH WEEKS OF LIFE)

When the basic organ structures of the embryo have been established and it is recognizable as a human being, it is called a *fetus* (see Fig. 14 – 1). During the fetal period, from 9 to 40 weeks, there is further growth and differentiation of the tissues and organs that began their development during the embryonic period. Growth is considerable: the fetus's CRL goes from approximately 30 mm to 300 mm. Its body proportions will undergo change, and its tiny organs will begin to function and supply a portion of its metabolic needs.

Fetal growth and differentiation is an extremely complex process, and the development of tissues and organs is asynchronous. Given these conditions, the fact that most infants are born normal is almost unbelievable.

Determining Fetal Age

Determining fetal age early in pregnancy is necessary for ongoing management of the prenatal period. The most common methods used to determine fetal age are:

- *Gestational age:* the age of the fetus as calculated from the LMP. This is the method most commonly used because the menstrual period is an event that the mother can remember or approximate.
- *Fetal age:* the age of the fetus as calculated from conception, or approximately 2 weeks after the LMP. This is the true age of the fetus, which begins its existence when the ovum and sperm fuse at conception.

9th to 12th Weeks

By 9 weeks the fetal head is so large that it constitutes half of its size. Fetal growth has become so rapid that between 9 and 12 weeks the CRL more than doubles. The face of the fetus has broadened, and the eyes are widely separated, although their lids remain fused.

Throughout this stage the legs and thighs are disproportionately small. By the end of 12 weeks, however, the upper limbs have reached normal human proportions. The lower limbs take longer to develop (Fig. 14 – 9).

The male and female external genitalia appear similar at nine weeks but reach full maturity and are distinguishable at 12 weeks. Production of red blood cells begins in the liver during the early weeks of this period, and this function is assumed by the spleen at 12 weeks.

13th to 16th Weeks

Rapid fetal growth occurs during this month. The length of the fetus will double. Its head now makes up one third of its length. The forehead is prominent, and the position of the eyes and ears becomes more anterior. Lanugo, or fine hair, grows on the forehead, and the fingernails are formed. For the first time the kidneys secrete urine, and the fetus begins to swallow amniotic fluid. The legs have become longer, and as skeletal ossification progresses, it can be seen on x-ray films at 16 weeks.

The fetus appears more human. Its mandible becomes recognizable as a chin, and the ears are placed higher on the head. At this time the placenta has been fully formed. (At the end of this period, the CRL is 112 mm, or 4.5 in; the weight, 105 g, or 3.7 oz.)

17th to 20th Weeks

Fetal growth slows, but its CRL increases by 50 mm and its lower limbs become fully formed. The fetal body becomes covered with lanugo, and its sebaceous glands secrete sebum, from which the *vernix caseosa* is formed. The vernix is a cheeselike material that covers the skin of the fetus to protect it from drying and hardening from exposure to the amniotic fluid.

Fetal movements are first felt by the mother between 16 and 20 weeks. This event is called *quickening*. At about this time, the fetal heart tones can first be heard with a fetoscope placed over the symphysis pubis. Brown fat, which becomes the site of heat production in the newborn, is formed. This specialized adipose tissue forms on various sites of the body to produce heat by oxidation of fatty acids.

At 20 weeks, the fetus is considered nonviable or previable, since it is too immature to survive out of the sustaining environment of the uterus. (At the end of this

Major Events of Fetal Period (9th to 40th Weeks)

Normal Events

Weeks 9 to 12

- Fetal head makes up one-half the fetal body.
- CRL doubles between 9 and 12 weeks
- Eyelids remain fused.
- Upper limbs develop to normal proportions, while the lower limbs remain less developed.
- Male and female genitalia are recognizable by 12 weeks.
- Production of red blood cells transfers from the liver to the spleen at 12 weeks.

Weeks 13 to 16

- Rapid fetal growth occurs.
- Fetus doubles in size.
- Lanugo begins to grow.
- Fingernails are formed.
- Kidneys begin to secrete urine.
- Fetus begins to swallow amniotic fluid.
- Fetus appears human.
- Placenta is fully formed.

Weeks 17 to 23

- Fetal growth slows.
- Lower limbs become fully formed.
- Fetal body is covered with lanugo.
- Vernix caseosa covers the body to protect the skin from amniotic fluid.
- Fetal movement is first felt by the mother around 20 weeks.
- Fetal heartbeat is first heard with a fetoscope.
- Brown fat forms.

Weeks 24 to 27

- Skin growth is rapid, and skin appears red and wrinkled.
- The eyes open, and eyelashes and eyebrows are formed.
- The fetus becomes viable at 27 weeks.

Weeks 28 to 31

- Subcutaneous fat is deposited.
- If the fetus is born at this time with immature lungs, respiratory distress syndrome may occur.

Weeks 32 to 36

- Weight gain is steady.
- Lanugo has disappeared from the body but remains on the head.
- Fingernails are growing.
- The fetus has a good chance of survival if born during these weeks.

Weeks 37 to 40

- Subcutaneous fat builds up steadily, and fetal contours become rounded.
- Fingernails and toenails are fully formed and extend beyond the ends of the fingers and toes.
- Both testes have descended in the male.
- The skull is fully developed and is larger than any other part of the body.

Possible Abnormal Events

- Mothers who use over-the-counter drugs indiscriminately are more likely to have infants with congenital malformations.
- Withdrawal seizure may occur in infants born to an alcoholic mother, and the newborn may experience fetal alcohol syndrome.
- Inadequate fetal growth may result from intrauterine infections, multiple pregnancies, and chromosome abnormalities.
- Intrauterine growth retardation may result from maternal narcotic use, cigarette smoking, and inadequate prenatal nutrition.
- Fetal growth retardation may result from placental insufficiency caused by such defects as placental infarction.
- Preterm birth is a major threat to survival when the mother is in a high-risk category.

period, the CRL is 160 mm, or 6.5 in; the weight, 310 g, or 10.8 oz.)

21st to 23rd Weeks

The fetus remains lean but is steadily gaining weight, and its body is assuming more human proportions. The skin remains red and wrinkled and is covered with vernix caseosa. The lungs are beginning to produce surfactant, and meconium begins to accumulate and reach the rectum. (At the end of this period, the CRL is 200 mm, or 8.1 in; the weight, 640 g or 1 lb, 4 oz.)

24th to 27th Weeks

The fetal skin grows rapidly. It appears wrinkled because of the absence of subcutaneous fat, and blood vessels close to the skin surface give it its red color. The face is

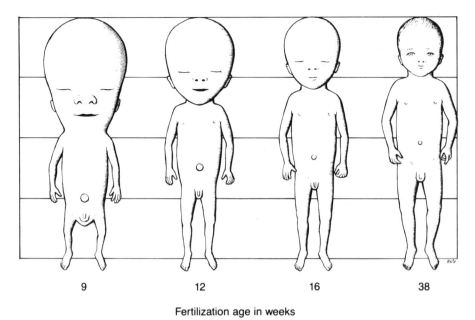

9 12 16 38

Fertilization age in weeks

Figure 14–9. Changing proportions of the body during the fetal period. By 36 weeks, the circumferences of the head and the abdomen are approximately equal. After this, the circumference of the abdomen may be greater. (Moore KL: The Developing Human. Philadelphia, WB Saunders, 1982)

maturing, the eyelashes and brows are formed, and the eyelids are now open. (At the end of this period, the CRL is 240 mm, or 9 in; the weight, 1080 g, or 2 lb, 6 oz.) Most fetuses are considered viable at about 27 weeks.

28th to 31st Weeks

Fetal contours are becoming rounder as a result of deposition of increasing amounts of subcutaneous fat (Fig. 14–10). The fetus will probably survive if born at this time, although its respiratory function may be too immature to permit life. (At the end of this period, the CRL is 275 mm, or 10.82 in; the weight, 1670 g, or 3 lb, 11 oz.)

32nd to 36th Weeks

At 8 months of gestation, the fetus's skin is still wrinkled, but it is steadily gaining weight. The lanugo has disappeared from its face but remains on its head. The vernix caseosa has become thick and continues to protect the skin from exposure to the amniotic fluid. The fingernails are fully grown. With good care the infant will survive if born at this time. (At the end of this period, the CRL is 310 mm, or 12.55 in; the weight, 2400 g, or 5 lb, 4 oz.)

37th to 39th Weeks

The fetus is becoming plumper and less wrinkled because of the increased accumulation of subcutaneous fat. In the male fetus the left testicle descends into the scro-

tum. Chances of survival for infants born during this period are excellent.

RELATED RESEARCH

Fertility Drug May Adversely Affect the Growing Fetus

Researchers at a large western university have found evidence that the fertility drug most commonly used in the United States may potenially interfere with normal fetal development.

It was discovered that the drug Clomiphene, normally used in the treatment of ovulatory failure in women desiring pregnancy, can produce malformations in the developing human reproductive system of the female, which involve the vagina, uterus, and fallopian tubes. Even though women stop taking the drug before attempting pregnancy, evidence shows that the drug remains in the body for weeks afterward.

The researchers feel that while it is possible that levels of Clomiphene in the body may fall below the threshold that would cause birth defects, their current findings, in conjunction with reports of reproductive tract deformities induced in rodents by the drug, raise concerns over the use of Clomiphene as a fertility drug.

Cunha GT: Fertility drug may adversely affect the growing fetus. J Hum Pathol 18:1132, 1987

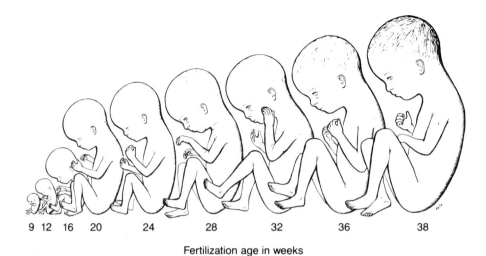

9 12 16   20   24   28   32   36   38

Fertilization age in weeks

Figure 14–10. Fetuses, about one-fifth actual size. Head hair begins to appear at about 20 weeks. Eyebrows and eyelashes are usually recognizable by 24 weeks, and the eyes reopen by 26 weeks. Fetuses born prematurely (22 weeks or more) may survive, but intensive care is required. The mean duration of pregnancy is 266 days (38 weeks) from fertilization, with a standard deviation of 12 days. In clinical practice, it is customary to refer to full term as 40 weeks from the first day of the last menstrual period (*LMP*), assuming that conception occurs 2 weeks after the onset of menses. Thus, when a provider refers to a pregnancy of 20 weeks, the actual age of the fetus is only 18 weeks. (Moore KL: The Developing Human. Philadelphia, WB Saunders, 1982)

40 Weeks

By the end of 40 weeks the fetus is fully developed. The fingernails and toenails are fully formed and extend beyond the fingers and toes. In the male both testes have descended into the scrotum. The skull is developed and is larger than any other portion of the body. (By 40 weeks, the CRL is 350 mm, or 14 in; the weight, 3300 g, or 7 lb, 4 oz.)

FETAL CIRCULATION

Fetal circulation is different from that of the newborn and infant. During fetal life, the fetal lungs do not act as respiratory organs; the gas-exchange function is wholly a placental function. Oxygenated blood flows from the placenta through the umbilical vein. Total blood flow through the umbilical cord has been estimated at approximately 125 ml/kg of body weight per minute, or approximately 500 ml/min in the average human fetus at term (Danforth 1986).

The blood flow continues through the umbilical vein and ductus venosus into the inferior vena cava (Fig. 14–11). It is within the vena cava that blood returning from the lower portion of the body is mixed. This blood then enters the right atrium, whereas blood from the inferior vena cava passes through the foramen ovale into the left

atrium. Its course continues into the left ventricle and through the aortic arch, where it is distributed to all organs except the lungs. Blood circulates through the head and upper extremities and to the trunk and lower extremities.

Venous blood from the upper body enters through the superior vena cava and flows into the right ventricle. Leaving the right ventricle, via the main pulmonary artery, the blood rejoins the aorta by way of the ductus arteriosus. The venous circulation returns to the placenta through the aorta and internal iliac and umbilical arteries, maintaining oxygenation of the placenta (see Fig. 14–4). The foramen ovale and the ductus arteriosus act as bypass channels, allowing a large part of the combined cardiac output to return to the placenta without flowing through the lungs. Approximately 55% of the combined ventricular output flows to the placenta, while 35% perfuses body tissues, the remaining 10% flowing through the lungs (Danforth 1986). Blood flow to the lungs is not for respiratory purposes but rather for nutrition.

Circulatory Transition from Fetal to Extrauterine Life

Blood continues to pass to and from the placenta up to the moment of birth. However, as soon as the baby is born and begins to breathe on its own, placental circulation ceases entirely.

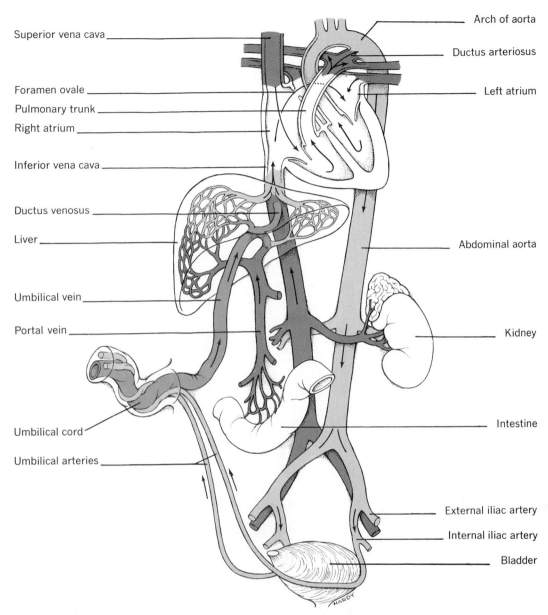

Superior vena cava

Foramen ovale

Pulmonary trunk

Right atrium

Inferior vena cava

Ductus venosus

Liver

Umbilical vein

Portal vein

Umbilical cord

Umbilical arteries

Arch of aorta

Ductus arteriosus

Left atrium

Abdominal aorta

Kidney

Intestine

External iliac artery

Internal iliac artery

Bladder

Figure 14–11. Fetal circulation. By a complex process, oxygen passes from the mother's bloodstream through the placenta and into the fetal blood. The course of blood in the fetus is indicated by arrows. Oxygenated blood travels to all fetal organs except the lungs.

The brain, gastrointestinal tract, kidneys, and, to a lesser degree, the liver of a full-term fetus are poised to function at birth. Transitions that take place during birth involve primarily the heart, lungs, and thermoregulation.

Respiratory efforts are made by most newborns within a few seconds of birth. At birth, the pulmonary alveoli are fluid-filled, and during delivery two important functions occur. Clamping the cord produces a drop in fetal arterial tension and a rise in blood carbon dioxide levels. As a result, the infant begins to gasp and, in conjunction with

neurologic and environmental stimuli, to breathe, air entering the alveoli with a positive intrathoracic pressure of up to 40 cm H_2O. As air enters the lungs, they expand and a rush of blood enters the pulmonary circulation. After the first few breaths there is almost complete lung expansion (Danforth 1986). This was not the case earlier in the century, when heavy maternal medication and general anesthesia were widely employed for delivery. The onset of breathing was frequently delayed for several minutes, during which tactile and thermal stimuli were applied, often combined with the administration of analeptics (Danforth 1986).

Venous return to the left atrium causes the foramen ovale to close, changing fetal circulation to adult-type circulation. When placental blood flow has ceased, functional closure of the ductus venosus occurs. Within 12 to 24 hours, the ductus arteriosus also closes.

Evaluation of the newborn at birth and shortly after is essential to the identification of problems that may affect its health during the postpartum period. The most important assessments include Apgar scoring, physical examination, and gestational maturity (see Unit V).

CHAPTER SUMMARY

Development of the fetus is a complex process. Even though combinations of genetic and environmental factors influence its growth and development, the process of becoming a unique individual occurs in a predictable sequence and in a predictable time.

The health status of mothers and the babies they carry is the most important single factor influencing the future health and well-being of all people. The provision of anticipatory guidance to women who are planning pregnancy, such as the preconception planning concept, could assist women in achieving a normal pregnancy and averting potential problems during the prenatal period. Women who are well-informed about the process of pregnancy and its progression are better prepared to deal with minor or major problems that may occur during the prenatal period and to seek prompt care.

STUDY QUESTIONS

1. Why are the first 8 weeks of life *in utero* so critical?
2. What are the major functions of the placenta, and how are these accomplished?

3. Explain the primary physiologic developments during the fetal period.

REFERENCES/BIBLIOGRAPHY

Battaglla FC, Meschea G: An Introduction to Fetal Physiology. Orlando, Academic Press, Harcourt Brace Jovanovich, 1986

Cunha GR: Fertility drug may adversely affect the growing fetus. J Hum Pathol 18:1132, 1987

Danforth DN, Scott JR (eds): Obstetrics and Gynecology, 5th ed. Philadelphia, JB Lippincott, 1986

Filkins K, Russon J: Human Prenatal Diagnosis. New York, Marcel Dekker, 1986

Kurjak, A: The Fetus as a Patient. Amsterdam-New York, Elsevier Science, 1985

Lavery JP: The Human Placenta: Clinical Perspective. Rockville, Aspen Publishers, Inc., 1987

Moore KL: The Developing Human, 3rd ed. Philadelphia, WB Saunders, 1982

Pritchard JA, MacDonald PC, Gant NF: Williams Obstetrics, 17th ed. East Norwalk, Appleton–Century–Crofts, 1985

Reeder SJ, Martin LL: Maternity Nursing: Family, Newborn, and Women's Health Care, 16th ed. Philadelphia, JB Lippincott, 1987

Sadler TW: Langman's Medical Embryology, 5th ed. Baltimore, Williams & Wilkins, 1985

Snell RS: Clinical Embryology for Medical Students, 3rd ed. Boston, Little Brown, 1983

SUGGESTED READINGS

Bernhardt J: Sensory capabilities of the fetus. MCN 12(6):44–46, 1987

Gantes M, Bartauius VM, Roberts J: The use of daily fetal movement records in a clinical setting. J Obstet Gynecol Neonatal Nurs 15(5):390, 1986

Smotherman WP, Robinson SR: Prenatal influences on development behavior is not a trivial aspect of fetal life. J Devel Behav Pediatr 8(3):171–176, 1987

15 nutritional aspects of pregnancy

LEARNING OBJECTIVES

After studying the material in this chapter, the student should be able to

- Identify steps to assess, maintain, and promote the nutritional status of pregnant women

- Identify and relate nutritional risk factors during pregnancy

- Use recommended dietary guidelines in helping pregnant women meet their nutritional needs

- Specify recommended daily intake of vitamins and minerals that are particularly important during pregnancy

- Offer appropriate nutrition counseling to pregnant women based on assessment of economic, religious, and cultural factors

KEY TERMS

Calorie

Joule

Kilocalorie

Megadose

Nutritional requirement

Pica

Recommended Daily Allowances (RDA)

Pregnancy is a unique period in the life cycle because at no other time is the well-being of one individual — the baby — so directly dependent on the well-being of another — the mother. The mother's nutritional status is an important determinant of her own well-being and the health of her fetus.

Nutritional care during pregnancy includes assessment and intervention to rehabilitate underweight and undernourished pregnant women and is necessary to ensure normal fetal growth and development. The nurse must appreciate the importance of nutrition and be knowledgeable about how the normal physiologic changes during pregnancy relate to nutritional needs.

This chapter presents basic information on the effects of maternal nutritional status on the course and outcome of pregnancy and describes daily nutritional requirements during pregnancy. Factors that affect women's dietary patterns during pregnancy are discussed, and nutritional risk factors are identified. Finally, an outline is given of the nursing process in the assessment of nutritional status and in interventions aimed at assisting the pregnant woman to improve her dietary pattern, reduce risks of complications, and help ensure delivery of a healthy newborn.

BASIS OF NUTRITIONAL CARE DURING PREGNANCY

Teamwork in Prenatal Nutritional Care

Effective implementation of nutritional care may involve a number of health professionals working together as a team. The entire health team plays a role in carrying out the nutritional care plan. There must be communication among the health team through progress notes in the patient's chart and through case conferences, where appropriate, so that the nutritional advice given to the woman is consistent.

The health care professionals comprising the team may include the physician, physician assistant, certified nurse midwife, registered nurse, nurse practitioner, public health nurse, registered dietitian, social worker, health educator, childbirth educator, community health worker, or nutrition aide. Additional providers may also be part of the interdisciplinary team, depending upon the specific needs of the population being served.

Selection of the most appropriate nutrition care provider must be made to meet the needs of the clientele and the type of practice. Nutrition services may be carried out by a nutritionist and/or a registered dietitian or by other health professionals in consultation with the nutritionist and/or dietitian.

All health professionals involved in the delivery of perinatal nutrition services should have the knowledge and

skills necessary to provide direct services to women with uncomplicated pregnancies or low-risk patients and to normal infants. For example, perinatal nutrition service providers should be able to:

- Evaluate current dietary practices.
- Counsel on nutrient needs and recommended diet during pregnancy and infancy.
- Refer, as necessary, to community resources such as social service and food assistance programs.
- Monitor and interpret clinical data pertinent to nutritional assessment of the woman.
- Identify risk factors.
- Seek consultation regarding, and refer as necessary, women considered to be at high nutritional risk.
- Provide information and advice on breast-feeding or alternative methods of infant feeding.
- Counsel on nutrient needs during lactation.

Much of this knowledge and many of these skills are necessary for the early identification, treatment, and referral of women with major nutritional problems.

Health care professionals who provide direct nutrition services for women with nutritionally high-risk conditions or for parents of infants with nutritionally high-risk conditions require specialized nutritional knowledge and advanced communication skills. To assure optimal outcome, direct services to high-risk clients should be developed and delivered by the nutritionist and/or registered dietitian and approved by the provider who has overall responsibility for assuring quality care.

In addition to having the knowledge and skills identified above for the uncomplicated pregnancy, the registered dietitian is uniquely trained to evaluate and manage the nutritional care of pregnant women with complex medical and surgical problems, such as diabetes mellitus, chronic renal disease, cardiac problems, and chronic lung disease. This would include: (1) screening for nutritional problems; (2) monitoring and assessing nutritional status; (3) developing and implementing complicated management plans; and (4) providing instructional resources for special dietary modifications (California Department of Health Services 1988). A registered dietitian will also be able to develop and assure continuity of nutrition care plans, including coordination and referral to local agencies with food and nutrition resources, as well as to provide follow-up services for clients and to monitor and evaluate results of nutrition intervention.

Importance of Nutrition During Pregnancy

Good nutrition is a product of lifelong eating patterns, and improved dietary habits during pregnancy cannot make up entirely for previous deficiencies. However, many pregnant women are highly motivated to change patterns for the good of their unborn child. Routine prenatal care also allows for ongoing nutritional guidance, reinforcement, and support. For these reasons, pregnancy is an excellent opportunity to assist women in choosing healthier diets for themselves and their families. If positive changes in eating habits become part of a lifestyle, they can contribute to improved family health for years to come.

The importance of adequate maternal nutrition to the course and outcome of pregnancy can be well appreciated when indicators of fetal development and perinatal mortality and morbidity are examined.

Adequate nutrition during pregnancy reduces the risk of maternal complications, ensures that tissue growth proceeds normally, and increases the likelihood that the newborn will attain an optimal birth weight. Mothers with nutritional deficiencies before and during pregnancy are more likely to experience certain complications, such as preeclampsia and anemia, and their infants have a higher perinatal morbidity and mortality caused by problems associated with low birth weight, malformations, and disturbances in cell development.

Inadequate maternal nutrition has a devastating effect on brain development in the fetus and newborn. The period of maximum brain growth in humans occurs late in fetal development. If the mother's nutrition is not adequate, the fetal brain will not develop fully and the number of brain cells will be low. The infant can never replace brain cells that did not develop *in utero,* although some researchers argue that the quality of brain cells can be improved by a good diet in infancy.

Birth weight is of major significance in both infant mortality and infant morbidity and is directly affected by maternal nutrition. Low birth weight is a known etiologic factor in cerebral palsy. There is also evidence that, as a group, children who were extremely undersized at birth have more frequent hospitalizations for illness, more hearing and visual disabilities, more behavioral disorders, and more learning problems when they enter school.

Numerous studies have reported a strong relationship between birth weight and maternal prepregnant weight and weight gain during pregnancy. This indicates the importance of nutritional guidance before pregnancy and early nutritional care during pregnancy. Some maternal factors have a direct impact on the nutritional status and birth weight of infants. For instance, smoking interferes with metabolic processes in the body, resulting in lower-birth-weight infants. Adolescent mothers are at higher risk of producing premature and low-birth-weight babies than women in their twenties. This probably reflects the fact that many adolescent mothers come from socioeconomically disadvantaged families and have especially poor nutritional patterns before and during their pregnancies. However, when adequate maternal weight gain

during pregnancy is achieved despite the presence of such risk factors, the chances that the infant will achieve optimal infant birth weight are increased.

The importance of nutrition during the childbearing year extends to the well-being of the infant in the first years of life. As mentioned before, brain cell development in the fetus can be decreased dramatically if the mother is poorly nourished. The infant's brain development can be arrested even further if it is malnourished in the early weeks of life. This may occur when impoverished families cannot afford infant formula and substitute other foods. However, infant malnutrition can also occur when the mother is too undernourished to produce sufficient amounts of high-quality breast milk.

Malnutrition among infants is a major contributor to infant mortality. Malnutrition in the very young does not usually kill outright but rather lowers resistance to infections and parasitic diseases that would not be life-threatening to a well-nourished infant. The most comprehensive investigation of infant mortality conducted in the Western hemisphere was carried out by the Pan American Health Organization (PAHO) in the early 1970s. Examining data on 35,000 infant deaths in 15 regions of North and South America, it found that *undernutrition* was associated with 34% of these deaths in Latin American communities. For most, death was due to diarrhea, measles, pneumonia, or some other disease for which malnutrition set the stage. Another third of the deaths was caused by prematurity, which is often a product of undernutrition in the mother.

Physiologic Changes During Pregnancy and Effects on Nutrition

The mother undergoes many complex physiologic adjustments during pregnancy. Some of these adjustments regulate maternal metabolism and promote optimal fetal growth and development. Others preserve maternal homeostasis and prepare the mother for labor, birth, and lactation. These physiologic changes affect the mother's appetite, digestion, absorption, and utilization of nutrients in many ways.

Hormonal Effects on Nutrition

During pregnancy, the placenta assumes a major role in the production of hormones. Some hormones are produced only during pregnancy, including human chorionic gonadotropin (HCG), human placental lactogen (HPL; also called human chorionic somatomammotropin [HCS]), and human chorionic thyrotropin (HCT). Other hormones that are normally present, such as progesterone and estrogen, are produced at higher levels during pregnancy, and have direct effects on metabolism and nutrition. For instance, progesterone causes a relaxation of the smooth muscles, including the gastrointestinal tract. This relaxation of the gastrointestinal tract reduces motility in the gut, allowing more time for the nutrients to be absorbed. Other metabolic effects of progesterone are increased maternal fat deposition and increased renal sodium excretion. Estrogen has a hygroscopic, or water-retaining effect. As a result, many pregnant women complain of excess fluid retention, which is regarded as normal. Morning nausea, which can have a significant impact on the mother's dietary intake, is believed to be caused in part by elevated HCG levels.

Metabolic Changes During Pregnancy

Some maternal physiologic adjustments have effects on overall metabolism and are the basis for the increased nutritional requirements and dietary allowances during pregnancy. These metabolic adjustments include:

- Increased plasma volume. Near the end of the first trimester of pregnancy, plasma volume begins to increase. By 34 weeks, it is about 50% greater than at conception, creating an increased need to carry nutrients and oxygenation.
- Progressive increases in blood lipids. Lipid levels, including serum triglycerides, cholesterol, free fatty acids, and vitamin A, increase during pregnancy. This is probably caused by the increase in circulating steroids, since cholesterol is a precursor for the synthesis of progesterone and estrogen in the placenta.
- Increase in red blood cells. Red cell production is stimulated during pregnancy, but because the increase is not as large as the expansion of plasma volume, hemodilution occurs. Plasma volume is increased by 50% at 34 weeks, whereas red blood cell volume has increased by only 20%.
- Increase in white blood cells
- Changes in renal function. There is an increased blood flow through the kidneys and an increase in the glomerular filtration rate to facilitate the clearance of waste products of baby and mother.
- Increase in cardiac output

These metabolic adjustments require an overall increase in requirements for nutrients and food energy. The next section discusses specific nutritional needs.

Nutrient Requirements During Pregnancy

During pregnancy, the mother must meet her own nutritional needs, in addition to the needs of the growing fetus, and additional demands from the growth of new tissue. Although this growth process means that requirements for all nutrients are increased during pregnancy, some nutrients are of particular importance in pregnancy. The following summary of requirements for food energy, protein, vitamins, and minerals during pregnancy is based on nationally recognized Recommended Dietary Allowances (RDA) (Neeson et al, 1983).

Energy Requirements

Additional calories are needed during pregnancy to support increased tissue synthesis by the mother and fetus and the additional metabolic cost incurred by this new tissue. Adequate intake of calories for energy is necessary for optimal protein utilization and tissue growth.

The generally accepted figure for the total energy cost of pregnancy is 80,000 kcal. When this figure is divided over the length of pregnancy, it averages out to an additional 300 calories per day above nonpregnant needs. Because caloric requirements are difficult to predict and vary widely among pregnant women, factors such as maternal age, activity, height, prepregnant weight, health, and stage of pregnancy must be considered. Because of differences in these parameters, individual caloric needs should be calculated by allowing a minimum of 36 kcal per kilogram of pregnant body weight. The pregnant adolescent's energy needs may be as high as 50 kcal/kg/day, depending on her daily activity levels and growth rate. Table 15–1 summarizes energy requirements during pregnancy.

Caloric expenditure is not distributed evenly throughout gestation. There is a slight increase during early preg-

Table 15–1   **Energy Requirements During Pregnancy**

Age in Years	Recommended Ratio kcal/kg Body Wt.	Nonpregnant Requirement (kcal/day)	Pregnant Requirement (kcal/day)
11–15	50	2200	2500
15–22	40	2100	2400
23–50	36	2000	2300

(Adapted from National Research Council: Recommended Dietary Allowances, 9th ed. Washington, DC, National Academy of Science, 1980)

Table 15–2   **Protein Requirements During Pregnancy**

Age in Years	Recommended Ratio g/kg Body Wt	Nonpregnant Requirement (g/day)	Pregnant Requirement (g/day)
11–15	1.7	46	76
15–18	1.5	46	76
19–50	1.3	44	74

(Adapted from National Research Council: Recommended Dietary Allowances, 9th ed. Washington, DC, National Academy of Science, 1980)

nancy, with a sharp increase near the end of the first trimester. This level then remains constant until term. During the second trimester, most of this extra caloric expenditure is devoted to maternal factors (blood expansion, growth of uterus, growth of breast tissue, and fat storage); during the last trimester, the caloric expenditure is due primarily to the growth of the fetus and placenta.

Protein Requirements

Protein is needed in increased amounts during pregnancy to provide sufficient amino acids for fetal development, for blood volume expansion, and for growth of maternal breast and uterine tissues. The current RDA for protein intake is an additional 30 g protein per day over nonpregnant needs, or a total allowance of 1.3 g/kg/day in an adult woman. It is important to remember that adequate protein intake without adequate calories should be avoided; if caloric intake is below the required amount, protein will be used for maternal energy needs rather than for its primary function of tissue building and maintenance (see Table 15–2 for recommended protein intake).

Vitamin Requirements

Generally requirements for all vitamins are increased during pregnancy (Tables 15–3 and 15–4). The accelerated energy and protein metabolism require increased

amounts of vitamins for tissue synthesis and energy production. One vitamin requiring special attention in pregnancy is folic acid (folacin).

Folic Acid (Folacin)

Folic acid or folacin is a vitamin that functions as a coenzyme in the synthesis of DNA. Clinical evidence of folic acid deficiency is usually first seen in tissues that have a rapid cell turnover, such as red blood cells. Folacin promotes fetal growth and prevents the macrocytic, megaloblastic anemia of pregnancy. The RDA for folacin is doubled during gestation from 400 μg/day to 800 μg/day. This amount can be provided by natural foods, such as dark green leafy vegetables, organ meats, eggs, milk, oranges, bananas, dry beans, and whole grain breads. However, this vitamin is very sensitive to high heat; overcooking foods may destroy as much as 80% of the folic acid activity. Many diets, even in developed countries, provide inadequate amounts of folacin. As a result, many authorities suggest that supplements of 400 μg/day to 800 μg/day of folic acid be prescribed for pregnant women. Supplementation is definitely in order for those pregnant women who are considered high-risk because of poverty, poor dietary habits, frequent or multiple pregnancies, chronic hemolytic anemia, and anticoagulant drug therapy. There is some evidence that a deficiency of

Table 15–3   **Recommended Intake of Fat-Soluble Vitamins**

Age in Years	Nonpregnant Intake			Pregnant Intake		
	Vitamin A (mcg RE)*	Vitamin D (mcg)	Vitamin E (mg TE)†	Vitamin A (mcg RE)	Vitamin D (mcg)	Vitamin E (mg TE)
11–14	800	10.0	8	1000	15.0	10
15–18	800	10.0	8	1000	15.0	10
19–22	800	7.5	8	1000	12.5	10
23–50	800	5.0	8	1000	10.0	10

* RE = retinol equivalents.
   800 = 4,000 IU (international units)
   1000 = 5,000 IU (international units)
† TE = tocopherol equivalents
(Adapted from National Research Council: Recommended Dietary Allowances, 9th ed. Washington, DC, National Academy of Science, 1980)

Table 15–4   Recommended Intake of Water-Soluble Vitamins

Vitamin	Age in Years			
	11–14	*15–18*	*19–22*	*23–50*
Nonpregnant Intake				
Vitamin C (mg)	50.0	60.0	60.0	60.0
Thiamin (mg)	1.1	1.1	1.1	1.0
Riboflavin (mg)	1.3	1.3	1.3	1.2
Niacin (mg)	15.0	14.0	14.0	13.0
Vitamin B-6 (mg)	1.8	2.0	2.0	2.0
Folacin (mg)	400.0	400.0	400.0	400.0
Vitamin B-12 (μg)	3.0	3.0	3.0	3.0
Pregnant Intake				
Vitamin C (mg)	70.0	80.0	80.0	80.0
Thiamin (mg)	1.5	1.5	1.5	1.4
Riboflavin (mg)	1.6	1.6	1.6	1.5
Niacin (mg)	17.0	16.0	16.0	15.0
Vitamin B-6 (mg)	2.4	2.6	2.6	2.6
Folacin (μg)	800.0	800.0	800.0	800.0
Vitamin B-12 (μg)	4.0	4.0	4.0	4.0

(Adapted from National Research Council: Recommended Dietary Allowances, 9th ed. Washington, DC, National Academy of Science, 1980)

folic acid may be associated with abruptio placentae, spontaneous abortion, preeclampsia, fetal malformations, especially neural tube defects, and subnormal infant development (Smithells 1980). Conclusive proof relating folic acid deficiency to adverse pregnancy outcome may never be possible from human studies. However, recommendations to pregnant women about folic acid intake must stress that the needs during pregnancy are increased and the intake in most diets is low.

Multiple Vitamin-Mineral Supplements

Since a prenatal vitamin-mineral supplement, in addition to iron and folic acid, is routinely recommended for prenatal patients, it is advisable that these supplements contain those nutrients whose intake by pregnant women is most likely to be inadequate. Therefore, it is recommended that a prenatal supplement contain at least vitamins B$_6$, D, E, C, folic acid, and pantothenic acid, and the minerals iron, calcium, magnesium, zinc, and copper.

It is important to note that the presence of moderate doses of calcium (especially calcium phosphate) and magnesium in a supplement may decrease iron absorption from that supplement, particularly when it is taken on an empty stomach (Biswas 1984, Seligman 1983). This could be related to a decrease in stomach acidity caused by some forms of calcium, which can occur when no food is present in the stomach (Recker 1985). It appears advisable to choose a prenatal supplement that does not contain large amounts of calcium or magnesium (greater than 250 mg and 100 mg, respectively), as well as one that does not contain the phosphate salt of calcium. In-

gestion of supplements with food may also be helpful because absorption of supplemental iron may be enhanced by the simultaneous ingestion of vitamin C and/or animal tissue. Considering the above information, guidelines for selection of a prenatal supplement are listed in the display.

If a woman is unwilling or unable to ingest sufficient calcium-rich foods to obtain the calcium required daily in pregnancy, calcium supplements may be recommended. If calcium supplements are required, consider the following guidelines for selection:

- They may be in the form of: calcium carbonate (40% elemental calcium), calcium citrate (24% elemental calcium), calcium lactate (14% elemental calcium), or calcium gluconate (9% elemental calcium).

- Calcium phosphate is not recommended because this form of calcium is poorly absorbed, and it interferes with iron absorption.

- The amount of calcium required from supplements depends on dietary intake. If supplemental calcium in dosages greater than 250 to 300 mg are required daily due to low dietary intake, it is recommended that the dosage be split into increments of 250 to 300 mg and each taken with a meal or snack to enhance absorption. Such dosages equal the amount of calcium in a serving from the milk-product group.

- Because of the mixed effects of calcium on iron and zinc absorption and retention, daily supplements with more than 100 g (1000 mg) of calcium is not recommended during pregnancy.

Guidelines for Selection of a Prenatal Supplement

- Contains a wide range of vitamins and minerals (particularly vitamins B$_6$ and D, E, folic acid, pantothenic acid, calcium, magnesium, iron, and possibly vitamin C, zinc and copper)
- Contains folic acid at the level of 0.4–0.8 mg/daily dose
- Contains iron at the level of 30–60 mg/daily dose
- Does not contain high levels of calcium and magnesium (greater than 250 mg and 100 mg, respectively)
- Does not contain calcium in the form of calcium phosphate
- Contains 5–10 mg of vitamin B$_6$/daily dose
- Contains vitamin E, zinc and copper at, or near, the RDA amounts of 15 IU, 20 mg, and 2 mg, respectively, if the iron content of the supplement exceeds 30 mg. (Higher amounts of zinc and copper should probably be avoided until further research indicates safety.)
- Contains vitamins C, D, and pantothenic acid at, or near, the RDA amounts of 80 mg, 400 IU, and 4–7 mg, respectively
- Reasonably priced and readily available

Adapted from: California Department of Health Services, Maternal and Child Health Branch. Nutrition During Pregnancy and the Postpartum Period: A Manual for Health Care Professionals, 1988

Women should be advised to use calcium supplements only if their diet is inadequate. Dietary sources are best, not only because they are well absorbed but other essential nutrients are present in foods.

Patients should be warned not to take more than the recommended daily dose of their prenatal tablet or recommended supplements. Some women concerned about their poor diet may decide to double or triple the recommended daily dose. This is of particular concern because an overdose of the fat-soluble vitamins A and D is possible at such levels of intake.

Vitamin Oversupplementation: "High Intake" and "Megadose"

Vitamin supplementation is a common self-care practice. Americans yearly spend over $1.5 billion on food supplements.

The terms *high intake* and *high dose* are used almost interchangeably when referring to large amounts of vita-

mins and minerals. High-dose intake of vitamins is often greatly in excess of the RDAs, which are the amounts judged "to meet the known nutritional needs of practically all healthy persons" (Biswas et al, 1984). *Megadose* refers to an amount that is at least ten times greater than the RDA. These excessive amounts are considered to be pharmacologic in strength; that is, they are so high that the vitamins or minerals act more as drugs than as nutrients. Since fat-soluble vitamins (A-D-E-K) tend to be stored in the liver and are excreted minimally in the urine, toxicity is a real danger for those ingesting high doses.

Vitamin A Toxicity

Vitamin A, which has received much publicity as a possible preventive agent for cancer, can cause toxicity in high doses. Side-effects of vitamin A toxicity include skin lesions, hair loss, headache, blurred vision, and diarrhea. The more serious toxic manifestations of vitamin A include liver, kidney, and bone damage. Vitamin A is a teratogen, and ingestion of high doses may lead to fetal abnormalities. Since prolonged intake of vitamin A at ten times the RDA or more can lead to severe toxicity, patients should be questioned about their use of vitamin A supplements.

Vitamin E Toxicity

Vitamin E in excessive amounts can interfere with vitamin K metabolism and blood coagulation. Depression and fatigue may occur after ingestion of 900 mg/day.

Vitamin D Toxicity

Vitamin D facilitates calcium and phosphorus absorption from the intestine. Some claim that megadoses of vitamin D will build stronger bones, especially if the vitamin is taken in a natural form, such as fish liver oil. However, vitamin D is perhaps the most toxic of the fat-soluble vitamins. Excess vitamin D causes calcium to be deposited in soft tissue, which can result in irreversible kidney damage. During pregnancy, excessive intake of vitamin D may contribute to the production of severe maternal and neonatal hypercalcemia.

Vitamin C Toxicity

Since vitamin C is a water-soluble vitamin, for many years most people considered large doses to be safe. However, megadoses of vitamin C may interfere with the normal metabolic process and can cause nausea, abdominal cramps, and diarrhea. In susceptible individuals, megadoses of vitamin C may precipitate kidney stones, interfere with copper metabolism, give inaccurate results in certain laboratory tests, adversely affect growing bone and, in pregnant women, cause neonatal bleeding. The value of consumption of large doses of vitamin C as therapy or for prophylactic purposes is questionable.

Mineral Requirements

Mineral requirements are also increased during pregnancy. This section discusses specific needs for iron, calcium, sodium, and zinc. (See Table 15–5 for recommended dietary intake of these minerals during pregnancy.)

Iron Requirements

Pregnancy imposes substantial demands for iron, primarily because of the markedly increased volume of the maternal blood supply and the growth of fetal and maternal tissues. Most iron in the body is in the form of hemoglobin, which is responsible for carrying oxygen to the body's cells, and the adequacy of the mother's iron store is reflected in the concentration of hemoglobin.

The "iron cost" of a full-term pregnancy with a single fetus has been calculated to be about 1000 mg. This means that approximately 3 mg *absorbed iron* is required *daily* during pregnancy. Both the fetus and the placenta effectively drain iron and folate from the mother, even if she is grossly deficient. This iron drain reaches a peak after the 20th week of pregnancy. Iron balance is also influenced by the mode of delivery: vaginal delivery is associated with a blood loss of at least 500 ml blood, which represents over 200 mg iron; cesarean section is associated with at least 1000 ml of blood loss, which represents more than 400 mg iron.

Although a portion of these needs could be met from the iron stores in the bone marrow, liver, and spleen, rarely are these sufficient to cover all the woman's needs without compromising her well-being. In men, iron stores range from 500 to 1500 mg, but in women, they tend to be much lower or even nonexistent because women tend to have diets low in iron and because blood is lost through menstruation.

Women with borderline iron stores will develop iron deficiency anemia if their iron intake is not supplemented during pregnancy. Even a woman whose nutritional status is excellent will complete a pregnancy with a deficit in available iron, if her dietary intake is not supplemented.

Nonpregnant women absorb only about 10% of the available iron in food. Thus, the dietary requirement of 18 mg/day for the nonpregnant woman produces an average of 1.8 mg/day for body use. During the second half of pregnancy, the efficiency of iron absorption from food increases to about 25%; in addition, the mother's iron loss is lessened by the cessation of menstrual blood flow. However, even with these physiologic adjustments, the increased iron requirement during pregnancy cannot be met by the iron content in typical American diets. The average American's diet contains only about 6 mg iron per 1000 calories. Thus, most authorities advise routine iron supplementation at levels of 30 mg to 60 mg ferrous iron daily throughout gestation and the early puerperium to replenish stores depleted by pregnancy. This iron supplement is given as 30 mg to 60 mg elemental iron or a simple ferrous salt, such as ferrous sulphate ($FeSO_4$), which is most readily absorbed.

Iron Deficiency Anemia. The most common nutritional disorder of pregnancy is iron deficiency anemia. Its symptoms include fatigue, anorexia, pallor, inability to concentrate, listlessness, and irritability. This condition

---

Table 15–5   **Recommended Intake of Minerals**

Mineral	Age in Years			
	11–14	*15–18*	*19–22*	*23–50*
Nonpregnant Intake				
Calcium (mg)	1200	1200	800	800
Phosphorus (mg)	1200	1200	800	800
Magnesium (mg)	300	300	300	300
Iron (mg)	18	18	18	18
Zinc (mg)	15	15	15	15
Iodine (mg)	150	150	150	150
Pregnant Intake				
Calcium (mg)	1600	1600	1200	1200
Phosphorus (mg)	1600	1600	1200	1200
Magnesium (mg)	450	450	450	450
Iron (mg)*	18	18	18	18
Zinc (mg)	20	20	20	20
Iodine (mg)	175	175	175	175

* An additional 30 to 60 mg of supplemental iron is needed daily in addition to dietary sources.
(Adapted from National Research Council: Recommended Dietary Allowances, 9th ed. Washington, DC, National Academy of Science, 1980)

causes a reduction in the capacity to do energy-requiring tasks because the iron deficiency imposes a limit on the body's ability to transport oxygen to the tissues.

There are three stages in the development of iron-deficiency anemia:

Stage 1. More iron is needed than the amount entering the body, and iron is mobilized from stores in the bone marrow, liver, and spleen. Continued depletion of iron stores causes a drop in the levels of serum transferrin, a protein that transports iron in the blood. Decreased saturation of serum transferrin during pregnancy (less than 15%) indicates that iron stores are inadequate. As a compensatory response to iron depletion, the efficiency of iron binding in the blood rises.

Stage 2. When iron stores are depleted, the marrow, in an attempt to conserve iron, produces fewer red cells. With continued iron depletion, the marrow is forced to produce red cells with lower levels of hemoglobin. Red blood cells produced during this stage are described as *normocytic* (normal in size) and *hypochromic* (pale in color).

Stage 3. Continued depletion leads to a deterioration in the quality and quantity of erythrocytes. The marrow is forced to produce smaller cells with less hemoglobin (i.e., *microcytic* and *hypochromic*). Cells of this kind are diagnostic of iron deficiency anemia.

In the prevention and treatment of iron deficiency anemia, there are two goals: correction of the deficit and replenishment of the iron stores. The iron in dietary iron supplements can be contained in one of several compounds. These vary according to the amount of available elemental iron they provide. The recommended supplemental intake is 30 to 60 mg/day elemental iron throughout pregnancy. The following calculations can be used to determine the amount of elemental iron provided by each compound.

$$\text{mg ferrous sulfate} \times 29\% = \text{mg elemental iron}$$
$$\text{mg ferrous gluconate} \times 12\% = \text{mg elemental iron}$$
$$\text{mg ferrous fumarate} \times 33\% = \text{mg elemental iron}$$

Iron is absorbed primarily in the stomach and upper duodenum. Iron supplements may cause gastrointestinal upsets, which can be minimized if the iron is taken with meals. Patients may also tolerate one form of dietary iron supplement more readily than another.

Calcium and Phosphorus Requirements

During pregnancy, extra calcium is required for fetal bone development. In the third trimester, the fetus accumulates calcium at an average rate of 300 mg/day. If calcium intake is inadequate, fetal needs will be met by demineralization of the maternal skeleton. Pregnancy is accompanied by extensive adjustments in calcium metabolism; hormonal factors, phosphorus, and vitamin D all positively affect maternal calcium retention. The recommended dietary requirement for calcium in pregnancy is an additional 400 mg/day over the nonpregnant need, for a total daily calcium intake of 1200 mg for the adult pregnant woman.

The requirement for phosphorus is similar to that for calcium; however, phosphorus is so widely available in foods that a dietary deficiency is rare. Calcium and phosphorus exist in a balanced ratio in the blood; this ratio can be disturbed by the amounts of calcium and phosphorus in foods. The American diet is high in phosphorus. High levels are found in most animal protein foods, and even greater amounts are found in processed foods, meats, and cola drinks. With the exception of dairy products, foods that are high in phosphorus contain only small amounts of calcium.

Sodium Requirements

Much has been learned in recent years about normal physiology of pregnancy. One result is that *sodium or salt restrictions are no longer advocated* for pregnant women. In years past, sodium restriction was recommended for pregnant women to prevent edema; this was thought to reduce the risk of eclampsia. However, it is now known that sodium metabolism is altered during pregnancy. In a normal pregnancy, the glomerular filtration rate is increased by approximately 50%. Compensatory mechanisms come into play to maintain fluid and electrolyte balance; the increased fluid normally retained during pregnancy actually increases the body's need for sodium. Although moderation in use of salt and other sodium-rich foods is appropriate for everyone, sodium restriction is not recommended during pregnancy. The recommended daily sodium intake is 2 to 3 g.

Zinc Requirements

The role of zinc in the synthesis of DNA and RNA makes it a highly important element in reproduction. Maternal zinc deficiency in rats has been shown to be highly teratogenic. In humans, the incidence of central nervous system malformations appears to be increased in areas where zinc deficiency is common. Marginal zinc deficiency has been documented in the United States. More recently, impaired taste acuity and subnormal growth in children have been associated with marginal zinc deficiency.

Marginal zinc deficiency may develop over a period of weeks. Therefore, it is important that zinc be supplied in the mother's diet daily. The RDA for zinc in pregnancy is 20 mg/day, an increase of 5 mg/day over the nonpreg-

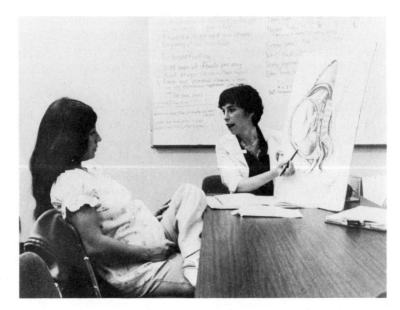

Figure 15–1. Nutrition teaching should assist the pregnant woman to appreciate the direct connection between good nutrition and fetal well-being. (Photo: Michele Vignes)

nant RDA. Zinc intake is closely related to protein intake in the diet, since animal proteins constitute the principal dietary sources of zinc. Meat, liver, eggs, and seafood (especially oysters) are the best sources of zinc. Milk, wheat germ, and legumes are good sources. The pregnant woman at risk for zinc deficiency is likely to have a dietary pattern that excludes complex carbohydrates (no legumes or whole grains) and dairy products and contains little or no meat. Those adhering to a strict vegan diet (no milk, animal protein, or eggs) are at risk for zinc deficiency. Diabetes also causes an increase in zinc losses.

IMPLICATIONS FOR NURSING CARE

The nurse's role in nutritional care of the pregnant woman involves careful assessment of nutritional status, intervention based on identified needs, and ongoing evaluation of the woman's nutritional status as pregnancy progresses. The nurse working in the outpatient setting has a particular responsibility in this area, especially if the setting does not allow for routine patient contact with a professional nutritionist. It is important to keep in mind the effect on the patient of the nurse's own positive attitude about nutrition. The nurse's enthusiasm, sensitivity, and awareness of the patient's needs contribute just as directly to effective nutritional counseling as her knowledge of principles and goals in nutritional care (Fig. 15–1).

Assessment of Nutritional Status

Data Used in Nutritional Evaluation

Cultural, socioeconomic, family, and developmental factors all come into play in forming nutritional habits. The nurse must collect this pertinent information as part of her assessment of a woman's nutritional status during pregnancy.

The nurse must rely on four types of data in her evaluation of the pregnant woman's nutritional status:

• Health history
• Physical examination
• Laboratory tests
• Dietary history

Each of these will be discussed in greater detail.

Health History

Assessment of the pregnant woman's nutritional status begins with a carefully taken health history, with special attention to obstetric history. These data help to identify nutritional problems that may be risk factors in the current pregnancy.

The health history is especially important in identifying factors that put pregnant women at nutritional risk.

Physical Examination

The physical examination is an important aspect of nutritional assessment. Probably the most important part of the physical examination is assessment of the prepreg-

(text continued on page 371)

Assessment Tool

Nutritional Assessment for Pregnant Women

Name _____ Date _____ Gestational age _____

Race _____ Language _____ Marital status _____

Date of birth _____ Education _____

Income needed _____ Food assistance needed _____

History
Previous Obstetric Record
Abortions: Yes _____ No _____ Elective _____ Spontaneous _____

Morbidity: LBW _____ Malf _____ Other _____

Mortality: Fetal _____ Neonatal _____

Physical Assessment
Age _____ Weight before pregnancy _____ Height _____

Present weight _____ Gain _____ Ideal weight _____ Under/over _____ pounds

Medical Assessment
Anemia, infections, diabetes, heart disease, liver diseases, tuberculosis, psychiatric illness, drug abuse, Rh incompatibility

Use of vitamins/mineral supplements _____

Vomiting _____ Frequency _____

Meals: Before _____ After _____ Duration _____ Pernicious _____

Potential Risk Factors Affecting Nutritional Status *(circle)*
underweight   overweight   severe nausea, vomiting   smoker   pica   adolescent

short interpartum period   birth control pills   income restricted   chronic disease (specify)

lactose intolerance   food allergy (specify)   strict vegetarian   lactating   twins

weight loss during pregnancy   fast weight gain

Other risk factors or problems _____

_____

_____

Drugs used: Tobacco   How much?   Exercise habits _____

Alcohol   How much?   Kind _____

Caffeine   How much?   Duration _____

                                                 Frequency _____

(continued)

Assessment Tool   (continued)

24-Hour Diet Recall

Time	Food Eaten	Amount	Time	Food Eaten	Amount

Education

Food Categories / Servings	Animal protein	Vegetable protein	Dairy products (calcium rich)	Whole grains, breads, and cereals	Vitamin C-rich foods	Green, leafy vegetables	Other fruits and vegetables	Fats and oils	Other foods
Summary									
Servings eaten									
Servings needed	2(4) 2		4	6	2	1–2	3	3 tsp	

Comments:

Suggestions made:
- Increase calories
- Decrease fat
- Decrease sugars
- Increase fiber
- Increase number of meals
- Ref. food programs
- Other _____

Mother's evaluation of her own diet: **Excellent**   Good   Fair   Poor
(circle one)

Changes mother feels she should make _____

_____

How the mother wants to feed the baby _____

nant and pregnant weight. The prepregnancy weight should be determined by history and is often used as a measure of nutritional status prior to conception. There are two commonly used methods of calculating ideal weight. One method is to refer to standard weight-for-height tables, which are calculated using actuarial data by insurance companies. A second method is to calculate ideal body weight using the rule-of-thumb assumption that the ideal weight for a woman 5 feet tall is between 90 lb and 110 lb and adding 5 lb for every inch over 5 feet. This formula provides a fair approximation of the woman's ideal weight. However, an ideal weight estimation should also consider genetic predisposition, age, preexisting maternal disease, and overall nutritional status. Often the pregnant women themselves can assist with their weight determination, though the nurse should keep in mind that they most often desire low weights for their heights because slenderness is highly valued.

Physical examination may also identify signs of nutritional deficiencies. Many signs of nutrient deficiency develop in exposed parts of the body — hair, face, neck, eyes, lips, gums, teeth, arms, hands, and lower extremities. Indicators of specific nutrient deficiencies that may be found in the physical examination in a pregnant or lactating woman who is nutritionally at risk are shown in Table 15–6.

Laboratory Tests

The nurse should remember that the findings of many laboratory tests are altered by normal gestation and must refer to standards for pregnant women when interpreting test results. If the standards for nonpregnant individuals are used, test results can falsely suggest deficiency states. For instance, blood levels of glucose, calcium, trace minerals, most amino acids, and nearly all water-soluble vitamins decline with pregnancy. Levels of other blood components, such as lipids and fat-soluble vitamins, rise during gestation. Table 15–7 summarizes the nonpregnant and pregnant normal ranges and the alterations that might be seen in nutritional deficiency.

Table 15–6   **Indicators of Nutrient Deficiency on Physical Examination**

Physical Finding	Nutrient Deficit
Significant nondependent edema	Protein
Filiform papillary atrophy of the tongue	Iron/folate
Diffusely enlarged and visible thyroid gland (goiter)	Iodine
Follicular hyperkeratosis of upper arms	Vitamin A
Diffusely swollen red interdental papillae of gums in a clean mouth	Vitamin C
Angular fissures and cheilosis of lips	Riboflavin

Dietary History

During the pregnant woman's first or second prenatal visit, the nurse should take a dietary history. The woman should receive a complete explanation of the purpose of this dietary history. The explanation gives the nurse an excellent opportunity to emphasize the importance of good nutrition during pregnancy and to encourage the patient to eat well. The nurse's goal is to determine if the pregnant woman's dietary intake is *adequate* in the *amounts* and *quality* of nutrients for her own needs and for the growth and development of her baby.

The dietary history is an indispensable part of nutritional assessment. In a busy clinic, however, it may be done hurriedly or overlooked altogether. The nurse must remember that the accuracy of the information she obtains depends on the patient's understanding of the reasons for the interview, her willingness to share this information with the nurse, and the importance the nurse places on this aspect of her assessment.

The 24-Hour Diet Recall.   A sample of the 24-hour diet recall is shown in the second page of the Assessment Tool. The nurse should first inquire about the patient's general pattern of daily activity and food intake, leading the patient through her usual routine from the time she gets up in the morning until she retires at night. The "24-hour diet recall" is then usually cross-checked with a food list to find out how food intake may vary throughout a usual week. The nurse should also ask about general food habits, overall frequency of food choices, patterns of preparation, seasoning, size of portions, and general likes and dislikes, rather than confining her questions to any specific day's food intake. This will assure the nurse of obtaining information about long-standing dietary practices as well as any short-term or recent changes. Use of the 24-hour diet recall in planning an adequate diet is discussed later in the chapter.

Factors Influencing Dietary Patterns

Preferences for, and emotional responses to food, socioeconomic background, cultural associations, and developmental status directly affect both attitudes toward nutrition and nutritional habits.

Meaning of Food and Food Consumption

Food and food consumption acquire meanings that, for most people, go well beyond the basic need for food as sustenance. Eating patterns develop very early, and food habits are among the most difficult patterns of behavior to change. Food in early childhood is associated with security and love. Attitudes and responses to food develop in relation to family and cultural practices. Children may be rewarded, punished, consoled, or controlled with food. For adults, eating is part of social interaction and is cul-

Table 15–7   **Laboratory Values Reflecting Nutritional Status in Pregnancy**

| Laboratory Test | Normal Range | | Findings in Deficiency |
	Nonpregnant	*Pregnant*	
Hgb/Hct	>12/36	>11/33*	<11/33*
Serum folic acid	5 to 21 ng/ml	3 to 15 ng/ml	<3 ng/ml
Serum Fe/Fe binding capacity	>50/250–400 ng/100 ml	>40/300–450 µg/100 ml	<40/450 ng/100 ml
Urinary acetone	Negative	Faint positive in A.M.	Positive
Fasting blood sugar	70–100 mg/100 ml	65–100 mg/100 ml	<65 mg/100 ml
2-hr postprandial blood sugar	<110 mg/100 ml	<120 mg/100 ml	—
Serum protein, total	6.5–8.5 g/100 ml	6–8 g/100 ml	<6 g/100 ml*
Serum albumin	3.5–5 g/100 ml	3–4.5 g/100 ml	<3.5 g/100 ml*
Blood urea nitrogen	10–25 mg/100 ml	5–15 mg/100 ml	<5 mg/100 ml
Urine urea nitrogen/total nitrogen ratio	>60	>60	<60
Cholesterol	120–220 mg/100 ml	200–335 mg/100 ml	—
Serum vitamin A	20–60 ng/100 ml*	20–60 ng/100 ml	<20 ng/100 ml
Serum carotene	50–300 ng/100 ml	80–325 ng/100 ml	<80 ng/100 ml*
Serum calcium	4.6–5.5 mEq/liter	4.2–5.2 mEq/liter	<4.2 mEq/liter or normal
Serum phosphate	2.5–4.8 mg/100 ml	2.3–4.6 mg/100 ml	No change
Alkaline phosphatase	35–48 IU/liter	35–150 IU/liter	No change
Serum ascorbic acid	0.2–2.0 mg/100 ml*	0.2–1.5 mg/100 ml*	<0.2 mg/100 ml*
Prothrombin time	12–15 sec	12–15 sec	Prolonged
Blood thiamine	1.6–4.0 ng/100 ml	—	Decreased
Urinary thiamine	>55 ng/g creatinine	—	<50
Blood lactic acid	5–20 mg/100 ml	—	Increased
Urinary riboflavin	>80 mg/g creatinine	—	<90*
N-methyl nicotinamide	1.6–4.3 mg/g creatinine	2.5–6 mg/g creatinine	<2.5 mg/g creatinine*
Kynurenic acid excretion	3 mg/24 hr	—	Increased
Xanthurenic acid excretion	3 mg/24 hr	—	Increased
FIGLU (Formimoglutamic acid) excretion (after 15 g L-histidine)	<3 mg/24 hr / 1–4 mg/24 hr	—	Increased / Increased
Serum vitamin B-12	330–1025 pg/ml	Decreased	Decreased
Methylmalonic acid	<10 mg/24 hr	—	Increased
Serum calcium	4.6–5.5 mEq/liter	4.2–5.2 mEq/liter	Normal
Serum thyroxine (T₄)	4.6–10.7 ng/ml	6–12.5 ng/ml	Decreased or normal

* Criteria from the Centers for Disease Control: Ten State Nutrition Survey, 1968–1970. DHEW Publication No. (HSM) 72-8134: 72-8133. Washington D.C., U.S. Government Printing Office, 1972
(Aubry RH, Roberts A, Cuenca VG: The assessment of maternal nutrition. Clin Perinatol 2(2):207, 1975)

turally defined as part of celebration, mourning, friendship, recreation, and gift-giving. Eating may become especially important at certain times in life for culturally or socially defined reasons; the saying that a pregnant woman is "eating for two" is one such example.

Socioeconomic Status

Socioeconomic status has a direct and profound effect on nutritional habits. When finances are strained, the food budget often is made up of the money that remains after fixed and more pressing costs, such as rent, transportation, and medicine, are met. Low-income families often cannot afford high-quality foods and purchase less expensive foods low in nutritional value but high in calories. Low-income families may also copy patterns of food buying advertised in the media; unfortunately, highly advertised items tend to be "prestige" food items that do not improve the overall nutritional value of the diet, such as coffee, soft drinks, and snack foods.

Employment patterns also directly affect nutritional status. As more women enter the work force, traditional food preparation patterns are giving way to the use of more "convenience" foods. Highly processed foods tend to contain food additives and preservatives with unknown long-term health effects. Diets that contain a lot of processed and convenience foods and "fast foods" tend to be higher in calories, fats, and sodium and lower in fiber than more traditional diets.

Cultural Influences on Dietary Patterns During Pregnancy

Food and food habits are prescribed culturally. Most cultures have a wealth of traditional dishes that use a variety of foods. This variety in traditional diets often leads to a well-balanced intake of essential nutrients. As people abandon traditional diets for more modern dietary patterns, they often end up with a less varied and less nutritious diet that is high in sodium, fat, and calories.

Some ethnic groups have developed dietary patterns in response to food intolerances that are relatively common among them. One common type is *lactose intolerance,* the symptoms of which include abdominal distention, nausea and vomiting, diarrhea, and cramping after consumption of milk. In the United States, lactose intolerance is common among blacks, Asians, Native Americans, and Mexican Americans, and milk consumption is low in the traditional diets of these groups.

Although it is instructive to examine dietary patterns among cultural groups in the United States for overall nutritional adequacy, most people are exposed to multicultural food patterns. People may adhere to their traditional food patterns at main meals, yet reflect mainstream cultural patterns in other meals or snacks. This underscores the importance of examining what families actually do in terms of food selection and preparation, rather than relying only on assumptions about cultural dietary patterns.

Mexican American Dietary Patterns

In the United States, particularly in the Southwest and West, Mexican Americans make up a major cultural subgroup among the childbearing population. Many Mexican Americans eat one "good" meal daily at noon; this is usually a hot meal that includes soup, beans, tortillas, and meat. Snacks may be taken throughout the day, especially if the main meal is delayed until the evening. Foods found in Mexican restaurants, such as tacos, enchiladas, and tamales, may not be a large part of a family's actual diet, especially if the mother is employed outside the home or if the family adopts the accelerated lifestyle common in the United States.

Milk is not typically consumed as a beverage, although it may be used occasionally in cooking. Vegetable and fruit consumption tends to be irregular; well-liked vegetables include peppers, lettuce, tomatoes, and corn. Overcooking vegetables often results in a loss of much of their nutritional value. Fruits commonly eaten are apples and bananas. Chilies, which are frequently used, may be an adequate source of vitamin C, but the ascorbic acid content of this food is often destroyed in processing. Sweets are consumed frequently. Fats, usually lard and butter, are frequently used in preparation, often by frying. Major nutrients that may be lacking in the Mexican American diet are vitamin A, vitamin C, and calcium. Iron consumption may be adequate because pinto beans, which are high in iron, form a significant part of the diet.

The pregnant Mexican American woman may be at nutritional risk for several reasons. First, she may not receive early prenatal care because of poverty, language and cultural barriers, or the belief that pregnancy is a normal state and does not require routine health care. For these reasons, dietary deficiencies may not be detected until late in pregnancy. If she snacks frequently on fast foods, sweets, or soft drinks, she may be taking in adequate calories but insufficient protein. The strong orientation toward the family and the high value placed on children in Mexican American culture may provide the opportunity for nutrition education for other family members and may be a strong motivator for the pregnant woman to improve her dietary habits.

Asian American Dietary Patterns

The largest Asian American populations in the United States are on the coasts, predominantly in larger cities. Asian American groups actually represent a variety of distinct and widely different ethnic groups, including Chinese, Japanese, and Southeast Asian. Among Asian peoples, food is an important aspect of the culture. For thousands of years, the Chinese have used foods along with herbs to improve and promote health and to treat disease. Traditional beliefs among Chinese and some Southeast Asian peoples divide foods into "hot" (Yang) foods, such as meat, eggs, and ginger, and "cold" (Yin) foods, such as winter melon, bananas, and fish. It is thought that these groups should be balanced in each meal, and certain types of foods will be prescribed or restricted on the basis of state of physical health.

Asian American diets include many vegetables, such as cabbage, snow peas, mushrooms, bean sprouts, and sweet potatoes, cooked quickly so that nutrient values are not lost. Food is usually purchased fresh and prepared the same day. White rice and noodles are the staples of the diet and may be eaten at every meal. Meat intake is moderate; fish and chicken may be used more often than red meat. Fresh fruit is often used. Milk and dairy products are rarely used in traditional diets. Asian Americans with less traditional diets may still avoid milk products because of lactose intolerance. Sweets are not commonly used.

Asian American diets often are very nutritious and contain adequate protein and nutrient levels. Calcium intake may be of concern, since milk intake is low. The pregnant Asian American woman who adheres to a more traditional diet may be in excellent nutritional status, except for calcium intake. Tofu (soybean curd) is an appropriate substitution; ½ cup of tofu contains the same amount of calcium as ½ cup of milk and the same amount of protein as two eggs. Asian Americans often regard the childbearing period as a very important time, and women may be motivated to make adjustments in their diets.

African American Dietary Patterns

Dietary patterns among African Americans vary widely according to region and socioeconomic status. Diets in middle-class or upwardly mobile African American families may be traditionally American and involve a high intake of red meats, starches, and snack foods. Poor families may spend food budgets on foods that are high in calories, fat, and carbohydrates and have extremely limited intakes of protein, fresh fruits, and vegetables. As income improves, families typically spend increasing amounts of the food budget for meat. African Americans may experience mild lactose intolerance and use little milk or dairy products in the diet. For many African Americans, "soul food" has strong cultural associations. This diet is based on one common in rural regions and relies heavily on foods available on subsistence farms, such as pork products, fried foods, gravies, field vegetables, and starches. Milk or dairy products are little used.

The pregnant African American woman may be at nutritional risk because of caloric imbalance in the diet. High intake of fats and carbohydrates, coupled with inadequate protein intake, contributes to obesity and may cause too-rapid weight gain during pregnancy. The high incidence of pregnancy-induced hypertension among poor African American women may reflect this dietary imbalance. Women living in extreme poverty are typically undernourished and at risk for inadequate weight gain during pregnancy.

Vegetarianism

Vegetarianism is widespread and diverse in the United States. This is due in part to the growth of "alternative lifestyles" that may involve various forms of vegetarianism, to the increased interest in fitness and health promotion, and to the increasing numbers of ethnic minorities for whom vegetarianism is a cultural norm. Generally, those adhering to vegetarian patterns can be classified in two broad groups.

Traditional vegetarians are those whose cultural or religious affiliation prescribes their diet, such as Seventh Day Adventists or Hindi sects. Groups with longstanding customs usually evolve relatively adequate diets through the consistent use of a wide variety of foods.

"New" vegetarians are those who have adopted vegetarian dietary patterns recently for reasons that are personal or philosophical, rather than religious or cultural. Dietary intake varies more widely in this group and may be associated with use of so-called health foods.

Within these two groups of vegetarians, there are also dietary subdivisions. There are many forms of vegetarianism, some more beneficial during pregnancy than others. *Vegans* are those who consume no animal foods of any kind. *Lacto-vegetarians* consume milk and dairy products but exclude meat, poultry, fish and seafood, and eggs. *Lacto-ovo-vegetarians* include both milk products and eggs in their diets. *Partial vegetarians* may exclude a specific type of animal food, usually meat, from their diet but may consume fish and poultry. *Fruitarians* are those who consume large amounts of fruit as a staple diet. *Macro-*

biotics consume highly restricted vegan diets, with the goal of achieving a diet of 100% cereals; this diet may result in severe nutritional deficiencies.

In general, a well-planned lacto-ovo-vegetarian diet, consisting of a variety of largely unrefined plant foods supplemented with milk and eggs, meets all known nutrient needs. Such a diet can be planned to meet calorie, nutrient, and protein requirements during pregnancy; as with other prenatal diets, iron and folic acid supplements are recommended. If a mother adheres to a vegan diet, consultation with a nutritionist or registered dietitian is advisable to ensure a safe calorie intake and adequate protein intake using grains, seeds, nuts, and vegetables.

Identifying Nutritional Risk Factors

Nutritional risk in pregnancy is currently identified by 18 factors established by the Maternal and Child Health Branch California Department of Health Services (1988) in conjunction with the American College of Obstetrics and Gynecology and the American Dietetics Association (1982). The recommended definition of maternal nutritional risk factors are listed in the box on pages 375 and 376. Some of these factors are discussed in this chapter while others are discussed in appropriate chapters in this text.

Adolescence and Pregnancy

The pregnant adolescent is likely to be at nutritional risk for several reasons. First, musculoskeletal growth in females can continue for 1 or 2 years after conception becomes possible. The pregnant adolescent must meet her own nutrient needs for growth and maturation in addition to those of the fetus. The increased demands for protein, calories, and nutrients are reflected in the recommended daily requirements for adolescents (shown in Tables 15–1 through 15–5). Adolescents also tend to have high activity levels, which poses additional nutritional demands.

Probably the most significant factors putting the pregnant adolescent at nutritional risk are ones related to psychosocial development. Adolescence is a time of striving for independence from parents and family and of increasing reliance on peers as a reference group. Good nutritional habits learned at home may be abandoned in favor of stops with friends at fast-food restaurants, junk food snacks, and erratic eating schedules. The influence of the media on adolescents also is powerful; advertisers of soda drinks, candy, and snack foods specifically aim at the teenage market. Advice from adults, especially parents, about nutrition may be threatening and is likely to be ignored. Another major factor influencing the nutritional status of the pregnant adolescent is concern with body and body image. Adolescents are preoccupied with their physical appearance and may engage in crash diets,

education materials for use with pregnant teenagers have been developed by various agencies and organizations across the United States to provide comprehensive services, often through an interdisciplinary team approach. *Nutrition and Adolescent Pregnancy: A Selected Annotated Bibliography* represents a joint effort of the public and private sectors — the Department of Health and Human Services (DHHS), the U.S. Department of Agriculture (USDA), and the March of Dimes Birth Defects Foundation (1986). This resource guide facilitates access to relevant references and educational materials that can help to improve the quality of care given to pregnant teens.

Caffeine and Alcohol Use in Pregnancy

Because of reports in the media and a general increase in interest in the health effects of diet, many pregnant women are concerned about the possible effects on the fetus of various food substances. The nurse should screen for caffeine and alcohol use and address any questions or concerns the mother may have. The nurse should recognize that *conclusive* research findings on the effects of substances on human pregnancy and birth are rare. Most preliminary work relies on animal research and retrospective studies of large numbers of pregnant women. Scientific evidence of a direct link between use of certain substances and problems in pregnancy may be tenuous at best. However, women can be advised that, since nearly all substances ingested by the mother affect her own health and potentially the health of her baby, it is wise to cut down on or avoid caffeine and alcohol during her pregnancy.

Caffeine. In 1980, the Food and Drug Administration issued a recommendation that pregnant women avoid, or use sparingly, foods and drugs containing caffeine. In part this recommendation was based on animal research that suggested that caffeine was associated with decreased intrauterine growth, skeletal anomalies, and low birth weight. However, as with all animal research, the applicability of those findings to humans is uncertain because of differences in mode and amount of the drug consumed and in its metabolism in the body. Two large retrospective studies have subsequently found no evidence of teratogenic effects of caffeine in humans. However, there was evidence that heavy coffee consumption (more than seven cups per day) may be associated with lower birth weight and increased incidence of premature rupture of membranes (Hogue 1981, Linn 1982).

On the evidence to date, caffeine appears to have little effect on pregnancy outcome. However, in view of the possible association between caffeine use and low birth weight and premature rupture of membranes, the nurse should encourage moderation in caffeine intake during pregnancy. Caffeine is found in many food and drug products, including coffee, tea, cola drinks, candy, and cough remedies.

Alcohol. In recent years, ethanol has been shown to be teratogenic in humans. *Fetal alcohol syndrome* is characterized by craniofacial abnormalities, delayed motor development, low birth weight and smallness for dates, and mental retardation. It occurs in 1 of 4000 to 5000 births. There is evidence that women who drink large amounts of alcohol (five or more drinks per day) regularly place their unborn children at increased risk for fetal alcohol syndrome, and the risk of congenital abnormalities and low birth weight is increased even among mothers who drink moderately (2 to 4 drinks per day). The risk of fetal alcohol syndrome appears to increase proportionately with increases in average daily intake of alcohol. The effects of very low consumption of alcohol have not yet been determined. Fetal alcohol syndrome is discussed further in Chapter 34.

The nurse should routinely screen for level of alcohol use among pregnant mothers and advise women of the potential risks to the fetus. Since safe intake levels have not been established, the safest practice is to abstain from all alcohol use during pregnancy. Women who are alcohol-addicted during pregnancy require specialized support and treatment for their condition.

Assessing Weight Gain During Pregnancy

Adequate prenatal care must include repeated measurements of body weight (Fig. 15–2). Adequate weight gain during pregnancy is essential to the continued good health of the mother and normal development of the fetus. Both prepregnant and pregnant weight are critical factors in the assessment of nutritional status. Prepregnant weight, fetal growth rate, and weight changes all

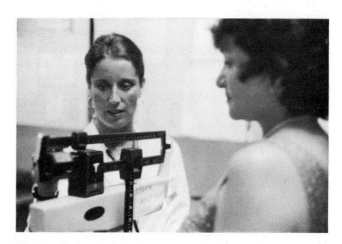

Figure 15–2. Assessment of the pattern of weight gain during pregnancy is an important nursing responsibility. (Courtesy of John B. Franklin Maternity Hospital, formerly Booth Maternity Center, Philadelphia)

reflect the woman's pattern of food utilization, particularly her calorie intake. The pregnant woman's weight at conception and her usual dietary practices and activity patterns must be evaluated before her optimal weight gain can be determined. The surest evidence of an adequate calorie intake is a steady weight gain. Weight loss or failure to gain weight during pregnancy places both mother and unborn infant at serious risk.

Nutritional excesses or deficiencies may exert stress on the body that can be sufficient to influence the infant's pattern of growth and birth weight and jeopardize both mother's and baby's physiologic homeostasis. Estimates of satisfactory weight gain for pregnant women are based on average weight gains observed in adult pregnant women in normal pregnancies. A satisfactory pattern of weight gain for the average woman is shown below:

10 weeks of gestation: 650 g (approx. 1.5 lb)

20 weeks of gestation: 4000 g (approx. 9.0 lb)

30 weeks of gestation: 8500 g (approx. 19.0 lb)

40 weeks of gestation: 12,500 g (approx. 27.5 lb)

Over the course of the pregnancy, a total weight gain of 25 to 30 pounds is recommended for nonobese pregnant women. During the second and third trimesters, a gain of about 1 pound per week is considered desirable.

Pregnant women are particularly susceptible to excess weight gain because of hormonal changes and increased appetite. Excess weight gain can usually be slowed if the woman is encouraged to satisfy her appetite with "high-quality" calories (*e.g.*, from cottage cheese, lean meats, fish, tofu, whole grains, fruits, vegetables) and avoid excess intake of fats and sugar.

However, restriction of food intake to reduce weight gain poses a serious threat. Women with low weight gain during pregnancy, especially those already 10% or more below the recommended weight for height, are at increased risk of delivering a low birth weight infant. If the mother's food intake is insufficient to provide for the fetus's need for energy, fetal growth and development will be impaired, because the mother's body does not mobilize or "burn" maternal skeletal muscle to provide additional needed energy to the fetus. With the exception of iron and folate, which the fetus claims from maternal stores, the fetus depends entirely on the mother's dietary intake to furnish nutrients and energy. For this reason, restrictive dieting to limit weight gain during pregnancy is *not recommended*.

The Underweight Woman With a Rapid Weight Gain

If the underweight woman tends to gain weight rapidly at the beginning of the first trimester, often as much as 1 pound per week, by 20 weeks of gestation she has gained 18 to 20 pounds. This pattern of weight gain is important to recognize because it is different from the one that health professionals usually associate with pregnancy. If the nurse sees *only* the standard recommendation of 2 to 3 pounds of weight gain during the first trimester, she then will be uncertain about how to manage the patient who shows rapid weight gain starting at the beginning of pregnant. It is important to remember that the baby will gain most of its weight in the last trimester. If the woman is advised to cut food intake at that point in an attempt to restrict her weight gain, the overall goal of producing a baby of optimum birth weight may be jeopardized. The nurse should also remember that the increased physiologic demand for food energy makes it difficult for most pregnant women to restrict calorie intake during the second and third trimesters of pregnancy; they are normally very hungry. The woman experiencing rapid weight gain in early pregnancy should be advised to satisfy her appetite with intake of high-quality foods in a regular pattern throughout the day and to keep her caloric intake within the recommended limit.

The Normal or Obese Woman With Excess Weight Gain

The nurse may encounter pregnant women who are at or above normal weight at the beginning of pregnancy but who, at some point, exceed the usual recommended gain of 1 pound per week during the last two trimesters. The nurse's assessment is first directed at determining the *cause* of the weight gain. The nurse should:

- Verify the prepregnancy weight.
- Take a 24-hour diet recall and calculate the woman's calorie and protein intake.
- Rule out excessive edema and hypertension.
- Check the woman's usual activity level, especially if her caloric intake does not appear to be excessive.
- Encourage the patient to increase her activity, primarily by walking. *Do not advise her to decrease calories or food intake.* Discourage *any* attempts at weight reduction by dieting: if fat is catabolized or "burned," ketonemia and ketonuria result, and these in turn can be life-threatening to the fetus and can cause intellectual impairment in the offspring.

The nurse should keep in mind that nondietary factors can also affect weight gain. For example, the woman could be eating the recommended 2400 kcal per day, but she might also have increased blood pressure and excess fluid retention, which could account for a weight gain of 3 pounds or more per week.

However, if pregnancy-induced hypertension and excess water retention are ruled out and the patient is gaining weight too fast, perhaps at a rate of 3 or 4 pounds every 2 weeks, the nurse must evaluate the patient's diet. If the patient's recommended intake is 2400 kcal but the

24-hour diet recall reveals an actual intake of 3000 kcal, the nurse should recommend that the patient reduce the amount of fat in her diet by decreasing, for example, the amount of oil used in food preparation and by using less salad dressing and margarine. The nurse should also double-check the size of food portions with the patient and should stress appetite control with high-quality sources of energy and protein.

The Woman With Insufficient or Slow Weight Gain

The nurse may also encounter pregnant women who consistently show slow weight gain that appears to be leading to insufficient total gain when calculated by weeks or trimesters. Weight gain during pregnancy is considered to be insufficient if the total gain is less than 20 pounds or if a satisfactory weight gain pattern has not been established by midpregnancy. The nurse's assessment is directed at determining the cause of the failure to gain weight. The nurse should:

- Verify prepregnant weight and determine if weight loss during the first trimester is due to nausea/vomiting. If the mother is frequently nauseated encourage her to eat dry toast or crackers in the morning before arising. She should also take small amounts of food frequently; the less she eats, the more her appetite will be depressed and the more likely it is that nausea will persist. The nurse can encourage her to take high-calorie, high-protein drinks, such as homemake milkshakes (milk, ice-cream, and fruit); drinking about 4 ounces every 2 hours often will ensure adequate protein and calories while stimulating the appetite.

- Check the woman's activity level against her daily dietary intake. Activities that require much walking, child care, and strenuous exercise of any kind require tremendous energy expenditures.

- Check for food intolerances that might be causing frequent stomach upsets, diarrhea, or decreased appetite.

- Check environmental influences, such as hot weather, disruptions in family circumstances, or significant changes in routine. These influences may be related to cultural practices. For example, a Hispanic woman living in a hot climate might drink rice water frequently to quench her thirst. Her reasoning might be that this is a healthy practice, since rice water is often given to babies. In fact, however, the carbohydrate level in rice water is sufficient to reduce her appetite for other food but does not provide enough nutrition to support weight gain.

- Check economic status and ability to buy food. Poor women are at particular risk for protein and iron deficiency. The low-income mother should be encouraged to participate in community food programs. (See section on Counseling the Low-Income Mother later in this chapter.)

- Assess the woman's emotional response to the pregnancy and to additional weight gain. If she is obese or disturbed about the pregnancy, she may be consciously or unconsciously limiting her weight gain. The nurse should reinforce that dieting during pregnancy is not recommended, because it deprives mother and fetus of nutrients needed for tissue growth and because weight loss is accompanied by maternal ketosis, a direct threat to fetal wellbeing.

Diagnosis

Nursing diagnosis in nutritional care focuses on identifying the causes of nutritional risks to maternal and fetal health. Once risk factors are identified, nursing care to reduce nutritional risk can be planned and implemented.

The following nursing diagnoses may be useful in nutritional care during pregnancy.

- Alterations in nutrition: Intake less than body requirements related to
  — Nausea
  — Lack of knowledge about nutritional requirements during pregnancy
- Alterations in nutrition: Intake more than body requirements related to
  — Increased appetite during pregnancy
  — Lack of knowledge about nutritional requirements during pregnancy
  — Decreased activity level
- Alterations in bowel elimination: constipation related to
  — Decreased peristalsis during pregnancy
  — Iron supplementation

Planning and Implementation

Using the 24-Hour Diet Recall to Plan an Adequate Diet

The 1988 MCH Daily Food Guide has been developed to ensure an intake of at least 80% of the RDA for pregnant and lactating women of average height (64 inches) and average weight (120 pounds prepregnant). The current MCH Daily Food Guide is based on computerized analyses of sample menus.

This means that the recommended number of servings from each group are actually the minimum during pregnancy; if the guide is followed and recognizing that each food group has more nourishing and less nourishing choices within it, will ensure an intake of at least 80% of the recommended RDAs. Therefore, this tool is the most practical and best available for the nurse to evalute how adequate the pregnant women's diet is. After the 24-hour recall has been completed, the food intake reported is compared with the Daily Pregnancy Food Group Guide (Table 15–8). Table 15–9 can be used in calculating nutrient intake from a mother's 24-hour diet recall, and Table 15–10 shows good sources of nutrients in which American diets are often deficient.

When comparing the patient's diet to the Daily Food Guide, the following factors must be considered:

Table 15–8   **Pregnancy Food Group Guide**

Food Group and Service Size	Servings per Day	Rationale
Protein Foods		
Meat, poultry, fish (2 oz), eggs (2); beans (1 cup cooked); nut butters (¼ cup) or nuts and seeds (½ cup); tofu (1 cup) or cottage cheese (½ cup)	4	To build tissues in mother and infant. These foods contain iron, protein, zinc, and many other nutrients.
Milk/Dairy Foods		
Nonfat, lowfat, or whole milk (1 cup); plain yogurt (1 cup); soymilk or tofu (1 cup); cheese (1.5–2 oz); nonfat milk powder (⅓ cup)	4	To build healthy bones and teeth. These foods are major source of calcium. They provide vitamins A and D, necessary for fetal development.
Grains **(Whole grains are best!)**		
Bread, rolls (1 slice); macaroni, rice, noodles (½ cup); hot cereal (½ cup); cold cereal (1 oz); wheat germ (1 tbsp)	6	To provide B vitamins for strong blood and nerves; iron and trace minerals; and fiber for optimal bowel function.
Vitamin C-Rich Foods		
Orange or grapefruit juice (½ cup); 1 orange or ½ grapefruit; bell peppers, greens, tomato, cantaloupe, broccoli, cabbage, cauliflower (1 cup)	2	To provide vitamin C (ascorbic acid) for connective tissue and resistence to infection and disease. Daily intake is necessary. Vitamin C intake is especially important for smokers. Whole fruits are preferable to juices; fruit drinks with added sugar should be avoided.
Green Leafy Vegetables		
Broccoli, Brussels sprouts, asparagus, cabbage, greens, red leaf or romaine lettuce, bok choy, watercress (1 cup raw or ¾ cup cooked)	1–2	To provide folacin and iron and vitamin A for soft skin and good eyesight. These foods also contain vitamins E, C, and K and natural fiber.
Other Fruits and Vegetables		
All fruits and vegetables not listed above, and their juices: apples, carrots, bananas, sweet potatoes, green beans, etc. (about ½ cup)	3	To promote general health. These foods contain many nutrients and fiber.
Fats and Oils		
Butter, margarine, Better-Butter, salad dressing, cream cheese, cooking fats, fatty cheeses	3 tsp.	For energy and healthy skin. These foods, however, should be used in *moderation*.

Table 15–9   **Approximate Nutritional Values of Common Foods**

Protein

7 g

1 oz lean meat, poultry, fish

1 egg

1 glass of milk

1 oz cheddar or pasteurized, processed cheese

¼ c cottage cheese

½ c dried beans or peas (cooked)

2 tbsp peanut butter

4 g

1 c whole grain cooked cereal

1 c bran flakes

1 c ice cream

½ c milk pudding

2 slices bacon

2 g

1 c ready-to-eat cereal

1 slice bread

1 serving cake, pie or cookies

1 g

½ c fruit or vegetables

Iron

3 mg

1 oz liver

3 oz lean, red meat

4–5 medium oysters

1 c dark greens

1 c green peas

½ c dried beans

1 tbsp blackstrap molasses

1 mg

3 oz fish

2 oz poultry

1 egg

4 prunes or ½ c prune juice

3 tbsp raisins

1 c fruit or vegetables (other than dark green)

2 slices whole grain or enriched bread

Calcium

300 mg

1 c milk

1–1.5 oz cheddar or swiss cheese

1–1½ c ice cream

3 oz sardines

½ c peanuts

1 c collard greens

1–1½ c kale, mustard, turnip greens

150 mg

1 oz pasteurized, processed cheese

3 oz salmon

1–1½ c dried beans

12 medium oysters

1 c broccoli

Vitamin A

10,000 IU

1 oz liver

½ c carrots

⅔ c pumpkin

1 (5 oz) sweet potato, cooked in skin

½ c dark leafy greens

½ cantaloupe (5-in diameter, orange-fleshed)

3,000 IU

3 raw apricots or ½ c canned halves

watermelon, 4 × 8-in wedge

½ c broccoli

½ c winter squash

1,000 IU

1 raw peach or 1 c canned

1 c fortified dry cereal

1 c green peas

1 raw tomato (2–2.5-in diameter)

½ c canned tomatoes

1 c green leafed lettuce

500 IU

1 c vitamin A—fortified milk

2 oz cheddar cheese

1 c ice cream

2 eggs

1 tbsp butter or fortified margarine

½ c green beans or limas

Ascorbic Acid (vitamin C)

50 mg

½ c orange or orange juice

½ c grapefruit or grapefruit juice

½ c lemon or lime juice

½ c fresh strawberries

¼ c cantaloupe (6.5-in diameter, orange-fleshed)

⅓ c broccoli

1 c fresh raw or lightly cooked cabbage

(continued)

Table 15-9   **Approximate Nutritional Values of Common Foods**   (continued)

Ascorbic Acid (vitamin C)

50 mg
⅓ c fresh cooked collard greens
½ c cooked dark-green leafy
  vegetables
½ raw green pepper

25 mg
1 c raw blackberries
watermelon, 4 × 8-in wedge
1 (5 oz) baked potato
1 tomato or 1 c tomato juice
1 baked sweet potato
½ c cauliflower

Thiamine (vitamin B₁)*

0.50 mg
2 oz lean fresh pork

0.25 mg
1 c oysters
3 oz liver
½ c green peas
1 c orange juice
1 c dried beans or peas
½ c peanuts

0.10-0.20 mg
3 oz tuna
3 oz lean beef
1 c milk
1 slice enriched or whole wheat
  bread
1 c enriched farina

Riboflavin (vitamin B₂)*

1.0-2.0 mg
1 oz liver

0.20-0.30 mg
½ c cottage cheese
8 oz plain yogurt
2 eggs
1 c dark-green vegetables

0.40-0.50 mg
1 c milk or yogurt
1 c oysters
1 c (40%) bran flakes

Niacin

10 mg
2 oz liver
2 oz poultry
3 oz tuna
½ c peanuts

5 mg
3 oz salmon
3 oz sardines
1 c oysters
3 oz lean beef, pork
2 tbsp peanut butter
1 c (40%) bran flakes

2-3 mg
3 oz ham
1 c fresh lima beans or
  black-eyed peas
1 c cooked corn
1 med. baked potato *or*
1 c cooked potato
1 c cooked enriched rice,
  spaghetti or noodles
1 c canned tomatoes or tomato
  juice

* For levels of B vitamins and iron in fortified cereals, check the labels

Calories.   Depending on the choice of foods within each group, the calorie intake based on the Daily Food Guide can range from 2000 to 3000 calories for the pregnant woman. Therefore, in order to consume adequate calories (most pregnant women need at least 2300), this can be obtained from increased servings of the food groups. But if foods not listed are eaten or methods of food preparation increase the calories from fats, the patient should be encouraged to make nutritious selections.

Protein.   Each serving recommended on the Daily Food Guide supplies approximately 14 g of protein, 2.4 mg of iron (supplementation needed), and 1.8 mg of zinc. However, light poultry, meat, fish, and tofu are lower in zinc than other foods in this group. In general, the Daily Food Guide provides about 150% of the RDA for protein. It is important to understand that the RDA level of protein must be exceeded in order to insure an adequate intake of B_6, iron, and zinc in the diet.

Calcium.   Each serving of the milk group supplies approximately 275 to 300 mg of calcium. Milk is also a good source of vitamin D. In addition, these foods supply protein, phosphorus, riboflavin, vitamins A, B_6, and B_{12}. For some women, this food group serves as primary sources of protein in the diet. If the recommended number of servings from this group is inadequate, the calcium intake is likely to be inadequate.

Table 15–10   **Food Sources of Nutrients**

Vitamins	*Minerals*
Vitamin B$_6$	**Iodine**
Bananas	Iodized salt
Whole grain cereals	Seafood
Chicken	**Magnesium**
Dry legumes	Bananas
Most dark-green leafy vegetables	Whole grain cereals
Most fish and shellfish	Dry beans
Muscle meats, liver and kidney	Milk
Peanuts, walnuts, filberts, and peanut butter	Most dark-green vegetables
Potatoes and sweet potatoes	Nuts and seeds
Prunes and raisins	Peanuts and peanut butter
Nutritional yeast	**Zinc**
Vitamin B$_{12}$	Shellfish
(Present in foods of animal origin only)	Meat
Kidney	Poultry
Liver	Cheese
Meats	Whole grain cereals
Milk	Dry beans
Most cheese	Cocoa
Most fish	Nuts and seeds
Shellfish	
Whole egg & egg yolk	
Folacin	
Liver	
Dark-green vegetables	
Dry beans	
Peanuts	
Wheat germ	
Vitamin D	
Vitamin D milk	
Egg yolk	
Saltwater fish	
Liver	
Vitamin E	
Vegetable oils	
Margarine	
Whole grain cereals	
Peanuts	

(From Science and Education Administration: Home and Garden Bulletin No. 72, Nutritive Value of Foods. Washington, DC, US Department of Agriculture, April 1981)

Folacin.   Each serving of dark green vegetables contributes significant amounts of folacin and magnesium; average is 75 μg/serving of folacin and 30 mg/serving of magnesium. If the pregnant woman avoids foods in the dark green vegetables, folacin is likely to be inadequate. In addition, these foods supply vitamins A, B$_6$, and E, riboflavin, iron, and fiber.

Vitamin C-rich Foods.   Each serving supplies about 60 mg of vitamin C. In addition, most foods from this group are good sources of folacin and vitamin A. Those foods that are particularly rich in vitamin A provide more than 2750 IU per serving. They include such foods as cantaloupe, mango, papaya, greens, bok choy, and spinach.

Breads and Cereals. This group is divided into two parts: whole grains and enriched products. Whole grain breads, cereals, and pastas provide significantly more magnesium, zinc, vitamins E and B$_6$, folacin, and fiber than enriched products. It is recommended that at least half of the bread and cereal servings eaten daily be made from whole grains.

Cultural Patterns

The Daily Food Guide can also be incorporated to meet the different cultural patterns of the pregnant woman. The sample menus shown in Figure 15–3 illustrate how cultural variations can be taken into account when a nutritionally adequate prenatal diet for an adult woman is being planned. All of these supply recommended daily allowances of calories, protein, vitamins A and C, and calcium. Iron intake for each plan is in an acceptable range (Mexican-American, 21.9 mg; black-American, 20.1 mg; Asian-American, 15.3 mg; and vegetarian, 12.0 mg), but iron and folic acid supplementation would still be recommended during pregnancy.

Teaching for Effective Self-Care

In nutritional care, as in many other aspects of maternity care, the main type of intervention required is teaching and counseling. In some settings, the nurse may work closely with a nutritionist to provide this care, while in other settings, the nurse has primary responsibility for providing nutritional information and encouragement to mothers regarding their dietary patterns.

Perhaps no area of prenatal care is so dependent on the pregnant woman's capacity for effective self-care as nutrition. The nurse's interventions must be aimed at informing and motivating women to make changes in their diets that will promote optimal health for themselves and their unborn babies. Many factors influence the effectiveness of nursing intervention to promote good nutritional self-care. The following sections provide some suggestions for the nurse engaged in this type of teaching.

A major way in which the nurse intervenes to promote optimal nutritional status during pregnancy is *by providing information and encouragement.* The goal of this intervention is to help women to make well-informed decisions about their diets during pregnancy. Teaching the maternity patient about nutrition should always be a high priority in nursing care and is especially important if the care setting does not allow for regular contact with a clinical nutritionist.

The effectiveness of the nurse's teaching depends to a large extent on sensitivity, rapport with the mother, and enthusiasm about healthy nutritional practices. She must schedule adequate time for teaching and have appropriate teaching aids available. If the nurse conveys by behavior and attitude that nutrition is boring, unimportant, or complicated, the mother may be less motivated to learn about improving her diet. Dietary patterns are often deeply ingrained habits that are difficult to change, and the pregnant woman should be encouraged to make changes one step at a time.

Visual Aids

The nurse can increase the effectiveness of her teaching by using attractive and informative teaching aids (Fig. 15–4). Pictures of foods in magazines may be useful in helping mothers estimate portion sizes, reinforcing information about food groups, and stimulating mothers to introduce more variety into their diet. Food group guides and nutrition information charts should be available so that both nurse and patient can refer to them readily.

Important Points

Some aspects of nutrition are especially important during pregnancy and may be of particular concern to mothers. The nurse should take special care to provide information and practical guidance in these areas.

Weight Gain. Many women do not welcome the increase in body weight and size that comes with pregnancy. However, they may accept it more readily if the nurse stresses that weight gain is the *only* way the fetus can be supplied with the nourishment it needs, and that some added body fat will be burned and provide necessary energy during lactation if the mother chooses to breastfeed.

Protein Intake. The nurse should stress the importance of meeting the daily requirement of 70 g to 80 g. Protein can be described as providing "building blocks" for her own tissues and for her fetus. For many women, dairy products will be a major source of protein. If a woman does not drink milk, the nurse can point out that milk can be used in preparation of foods such as soups, custards, and sauces and that cheese, yogurt, and icecream are alternative sources.

The nurse should review food groups with the woman, reminding her that meat, poultry, fish, eggs, and legumes are good sources of protein. The nurse can encourage economical ways to boost protein intake, such as creating complementary proteins by combining a small amount of complete animal protein with an incomplete plant protein; sample combinations are beans or pasta and cheese, eggs and whole-grain bread, poultry or fish and rice. Women who practice vegetarianism are often quite knowledgeable about nutrition; however, they should still carefully assess their protein intake and use supplements, such as high-protein drinks, if necessary.

Carbohydrate and Fat Intake. Carbohydrates and fats can be described as providing fuel for energy. The

Sample Menus From Various Cultures Giving An Adequate Diet

Pregnancy Guide — Number of servings to have each day

Meals	(X) Mexican	(0) Asian	(-) Black	(✓) Lacto-Ovo-Veget.	Protein (4)	Milk (4)	Grains (6)	Vit. C (2)	Green Veg. (1)	Other Fruits (3)	Fats & Oils (3 tsp)
Breakfast Time ___	2 corn tortillas 1 c beans 2 oz jack cheese on beans 1 c hot chocolate milk	1 c steamed rice ½ c tofu 2 oz fish Tea	½ c grits w/ 1 c milk 2 eggs 1 biscuit	1 c brown rice 1 tbsp honey 1 c milk 1 c orange juice	M X A 0 B – L ✓	XX ½ – ✓	X 00 – – ✓✓	 ✓✓			X 0 – ✓
Snack Time ___	quesadilla: corn tortilla w/1-2 oz melted cheese	2 oz cheese 1 peach or apple	1 orange or 1 c orange juice	1 piece toast 2 tbsp peanut butter	M A B L ✓	X 0	X ✓			 0	
Lunch Time ___	2 corn tortillas 1 c beans 1 c caldo (soup) w/2 oz chicken Salad: 1 green pepper, tomatoes, lettuce 1 c orange juice	1 c steamed rice 2 oz beef strips w/1 c fried vegetables: snow peas, broccoli, chinese cabbage 1 c milk custard	3 oz fried pork w/ 1 c black-eyed peas 1 c turnip greens 1 potato ½ c ice cream & 1 peach	1 c pinto beans ½ c rice Salad: ½ c spinach w/tomato, onion, cucumber, carrot 1 c milk	M XX A 0 B – – L ✓	X 0 ½ ✓	X 00 – ✓	XX 0 – – ✓	X 0 – ✓		X 0 – ✓
Snack Time ___	Peaches w/1 c cottage cheese	4 rice crackers 1 oz cheese 1 c orange juice	1 c buttermilk 4 crackers 1 banana	Hot sandwich w/2 pieces whole wheat toast and 2 oz cheese Peaches	M A B L ✓	X ½ – ✓	X 0 – ✓✓	XX 00		X – ✓	
Dinner or Supper Time ___	2 oz stewed chicken 2 corn tortillas 1 sweet potato Spinach, raw 1 carrot Mango juice	2 oz cashew chicken 1 c fried rice 1 c vegetables: bean sprouts, peppers, green onions, mushrooms 1 c tofu Tea	1 c meat & beans 1 c collard greens Cornbread Pudding made w/ ½ c milk	1 c rice 1 c lentils 1 stalk broccoli w/ 2 oz cheese or 1 c pinneaple	M X A 0 B – L ✓	X 0 ½ ✓	XXX 00 – ✓✓		X 0 – ✓	X ✓	X 0 – ✓
Bedtime Snack Time ___	1 c flan made w/ ½ c milk or 1 c hot chocolate	½ c nuts & seeds Peaches	1 piece toast 2 oz. cheese Strawberries	¼ c nuts and seeds on 1 c yogurt w/fruit	M A 0 B L ✓	½ – ✓	 – ✓	 –		0 ✓	

Figure 15–3. Sample menus from various cultures giving an adequate diet.

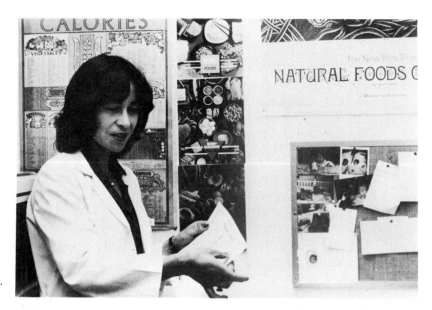

Figure 15–4. Attractive teaching aids are useful in nutrition teaching during pregnancy. (Photo: Michele Vignes)

woman should be encouraged to choose natural sources, such as fruits and whole grains, and to avoid processed foods high in sugar, because natural sources provide other needed nutrients without concentrated calories. The nurse can stress that this change in habits, if sustained, can be very helpful in weight control after pregnancy as well. The nurse can also point out that the typical American diet is high in fat and that the woman would be wise to choose low-fat or nonfat dairy products, to trim off fat from meats, and to substitute broiling or baking for frying.

Appetite Management. Women whose appetites are markedly increased during pregnancy may gain weight more rapidly than they would like because they feel hungry "all the time." The nurse should encourage women with this problem to take frequent small meals rather than one or two large meals a day. The woman should plan healthy, protein-containing snacks for herself and try to eat small amounts before she becomes very hungry.

Iron and Folic Acid Supplementation. Many women advised to take iron and folic acid supplements are not in the habit of taking vitamins or any medication on a regular basis and complain that remembering to take their prenatal vitamins is difficult. The nurse should encourage the woman to keep her vitamins in a place where she will see them, and to associate taking them with another daily activity, such as meals, brushing her teeth, or washing dishes.

"Giving Up" vs. "Cutting Down." Many women will be concerned about the effects of caffeine and alcohol in their diet but have difficulty giving up certain food habits. The nurse should explain that habits are often difficult to change and that cutting down gradually by setting realistic goals is often more effective than totally giving up favorite foods or beverages, feeling deprived, and then rebelling against the restriction. One strategy the nurse may use to help women who want to change habits but are experiencing difficulty is keeping a food diary for a few days. The woman simply keeps a log of what she eats, when, in what surroundings, and how she was feeling at the time. Keeping a food diary can allow a woman to "see" how her dietary intake is based on longstanding habits and what cues trigger her food habits. If a woman is motivated and will keep a food diary, this also provides an excellent diet recall with which to assess her progress.

Food Cravings. The nurse should reassure women that food cravings are not uncommon and that as long as the rest of her dietary intake is well-balanced, there is probably little harm in indulging occasionally. Some cultures hold specific beliefs about food cravings, such as a particular craving "marking" the baby physically. Although the nurse can gently provide accurate information and reassurance if a mother appears to be worried about a specific practice, she should be careful to do so without demeaning the mother's underlying cultural belief.

However, substances such as laundry starch, clay, or ice, which some pregnant women crave, may have detrimental effects on maternal health and indicate the need for systematic assessment and intervention. *Pica* is the practice of eating substances not ordinarily considered edible. It is most common in poverty stricken areas, where diets are likely to be inadequate. Pica is a learned practice, and women may have heard myths that eating some substances will produce a lighter-skinned newborn or an easier delivery. However, ingestion of such substances may interfere with iron absorption and contribute to iron-deficiency anemia, as well as causing hypokalemia, intestinal obstruction, and excessive weight gain. The nurse should correct any misinformation the woman may have, point out the potential risks associated with this practice, and encourage her to substitute other eating patterns.

Counseling Women at High Risk

Individual patients known to be at high nutritional risk, such as adolescents, impoverished women, or those with previously identified nutritional problems, will require additional time for individualized teaching and counseling.

The nurse must anticipate the need for referral to community programs, such as the Special Supplemental Feeding Program for Women, Infants, and Children (WIC), that provide nutritional assistance to low-income mothers and make herself thoroughly familiar with the services and programs available in her area. The nurse must plan to meet patients' learning needs by including time in routine prenatal visits for nutritional counseling and teaching, and by providing effective and appropriate printed materials and teaching aids. In settings where a nutritionist is available for prenatal care, the nurse and nutritionist should plan together how resources can be used most effectively to meet identified patient needs.

Counseling the Low-Income Mother

Low-income pregnant women are especially vulnerable to nutritional deficiency, particularly protein and iron deficiencies. Improving the quality of the diet on a restricted income requires specialized guidance about food buying, storage and preparation, as well as referral to programs designed to assure adequate provision of food to pregnant and new mothers. The nurse should ensure that the low-income mother is seen by a nutritionist and social worker whenever possible, and should encourage the mother to take advantage of these services. Local public health nurses are excellent sources of information for the nurse as well as the low-income mother.

Special Supplemental Feeding Program for Women, Infants and Children (WIC). This federally funded program is designed to provide supplemental foods to infants and children under 5 years of age and to pregnant, lactating, or postpartum women. People seen to be at nutritional risk by health care professionals can receive supplements of high-quality foods. This program requires that mothers also receive nutritional counseling and routine health care.

The eligibility criteria for the WIC program are as follows:

- Recurrent need for medical care
- Conformity with federal income guidelines
- Residence in a local agency's target area
- Determination by a health professional that "nutritional risk" is present

Evaluation of Nutritional Outcomes During Pregnancy

The nurse can use physiologic and behavioral indicators to evaluate the effectiveness of nutritional care during pregnancy. Adequate maternal weight gain during pregnancy, adequate maternal iron stores as reflected by hemoglobin and hematocrit levels before and after birth, and optimal infant birth weight are all measurable and objective indicators that reflect effective nutritional support during pregnancy. Behavioral outcomes may not be as readily measurable but may be just as important to consider when evaluating the effectiveness of nursing interventions directed at nutritional needs. The nurse can assess the woman's satisfaction with her management of her own diet and with her level of nutritional knowledge. Does she feel better informed about her own and her infant's nutritional needs? If she made changes in her own diet prenatally, does she feel positive about those changes? Is she motivated to continue with a healthier diet in the future? Truly effective nutritional care during pregnancy results in mothers establishing and *maintaining* healthier nutrition habits for themselves and their families into the childrearing years. The nurse plays a central role in the planning and delivery of that care.

CHAPTER SUMMARY

Adequate maternal nutrition is important in preventing perinatal morbidity and mortality and in achieving optimal fetal growth and development. Pregnancy causes significant changes in digestion and metabolism while increasing demands for specific nutrients, protein, and calorie intake. Maternal intake of iron and folic acid is especially important, and supplementation is commonly used to prevent iron deficiency anemia and to provide an adequate supply of these nutrients to the developing fetus. The mother's cultural background, socioeconomic status, and developmental level directly influence her dietary patterns and her overall nutritional status. The nurse must understand the need for a comprehensive nutritional assessment, including a healthy history, physical examination, and dietary history, and an ongoing assessment of maternal weight gain, to provide a basis for planning prenatal nutritional care. Major nursing interventions include ongoing assessment of maternal nutritional status, teaching mothers for effective self-care in relation to their dietary habits and providing support and encouragement.

STUDY QUESTIONS

1. Describe how the recommended dietary allowances for nonpregnant women and pregnant women differ.
2. What do U.S. nutrition studies show about the adequacy of dietary intake of iron and folic acid during pregnancy?
3. Why is the nutritional status of women prior to pregnancy important to pregnancy outcome?
4. Name good sources for each of the following nutrients: calcium, iron, zinc, vitamins C and D.
5. List the food groups and the number of servings from each group that should be included in the daily diet of a pregnant woman.
6. What should the nurse do when faced with a pregnant woman who uses megadoses of vitamin supplements?
7. State why sodium and calorie restrictions are not appropriate for most pregnant women.
8. What criteria would you use for the selection of prenatal vitamins?
9. What important considerations are needed if you advise calcium supplements during pregnancy?

REFERENCES/BIBLIOGRAPHY

American College of Obstetricians and Gynecologists and American Dietetic Association: Assessment of Maternal Nutrition. Chicago, American College of Obstetricians and Gynecologists, 1982

Biswas MK, Pernoll MJ, Mabie WC. A placebo-controlled comparative trial of various prenatal vitamin formulations in pregnant women. Clin Ther 6:763–769, 1984

California Department of Health Services, Maternal and Child Health Branch: Nutrition During Pregnancy and the Postpartum Period: A Manual for Health Care Professionals, 1988

Dubrick M: Dietary supplements and health aids: A critical evaluation. Part III. J Nutr Ed 15(4):123, 1983

Linn S, Schoenbaum S, Monson R, et al: No association between coffee consumption and adverse outcomes of pregnancy. N Engl J Med 306(3):141, 1982

National Research Council: Recommended Dietary Allowances (9th ed.) Washington, DC, National Academy of Science, 1980

Neeson J, Patterson K, Mercer R, et al: Pregnancy outcome for adolescents receiving prenatal care by nurse practitioners in extended roles. J Adolescent Health Care 4:94, 1983

Recker RR: Calcium absorption and achlorhydria. N Engl J Med 313(2):70–73, 1985

Smithells R, Sheppard S, Schorah C, et al: Possible prevention of neural tube defects by periconceptional vitamin supplementation. Lancet 1:339, 1980

Seligman PA, Caskey JH, Frazier JL, et al: Measurements of iron absorption from prenatal multivitamin-mineral supplements. Obstet Gynecol 61:356–362, 1983

16 nursing assessment of the pregnant woman

LEARNING OBJECTIVES

After studying the material in this chapter, the student should be able to

- Discuss the basic mechanism in all pregnancy tests and the various methods used to diagnose pregnancy

- Explain why early detection of pregnancy is important

- Understand and begin to recognize the presumptive, probable, and positive signs of pregnancy

- Demonstrate an understanding of the importance of prenatal assessment

- Describe the events of the first prenatal visit

- Explain the importance of the patient history in nursing assessment

- Describe the physical examination and identify some normal changes of pregnancy

- Know the basic laboratory studies performed for early pregnancy assessment and their significance

- Describe subsequent patient assessments

- Explain the role of the nurse in prenatal care

KEY TERMS

Amenorrhea	Nulligravida
Anencephaly	Nullipara
Ballottement	Parity
Colostrum	Parturient
Fetal age	Primigravida
Gestation	Primipara
Gestational age	Puerpera
Gravida	Viability
GTPAL	
Lightening	
Multigravida	
Multipara	

A great deal of attention during pregnancy is focused on labor and birth, the exciting and dramatic climax to 280 long days of waiting. However, equally important events occur during the prenatal period to ensure minimum risk at delivery and maximum health for the mother and baby.

The value of prenatal care provided in the outpatient setting cannot be overstated. At no other time in life does a healthy woman need health care with such regularity. Today, many women plan for pregnancy and prepare for the event by maintaining their health at a high level through good nutrition, exercise, and abstinence from cigarettes and drugs. A pregnancy under these ideal conditions has a better chance for healthy growth and development. Prenatal care does not guarantee a normal baby, but it can identify problems early so that they can be minimized or eliminated.

The intent of this chapter is to acquaint the nurse with the vocabulary of the prenatal period, to explain the tools used to assess the pregnant woman, to present comprehensive information on the assessment of the mother and fetus, and to present the nursing process as a holistic approach to prenatal care.

PREGNANCY DIAGNOSIS

A common maxim in the practice of obstetrics and gynecology is that *every woman who has been menstruating and misses a menstrual period is pregnant until proven otherwise.* Pregnancy must be ruled out in the initial phase of an amenorrhea workup even though the woman insists that she is not pregnant. A good question to ask women who have missed one or more periods is, "Have you been pregnant before?" If the reply is affirmative, the next question is, "Do you feel pregnant now?" If she feels pregnant, there is an 80% chance that she is indeed pregnant. Women who have never been pregnant may be less sensitive or knowledgeable about the early signs of pregnancy.

The earlier pregnancy is diagnosed, the safer it is for the mother and baby. During the first 12 weeks of pregnancy, the vital organ systems of the fetus are developing. Early diagnosis of pregnancy:

- Allows the woman wishing to continue her pregnancy to be counseled about potential insults to the developing fetus, such as x-ray exposure, vaccinations, medications, excessive alcohol intake, smoking, over-the-counter and illicit drugs, and occupational or other hazards

- Enables the woman contemplating abortion to consider her options in early pregnancy (abortion is safest for the woman when performed before 12 weeks of gestation)

- Permits early diagnosis of and intervention in an ectopic pregnancy, a common cause of maternal morbidity and mortality

Over the past decade, pregnancy testing has evolved from the slow and cumbersome biologic testing of animals to sophisticated blood tests that can diagnose pregnancy as early as 6 to 10 days after conception. A review of methods is presented in the accompanying display.

Clinical Changes of Pregnancy
Presumptive Evidence of Pregnancy

Pregnancy cannot be diagnosed on the basis of the presumptive signs; it can only be assumed until more concrete data are available.

- Abrupt cessation of menses in a healthy woman who previously had predictable menstrual periods suggests pregnancy. In a woman whose menses had been irregular, this symptom would be more difficult to evaluate. Some women experience spotting (light bleeding) during early pregnancy. Women who stop taking birth control pills may also have a variable period of amenorrhea.

- Nausea and vomiting, better known as "morning sickness," occur in about 50% of pregnant women. They begin between 2 and 6 weeks after conception and may spontaneously disappear at about 12 weeks. Some women continue to experience these symptoms for the duration of pregnancy.

- Bladder irritability occurs early in pregnancy when the enlarging uterus presses on the bladder, causing more

---

Methods of Pregnancy Diagnosis
Clinical changes

- Presumptive signs of pregnancy
- Probable signs of pregnancy
- Positive signs of pregnancy

Pregnancy tests

- Human chorionic gonadotropin tests
- Immunologic tests
- Radioimmunoassay
- Radioreceptor test
- New immunologic tests
- Home testing

Ultrasound diagnosis of pregnancy

frequent urination. As the uterus rises into the abdomen after 12 weeks, this symptom decreases, but it returns late in pregnancy.

- Breast tenderness is one of the earliest symptoms of pregnancy, and nipple tingling is thought to be the first clue to pregnancy for some women. Colostrum may be secreted early in multigravidas.
- Fatigue occurs in early pregnancy in response to increased hormone levels. Women often state they just cannot get enough sleep.

Probable Signs of Pregnancy

The probable signs of pregnancy include objective findings that can be detected by 12 to 16 weeks of gestation.

- Enlargement of the abdomen occurs as the fundus of the uterus rises out of the pelvis at 12 weeks of gestation. When enlargement progresses over a period of several weeks, it becomes a positive diagnostic sign. However, if other pregnancy symptoms do not corroborate the uterine signs, other causes, such as myomas, pseudocyesis, and neoplasms, need to be ruled out.
- Changes occur in the size, shape, and consistency of the uterus as it progresses from pear-shaped to globular. Later in pregnancy, the uterus becomes elongated as it grows upward.
- Intermittent painless uterine contractions can be palpated through the abdomen near the end of the first trimester. These Braxton Hicks contractions occur irregularly throughout pregnancy and may even occur in nonpregnant women.
- Ballottement, the rebound of a fetal part when displaced by a light tap of the examining finger through the abdominal or vaginal wall, suggests the presence of a fetus.
- Hegar's sign, a softening of the lower uterine segment, may be felt on bimanual examination.
- Chadwick's sign is a purplish hue, seen on speculum examination of the vagina and cervix.
- Sensation of fetal movement first occurs between 16 and 20 weeks when the woman notices a fluttering movement in the abdomen. If these sensations continue and become stronger daily, pregnancy is probable. By the time movement is felt, the diagnosis of pregnancy has probably been made.

Positive Signs of Pregnancy

The following signs are considered diagnostic of pregnancy:

- The fetal heartbeat can be heard and counted separately from the mother's by Doppler stethoscope as early as 10–12 weeks.
- The fetus can be recognized by ultrasound.

Pregnancy Tests

Pregnancy tests may be performed by a private physician or by a family planning or abortion clinic, or a home pregnancy test may be purchased. A first voided morning urine specimen should be collected when immunologic testing is to be done and the sample stored in the refrigerator until tested. It is most helpful when a woman has kept a menstrual calendar to record her menstrual periods, or when she is positive of the first day of her last menstrual period so that the timing of a pregnancy test can be accurate.

Human Chorionic Gonadotropin Tests

All laboratory systems used for pregnancy testing are based on the detection of human chorionic gonadotropin (HCG) in the maternal blood or urine. Soon after conception, the trophoblastic cells, responsible for the development of the placenta, begin producing HCG. After the fertilized egg has been implanted, the trophoblastic cells rapidly develop and produce increasing amounts of HCG. This hormone is essential to pregnancy maintenance and is found in the body only during pregnancy. By the time the first menstrual period is missed, HCG concentration is about 100 mIU/ml, and it doubles every 2 days until 10 weeks' gestation when it drops sharply. Eight weeks after a missed menstrual period (12 weeks of gestation), the HCG concentration in serum is over 10,000 mIU/ml.

Biologic Animal Bioassays

In 1927 Aschheim and Zondek first described the bioassay test for pregnancy, known as the A-Z test. The patient's urine was injected into an immature female mouse six times over a 2-day period; the animal was then killed, and its ovaries were examined for corpora lutea and corpora hemorrhagica, definitive signs of pregnancy. Although the test was 97% accurate, it required incubation, a steady supply of laboratory animals, and a large staff to maintain and examine the animals. It also required high levels of HCG and could not be used for early diagnosis. This and other early biologic tests were difficult to perform, expensive, and lacked the sensitivity of current testing methods.

Immunologic Tests

Developed in the late 1950s, immunologic (antibody) tests are still widely used as the tests of choice for large laboratories, small hospitals, and clinics where more sophisticated radioimmunoassay equipment is not avail-

NURSING ALERT

Errors in Pregnancy Testing

Some factors that influence the results of pregnancy testing are careless following of instructions, incorrect timing of the test reading, use of certain drugs by the woman, and careless handling of specimens. When pregnancy test results are reported as negative when the woman is in fact pregnant, they are called *false negative* results. When they are positive and pregnancy has not occurred, they are called *false positive* results. When either of these errors is suspected, the following causes should be considered:

False Negatives

- Error in reading
- Test performed too early or too late in pregnancy
- Urine too dilute
- Urine stored too long at room temperature
- Impending spontaneous abortion
- Missed abortion
- Ectopic pregnancy
- Interfering medication
- Too much antiserum

False Positives

- Error in reading
- Luteinizing hormone cross-reaction (test performed at time of ovulation or in a perimenopausal woman)
- Proteinuria, hematuria
- Persistent corpus luteum
- Recent pregnancy (test performed less than 10 days after abortion or full-term delivery)
- Detergent on glassware
- Drug interference (aldomet, marijuana, methadone, aspirin in large doses, phenothiazine)
- HCG treatment for infertility (injection within preceding 30 days) — affects serum tests only
- Tubo-ovarian abscess
- Thyrotoxicosis
- Trophoblastic disease (molar pregnancy or choriocarcinoma)
- HCG secreted by malignant tumor (ovary, breast, lung, kidney, gastrointestinal tract, sarcoma, malignant melanoma)

able. The immunologic tests have completely replaced the biologic tests because they are quicker, less expensive, and are standardized. Neither of these tests, however, is sensitive enough to detect HCG before the first menstrual period is missed.

Use of the immunologic tests is based on the ability of HCG in the woman's urine or serum to stimulate antibody production, which produces a demonstrable antigen–antibody reaction on a slide or in a tube. They are performed by mixing the woman's urine with a prepared serum containing antibodies to HCG. Then a carrier—either latex or particles for the slide test and erythrocytes coated with HCG for the tube test — is added to the mixture.

Positive reading: the HCG molecules from the urine bind with the serum anti-HCG antibodies, leaving no remaining anti-HCG antibodies. This leaves the red cells or latex particles in suspension, and the solution becomes cloudy because of their presence.

The end result is a cloudy suspension indicating absence of agglutination or agglutination inhibition (AI).

Negative reading: urine that contains no HCG does not bind to the anti-HCG serum, permitting the red cell or latex bodies that contain HCG serum to bind in clumps with the anti-HCG serum antibody. The end result is agglutinated latex particles or precipitated red blood cells, and the finding is that agglutination or macroagglutination is present.

The slide test can be completed and its results reported in 2 minutes. It is convenient and easy to read, but less sensitive than the tube test. The test will be negative if performed before 1 to 2 weeks after the last missed menstrual period, or 42 days of gestation. If the test is done at this date and is reported as negative, it should be repeated in 1 or 2 weeks. Often women are anxious to learn whether they are pregnant and seek verification too early for accurate interpretation of this test.

Table 16–1   **Slide and Tube Urinary Pregnancy Tests**

| Trade Name (Manufacturer) | Principle and End Point | | Sensitivity | Reaction Earliest | | Accuracy (%) |
	Positive	Negative		Time	Detection	
Slide Tests						
Pregnosis (Roche)	Milky white color	Macroagglutination	1.5–2.5 IU hCG/ml	2 min	5 days FMP	97.3–98.4 at 41 days LMP
UCG-Slide Test (Wampole)	Milky white color	Macroagglutination	2 IU hCG/ml	2 min	5 days FMP	97.0
Dap Test Macro (Wampole)	Macroagglutination	Milky white color	2 IU hCG/ml	2 min	4 days FMP	No claim
Pregnosticon Dri-Dot (Organon)	Milky white color	Thin agglutination	1–2 IU hCG/ml	2 min	5–7 days FMP	94.7–98.7 at 31–100 days FMP
Pregnosticon Slide Test (Organon)	Milky white color	Agglutination	1–2 IU hCG/ml	2 min	5 days FMP	98.1
Gravindex 90 (Ortho)	Milky white color	Agglutination	3–5 IU hCG/ml	2 min	No claim 5–7 days FMP	98.0
Pregnate (Fischer)	Milky white color	Agglutination	2–4 IU hCG/ml	2 min	7–10 days FMP (approx.)	98.4
Pregna β-Slide (International Diagnostics)	Greenish mixture	Agglutination	2 IU hCG/ml	2 min	No claim	99.5
Tube Tests						
Sensi-Tex (Roche)	Milky white color	Flocculation	0.25 IU hCG/ml	90 min	At or before MP	99.2
Placentex (Roche)	Milky white color	Flocculation	1.0 IU hCG/ml	+90 min	4 days FMP	98.1
UCG-Test (Wampole)	Ring	Mat	Undiluted 0.5 IU hCG/ml Diluted 1.3 IU hCG/ml	2 hr	4 days FMP	98.0
UCG-Quick-Tube (Wampole)	Ring	Mat	1.0 IU hCG/ml	2 hr	4 days FMP	98.0
UCG-Lyphotest (Wampole)	Ring	Mat	0.5–1.0 IU hCG/ml	2 hr	4 days FMP	98.0
Neocept (Organon)	Ring	Mat	0.2 IU hCG/ml	2 hr	At or before MP	No claim
Pregnosticon Accuspheres (Organon)	Ring	Mat	0.75–0.85 IU hCG/ml	2 hr	4 days FMP	98.9
Gravindex 90 (Ortho)	Ring	Mat	0.5 IU hCG/ml	90 min	4–7 days FMP	98.5
Pregna-β (International) Diagnostics	Ring	Mat	0.4–0.8 IU hCG/ml	2 hr	4 days FMP	98.0

Abbreviations:
  FMP — from missed period
  LMP — last menstrual period
  MP — missed period

The tube test requires 2 hours to complete and is sensitive to lower levels of HCG. It also has fewer false negative results (see Table 16–1).

Radioimmunoassay Test

The radioimmunoassay test (RIA beta-subunit HCG) is a highly specific and sensitive assay that can detect as little as 0.003 IU/ml of beta-HCG in the serum. It can detect pregnancy in the first week after conception (6 days) with almost 100% accuracy in 1 to 3 hours.

Radioreceptor Tests

The radioreceptor test (RRA) is the most recent addition to pregnancy testing. Radioactive HCG is used along with membrane receptors for HCG (prepared from bovine corpora lutea). Detection of the HCG molecule is accomplished by measuring its competition for specific receptor sites on the cell membrane. Biologically active HCG is detected even more accurately by this test than by the RIA. The test is now available as a kit that permits measurement of HCG within 1 hour. Except for the beta-subunit RIA, the RRA is the most sensitive pregnancy test now available.

The RIA and RRA test are not available in all women's health care settings. Sophisticated equipment and interpretation of the tests is available only in large hospitals or medical centers.

Home Pregnancy Testing
Advantages

- The accuracy of the test is high when the results are positive.
- The test is accessible, since kits are available at the local drug store.
- Confidentiality and privacy are assured.
- Earlier diagnosis may result in early prenatal care. When therapeutic abortion is intended, an earlier and safer procedure can be performed.
- The test results are easily readable when the test is performed accurately.

Disadvantages

- When the result is negative, a repeat test is necessary.
- Test instructions may not be followed correctly.
- When the test is positive the woman may be uncertain about what to do next.
- False positive and false negative results are possible.
- Pregnancy counseling may not be sought.
- Delay in seeking medical care for amenorrhea or pregnancy may occur.

New Immunologic Tests

A new breakthrough in pregnancy testing is on the horizon. Immunologic urine tests for detection of HCG that compare in sensitivity to the RRA test will soon be available. Involving neither radioactive materials nor complex equipment, the tests will give results in 1.5 to 2.0 hours and will be simple to use and interpret.

Home Pregnancy Tests

Home pregnancy test kits are available for sale over the counter. Like the immunologic tests performed in a clinic or laboratory, they are based upon detection of HCG in the

NURSING RESEARCH

Reducing Uncertainty: Self-diagnosis of Pregnancy

The purpose of this research was to discover how women make a self-diagnosis of pregnancy (to be later followed by their decisions about prenatal care). Data were collected from 30 pregnant women who were receiving care in a variety of health care settings. The researchers were looking for symptoms or cues the women experienced in early pregnancy that provided them the impetus to attempt to diagnose their pregnancy, and thus reduce their uncertainty.

The self-diagnosis process in this group of women was prompted for such reasons as (1) the need to make a decision regarding the continuation or termination of the pregnancy, (2) to seek early prenatal care when there was a previous problematic pregnancy, (3) a desire for pregnancy, and (4) the couple has been trying to conceive.

The cues triggering self-diagnosis of pregnancy were missed periods, lateness of period, changes in period, morning sickness, review of a previous pregnancy, breast tenderness, "just a feeling," vaginal spotting at the time of expected menses, and change in character of bleeding.

Even though the women were sure they were pregnant, all but four sought laboratory or professional confirmation. The four women who did not seek a pregnancy test were not sure of their pregnancy until 3 to 5 months gestation.

The authors sum up their findings by stating: "self-diagnosis is fundamental to the decision either to seek care or to engage in self-care activities. Understanding how individuals make diagnoses is an initial step in designing interventions to promote competence and confidence in the self-diagnostic process."

Patterson ET, Freese MP, Goldberg R: Reducing Uncertainty: Self-diagnosis of Pregnancy. Image, J Nurs Scholarship 18(3):105–109, Fall 1986

first voided morning urine specimen. Most are tube tests. In clinical trials, the tests were accurate in 97% of cases. Home pregnancy testing is of special benefit to women who:

- Have irregular menstrual periods
- Experience amenorrhea after stopping oral contraception
- Have problems with infertility
- Do not want to be pregnant

When the test is performed 2 weeks after the last menstrual period (LMP), it can provide fast and accurate information. However, the test must be performed with care and attention. When the test is negative, it should be repeated in 2 weeks to ensure that it was not done too early to detect the HCG. If the woman remains amenorrheic, she should seek medical care.

Ultrasound Diagnosis of Pregnancy

Pregnancy may be diagnosed and dated by ultrasonographic measurement of the intrauterine contents. It is not the diagnostic method of choice and is usually done only when a problem such as ectopic pregnancy or a blighted ovum is suspected. The procedure for ultrasound is simple, causes no discomfort to the patient (except that she must have a full bladder), and does not expose her to radiation.

The scanner can demonstrate a gestational sac or ring as early as 6 weeks after the LMP. The action of the fetal heart can be seen, and fetal movement can be detected. The fetal head and thorax can be identified and the gestational age estimated from the biparietal diameter.

For a description of the ultrasound and its many uses in pregnancy, see Chapter 17.

THE FOUR TRIMESTERS

It has been common practice to divide pregnancy into three equal parts, or *trimesters*. The 9 months of pregnancy are grouped into three periods of approximately 13 weeks each: weeks 1 to 13, 14 to 27, and 28 to 40. The events of pregnancy tend to group themselves into these time periods.

For patient-teaching purposes, this division may also be applied to the patient's interests and concerns. Early in her pregnancy she may be interested in discussing body changes, the early growth of the baby, and what she can do to control her nausea and vomiting or the other discomforts of early pregnancy. During the second trimes-

ter, she may be more comfortable discussing sexuality in pregnancy, exercise, and nutrition and will experience great excitement when the first fetal movements are felt. The third trimester is a time for anticipation of delivery, discussion of preparations for childbirth and breast-feeding, and touring the labor and delivery suite.

Physical symptoms also seem to group themselves by trimesters. Nausea and vomiting, increased fatigue, and frequency of urination are common in the first trimester. The second-trimester experience is usually more comfortable for the pregnant woman both physiologically and psychologically, whereas during the third trimester the woman experiences more discomfort from the growing uterus, increased urination, dependent edema, and problems with sleeping. In the latter half of the third trimester, she is anxious for the pregnancy to end. During the third trimester, the health care provider must be more alert for signs of pathology, such as preeclampsia, pregnancy-induced hypertension, and gestational diabetes.

Nevertheless, the trimesters are an arbitrary division, not meant to cluster the events of pregnancy rigidly but rather to arrange them for convenience when discussing the progression of events. When reporting or describing a stage of pregnancy or its duration, it is best to use the most precise and accurate information available, which is the gestational age of the fetus.

Current nursing literature commonly speaks of the "fourth trimester," which comprises the early postpartum weeks. The expression emphasizes the vulnerability of the mother during the early postpartum period, a subject previously ignored. This is a period when the new mother is busy adjusting to her baby, is usually very tired and somewhat anxious, and needs increased physical and emotional support.

THE FIRST PRENATAL VISIT

The first prenatal visit is important because it is at this visit that baseline data on the patient's health and the health of the present pregnancy are collected. A full patient workup is done including a complete history, physical examination, and collection of laboratory specimens. Possible pregnancy risk factors are also identified, and a long-term plan of care is formulated for reduction of risk to the mother and her infant.

During the first prenatal visit, the nurse has the opportunity to set the stage for a continuing relationship with the woman. When prenatal care is initiated at 6 weeks of gestation, the pregnant woman will make as many as 12 or 13 visits during the course of her pregnancy. During these weeks the quality of care provided and the support of the nurse will help make the pregnancy a positive growth experience.

The first prenatal visit is usually an extended one and may take 1 to 2 hours. Although details may vary from one setting to another, the events of this visit generally progress in the following order:

1. Orienting the patient to the setting
2. Collecting a health history
3. Assessing physical status
4. Performing a pelvic examination
5. Collecting specimens for lab work
6. Identifying risk factors
7. Teaching and counseling the patient

All these tasks are necessary if comprehensive data are to be collected and the patient fully informed.

Orienting the Patient to the Setting

When a pregnant woman first arrives for prenatal care, she is likely to be apprehensive, particularly if it is her first pregnancy. The first person she is likely to meet after registering for her appointment is the nurse. By introducing herself and greeting the patient, the nurse assures the expectant mother that she is welcome and important.

A brief description of the setting, information on its hours of operation, telephone numbers for contacting care providers, and an explanation of what happens during the first prenatal visit is enough for the patient to assimilate at this point.

Collecting the Health History

The setting for collecting the health history should be carefully chosen. It is essential to establish a climate conducive to information sharing.

The interview may be described as a conversation with a purpose. For the prenatal patient, a less formal "conversational" style of gathering information is appropriate. This method allows the nurse to guide the discussion and elicit important information, while establishing a relationship with the patient by expressing interest and concern.

In addition to providing information about the patient's health, the interview gives the nurse an opportunity to observe the patient's appearance and behavior. Observation can provide valuable information on the patient's feelings about herself and her pregnancy.

The health history is a brief biography and should elicit information about the patient's present and past health and her social, economic, psychologic, and sexual history. Most obstetric settings provide history forms that request

data similar to that obtained during a complete medical history, as well as data specific to the woman's reproductive history and her present pregnancy. Sample assessment tools are given here. It is important to know as much as possible about the patient, and such information should be usable by all members of the health care team. Records necessarily use standardized terminology, and the language used should have the same meaning and value to each professional who consults them. Not only must the information be complete; the reporting language must be consistent and appropriate as well.

When collecting data from patients, it is helpful to discuss with them the importance of the information and to explain terminology that may not be understood. The health history can be valuable for both the nurse and the patient. For this reason, the following section outlines the information needed to complete the prenatal history, as shown in the assessment tool beginning on page 417, and provides a specific rationale for its collection.

Demographic Data

Information obtained in the demographic portion of the history identifies the patient and her residence, telephone number, age, race, ethnic origin, religion, marital status, and occupation. Important information about the patient may be gained by exploring her replies and observing her behavior. See Table 16–2.

Menstrual History

The menstrual history is an important part of data collection, not only for pregnant women but for all female patients. During the reproductive years, it is important to know the age when menstruation first occurred (menarche), the regularity of periods, the duration and amount of menstrual flow, whether pain is associated with menses (dysmenorrhea), and whether uterine bleeding occurs between periods. (Since hormonal contraception produces an artificial menstrual cycle, the history should include only cycles when no oral or intramuscular contraception was used.) During this first prenatal visit, obtaining a menstrual history is essential to determine gestational age and expected date of delivery.

Calculating Date of Delivery

The average length of pregnancy, as calculated from the first day of the last menstrual period (LMP), is 280 days: 40 weeks, 10 lunar months, or 9 calendar months. The expected date of confinement (EDC), or the date of delivery, can be estimated by using Nägele's rule.

According to Nägele's rule, the EDC is calculated by adding 7 days to the date of the first day of the last normal menstrual period, and then counting back 3 months (first day of the LMP plus 7 days minus 3 months equals the EDC). For example, if a woman's last normal menstrual

Table 16–2   **Demographic Data**

Information	Rationale
Address	Obtaining the patient's address offers an opportunity to ask questions about her life style. In what part of town is her home located? Does she live in a house or an apartment? Does she live alone, or with friends, husband, or partner? Will she have trouble getting transportation to prenatal visits?
Age	Age of the expectant mother is extremely important. Teenagers and women over 35 are at greater risk for pregnancy complications.
Race/ Ethnic Origin	Congenital disorders and chromosome aberrations may be associated with race or ethnicity. Tay-Sachs disease, found in a segment of the Jewish population, is the most common metabolic disorder diagnosed prenatally. Sickle cell hemoglobin trait may be found in the black population. Culture may also influence a woman's attitude toward prenatal health care practices. There may be taboos related to the genitals, breasts, the use of contraception, or treatment by male health care providers.
Occupation	When a pregnant woman works, it is important to determine the kind of work she performs. • Does her job require strenuous activity? • Is her job sedentary? • Is she exposed to chemicals or other potential teratogens? For example, nursery and elementary school teachers may be exposed to children infected with rubella virus. Pregnant nurses working in newborn nurseries may be exposed to viral shedding from asymptomatic newborns. X-ray or radiation exposure may also present a problem.
Religion	Religious doctrines may influence medical care. Jehovah's Witnesses may refuse medical intervention necessary to maintain health or sustain life. Other religious faiths may prohibit abortion or contraception. The dietary rules of some religions may necessitate adjustments in the recommended nutrition plan to ensure adequate nourishment of the mother and fetus during pregnancy.

period began on February 4, her expected day of delivery would be November 11:

$$\text{February } 4 + 7 = \text{February } 11$$
$$\text{February } 11 - 3 \text{ months} = \text{November } 11 \text{ (EDC)}$$

Gestational calculators in the form of wheels can also be used to determine the EDC, weeks of gestation, and the estimated length and weight of the fetus for each week of gestation.

Dating Pregnancy When LMP Is Unknown

When the date of the LMP or conception is not known, a number of parameters can be used to determine the length of gestation. These include:

- Size of the uterus at the first prenatal visit, reported in terms of weeks of pregnancy (*e.g.,* 6 weeks' size)
- Presence of the uterus in the pelvis (indicates a pregnancy of *less than* 12 weeks of gestation)
- Presence of the uterus in the abdomen (indicates a pregnancy of *more than* 12 weeks of gestation)
- Date of the first positive pregnancy test
- Doppler detection of FHT; if present, gestation is at least 10 weeks
- Detection of fetal heart sounds with a fetoscope when the uterine fundus is located at the level of the umbilicus indicates a pregnancy of 20 weeks
- Fetal movement, or quickening (felt by 20 weeks of gestation by primigravidas; earlier in multigravidas)
- Sonography report (up to 18 weeks is the most clinically useful method to assess fetal age)

Present Pregnancy

The history of the present pregnancy deals with the progress of the pregnancy to date, symptoms being experienced, and the patient's feelings regarding the pregnancy. The following questions will elicit information essential to the nursing assessment and management of the patient.

- How is her general health? Her family's health?
- Was a pregnancy test performed, when, and was the result negative or positive?
- Was contraception used prior to this pregnancy? What kind? Were there side-effects? How long was it used, and when and why was it discontinued?
- Was this pregnancy planned? How does she feel about it?
- Has she experienced signs of early pregnancy, such as nausea and vomiting, breast tenderness, fatigue?
- Has she had any bleeding, spotting, or cramping since her last menstrual period?
- What was her prepregnant weight?
- Does she engage in any form of routine exercise?
- Is the father of the baby involved with the pregnancy? Is he offering support? What is his age, height, and weight, and does he have any significant medical history? What is his occupation?
- Does she smoke or drink alcoholic beverages? How many cigarettes per day? How many ounces of alcohol per day?

- Has she been exposed to teratogens or other substances (x-rays, chemicals) that may affect the fetus?
- Has she taken any over-the-counter drugs, street drugs, or prescription drugs since her last period? If so, what is the name of the drug and when, how often, and how much was taken?
- Has she been exposed to any contagious illnesses since her last menstrual period?

Previous Pregnancies

Pregnancy history can be recorded using the mnemonic *GTPAL:* G—gravida; T—term pregnancy; P—preterm birth; A—abortion; L—number of living children. If a woman has had six pregnancies, four term deliveries, one premature delivery, and one abortion, and has five living children, her previous pregnancy history would be reported as 6-4-1-1-5. If the premature delivery has resulted in the death of the infant, her history would be reported as 6-4-1-1-4.

The history of previous pregnancies provides important data that may be useful in the management of the present pregnancy, especially if problems or complications were experienced. Information obtained from the patient should include:

- Length of gestation
- Length of labor
- Type of delivery
- Fetal presentation
- Neonatal outcome
- Neonatal birthweight
- Complications of labor, delivery, and postpartum

Assessing Physical Status

Information collected for the health history provides 95% of the data needed to assess patient health. The remaining 5% is obtained from the findings of the physical examination and from laboratory assessments. A physical examination, guided by any information in the history that indicates a health problem, should be performed on all pregnant women at their first visit.

A complete physical examination should be performed on every pregnant woman. Physical findings will be different from the normal ones in those areas of the body where pregnancy changes are most dramatic. The physical assessment of these areas includes:

- Measurement of vital signs, height, and weight
- Palpation of thyroid
- Auscultation of maternal heart tones
- Inspection and palpation of the breasts
- Inspection and palpation of the abdomen
- Measurement of fundal height
- Auscultation of fetal heart tones
- Pelvic examination

Blood Pressure

Blood pressure is taken early in pregnancy to provide a baseline for the evaluation and comparison of readings that may become elevated later in gestation. A systolic increase of 30 mmHg or a diastolic increase of 15 mmHg above the baseline blood pressure is a significant abnormal finding.

Height and Weight

Height and weight assessment is important in pregnancy. A woman who has a short, square stature and broad, short hands may also have a small bony pelvis. As pregnancy progresses, she may appear large for dates when in fact this is an illusion created by the shorter distance from pubis to xiphoid. Conversely, a tall woman may appear smaller than her dates because of her long torso.

Prepregnant weight is used to assess sequential and total pregnancy weight gain. Even though a patient's weight gain follows the normal pregnancy curve, nutritional counseling is required to ensure that nutrient intake is adequate to meet the demands of the mother and baby. By 20 weeks of gestation, weight gain should be 10 pounds; at term the minimum recommended weight gain is 24 pounds.

Early loss of weight below the prepregnant level may mean that the patient has experienced significant nausea and vomiting. Referral to a nutritionist is imperative to avoid serious problems, such as dehydration and ketosis.

Weight gain considerably greater than average in late pregnancy (5 lb or more in 1 week) may indicate overeating or fluid retention. Rapid weight gain caused by fluid retention in conjunction with protein in the urine (proteinuria) and an elevated blood pressure (as defined above) may indicate that the patient is preeclamptic (*i.e.,* suffering from toxemia of pregnancy).

Early nutritional assessment and continued counseling throughout pregnancy are important for a healthy mother and baby.

Body Changes

Body changes that occur during pregnancy can be assessed on physical examination (Table 16–3).

Inspection and Palpation of the Breasts

Many physiologic changes occur in the breasts in preparation for milk production. These changes, all considered normal, include:

Table 16–3   **Body Changes in Pregnancy and Associated Problems**

Normal Changes	Related Discomforts	Potential Problems
Head and Neck		
Increased nasal vascularity	Epistaxis (nosebleeds)	
Chloasma (mask of pregnancy)	Cosmetic concern; may persist	
Epulis (gingival growth)	Bleeding gums, difficulty eating and keeping teeth clean	
Ptyalism (excessive secretion of saliva)	Nausea	Malnutrition
Enlarged thyroid gland, increased basal metabolic rate	Palpitations, fatigue	
Chest		
Increased circumference of chest wall	Hyperventilation, dyspnea	
Lateral movement of apex of heart		
Exaggerated splitting of first heart sound, loud third sound		
Systolic murmur in 90% of pregnant women; brachial blood pressure — highest when patient is sitting		Previous undetected cardiac disease
Breasts		
Enlargement of breasts, erection of nipples, darkening of areola, secretion of colostrum	Tenderness, tingling	Enlargement of supernumerary breast tissue in axilla
Abdomen/Pelvis		
Increase in uterine size; rising of uterus from pelvis at 12 to 13 weeks of gestation; decreased bladder tone	Increased frequency and urgency of urination	Nocturia; dysuria; costovertebral angle tenderness; protein, glucose, ketones in urine
Sensation of fetal movement at 18 to 20 weeks of gestation		Absence of fetal movement; lower abdominal pain
Increased white vaginal discharge		Increased risk for vaginal infection due to low pH
Back		
Increased lumbar curvature	Backache	
Extremities		
Palmar erythema	Itching hands	
Pressure on venous circulation of legs	Dependent edema of feet and legs	Varicosities

- Increase in size. The breasts enlarge and become "lumpy" because of the growth of the ductal system that produces the milk. Tenderness and sensitivity of the breasts may be experienced in the first trimester.
- Darkening and enlargement of the areola
- Erection of the nipples and leaking of colostrum late in the first trimester
- Appearance of venous pattern over the breasts
- Striae formation in breasts, which becomes excessively large

Changes in breast tissue make examination difficult, but it is still necessary. Considering that breast cancer will develop in one of every 11 women in the United States, the evidence in favor of regular breast examination, even during pregnancy, is convincing.

Women who practice breast self-examination will notice gradual tissue changes in pregnancy and will be able to identify changes that are not consistent. Women who do not routinely examine their breasts will be less aware of the changes that are occurring.

All pregnant women should have a breast examination

as part of their initial physical examination, and those not previously taught breast self-examination should be instructed in the technique. (See Chapter 18).

When questionable changes occur in breast tissue, further evaluation is needed. Recent lumps or masses; masses that feel hard or fixed; skin changes, such as dimpling, redness, edema, or ulceration; breast pain; nipple retraction or elevation; and rashes are all indications for referral.

Inspection and Palpation of the Abdomen

Prior to the ascent of the uterus from the pelvis into the abdomen early in pregnancy (12 weeks of gestation), a complete abdominal examination can be performed. The abdomen can be inspected, the bowel sounds and aorta auscultated, and the liver, spleen, kidneys, and gut palpated and percussed. As pregnancy progresses, the growing uterus fills the abdominal cavity, making external examination of the abdominal organs impossible.

At approximately 12 weeks of gestation, the uterus has grown large enough to rise from the pelvis and become an abdominal organ. After 12 weeks, the abdominal examination is performed at each prenatal visit, although for some assessments (*e.g.,* fetal lie), the fetus must be large enough for the examiner to palpate fetal parts; this portion of the examination, therefore, is initiated near term.

The abdominal examination can be performed by a nurse practitioner, nurse midwife, physician, or, with supervision, a student nurse. Nursing students working in outpatient obstetric settings can learn to perform this portion of the physical examination. The sequential manner in which the examination is performed makes it easy to learn and execute. However, experience with the examination and consistent validation of findings through immediate feedback are essential.

Preparation of the Patient

Correct preparation of the patient for the abdominal examination will increase her comfort and the efficiency of the examiner.

1. Explain the abdominal examination and its purpose to the patient.
2. Ask the patient to empty her bladder. A full bladder places upward pressure on the uterus, causing it to rise higher into the abdomen. Not only does this cause discomfort to the patient, but erroneous measurements can be made when the bladder is mistaken for the uterus.
3. Help the patient assume a comfortable position on the examination table. She should lie on her back with her hands at her sides and her abdomen bared. Elevate the head of the table slightly, and ask the patient to flex her knees. This will help ease the

tension of the abdominal muscles, allowing easier palpation.

Late in pregnancy, some women become dizzy or faint when lying on their backs. This condition, known as supine hypotensive syndrome, is caused by the weight of the uterus compressing the inferior vena cava and aorta that lie directly posterior to it. The flow of blood back to the heart decreases, cardiac output lessens, and the patient becomes faint. The patient should immediately be turned on her side so that the weight of the uterus will be shifted from the vessels. Relief to the patient is immediate.

Inspection of the Abdomen

Begin the examination by inspecting the skin of the abdomen. With the aid of a good light, note:

- The presence of scars, rashes, lesions, dilated veins, pulsations, irritation, and the condition of the umbilicus (late in pregnancy it may protrude and become sensitive)
- The presence of a linea nigra, striae, or fetal movement (after 18–20 weeks)
- The size, shape, and contour of the uterus

Palpation of the Abdomen

Abdominal palpation permits the examiner to feel fetal parts through the abdominal wall and the uterus late in pregnancy.

- Use warm hands and touch the abdomen lightly to reduce reflexive reaction.
- Keep the fingers together and use the palmar surface of the fingers.
- Use smoothly applied pressure to palpate the uterus, following the four steps of Leopold's maneuvers as described in the accompanying display, page 402.
- Be consistent. Following the four sequential steps of Leopold's maneuvers will help you to gain skill and improve the accuracy of your findings.

Measurement of Fundal Height

Measurement of fundal height provides information about the progressive growth of the pregnancy. The zero line of a centimeter-measuring tape is placed on the superior edge of the symphysis pubis and the tape brought over the abdominal curve to the top of the fundus. This is the McDonald's measurement (Fig. 16–1). After 20 weeks of gestation, the fundal height, measured in centimeters, approximates the weeks of pregnancy. For example, at 20 weeks, the uterus is at the umbilicus, and the fundal height measures approximately 20 cm; at 33 weeks the fundal height should approximate 33 cm.

Before 20 weeks of gestation, McDonald's measurements are not accurate, and the uterus is measured in finger breadths (FB) above the symphysis or below the umbilicus, rather than in centimeters. At 16 weeks, the fundus is located half-way between the symphysis and the umbilicus, approximately three finger breadths (3FB) above the symphysis. At 18 weeks the fundus is two finger breadths below the umbilicus. Figure 16–1 indicates fundal height at various stages of pregnancy.

Measurement of fundal height provides valuable information on the growth of the fetus and is an important part of the patient assessment at each visit. When performed by different care providers at each visit, however, measurements may be inconsistent. When measurements are not consistent with the gestational age of the fetus and fetal size cannot be determined by abdominal palpation, further assessment, such as sonography, may be indicated. (See Chapter 17.)

Auscultation of Fetal Heart Tones

Auscultation of the rate and rhythm of the fetal heartbeat gives an indication of its general health. The fetal heartbeat can first be heard with a fetoscope at 18 to 20 weeks of gestation; if a doppler ultrasound device is used, it can be detected as early as 10 weeks of gestation (Fig. 16–2). When the heartbeat is first heard, regardless of the instrument used, the experience of listening to the baby's heartbeat should be shared with the parents. It may be exciting for them to hear the baby's heart, and often the

(text continued on page 404)

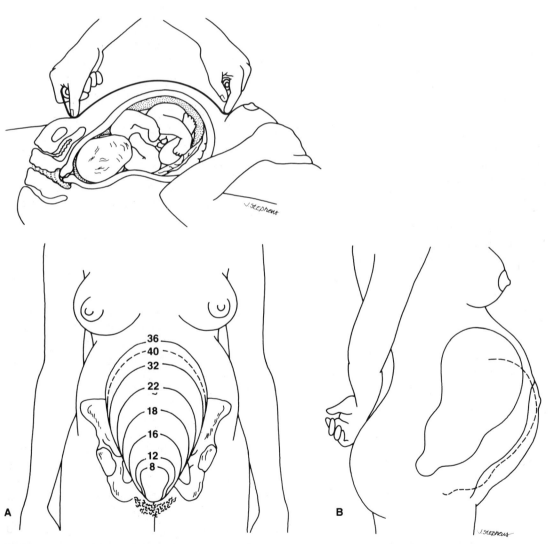

Figure 16–1. Measurement of fundal height. (Above) Procedure for measuring fundal height in centimeters (McDonald's measurement). (*A*) Fundal height at various weeks of gestation. (*B*) Lightening has occurred and the presenting part has settled into the pelvis. Fundal height decreases and the uterus rests anteriorly against the abdominal wall. In lay terms, "the baby has dropped." (Childbirth Graphics)

Leopold's Maneuvers

Leopold's maneuvers are performed late in pregnancy after the uterus becomes large enough to allow differentiation of fetal parts by palpation.

First Maneuver

Answers the question: *What is in the fundus? Head or breech?*
Finding: *Presentation*. This maneuver identifies the part of the fetus that lies over the inlet into the pelvis. The commonest presentations are *cephalic* (head first) and *breech* (pelvis first).

Performing First Maneuver

Facing the patient's head, use the tips of the fingers of both hands to palpate the uterine fundus.

- When the fetal head is in the fundus, it will feel hard, smooth, globular, mobile, and ballotable.
- When the breech is in the fundus, it will feel soft, irregular, round, and less mobile.

The *lie* of the fetus — the relationship between the long axis of the fetus and the long axis of the mother — can also be determined during the first maneuver. The lie is commonly longitudinal or transverse, but may occasionally be oblique.

Second Maneuver

Answers the question: *Where is the back?*
Finding: *Position*. This maneuver identifies the relationship of a fetal body part to the front, back, or sides of the maternal pelvis. There are many possible fetal positions.

Performing Second Maneuver

Remain facing the patient's head. Place your hands on either side of the abdomen. Steady the uterus with your hand on one side, and palpate the opposite side to determine the location of the fetal back.

- The back will feel firm, smooth, convex, resistant.
- The small parts (arms and legs) will feel small, irregularly placed, and knobby and may be actively or passively mobile.

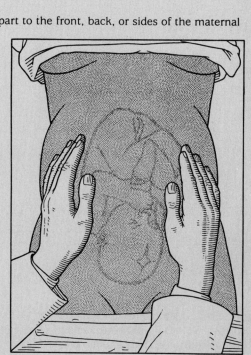

(continued)

Leopold's Maneuvers   (continued)

Third Maneuver

Answers the question: *What is the presenting part?*

Finding: *Presenting Part.* This maneuver identifies the most dependent part of the fetus—that is, the part that lies nearest the cervix. It is the part of the fetus that first contacts the finger in the vaginal examination, most commonly the head or breech.

Performing Third Maneuver

Place the tips of the first three fingers of each hand on either side of the patient's abdomen just above the symphysis, and ask the patient to take a deep breath and let it out. As she exhales, sink your fingers down slowly and deeply around the presenting part. Note the contour, size, and consistency of the part.

- The head will feel hard, smooth, and mobile if not engaged, immobile if engaged.
- The breech will feel soft and irregular.

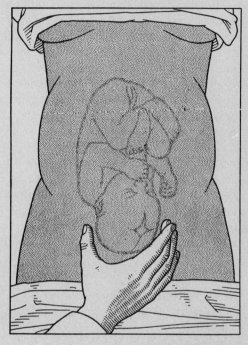

Fourth Maneuver

Answers the question: *Where is the cephalic prominence?*

Finding: *Cephalic Prominence.* This maneuver identifies the greatest prominence of the fetal head palpated over the brim of the pelvis. When the head is flexed (flexion attitude), the forehead forms the cephalic prominence. When the head is extended (extension attitude), the occiput becomes the cephalic prominence.

Performing Fourth Maneuver

Face the patient's feet. Gently move your fingers down the sides of the abdomen toward the pelvis until the fingers of one hand encounter a bony prominence. This is the cephalic prominence. If the prominence is on the opposite side from the back, it is the baby's brow, and the head is flexed. If the head is extended, the cephalic prominence will be located on the same side as the back and will be the occiput.

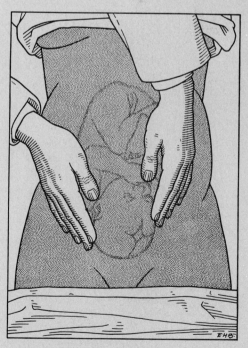

(Illustrations from Pritchard J, MacDonald P: Williams' Obstetrics, 16th ed. Norwalk, Conn., Appleton-Century-Crofts, 1980. Reprinted by permission)

pregnancy is validated for them at this time. The point of clearest heart tones for various fetal positions is shown in Figure 16–3.

The normal fetal heart rate (FHR) is 120 to 160 beats/min. When searching for heart tones, the normal rapid beat confirms that the examiner is hearing the fetal heartbeat rather than that of the mother. If the FHR is less than 100/min or more than 160/min with the uterus at rest, the fetus may be in distress. Regularity of the beat is a normal finding; irregularity is an abnormal finding.

The loudness of the fetal heart tones depends on the closeness of the fetal back to the mother's abdomen, as shown in Figure 16–3. The heartbeat will be muffled if the mother's abdominal wall is thick, as it is in obese women or when large amounts of fluid are contained in the amniotic sac, a condition known as hydramnios. Other sounds heard in the abdomen are funic souffle, caused by the rushing of blood through the umbilical arteries, and uterine souffle, caused by the sound of blood passing through the uterine blood vessels. The former sound is synchronous with the FHR; the latter is synchronous with the maternal pulse.

Failure to hear fetal heart tones may result from:

- Defective fetoscope or a noisy environment
- Early pregnancy (the fetus is too small)
- Fetal death (if fetal heart tones were heard previously and fetal movement has ceased, fetal demise is probable)
- Obesity in the pregnant woman
- Hydramnios
- Loud placental souffle that obscures the fetal heart tones
- Posterior position of the fetus (the back of the fetus is facing the mother's back)

More extensive techniques for assessing fetal well-being are discussed in Chapter 17.

Performing the Pelvic Examination

The pelvic examination is performed after the abdominal examination is completed. It provides a great deal of information about the normalcy of pelvic structures or the problems they might cause, the length of the pregnancy, the presence of infection, and the adequacy of the bony pelvis for delivery of the infant. The examination includes inspection and palpation of the external genitalia, speculum examination of the vagina and cervix, bimanual examination of the uterus and adnexa, and rectovaginal examination. A review of the anatomy of the genital tract (Chapter 5) will greatly facilitate understanding of the pelvic examination.

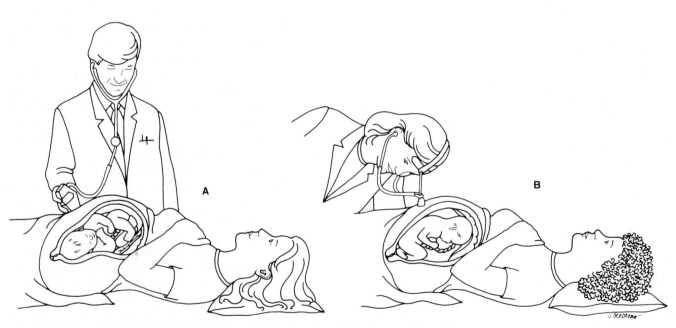

Figure 16–2. Auscultation of fetal heart tones. (*A*) Monitoring and counting fetal heart rate with an ultrasound stethoscope (Doppler ultrasound). May be heard at 8 to 11 weeks. (*B*) Monitoring fetal heart tone with a fetoscope. May be heard at 18 to 20 weeks. (Childbirth Graphics)

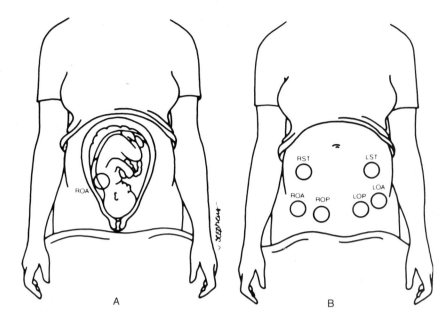

Figure 16–3. Points of maximum intensity for auscultation of fetal heart tones in specific fetal positions. (*A*) Heart tones are best heard through the fetus's back. (*B*) ROA = Right occipital anterior, LOA = Left occipital anterior, LOP = Left occipital posterior, ROP = Right occipital posterior, RST = Right sacrotransverse, LST = Left sacrotransverse. (Childbirth Graphics)

Preparation of Equipment

The following equipment is needed to perform a pelvic examination:

- Good light source
- Pair of plastic gloves
- Speculum
- Thayer-Martin media for a gonorrhea culture (if applicable)
- Pap bottle or card carrier with fixative
- Glass slides for the Pap smear
- Glass slides and KOH (potassium hydroxide) and saline solutions for preparation of a wet mount if vaginal infection is suspected
- Ayre spatula for Pap smear collection
- Sterile cotton swabs to collect secretions for specimens
- Other culture media as needed for specimens collected
- Lubricant, to be used for the bimanual and rectal examinations only

Preparation of the Patient

It is important that the patient's bladder be emptied before she is draped for the examination. A full bladder will cause discomfort during the bimanual examination and will also hinder palpation of the uterus for size. The patient should be nude from the waist down, but she may prefer to wear her shoes to protect her feet in the stirrups. She is placed in the lithotomy position with her feet in the stirrups and her buttocks positioned slightly over the

edge of the table with her legs spread wide apart (Fig. 16–4). The patient should be instructed to put her arms at her sides or fold them under her breasts. When her head is resting on her elevated arms, the abdominal muscles become taut and examination is difficult.

The patient should be told what will be happening during the examination and what she may expect to feel as it proceeds. Her past experience with pelvic examinations should be explored and reassurance given that procedures will be explained to her. Helping the patient to relax by demonstrating deep, slow breathing is often effective in achieving cooperation.

Some patients are helped by seeing the speculum and getting an explanation of its use; however, the opposite might be true for other women. For women interested in seeing their genitals, a long-handled mirror can be provided. In some cases, it may be necessary to allow the patient to insert the speculum herself, with direction from the examiner. This is sometimes helpful with teenage patients who are fearful of being hurt. A wide variety of reactions to the examination can occur, and the attitude of the nurse will greatly influence the quality of the experience for the patient, not only in the present examination, but in future ones as well. When the equipment for the pelvic examination is ready and the patient has been prepared, the various steps of the examination will be performed in the following order:

1. Inspection and palpation of the external genitalia
2. Speculum examination and specimen collection
3. Bimanual examination, including pelvimetry
4. Rectovaginal examination

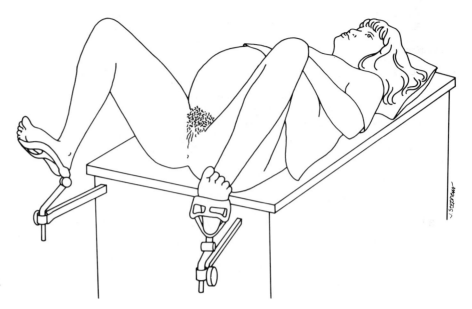

Figure 16–4. Lithotomy position. (Childbirth Graphics)

Inspection and Palpation of the External Genitalia

This is the first step of the pelvic examination and is especially important during pregnancy (Table 16–4). If abnormalities such as vulvar varicosities, fungal infection, pediculosis, or hemorrhoids are found, they can be treated or palliated before labor and delivery. Infections identified in the prenatal period should be treated early to prevent exposing the fetus to infection at birth.

The Speculum Examination

Prior to the speculum examination, the patient should be queried about the use of vaginal medication or a douche in the past 24 hours, since vaginal and cervical secretions are washed away or altered by these intrusions. If they have been used recently, collection of the Pap and gonorrhea smears and wet mount slides should be deferred until the next visit, and the patient should be cautioned against using medication or a douche prior to a pelvic examination.

The speculum is made up of two blades and a handle (see the display, page 409). The posterior blade is fixed, and the anterior blade is movable. The blades are held together by a thumbscrew on the handle. Loosening the thumbscrew permits the blades to be separated. The anterior blade is hinged and is controlled by a thumbpiece on its side. This permits it to be elevated, causing separation of the blades and allowing visualization of the vagina. When visualization is adequate, the thumbscrew is tightened to lock the blades in position. Elevation of the anterior blade is also useful for a clearer view of the cervix and better access to it during IUD insertion and cervical or endometrial biopsy.

When the speculum is being introduced into the vagina, the thumbscrew should be loosened and the blades should be closely approximated.

Method of Examination

The speculum examination is performed in the following manner.

1. Select the speculum appropriate for the patient. Warm it and lubricate it with warm water.

2. Place the index and middle fingers 1 inch into the vagina. Spread the fingers, exerting a downward pressure on the perineal body.

3. Ask the patient to bear down while you insert the closed speculum in an oblique plane until it is beyond the hymenal ring (Fig. 16–5A). *Downward pressure* during insertion is extremely important to ensure that the sensitive anterior structures (urethra and clitoris) are not traumatized.

4. Withdraw the fingers, turn the speculum to the horizontal plane, and advance it slowly, maintaining downward pressure, until resistance is met (Fig. 16–5B).

5. The shorter upper blade should be in front of the cervix and is lifted with the thumblever. Maneuver the speculum so that when the blades are fully opened, the cervix comes into view (Fig. 16–5C).

6. If the cervix is not seen, withdraw the speculum about halfway and reinsert it on a different plane. When the cervix is visualized, secure the blades in position by tightening the thumbscrew. Then proceed with the examination as outlined in Table 16–5.

Table 16-4 Inspection and Palpation of the External Genitalia

Organ or Structure	Action	Normal Findings	Pregnancy Changes	Abnormal Findings
Inspection				
Mons Pubis	Adjust the light and sit on a stool at the foot of the table facing the patient's perineum. Inspect the external genitals.	Mature secondary sexual characteristics	None	
		Skin covered by inverse triangle of curly hair (female escutcheon)	None	Pediculosis pubis (crab lice) or nits (eggs on hair shafts). Pruritus (itching), excoriation from scratching, folliculitis (infected hair follicle)
Labia Majora		Lie in close opposition in nulliparous women, may gap widely in multiparous ones; feel soft, have moist inner surface	Inner surface drier and skinlike	Pruritus, excoriation from scratching, lesions, vesicles, varicosities, discharge between folds from vaginal infection, Bartholin's gland tenderness, edema, redness
Inspection and Palpation				
	Tell the patient she will be touched. With gloved fingers, separate the labia majora, exposing the labia minora.			
Labia Minora		Hidden under labia majora in nulliparous women, project beyond labia majora in multiparous women; vary greatly in size and shape; feel soft	None in multiparas	Redness caused by vaginal infection or allergic reaction to douches, perfumed soap; wartlike growths, lesions
Clitoris	Observe the clitoris and retract its prepuce.	Small, erectile, highly vascular body, rarely exceeds 2 cm in length, covered by retractable prepuce	None	Clitoral hypertrophy, fixed prepuce that cannot be retracted (may interfere with sexual stimulation), lesions, chancres of sexually transmitted diseases
Urethral Meatus	Spread the labia with the index and second fingers of the gloved hand, inspect the urethra.	Vertical slit with pinkish, puckered appearance	None observable; dilatation of urethral canal due to increased progesterone	Polyps, growths, discharge, caruncle, erythema
Skene's Ducts (on either side of urethra at 4 and 8 o'clock)	Insert the index finger of the right hand 1 inch into the introitus, and gently press upward on the urethra. This is called "milking."	Duct may or may not be observable; no discharge	None	Yellowish-white discharge oozing from Skene's duct (gonorrhea culture needed)
Vaginal Musculature	As the fingers are withdrawn from the vagina, gently spread the vaginal orifice. Holding your fingers steady, ask the patient to cough.	Firm or relaxed muscle tone	More relaxed muscle tone, particularly in multigravidas	Cystocele (prolapse of bladder that protrudes in anterior vagina); rectocele (prolapse of rectum into posterior vagina)

(continued)

Table 16-4 **Inspection and Palpation of the External Genitalia** (continued)

Organ or Structure	Action	Normal Findings	Pregnancy Changes	Abnormal Findings
Inspection and Palpation				
Pubococcygeal Musculature	Insert the fingers further into the vagina and ask the patient to tighten her muscles around your finger. (These are the muscles used to stop the stream during urination.)	Tight muscle control	More relaxed muscle tone, particularly in multiparous women	Loss of bladder tone as a result of pregnancy; leaking of urine, especially in older women, when perineal muscle tone is not maintained
Bartholin's Glands	With the fingers in the vagina, sweep them laterally on either side of the posterior fourchette to palpate the Bartholin's glands at 4 and 8 o'clock.	Glands not felt	None	Gland enlargement from infection, usually unilateral, exudate from duct, reddening of skin; may be extremely painful, with patient unable to walk
Perineum (area between the vagina and anus)	Remove the gloved hand from the vagina and use both hands to spread the buttocks apart to observe the perineum and anus.	No lesions; possibly episiotomy scar from previous delivery	None	Lesions, cysts, infection
Anus		Darker skin	None	Hemorrhoids, inflammation, lesions, fissures

Specimen Collection

Before the speculum is removed from the vagina, Pap, gonorrhea, and vaginal smears should be collected as indicated in Table 16-4.

Papanicolaou Test. The Papanicolaou (Pap) test is a cervical smear performed to screen for cervical cancer or the presence of precancerous cells.

Gonorrhea Culture. A gonorrhea culture is a cervical smear used to test for gonorrhea. The gonococcus is a fragile, anaerobic organism. It will not grow in the presence of oxygen or survive when it is cold. Thus, special handling of the gonorrhea smear is necessary. The Thayer–Martin plate on which the smear is collected should be placed within 10 to 15 minutes in an anaerobic, warm atmosphere.

Vaginal Smear. A vaginal smear is collected when there are symptoms of a vaginal infection or one is suspected. Vaginal infections are common in pregnancy because of disturbances of the vaginal ecology by changing hormone levels. These disturbances include an overabundance of vaginal glycogen, increased physiologic discharge, and local tissue edema caused by increased vascularity.

Many women may be unaware of or uninformed about symptoms of vaginal infection. Prior to the pelvic examination, it is appropriate to ask whether the patient has experienced symptoms such as excessive vaginal discharge, odor, itching, dyspareunia, or burning with urination (caused when urine runs over irritated vaginal tissue). If symptoms are present, or the vagina looks red and inflamed upon inspection, a microscopic examination of the discharge is done to identify the infecting organism. This is called a *wet mount* and identifies the presence of *Candida* (yeast), *Trichomonas,* and *Gardnerella,* now commonly known as *bacterial vaginosis.* Herpes vaginitis cannot be identified by wet mount. It is a viral infection, and special testing by serologic antibody screen, special media, or (less effectively) Pap smear is necessary for its identification.

During the speculum examination, vaginal discharge is collected on a cotton swab or wooden spatula and spread on slides. A KOH (potassium hydroxide) 10% slide is used to identify the pseudomycelia (treelike) signs of *Candida,* and a warm saline slide is used to identify the

Speculum Types

- *Virginal speculum:* smallest available and has short, narrow, and flat blades. It is used in young women and in women who have had little or no sexual intercourse.
- *Graves speculum:* available in standard and large sizes. The standard size is appropriate to use in examining multiparous women and in sexually active women.
- *Pederson speculum:* longer than the Graves but is flatter and narrower. It is used for women who are nulligravid, multigravid, or sexually active and have tight musculature. It is also useful in examining postmenopausal women with contracted vaginas.
- *Plastic speculum:* available in three sizes — small, medium, and large. It is not routinely used in all health care settings.

Advantages of Plastic Speculum:
- Disposable
- Transparency permits a better view of the vaginal tissue
- Can be used in self-care examination

Disadvantages of Plastic Speculum:
- Harder to insert into a dry vagina when only water can be used as a lubricant
- May be uncomfortable for the patient, and distort the shape of the cervical os, and expose the columnar cells of the cervical canal, causing them to appear everted onto the exterior cervical surface

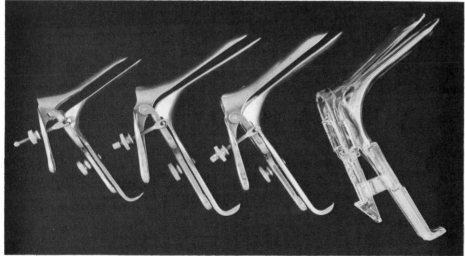

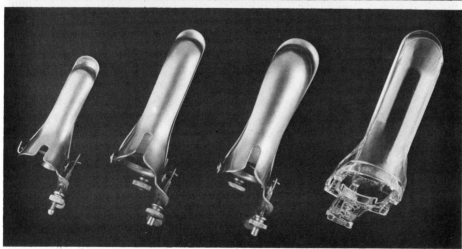

Specula. From left to right: small metal Pederson, medium metal Pederson, medium metal Graves, and large plastic Pederson.

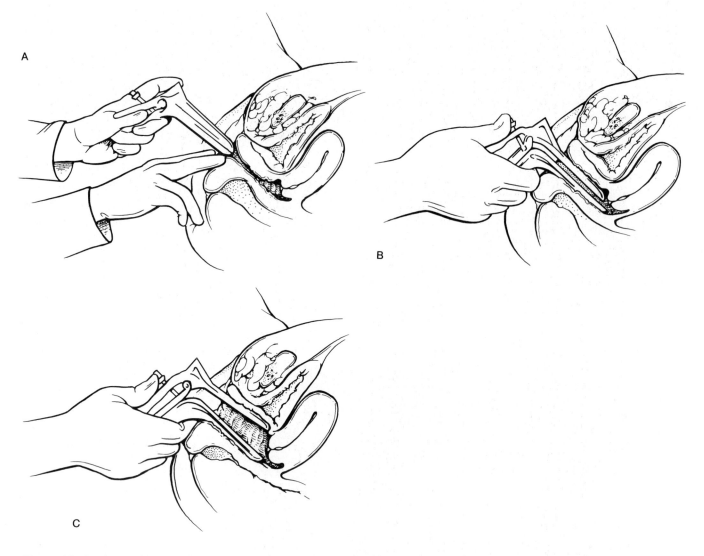

A

B

C

Figure 16–5. Speculum examination. (*A*) Insertion. (*B*) Advance. (*C*) Opening the speculum to allow examination of the cervix.

motile trichomonad. The organisms, the symptoms they cause, and their diagnoses are covered in Chapter 20.

Bimanual Examination

Some of the most vital information gathered during an obstetric or gynecologic physical assessment is obtained during the bimanual examination (Table 16–6). As the uterus, ovaries (and their surrounding tissues, the adnexae), the pelvic ligaments, and the rectum are palpated, a complete picture of the woman's reproductive organs can be drawn (Fig. 16–6).

During pregnancy the examiner is concentrating on findings that provide information about the pregnancy, such as:

- The size of the uterus in weeks (*e.g.,* 8 weeks' size), the shape of the uterus, its position, its softness or firmness, its location
- The condition of the cervical os: closed or open, soft or firm, thick or thin (the latter condition, known as *effacement,* is an early sign of labor); and its position: posterior or anterior
- The presentation (after 27 weeks) of the fetus and the status of its descent into the pelvis in late pregnancy (station)

The examination should be learned and performed in a consistent manner.

Some points to remember are:

Table 16-5   Procedures in the Speculum Examination

Procedure	Pregnancy Changes	Abnormal Findings
With the light placed for optimum visualization: 1. Inspect the cervix via the speculum	Nulliparous cervical os appears small and round; parous os is slitlike and may have scars from tears during previous delivery. Bluish, friable cervix (bleeds easily); white discharge	Dilated os; yellowish, greenish, or foul-smelling discharge at cervical os; inflammation
2. Collect specimens: *Cervical:* Pap smear; gonorrhea or other cervical smears if infection suspected	Increased amount of white, normal discharge	Blood from os, lesions, irregular configuration of ectropion
Vaginal: Wet mount of saline and KOH to diagnose suspected vaginal infections	Bluish vagina	Abnormal-appearing discharge, lesions, cysts
3. Remove the speculum in the following manner. Loosen the thumbscrew. Maintaining a downward pressure, rotate the speculum as you slowly withdraw it. Hold the thumb lightly on the thumbscrew to allow you to see the vaginal walls between the blades. As the speculum is withdrawn, it gradually closes and it will be fully closed as it is withdrawn at an oblique angle.	Pinkish-blue color rugae	Structural abnormalities, inflammation, lesions, white plaques, contact bleeding

(A) Normal nulliparous cervix. (B) Normal parous cervix.

- The patient's hands should be at her sides to maintain abdominal relaxation
- Palpate with the flat part of the fingers; they are more sensitive than the fingertips.
- Slow, relaxed, firm movements will avoid pain to the patient and help her relax her abdominal muscles.
- If the patient becomes tense, relax your hand and reassure her that the examination should not be painful, although she may experience a feeling of pressure.

A gentle vaginal or speculum examination is performed when there is vaginal bleeding in the third trimester and only with medical consultation. The bleeding may be caused by placenta previa (a placenta lying over the internal cervical os). A finger placed through the os into the placenta may cause the patient to hemorrhage or exsanguinate.

Pelvimetry

Pelvimetry is the measurement of the dimensions and proportions of the bony pelvis in order to assess whether it is large enough to accommodate the delivery of an infant. A normal vaginal delivery can occur only when the bony pelvis is large enough for the largest diameter of the infant, the head, to pass through it.

Pelvic measurements are usually obtained as part of the initial pelvic examination. When the bimanual portion of the examination is completed and while the fingers are still placed in the vagina, the fingers are moved over the landmarks of the bony pelvis and their size is approximated. The assessment is subjective, and its accuracy depends upon the skill and experience of the examiner. Although precise measurements cannot be made, the adequacy of the proportions and the dimensions of the pelvis can be quite accurately estimated.

Currently, if done at all, pelvimetry is delayed until late in pregnancy. It is considered more comfortable for the patient, since the pelvic tissues are softer and the capacity of the pelvis in relation to the size of the fetus can be more accurately assessed at this time. It is not crucial to assess the adequacy of the pelvis early, and since nothing can be done about it, some argue it is unnecessary. If the pelvis is assessed as borderline (*i.e.*, it may or may not be adequate), the patient will be given a trial labor. Sometimes,

Table 16–6   **Bimanual Examination**

Procedures	Pregnancy Changes	Abnormal Findings
1. Remove the glove from the left hand and lubricate the first two fingers of the right hand. Insert the lubricated finger into the vagina, maintaining *downward pressure*. With the fingers well into the vagina rotate the hand until the palm is up. The thumb is kept vertical in the midline, while the other two fingers curve out of the way.		
Cervix		
2. Place the left hand on the abdomen halfway between the symphysis and the umbilicus. Push the vaginal hand forward and backward until each of the fingers is in a lateral fornix with the cervix in between. Palpate the cervix; it should be freely movable.	Cervix 1.5–2.0 cm long; firm until term, then soft, elastic, and thick. External os closed (nullipara) or admits one fingertip (multipara). Internal os closed.	Roughened areas, edema, bleeding, dilatation before at term, tenderness with movement. Short or irregular length; soft and pliable <37 weeks; internal os open <37 weeks
Uterus		
3. Determine uterine position by passing the fingers along the front and back of the cervix. With the first two fingers over the cervix, push it upward, lifting the uterus into the abdomen. Palpate the uterus between the vaginal and abdominal hands by moving the uterus from side to side with one finger in the lateral fornices so that the surface of the uterus can be felt (Fig. 16–5*A*)	Shape changes from globular to ovoid. Uterine size depends on age of gestation. Feels softer than nonpregnant uterus. Irregular, painless Braxton Hicks contractions may be felt. Becomes an abdominal organ at 12 weeks.	Tenderness with movement, myomas (fibroids) felt as firm irregularities on its surface. Deviations to either side may be due to pelvic masses or adhesions.
4. To palpate the adnexa, place the vaginal fingers palm upward in the right lateral fornix and the abdominal hand in the area of the right iliac crest. The hands are brought together and moved together toward the midline. The vaginal fingers will feel the ovaries slip between the fingers while the abdominal hand is pushing them downward. Repeat on the left side (Fig. 16–5*B*). In some women the ovaries are not palpable even in the nonpregnant state.	When the uterus becomes an abdominal organ, the ovaries cannot be palpated.	Tenderness, cystic masses, firm masses, enlargement (normal size 4 × 6 cm)

vaginal delivery will be possible in such cases because of the give and take of the softening pelvic joints and the ability of the infant's cranial bones to overlap during delivery. Moreover, smaller infants can often be delivered successfully through a borderline pelvis. The characteristics of the different types of pelves and their measurements are shown in Figure 16–7.

Rarely, x-ray pelvimetry is used to determine precise pelvic measurements. When the genetic effect of radiation on the fetus was first demonstrated, its use in pregnancy dropped sharply. The use of trial labors and the decline in the use of midforceps delivery, which required knowledge of the precise structure of the pelvis, have also reduced the popularity of x-ray pelvimetry. It may, however, be used when:

- It is necessary to diagnose breech position during active labor
- Fetal position is unclear

Whenever x-ray pelvimetry is to be used, the patient should be consulted and informed.

Collecting Specimens for Laboratory Tests

Collection of specimens for laboratory tests during the first prenatal visit is an important part of the assessment of the pregnant woman. The nurse performs an initial assessment of the patient's blood pressure and height and weight and collects a clean-catch urine specimen so

A   B

Figure 16-6. Bimanual examination. (*A*) Palpation of the uterus. (*B*) Palpation of the adnexa.

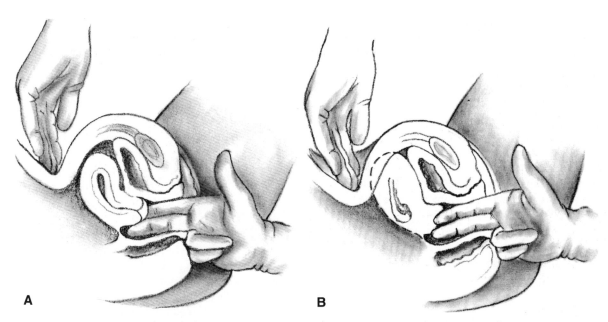

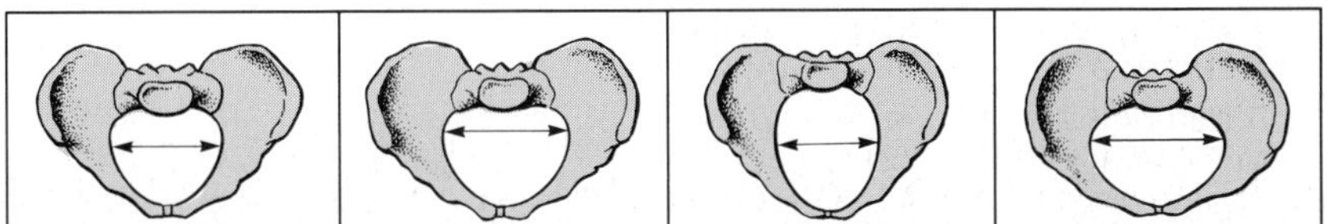

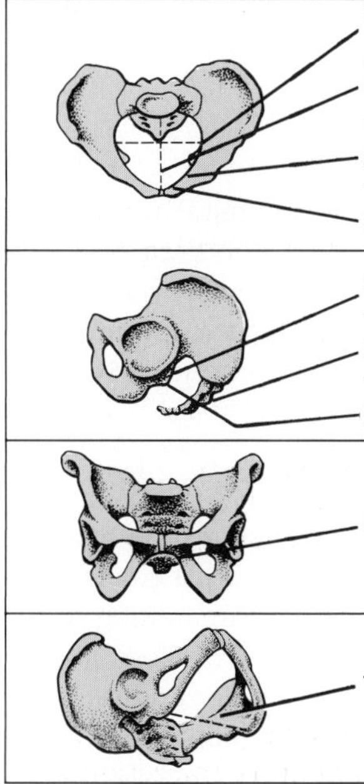

	Gynecoid	Android	Anthropoid	Platypelloid
Bone structure	Medium	Heavy	Medium	Medium
Widest transverse diameter of inlet	12.0 cm	12.0 cm	< 12.0 cm	12.0 cm
Anteroposterior diameter of inlet	11.0 cm	11.0 cm	> 12.0 cm	10.0 cm
Side walls	Straight	Convergent	Narrow	Wide
Forepelvis	Wide	Narrow	Divergent	Straight
Sacrosciatic notch	Medium	Narrow	Backward	Forward
Inclination of sacrum	Medium	Forward (lower 1/3)	Wide	Narrow
Ischial spines	Not prominent	Prominent	Not prominent	Not prominent
Suprapubic arch	Wide	Narrow	Medium	Wide
Transverse diameter of outlet	10.0 cm	< 10.0 cm	10.0 cm	10.0 cm

Figure 16-7. Characteristics of four types of pelves. (Reproduced with permission from Benson RC (ed): Current Obstetric and Gynecologic Diagnosis and Treatment, 4th ed. Los Altos, CA, Lange Medical Publications, 1982)

that the dipstick reading will be available to the health care provider before the patient assessment. During the pelvic examination, vaginal, gonorrhea, and Pap smears are collected, and, along with prenatal blood studies and urine for microscopic examination, are sent to the laboratory. Results of these tests are evaluated on the second prenatal visit. The laboratory tests and procedures used in assessing the pregnant patient are listed in Table 16–7. If the test results are normal and the woman does not present later problems, routine monitoring of blood pressure and weight, urine dipstick testing at each visit, and anemia screening every trimester will probably be the only tests required for the duration of the pregnancy.

The following tests are used for screening and pregnancy monitoring. When abnormal or inconclusive results are reported, additional tests may be required.

Blood Tests

Blood tests are used to identify blood group and type and to screen for anemia, antibodies, infection, and blood hemoglobinopathies (abnormal forms of hemoglobin such as sickle cells) and diabetes.

Hemoglobin and Hematocrit

A hemoglobin (Hgb) or hematocrit (Hct) test is used to detect anemia. A Hgb reading below 10.5 g/100 ml or a Hct below 32% indicates anemia in the pregnant woman. The commonest causes of anemia are previous heavy menstrual periods and a diet low in iron. When pathologic causes of anemia have been excluded, iron supplementation and diet counseling are indicated.

Blood Type

Blood type, Rh, and antibody titer tests identify blood types as O, A, B, or AB and as having a positive or negative Rh factor. Eighty-five percent of the population has a positive Rh factor (Rh+); 15% have a negative Rh factor (Rh−). When the mother's blood is identified as Rh− during pregnancy, the factor of her mate must be obtained. When the father's Rh factor is negative, so is the fetus's, and no problems will arise. If, however, the father's blood is Rh+, the fetus's may also be Rh+. The combination of an Rh− mother and an Rh+ fetus may cause the mother's body to react to the fetus as a foreign object, producing antibodies against it and placing it at risk for erythroblastosis fetalis. (See Chapter 19 for more information on this condition.)

To determine whether the Rh− mother is producing antibodies against her Rh+ infant's blood, Rh antibody titer tests are performed on the mother's blood periodically during pregnancy. If antibodies are detected, as in-

dicated by a rising titer, the patient is considered to be at high risk. Although Rh is the commonest type of blood antibody, other less common types can also cause fetal hemolytic disease and can be detected by antibody titer. (See Chapter 19.)

Rubella Screening

Rubella screening is done to determine whether the mother has had rubella (German measles). Past infection can be documented by the presence of antibodies to rubella in her blood. It is very important to counsel women who are not immune to avoid contact with suspected cases of rubella. If contracted in early pregnancy (the first 12 weeks), the disease may cause grave effects in the fetus, including blindness, deafness, mental retardation, and cardiac defects.

Susceptible women are not immunized during pregnancy, but rubella vaccine is given early in the postpartum period to prevent future infection. The vaccine is safe to use in breastfeeding mothers.

Serology

Serology (the Venereal Disease Research Laboratory [VDRL] and fluorescent treponemal antibody absorption [FTA-ABS]) tests are used to screen and diagnose women with syphilis. The spirochete *Treponema pallidum,* the organism responsible for the disease, crosses the placenta and infects the infant. When the mother is treated before 18 weeks of gestation, the spirochete is usually eradicated from fetal tissues, causing minimal or no damage. If the mother is not treated until after 18 weeks, there may be evidence of a syphilitic infection in the newborn. When untreated, the disease may cause prematurity, intrauterine death, or congenital syphilis.

Hemoglobin Electrophoresis

This blood test is utilized to detect genetic hemoglobin disorders such as sickle cell anemia (SS disease), sickle cell-hemoglobin C disease (SC disease), and thalassemias. These are recessively inherited diseases encountered primarily in the black population. Black women are routinely screened for these disorders.

Hepatitis B

Many prenatal clinics are also screening the blood of pregnant women for hepatitis B. During pregnancy this virus has been identified as the most threatening to the fetus and neonate. Inoculation and transmission of hepatitis B infection is through sexual contact and blood or parenteral exposure. Transmission of hepatitis B from mother to infant occurs through blood contact during the intrapartum and postpartum periods. Women at most risk for transmitting the virus are those:

Table 16-7 **Elements of Prenatal Assessment in Initial and Subsequent Visits**

Assessment	Rationale
Initial Visit:	
Health History: Collect demographic data and detailed health history, present health, and menstrual/obstetric history, present and past pregnancy symptoms or problems.	To obtain data about possible influences (ethnic/cultural factors, work status) and status of present pregnancy (use of drugs, smoking, dietary practices).
Psychosocial Assessment: Assess and record patient's and partner's attitudes toward pregnancy, emotional and financial impact on family, expectations for pregnancy.	To identify patients unprepared for life changes associated with pregnancy or who need early referral to additional resources.
Physical Examination: Record height, weight, prepregnant weight, blood pressure, pulse, temperature. Examine body systems: skin, head (eyes, ears, nose, neck, throat), chest (breasts, lungs, heart, back), extremities, abdomen, pelvis (bimanual examination, laboratory tests including Pap smear, gonorrhea smear, wet mount).	To assess maternal health and fetal growth, and to ensure that abnormal findings are promptly identified and treated. Early pelvic examination allows for immediate determination of uterine size, presence of vaginal or pelvic infection or structural abnormalities which may affect pregnancy. However, pelvic examination may be deferred to later visit if necessary for patient comfort; teenagers frequently refuse an initial pelvic examination.
Subsequent Visits	
Pregnancy Status—Ongoing: Assess and record presence of common pregnancy discomforts (nausea, vomiting, backache, constipation, heartburn, headache, varicosities). Assess for abnormal signs (bleeding, lack of fetal movement after quickening, elevated blood pressure, excessive weight gain or loss). Review dietary intake of iron, iron supplementation, 24 hour dietary recall (protein, 4 servings; milk products, 4 servings; bread, cereals, 4 servings, vitamin C-rich fruits and vegetables, 1 serving; dark green vegetables, 1 serving; other fruits and vegetables, 1 serving). Review weight gain.	To check for symptoms causing maternal discomfort and prescribe care. To check for factors that may inhibit adequate nutrient intake, and enable early detection and correction of dietary problems adversely affecting maternal weight gain.
Physical Examination—Ongoing: Check blood pressure, edema, fundal height, fetal heart tones (record date first heard with fetoscope); perform Leopold's maneuvers. Date and record when first fetal movements felt.	To rule out presence of hypertension. To monitor growth rate of fetus and confirm gestational age; if uterine fundus is palpated at the umbilicus and FHT heard just above the symphysis, pregnancy is confirmed to be at 20 weeks of gestation. First detection of fetal movement usually at 19–20 weeks in primigravida, 17–20 weeks in multigravida.
Laboratory Tests—Ongoing: Perform routine urine dipstick tests for glucose, protein, ketones. Perform complete blood count or Hgb, Hct tests each trimester. Perform Rh antibody screen at 24–28 weeks if Rh negative or previous sensitization. Repeat tests for STDs as indicated. Perform blood glucose screen at 24–28 weeks.	To check for glucosuria, proteinuria (possible urinary tract infection, early preeclampsia), ketonuria (indicates inadequate caloric intake). Blood studies will indicate iron deficiency anemia (Hgb of 11 g/dl if other causes have been ruled out). To identify rising titers signalling maternal sensitization. To ensure absence of sexually-transmitted infection at time of delivery. To identify gestational diabetes.
Psychosocial Assessment—Ongoing: Assess patient concerns about physical and emotional changes, plans for meeting learning needs, plans for childbirth.	To identify needs for support, counseling and anticipatory guidance. To provide referral for childbirth or parenting preparation as needed and desired.
Physical Examination After 38 Weeks of Gestation: Assess and record signs of impending labor: lightening, engagement, cervical status.	To document normal progression toward delivery between 38–40 weeks' gestation. Primigravidas experience lightening about 2 weeks before delivery; multigravidas usually just before or during labor. Cervical check allows detection of cervical softening, effacement, dilatation, station, and presenting fetal part.

- Of Asian, Pacific Island, or Alaskan Eskimo descent, whether immigrant or U.S. born
- Born in Haiti or sub-Saharan Africa
- With a past history of acute or chronic liver disease or hepatitis
- Who have frequent occupational exposure to blood in medical or dental settings
- That have home contact with an HB carrier or hemodialysis patient
- Who have multiple episodes of sexually transmitted disease
- Who are bi/homosexual, or heterosexual with multiple partners
- Who have been rejected as a blood donor

- Who use illegal IV drugs
- Work or reside in an institution for the mentally retarded
- Work in a hemodialysis unit
- Exhibit symptoms of fever, headache, anorexia, pharyngitis, and/or abdominal pain
- Who are military personnel or foreign travelers

HIV Testing

The Morbidity and Mortality Weekly Report (MMWR) of December 6, 1985, discusses the Centers for Disease Control recommendations for prevention of human immunosuppression virus transmission during the prenatal period. It is advised that women who are pregnant, or those that may become pregnant, be offered counseling and testing for the HIV antibody.

The women for whom these recommendations apply belong to one of the following groups:

- Those with evidence of HIV infection
- Those who have used intravenous drugs for nonmedical purposes
- Those born in countries where heterosexual transmission is high
- Those who engage in prostitution
- Those who are, or have been sex partners of intravenous drug abusers, bisexual men, male hemophiliacs, men born in countries where heterosexual contact may play a major role, and men who have evidence of HIV infection.

Urine Tests

Urine collected for testing should always be a midstream specimen. The purpose of urine testing is to detect the presence of urinary tract infection and substances in the urine that may indicate a problem.

Protein should not be present in the urine. Small amounts (traces) may be found when the specimen is contaminated by vaginal secretions or blood. Large amounts of protein may indicate kidney disease or preeclampsia.

Glucose found in the urine on one occasion may indicate the normal stress of pregnancy on the renal threshold. When large amounts appear in the urine on more than one occasion, further testing should be done, as discussed in Chapter 20.

Ketones are products of fat metabolism found in urine only during fasting, after heavy exercise, or when pregnant women cannot maintain food intake because of nausea or vomiting. Since these substances may be deleterious to the fetus, the spilling of ketones should be prevented by adequate nutritional and fluid intake.

Bilirubin is a product of red blood cell destruction. Its presence in the urine suggests liver or gallbladder disease, or breakdown of red blood cells.

Blood in the urine (hematuria) suggests urinary tract infection, kidney disease, or vaginal contamination of the specimen.

White blood cells at amounts greater than 4/HPF (high-powered field) indicate a urinary tract infection.

Bacteria in the urine (bacteriuria) indicates urinary tract inflammation. A urine culture is done to diagnose urinary tract infection and to identify the organism responsible. A culture is considered positive for urinary tract infection when the colony count exceeds 100,000 (10^5). For laboratory values of the blood and urine tests, see Table 18–7.

Diabetes Screening

Screening for gestational diabetes is a standard part of prenatal care for all women. Testing is done at 24–28 weeks because the hormonal effects that block insulin utilization and result in elevated blood glucose are clearly detectable at this time. A blood sample is drawn 1 hour after 50 g of a glucose drink are administered to the woman. An abnormal result of > 135 mg/dl indicates the need for further screening (see Chapter 20).

Identifying High-Risk Patients

Pregnancy presents a risk of morbidity and mortality over that of the nonpregnant state. High-risk factors, therefore, must be identified as early as possible. Useful scoring systems have been developed to identify high risk in pregnancy. The Prenatal Risk Indicator Form (see the accompanying display) is used in the prenatal setting for early identification of problems.

All the information needed to complete the Prenatal Risk Indicator Form is obtained during the prenatal history and physical examination. Completion of the form and scoring can be done before or after the charting of the first visit. When indications of risk are identified, they should be shared with the patient during her next visit. Her cooperation in modifying risk factors or preventing their exacerbation may enhance the outcome of the pregnancy. (Nursing care of the patient with an at-risk pregnancy is addressed in Chapters 19 and 20.)

Adolescent Pregnancy. Typically adolescent pregnancy is an unplanned and unintended event. Reasons for teen-age pregnancy are multiple and complex. The teenager who becomes pregnant may, or may not, become rebellious, is typically concerned about the reactions of other people to her pregnancy, and is often in personal turmoil. She may be economically disadvantaged, less future-oriented, and perhaps less cooperative in planning her own care. She may resist supplemental medications (iron and vitamins) and nutritional advice and may have

ASSESSMENT TOOL

Prenatal Risk Indicator Form

Risk Score	Risk Indicator
	Demographic Factors
2	Maternal Age: 15 or under, 35 or over
1	Parity: Nulliparous
2	grand multipara
1	Race: Nonwhite
1	Marital status: Single
1	Economic status: Dependent on public assistance
2	Prenatal care: First visit after 27 weeks
	or less than 5 visits
	Obstetric Factors
1	Infertility factors: less than 2 years
2	more than 2 years
1	Previous abortion: one
2	two or more
	Premature or low birth weight infant:
1	history of one
5	history of two or more
7	this pregnancy
	Previous excessive size infant:
1	one
2	two or more
5	Previous perinatal loss: one
7	two or more
7	Postterm, beyond 42 weeks: this pregnancy
5	Previous cesarean delivery
1	Previous congenital anomaly
7	Incompetent cervix
5	Uterine anomaly
2	Contracted pelvis
1	Abnormal presentation: history of
7	this pregnancy
7	Rh negative, sensitized
7	Polyhydramnios
1	Preeclampsia, mild, history of
3	this pregnancy
2	Preeclampsia, severe, history of
7	this pregnancy
1	Multiple pregnancy: history of
7	this pregnancy
	Miscellaneous Factors
1	Nutrition: more than 20% overweight prepregnancy
5	massive obesity
2	more than 10% underweight prepregnancy

(continued)

417

ASSESSMENT TOOL   (continued)

Risk Score	Risk Indicator
3	poor nutrition
5	inadequate weight gain
3	(less than 12 lb)
	excessive weight gain
	(more than 48 lb)
1	Smoking more than one pack/day
1	Drug or alcohol abuse: history of
2	this pregnancy

Medical Factors

Risk Score	Risk Indicator
1	Anemia: 8–10 g hgb
2	under 8 g hgb
2	Sickle cell trait
7	Sickle cell disease
2	Hypertension: mild
7	severe
2	Heart disease: Class I or II
5	Class III or IV
7	Heart failure: history of
7	this pregnancy
3	Diabetes: gestational
7	overt
1	Thyroid disease: history of
7	this pregnancy
	Veneral disease
1	gonorrhea or syphilis: history of
5	this pregnancy
3	Cervical neoplasia
	Urinary tract infection
1	afebrile: history of
3	this pregnancy
	Urinary tract infection,
2	febrile: history of
5	this pregnancy
	Psychiatric or neurologic problem:
1	history of
1	this pregnancy
	Other medical condition (e.g., pulmonary disease, severe influenza):
1	history of
5	this pregnancy

(continued)

ASSESSMENT TOOL   (continued)

Risk Score

_____ At first visit

_____ At 36 weeks

_____ On admission to labor and delivery

Risk factors have been assigned a weighted number from 7 (highest) to 1 (lowest).
A total score of 7 or more places the woman in the high-risk category. Patients identified as high risk should be referred for consultation or intensified prenatal care.

(Edwards L. et al: Simplified antepartum risk-scoring system. Obstet Gynecol 5(2):238, 1979. Reprinted with permission from The American College of Obstetricians and Gynecologists.)

difficulty describing symptoms, past illnesses, and treatment. She is also more inclined to be late for or miss prenatal appointments. For more comprehensive information on adolescent pregnancy and its associated psychological and perinatal risk see Chapters 15 and 20.

Over-35 Primigravida. The primigravida over 35 years old is at the other extreme from the adolescent primigravida. She is more likely to be married and to place a high value on her pregnancy, since the couple has usually made the decision to become parents after much soul-searching. She is often better educated than the average woman and holds a responsible job. Because of her intense interest in her own pregnancy, she will be well-read and informed about pregnancy. She may be very anxious, but for different reasons than the teenager. The pregnancy might be her one chance to bear a child, and she is fully aware of the risks involved. She is probably aware of the need for an amniocentesis to rule out genetic abnormalities in the fetus and the availability of abortion if the fetus is defective. (The psychosocial aspects of delayed childbearing and the process of psychological adaptation to pregnancy are addressed in Chapters 11 and 12.)

Teaching and Counseling

When the history and physical examination are completed, the expectant mother should be assured, when appropriate, that her pregnancy appears to be progressing well. Results of the laboratory studies will generally be available in 3 days and abnormal findings are followed up as soon as possible. The nurse should reassure her (especially if she is a teen-ager) that complete physical and pelvic examinations will not be repeated at subsequent visits unless there are special problems or verification of normal progress is needed.

SELF-CARE TEACHING

Warning Signs of Pregnancy Complication

The nurse should advise the patient that if she experiences the following symptoms, she should call her physician or clinic immediately.

- Vaginal bleeding
- Swelling (edema) of the face
- Continuous and severe headache
- Blurring or dimness of vision
- Abdominal pain
- Persistent vomiting
- Chills or fever
- Dysuria (painful urination)
- Fluid escaping from the vagina

Supplemental iron and prenatal vitamins are usually prescribed. A brief explanation or a handout that contains information on the nutritional needs of the pregnant woman may be helpful to the patient who is unaware of the importance of good nutrition in pregnancy. (Nutritional aspects of pregnancy are further discussed in Chapter 15.)

The nurse must also instruct the patient about warning signs that require immediate care. If the patient's pregnancy is jeopardized, warning signs will alert her to seek immediate care. Without alarming the patient, explain to her that if any of the following symptoms occur, day or night, she should call her care provider (see the Self-Care Teaching display, above).

Since the first prenatal visit is usually long, it is best to limit the information given the patient to the answers to her own initial questions. She will probably need to ask questions about her care provider and the care that she will receive — for example:

- Will she be able to express her concerns and discuss issues about which she has strong feelings, such as the use of forceps or episiotomy at delivery?
- Will her partner be allowed to attend prenatal visits and participate in labor and delivery?
- Will a pelvic examination be done on each visit?

Many questions can be answered frankly and fully. The patient's comfort in asking these questions on her initial contact and her impression of the setting may set the tone for future visits.

Nursing care of the expectant couple, emphasizing patient teaching, is fully discovered in Chapter 18, and the process of psychological adaptation of both partners to pregnancy is addressed in Chapter 12.

The nurse should answer any questions the patient has regarding the visit or her care, set a date for her next appointment, and encourage her to call if she has concerns before that time.

SUBSEQUENT PRENATAL VISITS

Schedules for return prenatal visits may be adapted to suit the needs of individual patients, especially those with physical or emotional problems. However, the usual schedule of visits is the following:

- Every 4 weeks until 28 weeks of pregnancy
- Every 2 weeks until 36 weeks of pregnancy
- Every week until delivery

During subsequent visits, when the patient is more comfortable and less distracted, further information about the setting and its resources can be given. Information can be shared about support services, such as Lamaze and other childbirth classes, nutritional counseling, dental care, psychological support, referral for food supplements, and other resources. The policies of the facility regarding labor, delivery, and postpartum care can be discussed as the patient indicates interest or as these issues become pertinent.

In coming to the health care setting, the pregnant woman and her partner are placing their trust in the care providers. Many times they have specific ideas about what is important in pregnancy management. Some will be interested in childbirth alternatives, and some, for religious or cultural reasons, may be reluctant to participate in certain aspects of prenatal care (such as that involving a male care provider). It is important that patient wishes be recorded so that members of the health care team are not only aware of the patient's desires but also, for ethical and legal reasons, are willing to make their practice conform to the patient's preference.

Often the husband or partner cannot participate in the prenatal visits because of his work schedule. If the woman has no other support person, it is doubly important for the nurse to spend time with her at each visit, discussing the events of pregnancy, answering questions, and providing continuity of support.

The history-taking and the examination that occur during follow-up prenatal visits are structured to obtain comprehensive information on the physical and emotional condition of the mother and her developing fetus. When deviation from the normal development occurs, immediate assessment can be made or planned. Table 16–7 outlines the procedures for maternal/fetal well-being assessment throughout a normal pregnancy.

Chapter 18 focuses on the process of nursing care in a normal pregnancy, including diagnosis based on systematic assessment, planning and implementing care, and evaluating outcomes. This process of ongoing assessment and diagnosis will identify a small number of patients who, while initially thought to be low-risk, will go on to develop complications of pregnancy. If the care provider is sensitive in explaining to the woman the problems identified, the care that will be provided, and the possible outcomes, the patient is more likely to be able to absorb this information and will feel she has adequate support with which she can cope with the at-risk situation, make decisions, and care for herself to achieve the best possible outcome.

CHAPTER SUMMARY

Prenatal assessment by the nurse provides baseline data that are valuable in health maintenance during pregnancy and can contribute materially to a successful outcome. Initial assessment calls for a detailed and meticulously recorded history, a comprehensive physical examination, an array of laboratory tests, and recording of findings. The initial prenatal examination is more than a guide. It establishes the psychophysical basis on which the management of the pregnancy is to proceed.

Prenatal assessment allows the nurse to establish rapport with the pregnant woman. It should be a shared experience involving empathy and mutual interest in a successful outcome. Each of the many steps taken in the prenatal assessment provides the nurse with an opportunity to share her knowledge and to explain, to teach, and to counsel.

STUDY QUESTIONS

1. What are the advantages of early diagnosis of pregnancy?
2. What are the positive signs of pregnancy and when can they be detected?
3. What specific hormone must be present for laboratory diagnosis of pregnancy, regardless of the type of test performed?
4. What is the chief objective of prenatal care?
5. According to Nägele's rule, what is the patient's EDC when the first day of her last menstrual period was January 16?
6. A pregnant woman has had three previous pregnancies, one abortion and one premature delivery, and has two living children. How would this information be recorded using the GTPAL system?
7. Why is it important to ask the patient to empty her bladder before performing an abdominal examination?
8. The patient is at 20 weeks of gestation. Auscultation fails to discern fetal heart tones. What does this signify?
9. The pubococcygeal muscle lacks tone on examination. What does this indicate?
10. Blood pressure and weight are baseline data used in assessing a patient's progress. If they appear to be normal, is it necessary to perform blood and urine laboratory tests? Why?
11. What is meant by the fourth trimester?
12. What is the significance of perineal scar tissue, discovered when examining a patient?

REFERENCES/BIBLIOGRAPHY

A Directory of Volunteer Organizations in Maternal and Child Health, Maternal Center for Education in Maternal and Child Health, Washington DC, 20057, December 1985

Artal R, Boelime T: Hepatitis B: The nurse–midwife's role in management and prevention. Nurse–Midwifery 30:79–87, 1985

Barger MF, Lops VR, Fullerton JT, et al: Protocols for Gynecology and Obstetrics Health Care. Orlando, Grune & Stratton, 1988

Carpenito LJ: Nursing Diagnosis: Application to Clinical Practice, 2nd ed. Philadelphia, JB Lippincott, 1987

Cobett MA, Meyer JH: The Adolescent and Pregnancy. Boston, Blackwell Scientific Publication, 1986

Knor ER: Decision Making in Obstetrical Nursing. Toronto, BC Decker, 1987

Lavery JP: Obstetric problems. In Lavery JP, Sanfilippo JS (eds): Pediatric and Adolescent Obstetrics and Gynecology. New York, Springer–Verlag, 1985

Littlefield VM: Health Education for Women: A Guide for Nurses and Other Health Professionals. Norwalk, Appleton-Century-Crofts, 1986

McGee EA, Schiller L: Pregnancy and parenting: Psychologic perspectives, In Lavery JP, Sanfilippo JS (eds): Pediatric and Adolescent Obstetrics and Gynecology, New York, Springer–Verlag, 1985

Minkoff H, Nanda D, Menez R, Fikrig S: Pregnancy immunodeficiency syndrome or AID's related complex. Obstet/Gynecol 69(3):285–287, 1987

Neural Tube Defects (pamphlet). American College of Obstetrics and Gynecology, Washington DC, 1985

Patteron ET, Freese MP, Goldberg R: Reducing uncertainty: Self-diagnosis of pregnancy. Image J Nurs Scholarship 18(3):105–109, 1986

Tanner J: Growth at Adolescence. Oxford, England, Blackwell Scientific Press, 1962

Whitley N: A Manual of Clinical Obstetrics. Philadelphia, JB Lippincott, 1985

SUGGESTED READINGS

Cohen AW: Movement is a yardstick for fetal well-being. Contemp OB/GYN 26(2):61–72, 1985

McFarlin BL, et al: Concurrent validity of Leopold's maneuvers in determining fetal presentation and position. J Nurse Midwifery 30(5):280–284, 1986

Miller S: Prenatal nursing assessment of the expectant family. Nurse Practit 11(5):40–52, May 1986

Mueller LS: Pregnancy and sexuality, J Obstet Gynecol Neonatal Nurs 14(6):289–294, 1985

Paolone AM, Worthington S: Caution and advice on exercise during pregnancy. Contemp OB/GYN (Special Issue: The Active Woman) 25:150–162, 1985

Poole CJ: Fatigue during the first semester of pregnancy. J Obstet Gynecol Neonatal Nurs 15(5):375–379, 1986

Rising S: Childbearing its dilemmas. In Kjervik D, Martinson IM (eds): Women in Health and Illness: Life Experience and Crisis pp 67–69. Philadelphia, WB Saunders, 1986

Slager–Earnest SE, Hoffman SJ, Anderson Beckman CJ: Effects of a specialized prenatal adolescent program on maternal and infant outcomes, J Obstet Gynecol Neonatal Nurs 16(6):422–428, 1987

Taubenheim AM, Silbernagel T: Meeting the needs of expectant fathers. Maternal–Child Health 13(2):110–113, 1988

Wawrzyniak MN: The painless pelvic, Am J Maternal/Child Nurs 11(30):178–179, 1986

17 assessment of fetal well-being

LEARNING OBJECTIVES

After studying the material in this chapter, the student should be able to

- Describe the four major modalities used for assessment of fetal well-being and when they are typically used

- Explain why estimation of gestational age is an important component of prenatal care

- Explain what information can be gained from amniocentesis, biophysical profile, ultrasonograph, and fetal movement and heart rate studies

- Describe nursing responsibilities related to assessment of fetal well-being

KEY TERMS

Ultrasonography

Biparietal diameter

Crown–rump length

Kick count

L/S ratio

Biophysical profile

Nonstress test

Contraction stress test

Reactivity

Assessment of fetal health should ideally begin before conception occurs. Prospective parents would be wise to prepare themselves physically and psychologically for pregnancy and parenthood. Nurses who provide family planning advice need to emphasize the importance of both prospective parents being physically healthy, eating a nutritious diet, and avoiding all drugs, cigarettes, and alcohol when planning to conceive. Women who take prescription drugs or have a preexisting health problem should consult with their health care provider prior to conception.

This is especially important for women with disorders that contribute to perinatal problems, such as diabetes mellitus, which is associated with a higher incidence of congenital anomalies, or preexisting hypertension, which is associated with placental insufficiency and intrauterine growth retardation. Evidence supports the role of pre-pregnancy counseling and care in the reduction of risk for congenital anomalies. In addition, patients with previous children with genetic or structural defects may benefit from evaluation and counseling regarding recurrence risks. Parental chromosomal analysis may be indicated to detect abnormalities that may affect future fetuses (see Chapter 9 for discussion of genetic screening and counseling).

Knowledge of the ramifications of health problems, combined with early prenatal care, will do a great deal to ensure the well-being of both the parents and the newborn infant.

ASSESSING FETAL HEALTH

In most situations assessment of fetal health includes monitoring of maternal weight gain, uterine growth, fetal activity, and fetal heart rate at each antepartum visit. In approximately 20% of all pregnancies, there is a need for further assessment. Indications from the family's health history or the mother's past or present pregnancy history identify the patients in need of further assessment. The antepartum nurse plays an important role in identifying such patients, performing many types of assessments, and providing information and support to families.

Antepartum assessment of fetal health involves the use of simple, noninvasive techniques that can reassure both the health care provider and the expectant parents that the fetus is growing appropriately. When deviations from the norm occur, early detection, consultation, and support of the expectant parents by the nurse may avert or reduce physical and emotional stress.

Four major modalities are currently used to assess fetal well-being:

- Inspection of uterine growth and auscultation of fetal heart rate

- Ultrasonography to estimate gestational age, assess fetal growth, and diagnose intrauterine problems
- Assessment of fetal heart rate response to changes in oxygenation levels, and assessment of fetal movement
- Direct assay of amniotic fluid

Inspection of uterine growth by fundal height and auscultation of fetal heart rate are done throughout the prenatal period. Ultrasonography may be used early in pregnancy to estimate gestational age, and later to rule out fetal, placental, or uterine problems. Assessment of fetal movement may be done throughout the second and third trimesters on a fairly routine basis, while assessment of fetal heart rate responses to contractions or to fetal movement will be done in the second or third trimester if there is a question of fetal status. Direct assay of amniotic fluid through amniocentesis is performed early in pregnancy for genetic screening, and later to evaluate fetal maturity or to rule out a complication like intrauterine infection. The following section discusses these major fetal assessment modalities in more detail as they are likely to be used in each trimester of pregnancy.

Nursing assessment of the fetus begins with a careful, detailed health history of the mother, father, and the family of each parent extending back three generations. The history should also include the maternal menstrual and obstetric history, maternal and paternal exposure to teratogens, and the parents' ethnic or racial backgrounds.

Objective methods used to assess fetal well-being are also important assessment tools. These include auscultation of fetal heart rate, measurement of fundal height, the monitoring of quickening and fetal movement, and ultrasonography. The nurse's role in performing these functions is discussed below.

First-Trimester Fetal Assessment

Methods of fetal assessment in the first 13 weeks of pregnancy primarily involve confirmation of the pregnancy and estimation of gestational age. Information collected during these visits will be added to the health history and physical assessment data gathered about the mother (*e.g.,* weight, findings from the bimanual examination of the uterus) to establish a complete data base for the pregnancy.

Auscultation of Fetal Heart Rate

Since fetal heart tones cannot be heard with a DeLee–Hillis fetoscope until about 20 weeks of gestation, the ultrasound stethoscope, or Doppler ultrasound, provides another method of fetal assessment during the first trimester (Fig. 17–1). The ultrasound stethoscope, or Doptone, is a hand-held, battery-operated device that utilizes ultrasound and the Doppler effect to detect motion. The

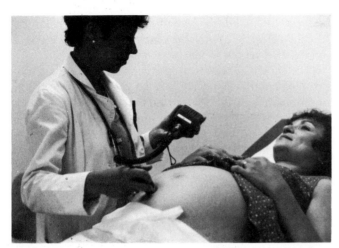

Figure 17–1. Doppler ultrasound monitoring of fetal heartbeat. (Courtesy of John B. Franklin Maternity Hospital, formerly Booth Maternity Center, Philadelphia)

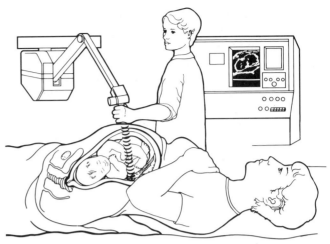

Figure 17–2. Ultrasonography. (Childbirth Graphics)

single transducer on the Doptone sends out a continuous beam of high-frequency sound waves. This beam, when directed through to the fetus, is reflected back from fetal tissues to varying degrees. Moving structures or objects, such as the valves of the fetal heart, reflect sound waves at different frequencies, which the transducer interprets and translates into an audible sound, such as the fetal heart rate. Gross movements of fetal extremities can also be heard as quick, harsh sounds. The Doptone, like other ultrasound devices, requires the use of mineral oil or gel to improve sound conduction.

Between 10 and 12 weeks of gestation, the fetal heart rate (FHR) can first be heard using the Doptone. It is usually found midline in the suprapubic region. The FHR is normally between 120 and 160 beats/minute and can be distinguished from the slower maternal heart rate by palpating the mother's pulse at the same time.

Parents may enjoy hearing the fetal heart rate, and a speaker is attached to most Doptones, allowing the sound to be amplified into the room. This can also be an opportunity for parents to begin attachment to their baby. Use of the Doptone during the first trimester has become routine in most antepartum clinics. Although it is not specifically diagnostic of fetal health, it does confirm fetal life.

Ultrasonography

Ultrasonography is a noninvasive procedure using ultrasound waves to provide imaging of the fetus, placenta, and uterus (Fig. 17–2). Serial sonograms will also reflect time-dependent changes in structure. Advances in the development of ultrasound equipment have rapidly moved it from the research laboratory into labor units and outpatient settings. The first scanning methods used a static B-scan, which provided a two-dimensional image in cross section. Now, real-time (B-scan) ultrasound pro-

vides continuous cross-sectional motion pictures of internal structures. Ultrasound can accomplish the following (Queenan and Warsof 1985):

- Estimate gestational age
- Locate the placenta
- Monitor fetal growth and movement
- Detect multiple gestations
- Identify certain congenital malformations

During the first trimester, purposes of ultrasound use include

- Assessment of gestational age
- Evaluation for congenital anomalies
- Diagnostic evaluation of vaginal bleeding
- Confirmation of suspected multiple gestation
- Evaluation of fetal growth
- Adjunct to prenatal testing (amniocentesis, chorionic villus sampling)
- Diagnostic evaluation of pelvic mass

As early as 4 weeks after the last menstrual period (LMP), a gestational sac implanted within the endometrial cavity can be detected by a static scanner. With use of a real-time scanner, cardiac activity is readily identifiable by 7 weeks post-LMP. Identification of the gestational sac or fetal cardiac activity documents the presence of the fetus.

The most common use of ultrasound during the first trimester is to assess gestational age. Because of the rapid rate of growth in the first trimester, accuracy in dating a pregnancy is believed to be highest between 7 and 13 weeks after the LMP. The crown–rump length (CRL) of the embryo or fetus is measured using real-time sonography.

Sonographs use a chart of CRLs measured in millimeters to estimate gestational age (Table 17–1). Between

Table 17–1   **Average Size of Embryo and Fetus by Crown–Rump Length (CRL)**

Age	CRL
2 weeks	1.5 mm
3 weeks	2.5 mm
4 weeks	5.0 mm
5 weeks	8.5 mm
7 weeks	20.0 mm
2 months	33.0 mm
3 months	95.0 mm
4 months	135.0 mm
6 months	230.0 mm
9 months	335.0 mm

7 and 13 weeks, the assessment of gestational age is accurate to within 1 to 3 days with 95% confidence. During the second trimester normal biological differences in fetal growth contribute to making ultrasound slightly less accurate in assessing gestational age.

A full bladder may improve ultrasonic resolution in women at 20 weeks of gestation or earlier. The full bladder serves as an anatomical landmark and elevates the uterus out of the pelvis for better visualization. If a full bladder is desirable, women should drink at least 1 liter water 1 to 2 hours before the examination. During the procedure, the woman will be placed on her back. It is important to ensure comfort, since the examination could last as long as 30 minutes. Mineral oil or gel is smeared over the abdomen to act as a conductive medium for the ultrasound and to reduce friction from the transducer as it is moved across skin. The procedure is painless, although many women report discomfort from the pressure of a full bladder.

The nurse should explain to the woman that in most cases she will be able to see an image of her baby on the machine's monitor. The ultrasonographer can point out identifiable structures, such as the head, extremities, or moving heart valves. Pregnant women are usually delighted to have a first glimpse of the baby. When ultrasound is used as an adjunct to prenatal diagnosis, visualization of the fetus may contribute to the difficult decisions parents face regarding termination or continuation of the pregnancy in the event a congenital or chromosomal defect is detected. Nurses should be sensitive to these issues and support the parents' decisions about visualization of their infant via ultrasound.

Second-Trimester Fetal Assessment

As the fetus continues to grow, many dramatic changes occur between the 14th and 26th weeks of pregnancy. With the uterus expanding, the expectant mother begins to "show," announcing her pregnancy to the out-

side world. In addition, the thinner walls of the enlarging uterus combined with the activity of the growing fetus enable the mother to feel fetal movement. These changes will affect the methods of fetal assessment as well.

Assessment of the height of the uterine fundus has long been used to monitor fetal growth. Recent studies support the value of this time-honored measurement as an indicator of fetal growth. Once the uterus is palpable abdominally (usually by 12 weeks after LMP), the location of the fundus in relation to the symphysis pubis can be identified and is referred to as fundal height, usually expressed in centimeters.

Measurement of Fundal Height

From 16 to 20 weeks of gestation (beginning when the fundus is palpable abdominally) until the end of pregnancy, the fundal height should be measured and recorded on the uterine growth chart at each antepartum clinic visit, or weekly if the pregnant woman becomes hospitalized for any reason. The measurement (known as *McDonald's measurement*) is simple to do and is often a nursing responsibility. However, the reliability of the uterine growth chart will be affected if a consistent method of measurement is not used, and accuracy will be less than desired when different examiners are involved. Measurements should always be done with the mother in the same position and having an empty bladder (Engstrom 1988).

Using a nonstretching but flexible metric measuring tape, the examiner places the zero line of the tape on the superior border of the symphysis pubis. It should then be stretched across the contour of the abdomen at the midline to the top of the fundus. This measurement in centimeters is graphed on the uterine growth chart on the line that corresponds to the number of weeks of gestation, as previously determined. After 20 to 22 weeks of gestation, the fundal height in centimeters is expected to approximate the gestational age in weeks. There should be a consistent increase in uterine size at each visit for a smooth growth curve that indicates adequate interval growth. When the measurement is consistently 1 to 2 cm greater or less than expected, there is usually no cause for concern; individual variation, such as short stature, may be the reason. However, if the measurement has been done in a consistent manner, a less than 2 cm or greater than 6 cm increase of fundal height in 4 weeks calls for further evaluation.

Some causes of fundal height greater than predicted for gestational age include

- Multiple gestation
- Polyhydramnios
- Fetal macrosomia

Lower fundal height than expected can indicate

- Abnormal fetal presentation
- Growth-retarded fetus
- Congenital anomalies
- Oligohydramnios

Discrepancy of uterine size and gestational age can also suggest incorrect dating of the pregnancy.

Assessing Fetal Heart Rate

During the second trimester, assessing the FHR continues to be a part of each antepartum assessment. As the fetus nears 20 weeks of gestation, the fetoscope may be employed rather than the Doptone. Use of the fetoscope may lengthen the time necessary to locate and hear the FHR, since the sound produced is soft, similar to that of a watch ticking beneath a pillow. To avoid anxiety to the mother during the search for the heart tone, explain that it is the use of the less sophisticated fetoscope, and not a problem with the baby, that is causing the delay (Fig. 17–3). (See Chapter 16 for a more detailed description of this procedure.)

Fetal Movement/Quickening

An additional parameter used to confirm gestational age is fetal movement, or quickening. For most primigravidas, fetal movement is first detected between 18 and 20 weeks after the LMP, whereas secundigravidas and multigravidas may experience fetal movement as early as 16 weeks. As the primigravida approaches the midpoint of her pregnancy, she should be advised to expect a light,

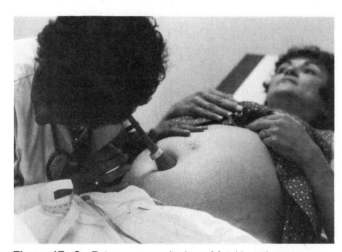

Figure 17–3. Fetoscope monitoring of fetal heartbeat. (Courtesy of John B. Franklin Maternity Hospital, formerly Booth Maternity Center, Philadelphia)

fluttery feeling that may be fetal movement but is often mistaken for intestinal gas. The mother should be asked to record the date when she first notices this sensation. (The experienced mother can be advised that she may feel movement earlier than with the first baby, since she is more sensitive to the movement.) The date can then be compared with her LMP to assess the accuracy of the dating of the pregnancy.

Ultrasonography

Ultrasound is used during the second trimester for the following reasons:

- To assess gestational age
- To diagnose multiple gestations
- To assess fetal growth
- To identify structural abnormalities of the fetus (*e.g.,* hydrocephaly)
- To guide procedures such as amniocentesis and fetoscopy
- To assess placental location

When gestational age must be verified during the second trimester, ultrasound is used. After 14 weeks of gestation, the widest transverse diameter of the fetal head, known as the biparietal diameter (BPD), is used as a means of assessing gestational age. Ultrasonographers believe that the optimal time for determining gestational age by BPD is between 16 and 20 weeks of gestation. At this time the 90% confidence limits are plus or minus 1 week. After 26 weeks of gestation, BPD is not believed to predict gestational age as accurately. The most reliable ways to assess gestational age using ultrasound are CRL measurement between 7 and 13 weeks of gestation and BPD measurement between 16 and 20 weeks. Sonography is recommended at this time as a baseline evaluation for all pregnancies that are at risk for complications. The nurse should review clinical parameters for gestational age assessment, including

- Detection of fetal movement by mother
- Audible fetal heart tones
- Fundal height measurement

The accuracy of gestational age estimation by ultrasound is enhanced by early evaluation.

When there is concern that the growth of the infant may be excessive or less than expected, serial or repeated sonograms will indicate whether growth is appropriate for gestational age or whether there is evidence of multiple pregnancy or abnormal amounts of amniotic fluid. Generalized fetal edema (fetal hydrops) may be noted in the Rh-immunized infant.

Third-Trimester Fetal Assessment

During the last trimester of pregnancy (weeks 28 to 40), the monitoring of fetal growth, FHR, and fetal activity continues. The uterine growth curve should continue to show positive interval growth. As the antepartum visits increase in frequency, a continuation of 1 cm/week growth of fundal height through 36 weeks of gestation is expected. In the primigravida, the fetus will begin to descend into the pelvis after 38 weeks, and the fundal height may decrease 2 to 4 cm when "lightening" has occurred. At this time the mother will usually report more pressure or weight in her pelvis or lower back but easier breathing because diaphragmatic pressure has decreased.

Monitoring Fetal Movement

Many antepartum health care providers advocate daily maternal monitoring of fetal movement during the third trimester. Starting after 28 weeks of gestation, mothers are asked to complete a fetal movement or kick count chart each day (Fig. 17–4).

At some time each day, the woman is asked to lie down, preferably on her side and to palpate her abdomen to help detect fetal movement. Counting continues until a total of 10 movements have been felt. Most women report perceiving ten movements in 20 minutes to 2 hours. When ten movements have not been felt in 3 hours, the health care provider should be notified; in some cases further FHR evaluation may be performed. Variations in fetal activity and sleep patterns occur, so that 3 hours is believed to be adequate time in which to expect ten fetal movements. Other methods include counting fetal movements for 30 minutes 3 times a day (Gantes et al 1986).

Studies of high-risk pregnancies have reported decreased perinatal morbidity and mortality when the women monitor fetal activity. On the basis of these studies, many antepartum health care providers feel that fetal movement recording should be routine for all high-risk pregnant women.

The antepartum nurse can teach mothers this simple yet effective method of fetal monitoring. Sharing the following information with the mothers will help them to understand what is happening and be more aware of the activities of their babies.

- Fetal activity often increases after meals or light massaging of the abdomen.
- A short walk can also make the baby more active.
- Babies normally have periods of sleep throughout the day, usually lasting 20 minutes.
- During the last 2 to 3 weeks before delivery, activity normally decreases as the fetal presenting part becomes engaged and there is less room to move around.

It is important to use a reassuring, calm approach when explaining self-monitoring to the mother. The nurse can explain to her that this is a way she can take part in maintaining the health of her baby before it is born. The value of reporting decreased fetal activity cannot be too strongly stressed. Intrauterine fetal death is often preceded by several days of decreased fetal movement.

Ultrasonography

During the third trimester, sonography is often used to determine fetal position or estimate fetal size. When a sonogram has not been done previously, it is difficult to make an assessment of gestational age at this time. It is helpful when fetal growth can be assessed by comparing previous sonographic measurements with current fetal size. Head circumference, abdominal circumference, and femur length are the most common measurements taken to estimate fetal weight and interval growth during the third trimester.

MONITORING FETAL WELL-BEING

The field of perinatology has been concerned with maintaining the health of the mother and the infant during the pregnancy. Electronic and chemical tests allow the clinician to "observe" the infant *in utero*. Although these tests provide different information, they all indicate in some way whether the maternal-placental-fetal unit is intact and functioning. From this information, the clinician can decide whether the pregnancy can safely be continued or whether intervention is indicated.

From a philosophical perspective, there are opposing opinions on the use of technology in obstetrics. Proponents cite the many infants who survive because early detection of problems leads to timely medical intervention and management. Those opposed feel that obstetricians and pediatricians begin a process they cannot end. That is, early detection often results in the delivery of a preterm baby who requires life support systems for an extended period of time. However, life support does not ensure the recovery of the infant, and in the process of life support there are added risks that may result in the infant's long-term disability. Once the process of life support is begun, the ethical question arises as to who, if anyone, has the right to stop it.

This section discusses the available means of testing for fetal well-being, and the positive aspects are emphasized. The nurse should keep in mind that not all people — parents or clinicians — would agree with this emphasis. Nurses are the members of the health care team most frequently responsible for explaining and performing the recommended tests. Parents will usually ask the nurse's

Kick Counts

Instructions

An easy way to check the health of your baby is to count the number of times the baby kicks once each day. At the same time every day, after you have eaten, record the amount of time it takes for your baby to kick ten times.

For example, on Monday, you begin to count your baby's kicks at 10:00 A.M. By 10:30 A.M. your baby has kicked ten times. You fill in the chart like this:

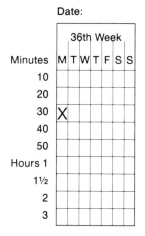

Remember that every baby is an individual. They have times when they sleep and times when they are active. If you start counting and the baby isn't kicking, stop, walk around for 5 minutes, and then count again (Hint: Count baby's kicks after you have eaten).

At the end of 3 hours, if your baby has not kicked ten times, call the delivery room at the hospital.

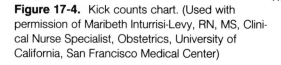

Figure 17-4. Kick counts chart. (Used with permission of Maribeth Inturrisi-Levy, RN, MS, Clinical Nurse Specialist, Obstetrics, University of California, San Francisco Medical Center)

DATE:

Minutes	28th Week	29th Week	30th Week	31st Week

DATE:

Minutes	32nd Week	33rd Week	34th Week	35th Week

DATE:

Minutes	36th Week	36th Week	38th Week	39th Week

DATE:

Minutes	40th Week	41st Week	42nd Week	43rd Week

advice. Nurses must be aware of their own prejudices and biases and support the family in considering all the factors in their attempt to arrive at the best decision for both mother and infant.

Amniocentesis

Amniocentesis is the aspiration of fluid from the uterus through an abdominal puncture for the purpose of fluid analysis (Fig. 17–5). This testing may be conducted at any time during pregnancy. When the procedure is advised in the first half of pregnancy (14 to 20 weeks), it is usually for the purpose of studying genetic makeup and determining developmental abnormalities. The procedure is discussed in more detail in Chapter 9, Genetics and Genetic Counseling. Amniocentesis is done in the third trimester usually for the purpose of determining fetal lung maturity or blood group or of detecting amnionitis.

Once the fluid is obtained, laboratory testing will depend on the maternal complication. For example, in the case of the Rh-negative mother, the fluid will be used to test for elevated bilirubin levels, which would indicate the presence of hemolytic anemia. Culture and sensitivity tests are done on the fluid if amnionitis is suspected. Fetal lung maturity tests are indicated with any maternal or potential fetal problem indicating early delivery of the infant. These include determinations of the L/S ratio (see following paragraph) and tests for the presence of phosphatidylglycerol (PG).

Lecithin–Sphingomyelin Ratio (L/S Ratio)

Since most neonatal morbidity and mortality results from pulmonary immaturity and respiratory distress, reliable indicators of fetal lung maturity are essential in predicting postdelivery status of the infant. Assessment

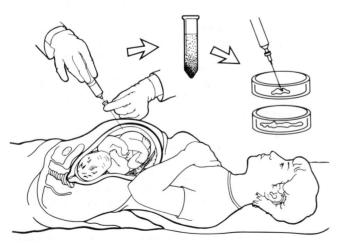

Figure 17–5. Transabdominal amniocentesis. (Childbirth Graphics)

of the L/S ratio from amniotic fluid is the oldest and most reliable of the tests available today. Lecithin and sphingomyelin are phospholipids produced by the lung tissue. These lipids mix with amniotic fluid in the lung to reduce the surface tension and protect against alveolar collapse. These phospholipids have a detergent quality and are also known as surfactants. If an adequate amount of both factors is present at birth, neonatal breathing will result in expanded alveoli. If an inadequate amount is available, varying numbers of alveoli will collapse, and the neonate may develop respiratory distress syndrome (RDS) of proportionate severity.

Lecithin and sphingomyelin are reported as a ratio. Depending upon the laboratory analysis used to determine the amounts of lecithin and sphingomyelin present, different ratios indicate lung maturity. In most centers, the ratio 2:1 (*i.e.*, twice as much lecithin as sphingomyelin is present) is used as a level indicating maturity. There is less lecithin than sphingomyelin until 30 to 32 weeks of gestation, and then the concentrations become equal. The amount of lecithin rapidly increases after 35 weeks, whereas the amount of sphingomyelin remains constant. Thus, laboratory results are often reported as an L/S ratio of, for example, 2 (the constant level of sphingomyelin being understood).

There are two forms of lecithin, stable and unstable. Stable lecithin does not become functional until 35 weeks of gestation. Hypoglycemia, hypoxia, and hypothermia may break down the unstable form of lecithin, increasing the infant's susceptibility to RDS.

In the event of an obstetric emergency requiring immediate decisions about delivery, a "shake test" may be done to establish fetal lung maturity. This is a bedside test of the L/S ratio. The test relies on the fact that the detergent action of the phospholipids causes a stable foam to form. Amniotic fluid is agitated in a test tube with saline and ethanol. It is examined after sitting for 15 minutes for the presence of small, stable bubbles resting on top of the fluid: their presence is associated with mature fetal lung. Since false negatives are common, this test is used only as an immediate indicator, with more accurate fluid analysis being established by standard testing in the laboratory.

Phosphatidylglycerol (PG)

As research has continued on the physiology of fetal lung maturity, many other phospholipids and fatty acids have been identified. The presence of phosphatidylglycerol (PG) and phosphatidylinositol (PI) has been found to correlate with fetal lung maturity. Preliminary studies have shown that in prematurely born neonates without RDS, PG could be isolated from gastric, pharyngeal, and tracheal aspirates within 4 hours after birth. Infants with RDS had no detectable PG.

PG is used in conjunction with the L/S ratio. If the L/S

ratio is 2 and the PG is positive, there is strong evidence of fetal lung maturity. PG may provide stability that makes the infant less susceptible to RDS when experiencing hypoglycemia, hypothermia, or hypoxia.

Some research is being done on using PI in the same manner as PG. The presence of PI is also a reliable indicator of fetal lung maturity (Gabbe 1985).

Biophysical Profile/Ultrasonography

Real-time ultrasound may also be used to perform a biophysical profile of the fetus. This procedure involves evaluation of such selected parameters as fetal movement, fetal tone, fetal breathing movements, amniotic fluid volume, and placental maturation. These parameters are assessed and scored numerically by a specially-trained sonographer. Higher scores provide evidence of fetal well-being, while low scores indicate the need for further evaluation (see Table 17–2). Biophysical profiles are most frequently used as an adjunct to nonstress and contraction stress testing. Common indications for fetal assessment using biophysical profile include the following (Dauphinee 1987):

- Hypertensive disorders
- Diabetes mellitus
- Post-dates pregnancy (possible postmaturity)
- Suspected intrauterine growth retardation

Electronic Fetal Heart Rate Monitoring

Fetal monitors are frequently used during labor to watch for changes in the fetal heart rate and pattern. This use of fetal monitors is discussed in Chapters 23 and 25.

Table 17–2 Biophysical Profile

Variables	Normal (score = 2)	Abnormal (score = 0)
Fetal breathing movements	One or more episodes in 30 min, each lasting ≥ 30 sec	Episodes absent or no episode of ≥ 30 sec in 30 min
Gross body movements	Three or more discrete body/limb movements in 30 min (episodes of active continuous movement considered as a single movement)	Less than three episodes of body/limb movements in 30 min
Fetal tone	One or more episodes of active extension with return to flexion of fetal limb(s) or trunk; opening and closing of hand considered normal tone	Slow extension with return to flexion; movement of limb in full extension, or fetal movement absent
Reactive fetal heart rate	Two or more episodes of acceleration (≥ 15 beats per min) in 20 min, each lasting ≥ 15 sec and associated with fetal movement	Less than two episodes of acceleration or acceleration of < 15 beats per min in 20 min
Qualitative amniotic fluid volume	One or more pockets of fluid measuring ≥ 1 cm in two perpendicular planes	Pockets absent or pocket < 1 cm in two perpendicular planes

Score	Interpretation	Recommended Management
10	Normal infant, low risk for chronic asphyxia	Repeat testing at weekly intervals; repeat twice weekly in diabetic patients and patients ≥ 42 weeks
8	Normal infant, low risk for chronic asphyxia	Repeat testing at weekly intervals; repeat twice weekly in diabetic patients and patients ≥ 42 weeks; oligohydramnios is indication for delivery
6	Suspected chronic asphyxia	Repeat testing within 24 hrs; oligohydramnios or repeat score ≤ 6 is indication for delivery
4	Suspected chronic asphyxia	Indications for delivery are ≥ 36 weeks and favorable cervix; if < 36 weeks and lecithin/sphingomyelin ratio < 2.0, repeat test in 24 hrs; repeat score ≤ 6 or oligohydramnios is indication for delivery
2	Strong suspicion of chronic asphyxia	Extend testing time to 120 min; persistent score ≤ 4, regardless of gestational age, is indication for delivery

Reprinted with permission from Manning FA, Morrison I, Lange IR et al.: Fetal assessment based on fetal biophysical profile scoring: Experience in 12,620 referred high risk pregnancies. Am J Obstet Gynecol 151:345, 1985

In this chapter, discussion is limited to the use of the electronic fetal monitor in evaluating fetal status before the onset of labor when a complication of pregnancy is present (Fig. 17–6). This type of testing has its own specific procedures and interpretation.

Electronic monitors allow observation of the fetus by indicating the response of the fetal heart rate to fetal movement or to spontaneous or induced contractions. Contractions "stress" the fetus by reducing uterine perfusion. Variations in fetal heart rate in response to con-

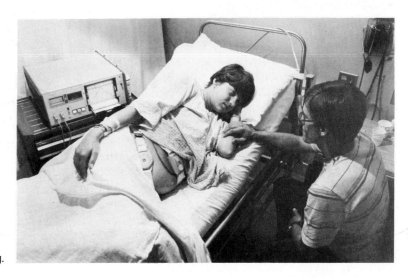

Figure 17–6. Electronic fetal monitoring.

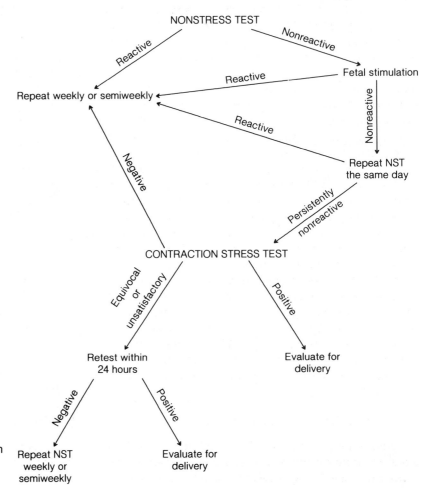

Figure 17–7. Scheme for performing antepartum testing with the nonstress test and the contraction stress test. (Dauphinee J: Antepartum testing: A challenge for nursing. J Perinatal Neonatal Nurs 1(1): 41, 1987)

tractions may be detectable on the monitor if a fetus is already compromised by any of the following factors:

- Fetal disease
- Placental disease
- Maternal disease
- Cord compression

Nonstress Test

The least invasive test of fetal well-being, the nonstress test (NST), is the one usually done first. The nonstress test indirectly assesses placental respiratory function by observation of the fetal heart rate in response to fetal movement. Adequate perfusion is necessary to maintain the integrity of the central nervous system and reflex responses that control the fetal heart rate. The healthy fetus responds to fetal movement with an acceleration of heart rate. Different facilities require various schemes of heart rate accelerations to constitute a negative or "reactive" test result, indicating healthy placental respiratory function. The most common scheme requires two fetal heart rate accelerations occurring within a 10-minute period, with each acceleration increasing heart rate at least 15 bpm and sustained for at least 15 seconds.

The nurse will most frequently be responsible for administering the NST. The external electronic fetal monitor is applied as described in Chapter 25. The resulting tracing is observed and interpreted. The baseline fetal heart rate is identified and any periodic patterns present are noted. The uterine activity tracing is observed for contractions. The NST is interpreted as reactive or negative for placental respiratory malfunction when the criteria for reactivity described above are obtained. The fetal heart rate should otherwise be *normal*. It is most important to interpret the entire tracing. If an abnormal rate (less than 120 bpm or more than 160 bpm is noted or decelerations (early, variable, or late) are seen, the test requires follow-up evaluation even though the NST itself is reactive.

When performing the NST, the nurse should continue monitoring for at least 40 minutes before the test is judged nonreactive, to account for normal period of fetal sleep. The NST is nonreactive or positive when criteria for reactivity are not met. It is important to remember that the NST is a screening procedure; thus, a nonreactive test must be followed with further evaluation the same day to determine fetal status (Fig. 17–7). Other tests that may be used include the contraction stress test (CST), described below, or the biophysical profile (BPP), described previously.

Contraction Stress Test (CST)

Uterine perfusion through the spiral arteries is decreased through a contraction and thus stresses the fetus with diminished oxygen delivery. The fetus with limited

NURSING RESEARCH

A Comparison of Two Methods of Breast Stimulation Stress Testing

Breast stimulation is increasingly used as a method of inducing uterine contractions for testing fetal response. A study was conducted to test the efficacy and safety of two methods of breast stimulation: (a) manual rolling of the nipple, and (b) application of moist hot pads to the nipple before stimulation.

A sample of 54 patients with perinatal conditions that required stress testing for assessing fetal well-being were randomly assigned to one of two groups. Both groups were observed for baseline data on uterine activity and fetal heart rate for 10 minutes. One group then received application of a warm compress to both breasts for 5 minutes, followed by unilateral nipple stimulation. If uterine response was inadequate, this was followed by bilateral breast stimulation, followed by a 10-minute recovery period. The second group followed the same protocol without the application of warm compresses.

Application of moist heat did not appear to improve the effectiveness or safety of the breast stimulation stress testing. Both methods achieved effective levels of uterine activity, and both resulted in similar infrequent occurrences of exaggerated uterine activity. These findings suggest that, regardless of the exact method of breast stimulation, the nurse should remain with the patient throughout the procedure to assess uterine and fetal responses to breast stimulation and that nurses doing breast stimulation stress testing should take responsibility for developing a uniform safe protocol for such testing.

Moenning R, Hill W: A randomized study comparing two methods of performing the breast stimulation stress test. J Obstet Gynecol Neonatal Nurs 16(4):253–258, 1987

reserve responds with late decelerations while the healthy fetus maintains a normal baseline without decelerations. At least three contractions in a 10-minute period must be observed in order to observe the fetal response to stress. Contractions may be occurring spontaneously with adequate frequency; more often, stimulation will be required by an intravenous oxytocin infusion. This is called the oxytocin challenge test (OCT). Contraction stimulation can often be induced by nipple stimulation.

Outcome

Regardless of the type of test performed, the expected outcome is the same. The monitor is placed on the patient as shown in Figure 17–6. The transducer is adjusted to achieve the best possible tracing of the fetal heart rate (that is, one without interruptions in the pattern tracing). Once a good tracing is achieved and the patient is in a comfortable position, a "baseline strip" is run. This provides a reading of the activity of the uterus and the infant without intervention or manipulation. The baseline will help determine the need for additional uterine stimulation.

Uterine contractions can often be induced by nipple stimulation and consequent prolactin release. The patient is instructed to rub one nipple gently through her light clothing for 2 minutes or until a contraction begins. Stimulation is then stopped and restarted after 5 minutes if by that time the contraction frequency is inadequate. If nipple stimulation is unsuccessful, intravenous infusion of low-dose oxytocin is begun at 0.5 mU/min and increased by 0.5 mU/min every 15 minutes until the desired number of contractions is achieved. The goal for all three methods is to achieve three contractions within 10 minutes, lasting 40 to 60 seconds each (Mayberry and Inturrissi–Levy 1987).

IMPLICATIONS FOR NURSING CARE

Ongoing assessment and monitoring of fetal well-being is an essential component of prenatal care and has long been a major nursing responsibility in many settings. Such basic assessment techniques as auscultation of fetal heart rate and monitoring uterine growth provide essential information about fetal status and the progress of pregnancy. However, new technologic advances have contributed new diagnostic and clinical assessment tools. With these new tools come new nursing responsibilities.

Electronic fetal monitoring (EFM), especially its application in the antepartum evaluation of fetal status, has had a major impact on nursing practice. For example, the nursing skills required for practice have rapidly expanded beyond the standard intrapartal use of EFM to include interpretation of antepartum tests. This rapid expansion in practice responsibilities requires the nurse to continually update clinical knowledge. The nurse must also evaluate innovations in biomedical technology carefully from a nursing perspective by asking such questions as, What nursing functions will be changed because of this new technology? What new knowledge and skills are needed? What standardized procedures should be developed and tested? What are the costs of this new technology and how do they weigh against the benefits? Will the technology generate information that will clearly improve patient outcomes by reducing risk, or will the procedure generate additional risks?

Finally, the perinatal nurse must constantly keep in

RELATED RESEARCH

Percutaneous Umbilical Cord Sampling

Percutaneous umbilical blood sampling (PUBS) is an as yet experimental method for assessment and management of such fetal disorders as erythroblastosis fetalis and congenital infections. This procedure involves passing a fine needle through the maternal abdomen and uterine wall into a vessel in the umbilical cord under the guidance of ultrasonography. PUBS can be done at or after 16 weeks of gestation.

Because of the mobility of the umbilical cord, the puncture is made close to the placental insertion. A fetal blood sample is aspirated and can be tested for complete blood count, type and antibody screen, and direct and indirect Coombs and karyotype if indicated. Since fetal RBCs are larger than maternal RBCs, mean corpuscular volume is used to verify that the sample is fetal in origin.

Potential complications include infection (1%); preterm labor with premature rupture of membranes (0.2%), placental abruption, laceration, or thrombus of an umbilical vessel; and transient fetal arrhythmias. Cord bleeding appears to occur in almost 20% of cases but is self-limiting.

Although PUBS is experimental and presents certain risks, it offers more precise diagnosis and the possibility of treating some fetal conditions (for instance, treatment of erythroblastosis fetalis by direct intravascular fetal transfusion). As this technology develops, nurses should remain well informed in order to provide optimum care and support for high-risk perinatal patients and their families.

Dunn P, Weiner S, Ludomirski A: Percutaneous umbilical blood sampling. J Obstet Gynecol Neonatal Nurs 17(5):308–316, 1988

mind that "a major challenge to nurses is to balance the impact of instrumentation and monitoring with the primary nurse–patient relationship. Although these techniques augment practice, they should never replace thoughtful analysis and the therapeutic process of human interaction" (Gibes and Angelini 1987).

CHAPTER SUMMARY

The health status of mothers and the babies they carry is the most important influence on the future health and well-being of human beings. The provision of good health care in the prenatal period may avert potential problems.

Nurses in prenatal settings can effectively monitor fetal growth and well-being, teach, and offer anticipatory guidance to pregnant women and their families. To do this the nurse must be knowledgeable about the normal growth of the fetus; such methods as McDonald's measurements and ultrasonography to assess fetal growth; the use of Leopold maneuvers; the normal growth curve of the uterus and its relationship to the mother's diet; and methods of assessing fetal heart rate and fetal responses to changes in oxygenation, such as nonstress and contraction stress testing.

However, technological advances in this area are occurring at a rapid rate, often outstripping the professional ability to completely master new technology or consider the ethical and psychological implications. The nurse must continually update both knowledge and understanding and still remain family-centered in the care of families who require more intensified fetal assessment.

STUDY QUESTIONS

1. Describe two procedures to estimate gestational age early in pregnancy. Explain why estimation of gestational age is an important part of prenatal care.
2. How would you instruct a patient in preparation for ultrasonography?
3. A mother at 32 weeks gestation is concerned because she has not felt fetal movement for 2 to 3 hours. What would you advise her to do?
4. Describe three tests that may be performed on amniotic fluid.
5. In an emergency, fetal lung maturity may be determined at the bedside by performing the shake test. Explain this testing method and the expected result.
6. Discuss the differences between the nonstress test, the nipple stimulation test, and the oxytocin challenge test.

REFERENCES/BIBLIOGRAPHY

Dauphinee J: Antepartum testing: A challenge for nursing. J Perinat Neonatal Nurs 1(1):29–49, 1987

Engstrom J: Measurement of fundal height. J Obstet Gynecol Neonatal Nurs 17(3):172–179, 1988

Gabbe S: Fetal lung maturity. In Queenan J (ed): Management of High-Risk Pregnancy. Oradell, NJ, Medical Economics, 1985

Gantes M, Schy V, Bartasius M, Roberts J: The use of daily fetal movement records in a clinical setting. J Obstet Gynecol Neonatal Nurs 15(5):390–394, 1986

Gibes R, Angelini D: Editorial: Monitoring and instrumentation. J Perinat Neonatal Nurs 1(1):vii, 1987

Mayberry L, Inturrissi–Levy M: Use of breast stimulation for contraction stress tests. J Obstet Gynecol Neonatal Nurs 16(2):121–126, 1987

Queenan J, Warsof S: Ultrasonography. In Queenan J (ed): Management of High-Risk Pregnancy. Oradell, NJ, Medical Economics, 1985

SUGGESTED READINGS

Dauphinee J: Antepartum testing: A challenge for nursing. J Perinat Neonatal Nurs 1(1)29–49, 1987

Harmon J, Barry M: Antenatal testing—mobile outpatient monitoring service. J Obstet Gynecol Neonatal Nurs 18(1):21–24, 1989

Milne L, Rich O: Cognitive and affective aspects of the responses of pregnant women to sonography. Matern Child Nurs J 10(1):16–39, 1981

Oakley A: The history of ultrasonography in obstetrics. Birth 13(1):8–16, 1986

18 nursing care of the expectant couple

LEARNING OBJECTIVES

After studying the material in this chapter, the student should be able to

- Explain the rationale for anticipatory guidance

- Identify two aspects of pregnancy for which anticipatory guidance will be needed

- Recognize the importance of individualizing teaching and counseling for each woman or family

- Recognize the importance of making referrals when indicated

- Identify situations that require referrals

- Identify symptoms that clients must be taught to report

- Distinguish between true and false labor

- Identify risks related to employment, travel, sports, and exercise during pregnancy

- Identify the benefits of sports and exercise during pregnancy

- Teach clients to perform breast self-examination and prepare for breast-feeding

- Identify causes, assessment data, interventions, and expected outcomes for the common discomforts of pregnancy

KEY TERMS

Anticipatory guidance

Kegel exercise

Tailor sitting

Pelvic tilt

Pubococcygeus muscle

The prospects of a smooth pregnancy and the birth of a healthy baby are aided considerably by early and thorough prenatal care. Since childbearing is an essentially normal process for most women, much prenatal care centers on education aimed at maintaining well-being. Thus patient education is a major component of perinatal nursing care.

The nurse is not simply the administrator of another health care provider's orders. She may have more contact with patients and their families than any other health care provider and thus must undertake needed patient teaching. Because of the time spent with women in the obstetric setting, the nurse is in a unique position to assess women's physical and psychosocial needs and decide whether referrals are needed. In answering the many questions that women raise about their pregnancies, their growing fetus, labor and delivery, breast-feeding, and the postpartum period, the nurse contributes directly to the quality of the individual experience as well as to health outcomes for the entire family.

With her knowledge of the needs of the pregnant woman and the many services offered by health care organizations and the community, the nurse can inform patients of the resources available to them. Such intervention, especially early in pregnancy, can significantly enhance perinatal care for the pregnant woman and her family.

This chapter focuses on nursing care in the prenatal period, with an emphasis on patient education. The chapter begins with the concerns encountered during the 9 months of gestation and the nurse's role in anticipatory guidance and patient education. Nutrition, sexuality, and psychosocial adaptation to pregnancy are dealt with in detail in other chapters and addressed only briefly here. This chapter emphasizes teaching and guidance related to exercise, work, travel and leisure, signs of complications, and preparation for parenting.

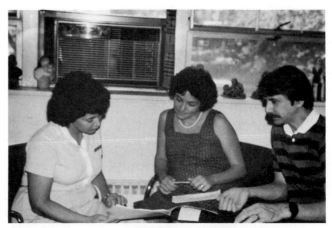

Figure 18–1. The nurse provides nursing care for the pregnant woman and her partner. Assessment of both the mother and her partner is an important first step for future teaching. (Courtesy of John B. Franklin Maternity Hospital, formerly Booth Maternity Center, Philadelphia)

sessments to determine if the pregnant woman is continuing within appropriate parameters. Elements of prenatal assessment at subsequent visits are listed in the same display in Chapter 16. They include ongoing assessments of pregnancy status, physical examination, laboratory tests, and ongoing psychosocial assessment.

Assessment of the entire family unit may be necessary to provide effective care. The concerns of the father or partner throughout the pregnancy should be within the scope of the nurse's time and attention, since the long-term health of the family unit may rest on the degree to which both parents adapt positively to the demands of pregnancy, birth, and the first year of parenting (Fig. 18–1). The process of psychosocial adaptation to pregnancy is discussed in Chapter 12. Some important points will be highlighted here, since they relate to the process of identifying patient needs and implementing nursing care to meet those needs.

Assessment

The process of assessment throughout pregnancy as an essential component of nursing care was addressed in Chapter 16. Once the woman's pregnancy has been established, a variety of assessments are made at the first visit and subsequent prenatal visits. Elements of prenatal assessment at the initial visit are listed in a display in Chapter 16 and include such things as health history (present, menstrual/obstetric, and previous pregnancies), psychosocial assessment (attitudes, emotions, financial impact, and expectations), and complete physical examination. Subsequent visits include continuing as-

Diagnosis

Nursing diagnosis in the care of the expectant couple tends to focus on identifying patient learning needs as pregnancy progresses as well as supporting self-care behaviors associated with optimal psychosocial and physical adaptation to pregnancy. The following are nursing diagnoses that reflect possible problems that may arise during the pregnancy:

- Altered health maintenance related to physical adaptations to pregnancy

- Anxiety related to anticipated role changes during pregnancy
- Altered comfort: discomforts of pregnancy
- Self-care deficit related to activity, exercise, and breast care during pregnancy

While perinatal care usually involves essentially healthy families, the nurse must also be alert for emergence of potential or actual complications so she can notify the physician or nurse-midwife about problems. Such complications include problems such as preterm labor, pregnancy-induced hypertension, vaginal bleeding, and family violence.

The nurse is responsible for monitoring for potential complications and for teaching the pregnant woman and her family to be aware of the signs and symptoms of these complications.

Planning and Implementation

The nurse works with the pregnant woman and her support person to plan and implement care based on identified patient needs throughout the pregnancy. However, as pregnancy progresses, patient and family needs shift, and the nurse will not always be in a position to provide information precisely when the family needs it. The nurse uses knowledge about the kinds of concerns patients have at various points during pregnancy to anticipate the needs of the individual woman and her support person and to help plan and implement patient teaching. This provision of the appropriate information to the couple at the appropriate time is *anticipatory guidance.*

Prenatal classes are a cost-effective way to provide education and anticipatory guidance for clients. Prenatal classes are discussed at the end of this chapter. In order to meet the needs of each family during pregnancy, however, there must be constant reassessment of needs and reinforcement of teaching at individual prenatal appointments.

Promoting Health Maintenance with Informational Support

A family must have certain information in order to understand the events of pregnancy, participate in their own care, prepare for the expected changes, share their individual concerns, and, ultimately, experience a positive physical and emotional outcome. The nurse has about 7 months to impart this information.

The learning needs of pregnant women and their fami-

lies vary greatly. Such factors as age, educational level, socioeconomic status, marital status, culture, religion, parity, and, perhaps the most important, the interest of the woman and her family will all influence their learning needs. What is taught to one family may be inappropriate for another.

Anticipatory guidance, then, must start with the learner's level of understanding. The nurse must also take into account the woman's immediate concerns (see Trimester Concerns later in this chapter). Assessing the woman's social surroundings and history can help to illuminate potential problems. The emotional dimensions of the nurse–patient interaction must also be considered.

Patients often see health care providers as authority figures. Nurses will be expected to answer questions as well as impart knowledge. It is more realistic, however, for the nurse and the patient to interact to find solutions. The nurse brings knowledge of the anatomy, physiology, and psychology of pregnancy and the process of gestation. The family brings its unique understanding of the significance of the pregnancy within that social system as well as the role-defining experiences each member has had. The nurse's task is to promote an exchange of knowledge during counseling sessions.

The nurse should also understand her role as a counselor and recognize that she must examine her own biases and perceptions. The nurse should not force the patient into any particular course of action. The nurse's own beliefs, such as the belief that the father should be actively involved in pregnancy or that all children must be breast-fed, must be examined and steps taken to avoid imposing these beliefs on the expectant family. Nurses must realize that even if they have difficulty with the family's decision, the decision is the *family's.* If the nurse wishes to present alternatives for consideration, the alternatives must be compatible with the family's way of life or they will be disregarded.

There are two main issues around which the nurse organizes anticipatory guidance and patient teaching during pregnancy:

- Trimester concerns
- Personal concerns

Learning readiness is the nurse's basic guide to both areas. The remainder of the chapter deals with these issues.

Expected Outcome: The pregnant woman and her support person verbalize an understanding of teaching involving their concerns and demonstrate learning by maintaining or acquiring useful self-care behaviors.

Addressing Specific Physical/Psychosocial Adaptations

Trimester Concerns

Pregnant women and their partners have different concerns at various stages of pregnancy. The nurse must deal with their immediate concerns first. Then she can present additional information anticipating their other concerns.

Time in the first trimester should be devoted to exploring the parents' reactions to the pregnancy: how it will change their daily lives, who will be responsible for infant care, and the need for mutual support as well as a sharing of the workload.

In the second trimester couples are making a transition from acceptance of the pregnancy to preparations for labor and delivery and a new baby. Discussions should focus on this transition and investigate birth plans and options.

In the third trimester, concerns turn to the imminent delivery and care of the infant. Couples may tour the labor and delivery rooms and nursery or other facilities they will use (Fig. 18–2). Decisions about infant care practices are a major concern at this time.

The nurse should address the pregnancy as part of the family's total situation. The couple must be allowed to express their doubts and fears and insecurities. Parents usually know what society expects of them but not what will happen if they alter the typical family structure and,

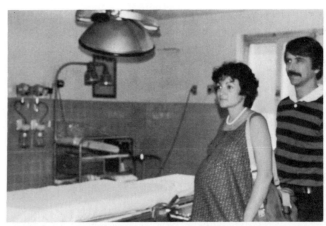

Figure 18–2. In the third trimester the pregnant woman and her partner tour the facility where their baby will be born. (Courtesy of John B. Franklin Maternity Hospital, formerly Booth Maternity Center, Philadelphia)

for example, have the father stay home with the baby. Beyond anticipating societal pressures, the mother in this instance may need anticipatory counseling to help her recognize and overcome her guilt at not being a mother 24 hours a day.

Delivering the facts of pregnancy is only part of the nurse's job. A challenging and rewarding part of her role is helping the couple to identify their needs, verbalize their feelings and concerns, seek solutions, and work toward goals.

Personal Concerns

The nurse's ability to provide anticipatory guidance is related to her knowledge and assessment of the individual needs of the woman and her family. The following issues are some of those the nurse will encounter in prenatal counseling. Each of these issues is discussed in depth in Chapter 12 and are reviewed briefly here.

Age-Related Issues

A woman's age can have a significant impact on her emotional and psychological approach to the pregnancy as well as her medical risk factors. Pregnant adolescents require an extensive environmental support system to promote optimal health and psychological and social potential for both mother and child. Each pregnant adolescent must be assessed individually, since young women between 12 and 19 years old vary greatly in their progression through the developmental tasks of adolescence. Physical development, attitudes toward health, and interest in or ability to seek prenatal care will all influence the outcome of the pregnancy. Emotional support, financial resources, self-esteem, and ability to formulate personal goals must be assessed. Short-term and long-term plans must be developed for each pregnant teen-ager, with

---

Trimester Concerns

First Trimester

- Nausea and vomiting
- Effects of drugs on the fetus
- Changes in body image (especially for teen-agers)
- Family reactions
- Nutritional needs
- Genetic tests

Second Trimester

- Weight gain
- Common discomforts
- Sexual activity: Will it hurt the baby? Am I still attractive?

Third Trimester

- Preparation for labor and delivery
- Preparation for breast-feeding
- Concerns about immediate care of baby

constant reevaluations as the pregnancy progresses (see Chapter 10).

"Elderly primigravidas" are another population with specific age-related concerns. (The nurse should recognize that some women are sensitive about the term itself.) Generally defined as primiparous women of age 35 or older, this group's primary age-related issue is the need for genetic counseling. A couple may refuse genetic

NURSING RESEARCH

First Pregnancy After 35

A descriptive study was conducted to explore women's experiences of a first pregnancy after age 35. Twelve primigravidas between 24 and 34 weeks of gestation were interviewed about their experiences. Interviews were semistructured in nature, and lasted 60 to 100 minutes. Interviews were audio-recorded and transcribed; transcripts were then analyzed for themes, using grounded theory methods for qualitative data.

Findings suggest that older first-time expectant mothers experience distinct phases in their adaptation to pregnancy. "Planning for pregnancy" was the period during which women attempted to become pregnant "at the right time," and planned change was the dominant concept. "Seeking safe passage" (conception through 20 weeks) was a period in which women worked to attain an optimal outcome for self and fetus, and the dominant concept was control over their lives and their pregnancies. "Accepting the pregnancy" was a phase in which women recognized they were entering a major life transition and in which they tried to savor the moment as real *now*. Finally, "anticipating the future" was a phase predominant in the last half of pregnancy in which the major concept was uncertainty about how to combine their new role as mother with their established role as working woman.

The tendency for these women to describe pregnancy and motherhood as a "project" and to engage in much planning and goal-directed behavior has implications for nursing care. Anticipatory guidance may be needed to alert the woman to predictable changes and potential ways for managing the needed adaptation over time. The nurse can reinforce planning and goal directedness while reminding women that some aspects of pregnancy and parenting are not predictable and that uncertainty is a natural response. Finally, women may require support in deciding what aspects of their life-styles they want to retain and what aspects they will let go until they have established themselves securely in the parental role.

Winslow W: First pregnancy after 35: What is the experience? MCN 12(2):92–96, 1987

counseling or genetic tests — that is their right. But the nurse is obligated to raise the subject and must provide them with information about genetic risks. Other age-related issues that may be of concern to the woman are general health status, previous obstetric history, career and lifestyle interruptions, and changes in the couple relationship resulting from postponed motherhood (see Chapter 11).

Social and Marital Issues

Variations in social and marital situations require independent assessments and variations in the anticipatory guidance provided. The concerns of single mothers may differ from those of partnered mothers. Furthermore, a single mother's concerns will differ depending on whether she is single by choice, divorce, or widowhood or because the father chose not to be involved in the pregnancy. Single mothers may have difficulty deciding whether to continue the pregnancy alone or with minimal support from the father. It may be difficult to find family and social support, and legal and financial questions also worry single gravidas (Tilden 1983).

Expectant couples who have a child or children are concerned about sibling issues. Newly partnered couples who have children from previous relationships will also express concerns about sibling acceptance of a new baby. These couples and their children can often be helped by referral to hospital or clinic classes or community mental health seminars dealing with sibling preparation for a new baby.

Pregnant women may also express concern about their partner's level of involvement in the pregnancy. A father's developmental progression through the pregnancy does not always parallel the mother's, and although this is not unusual, it can be a cause for concern and a source of strife (see Chapter 12, Individual and Family Adaptation to Pregnancy).

Pregnant women in lesbian relationships will have specific concerns. The decision to conceive will have been conscious and generally (but not always) presupposes a decision to continue the pregnancy and parent the child. But problems surrounding disclosure to family, societal disapproval, and changes in the couple relationship indicate the need for a strong support group for the woman and her partner.

Previous Obstetric History

Women who have had previous obstetric complications or losses will bring many anxieties to the current pregnancy. Their concerns may arise from popular myths and misconceptions or from admonitions from previous health care providers. The nurse's role is to obtain an accurate and detailed health history, including an obstetric and gynecological history, and perform a social and psychological assessment to ascertain the basis of the woman's concerns and formulate appropriate education and counseling plans. These women and their families must be particularly encouraged to call the health care provider when questions and concerns arise.

A woman with a history of one or more spontaneous abortions, late (second-trimester) therapeutic abortions, or a cervical conization may be fearful of spontaneous abortion or preterm labor. Some women verbalize their concerns, whereas others are afraid to ask questions; thus, a nurse must be alert for unexpressed concerns when women present with such histories. Occasionally a woman's partner is unaware of her obstetric history, and she is anxious that her privacy be maintained. The nurse must ensure confidentiality and not refer to this history in a joint session without the woman's approval.

Women with histories of obstetric complications such as preterm labor, placenta previa, or preeclampsia will be fearful of recurrences. They must be advised of risks as well as reassured of close observation and diagnostic and preventive measures where possible. Families that have experienced the loss of a fetus or neonate or the anxieties of a premature birth will have many concerns during the pregnancy and will require additional time for sensitive listening and support.

Psychosocial Risk Factors

Women who suffer from chronic or debilitating diseases and handicapped women will have concerns about the effects of their disease or medications on the pregnancy and fetus as well as the effect of the pregnancy on their health status. They may fear alterations in body image and immobility. They may also worry about their ability to care for an infant, to breast-feed, or to parent a child. Communication with the partner and social and emotional support must be encouraged. Social service referrals may be indicated.

Women who approach pregnancy without social support—whether this is the result of the absence or indifference of the partner, lack of parental figures or relationship, minimal social contacts, or relocation to a new community—will require support and assistance from the health care provider. The nurse must also be aware that family violence may begin during pregnancy and be watchful for women who may be at risk (see section later in this chapter). The nurse must be on the alert for these needs and encourage the woman to seek appropriate outlets in social groups, community organizations, or prenatal classes and through social and psychological referrals where necessary.

In conclusion, in order to provide anticipatory guidance to pregnant women and their partners, the nurse must have theoretical knowledge of the physiologic and psychological changes of pregnancy, women's common concerns, and situations in which specific teaching is

needed. But that information could also be obtained from a comprehensive book on the subject. The nurse's true value in prenatal care often lies in her ability to develop a trusting relationship with the woman and her family in order to assess their unique needs and formulate and implement an appropriate plan, thus moving the nurse–patient relationship from the trusting realm to the therapeutic realm.

Referrals

It is not unusual for expectant women and their families to need referrals to other physicians, counselors, or social agencies during the course of the pregnancy. Sometimes the physiologic, psychological, or financial stresses of pregnancy can precipitate a crisis. At other times the changes of pregnancy or the anxieties of additional responsibilities can cause a woman or family struggling with chronic illness or other problems to need help beyond the usual prenatal care and education.

Through nursing assessments the nurse will determine when a family needs a referral for additional assistance. Patients do not always ask for help outright, so the nurse will have to make suggestions based on her knowledge of normal adaptation to pregnancy and her ability to observe and assess the family's coping mechanisms as their situation changes. Offices and clinic facilities that provide prenatal care will usually have a protocol book that can assist the nurse in determining when specific conditions require a referral.

It is essential for the nurse to be aware of resources available in the community. Facilities providing prenatal care usually have referral lists for women with specific needs, but cases will always arise that are not covered by the referral list. If a woman or family needs a service that is not supplied by any of the agencies on the list, the nurse must find an agency that does supply it and promptly contact the family to make the referral.

Some women have difficulty entering the health care system for a condition other than pregnancy. They may be disinclined to follow up on a referral, particularly if they are in a state of disequilibrium, are denying the problem, are embarrassed, or think that further care will not do any good anyway. In these situations the nurse can further assist by arranging an appointment (and transportation if necessary) and should find out afterwards whether the patient kept the appointment. If patients habitually break appointments, further assessment must be done to ascertain why. The nurse must carefully document her interventions and counseling of the patient to seek additional help.

Counseling Referrals.   Certain problems identified during the nursing assessment or reported by the patient call for a counseling referral: marital, sexual, and work-related difficulties; troubles with children; adolescents' difficulties with family or partner; problems with developmental adaptation to pregnancy; and substance abuse or dependency. Psychologists, professional counselors, psychiatrists, community support groups, and crisis-prevention agencies are all appropriate resources to utilize.

Nutrition Referrals. The physiologic changes of pregnancy make great nutritional demands on the pregnant woman (see Chapter 15). Clients should be referred to a nutritionist if they begin the pregnancy extremely far under or over their ideal weight, if weight gain during pregnancy is insufficient or excessive, if intake is largely empty calories or is poorly balanced, or if a previously existing nutritional or metabolic disease might be exaggerated by pregnancy.

Adolescents frequently require nutrition referrals for poor eating habits or dieting prompted by concern about their appearance. Families will also benefit from such referrals if low income interferes with eating healthy foods. Nutritionists can give advice about obtaining wholesome food on a limited budget. This is especially valuable when there will soon be another mouth to feed. Women from other cultures may not eat well because they cannot find their customary foods; they too should be referred to a nutritionist for assistance.

Social Referrals. When pregnancy places financial burdens on the family that they are unable to deal with or work out successfully, a social work referral is needed. Social workers can help these families deal with the bureaucratic systems that supply food stamps, welfare, and housing; with school placement and counseling; and with other problems as they arise. Teenagers, single women, and unemployed and low-income women and their families are particularly likely to need to be referred to social workers.

Genetic Counseling Referrals. Health care providers are responsible for informing expectant parents of their genetic risks and of the prenatal genetic diagnostic tests available (see Chapter 9). It is important to inform a couple of the genetic tests available to them, regardless of their age and risk factors. It is the couple's choice to obtain or decline testing. Couples must be given clear and accurate explanations early in the pregnancy so that they can make timely and informed decisions. Health care providers must document the counseling given.

Expected Outcome: The pregnant woman and her family utilize the nurse as a resource person for needed services and information, and are active participants in health maintenance and promotion.

Providing Support for Common Discomforts

During the 9 months of pregnancy, many changes occur in a woman's body as a result of hormonal influences and the body's response and adaptation to the gestational process. Changes such as stronger fingernails, hair with fuller body, or larger breasts are often appreciated by the woman or her partner. Other changes, such as nausea or breast tenderness, are unpleasant for the woman but usually short-lived. Still other changes, such as hemorrhoids or varicosities, usually occur later in the pregnancy and may get worse over time.

Responses to the discomforts of pregnancy vary, depending on the severity of the symptoms, the significance of the symptoms for each woman, and individual tolerance for discomfort. The nurse's role is to do a nursing assessment for the specific complaint, reassure the woman, make appropriate nursing interventions, and provide the necessary education. Often a patient will only need reassurance that her discomfort is a temporary and normal phenomenon of pregnancy. Frequently a patient will need detailed teaching about preventive measures, and occasionally one will need careful instructions about warning signs to report.

The following pages provide nursing care plans for the discomforts of pregnancy. The nurse can use the accompanying Nursing Care Plan as a reference source when counseling patients.

Expected Outcome: The pregnant woman and support person/family will implement safe and appropriate self-care during common pregnancy discomforts that results in reduction of symptoms and continued self-care behaviors.

Supporting Self-Care

One of the characteristics of perinatal care is that, by and large, the nurse is working with a healthy population that requires only guidance about appropriate self-care. The following section addresses some common self-care needs of pregnant women and their partners throughout pregnancy. Since the patient is in the best position to care for herself appropriately, if she is well informed, teaching again is a central component of the nurse's care.

Activities During Pregnancy

Pregnancy is a normal physiologic event and should not require a woman to alter her lifestyle drastically. However, most pregnant women and their partners do wonder

(text continued on page 468)

NURSING CARE PLAN

The Woman With Common Discomforts of Pregnancy

Nursing Diagnosis (Patient Problem) and Assessment Data	Nursing Interventions	Rationale
Nursing Diagnosis: *altered comfort: nausea and vomiting*		
• Patient c/o nausea and/or vomiting, especially in the morning	Reassure the patient that nausea and vomiting usually resolve spontaneously after the first trimester. Occur in 50%–80% of women.	In the absence of other problems, nausea/vomiting thought to be related to these physiologic changes in first trimester:
		• Increased levels of progesterone (decreases gastric emptying time)
		• Increased levels of human chorionic gonadotropin
		• Decreased gastric secretion of hydrochloric acid and pepsin. May be accompanied by fatigue, dizziness, hot flashes, constipation, sleep disturbances
	Advise the patient to avoid greasy, spicy foods. Avoid odors that predispose to nausea (use fan while cooking). Eat 6 small meals a day instead of 3 large ones. Increase protein snacks (cheese, nuts, eggs). Eat foods high in carbohydrates (better tolerated). Eat dry, unsalted crackers before arising in morning. Drink fluids between meals (decreases dehydration). Avoid liquids with meals. Sip carbonated water (not sweet sodas) to prevent onset of nausea. Try spearmint, peppermint, or raspberry tea. Take iron tablets and vitamins after meals or bedtime. Try 50 to 100 mg/day vitamin B_6 (after a meal) to reduce nausea. Have yogurt, cottage cheese, juice, or milk when awakened by nocturia to decrease nausea in morning. Take frequent fresh air walks, especially after meals. Maintain good posture (to relieve pressure on stomach) Avoid sudden movements.	Self-care measures designed to decrease gastric irritability while maintaining intake are recommended. No one measure works for all women, so patient should try several techniques.
	Caution the patient to avoid over-the-counter antinausea medications or any medicines without consultation with health care provider.	Some preparations are not regarded as safe for use in pregnancy, or may cause undesirable side-effects.

(continued)

NURSING CARE PLAN (continued)

The Woman With Common Discomforts of Pregnancy

Nursing Diagnosis (Patient Problem) and Assessment Data	Nursing Interventions	Rationale

Expected Outcome:

The pregnant woman verbalizes understanding of self-care measures and the fact that she feels better with one or several of the measures, as evidenced by reduced/no nausea and vomiting.

Nursing Diagnosis:
altered nutrition: less than body requirements related to nausea/vomiting

• Weight loss • Dehydration • Decreased skin turgor • Ketonuria	Assess and document the extent of nausea and vomiting and signs and symptoms of dehydration.	These signs indicate significant dehydration and inadequate maternal intake.
	Assess emotional response to pregnancy.	Significant emotional ambivalence about pregnancy may be contributing factor.
	Assess possibility of other diagnostic problems — stomach or gastric ulcers, cholecystitis, pancreatitis, hepatitis, gastroenteritis, appendicitis, or intestinal flu.	Other conditions should be ruled out if nausea is severe and persistent.
	Evaluate diet for adequacy of food intake and quality of nutrients.	Inadequate intake of nutrients and liquids can inhibit optimal weight gain. Low maternal blood glucose can further exacerbate nausea/vomiting.
	Review self-care measures (listed above) and emphasize importance of adequate dietary intake.	

Expected Outcome:

Pregnant woman demonstrates an improvement in nutrition as evidenced by regaining weight loss and continuing to maintain appropriate gains for trimester.

Nursing Diagnosis:
altered comfort: discomfort related to breast fullness and tingling

	Assess whether discomfort is generalized or local. Assess for injury. Assess for supernumerary breast and axillary tissue involvement. Assess for leaking of colostrum, which may cause cracked nipples.	In the absence of evidence of injury or infection, symptoms are probably caused by: • Fat deposition, caused by estrogen, and development of stromal tissue and ductile system.

(continued)

NURSING CARE PLAN (continued)

The Woman With Common Discomforts of Pregnancy

Nursing Diagnosis (Patient Problem) and Assessment Data	Nursing Interventions	Rationale
		• Development of lobules, alveoli proliferation and secretion, and breast swelling, caused by progesterone
		• Increased vascular supply to breasts
	Reassure the patient that breast changes and discomforts are natural; fullness will continue throughout pregnancy, but tenderness usually resolves after first trimester.	
	Teach the patient anatomy and physiology of breast changes; breast self-examination; breast-feeding preparations at onset of third trimester.	
	Advise the patient to wear support bra with wide adjustable straps and smooth interior to decrease irritation.	Increased breast size requires additional support.
	Avoid pressure on breasts.	
	Avoid use of soap on nipples	Soap dries sensitive skin, predisposes to cracking.
	Resume regular breast self-examination after tenderness subsides.	

Expected Outcome:

Patient uses appropriate techniques to reduce discomfort and promote breast health, as evidenced by clean, dry nipples without cracks or sores and no complaints about breast discomfort.

Nursing Diagnosis:
altered urinary elimination pattern related to urinary frequency/urgency

	Assess for urinary tract infections (urethritis, cystitis, pyelonephritis):	In the absence of other problems, frequency/urgency may be caused by: Stretching of the base of the
	• Urinalysis	bladder by the enlarging uterus in the first trimester, producing a
	• Urine culture	sensation of fullness; reduction in
	• Fever or chills	bladder capacity through pressure of enlarging uterus on bladder;
	• Costovertebral or suprapubic tenderness	compression of bladder by presenting part in third trimester; excessive
	Assess diet for excessive coffee, tea or cola intake.	fluid intake; promotion of urine output by kidneys when woman is in
	Assess for diabetes: excessive thirst, abnormal blood glucose levels.	supine position (nocturia); urinary tract infection; diabetes

(continued)

446

The Woman With Common Discomforts of Pregnancy

Nursing Diagnosis (Patient Problem) and Assessment Data	Nursing Interventions	Rationale
	Advise the patient to maintain hydration during daytime but decrease fluid intake in the evening to reduce nocturia; void when the urge occurs to avoid bladder distention and urinary stasis; limit intake of caffeinated beverages (tea, coffee, cola); do Kegel exercises to strengthen pelvic floor muscles and decrease urinary leakage	Self-care measures eliminate most annoying symptoms (nocturia) while maintaining optimal hydration.
	Teach the patient the signs of urinary tract infection (urgency or burning) and the importance of prompt medical attention should the signs occur.	Urinary tract infections are associated with increased risk of preterm labor.

Expected Outcome:

Pregnant woman maintains appropriate urinary elimination as demonstrated by using appropriate techniques to reduce frequency and nocturia and verbalization of the signs of urinary tract infection requiring prompt medical attention.

Nursing Diagnosis:
fatigue related to pregnancy

• Patient c/o lack of energy, unusual need for sleep	Assess nutrition for anemia or inadequate caloric intake. Assess hemoglobin (Hgb) and hematocrit (Hct). Assess psychosocial status for anxiety and depression. Assess exercise regimen. Assess activity level and amount of rest. Assess whether fatigue is appropriate for trimester of pregnancy.	In the absence of other causes, probably due to: • Increased hormonal production; possible role of ovarian hormone relaxin • Increased demands on cardiopulmonary systems in last trimester • 25% increase in basal metabolic rate • Inadequate nutrition • Anemia • Lack of exercise • Excessive activity • Excessive weight gain • Psychogenic causes • Infection • Incorrect posture

(continued)

The Woman With Common Discomforts of Pregnancy

Nursing Diagnosis (Patient Problem) and Assessment Data	Nursing Interventions	Rationale
	Reassure the patient that fatigue is a normal and temporary aspect of pregnancy. Advise the patient to take frequent rest periods (lie down during coffee breaks, *etc*); get adequate exercise; increase social stimulation (when appropriate) with family, friends, or groups; decrease activities that may cause overexertion; explore opportunities to participate in activities she enjoys; get assistance with child care if possible; practice deep breathing and relaxation exercises.	

Expected Outcome:

Patient demonstrates an understanding of the causes of fatigue as evidenced by using appropriate techniques to reduce fatigue.

Nursing Diagnosis:
altered comfort related to leukorrhea (vaginal discharge)

	Assess type, color, amount, and odor of discharge. Assess whether patient suffers from pruritus. Assess for partner's complaints of symptoms or new or multiple partners. Evaluate for *Candida albicans* or sexually transmitted infection.	In the absence of other problems, probably caused by: • Increased production of cervical mucus, recognized as a profuse, thin, white or yellowish vaginal discharge, caused by estrogen • Increased cervical vascularity and desquamation
	Reassure the patient that increased discharge is a normal process of pregnancy.	
	Advise the patient to use good perineal hygiene; keep vulva dry by using hairdryer after washing and dusting with cornstarch; use external vinegar and water rinse; wear loose cotton undergarments; avoid pantyhose and tight clothing; use perineal pads and change them frequently; report pruritus and foul odor.	Self-care measures are designed to decrease perineal dampness.

(continued)

NURSING CARE PLAN (continued)

The Woman With Common Discomforts of Pregnancy

Nursing Diagnosis (Patient Problem) and Assessment Data	Nursing Interventions	Rationale
	Caution the patient to avoid douching, tampons	Both practices further disturb vaginal flora and may increase risk of infection.

Expected Outcome:

Patient demonstrates an understanding of the causes of leukorrhea, recognizes signs of vaginal infection, and uses appropriate prophylactic techniques.

Nursing Diagnosis:
altered sexuality patterns

• Patient complains of decreased libido or decrease in partner's libido • Physical discomfort or aversion to intercourse	Assess reasons for changes in libido: physical discomforts or emotional origins. Assess couple's psychological response to pregnancy. Assess couple's communication skills and ability to cope with and resolve the perceived difficulties. Reassure the patient and her partner that variations in sexual interest occur in pregnancy, and that they can enjoy their usual sexual activities unless their health care provider *specifically* contraindicates sexual activity for them. Advise the patient and her partner that good communication between partners is essential. Cuddling, kissing, and stroking will often provide emotional satisfaction and also fulfill some physical needs. Massage is another alternative or adjunct form of sexual expression. Variations in position during intercourse may become necessary for comfort as pregnancy progresses (*e.g.,* intercourse with the woman on top or with the man entering from behind). Mutual masturbation and oral sex are other adjuncts or alternatives to sexual activity if intercourse becomes too uncomfortable. Refer couple for sexual or couple counseling, if self-care practices are not effective.	In the absence of other causes, probably due to: • Complicated interplay between physiologic discomforts and hormonal and emotional changes. In the first trimester, decreased libido may be due to fatigue, nausea and vomiting, breast tenderness, and ambivalence toward the pregnancy. The second trimester is usually characterized by an increase in libido. There is often a decrease in libido at the end of the third trimester, usually related to physical discomforts, fatigue, and anxiety. • Problems in the couple relationship: Fear that intercourse will harm the embryo/fetus; progress through psychosocial tasks of pregnancy; changed body image; discomfort from relaxation of pelvic joints and ligaments; painful contractions from orgasm (third trimester).

(continued)

NURSING CARE PLAN (continued)

The Woman With Common Discomforts of Pregnancy

Nursing Diagnosis (Patient Problem) and Assessment Data	Nursing Interventions	Rationale

Expected Outcome:

Patient and partner demonstrate an understanding and acceptance of causes of changes in libido by communicating concerns to one another in an attempt to enhance mutual understanding.

Nursing Diagnosis:
ineffective individual coping related to mood changes:

• Patient c/o marked mood swings, unusual withdrawal or teariness	Assess woman's emotional stability and coping mechanisms and compare with prepregnant emotional stability, if known. Assess couple's communication skills, attitude toward pregnancy, and progression through developmental tasks of pregnancy. Assess the support system available to the woman or couple in family, friends, church, community, and workplace. Assess woman's nutritional status with regard to fatigue, anemia, and caloric intake. Assess for dependence on drugs, alcohol, and other substances. Reassure the patient and her partner that mood swings are a normal component of pregnancy. Encourage the patient or couple to discuss their feelings with a trusted person; continue activities that bring enjoyment; take time for good grooming, rest, sleep, and exercise. Refer the patient or couple for counseling if appropriate.	In the absence of other causes, may be due to: • Depressant effect of progesterone on the central nervous system • Prominence of physical and emotional changes of pregnancy to the pregnant woman • Marked introversion, often secondary to developmental tasks of pregnancy • Lack of support system for woman and partner • Physical discomforts of pregnancy, fatigue • Anxiety • Changed body image

Expected Outcome:

Patient and partner demonstrate an understanding and acceptance of the causes of mood changes as evidenced by maintaining and using appropriate techniques to reduce negative effects of mood changes.

Nursing Diagnosis:
altered comfort: heartburn

• Patient c/o "heartburn" especially at night or when lying down	Assess nutritional status and habits. Assess psychosocial status for	In the absence of other causes, probably due to:

(continued)

NURSING CARE PLAN (continued)

The Woman With Common Discomforts of Pregnancy

Nursing Diagnosis (Patient Problem) and Assessment Data	Nursing Interventions	Rationale
• Patient complains of belching or gastric "fullness"	tension or depression. Assess previous medical history for gastrointestinal illness, cholecystitis, or hiatal hernia. Reassure the patient that normal pregnancy changes are causing the heartburn. Advise the patient to: eliminate greasy, spicy foods from diet; eat small bland meals; eat 6 small meals a day, not 3 large ones; eat slowly and chew thoroughly; chew gum (sometimes helpful); avoid coffee and cigarettes because they irritate the stomach; drink 8 glasses of fluids a day; drink hot tea; avoid sodium bicarbonate. Advise the patient to avoid lying down, bending or stooping after eating; wear clothes that fit loosely around the waistline; when heartburn occurs, sip water, milk, or carbonated water, or eat 1 tablespoonful of yogurt, heavy cream, or half-and-half; do flying exercise to decrease heartburn (see Fig. 18-3). Advise the patient to try antacids (without phosphorus) if necessary—aluminum hydroxide; Gelusil; Amphojel; calcium carbonate; Tums; magnesium hydroxide; Maalox; Mylanta; Riopan. Caution patient to avoid heartburn medicines containing aspirin (Alka Seltzer, Fizrin), heartburn medicines containing sodium (baking soda, soda mint, Eno, Fizrin, Rolaids, Alka Seltzer).	• Relaxation of smooth gastrointestinal muscles and cardiac sphincter of stomach by progesterone, allowing gastric reflux of stomach contents to lower esophagus • Displacement of stomach and duodenum by enlarging uterus • Decreased hydrochloric acid and pepsin secretion in the stomach, caused by estrogen • Emotional factors Self-care measures to decrease gastric activity and promote stomach emptying are recommended.

(continued)

NURSING CARE PLAN (continued)

The Woman With Common Discomforts of Pregnancy

Nursing Diagnosis (Patient Problem) and Assessment Data	Nursing Interventions	Rationale

Expected Outcome:

Patient demonstrates an understanding of the causes of heartburn as evidenced by using appropriate techniques to decrease heartburn.

Nursing Diagnosis:
altered comfort: excessive salivation

	Nursing Interventions	Rationale
	Assess nutrition for iron deficiency or excessive starch intake. Observe for specific oral lesions (salivary calculus, syphilis). Assess emotional status (hysteria). Assess for tonsillitis and stomatitis. Assess previous medical history or current status for gastric, pancreatic, or hepatic disorder. Reassure the patient that this is a pregnancy-related situation that will resolve. Advise the patient to: • Suck hard candy • Avoid excessive starch intake • Practice good oral hygiene • Maintain good nutrition	In the absence of other causes, probably due to: • Salivary gland stimulation by starch intake • Increased acidity of saliva, leading to gland production of saliva • Difficulty in swallowing caused by nausea, contributing to the sensation of increased saliva • Unusual food cravings or pica • Oral infections or lesions

Expected Outcome:

Patient understands the cause of excessive salivation as demonstrated by using appropriate techniques to decrease salivary excess.

Nursing Diagnosis:
altered bowel elimination: flatulence

	Nursing Interventions	Rationale
	Assess nutrition status with regard to intake of gas-forming foods. Assess bowel habits. Assess exercise and activity levels. Assess for abdominal pain, eructation, bloating, distention, or passing excessive flatus. Assess antacid use (baking soda will cause flatulence).	In the absence of other causes, probably due to: • Ingestion of gas-forming food • Acrophagia (air-swallowing), ptyalism, or nausea • Decreased motility of gut • Decreased exercise

(continued)

452

NURSING CARE PLAN   (continued)

The Woman With Common Discomforts of Pregnancy

Nursing Diagnosis (Patient Problem) and Assessment Data	Nursing Interventions	Rationale
	Reassure the patient that flatulence is a pregnancy-related phenomenon and will not harm her or the fetus. Advise the patient to avoid gas-forming foods (cabbage, beans, fried foods) and large meals; chew food thoroughly; decrease salivation by not chewing gum or smoking; change position frequently; have regular bowel habits; exercise regularly.	• Uterine compression of gut • Constipation • Fecal impaction

Expected Outcome:

Patient understands the causes of flatulence as evidenced by using appropriate techniques to decrease flatulence.

Nursing Diagnosis:
altered comfort: headache

	Assess symptoms to determine whether headache is a normal phenomenon of pregnancy or a warning sign of pregnancy complications: Type of headache (front, side, back of head); difference from usual headaches; visual disturbances (frequency of occurrence); causative factors (fatigue, bad lighting, eye strain, stuffy office, emotional stress, poor nutrition, dehydration). Assess for other toxemia or pre-eclampsia symptoms: proteinuria, weight gain, elevated blood pressure, edema, exaggerated reflexes (hyperreflexia), and so on. Assess for sinusitis, upper respiratory infection, and allergies. Assess previous attempts at relief and their effectiveness. Assess previous medical history and family history for renal cardia or vascular disease.	In the absence of other causes, probably due to: • Increased circulating volume and heart rate (contribute to dilation and distention of cerebral arteries) • Vascular congestion of nasal turbinates from tissue edema • Emotional tension, causing spasm of sternocleidomastoid muscles of the neck and shoulders • Fatigue • Second-trimester decrease in blood pressure

(continued)

The Woman With Common Discomforts of Pregnancy

Nursing Diagnosis (Patient Problem) and Assessment Data	Nursing Interventions	Rationale
	Explain the blood mechanisms that may be responsible for headache. Reassure the patient that symptoms are temporary and will respond to treatment.	
	Advise the patient to increase rest and relaxation; engage in activities that are relaxing and rewarding; perform relaxation exercises; make dietary changes if causative foods or food allergies are isolated (cheeses, red wines, and shellfish can cause headaches); adjust salts and sugars in diet for relief of symptoms; avoid long periods without eating.	Self-care measures to reduce tension and dehydration are recommended.
	Maintain hydration. Apply cool wet cloth to forehead and back of neck; massage neck, shoulders, face, and scalp; take slow walks in fresh air; arrange for child care help if appropriate; try acetaminophen (Tylenol; 2 tablets every 4–6 hr) after the first trimester if headache is severe.	
	Caution the patient *not* to use drugs without the health care provider's knowledge.	*No* drugs should be used during pregnancy unless necessary and prescribed by care provider.
	Teach the patient to report signs of toxemia and preeclampsia: severe, frequent, or long-lasting headaches; blurry vision or spots of bright lights before eyes; edema of face, hands, or legs in the morning; scanty concentrated urine.	

Expected Outcome:

Patient understands the causes of headaches and uses appropriate techniques to reduce headaches as evidenced by a decrease in headaches.

Nursing Diagnosis:
altered comfort: round ligament pain

	Assess cause of onset (exercise, sudden movement, *etc.*) and site of	In the absence of other causes, probably due to

The Woman With Common Discomforts of Pregnancy

Nursing Diagnosis (Patient Problem) and Assessment Data	Nursing Interventions	Rationale
	pain (unilateral or bilateral). Assess uterine activity to distinguish round ligament pain from preterm labor; rhythmic uterine tightening and relaxing and sensation of pelvic pressure are symptomatic of preterm labor. Assess for other possible causes of pain: corpus luteal cyst rupture, ectopic pregnancy, Braxton Hicks contractions, constipation, appendicitis, inguinal hernia. (See all interventions under Backache.)	• Stretching of round ligaments caused by uterine growth (round ligaments extend bilaterally from anterior and inferior to the oviducts through the inguinal cava to insert in the superior portion of the labia majora).
	Reassure the patient and explain the cause of round ligament pain	
	Advise the patient to avoid sudden jerking or twisting movements	Sudden jerking or twisting of the torso pulls on these ligaments, causing unilateral or bilateral pain in the lateral lower abdominal wall.
	Rise slowly from recumbent position. Apply local heat to the area of discomfort. Do total body relaxation exercises. Avoid excessive exercise, standing, and walking.	

Expected Outcome:

Patient understands the causes of round ligament pain as demonstrated by use of appropriate techniques to reduce occurrences of round ligament pain.

Nursing Diagnosis:
activity intolerance related to dyspnea (shortness of breath)

	Assess frequency of occurrence of dyspnea, its associations (exercise, sleep, supine position, etc.), and its manifestations (dizziness, fainting, etc.).	In the absence of other causes probably due to:
	Assess nutrition and Hgb/Hct for anemia. Assess whether client hyperventilates. Assess for thoracic deformities and previous medical history of asthma or pulmonary disease.	• Compression of vena cava by gravid uterus, decreasing venous return to the heart and causing arterial hypotension; further compromise of circulatory status by lying in supine position (supine hypotensive syndrome)
		• Prevention of maximum lung expansion by enlarging uterus

(continued)

NURSING CARE PLAN (continued)

The Woman With Common Discomforts of Pregnancy

Nursing Diagnosis (Patient Problem) and Assessment Data	Nursing Interventions	Rationale
	Reassure the patient by explaining the physiologic reasons for dyspnea in pregnancy. Advise the patient to:	• Increased awareness of breathing
	• Sit and stand up straight • Rest after exercise • Avoid overexertion • Sleep and rest in left lateral position or semi-Fowler's position with head elevated	

Expected Outcome:

Patient demonstrates an understanding and acceptance of the causes of dyspnea as evidenced by using appropriate techniques to decrease dyspnea.

Nursing Diagnosis:
altered comfort: backache

	Assess posture, lifting techniques, type of footwear worn, and so on. Assess activity level and rest periods. Assess for acute back muscle strain and anatomical musculoskeletal defects.	In the absence of other causes, probably due to: • Increased weight of growing uterus, which pulls spine forward and changes center of gravity, thus leading to compensatory lordosis and muscle strain • Lack of support from lax abdominal muscles, which contribute to compensatory lordosis • Relaxation of pelvic ligaments and body joints, caused by estrogen and relaxin • Fatigue and muscle tension • High-heeled shoes, which cause postural changes and low back strain • Excessive weight gain, which increases strain on back muscles • Exaggerated lordosis, which may cause aching and numbness of the upper extremities

(continued)

NURSING CARE PLAN   (continued)

The Woman With Common Discomforts of Pregnancy

Nursing Diagnosis (Patient Problem) and Assessment Data	Nursing Interventions	Rationale
		• Increased intercostal respiration and expansion of thoracic cage, which may contribute to upper back pain
	Advise the patient to avoid overexten-sion and fatigue; rest frequently in recumbent position; wear comfort-able, low-heeled shoes; apply local heat to backaches; get regular daily exercise; have friend give back massage; elevate one leg on stool or box while standing; perform total body relaxation exercises; avoid lifting small children; have toddlers climb onto lap.	Self-care techniques to relieve back strain and promote flexibility and good posture are recommended.
	Teach the patient to exercise; maintain good posture, especially pelvic cradle posture; do pelvic tilts several times daily; sit in tailor position; use proper lifting techniques.	

Expected Outcome:

Patient understands the causes of backache and uses appropriate techniques to reduce backache as evidenced by improved posture and verbalization that backaches have decreased.

Nursing Diagnosis:
altered bowel elimination: constipation

	Assess diet for fiber, fluid, and iron intake; assess exercise; assess prepregnant and current bowel habits (irregularity, impaction); as-sess psychological status (depression, anxiety); assess for other possible causes of bowel changes (irritable colon, atonic colon).	In the absence of other causes, probably due to:
		• Relaxation of muscle tone and decreased peristalsis, caused by progesterone, which allow increased water resorption from the bowel.
	Reassure the patient that constipation is pregnancy-related and will resolve.	• Pressure from the uterus on the colon and rectum
		• Decreased physical exercise
		• Decreased fluid intake; inadequate roughage in diet
		• Changes in eating habits, especially increases in calcium and iron intake
		• Stress
		• Fecal impaction

(continued)

The Woman With Common Discomforts of Pregnancy

Nursing Diagnosis (Patient Problem) and Assessment Data	Nursing Interventions	Rationale
	Advise the patient to increase fluid intake (6–8 glasses/day) and drink warm liquids on arising in the morning; increase exercise; increase fiber intake by eating whole-grain breads and cereals (bran), raw, unpeeled or dry fruits and vegetables; establish regular bowel habits; take time for bowel movements, neither forcing them nor resisting the urge.	Self-care measures to increase roughage and promote normal bowel function.
	Use extra bulk such as Metamucil, 1 tsp/day as needed; use a stool-softener such as Colace, 150 to 200 mg/day for 5 to 10 days, or a mild laxative such as milk of magnesia; raise feet on stool or box during bowel movement to decrease straining; caution the patient to avoid mineral oil as a laxative because it prevents absorption of fat-soluble vitamins from the gut.	

Expected Outcome:

Patient understands the causes of constipation and uses appropriate techniques to reduce constipation as evidenced by patient's verbalization of decreased constipation and comfort with bowel movements.

Nursing Diagnosis:
altered comfort: pain from varicosities

	Assess whether varicosities are associated with mild discomfort or severe pain. Assess previous history and family history of varicosities. Assess levels of activity, exercise, and rest. Assess and document extent of varicosities. With patient supine, observe for signs of venous stasis (pitting, stasis, pigmentation, or ulceration). With patient standing observe for dilated veins in legs.	In the absence of other causes, probably due to: • Increased blood volume, putting additional pressure on venous circulation • Increased pressure from enlarging uterus, which restricts venous return from legs and perineum, causing vulvar and leg varicosities and hemorrhoids • Congenital predisposition to weakness in the vascular walls

(continued)

NURSING CARE PLAN (continued)

The Woman With Common Discomforts of Pregnancy

Nursing Diagnosis (Patient Problem) and Assessment Data	Nursing Interventions	Rationale
		• Inactivity and poor muscle tone • Prolonged standing, which causes venous pooling in lower limbs and pelvis • Obesity
	Reassure the patient by explaining the cause of varicosities. Explain that varicosities will not resolve during pregnancy, but steps can be taken to control symptoms (throbbing) and progress of condition.	
	Advise the patient to rest in the recumbent position with legs elevated *above* the level of the body twice a day or more; wear support hose. To put on properly, the patient should lie flat and raise legs to drain the veins, rolling stocking on while legs are still elevated. Hose should be put on *before* arising in the morning. Wear loose clothing and avoid round garters and tight knee-highs. Refrain from crossing legs at the knee; get up and move around every hour if sedentary; get regular exercise or walk each day; wear comfortable shoes to decrease the strain on legs when walking or standing; wear a pelvic pad supported by a T-binder for support of vulvar varicosities.	Self-care measures designed to decrease venous pooling and promote comfort.

Expected Outcome:

Patient uses appropriate techniques to reduce the discomfort and progress of varicosities as evidenced by verbalization of less discomfort and evidence of reduction of progress of varicosities.

Nursing Diagnosis:
altered comfort: hemorrhoids

	Assess nutrition for fiber, fluid, and iron intake. Assess exercise activity. Assess prepregnant and current bowel habits. Reassure the patient	In the absence of other causes, probably due to: • See all causes under varicosities

(continued)

The Woman With Common Discomforts of Pregnancy

Nursing Diagnosis (Patient Problem) and Assessment Data	Nursing Interventions	Rationale
	by explaining the causes and ways of preventing hemorrhoids.	• Relaxation of the smooth muscle of the bowel, contributing to constipation and straining at stool, the latter of which predisposes the patient to hemorrhoid formation
	Advise client to avoid constipation (see interventions under Constipation); take warm or cool sitz baths (whichever is most soothing) and, if possible, use a finger to gently replace the hemorrhoid into the anal canal.	
	Cleanse the anus carefully after defecation; place petroleum jelly in the rectum after defecation; apply cool witch hazel compresses for comfort as necessary; refrain from straining during bowel movements, since this exacerbates the problem.	
	Teach clients to lie in knee–chest position for up to 15 min/day. Do Kegel exercises to strengthen perineum and help prevent and control hemorrhoids. Caution the patient to consult her health care provider before using any hemorrhoidal medications.	

Expected Outcome:

Patient understands the causes of hemorrhoids and uses appropriate techniques to control and prevent hemorrhoids as evidenced by controlled hemorrhoids on inspection and palpation.

Nursing Diagnosis:
altered comfort: leg cramps

	Assess diet for excessive or inadequate dairy product intake or excessive soft drink intake.	In the absence of other causes, probably due to:
	Assess for other possible cause of leg pain, such as phlebitis (skin warm to touch, palpable thrombus, positive Homan's sign).	• Disturbance in the body's calcium–phosporus ratio (increased phosphorus predisposes to leg cramps); excessive intake of dairy products, which increases both calcium and phosphorus levels; inadequate intake of dairy products, which decreases calcium levels; high soft

(continued)

NURSING CARE PLAN (continued)

The Woman With Common Discomforts of Pregnancy

Nursing Diagnosis (Patient Problem) and Assessment Data	Nursing Interventions	Rationale
		drink intake, which increases phosphorus levels
		• Fatigue or muscle strain in the extremities
		• Blood vessel occlusion in the legs
		• Sudden stretching of the leg and foot (pointing the toes)
	Advise the patient to limit intake of dairy products to 4 servings/day or take calcium supplements if intake is inadequate (chewable calcium carbonate tablets, 1 g 3 times/day); decrease the amount of phosphorus in the diet (e.g., by decreasing intake of soft drinks), and take antacids containing aluminum hydroxide (e.g., Amphojel) to bind the phosphorus; dorsiflex foot (point toes toward head) when cramping occurs; avoid toe-pointing stretch of legs; apply local heat to sore leg muscles; keep legs warm; stretch calf muscles before bedtime; take a warm bath before bedtime; loosen heavy covers at end of bed; elevate and support legs on pillow at night; stand on affected leg to straighten muscle; get regular exercise, particularly walking.	
	Caution the patient not to massage the calf because of the risk of undetected thrombus.	
	Teach patient signs of possible thrombus (all above) and to report such signs to care provider immediately.	

Expected Outcome:

Patient understands the cause of leg cramps and uses techniques to prevent leg cramps as evidenced by patient's verbalization of decrease in leg cramps.

(continued)

NURSING CARE PLAN (continued)

The Woman With Common Discomforts of Pregnancy

Nursing Diagnosis (Patient Problem) and Assessment Data	Nursing Interventions	Rationale
Nursing Diagnosis: *disturbance in self-concept: body image related to physical changes*		
	Observe for pigment changes of face, abdomen, and breasts (areola will darken).	Common skin changes include: *Linea nigra* of abdomen, a single thin, dark line from pubis to umbilicus: hormone-related.
		Chloasma of face (mask of pregnancy), darker pigment, predominantly on forehead and cheeks.
		Striae gravidarum (stretch marks) over abdomen, buttocks, or breasts due to inelasticity of skin: probably genetic component.
		Acne: probably due to increased progesterone and increased activity of sweat and sebaceous glands as a result of increased circulation.
	Reassure the patient that although pigment changes cannot be prevented, the pigmentation will gradually fade after birth. Stretch marks will fade from red or purple to faint silvery lines. Advise the patient to apply moisturizing lotions or oils to abdomen, breasts, buttocks, although these measures alone will not prevent striae if a woman is genetically predisposed to them.	
	Advise the patient to stay out of the sun or wear a strong sunscreen to prevent further darkening of chloasma. Reassure the patient experiencing acne that it may decrease after the first trimester. Advise the patient experiencing acne to thoroughly cleanse the skin with soap and water and to apply topical astringents.	

Expected Outcome:

Patient understands the causes of skin changes as demonstrated by using appropriate techniques to decrease skin changes where possible and verbalization of acceptance where not possible.

(continued)

The Woman With Common Discomforts of Pregnancy

Nursing Diagnosis (Patient Problem) and Assessment Data	Nursing Interventions	Rationale

Nursing Diagnosis:

altered comfort: Braxton Hicks contractions

• Patient complains of rhythmic tightening of uterus • Patient expresses concern about distinguishing true and false labor	Assess frequency, strength, regularity, and associated symptoms of Braxton Hicks contractions to distinguish from preterm labor or true labor. Reassure the patient that these contractions are a normal part of pregnancy and a preparation for labor. Advise the patient to rest in the left lateral recumbent position; try walking or exercising, which may make the contractions cease. Teach client to distinguish Braxton Hicks contractions from preterm labor (see the display in the section on True Labor) and to call health care provider if signs of preterm or true labor occur.	Probably caused by increased estrogen levels and distention of the uterus Patient needs to be able to assess own labor status correctly to avoid unnecessary or overly delayed trips to labor unit.

Expected Outcome:

Patient verbalizes an understanding of the causes and distinguishing attributes of Braxton Hicks contractions as demonstrated by informing health care provider of contractions resembling the true labor process. Patient utilizes appropriate techniques to alleviate the discomfort of the contractions.

Nursing Diagnosis:

altered nutrition: potential for more than body requirements related to food cravings

	Assess nutritional status for weight gain and anemia. Observe for bizarre eating habits. Assess for cultural or socioeconomic factors that might predispose a woman to indulge in pica. Assess for emotional and psychological factors that might contribute to pica. Advise the patient to eat well-balanced meals; gain appropriate amounts of	In the absence of other causes, probably due to: • Increased calorie intake required by physiologic changes of pregnancy; women's choice of foods that most appeal to them • Etiology unknown in the case of pica, a craving for substances such as clay, laundry starch, plaster, soap, toothpaste, or ice scraped from freezer

(continued)

NURSING CARE PLAN   (continued)

The Woman With Common Discomforts of Pregnancy

Nursing Diagnosis (Patient Problem) and Assessment Data	Nursing Interventions	Rationale
	weight; take iron and vitamin supplements.	
	Counsel the patient experiencing pica. If nutritional status is adequate and the substance eaten is not harmful, counseling alone is necessary. If pica is interfering wth nutrition, iron and vitamin supplements must be given.	
	Refer the patient to nutritionist for counseling; social worker for financial aid if necessary; counseling for emotional needs if necessary.	

Expected Outcome:

Patient demonstrates an awareness of the possible harmful effects of her food habits on her nutritional status by decreasing her intake of nonfood items and eating well-balanced meals with appropriate weight gain, absence of anemia, and general good health and feeling of well-being.

Nursing Diagnosis:
activity intolerance: dizziness and fainting

• Patient complains of lightheadedness on arising • Patient complains of dizziness, loss of balance	Assess cause of dizziness and associated factors. In first trimester, dizziness can be due to nausea and vomiting, hypoglycemia, lower blood pressure in second trimester, or ectopic pregnancy. In last trimester, dizziness can be due to position changes, hypoglycemia, or preeclampsia. Also consider ocular or neurologic causes. Assess nutritional status for anemia, hypoglycemia, and excessive nausea and vomiting. Assess emotional status (anxiety). Assess for infection (fever, chills, pain). Reassure the patient by explaining the possible causes of dizziness. Advise the patient to rise slowly from sitting or lying positions; lie on either side rather than on the back when recumbent; eat smaller, more	In the absence of other causes, probably due to: • Increased total blood volume, beginning at 10 to 14 weeks of gestation and peaking at 34 to 36 weeks • Anemia, which decreases the oxygen-carrying capacity of red blood cells, causing less oxygen to be supplied to the brain • Compression of the vena cava by the uterus in the supine position, causing decreased blood return to the heart and brain (supine hypertension) • Lower blood pressure in second trimester • Pooling of blood in lower extremities, causing dizziness on sudden change from supine or sitting position to standing.

(continued)

The Woman With Common Discomforts of Pregnancy

Nursing Diagnosis (Patient Problem) and Assessment Data	Nursing Interventions	Rationale
	frequent meals to prevent hypoglycemia; avoid crowds and crowded areas; avoid hyperventilation; get sufficient rest; assess factors in her life that may be distressing to her; take iron and vitamin supplements. Teach the patient to sit down or lie in left lateral position when she feels slightly dizzy to avoid falling if she faints. Refer to nutritionist or counselor if appropriate.	• Hyperventilation (increased levels of CO_2 in the blood) • Hypoglycemia • Emotional factors • Fatigue • Infections

Expected Outcome:

Patient uses appropriate techniques to reduce dizziness as evidenced by less frequent episodes of dizziness.

Nursing Diagnosis:

anxiety related to epulis (bleeding gums) and epistaxis (nosebleeds)

	Assess oral hygiene and observe for swollen, reddened gingiva that bleed when touched.	In the absence of other causes, probably due to:
	Assess blood pressure to rule out hypertension as a cause of the nosebleed.	• Hypertrophy and hyperemia of the gingiva and nasal mucosa, probably related to estrogen levels
	Reassure the patient that these are normal phenomena of pregnancy and will resolve spontaneously after delivery.	
	Advise the patient to maintain good oral hygiene; use a soft toothbrush; brush from gums toward teeth; floss gently; use warm saline mouthwashes to relieve discomfort; get regular dental checkups and hygienist treatments; maintain a well-balanced diet, including fresh fruits and vegetables; cut hard food (apples, carrots) into small pieces before chewing. Refer to a dentist for serious gum conditions.	Self-care measures to reduce trauma and promote good oral health are indicated.

Expected Outcome:

Patient addresses feelings of anxiety as evidenced by discussing her anxiety with the nurse and verbalizing her acceptance of discomfort and using appropriate techniques.

(continued)

NURSING CARE PLAN (continued)

The Woman With Common Discomforts of Pregnancy

Nursing Diagnosis (Patient Problem) and Assessment Data	Nursing Interventions	Rationale
Nursing Diagnosis: *sleep pattern disturbance: insomnia*	Assess usual sleep habits (somnolence during the day). Observe for fatigue and irritability. Assess emotional status (anxiety or depression). Assess nutritional habits (late meals, stimulants, evening fluid intake, calcium–phosphorus).	In the absence of other problems, insomnia may be related to: • Inability to find a comfortable position because of the enlarged abdomen • Excessive anxiety about the pregnancy or other concerns. Nocturia and subsequent inability to resume sleep • Fetal activity • A large meal prior to bedtime, indigestion, heartburn • Leg cramps • Dyspnea
	Reassure the patient that insomnia is not unusual in late pregnancy.	
	Advise the patient to avoid late, large meals; stimulants such as caffeine, tea, and cola drinks before bedtime; decrease fluid intake in the evening, but maintain adequate intake (6–8 glasses) during the day; get daily exercise; take measures to prevent leg cramps (see interventions under Leg Cramps); sleep with pillows propped to elevate head and chest to avoid heartburn and dyspnea; place a pillow between the legs to support them when in the lateral recumbent position; take an evening stroll in fresh air. Sleep with the window open. Caution the patient not to use sleeping medicine without consulting health care provider.	

Expected Outcome:

Patient understands the causes of insomnia and uses appropriate techniques to reduce insomnia as evidenced by her verbalization that insomnia is reduced and she feels well rested.

(continued)

NURSING CARE PLAN   (continued)

The Woman With Common Discomforts of Pregnancy

Nursing Diagnosis (Patient Problem) and Assessment Data	Nursing Interventions	Rationale
Nursing Diagnosis: *fluid volume excess: edema*	Assess and document amount and location of edema.	In the absence of other causes, probably due to:
	Assess nutrition for salt, protein, and fluid intake.	• Increased sodium and water retention and increased capillary permeability, probably related to hormones
	Assess rest and activity levels.	• Increased venous pressure
	Assess for other symptoms of pre-eclampsia (proteinuria, hypertension, weight gain, hyperreflexia, scanty urine output). Also consider other renal or cardiac impairments.	• Decreased venous return from dependent structures
	Reassure the patient that physiologic edema is a normal phenomenon of pregnancy.	• Varicose veins with congestion
	Advise the patient to increase rest periods, lying on the left side; elevate legs when sitting; wear support hose (see interventions under Varicosities); restrict intake of salty foods (potato chips, pickles, canned soups, etc.), but not to adopt a salt-free diet; salt may be used in cooking. Increase intake of protein foods (decreased protein contributes to fluid retention in tissues); decrease intake of carboyhdrates (especially simple sugars) and fats, since they also cause fluid retention in tissues; drink 6 to 8 glasses fluid/day to aid in natural diuresis.	• Dietary protein deficiency
	Teach the patient to report signs of toxemia and preeclampsia: generalized edema, weight gain, headaches, flashing lights, decreased urine output.	• Increased dietery intake of sodium

Expected Outcome:

Patient understands the causes of edema and uses appropriate techniques to decrease edema, as evidenced by a decrease in edema.

whether they can continue their usual activities throughout the pregnancy. This section will examine common concerns about employment, travel, leisure activities, and exercise during pregnancy.

Employment

Many women comfortably continue working throughout their pregnancies. Two judgments are necessary: is the work environment safe for a developing fetus, and can the pregnant woman carry out work commitments without undue stress and fatigue or physical injury? If a pregnancy becomes complicated, the patient must discuss modifications of work plans with her health care provider. In counseling women about job safety, the nurse's role is to assist each woman in obtaining information about particular toxic substances or other hazards and to support her in seeking pregnancy-indicated work transfers when necessary.

Environmental Safety. Pregnant women should not work in environments where they are exposed to hazardous substances. If necessary, the pregnant woman should be transferred to another work area for the duration of the pregnancy. If there is any question about the safety of a particular substance, major medical centers often have teratogen registries that compile information and make it available to the public on request.

Pregnant women need to be particularly careful of substances that have been identified as toxic, such as carbon monoxide, mercury, lead, nitro compounds of anesthetic gases, x-rays and radioactive substances, benzene, turpentine, and other industrial cleaning agents. When in danger of exposure to any of these agents — for example, when doing household cleaning — the pregnant woman should be particularly careful about wearing gloves and ensuring that the area is well ventilated.

One environmental hazard that may easily be overlooked is toxoplasmosis, a parasitic infection caused by *Toxoplasma gondii*. The disease can be acquired through contact with infected cat feces or by eating raw or undercooked meat that has been infected with the organsim. Congenital infection can occur when toxoplasmosis is acquired during pregnancy. The pregnant woman who owns a cat should be warned against coming into contact with its waste products. She should avoid emptying or cleaning cat litter boxes and eating raw or undercooked meat. She should be advised to report symptoms of fatigue, muscle pain, or enlarged lymph nodes to her care provider so that diagnostic tests can be done.

Fatigue and Injury. Pregnant women who continue full-time employment must have adequate breaks to rest and obtain nourishing snacks. Women employed in positions requiring constant standing and walking or lifting of heavy objects may require transfers to less physically demanding positions during the pregnancy. Women performing sedentary jobs should get up and walk around once every hour.

Women in positions requiring delicate balance, such as scaffold or stepladder work, may be unable to safely continue in those positions as the pregnancy progresses and the growing uterus alters their center of gravity and sense of balance. Women operating heavy equipment or working in jobs where severe injuries are a risk should exercise caution and request transfers where necessary.

Video display terminals in the workplace are currently the cause of some concern, but there is little conclusive evidence that they pose a danger to the fetus. Patients using them should, however, be urged to maintain a stringent rest break schedule.

Travel and Leisure

There are few absolute restrictions on travel and leisure activities during pregnancy. However, certain precautions are advised to prevent injury to mother or baby or undue fatigue to the mother.

Travel. In general, the second trimester is the best time to take trips: the woman is usually feeling her best and enjoying a good energy level. Families may want to consider distance from health care facilities in planning a trip. It may not be the best time to do backwoods backpacking, but one can consider car camping and day hikes. On the other hand, experienced backpackers can continue their usual activities, with appropriate adjustments in pack weight and altitudes hiked for the pregnant woman.

Pregnant women traveling by air should check for any airline restrictions on air travel in late pregnancy. When traveling by air, car, or bus, the pregnant woman should avoid sitting for long periods. A stretch or walk should be scheduled every hour.

Safety belts should be worn at all times. The shoulder strap should fit comfortably over the shoulder and across the chest. The waist strap should be placed under the abdomen, low and comfortably snug on the hips and upper thighs.

Sports and Recreation. It is safe for a pregnant woman to continue her usual recreational activities unless informed of a specific medical contraindication. If she is proficient in activities requiring strength and agility, she may continue those activities during pregnancy. Modifications may be necessary as the weight of a growing uterus decreases endurance and alters balance. For example, pregnant women should decrease their jogging speed and let their partners dive for the low tennis balls.

Women who are extremely athletic and active generally know the risks of their particular sports. There are a few activities contraindicated in pregnancy because of the risks to the fetus. Scuba diving is unsafe because of depth pressures. High-altitude activities are not recommended because of the risks of hypoxia and hypothermia. When in doubt, the woman should ask her health care provider about the safety of her activities.

Normally sedentary women should not take up demanding sports while they are pregnant. This is not the year to learn downhill skiing or wind surfing. It is safe, however, to start an exercise regimen during pregnancy.

Exercise During Pregnancy

It is important for pregnant women to have a regular exercise program. Regular exercise will not only help them feel fit and energetic but will also help to prevent or ameliorate such discomforts as constipation, hemorrhoids, varicosities, and insomnia. The woman should begin slowly, with the proper guidance, and should listen to signals from her body. Any muscle cramping indicates overexertion, and the woman should rest until it resolves. The exercise regimen should focus on three areas: posture, cardiovascular fitness, and pelvic muscle strengthening.

Posture

Maintaining good posture in pregnancy is essential for the prevention of backaches, compression of abdominal and pelvic organs, and stress on muscles and ligaments.

Physiologic changes of pregnancy shift the center of gravity forward. The weight of the growing uterus tilts the pelvis forward, shortening the back muscles and allowing the abdominal muscles to weaken. To compensate for the altered center of gravity, pregnant women often lean backward, exaggerating the lumbar curve (lordosis) and further shortening and stressing the back muscles.

Maintaining good posture requires a constant effort, but as awareness of correct position improves, it will become more natural. The nurse should encourage women to practice good posture because the reward is improved comfort and ease of breathing with less backache and heartburn.

Good posture means more than standing up straight. It involves good body alignment in every position: standing, sitting, lying on one's back, side, or abdomen, sitting on a stool or at a desk, lifting a child, working at a counter, sitting on the floor, vacuuming the rug, or cleaning the tub.

Pelvic Tilts. Pregnant women can learn to improve their posture by developing an awareness of proper pelvic tilting. Since the pelvic girdle supports the spinal column, correct alignment of the spinal column requires correct pelvic girdle alignment.

To do a pelvic tilt, the woman stands with her head held high, her shoulders back and down, and her hips level and parallel to the ground. She tilts back the pelvis by pulling

her buttock muscles down and pulling her abdominal muscles up. Initially this will be easier to do if she bends her knees slightly while tightening her buttock and abdominal muscles. When the tilt is done properly, the back will be flattened, with the usual lumbar curve ironed out.

The woman can practice the exercise by alternately holding the correct pelvic tilt and relaxing into her previous posture. In doing so she will receive positive reinforcement, since the pelvic tilt position feels better.

It is also important to strengthen the abdominal muscles when pregnant. These muscles give support to the growing uterus and must be strong to prevent the weight of the gravid uterus from pulling forward. Thus, strong abdominal muscles are necessary to maintain proper pelvic tilt. The correct pelvic tilt can be held when standing, walking, or lying supine with knees bent or supported by a pillow. The same principles of back and pelvic alignment apply for other positions also.

When sitting, the lumbar spine must be adequately supported to avoid slouching. The feet must be supported in front of the body, either on the floor or elevated on a stool. Chairs with high backs and arm rests are most comfortable because they brace the head and shoulders.

Lying prone is helpful in pregnancy because it stretches the muscles anterior to the hip joints, as long as the lumbar curve is not concurrently exaggerated. Inserting a pillow under the pelvis helps to straighten the back and allow the abdominal muscles to relax. Women frequently ask if they can lie on their stomachs when pregnant, and they should be encouraged to do so until it is no longer comfortable for them.

The importance of the pelvic tilt cannot be overemphasized. It is the hallmark of good posture and a prerequisite to comfort during pregnancy.

Tailor Sitting. Tailor sitting is encouraged antepartally to stretch the muscles and ligaments of the inner thighs, round out the lower back, and promote relaxation of the pelvic floor (Noble 1982). The woman sits on the floor with back straight, knees bent, and either the legs crossed at the ankles or the soles of the feet held together. The knees should not be pressed toward the floor but instead gently encouraged to drop toward it through alternate contraction and relaxation of the thigh muscles. This exercise is contraindicated if a woman experiences pain from separation of the symphysis pubis.

When in the tailor position, the woman can do shoulder rotations to alleviate upper backache. She can also do "flying exercises" to stretch her torso and relieve pressure on compressed organs, as shown in Figure 18–3.

Pregnant women should be encouraged to join prenatal classes in exercise, yoga, and relaxation. Through these classes women will learn other exercises to improve their posture and relieve the aches and discomforts of pregnancy.

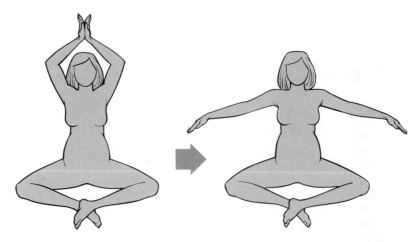

Figure 18-3. Flying exercise to decrease heartburn. Sitting cross-legged, the woman raises and lowers her arms quickly, bringing the backs of her hands together over her head. This is repeated several times.

Cardiovascular Fitness

The goals of cardiovascular exercise are to improve circulatory and respiratory performance, tone the body, and build up physical endurance. Pregnant women should be encouraged to pursue these goals. An additional advantage of cardiovascular exercise is the improved ability of the body to adapt to the physiologic changes of pregnancy, including a reduction in many common discomforts, such as constipation, hemorrhoids, varicosities, leg cramps, edema, insomnia, and backache.

Pregnant women can achieve cardiovascular fitness through many of the activities they regularly enjoy, such as swimming, bicycling, walking, jogging, or aerobics classes. The important rules are to begin exercising slowly, modify exercise goals according to their abilities, and do no exercise that causes pain.

A woman who is in good physical condition has a great psychological advantage in pregnancy: she knows and trusts the strengths and abilities of her body, and this attitude can give her confidence for her labor and delivery.

Pelvic Muscle Strengthening

The pelvic floor, or perineum, is the structure that supports the contents of the pelvic girdle. The growing weight of the uterus during pregnancy places increasing stress on the pelvic floor muscles. These muscles are not routinely exercised, and the lack of muscular activity delays the return of blood to the heart from the lower extremities, resulting in pelvic congestion. In the pregnant woman this perineal congestion is manifested in the discomforts of hemorrhoids, vulvar varicosities, and edema.

Kegel Exercises. Kegel exercises, which involve alternating contraction and release of the pubococcygeus muscle strengthen the pelvic floor muscles and are easy to do. Like pelvic tilts, however, results are realized only when the exercises become a conscious, routine process.

The benefits of Kegel exercises include prevention of the discomforts of pelvic congestion, enhanced sexual enjoyment (Nobel 1982), and a more rapid postpartum recovery of the pelvic floor (Henderson 1983).

The pubococcygeus muscle is contracted when one is trying to prevent the flow of urine or a bowel movement. Pubococcygeal contraction does *not* involve contraction of thigh or buttock muscles. Trying to prevent the flow of urine while urinating will help the woman to identify the correct muscles. Practicing muscle contractions with two fingers inserted in the vagina or during sexual intercourse will enable her or her partner to gauge the increasing strength of her contractions.

The Kegel exercises can be practiced at any time — sitting, standing, or lying down — and with practice a woman will recognize the increased strength of her pelvic floor muscles. They should be initiated as early as possible in pregnancy to help prevent perineal congestion. The alternation of contraction and release helps women recognize when the pelvic floor is relaxed, important knowledge during delivery (Noble 1982). The steps for the Kegel exercises are listed in the accompanying self-care teaching display, page 471.

Perineal Massage. Although not a true exercise, massage of the perineum contributes to a softening of the tissues and relaxation of the pelvic floor. This is done to decrease resistance to pressure during delivery, with the hope of reducing the need for an episiotomy. (See the accompanying self-care teaching display, opposite page.)

While leaning comfortably against some pillows, the woman should use her fingers to rub some vegetable oil gently into her perineum and lower vaginal wall. The woman or her partner can stretch the vaginal tissue by inserting their fingers 2 to 3 inches into the vagina and gently and rhythmically sliding the fingers down toward the rectum and then back up. The woman should concentrate on relaxing her muscles against this gentle pressure. Pressure can be slowly increased over time, just up to the point of discomfort or "stinging."

SELF-CARE TEACHING

Kegel Exercises

After childbirth the pubococcygeal muscles need to be strengthened by Kegel exercises. In 1952 Arnold Kegel developed a series of exercises for women whose pubococcygeal muscles were so slack that they were losing urine when they coughed or sneezed. This may be a problem for older women who lack muscle tone and for postpartum women as well. Regular practice of the Kegel exercises can restore muscle tone in about 6 weeks. The pelvic floor muscles contract during orgasm, and, just like any muscle, they work better when they are in better shape. Thus, there is a sexual benefit when muscle tone improves.

The steps for the Kegel exercises are as follows:

1. Locate the muscles surrounding the vagina by sitting on the toilet and starting and stopping the flow of urine.
2. Test the baseline strength of the muscles by inserting a finger in the opening of the vagina and contracting the muscles.
3. Exercise A — Squeeze the muscles together and hold the squeeze for 3 seconds. Relax the muscles. Repeat.
4. Exercise B — Contract and relax the muscles as rapidly as possible 10 to 25 times. Repeat.
5. Exercise C — Imagine sitting in a pan of water and sucking water into the vagina. Hold for 3 seconds.
6. Exercise D — Push out as during a bowel movement, only with the vagina. Hold for 3 seconds.
7. Repeat exercises A, C, and D ten times each, and exercise B once. Repeat the entire series three times a day.

Additional benefits from the Kegel exercises are increased vaginal lubrication during sexual arousal, relief of constipation, increased flexibility of episiotomy scars, and stronger gripping of the base of the penis during intercourse.

SELF-CARE TEACHING

Reducing the Need for Routine Episiotomy

Pregnant women interested in avoiding "routine" episiotomy can be encouraged to adhere to the following regimen:

- Eat a nutritious diet not only for your own and the baby's health but to promote healthy, pliable tissues.
- Seek prompt treatment of vaginal infections.
- Use good perineal hygiene by avoiding douching (which should not be practiced during pregnancy in any case) and the use of perfumed sprays on the genitals; wear loose cotton underwear to permit passage of air to the perineum to promote dryness and healthy tissue.
- Develop perineal muscular awareness through Kegel exercises.
- Perform perineal massage and stretching to increase the suppleness of perineal tissues and to familiarize yourself with the sensations of perineal pressure and stretching.
- Discuss with your care provider your desire to deliver the baby over an intact perineum, if possible, in order to obtain provider support and receive additional instruction.
- Attend childbirth education classes that teach gentle pushing and various positions for birth.

Perineal massage should be done for 5 minutes a day in the last 6 weeks of pregnancy. Doing it in combination with pelvic floor contractions will help the woman to develop an awareness of pelvic tension and relaxation that will assist her in labor and delivery.

Breast Care

Breast care during pregnancy has two facets: it is important to begin and/or continue a regimen of regular breast examination, and for women wishing to breast-feed it is advantageous to begin breast preparation during the third trimester.

Breast Self-Examination

Ninety percent of breast cancers are found by the woman or her partner. For this reason it is important that women understand the importance of examining the breasts on a monthly basis. (See the accompanying display on page 472.) During pregnancy there is no special time of the month that is best to perform the examination. (In nonpregnant women, 5 days after cessation of menses is the optimum time to detect changes.)

Breast-feeding Preparation

Women are taught about breast-feeding during pregnancy so that they will know how to handle their breasts, how it will feel to have an infant sucking, and how to express milk. Pregnancy is also a good time to teach the importance of proper nutrition during lactation.

It is difficult to breast-feed properly if the woman's partner and friends are not supportive or if the woman is only breast-feeding to please her partner. Exploration of

NURSING RESEARCH

Teaching Breast Self-Examination

This study investigated the effect of routine teaching of breast self-examination (BSE) during office visits on a sample of 121 women who reported performing BSE less than four times a year. Subjects were randomly assigned to two experimental groups, one of which received "routine" instruction that focused on the basics of BSE; a second group received more individualized teaching, dealing with perceived barriers to performing BSE and including reinforcement of perceived benefits as well as of development of BSE skill. An additional 81 women who reported performing BSE more than four times a year served as a comparison group.

Data analysis revealed no difference in frequency of BSE between the two experimental groups; all reported greater frequency of BSE and increased confidence in BSE skill. Belief that BSE would provide peace of mind was the greatest predictor of practice.

This study challenges the commonly held view that individualized instruction is more effective in promoting positive health practices. In addition, the finding that a positive motivator, that is, peace of mind, was most often related to practicing BSE brings into question the frequent assumption that the fear that results from emphasizing health risks will more adequately motivate women to perform measures aimed at detecting tumors.

Nettles–Carlson B, Field M, Friedman B, Smith L: Effectiveness of teaching breast self-examination during office visits. Res Nurs Health 11(1):41–50, 1988

attitudes toward breast-feeding must begin early in the pregnancy. Was the mother or father breast-fed? Have their previous children been breast-fed, and how was that experience? For best results women should choose freely how to feed their babies.

Breast preparation is not difficult. It consists of three exercises, described in the accompanying self-care teaching display.

Breast preparation should begin at 28 weeks of gestation, and the exercises should be practiced twice a day. It is not absolutely essential that women do manual expression of colostrum, but it is helpful for later breast-feeding. Breast preparation is contraindicated in women at risk for premature labor.

Many supportive resources are available for women who want to breast-feed: prenatal and postpartum classes; local community groups, whose members answer questions and make home visits to assist the new mother; and literature. Pregnant women should be en-

couraged to take advantage of these resources. See Chapter 37 for an in-depth discussion of breast-feeding techniques.

Expected Outcome: The pregnant woman demonstrates appropriate self-care measures by performing sound prenatal exercises, by remaining active at work and through travel without fatigue and injury, and by performing breast self-examination and preparations for breast-feeding.

SELF-CARE TEACHING

Preparation for Breast-feeding

The nurse can instruct the patient in breast preparation as follows:

- **Nipple rolling**—Roll the nipples between two fingers like radio dials to help toughen the nipple before it is exposed to the infant's sucking
- **Massaging breasts**—Using your hands, gently massage breasts to provide stimulation prior to manual expression of colostrum.
- **Manual expression of colostrum**—Colostrum, the sticky, clear or yellowish secretion of the breasts during pregnancy and prior to lactation, can be expressed. Place fingers or thumb and fingers on the breast 1 inch above and below the nipple. Push the breast in toward the chest and then squeeze the fingers in together.

Monitoring for Complications

Women vary in their knowledge of normal and abnormal occurrences in pregnancy, in their attitudes toward obtaining health care, in their tolerance for pain and discomfort, and in their handling of anxiety when problems are suspected. The nurse must assess the woman's understanding of the physical changes of pregnancy and her motivation to seek health services should a complication arise. Then the nurse and patient develop a teaching plan that includes the signs and symptoms of complications of pregnancy. Some patients will need only a list of symptoms to report; others will demand a rationale for every item on the list. The nurse must be prepared to meet the learning needs of each patient.

SELF-CARE TEACHING

Breast Self-Examination

Inspection in the Shower

It is easier to examine your breasts when your hands are soapy. With your right hand behind your head, examine your right breast with your left hand, using a grid or circular motion. Reverse the procedure to examine the other breast.

Inspection in a Mirror

Stand in front of a mirror for further inspection:

A. With arms at sides, look for
   • Changes in size and shape of breasts
   • Changes in skin: dimpling, puckering, scaling, redness, swelling
   • Changes in nipple: inversion, scaling, discharge, erosion, nipples pointing in different directions
B. Holding arms over the head, inspect closely in the mirror for masses, breast symmetry, puckering.

C. Press hands firmly on hips, bow slightly forward. Inspect in mirror for lumps or pulling of the skin.
D. Each breast should be a mirror image of the other. If you think you detect a lump in a breast, check the other side to see if it feels the same. If so, this is undoubtedly normal tissue. Examine, using the circular or grid motion as in the shower.
E. Gently squeeze the nipple of each breast between your thumb and index finger to check for signs of discharge or bleeding.

Inspection Lying Down

Lying flat on your back, with your right hand under your head and a pillow or towel under your right shoulder, use your left hand to gently feel your right breast, using concentric circles to cover the entire breast and nipple. Repeat on your left breast.

(Art courtesy Childbirth Graphics)

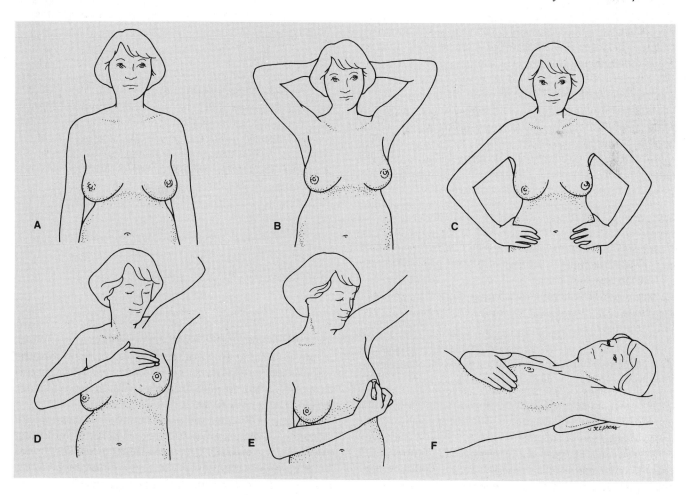

Signs and Symptoms to Report Promptly

The following section highlights signs and symptoms that the patient must report at once. Details of pregnancy complications can be found in Chapter 19. The intent here is to make the patient aware of the kinds of problems that can occur and the need for early reporting of symptoms. Early reporting will lead to early identification of complications and timely intervention and will maximize the changes for a favorable pregnancy outcome.

Vaginal Bleeding

Any sudden onset of frank, profuse vaginal bleeding should be reported immediately. Such bleeding is different from the light pink spotting that results from a causative action, such as sexual intercourse or a vaginal examination. Vaginal bleeding can be a sign of ectopic pregnancy or threatened abortion in the first trimester or threatened abortion, placenta previa, or abruptio placentae in the second and third trimesters.

Dizziness

Also to be reported is sudden and extreme dizziness associated with pelvic or uterine pain. These symptoms may indicate the presence of ectopic pregnancy or abruptio placentae, where blood is trapped in the abdominal cavity or between the placenta and uterine wall and does not present vaginally.

Preterm Labor Symptoms

Patients should be taught the signs and symptoms of *preterm labor* (PTL), the name given to labor between 28 and 36 weeks of gestation. PTL recognized early and monitored appropriately may be stopped; and even if it cannot be stopped, early detection will allow preparations to be made for the birth of a premature baby.

The following symptoms of PTL should be reported at once to the health care provider:

- Rhythmic tightening (or contracting) of the uterus, as distinguished from irregular Braxton Hicks contractions
- Any constant low abdominal cramping
- Constant low backache
- Leakage of fluid from the vagina. Patients may notice fluid leaking from the vagina and believe it to be urine. It may in fact be urine, but the only way to be sure is to examine it to rule out amniotic fluid leakage.

The point to be emphasized is that any possible symptom of PTL should be evaluated. The patient cannot necessarily distinguish contractions at home, and the nurse cannot distinguish them over the telephone. Teaching the patient to recognize PTL symptoms and report them if they occur is preventive medicine at its best.

SELF-CARE TEACHING

Signs and Symptoms to Report Promptly

- Vaginal bleeding—any sudden onset of frank, profuse vaginal bleeding; this differs from pink spotting.
- Dizziness—sudden and extreme dizziness associated with pelvic or uterine pain
- Preterm labor symptoms—between 28 and 36 weeks:
  - Rhythmic tightening of uterus, as distinguished from Braxton Hicks contractions
  - Any constant low abdominal cramping
  - Constant low backache
  - Leakage of fluid from vagina
- Rupture of membranes—any sudden gushing or slow leaking of fluid from vagina
- Preeclampsia symptoms:
  - Generalized edema, particularly in face, hands, lower extremities, and sacral area
  - Rapid weight gain over several days or a week
  - Headaches
  - Visual disturbances
  - Dizziness
  - Nervousness, irritability
  - Decreased or scanty urine output
  - Vomiting
  - Epigastric pain
- Decrease in or absence of fetal activity—any marked, abrupt decrease in fetal activity or absence of fetal activity for 24 hours
- True labor:
  - Expulsion of mucous plug (pink mucus from the vagina)
  - Rupture of membranes (leaking or gushing of fluid)
  - Contractions

Rupture of Membranes

Any sudden gushing or slow leaking of fluid from the vagina must be reported. The amniotic fluid is enclosed in a sac that surrounds and protects the fetus. Once that sac breaks, the fetus can be at risk for infection.

Leaking of fluid or rupture of membranes can precede labor in a term pregnancy. Health care providers must know when the leaking begins. Delay of delivery more than 24 hours after membrane rupture may mean a risk of infection to the fetus.

Leaking of fluid prior to term must be reported immediately. The risks in this situation are infection and preterm labor.

Any woman experiencing an outbreak of genital herpes must report leaking of fluid immediately so that appropriate measures can be taken to protect the baby from infection.

Preeclampsia Symptoms

Early warning signs of preeclampsia will frequently be noted at a prenatal visit. Edema or rising blood pressure will alert the nurse that the patient should be told to report the following occurrences.

- Generalized edema, particularly in face, hands, lower extremities, and sacral area
- Rapid weight gain over several days or a week
- Headaches
- Visual disturbances, such as double vision, blurred vision, silver lights, or flashing lights
- Dizziness
- Nervousness, irritability
- Decreased or scanty urine output
- Vomiting
- Epigastric pain (an ominous and late sign)

Decrease in or Absence of Fetal Activity

Any marked, abrupt decrease in fetal activity or absence of fetal activity for 24 hours must be reported immediately. A significant decrease in fetal activity can be a sign of fetal distress, and cessation of activity could indicate fetal demise.

True Labor

True labor is unmistakable when it starts abruptly and progresses rapidly. However, not all women experience labor that way. Women in late pregnancy can become discouraged when they experience false labor or when the first stage of their labor is prolonged. Information given in birth preparation classes should be reinforced by the nurse to help the couple distinguish true from false labor and conserve their energy accordingly (Table 18–1). Frequently the nurse will counsel couples by telephone to help them identify their labor signs.

True labor can begin in one of three ways or a combination of the three.

Expulsion of Mucous Plug.   The mucous plug may be expelled from the cervix at the onset of labor as a result of cervical dilatation, appearing as pink mucus from the vagina ("show" or "bloody show"). It can, however, also appear 1 or 2 weeks before the onset of actual labor.

Rupture of Membranes.   Rupture of the amniotic membranes may be signaled by a leaking or gushing of fluid. Patients should report the character of the fluid; amniotic fluid is usually clear or slightly bloodtinged. Discolored greenish fluid or frank blood should be reported immediately. When labor does not occur spontaneously after the rupture of membranes, many clinicians will choose to induce labor within 12 to 24 hours.

Contractions.   Uterine contractions may begin as backache and progress over the abdomen, causing the uterus to become firm. True labor contractions occur at a regular rate and gradually increase in duration, strength, and frequency.

In false labor, contractions generally occur over the abdomen and can sometimes be relieved by walking. Passage of the mucous plug and membrane rupture do not occur. False labor consists of Braxton Hicks contractions, which are irregular in duration, strength, and frequency. Occasionally a woman finds false labor so uncomfortable that she is unable to sleep or rest. In such instances a mild sedative may be prescribed. (See the accompanying table on the qualities distinguishing true labor from Braxton Hicks contractions.)

Threats to Health

The nurse must recognize that many pregnant women and their families live in circumstances where the major threats to health are not complications of pregnancy but

Table 18–1   Distinguishing True Labor From Braxton Hicks Contractions

Parameter	True Labor Contractions	Braxton Hicks Contractions
Intervals	Regular	Irregular
Frequency	Gradually increasing	Inconsistent
Intensity	Gradually increasing	Variable
Location	Primarily in the back	Over abdomen
Aggravating/alleviating factors	Intensified by walking	Sometimes relieved by walking
Bloody show	Usually present	Not present
Rupture of membranes	Sometimes present	Not present

social conditions that place them at significant psychological and physical risk. The following section addresses one such threat: family violence during pregnancy.

Family Violence: Battered Pregnant Woman

Domestic violence has become a major health problem in the U.S. (Valente 1986); it is a problem that crosses socioeconomic lines. Estimates vary, but each year at least 2 million women are battered by their intimate partners; this figure may actually be as high as 6 million. Battering during pregnancy probably represents about 10% of those cases (Chez 1989).

Available information provides no clear picture of the objective perinatal risks associated with battering during pregnancy. However, the subjective risk perceived by pregnant women in abusive relationships is always high. The woman usually feels helpless and depressed because she can not break out of the abusive relationship, in part because in most cases there is a history of love and loyalty in the relationship, intensifying the woman's ambivalence. However, the physical risks she faces, as well as the risk to her other children, may precipitate a call for help. Men who batter women often physically and/or psychologically abuse children as well (Schecter and Gray 1988).

The nurse must be alert to subtle cues in the patient's history or physical examination that suggest physical abuse. Repeated accidents with physical injury; overt de-

NURSING RESEARCH

Intervention Strategies for Battering During Pregnancy

Battering during pregnancy is an under-reported crime and a major health problem affecting significant numbers of women. Battering often escalates during pregnancy or the postpartum period. Interviews with 290 healthy pregnant women revealed that 23% had been battered before or during the current pregnancy. Of those, most were unaware of resources available for battered women. The most frequently cited resource mentioned was their family. Another 9% demonstrated behaviors suggestive of battering (crying, anxiety, and ambivalent answers, such as "Not recently" or "Don't all men hit?") Of the women battered, only 8% had sought treatment for injuries.

Perinatal care-givers can intervene to prevent battering through discussions about family violence in childbirth and parenting classes, designing and testing programs to identify families at risk for violence, and providing community education.

Helton A, Snodgrass F: Battering during pregnancy: Intervention Strategies. Birth 14(3)142, 144, 1987

pression; alcohol/drug use; missing prenatal care appointments with subsequent appearance of healing physical injuries; or any injury to the head, neck, abdomen, genitalia, or breasts that occurs at home should be evaluated further. Cigarette burns, trauma to the face, or multiple injuries at different phases of healing are potentially important clues to battering (Chez 1989).

Upon recognizing injuries that are suggestive of family violence, the nurse must interview the patient in a supportive, nonthreatening way in a setting that assures privacy. The nurse can ask the woman gently and directly if she is in a relationship with anyone who threatens or physically hurts her. Many women will respond honestly; those who cannot will nevertheless have heard the offer of assistance and may accept it at another time (Chez 1989).

If the woman reports physical abuse, the nurse's first priority is to facilitate care for emotional and physical injuries, including assessment of fetal status if the woman expresses worry in this regard. The nurse must also remember that documentation should be complete, since patient records may eventually become part of a legal action if required by state law.

The nurse's second priority is to assist the patient in accessing assistance through a domestic violence program. The nurse may make this referral, with consent of the patient, or if the patient is unwilling to take that step, the nurse should give the patient information on how to access such assistance herself. A domestic violence hotline for the U.S. (1-800-333-5723) will provide the patient with information about community resources appropriate to her needs, including bilingual and telecommunication services for the deaf (Chez 1989). Counseling the patient regarding her situation and assisting her to make a change in her situation is beyond the usual scope of perinatal nursing practice and is better handled by specialized programs and care providers. However, the nurse can provide significant support by acting as a catalyst for change by being alert to women who may be at risk, by taking the initiative to ask about battering when there is reason to ask, and by providing support, encouragement, physical comfort, and needed information about available help to women who need it.

Expected Outcome: The pregnant woman expresses satisfaction with health teaching and maintains a normal pregnancy without psychosocial or physical complications.

Leading Prenatal Classes

The pregnant woman and her partner should be provided with information about prenatal classes at the first prenatal visit. Class participation should be encouraged according to trimester concerns. The subjects listed in the accompanying display (below) should be discussed in such classes or the same information should be provided in some other way if the facility does not have the resources for group classes.

Topics can be combined where appropriate. For example, a first-trimester class could cover orientation to the facility, nutrition, adaptation to pregnancy, and interventions for the common discomforts of pregnancy. A breast-feeding class in the early third trimester could re-emphasize the nutritional needs of pregnancy.

Classes dealing with early adaptation to pregnancy may be more successful if mothers and partners meet separately. Men might be more likely to raise intimate subjects when only other men are present, and the same might be true of women. Some women may be uncomfortable and embarrassed about practicing breast-feeding preparation with men present.

Some couples will need help in choosing birth preparation classes if confronted with many alternatives (see Chapter 21). Nurses must explain the differences among classes and encourage couples to call the childbirth educator for additional details. They should also consider the time, location, and cost of classes.

Preparation for Cesarean Birth

Approximately one out of every four to five births in the U.S. today occurs through cesarean delivery. Childbirth preparation classes usually provide information on cesarean birth. It is important for the nurse to anticipate questions and concerns about the possibility of needing a cesarean delivery.

Cesarean birth may be anticipated or unanticipated. Unanticipated cesarean birth may be caused by failure to progress in labor, cephalopelvic disproportion, an abnormal presentation, fetal distress, or a maternal or fetal contraindication to labor, such as a recent outbreak of herpes. A cesarean birth may be anticipated if the woman has had a previous cesarean birth or if there is a known abnormal presentation or contraindication to vaginal birth.

Couples must receive information about hospital procedures for cesarean deliveries. Unanticipated cesarean births can happen very suddenly, and the more information a couple has in advance, the better prepared they will be. The information should include hospital policies on

- Presence of partners or support persons in the operating room
- Electronic fetal monitoring
- Oxygen administration to the mother
- Intravenous fluid administration to the mother
- Abdominal preparation
- Catheterization
- Anesthesia alternatives and administration
- Immediate postoperative activities for mother, partner or support person, and baby
- Maternal recovery

The nurse should also discuss emotional and psychological responses to cesarean deliveries. (See Chapter 26 for further discussion of cesarean birth.)

Preparation for Parenting

It is not possible to "teach" a couple prenatally all the parenting skills they will need, but parents must consider many choices before the birth of a baby. The nurse must be alert to possible parenting problems and make assessments and interventions or referrals where necessary. (See Chapter 36 for a full discussion of adaptation to parenthood.)

During the last several months of pregnancy, the nurse must assess whether the couple is realistically planning for the arrival of their new baby. The nurse must also determine whether the couple will be receiving the support they need during early parenting. Has the couple been preparing their home for a new arrival? Are there financial or emotional constraints preventing a couple from obtaining necessary baby items? Have they procured a safe infant car seat? Who is available to assist the parents in the first few weeks postpartum? The nurse must help the couple to realize that this may be an extremely exhausting time. Couples often need help setting limits for visiting relatives — parents should learn to do baby care while the doting relatives help with the cooking and cleaning. Visiting guests should bring food and expect to help in the cleanup. Parents must learn to set these limits to prevent fatigue and overexhaustion.

The nurse must assess whether the partners are receiving the support they need from each other and whether they need additional support from community

Topics for Prenatal Classes

- Orientation to the facility providing prenatal care
- Nutritional needs
- Physiologic and psychological adaptation to pregnancy
- Adaptation to pregnancy
- Sibling preparation
- Breast-feeding preparation
- Labor and delivery preparation and refresher classes
- Cesarean delivery classes
- Infant care
- Postpartum support groups

NURSING RESEARCH

Parents' Prenatal Expectations and Actual Experiences in Parenting

A study was conducted to determine how parents' prenatal expectations of their parenting role compared with their actual experiences after their baby was born. Thirty-three middle-class primigravidas and their partners were recruited from childbirth preparation classes and were asked to estimate how much of their time they would be spending with their infant in such activities as feeding, bathing, and diapering. Parents were then visited in their home 3 weeks after the birth and were again asked to estimate the time actually spent in these activities.

Prenatally, mothers expected to spend more time with their infant than did fathers. At 3 weeks postbirth, mothers were spending more time with their infant than they had expected whereas fathers were spending considerably less time with their infants than they had expected. Thus, expectations for parenting are not realized by either parent, raising the potential for feelings of being overworked and stressed among mothers and feelings of disappointment, incompetence, and being left out among fathers. Anticipatory guidance may be increasingly important in helping parents establish realistic expectations and learn how to implement their roles in a workable and mutually satisfying way during the early weeks of parenting.

Humenick S, Bugen L: Parenting roles: Expectation versus reality. MCN 12(1):36–39, 1987

NURSING RESEARCH

Primiparas' Concerns About Learning Infant Care

A study was conducted to determine if pregnant women's desire to learn infant care changes during pregnancy. The existing literature presents considerable conflict about the most appropriate timing of infant care teaching during pregnancy, with some experts suggesting late pregnancy and others suggesting that the woman is primarily concerned about labor and birth at that point and that infant care teaching is best done earlier in pregnancy. One hundred and eighty-nine first-time expectant mothers were interviewed about infant care and their own learning needs. Interviews were audiotaped and transcribed, and transcripts were analyzed using content analysis techniques.

Findings suggest that desire to learn infant care was significantly higher late in pregnancy; however, overall concern for learning infant care was only 5% of the total concerns expressed. This probably reflects the fact that while pregnant women have more choices to make regarding their antenatal care and strategies for coping with labor and birth, their predominant concerns focus on maintaining maternal health and learning about labor and birth. These findings suggest that teaching infant care practices in late pregnancy may not be optimal because desire to learn may be low relative to other concerns. Additional study is needed to determine what factors influence desire to learn infant care and what time period would be optimal to provide teaching.

Bliss–Holtz J: Primiparas' prenatal concern for learning infant care. Nurs Res 37(1):20–24, 1988

resources. Can parents get occasional child-care relief from friends, neighbors, or day-care facilities? Are there community classes or support groups available for parents' specific learning needs? Are there exercise classes that permit mothers to bring their infants? These are some of the questions the nurse must anticipate.

Couples who are at high risk for parenting difficulties can often be identified during the 9 months of gestation. Good prenatal care includes nursing assessments of these potential problems and interventions to provide the necessary assistance.

Couples who do not communicate well or who show overt troublesome behavior, such as anger, hostility, continued denial of the pregnancy, or failure to prepare for the baby, are at increased risk for postpartum adjustment problems. If one or both parents are abnormally uninvolved in the pregnancy or extremely overstressed by it, they will need intervention. Couples who have no family, friends, or community support, as well as couples sub-

jected to abuse as children, will be at a higher risk for parenting problems. The nurse must be alert to these risk factors.

Evaluation

Evaluation of prenatal care is usually done on the basis of perinatal outcomes; outcomes such as incidence of complications, maternal weight gain, infant birth weight, and maternal/neonatal morbidity and mortality are often referred to as "hard" outcomes, meaning they are easily and routinely measured and are easy to quantify. The quality of nursing care in the prenatal period is directly reflected in these outcomes, as repeated studies have shown. The fact that prenatal care "works" is hardly questioned; indeed, the question more commonly asked in evaluating the effectiveness of prenatal care is not "whether?" but "when?", since most complications still occur in women who have delayed or no prenatal care because they have inadequate access to it (American Nurses Association 1987).

However, effectiveness of nursing care is also reflected in "soft" outcomes, such as the comfort and ease of parental adaptation to pregnancy, the effectiveness with which parents care for themselves, and the extent to which psychosocial risk factors fail to produce actual trauma because they were recognized and counterbalanced by appropriate and supportive care. In many ways nurses are still the "invisible" providers in prenatal care; additional research demonstrating the effectiveness of prenatal nursing care in producing positive outcomes is needed before the extent of nursing care in the prenatal period will become more evident and valued.

CHAPTER SUMMARY

When working with expectant couples, the nurse must assess the meaning and significance of the pregnancy to each family. Each family member carries a previous history as well as current concerns and expectations into the new pregnancy. Individual members have a variety of learning needs that test the nurse's insights, knowledge, and skills in counseling. The pregnant woman's needs are many and rapidly changing. For instance, she may need anticipatory guidance about the dramatic physical and emotional changes she will experience in early pregnancy; discussion of the more stable second trimester, which is normally the most comfortable; and discussion about the eventful third trimester, when labor and delivery will be uppermost in the consciousness of the mother and her family.

Although most families share some general concerns associated with the trimesters of gestation, many other concerns will be specific to each family. When assessing the family's needs, the nurse must use her knowledge of the physiologic and psychological processes of pregnancy as a framework. The nurse must be prepared to answer a myriad of questions and to use her judgment in deciding how the information can best be conveyed to the expectant woman and her family.

STUDY QUESTIONS

1. Define anticipatory guidance.
2. What factors influence a woman's or a family's learning needs in pregnancy?
3. The nurse must address the pregnancy in the context of the total family situation. Explain what this means.
4. How can a woman's age affect her approach to the pregnancy?
5. List five reasons why a woman or couple would need a referral. What referrals would be appropriate for these reasons?
6. List five signs or symptoms that a woman should report at once.
7. List seven characteristics that distinguish true labor from false labor.
8. Identify matters of concern to pregnant women employed outside the household.
9. List clues that may suggest a woman has been battered during pregnancy. Describe the nurse's course of action upon observing such clues.
10. A patient has a question about exercising during pregnancy. What points is it important to assess prior to your counseling?
11. Explain the value of the following antepartum exercises:

    pelvic tilt
    Kegel
    tailor sitting
    perineal massage

12. Describe how to teach breast self-examination and prenatal preparation for breast-feeding.

REFERENCES/BIBLIOGRAPHY

American Nurses Association: Access to Prenatal Care: Key to Preventing Low Birth Weight. Kansas City, MO, 1987

Brucker M: Management of minor common discomforts in pregnancy: Part II—Managing minor pain in pregnancy. J Nurse Midwife 33(1):25–29, 1988

Brucker M: (1988) Management of minor common discomforts in pregnancy: Part III—Managing gastrointestinal problems in pregnancy. J Nurse Midwife 33(2):67–72, 1988

Chez R: If you suspect a patient is a victim of violence. Symposium, Contemp OB/GYN 29(6):132, 1987

Chez R: Battered pregnant women. Genesis 11(1):15–16, 1989

Dilorio C: Management of nausea and vomiting in pregnancy. Nurse Pract 13(5):23–28, 1988

Henderson JS: Effects of a prenatal teaching program on postpartum regeneration of the pubococcygeal muscle. J Obstet Gynecol Neonatal Nurs 12(6):403, 1983

Horan M: Discomfort and pain during pregnancy. Mat Child Nurs J 9(4):267, 1984

Littlefield VM: Women as Victims: Education for Prevention: Health Education for Women. East Norwalk, Appleton–Century–Crofts, 1986

Noble E: Essential Exercises for the Childbearing Year. Boston, Houghton Mifflin, 1982

Richards D: Guidelines for exercise during pregnancy. Occup Health Nurs (October):508–509, 1985

Schecter S, Gray LT: A framework for understanding and empowering battered women. In Strause MB (ed): Abuse and Victimization Across the Life Span. Baltimore, Johns Hopkins University Press, 1988

Smith L: Evaluation and management of muscle contraction headache. Nurse Pract 13(1):20–27, 1988

Tilden VP: Perceptions of single vs. partnered adult gravidas in the mid trimester. J Obstet Gynecol Neonatal Nurs 12(1):40, 1983

Valente C: Working with the physically abused woman. In Kjervick DK, Martinson IM (eds): Women in Health and Illness. Philadelphia, WB Saunders, 1986

SUGGESTED READINGS

American Nurses Association: Access to Prenatal Care: Key to Preventing Low Birth Weight. Kansas City, MO, 1987

Chez R: Battered pregnant women. Genesis 11(1):15–16, 1989

Tiedje L, Collins B: Combining employment and motherhood. MCN 14(1):29–34, 1989

19 complications of pregnancy

LEARNING OBJECTIVES

After studying the material in this chapter, the student should be able to

- Describe complications associated with physiologic changes in pregnancy

- Enumerate psychosocial factors that may place women at risk for pregnancy complications

- Identify the physical findings associated with specified pregnancy complications

- Identify essential adjustments in nursing management based on the assessment of a specified complication

- Demonstrate an understanding of the nurse's role in anticipatory guidance and health teaching when pregnancy is at risk

KEY TERMS

Abortion

Abruption

Antibody titer

Eclampsia

Ectopic pregnancy

Erythroblastosis

Fetal-maternal immunization

Hemoglobinopathy

Hydrops fetalis

Hyperbilirubinemia

Hyperemesis gravidarum

Placenta previa

Sensitization

Thalassemia

Tocolysis

Complications may occur at any point during pregnancy. They may result from preexisting medical problems or from the pregnancy itself. Because of the complex connections between maternal problems and the normal physiologic changes that occur during pregnancy, close prenatal surveillance is vital. Clinical research has repeatedly found that, regardless of complications, early and consistent prenatal care results in improved health for both mother and infant.

The normal physiologic changes that occur in the woman's body during the 9 months of gestation set the specialty of maternity care apart from all other areas in nursing. The objective of prenatal care is to monitor specific parameters with the goal of averting or minimizing problems. To achieve this goal, the nurse must be knowledgeable about the physiology of pregnancy and the numerous changes that can occur, and must recognize the significance of deviations from the normal. Nurses prepared to work in high-risk settings can provide guidance and expedite care by monitoring laboratory studies, collecting specimens, referring patients for special care or treatments, and by patient support through teaching and encouragement.

The nurse must also be able to translate that knowledge into pragmatic teaching that patients will understand. Anticipatory guidance is used daily to direct the nurse's teaching of events pertinent to each trimester, to reduce fear of the unknown, and to increase family members' abilities to participate in maintaining their own health.

Health teaching offered over time in a positive and informal manner allows comfort and trust to develop between the nurse and the pregnant woman and her family. Honesty and directness foster confidence and compliance. These principles are especially important when problems arise during pregnancy.

AT-RISK PREGNANCY

Students of maternity nursing often hear the terms *high risk* or *at risk* and must be aware that pregnancy is normal until proved otherwise. Since the specialty of obstetrics has closely defined what is normal, all factors outside these parameters are referred to as risk factors. Some of these factors, such as genetic susceptibility, hypertension, or anemia, may be identified from the patient's history and physical examination, or from laboratory findings.

Factors that alter the physiologic process of pregnancy may seriously affect the health of the mother and infant. Maternal problems such as diabetes, heart disease, and anemia may compromise the quality of the pregnancy and the fetal outcome. Poverty, malnutrition, the fact that a pregnancy is unwanted, and increased maternal age can also lead to pregnancy complications and are thus referred to as risk factors.

Most women with high-risk pregnancies start their pregnancy expecting a normal prenatal course but later experience risk factors such as bleeding, inconsistent uterine growth, or anemia. The purpose of good prenatal care is to identify the at-risk group of women and initiate early intervention to prevent or alleviate problems.

Rapid technologic advances have changed the practice of obstetrics and maternity nursing. Protocols and screening methods have been devised to identify the woman at risk for pregnancy-related problems. The term *at risk* emphasizes the obstetric approach to prevention; that is, to screen patients, identify problems, and tailor management to promote optimal pregnancy outcome.

Ultrasound was first used as a diagnostic tool in maternity care and screening before it was used for other contemporary applications. Biochemical and biophysical fetal monitoring has greatly improved infant survival rates.

The art of maternity care is often overshadowed by the urgency of complications and the marvels of technology. John Naisbitt in *Megatrends* discusses the need for maternity care to maintain a ''high-touch'' quality; when pregnancy becomes complicated, care rapidly becomes ''high-tech.'' Procedures necessary to facilitate optimal care may be alienating, frightening, and mysterious to the mother and family. The nurse plays the role of mediator and equalizer by translating ''high-tech'' into humanistic terms.

Procedures are tools that give health care providers the means by which they can arrive at decisions and make diagnoses. Therefore, the term *at risk* connotes a continuing alertness to patient cues. Although this chapter focuses on complications, even when a pregnancy has complications the nurse should be mindful of the ordinary concerns of the family, such as breast-feeding, nutrition, and sibling adjustment, and maintain the art of caring.

NAUSEA AND VOMITING/ HYPEREMESIS GRAVIDARUM

One of the most common and best-known symptoms of early pregnancy is nausea and vomiting, generally called *morning sickness*. This uncomfortable dyad of symptoms occurs in about 50% of all pregnancies and is often experienced with or without food intake at any time of the day. One or both of these symptoms may continue until about 12 weeks of gestation, at which time they normally disappear or decrease in severity.

In *hyperemesis gravidarum,* vomiting is severe enough to cause electrolyte, metabolic, and nutritional imbalances even in the absence of a specific medical problem.

Etiology

Many causative factors for nausea and vomiting in pregnancy have been identified, including hormonal, histaminic, and psychogenic as well as factors related to vitamin utilization. Current theory postulates that the rapidly increasing levels of human chorionic gonadotropin (HCG) in early pregnancy induce emesis. That this theory is valid is suggested by the fact that women carrying multiple pregnancies and those with hydatidiform moles have extremely high levels of HCG and also experience exaggerated symptoms of nausea and vomiting. However, the theory remains unproved, and the causative factors of the illness have not yet been positively identified. Although psychological factors were once considered unimportant or irrelevant in pregnancy-related nausea and vomiting, their role is now generally accepted. Studies have reported a relationship between the woman's feeling about pregnancy and vomiting during pregnancy. Ambivalence toward the pregnancy and, ultimately, the child or a negative reaction to the initial fetal movements may be contributing factors.

Treatment

Continued vomiting results in dehydration. This will ultimately decrease the circulating volume of blood, causing hypovolemia (decreased blood volume). Laboratory studies will reveal hemoconcentration and, in severe cases, loss of hydrogen, sodium, potassium, and chloride, which will result in hyponatremia (decreased sodium in the blood) and hypokalemia (decreased potassium in the blood). During pregnancy, gastric acid secretion normally is reduced because of increased estrogen stimulation. This places the woman at risk for alkalosis rather than the acidosis that usually occurs in an advanced stage of dehydration. When dehydration has occurred, hospitalization is required to correct fluid and electrolyte deficits by intravenous infusion. Treatment should continue until vomiting is controlled.

When hospitalization is required for severe symptoms, treatment goals are to hydrate the patient, establish electrolyte balance, and provide vitamin supplementation.

These goals are accomplished by restricting oral intake and beginning parenteral administration of fluids supplemented with electrolytes and vitamins. This treatment provides rest for the gastrointestinal tract that has become overstimulated by severe vomiting.

Implications for Nursing Care

It is important for the nurse to determine factors in the woman's life that may be contributing to her symptoms. Such questions as the following generally supply infor-

mation that provides insights into the woman's life-style and into how she feels about what is happening to her. How do you feel about this pregnancy? Was it planned or unplanned? Do you have a partner, and is he supportive? Do you have adequate housing and money for food? Is your family supportive? Do you have social contacts, and are you able to get out with friends? Do you participate in any activities that you enjoy, such as clubs, groups, or the like? Are you getting exercise, especially outdoors?

Beginning as "morning sickness," hyperemesis gravidarum insidiously progresses from a mild to a severe state. The nurse can assess the severity of symptoms by the following methods:

- Compare the woman's prepregnant weight with her current weight.
- Compare actual weight gain with the expected weight gain for the week of gestation.
- Review the woman's dietary intake in the preceding 24 hours.
- Compare the woman's usual eating habits with her current intake.
- Determine whether the woman is ingesting substances that are not foods, such as starch, clay, toothpaste, and so on, which would indicate pica.
- Perform a dipstick urine test for the presence of ketones.
- Examine skin turgor.
- Examine the tongue for a red, shiny appearance that may indicate anemia.

Mild nausea and vomiting may respond to dietary adjustment and vitamin supplementation. A dietary history will provide the information needed to counsel the woman about the types and amounts of foods she needs to maintain adequate nourishment for her own and her infant's nutritional needs. The suggestions in the accompanying Self-Care Teaching display (page 484) may assist the woman to decrease or eliminate gastric upset, nausea, and vomiting.

Symptoms vary widely, and there is a risk of increasing dehydration. When conservative measures of dietary counseling and psychological support do not bring relief or resolution of nausea and vomiting, the following criteria are used to diagnose hyperemesis gravidarum:

- It occurs during the first 16 weeks of gestation.
- It is accompanied by disturbances of appetite.
- It causes alterations in nutritional status, as evidenced by weight loss, electrolyte imbalance, and ketosis with ketonuria.
- It is intractable in nature.

In women who are not seriously dehydrated, hospitalization may be avoided by the administration of intrave-

SELF-CARE TEACHING

The Patient With Gastric Upset and Nausea and Vomiting

- Eliminate fried foods.
- Avoid spicy foods.
- Eat bland, low-fat foods.
- Increase intake of carbohydrate foods.
- Avoid rich meats, such as beef and pork.
- Avoid an empty stomach by eating small amounts of food every 2 hr.
- Eat dry crackers or toast on arising in the morning.
- Take most nourishment in liquid form, such as soups, eggnog, high-protein fluids.
- Discontinue prenatal vitamins and iron until vomiting is controlled.
- Take a 50-mg supplemental dose of vitamin B_6 twice daily (not on an empty stomach).

nous fluids in the outpatient setting. Administration of 1000 ml lactated Ringer's solution corrects dehydration, restores electrolyte balance, and may interrupt or relieve the nausea and vomiting cycle.

Carefully monitoring and recording the patient's fluid intake and urinary and vomitus output is important. Oral hygiene measures are important because the patient's mouth will become excessively dry from lack of oral fluid intake. After vomiting episodes, the mouth should be rinsed. Bed linen or gowns should be changed as necessary.

When vomiting begins to decrease in response to treatment, limited amounts of liquids, such as tea or ice chips, and bland foods, such as crackers or toast, may be given at intervals of 2 to 3 hours. Depending on the patient's response to these foods, her diet can be increased gradually until she is able to eat a regular diet. During this time, it is also important to provide a quiet and restful atmosphere to promote needed rest and sleep.

During the patient's hospitalization, the nurse should be cognizant of her psychologic needs and be supportive and accepting. Helping the woman to recognize her feelings and creating an atmosphere in which she can verbalize them through listening and nonjudgmental behavior will aid her in resolving some of her fears and concerns.

Following intravenous therapy, the patient should be given specific instructions for progressing to oral fluid intake. The nurse should follow-up by telephone to assess whether the patient is ready to progress to a more standard diet or whether reevaluation is needed. Appropriate referrals to a social worker, psychologist, or public health

nurse or to a supplemental food plan may help to improve the woman's situation and interrupt the nausea and vomiting cycle.

After her symptoms subside and she is discharged from the hospital, the patient should be followed closely in the outpatient setting. A single provider of care who is knowledgeable about the patient and has established a good relationship with her should care for her consistently and be alert to subtle changes that may presage further problems. When nausea and vomiting persist throughout pregnancy (even though controlled), those symptoms disappear rapidly following delivery.

ANEMIA IN PREGNANCY

It has been estimated that 56% of all pregnant women have some degree of anemia, the percentage varying according to geographic location and socioeconomic grouping. Anemia may be caused by a number of conditions in pregnancy, which result from nutritional deficiency, hemolysis, or blood loss.

The normal physiologic changes of pregnancy cause increases in blood volume and red blood cell production. A total of 750 to 1000 mg of absorbed iron or the equivalent of four or more units of transfused blood is needed to meet the increased iron needs of pregnancy. During the second trimester, a drop in hemoglobin and hematocrit levels can be expected. This results from a 50% increase in plasma volume, which, along with retention of intracellular fluid, causes physiologic hemodilution during pregnancy. Consequently, anemia in pregnancy is defined as a hemoglobin of 10 g or less during the second and third trimesters. This low figure reflects the hemodilutional effect. Additionally, hemoglobin levels are influenced by the following factors:

- Rate of erythrocyte breakdown and iron reutilization by the bone marrow
- Dietary intake of iron (inadequate diets can provide only 10 to 18 mg of iron daily; the normal requirement during pregnancy is 30 to 60 mg of elemental iron)
- Ability of the gastrointestinal tract to absorb iron (normally only about 10% of intake is absorbed, but this increases to 20% when iron deficiency exists)
- Loss of 200 to 250 mg of iron from blood loss at the time of delivery

Because of these dynamic factors, regular screening for the presence of anemia during pregnancy is routine. A complete blood count (CBC) is performed at the first prenatal visit, at 28 and 36 weeks of gestation, at the time of hospital admission, and on the first postpartum day. Additional testing is performed if low hemoglobin levels are found.

NURSING CARE PLAN

The Woman With Possible Hyperemesis

Nursing Diagnosis (Patient Problem) and Assessment Data	Nursing Interventions	Rationale
Probable Complication: *hyperemesis*		
• Patient complains of constant nausea and vomiting without relief from self-care measures. (See Nursing Care Plan: Women with Common Discomforts of Pregnancy, Chapter 18).	Obtain a nutritional history. Weigh the patient. Check the patient's state of hydration. Confirm that laboratory tests to detect electrolyte deficits or acidosis have been obtained.	Precise determinations of amounts of nutrients and fluids ingested by the patient are needed. Prompt detection of abnormal laboratory values will permit early diagnosis and intervention.
• Poor skin turgor, contracted urine, ketosis/acidosis by dipstick	Explain the need for intravenous fluids.	Intravenous fluids containing sodium, potassium, chloride, bicarbonate, glucose, and water are needed until vomiting is controlled.

Expected Outcome:

Woman responds to treatment for hyperemesis as evidenced by diminishing nausea or vomiting, adequate hydration, and maintenance of appropriate weight gain.

Nursing Diagnosis:
fear related to persistent nausea/vomiting and hospitalization

	Prepare the patient for hospitalization. Offer reassurance and support.	Hospital treatment is sometimes required to control vomiting, restore electrolyte balance, correct dehydration, and prevent starvation. Reassurance that treatment should lessen symptoms and support fetal health may reduce patient anxiety.

Expected Outcome:

Woman understands risk and need for treatment as demonstrated by the type of questions asked and statement of her desire for treatment and hospitalization.

Nursing Diagnosis:
ineffective individual coping related to at-risk pregnancy

• Family members ridicule or down-play physical condition.	Refer the patient for psychological counseling when appropriate.	Patients experiencing intractable vomiting may be helped by professional psychological intervention.
• Mother insists on early discharge to return to family responsibilities regardless of physical condition.	Refer to a social worker when appropriate.	Social problems may contribute to stress and hyperemesis.

(continued)

The Woman With Possible Hyperemesis

Nursing Diagnosis (Patient Problem) and Assessment Data	Nursing Interventions	Rationale

Expected Outcome:

Woman responds to nursing support and counseling as evidenced by making and keeping further appointments for follow-up or psychological or sociological counseling.

Etiology

The etiology and severity of anemia determines the risk to the woman and her developing fetus. Maternal morbidity is uncommon unless the hemoglobin level falls below 6 g; however, it is possible that subtle complications, such as delayed wound healing, infection, and postpartum hemorrhage, may occur with less severe reduction of hemoglobin.

Mild anemia of 11 g poses no threat to the mother or infant but is an indication that the nutritional state of the mother is less than optimal. When the mother intends to breast-feed, it is important for her hemoglobin level to be maintained at 12 g or above so that her body will be provided with the nutrients and oxygen required for successful breast-feeding. (See Chapters 15 and 16 for further discussion of nutrition and screening.)

Causes of Anemia

- Nutritional deficiency
    Iron deficiency
    Megaloblastic anemia (includes folic acid deficiency and B_{12} deficiency)
- Blood loss, acute and chronic
- Hemolysis (increased destruction of red blood cells)
    Congenital sickle cell anemia
    Thalassemia
    G6PD (glucose-6-phosphate dehydrogenase) deficiency, an enzyme deficiency

---

Iron Deficiency Anemia

Iron deficiency anemia results from reduced hemoglobin production caused by depletion of iron stores. Depleted iron stores may result from an inadequate dietary intake of iron, malabsorption, blood loss, or hemolysis. When iron deficiency anemia has been diagnosed, it is usual to assume that the hematologic system is normal but lacks available iron to meet its needs — that is, it will respond when iron intake is increased. When other values of the CBC are abnormal but do not reflect iron deficiency, further anemia work-up is indicated.

When anemia is remarkable — that is, the hemoglobin level is less than 10.5 g *in the first trimester* — the patient may experience fatigue, headache, and tachycardia. Severe iron deficiency is uncommon. It may cause brittle fingernails, cheilosis, or a smooth, shiny, red tongue. Women with these symptoms are often lacking in other nutrients as well as iron.

Treatment

Supplements of iron and vitamin C are standard treatment for iron deficiency anemia; however, they should never be considered a substitute for good nutrition. The usual recommended dosages for supplementation are:

Ferrous sulfate, 320 mg orally, three times a day
Vitamin C, 500 mg orally, daily

Supplemental iron may cause gastrointestinal upset accompanied by either constipation or diarrhea. To minimize this reaction, especially in early pregnancy when there is a tendency for nausea, advise the patient to take the iron preparation with or following meals. However, maximum absorption occurs when iron is taken with orange juice between meals, and this method may be best suited for use after the first trimester. Also advise the patient that the iron in the pills is not fully absorbed and some will be excreted in the feces, causing them to become dark green or black. The presence of dark stools, as noted by the patient, is an indication of her compliance.

Implications for Nursing Care

Depending on the health care setting, the nurse may develop a dietary plan with the assistance of a nutritionist. Evaluation of the diet for the past 24 hours will provide a baseline from which a diet, including more iron-rich foods, can be planned. Chapter 15 contains more detailed nutritional information referring to anemias of pregnancy.

As a general counseling rule, the redder the meat and the greener the vegetable, the richer it is as a source of iron. Vitamin C, a nutrient essential for the optimal absorption of iron, is abundant in dark green fresh vegetables and citrus fruits. Vitamin C is chemically unstable and readily breaks down when heated. Therefore, fresh, uncooked vegetables are an important source. Since vitamin C is not stored in the body, sufficient quantities must be eaten each day to fulfill daily requirements.

The body responds to supplemental iron in about 7 to 15 days by increasing its production of young red blood cells (reticulocytes). When the patient has taken the recommended dose of iron, the red blood cell response can be measured in about 2 weeks by an elevation in the percentage of reticulocytes, as reported by the laboratory reticulocyte count. An early response validating iron ingestion may be an increase of 0.5%. This will elevate to as much as 3% by 10 to 15 days. Relaying this information to the patient will encourage her to keep taking the pills.

Folic Acid Deficiency

Folic acid deficiency is discussed in Chapter 15, Maternal Nutrition in Pregnancy.

HEMOGLOBINOPATHIES

Hemoglobinopathies are a group of diseases caused by genetic defects of polypeptide synthesis resulting in the production of abnormal hemoglobin. Disorders of the blood are not uncommon in pregnancy and can affect any of the four basic components of blood: erythrocytes or red blood cells, white blood cells, platelets, or plasma. In the hemoglobinopathies that are to be discussed, the most commonly affected component is the red blood cell.

Red blood cells are produced in the bone marrow and have a lifespan of 120 days. When they become old or

defective, they are filtered out of the blood stream and broken down by the spleen, liver, and lymph glands. The iron they contain is not lost but is resorbed back into the body for reuse. As red blood cells are lost from the system through attrition, they must be replaced to maintain homeostasis. The bone marrow busily produces new red blood cells to replace and maintain the full complement of cells. The new red blood cells — called *reticulocytes* — are not quite mature and are larger than mature cells. Laboratory measurements of the ratio between reticulocytes and normal mature red blood cells are useful in assessments of the body's response to iron therapy, blood loss, or anemia of other blood disorders.

In many blood disorders, the hemoglobin molecule within the red blood cell is most affected.

The function of hemoglobin is to carry oxygen to the tissues. The hemoglobin molecule is composed of four heme groups (the iron-containing portion of the molecule) and a globin (protein constituent). Abnormalities of the heme and globin molecules can occur, although those of the heme are relatively rare and are manifested only when B_6 deficiency, lead poisoning, or copper deficiency exists. Important in pregnancy, however, are alterations or abnormalities in the synthesis of the globin molecule. These abnormalities can be in the structure or the production of globin.

Fetal hemoglobin (Hb F), the hemoglobin contained in the fetus, differs from adult hemoglobin and can release oxygen at a lower *p*H and oxygen tension. This ability facilitates the diffusion of oxygen from mother to fetus. At birth, the neonate's blood contains 60% to 80% Hb F. By 2 years of age, Hb F accounts for less than 2% of the child's total hemoglobin.

Thalassemia

Thalassemia is a genetic disorder that affects the red blood cells of hemoglobin. It is most commonly found in people in Mediterranean origin, in Asians (especially Chinese), and in people of African ancestry, including West Indian and American blacks. In the United States there are approximately 1000 cases of thalassemia each year, and these result in approximately 50 deaths.

Etiology
Each individual inherits two genes (one from each parent) that control the production of alpha- and beta-globin chains. In thalassemia the hemoglobin chains are not structurally abnormal, but the production of either alpha or beta chains is decreased. When this occurs, synthesis of the defective chain is impaired, and the precipitation of normal chains disrupts red blood cell function. The degree of defective production in the individual depends on whether thalassemia genes are inherited from one or both

parents. The condition of having inherited a thalassemia gene from one parent is called *thalassemia trait.*

Alpha-Thalassemia

In the homozygous form of thalassemia, the affected fetus has received an alpha-thalassemia gene from each parent. As a consequence, no alpha chains are produced, and the fetus is unable to synthesize normal Hb F. Intrauterine death usually occurs, with the fetus exhibiting the clinical features of hydrops fetalis.

Individuals inheriting one alpha-thalassemia gene (heterozygous inheritance) experience only a mild-to-moderate chronic anemia and may be unaware they are carrying the trait.

Beta-Thalassemia

The homozygous form of beta-thalassemia is also called *thalassemia major, Cooley's anemia,* or *Mediterranean anemia.* In this disease the fetus has inherited a beta-thalassemia gene from each parent, has no beta chains, but does have an excessive number of alpha chains. The disease is characterized by severe hemolytic anemia caused by the precipitation of alpha chains within abnormal red blood cells. An infant born with Cooley's anemia will be severely anemic and can only survive by frequent blood transfusion. Female children who survive to reproductive age are often sterile.

Beta-Thalassemia Trait (Beta-Thalassemia minor)

This condition results when a person inherits one gene for normal beta-globin and one beta-thalassemia gene (heterozygous inheritance). The inherited beta-thalassemia gene causes decreased production of beta-globin chains, but this condition is of minor consequence and is not considered a disease. It causes no physical or mental problems to carriers, who need no treatment and have a normal life expectancy. However, when the condition is diagnosed, carriers should be referred for genetic counseling, if they are considering the possibility of having children.

Treatment

It is now possible to diagnose fetal beta-thalassemia prenatally. This is accomplished through fetoscopy, fetal blood sampling, and column chromatography at 16 to 20 weeks of gestation. Risk to the fetus is not insignificant, ranging from 5% to 10%. The skill of the physician performing the procedure has a major influence on the outcome.

Fetal alpha-thalassemia can also be diagnosed by DNA analysis of amniotic fluid cells obtained by amniocentesis. This test seeks evidence of alpha-globin gene deletion, the cause of this disorder.

When the father of the baby is also diagnosed as having beta-thalassemia minor (trait), the baby is at risk for developing severe disease. Their infant has a 25% chance of hemozygous disease, a 50% chance of heterozygous disease, and a 25% chance of being unaffected. The couple will need supportive genetic counseling and nursing care. They will have major decisions to make about the present pregnancy and plans for future babies.

Implications for Nursing Care

When a pregnant woman is unaware that she has beta-thalassemia and is told that she is carrying this trait (and possibly transmitting it to her infant), she will need sensitive and empathetic support. Although the disease need not disrupt her health or life, she must be aware of its possible ramifications.

When the diagnosis is made, the nurse should stress to the patient the need to have the father of the baby screened for thalassemia. If he is not carrying the gene, the couple should be referred to a genetic counselor to obtain information about the odds that their baby, and future babies, will carry the trait.

During the prenatal period, the nurse should carefully assess the patient through the interim history, physical findings, and patient symptoms. Signs of urinary tract infection, of chest colds that might progress to pneumonia, and of pulmonary congestion should be identified early and lead to swift and appropriate medical intervention.

Since the woman generally is not ill, normal prenatal activities, counseling, and classes are continued. The necessity for increased rest should be stressed and arrangements made for help at home, if this becomes necessary.

Sickle Cell Disease

Sickle cell disease (sickle cell anemia) is an autosomal dominant heritable disorder limited to blacks, transmitted to the offspring by either the father or mother (heterozygous form), or by both (homozygous form). Approximately 0.3% of black people in the United States, or 50,000 people, suffer from sickle cell anemia (Hb SS).

Etiology

The term *sickle cell disease* originates from the characteristic sickle shape of the circulating red blood cells of affected persons. This abnormal hemoglobin results from alteration of the beta chain. Homozygous (SS) persons have inherited the Hb S gene from each parent, resulting in up to 95% of their hemoglobin being of the Hb SS type; normal adult hemoglobin (Hb A_1), makes up the remainder.

Heterozygous carriers (who are said to have *sickle cell trait*) have a mixture of about 65% normal Hb A_1 and 35%

sickle Hb S hemoglobin in their red blood cells. These carriers of the gene are asymptomatic and experience few problems, with the exception of increased numbers of urinary tract infections and possible sickling at high altitudes. About 8% of the black population have the trait and live full, productive lives with a normal life expectancy. In these people, over 40% of the hemoglobin must be affected before they are symptomatic for more than persistent anemia.

Sickle cell disease begins in infancy and is associated with a lifelong history of anemia, chronic illness, and abdominal and joint pain. Many sufferers die before they reach reproductive age, whereas others are incapable of normal sexual activity because of the disorder.

Maternal/Fetal Implications

During pregnancy, women with sickle cell disease (Hb SS) experience higher rates of spontaneous abortion, stillbirths, neonatal deaths, and premature labor. Fetal wastage is high: one third to one half of all known pregnancies terminate for these reasons. The cause of the perinatal loss is unknown, and placentas from these births exhibit no damage from sickling or infarcts. No increase in congenital anomalies is reported, although intrauterine growth retardation is common.

Anemia is the cardinal finding (100%) in pregnant patients with sickle cell disease. The anemia becomes increasingly severe as pregnancy progresses. About 10% to 20% of affected women have acute crises during pregnancy. These may occur at any time. Pregnancy places women at particular risk for infection, which accounts for 50% to 60% of the morbidity experienced during pregnancy. Common infections include urinary tract infection, pneumonia, and postpartum endometritis. These problems are especially severe in these women and result from stagnation of oxygenated red blood cells in the viscera, which leads to deoxygenation and sickling. Again, this becomes a vicious cycle that may lead to crises. Not infrequently, cardiomegaly, congestive heart failure, and pulmonary infarction occur. A maternal mortality rate of 25% demonstrates the seriousness of sickle cell disease.

Women with sickle cell trait may never exhibit any symptom but anemia. Anemia is chronic and may be profound, depending on the percent of Hb S present. Spontaneous abortions and infections are still the primary concern for pregnant women who carry the trait, although most trait carriers have uneventful pregnancies.

Treatment

There is no current standard treatment other than supportive measures for sickle cell disease. The woman with sickle cell disease is followed prenatally in a high-risk clinic or private practice where her condition is closely supervised. When infection or other problems arise, the woman is hospitalized immediately.

In the outpatient prenatal setting, initial laboratory assessment is performed to specifically define the woman's hemoglobinopathy, using Sickledex and hemoglobin electrophoresis. Iron and folate stores and reticulocyte counts are assessed, and screening for hemolysis is completed. Dietary counseling and folic acid supplements are provided. Iron therapy is not necessary, since iron deficiency is not a characteristic of this disease. Frequent monitoring for infection is indicated to facilitate immediate treatment to decrease morbidity.

Implications for Nursing Care

Initial history-taking by the nurse will identify women with the disease or the trait, either through the patient's knowledge of its existence or through a family history of disease. Hemoglobin electrophoresis differentiates between sickle cell disease and sickle cell trait. When less than 40% of a woman's total hemoglobin is sickle cell hemoglobin (Hb S), that woman carries the sickle cell trait (SC-A), which she may or may not be aware of. In women with sickle cell disease, over 90% of the total hemoglobin is Hb S.

The initial patient history should document problems or complications that have been, or are being, experienced by the patient. Interim histories should routinely include queries about even the most minor problems.

As soon as sickle cell trait is diagnosed in the mother, the father should be screened for the trait. If he also has the trait, the fetus has a 25% chance of having the disease. Referral to genetic counseling is imperative for couples that may pass on the trait or the disease to their offspring.

Nurses play an important role in teaching patients about their pregnancies, in helping them to maintain optimal health through nutrition counseling, and in monitoring signs of problems. The nurse can intervene in the following ways:

- Ensuring that genetic counseling is made available
- Encouraging frequent prenatal visits for ongoing monitoring
- Obtaining urine cultures once a month, whether or not the patient is symptomatic
- Stressing to the patient the importance of taking her daily dose of folic acid (1–5 mg)
- Assisting with hospital admission when necessary
- Counseling the couple in family planning methods and permanent sterilization or abortion, if requested.

Glucose-6-Phosphate Dehydrogenase Deficiency (G6PD)

About 10% of the black population of the United States is affected by glucose-6-phosphate dehydrogenase (G6PD) deficiency. The disease is characterized by a sex-linked red blood cell enzyme (G6PD) deficiency that is carried on the X (female) sex chromosome. G6PD is an important enzyme in the production of normal red blood cells. When it is deficient, the membrane of the cell is not maintained, and when the cell is exposed to a host of oxidant drugs, it is destroyed (hemolyzed) and removed from the circulation by the spleen.

Maternal risk for women with this enzyme deficiency is primarily related to the increased incidence of urinary tract infections. Risks to the fetus include neonatal jaundice, hydrops fetalis (erythroblastosis), and intrauterine death.

Treatment

Successful treatment of G6PD-related anemia in the pregnant patient is through iron and folic acid supplementation, nutrition counseling, and avoiding oxidizing drugs.

Implications for Nursing Care

When taking the prenatal history, the nurse should be alert to patient reports of episodes of jaundice of unknown origin. Many patients are unaware that they have G6PD deficiency because they have never ingested an oxidizing drug or have not sought medical help when these occasions arose.

When the pregnant patient is unaware that she has G6PD deficiency, she will require careful counseling about its signs and symptoms during and after pregnancy. The nurse must make the patient aware of the drugs that she should avoid by supplying her with a complete list of their names. She should also point out that many drugs that precipitate G6PD are sold over the counter at drug stores, such as acetaminophen, phenacetin, salicylates, and some sulfa drugs. It may be difficult for the patient to find appropriate drugs to deal with everyday problems such as headache (salicylates should not be used in pregnancy) or, more importantly, urinary tract infections that are normally treated with sulfa drugs.

Since this is a female-linked disorder, the father of the baby need not be tested.

HEMOLYTIC DISEASE OF THE FETUS/NEWBORN

In 1.5% of all pregnancies, hemolytic disease of the fetus or newborn occurs. It is caused by an immune reaction by the mother's blood against the blood group factor on the fetus's red blood cells. When the fetus inherits a blood group antigen from the father, which the mother does not possess, the mother's body forms an antibody against that particular blood group antigen, and hemolytic disease begins. Hemolytic disease can result from ABO incompatibility or, more commonly, Rh incompatibility.

ABO Incompatibility

ABO incompatibility occurs in about 20% of all pregnancies. To understand the dynamics that can occur between a mother and her developing fetus when their blood types are different, an understanding of the blood groups is important.

Etiology

There are four major blood groups that belong to the ABO blood group system. These are blood types A, B, AB, and O. Red blood cells have either antigen A, B, or AB, or no antigen on the surface of the cells. Type A blood has A antigen, B has B antigen, AB has A and B antigens, and O contains no antigen. The antigens are all capable of producing antibodies. Plasma contains reciprocal antibodies. For example, a group A person will have anti-B antibody; group B will have anti-A antibody, group AB will have no antibody, and group O will have both anti-A and anti-B antibodies.

Theoretically, maternal and fetal blood do not mix; actually, small hemorrhages can occur across the placenta in both directions. The Kleihauer–Betke staining technique provides a method of testing to determine the presence of fetal cells in the maternal circulation. Using this technique, numerous studies have shown that the incidence of transplacental hemorrhage increases as pregnancy progresses. At the time of delivery there appears to be a large transfer of red blood cells from the fetus to the mother, and it has been determined that most fetal-to-maternal immunizations occur at this time.

About half the cases of ABO incompatibility are in blood group O mothers who are carrying a group A or B fetus. The group O mother has naturally occurring anti-A and anti-B antibodies in her plasma that may cause maternal sensitization against the fetal blood antigen and cause some degree of erythroblastosis. However, because the anti-A and B immune bodies are not passed easily from mother to fetus, only 10% of those pregnancies identified as ABO incompatible actually develop hemolytic disease.

Maternal/Fetal Implications

The hemolytic response of the fetus is usually mild, and mild-to-moderate hyperbilirubinemia is evident in the newborn. Phototherapy usually suffices to effectively resolve the jaundice in the newborn. (See Chapters 32 and 34 for discussion of phototherapy and other treatment for hyperbilirubinemia.)

All pregnant women should be screened with an anti-body titer between 28 and 32 weeks of gestation. However, since hemolytic disease from this type of incompatibility is almost always mild, no prenatal treatment is indicated.

Rh Incompatibility

Rh incompatibility is clinically the most important form of blood incompatibility, making up over 75% of cases.

Etiology

Rh is a genetically determined factor present in red blood cells. A complex system, the Rh factors appear to have three loci — C, D, and E — within the cells. These factors are so closely linked they behave in an integrated fashion, as if they were a single gene. There are several different sets of notations for the Rh factors, but the most familiar is the D designate, or Du factor. This means that if a person is D-positive, the D factor is present on the surface of red blood cells. Rh(D)-negative denotes the absence of the D, or (CDE), factor on red blood cells.

When an Rh-negative mother carries an Rh-positive fetus, the antibodies she develops against her infant's blood group antigen may cause varying degrees of fetal anemia and jaundice after birth. Fetal anemia presents the major problem when, because the fetus manufactures blood at an accelerated rate to compensate for its anemia, many erythroblasts (immature red cells) pass into the fetal circulation prematurely. When these cells are identified on peripheral blood smears, erythroblastosis fetalis is diagnosed.

Maternal/Fetal Implications

When a pregnant woman is Rh negative, she has no D antigen on the surface of her red blood cells. If the blood of her fetus is Rh positive, the mother may become sensitized to it. Less than 0.5 ml Rh-positive blood gaining entrance into the maternal circulation will sensitize the mother to her baby's blood. The first exposure causes a response with IgM antibodies. These antibodies are large molecules that are unable to cross the placenta. In conjunction with the high levels of circulating corticosteroids and a tendency toward immunologic tolerance during pregnancy, they offer protection against sensitization. With repeated transplacental hemorrhages, the mother's body will respond by forming IgG antibodies, which are small enough to cross the placenta and enter the fetal circulation. The IgG antibodies coat the Rh-positive fetal red blood cells, causing their hemolysis. A schematic depiction of this process is shown in Figure 19–1.

Treatment

On the first prenatal visit, all pregnant women are screened for blood type, Rh factor, and for the presence of antibodies. Obtaining antibody titers is especially critical in multiparous women or those with a history of previous abortions, stillbirths, or ectopic pregnancies, because these women may have been exposed to transplacental hemorrhage previously. A critical titer level, that is, the level below which fetal death does not occur is established by laboratory analysis. In the case of a first immunized pregnancy, when the titer does not reach this level, the woman is usually delivered at term. This reduces the time the infant is exposed to sensitized maternal cells but ensures that the infant is mature. Antibody titers are watched from 24 weeks of gestation on; stable or declining titers are reassuring, while an increasing titer raises concern about fetal status. When the critical antibody titer is reached during pregnancy, amniotic fluid analysis provides more accurate information about the condition of the fetus.

Amniocentesis is performed in sensitized women to determine the level of bilirubin in amniotic fluid. Tests of amniotic fluid begin at 28 weeks or whenever antibody levels become critical. Depending on previous laboratory results, amniocentesis is repeated every 1 to 3 weeks. Generally, when the concentration of bilirubin rises before 32 weeks of gestation, an intrauterine transfusion is performed. After 32 weeks, the infant is delivered, transfused, and managed for prematurity.

The sensitized fetus is at risk to develop a progressive syndrome called erythroblastosis fetalis. This occurs when fetal blood reacts with the mother's Rh-negative antibodies to break down Rh-positive fetal red cells, causing hemolytic anemia. The destruction of fetal red blood cells releases bilirubin into the amniotic fluid, which is the basis for fetal jaundice. Marked anemia leads to cardiac decompensation, cardiomegaly (enlargement of the heart), and hepatosplenomegaly (enlargement of the liver and spleen). Because of liver and heart dysfunction, progressive edema results in ascites and generalized edema, referred to as *hydrops fetalis*. At this stage of involvement, intrauterine transfusion is of little use and the infant is at serious risk for intrauterine or neonatal death. (See Chapter 34 for an in-depth discussion of care of the infant with erythroblastosis fetalis).

Rh Immune Prophylaxis

Until the 1980s, the pregnancy outlook for an Rh-negative woman with an Rh-positive partner was almost predictable. No difficulty was usually experienced during the first pregnancy, but the mother became sensitized with Rh-positive red blood cells during delivery of the first infant. During the second sensitized pregnancy, the fetus

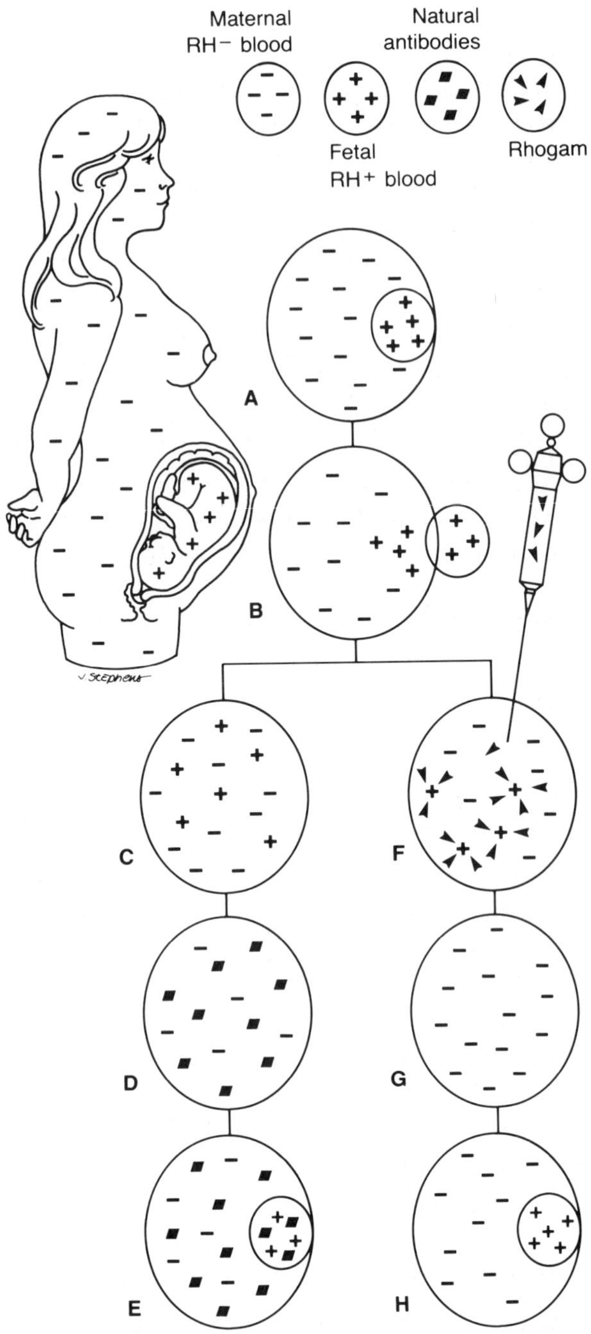

Figure 19–1. Rh disease and its prevention. *(A)* When a primigravida has Rh-negative blood and the father's blood is Rh positive, the blood of the fetus may also be Rh positive. *(B)* When the Rh-positive infant is delivered, small amounts of its blood may escape into the maternal circulation. *(C)* Immune globulin (RhoGAM) is not administered to the mother, so Rh-positive blood cells remain in her circulatory system. *(D)* The mother's natural antibodies are released to destroy the foreign Rh-positive cells, and she becomes permanently sensitized. *(E)* With a subsequent pregnancy with an Rh-positive fetus, the mother's body contains antibodies against her fetus. Erythroblastosis fetalis may result. *(F)* To avoid this potentially fatal disease in the fetus, immune globulin should be given after the first pregnancy. Once sensitization takes place, it can never be reversed, even with immune globulin. *(G)* An injection of immune globulin after the first pregnancy causes destruction of the Rh-positive cells in the mother's blood and prevents maternal sensitization. *(H)* In a subsequent pregnancy with an Rh-negative infant, the maternal blood is free from anti-Rh-negative antibodies. (Childbirth Graphics)

became sensitized from the mother's antibodies and developed some degree of erythroblastosis fetalis. The life of the fetus was in danger by the third trimester, at which time the fetus was likely to develop hydrops fetalis. A third pregnancy resulted in early fetal sensitization and a high rate of fetal mortality. Women in this category were advised against further pregnancies.

During the 1960s, microbiologists came to understand that when an antigen and its corresponding antibody are injected simultaneously, the individual does not become sensitized to the antigen. Research showed that injecting

Rh-immune globulin (RhoGAM) within 72 hours of maternal exposure to antigens protected against Rh immunization of the mother. Without maternal sensitization and the development of Rh antibodies, sensitization during subsequent pregnancies did not occur. Theoretically, this method of prophylaxis should be almost 100% effective. Unfortunately, sometimes it fails to prevent immunization of the mother.

- The dose of Rh-immune globulin may be too small; the standard 300-μ dose will protect against 30 ml Rh-positive fetal whole blood during transplacental hemorrhage.

- The Rh-immune globulin may not be administered, as after a first pregnancy resulting in early spontaneous abortion without hospitalization.
- The potency of a vial of Rh-immune globulin may be decreased.
- The patient may be already immunized by an early transplacental hemorrhage.

Because immunization of the mother can occur from transplacental hemorrhages at any time after 8 to 10 weeks of gestation, Rh-negative women should receive Rh-immune globulin under the following conditions:

- As prophylaxis in an unsensitized woman at 28 weeks
- After a spontaneous abortion—the risk of transplacental hemorrhage is low if a dilation and curettage is not performed
- After an induced abortion with uterine manipulation
- In pregnancy when early separation of the placenta occurs
- During amniocentesis, where the risk of transplacental hemorrhage depends on the location of the placenta and the skill of the operator
- In nonpregnant women, following a mismatched blood transfusion

The standard dosages of Rh-immune globulin are:

1. 50-μg, which is indicated for
   - Spontaneous abortion
   - Induced abortion
   - Ectopic pregnancy
   - Amniocentesis
2. A 300-μg dose is indicated for
   - Premature delivery
   - Term delivery

Implications for Nursing Care

With the advent of Rh-immune globulin, more and more of the focus of nursing care for the Rh-negative mother is on monitoring laboratory values during pregnancy.

During the prenatal period, monitoring the Rh-negative mother for Rh antibody titer is performed at 24, 28, 32, 36, and 40 weeks. Even when titer tests are negative, the American College of Obstetricians and Gynecologists recommends that Rh-immune globulin be administered at 28 weeks to protect against the effects of early transplacental hemorrhage. It is the nurse's function to ensure the patient is crossmatched with Rh-immune globulin. Coordination with the laboratory for the injection "set-up" is necessary. The patient returns for intramuscular

injection after the immune globulin becomes available from the laboratory.

If a mother becomes immunized, her management focuses on close monitoring of fetal well-being, as reflected in Rh titers, amniocentesis results, and sonography. The mother may exhibit no effects, whereas the infant may become progressively anemic.

The woman and her family must be given informative, clear explanations of the problems. The mother's anticipated care must be discussed so that she can participate in it fully. Discussion of current testing and treatment is often reassuring to the family that feels helpless and often guilty about the threat to the unborn infant. The nurse should closely observe and assess family dynamics and intervene with support and counseling as appropriate.

When in labor the Rh-negative mother should be crossmatched for Rh-immune globulin to be given (depending on the protocol of the setting) within 72 hours after delivery. The nurse should be aware that disruptive events, such as placental abruption, may warrant a dose of Rh-immune globulin greater than the usual 300 μg.

If the mother has become sensitized and some degree of erythroblastosis fetalis is evident, the labor nurse should alert the neonatal team to be present at delivery to care for the newborn. Rh-negative blood will be available so that the infant can be transfused at once. Immediate laboratory studies will be done to determine the infant's hemoglobin and hematocrit levels and blood type. If type-specific blood is not used for the transfusion, type O Rh-negative blood may be used. This blood does not contain antibodies and does not hemolyze the infant's blood.

If the infant is hydropic, he or she must be immediately transferred to the nursery intensive care unit for evaluation and care. (See Chapter 34.)

The nurse plays an important role in informing the family, in terms they can understand, about the condition of the infant.

INCOMPETENT CERVIX

An incompetent cervix is unable to support the increasing weight of a pregnancy. As pregnancy progresses, dilatation and effacement of the cervix occur and may result in spontaneous abortion.

Etiology

The cervix is primarily composed of connective tissue that has a fibromuscular junction located between the cervix and the body of the uterus. This junction is the internal os of the cervix and the portion weakened by trauma. Factors that predispose to cervical incompetence are the following:

- Previous second-trimester spontaneous abortion
- Previous difficult delivery
- Cervical conization or biopsy

Once the cervix has been sufficiently damaged by one or more of these factors, pressure from subsequent pregnancies may cause the internal os to dilate. This dilatation is usually painless, and the patient may be unaware of what is happening. However, some women experience uterine contractions between 16 and 20 weeks of gestation that may be noticed as low back pain. When a patient complains of pain to her care-provider, a bimanual examination should be performed to check for dilatation of the internal os.

Treatment

When incompetent cervix is verified, a cerclage procedure to place an encircling suture around the cervical os is performed. A cross-section of the cervix after cerclage (McDonald's procedure) is shown in Figure 19–2. The suture is left in place until close to term. It is then removed, and labor allowed to begin spontaneously. This procedure must be repeated with each pregnancy. Even though it is simple to place the suture, the procedure is not without risk. Bed rest for 24 hours must be maintained to quiet an irritable uterine response to cervical manipulation; patient activity is increased gradually over the period of a week. Scarring and stenosis of the os occasionally result from the suturing and render the cervix incapable of dilating after the suture is removed. When this happens, a cesarean delivery is necessary.

The Shirodkar procedure also uses a purse-string ligature to maintain a closed cervix during pregnancy. When the woman wants and anticipates future pregnancies, the ligature can be left in place permanently, and subsequent births can be by cesarean delivery.

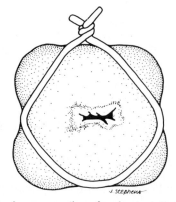

Figure 19–2. A cross section of an incompetent cervix showing a cerclage suture in place. The suture is removed at term to allow cervical dilatation and delivery. (Childbirth Graphics)

Implications for Nursing Care

The nurse may be alerted to the risk of incompetent cervix by reviewing the patient's history for significant factors, such as

- Previous preterm delivery
- History of middle-trimester abortion
- History of surgical or obstetric trauma to the cervix

In general, dilation associated with incompetent cervix is a silent event. Following cervical suturing the patient is maintained on bed rest for several days and will be slowly ambulated to increase activity. This will allow time for the nurse to explore the patient's reaction to the procedure and to respond to her queries. Listening to the fetal heart tones may reassure the patient and her family that the baby is doing well.

FIRST-TRIMESTER BLEEDING/ABORTION

Vaginal bleeding occurs in approximately 50% of all pregnancies, and pregnancy loss with early bleeding episodes is a primary concern in the first trimester.

Etiology

The incidence and cause of early pregnancy loss is difficult to determine, but the rate of spontaneous abortion may be as high as 20% or more. The rate is highest during the first 10 weeks of gestation and decreases to 3% by the 20th week. When bleeding occurs in the second and third trimesters, the risk to the mother and infant is much greater. Despite the numerous influences that may cause early pregnancy loss, most pregnancies proceed to term without difficulty.

Abortion is the termination of pregnancy before the conceptus reaches 20 weeks of gestation, a mass of 500 g, or a crown–rump length of 18 cm. In about 60% of spontaneous abortions, the causes are multiple and include abnormal embryonic development, chromosomal defects, and inheritable disorders. Maternal factors that can cause abortion are abnormal uterine development, systemic disease, endocrine or nutritional problems, and immunologic deficiencies. Environmental factors, such as drugs, radiation, or trauma, also play a role in pregnancy loss.

Types of Abortion

Threatened Abortion.   The pregnant woman experiences slight bleeding that may persist for several weeks and is accompanied by uterine cramping and pain. No cervical dilatation or effacement occurs, and no tissue is passed. If the bleeding persists, little can be done except to advise bed rest for 48 hours.

(text continued on page 497)

NURSING CARE PLAN

The Woman Experiencing Spontaneous Abortion

Nursing Diagnosis (Patient Problem) and Assessment Data	Nursing Interventions	Rationale
Probable Complication: *spontaneous abortion* • Vaginal bleeding is present in first 20 weeks • History of abortion • Complains of cramping and lower abdominal pain	Assess history of past pregnancies, length of bleeding, its amount (number of pads and their saturation), the appearance of the blood or discharge: Does it contain tissuelike material? Are uterine contractions being experienced? How often, how intense, what pattern, and what has the woman done at home to control contractions? Advise patient to seek immediate care if tissuelike material is passed. Prepare the patient for pelvic examination. Carefully explain the cause of abortions and possible outcomes.	Management will include careful speculum examination to assess cervical dilatation, amount of bleeding, extrusion of tissue from cervical os. Sonography may be ordered to assess fetal viability when bleeding persists. Suction evacuation of the uterus may be necessary when abortion is inevitable or incomplete.

Expected Outcome:

Woman seeks professional care and responds to treatment by maintaining pregnancy. Woman responds to nursing teaching regarding diet, rest, and iron supplementation as evidenced by her verbal confirmation of interventions and rationale and physical recovery from abortion.

Nursing Diagnosis: *grieving related to pregnancy loss*	Reassure the couple that the bleeding is not the result of any maternal behavior. Offer emotional support and advice about convalescence. Recommend several days of rest.	Parents should take time to recover and acknowledge their loss, as well as to recover from physical stress.
	Offer contraceptive counseling to delay pregnancy until the woman has recovered.	Early conception before maternal physical and psychological recovery may predispose to later problems.

Expected Outcome:

The patient and family demonstrate behaviors associated with normal grieving without signs of morbid grief reaction.

(continued)

The Woman Experiencing Spontaneous Abortion

Nursing Diagnosis (Patient Problem) and Assessment Data	Nursing Interventions	Rationale
Potential Complication: *infection*		
	Suggest avoidance of intercourse until after the next menses. Condoms can be used when necessary.	Vulnerability to uterine infection is increased at this time.

Expected Outcome:

Woman remains free of signs of infection through the first subsequent menstrual period.

Potential Complication: *anemia*		
	Recommend iron supplementation, increased dietary intake of iron.	Rebuild the woman's iron stores, which may be depleted by heavy bleeding.

Expected Outcome:

Woman responds to iron supplementation by maintenance of normal blood values.

Potential Complication: *maternal sensitization*		
• Rh-negative mother	RhoGAM is ordered and given to all Rh-negative women after abortion.	Leakage of fetal blood into the maternal circulation is possible. RhoGAM is given to prevent maternal sensitization, and resulting complications in later pregnancies.

Expected Outcome:

Woman accepts and understands need for RhoGAM.

Nursing Diagnosis: *fluid volume deficit related to heavy vaginal bleeding*		
	Obtain orders for IV fluids. Monitor vital signs; obtain lab studies (CBC, type, and cross).	Hemorrhage and shock are rare but serious complications of SAB.

(continued)

NURSING CARE PLAN (continued)

The Woman Experiencing Spontaneous Abortion

Nursing Diagnosis (Patient Problem) and Assessment Data	Nursing Interventions	Rationale
	Prepare for surgery.	Dilation and curettage may be necessary to stop bleeding.

Expected Outcome:

Woman maintains fluid volume balance as demonstrated by maintenance of normal vital signs and hydration.

Inevitable Abortion. When the abortion reaches the inevitable stage, the cervix is soft and its os is dilated, bleeding may be profuse, and abdominal cramping begins to resemble the pain of labor. Fetal size is consistent with dates, but its loss is certain.

Incomplete Abortion. When the products of conception are only partially evacuated during abortion, the abortion is incomplete. Tissues that remain in the uterus contain portions of the fetal membrane or placenta. Bleeding and cramping continue and become more severe. Prolonged retention of the tissues predisposes the woman to infection, and immediate medical intervention is needed.

Complete Abortion. When the entire products of conception (fetus and placenta) are passed, abortion is considered complete. Following the abortion, there is relief from pain and the bleeding usually stops. This type of abortion is more likely to occur early in gestation.

Missed Abortion. When the fetus dies *in utero* but remains, along with the placenta and tissues, in the uterus, a *missed abortion* has occurred. Pregnancy symptoms abate, but amenorrhea continues. When the patient is unaware that a missed abortion has occurred and it is not detected within about 2 months by the health care providers, coagulopathy may occur, causing life-threatening illness.

Treatment

When pregnancy has been diagnosed, the presence of uterine bleeding, uterine contractions, and uterine pain are ominous signs and must be considered as indicating a threatened abortion, until proved otherwise. Even when a woman possesses these signs, the diagnosis of inevitable abortion may be difficult to make. Ultrasound is highly reliable in determining the presence of a viable gestational sac but cannot predict the continued viability of the pregnancy.

For the clinician, the pregnant woman, and her family, early vaginal bleeding calls for "watchful waiting." When the cervical os is determined to be closed by vaginal examination, treatment is conservative. Women are usually advised to maintain bed rest — the decreased physical activity *may* help to maintain the pregnancy. Equally important, the woman feels that she is doing everything possible to avert the loss of her pregnancy. When bleeding persists, weekly sonograms are continued to ascertain whether the pregnancy is still viable.

Many abortions occur at home. In those where the products of conception are contained within an intact sac, complete membranes are present, and bleeding has stopped, no surgical intervention is indicated.

Inevitable and incomplete abortions are managed by evacuation of the uterus in the simplest, safest, and most effective manner. Before 12 weeks of gestation, this is accomplished by suction curettage followed by sharp curettage to ensure that all gestational tissue has been removed from the uterus. The tissue specimen from the evacuation must be carefully examined for completeness. When there is doubt about its completeness or normalcy, it should be sent to the histology laboratory for further examination.

Implications for Nursing Care

The woman and her partner benefit from considerate and careful explanation of the nature of the abortion and its possible future ramifications. When the nurse is in-

497

SELF-CARE TEACHING

The Patient Who Has Had a Spontaneous Abortion

- Bleeding should be minimal—heavy bleeding may indicate retained tissue or infection
- A scant dark discharge may persist for 1 to 2 wk
- To avoid infection, abstain from intercourse until bleeding has stopped

volved before medical intervention is necessary, she can advise the couple that bed rest is the major factor in retaining the pregnancy. She should also assure them that abortions are common and that most have no relationship to maternal behavior.

Regardless of the means, the patient who has recently aborted needs emotional support and advice about her convalescence. As with normal labor and delivery, several days of rest are necessary to recover. Iron supplementation should be advised when large amounts of blood have been lost. See the Self-Care Teaching display on this page.

When the patient is Rh-negative, the necessity for an intramuscular dose of 50 μg Rh (D antigen) immune globulin is explained and the dose is given. When necessary, contraceptive advice can be offered to couples who may want to delay or avoid another pregnancy.

ECTOPIC PREGNANCY

In ectopic pregnancy the fertilized ovum implants outside the cavity of the uterus—in the fallopian tube in 95% of the cases. Other rare implantation sites are the abdomen, cervix, ovary, and the wall of the uterus. Ectopic pregnancy is a life-threatening condition presently responsible for 12% of maternal mortality, up from 6% a decade ago.

Etiology

This increase can be accounted for by the growing number of reproductive-aged women who have pelvic inflammatory disease (PID), have had tubal surgery, or use the IUD (see Chapter 8). All of these can lead to tubal adhesions and delays in ovum transport.

When ectopic pregnancy occurs, the woman first experiences symptoms of bleeding and pelvic pain soon after the first missed period, when she may still be unaware of her pregnancy. The space within the lumen of the tube is small, and the growth of the embryo quickly distends the tube to capacity, causing it to rupture within the first 12 weeks of pregnancy. During pregnancy, the

NURSING ALERT

The Patient With Possible Ectopic Pregnancy

The nurse must be alert to the possibility of an ectopic pregnancy in a woman who reports a missed menstrual period, spotting, pelvic pain and who has a history of IUD use or pelvic inflammatory disease. A serum pregnancy test should be performed, and sonography may be ordered to detect uterine contents.

Should the patient complain of faintness and shoulder pain, the nurse must alert the physician immediately. These are signs of internal bleeding irritating the phrenic nerve, and signal a possible ruptured ectopic pregnancy. Monitor vital signs, obtain orders of IV fluids, blood type and crossmatch, and facilitate transfer for immediate surgery.

tubal environment becomes highly vascular, and hemorrhage resulting from tubal rupture is considerable and life-threatening.

Treatment

When ectopic pregnancy is diagnosed before it has become critical, life-threatening bleeding and emergency surgery can be avoided. Women who seek early gynecologic care when they experience amenorrhea associated with pain or bleeding can be diagnosed before the condition becomes an emergency. Correct diagnosis can be made by pregnancy testing in conjunction with sonographic identification of a gestational sac outside the uterus. These findings will also help to rule out pelvic infection, appendicitis, and ovarian cysts, which commonly present with the same symptoms.

Management of ectopic pregnancy consists of surgical removal of the affected tube. If the uninvolved tube is patent, saving the involved tube is not essential, since fertility is preserved in the remaining tube.

Implications for Nursing Care

In a prenatal health care setting, the nurse may be instrumental in identifying women who are at risk for ectopic pregnancy. A history of pelvic infection, IUD use, or tubal surgery should alert the nurse to the risk. In conjunction, the symptoms of amenorrhea, abdominal pain, spotting, and the presence of a pelvic mass located in the area of the adnexa make immediate referral for medical intervention imperative. In women who are experiencing internal hemorrhage, symptoms of ectopic pregnancy also include vertigo, shoulder pain (from diaphragmatic irritation of the phrenic nerve caused by intraperitoneal blood, which is dispersed in the abdomen when the patient is lying down), a decreasing blood pressure, and increased pulse rate. These symptoms signal an emergency situation.

The nurse should swiftly refer the patient to a physician when she has the slightest suspicion of an ectopic pregnancy. Not until the pregnancy is diagnosed can she provide presurgery counseling or discuss what her suspicions might be. When the patient has been informed by the care-provider that she has an ectopic pregnancy, the nurse should be available to talk with the patient to help her to understand what is happening and what the treatment will be. She is also in a good position to reassure the woman that although she will only have the use of one tube after surgery, she will still be fertile because the other tube remains intact. When possible, the nurse should visit the patient after the operation to offer her support.

HYDATIDIFORM MOLE

Bleeding in early pregnancy may also result from the growth of a hydatidiform mole, a developmental anomaly of the placenta. Hydatidiform mole occurs about once in every 2000 live births in the United States. It is found more frequently in Asia, the South Pacific, and the Philippines. In 85% of the cases the mole is benign and needs only close follow-up.

Etiology

The mole, which is a placental tumor, develops after a pregnancy has occurred. For unknown reasons, the embryo dies *in utero* but the placenta continues to grow rapidly. The trophoblastic cells continue to grow, become aggressive, and form an invasive tumor. The tumor (mole) is characterized by proliferation of placental villi that become edematous and form grapelike clusters; absence of blood vessels; and absence of a fetus and amniotic sac within the uterus. Since trophoblastic cells are responsible for the production of HCG, a pregnancy test will register positive even though the fetus is dead. High amounts of HCG in the blood also cause the woman to experience exaggerated symptoms of pregnancy, including the following:

- Severe nausea and vomiting
- Signs of preeclampsia, such as elevated blood pressure and proteinuria (these may help to diagnose the mole)
- Hyperthyroidism (about 8% to 10% of cases)

Symptoms due to molar mass include the following:

- Absence of fetal movement or heart beat
- Passage from the vagina of grapelike clusters

- Uterine size larger than expected for dates (50% of cases)
- Anemia out of proportion to blood loss
- Adnexal masses caused by luteal cysts
- Pulmonary embolism from large amounts of trophoblastic tissue transported to the lungs (rare)

Treatment

Diagnosis of molar pregnancy by sonography is 98% accurate. As soon as the diagnosis is made, the uterus should be evacuated by suction (vacuum) curettage. Sharp curettage should follow to ensure that the molar tissue has been removed completely.

Following curettage, the patient is monitored regularly for HCG levels to ensure that no molar tissue remains. HCG levels are obtained at weekly intervals, and in uncomplicated cases, the HCG value should return to 0.1 mIU/ml by the 10th to 14th week after evacuation. To ensure long-term remission of growth, HCG levels are monitored once a month for a year. Pregnancy is contraindicated during this period because the high levels of HCG associated with it could stimulate the growth of any remaining molar tissue. Birth control pills are the method of choice for contraception, since they suppress pituitary luteinizing hormone (LH), which may interfere with HCG monitoring.

Not all hydatidiform moles follow such a benign course. Some 15% continue to proliferate and become invasive; 5% develop choriocarcinoma. These are life-threatening events and require chemotherapy, constant vigilance, and expert medical attention.

Implications for Nursing Care

In a prenatal setting, the most important contribution the nurse can make to the assessment of the patient is history-taking and the physical examination. Molar pregnancy is relatively rare and its diagnosis is elusive. However, a history of amenorrhea, the presence of symptoms described above, and the physical finding of an adnexal mass should alert the nurse to inform the physician immediately.

Women with molar pregnancy and their families need to understand and deal with the possible consequences of the disease and the necessity for a long and tedious course of treatment. The nurse can discuss with them and help them deal with the many issues surrounding pregnancy loss, recognition that the pregnancy was abnormal, and the need to postpone a subsequent pregnancy. The woman will need to be able to discuss her grief, anger, or fear. Fifteen percent of patients with hydatidiform mole will progress to either an invasive mole or choriocarcinoma. Therefore, the nurse should carefully explain the symptoms that may indicate exacerbation of the mole.

These include irregular vaginal bleeding, spitting up blood, severe and persistent headaches, and persistent secretion from the breasts (galactorrhea).

SECOND-TRIMESTER BLEEDING

Many bleeding problems originate in the first trimester but may continue into the second trimester. An example of this is the hydatidiform mole in which pregnancy loss occurs in the first trimester but diagnosis may not be made until well into the second trimester. As many as 15% of spontaneous abortions happen in the second trimester. There are common problems of the second trimester that may have their origins in the growth and development of the placenta and fetus during the first trimester. Among these is placenta previa.

Placenta Previa

Growth of the placenta within the uterus normally takes place in the upper body of the uterus, well away from its lower segment. In placenta previa, on the other hand, the placenta implants and develops in the lower uterine segment and encroaches on or covers the internal cervical os. When labor begins and the cervix dilates, the placenta is torn from its implantation site and exposes open, bleeding blood vessels.

Classification of placenta previa is based on the proximity of the placenta to the cervical os, which is the direct determinant of the risk of hemorrhage to the pregnant woman. Four degrees of placenta previa are recognized, as shown in Figure 19–3.

- *Total:* the placenta completely covers the internal cervical os
- *Partial:* the placenta partially covers the internal os (central)
- *Marginal:* the edge of the placenta lies at the border of the os
- *Low-lying:* the placenta is very near the region of the os

During labor, the classification of previa may change as cervical dilatation progresses.

Etiology

The incidence of placenta previa is one in 300 deliveries. Among the important factors that place women at risk for placenta previa are the following:

- Age greater than 35 and multiparity. The effect of age is the most important and accounts for one third of the cases. Of women experiencing placenta previa, 80% are multiparous.
- Prior placenta previa. The incidence of placenta previa among women who have already had one is 12 times the general incidence.

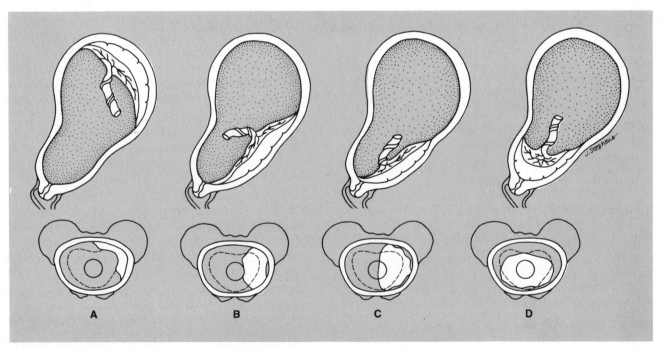

Figure 19–3. Placental positions. *(A)* Normal position. *(B)* Low implantation. *(C)* Partial placenta previa. *(D)* Total placenta previa. (Childbirth Graphics)

- Incidence increases in women who have recently had a dilatation and curettage.

The etiology of placenta previa is not known. It is believed that when the development of the vasculature in the uterine fundus is deficient for any reason, the placenta implants at a lower level, where the blood supply is more conducive to its growth. A large, thin placenta may develop in an attempt to increase perfusion. Fetal erythroblastosis and multiple pregnancy may also give rise to a large placenta that may approach a previa condition. Factors that predispose to low placental implantation include previous uterine scarring, the presence of uterine tumors, faulty implantation, endometritis, and large placentas. Low placental implantation may lead to abnormal fetal presentations because of fetal accommodation to the altered space. The pathophysiologic process underlying placenta previa appears to be related to conditions that alter the normal function of the uterine decidua and its vascularization.

The cardinal sign of placenta previa is painless vaginal bleeding in women carrying pregnancies until midterm or later. Bleeding occurs without warning and often happens during sleep without a precipitating factor.

The degree of placental placement over the internal os determines the severity of the bleeding and the onset of the initial episode. Women with central previa will have the first onset of bleeding by 28 to 30 weeks of gestation. The first episode of bleeding is never severe enough to be fatal to the mother or infant. The amount of bleeding varies, and bleeding may cease for some time after the initial episode. In about 90% of women, however, there will be a subsequent, life-threatening hemorrhage.

Diagnosis of placenta previa is safest and is 97% accurate when the location of the placenta is determined by sonography. When the placenta is determined to be normally placed, placenta previa is not the problem and other causes of bleeding must be investigated. When the placenta can be clearly visualized, the radiologist can frequently determine the degree of previa. This information is extremely important to the continued management of the patient.

Treatment

When an episode of bleeding occurs in a patient who is in the late second trimester or early third trimester, a conservative approach to treatment is usually taken. The risk associated with delivery at this stage is considerable, since the infant weighs less than 2500 g and pulmonary maturity is still weeks away.

The patient is admitted to the hospital and placed on strict bed rest. She is carefully observed for further bleeding. It is essential that nothing be placed in the patient's vagina, since further bleeding could easily be caused by manipulation of the cervix. When bleeding stops, the pa-

tient may be kept a further 24 hours in the hospital and ambulated. If no further bleeding occurs, she may then be discharged, provided she follows certain precautions:

- She has immediate transportation to the hospital available at all times.
- She reports to the hospital at once if there is further bleeding.
- She will not have intercourse or place anything in her vagina until after delivery.

Implications for Nursing Care

See Chapter 28 for discussion of inpatient nursing care of women with bleeding (placenta previa, abruptio placentae) in pregnancy.

MULTIPLE GESTATION

The incidence of 1 in 200 births of monozygotic (identical) twins is the same throughout the world. The prevalence figure for fraternal twins, calculated from records of live births in the United States, is 1 in 80. However, studies using diagnostic ultrasound during the first trimester of pregnancy indicate that the conception rate of twins is two to four times greater than the number of twins born. This phenomenon occurs because one fetus fails to develop and becomes resorbed during the second trimester.

Etiology

Identical twins develop genetically from the "splitting" of a monozygote. In humans, the splitting occurs before the 15th day of conception. After this time, splitting cannot occur because of the advanced development of the embryo. Since, in monozygotic twinning, two embryos develop from the identical genetic material of one sperm and one egg, monozygotic twins are always of the same sex and are said to be mirror-images of each other. They develop within a common chorionic sac and have a common placenta, although each develops its own amnion and umbilical cord.

Fraternal twins develop from two ova that are fertilized at the same time. The tendency to have fraternal twins is hereditary and may be passed by either the father or mother, but is expressed only by daughters. Secretion of higher levels of follicle-stimulating hormone (FSH) in these daughters results in occasional multiple ovulations and conceptions. Although from the same genetic pool, fraternal twins have separate gestational sacs and placentas and develop as differently as other siblings.

Another possible variation in "splitting" may produce triplets and quadruplets. Occasionally the splitting process is incomplete and conjoined twins result. This occurs in 1 in 50,000 pregnancies.

The incidence of multiple gestations has increased in recent years because of the increased use of fertility drugs. High doses of these drugs cause multiple ovulations (and possible conceptions).

Maternal/Fetal Implications

Perinatal mortality resulting from twin births is as high as 14%, the greatest mortality resulting from premature birth. Twins sharing the same amniotic sac may entangle umbilical cords, causing the death of one fetus. In monozygotic twins, direct communication of fetal blood vessels may occur, resulting in a "transfusion syndrome." When this happens, one infant, called the *recipient twin,* is large, edematous, and polycythemic. The second, *donor* twin remains small and anemic because its blood is being shunted to its sibling. If the small twin survives, it will require postdelivery transfusion. The transfusion syndrome increases the probability that both twins will suffer permanent, debilitating sequelae. If the donor twin dies *in utero,* the surviving twin will develop normally. After death, the donor twin becomes progressively compressed *in utero* and assumes a fossil-like configuration known as *fetus papyraceus.*

Nursing care of mothers with twin pregnancies should be focused on monitoring prenatal events and maintaining optimum maternal health. During prenatal assessment, there are indicators of multiple pregnancy, including

- Excessive nausea and vomiting
- Larger uterine size than expected, especially after 20 weeks of gestation
- Polyhydramnios (excessive amniotic fluid in the uterus)
- A rapid drop in hemoglobin value
- Signs of developing pregnancy-induced hypertension
- Palpable small fetal parts in all quadrants of the abdomen
- Fetal movement felt in all quadrants by the mother

Fetal heart beats at two different sites and at two different rates are a strong indication of twins, but are difficult to detect even during late pregnancy. If twin pregnancy is suspected, regardless of the gestational age, diagnosis should be confirmed by ultrasound.

Prenatal care of a woman with a twin pregnancy requires knowledge of the problems that may arise and an alertness to early signs of problems. The mother is at risk for the six Ps: *P*reeclampsia, *P*rimary anemia, *P*ressure, *P*lacenta previa, *P*rematurity, and *P*ostpartum hemorrhage. Additionally, a seventh P, *P*sychological concern, is equally important.

Treatment

In addition to the usual monitoring of prenatal care, special attention to the following aspects of care is imperative.

- Determination of maternal weight gain
- Evaluation of blood pressure
- Prevention of anemia by dietary and iron supplementation
- Frequent evaluation of the hemoglobin and hematocrit
- Administration of nonstress testing to assess fetal response, beginning at 37 weeks
- Evaluation of fetal lung maturity at 36 or 37 weeks
- Ultrasound determinations, in late pregnancy, of size and positions of the fetuses

Women who are at risk for hypertension or other problems may be placed on bedrest in an attempt to increase uterine perfusion (to supply more oxygen and nutrients to the fetuses), to increase fetal weight, and to prolong the length of pregnancy to allow greater fetal maturity.

Implications for Nursing Care

The pregnant woman can do much to improve the quality of her pregnancy and enhance its outcome. It is a function of nursing care to supply the woman with information to help her achieve these goals. The pregnant woman should be advised to

- Rest several times each day, for about a half-hour, in the left lateral recumbent position. This position lifts the uterus from the major blood vessels that lie directly behind it and results in increased blood flow to the uterus. The placenta receives increased amounts of maternal blood, transmission of nutrients and oxygen to the fetuses is increased, and excretion of waste products is facilitated. This position also helps to increase kidney function and aids removal of excess water from the body.

- Avoid excessive intake of salt. Excessive salt accumulated in the body, especially during pregnancy, causes fluids to be retained in the interstitial spaces. Generalized edema may result and cause edema of the hands and feet and increase the workload of the heart and kidneys, with a possible end result of increased blood pressure.

- Increase intake of fluids to eight glasses a day. Increased ingestion of fluids in conjunction with resting in the left lateral recumbent position, helps to flush fluids from the body. Since kidney function is enhanced, more fluids reach the bladder to be expelled more frequently. As a result, the woman may complain of urinary frequency. When no urinary tract infection exists, she can be reassured that this is not only healthy but helpful.

- Maintain adequate nutrition. Requirements for calories, protein, minerals, vitamins, and essential fatty acids are increased in women carrying twins. Increased nutrient needs of the fetuses require an additional 300 kcal or more of food and energy sources. These should be high-quality calories such as those found in a well-rounded diet that contains all the food groups. Nutritional counseling is extremely important for these women and should be supplied by the nurse or the nutritionist, as appropriate. Since there are two babies and the mother's additional needs to consider, nutritional counseling must be explicit, careful, and thorough.

- Monitor contractions. Self-evaluation of uterine contractions for detection of preterm labor is discussed later in this chapter.

When the expectant mother has been properly coached about what she can expect during the prenatal course, she is more likely to follow suggestions supplied by the nurse. Most women are intent on doing whatever is necessary to increase the likelihood of healthy, mature infants.

As term approaches, the mother will be anxious about the method of delivery to be used. In twin pregnancies, this depends on many factors, including the following:

Mother's previous obstetric history

Mother's health

Week of gestation that labor begins

Estimated size and presentation of infant

Progress of labor

Intrapartum aspects of care are discussed in Chapter 28.

PRETERM AND POST-TERM LABOR

As pregnancy nears completion, prelabor changes may be noted by the patient and clinician. Mild, irregular contractions affect the dilatation, effacement, position, and consistency of the cervix. The actual mechanisms that initiate the labor process are still not understood, but labor normally occurs between 37 and 42 weeks after the last menstrual period (LMP). However, 10% of pregnant women experience labor before the 37th week of gestation, and 5% to 8%, after the 42nd week. Since early and late delivery both pose risks to the infant, the terms used to designate these phenomena have been changed in an

attempt to provide more accurate descriptions. The terms *preterm labor* and *post-term labor* are now used widely. Yet they remain unsatisfactory, because it is often difficult to calculate the beginning of pregnancy when the LMP is unknown. Great care must be used when attempting to correlate early pregnancy findings based on the LMP and uterine size as determined clinically and sonographically.

Preterm Labor

Labor that begins before the 37th week of pregnancy is known as *preterm* labor. Preterm birth, therefore, refers to any delivery between 20 and 37 weeks of gestation.

Preterm labor and birth is the greatest single problem in contemporary obstetrics; 75% of perinatal mortality and 85% of neonatal deaths are attributable to complications resulting from preterm delivery. Among those preterm infants who survive, long-term sequelae and motor and intellectual handicaps are found. Preterm labor occurs in 6% to 7% of pregnant women in the United States; the incidence is 10% to 11% among the black population. This higher incidence is believed to be related to socioeconomic factors rather than racial ones.

Etiology

Although the cause of preterm labor is still unknown, multiple medical and social factors have been related to an increase in preterm births (see the display below).

Risk Factors for Preterm Labor and Birth

Medical Factors

DES exposure

Uterine anomaly

Prenatal bleeding

Multiple gestation

Previous preterm labor or birth

Cervical dilatation >2 cm by 32 wk.

Previous cone biopsy/incompetent cervix

Multiple spontaneous or therapeutic abortions

Social Factors

Poor nutrition

Alcohol abuse

Drug addiction

Cigarette smoking

Restricted access to prenatal care

In addition, recent research suggests that a variety of social and physical factors may place a woman at increased risk for preterm labor. These factors provide the basis for risk reduction strategies that may assist in extending the length of gestation in about 50% of women assessed to be at risk for preterm labor (Creasy 1984).

Risk Reduction Strategies for Preterm Labor

When a woman has been assessed as at risk for preterm labor, the following strategies should be implemented to increase her chances of delivering a mature infant.

The pregnant woman should be counseled to

- Recognize the signs and symptoms of preterm labor and to seek obstetric care immediately when they occur
- Maintain a schedule of regular weekly prenatal check-ups to allow ongoing assessment of cervical status and uterine activity
- Curtail work activities and maintain bed rest as prescribed
- Refrain from sexual intercourse and orgasm (sexual stimulation and uterine contractions associated with orgasm may trigger labor)
- Restrict travel outside her immediate community in case labor ensues
- Optimize her health by maintaining an adequate diet, taking prenatal vitamins or iron, practicing good hygiene, and avoiding people with infectious diseases

Obstetric practices to delay labor in high-risk pregnant women include the following:

- Patients with multiple gestations are placed on bed rest during the last trimester to extend gestation as long as possible.
- Patients with known placenta previa are placed on bed rest. If bleeding occurs without fetal jeopardy, blood replacement may be indicated to maintain optimal maternal status until delivery.
- Patients with a history of pregnancy losses due to incompetent cervix should have surgical therapy (cerclage) early in the second trimester to avoid spontaneous cervical dilatation.
- Patients with symptomatic leiomyomas are placed on bed rest and given analgesics for pelvic pain; surgical intervention is delayed as long as possible.
- If labor ensues, attempts to suppress it should include hospitalization, IV hydration, and tocolytic therapy.
- Fetal maturity must be carefully evaluated before delivery is allowed.

Preterm labor is differentiated from "false labor" or Braxton Hicks contractions in that the uterine contractions of preterm labor result in cervical change. However, if a woman is experiencing painful uterine contractions without evidence of cervical change, she should be closely monitored; if contractions continue for 1 hour and begin to produce cervical effacement, threatened preterm labor is diagnosed (Creasy 1984).

Maternal Implications

Maternal risks in preterm labor and birth, at least in terms of physical problems, are not considered high. Risks are, however, associated with a variety of treatment modalities for preterm labor, such as tocolytic therapy and prolonged bed rest.

The emotional stress of preterm labor and worry about fetal status is significant, not only for the mother but also for her partner and their entire family. It is not uncommon for parents to feel anger and guilt, alternately blaming themselves and the pregnancy or fetus for this profound disruption of their lives. The woman is likely to become anxious and depressed, if her preterm labor is only minimally controlled with tocolysis. Preterm labor causes the woman to focus intently on her body and its failure to perform normally, since she must closely monitor uterine activity during the course of therapy; this can be especially stressful when she has few diversions with which to occupy her mind during hospitalization.

Stress may be intensified in families in which the woman must be hospitalized for an extended period after being managed at home on bed rest for some time. These couples have already experienced considerable disruption in their daily lives, including their household routines, income (if the woman was forced to give up paid employment), and emotional and sexual relationship. The woman is likely to worry about her partner and how he is managing at home, especially if there are other children. His stress may, in fact, be significant if he is employed and has little or no assistance in managing the household and little social and emotional support in coping with the threat of his partner and their unborn infant.

Families may also experience intense stress when the mother's physiologic condition is deteriorating. Situations where preterm delivery is needed to improve maternal status but will directly threaten chances for fetal well-being may be especially difficult for families whose religious or moral beliefs prohibit placing the unborn in jeopardy.

Fetal/Neonatal Implications

Preterm labor and birth pose great risk to the fetus and neonate, and neonatal outcomes depend in large part on the quality of perinatal care. Mortality is increased among preterm infants and is especially high among those born at less than 32 weeks of gestation. As mentioned before, prematurity is responsible not only for nearly two-thirds of neonatal deaths but for increased long-term morbidity as well.

The major threat to neonatal survival is respiratory distress syndrome resulting from lung immaturity. Other threats include immaturity of other organ systems, lack of fat storage, problems in thermoregulation, and increased risk of intracranial trauma and hemorrhage during delivery. (See Chapters 33 and 34 for further discussion of the care of the preterm infant.)

Treatment

Once the patient is identified as at risk for preterm labor, her management includes increased rest, increased fluids, good nutrition, increased prenatal surveillance and, if indicated, tocolytic therapy.

Increased prenatal surveillance minimally consists of biweekly prenatal visits with cervical examination. In the very high-risk patient, it may consist of daily at-home monitoring with a portable tocodynamometer for the detection of contractions. Home monitoring combined with daily telephone follow-up by the perinatal nurse or weekly public health nursing visits seem to improve patient reporting and early detection of symptoms (Iams et al 1987).

Therapy to suppress preterm labor may be successful, but should be initiated before moderate cervical change has occurred. Once the cervix has effaced beyond 60% and reached 4 cm of dilatation, the chances of arresting labor for any significant duration are diminished.

Because of the specialized care required by the preterm neonate, maternal transport to a tertiary care center may be arranged so that optimal care during delivery and intensive neonatal support are available.

Therapy to suppress preterm labor includes bed rest and the use of drugs called tocolytic agents. Beta-sympathomimetic agents are most commonly used for tocolysis. Central nervous system depressants may also be used intravenously. Ethanol, or magnesium sulfate may be used in combination with other tocolytic drugs, or when there are contraindications to their use. These agents are discussed in more detail in Chapter 28.

When preterm labor can be suppressed by hospitalization and tocolytic therapy, the mother may be discharged home on a regimen of bed rest and oral tocolytics. Some settings are now using telemetric antenatal monitoring, which allows the mother to monitor uterine activity for periods of time at home and transmit findings via telephone to a receiving station in the inpatient setting, where the data are analyzed by a physician or nurse; if worrisome levels of uterine activity are detected, phone contact can be made immediately with the mother to advise changes in her home regimen or immediate evaluation and possible hospitalization. (Inpatient aspects of preterm labor treatment are discussed in Chapter 28.)

Implications for Nursing Care

There is general agreement that improved neonatal outcomes are more likely if emphasis is placed on identifying women who are at risk for preterm labor, teaching them how to recognize early signs, and treating them when preterm labor is suspected. For this reason, all pregnant women should be instructed on how to recognize warning signs of preterm labor. Thus, an important nursing responsibility is patient education regarding signs and risk factors for preterm labor.

Once preterm labor is diagnosed and treatment is started, an important element of nursing care is the ongoing support of the woman and her family, since treatment may last 10 to 15 weeks, depending on the time of diagnosis.

When the woman first experiences the import of preterm labor, she is anxious for her own welfare and for that

SELF-CARE TEACHING

Preterm Labor Symptoms

The following symptoms should be reported to the careprovider without delay:

- Uterine contractions that may be felt as abdominal tightening with or without pain
- Menstrual-like cramping, often rhythmic and felt just above the pubic bone
- Pelvic pressure or fullness noted in pelvic area, back, or thighs
- Intestinal cramps with or without diarrhea
- An increase in vaginal discharge; the consistency may change from mucousy to watery
- A general feeling that something is wrong

If you feel any of the warning signs follow the following steps:

- Lie down and place a pillow at your back so that it tilts you on to your left side.
- Place your fingertips on each side of your abdomen (about the level of your umbilicus) so that you can press and feel differences between tightness and relaxation of the uterus.
- If you feel tightening, you are having a contraction. Use your watch to time the length of the tightening and the minutes until another tightening occurs.
- If, after an hour, you continue to have four or more contractions per hour, call your doctor immediately or go to the labor and delivery unit.
- If you have a large amount of clear fluid or pink or brown discharge call your doctor immediately.

NURSING CARE PLAN

The Woman at Risk for Preterm Labor

Nursing Diagnosis (Patient Problem) and Assessment Data	Nursing Interventions	Rationale
Nursing Diagnosis: *altered health maintenance related to self-care and risk factors for preterm labor*		
	Discuss with the patient the findings from her history that may cause early labor.	Although the woman with a high-risk score will not always deliver preterm, she must be made aware of the possibility. She will need to participate in her care by self-monitoring and maintaining frequent prenatal visits.
	Provide handouts on preterm labor and discuss its signs and symptoms.	When the cervix is dilated more than 2 cm, or is over 60% effaced, a diagnosis of preterm labor is made.

Expected Outcome:

The patient verbalizes an understanding of the treatment regimen for preterm labor, and demonstrates ability for appropriate self-care at home with assistance.

Potential Complication:
preterm labor

• Patient complains of pelvic heaviness, cramping, backache, or increased vaginal discharge. • Cervical dilatation is greater than 2 cm.	Advise bed rest at home and list events that might precipitate contractions. Assess patient's ability to identify contractions. Assess patient's ability to identify contractions. Assist patient to identify support systems to be used at home. Advise patient about dosage, scheduling, and side effects of drugs she is to take. Provide referral to public health nurse for support and teaching.	Bed rest is needed to counter the effects of gravitational pull, increase blood perfusion, and reduce uterine activity. Patient must know how to assess contractions, what restriction of activities is necessary, and how to take medications. She must be aware of the importance of monitoring contractions and the necessity of weekly prenatal visits. Additional support may be needed to enable women to maintain this regimen until delivery is safe.

Expected Outcome:

Patient complies with treatment regimen and delivers healthy, full-term baby.

of the unborn baby. The psychologic stress with an increase in catecholamines further compromises the pregnancy (Carney 1984). The nurse should provide realistic support, providing information about what is occurring and reassurance that all that can be done is being done. After the initial shock, the woman feels anger and guilt. She is angry this is not the idealized pregnancy she had imagined. She feels guilty because she invariably believes she did something to cause labor. The nurse needs to first be a good listener and then provide appropriate information.

If the woman is receiving beta-sympathomimetics, she should be informed that the medication may cause her to feel emotionally labile. (See Chapter 28 for a discussion of tocolytic therapy.) This is sometimes difficult to handle when the experience of preterm labor is, in itself, emotionally difficult.

For women on long-term treatment, the medication routine, the bed rest, and perhaps the home monitoring routine, cause them to feel they have lost control over their body and their independence. Hostility or passive-aggressive behavior in the form of noncompliance may be an initial reaction.

Home-based therapy usually leads to social isolation, boredom, and depression. Daily or weekly contact gives the nurse an opportunity to suggest ways to relieve the woman's isolation. Most importantly, women should be encouraged to use the telephone to keep in contact with friends and family on a daily basis. They should invite close friends to their home, so that the patient can rest and visit from a couch, instead of her bed, for a change of environment.

The nurse should also be alert for counseling needs concerning changes in the patient's relationship with her husband or needs for child care when bed rest at home is required.

Post-term Labor

Post-term labor refers to labor that occurs after 42 weeks of gestation. The terms *postdate* and *postmaturity* are also used. Postmaturity is identified by specific characteristics that can be found on physical and neurologic examination of the newborn, and therefore it cannot be determined until after the delivery. Postmaturity, which occurs in 20% to 40% of pregnancies exceeding 42 weeks, poses known risks to the fetus. Because of these risks, accurate dating of the pregnancy is important and, as with preterm labor, attempts should be made to correlate LMP and clinical uterine size with support from sonography. Pregnancy can be dated most accurately when dating is begun early.

In pregnancies that extend beyond 42 weeks, the incidence of fetal distress and sudden fetal death rise sharply. Infants who are also small for gestational age (SGA) or large for gestational age (LGA) are especially at risk; the highest rate of fetal death occurs during labor secondary to meconium aspiration (see Chapters 33 and 34).

Treatment

Once the pregnancy is thought to be past 40 weeks of gestation, close surveillance of the fetus begins. Every 5 to 7 days, fetal well-being is evaluated to determine whether the pregnancy can safely be continued. Tests vary depending on the facilities available, but include those discussed in Chapter 17.

The cervix is examined weekly to determine its preparedness for labor. As the cervix prepares for labor, or "ripens," it moves from a posterior to a midposition, its consistency softens, effacement greater than 50% occurs, and dilatation of the cervical os measures 1 to 2 cm. Labor can be induced at this time if necessary.

Implications for Nursing Care

When testing for fetal well-being begins, the nurse needs to reassure the mother. The patient is anxious to deliver, and is concerned for the health of her infant. Testing requires frequent visits to the health facility, blood tests, and fetal monitoring. Without being caused anxiety, the patient needs to understand the importance of keeping these appointments. The patient should be given anticipatory guidance about what tests are to be performed, why they are necessary, and what the anticipated outcome will be.

When the patient has not delivered by the end of the 42nd week, she will be admitted to the hospital for induction of labor (see Chapter 26 on labor induction). The nursing emphasis in labor induction is on close monitoring of oxytocin drip, on maintaining uterine contractions at a safe level, on supporting the mother, and on closely monitoring fetal well-being, with continuous internal fetal monitoring being preferred.

The procedure for induction of labor is the same as that discussed in Chapter 26 for oxytocin intravenous infusion. If there is any indication of fetal distress during induction, the neonatal team should be present at delivery. Since meconium aspiration is the most common problem, any evidence of meconium-stained fluid calls for laryngoscopic examination of the vocal cords for evidence of aspiration. A high cesarean delivery rate can be expected because of failed induction secondary to cephalopelvic disproportion, unripe cervix, or fetal distress.

Following delivery, the infant should be observed for signs of hypoglycemia, respiratory distress, and seizures.

HYPERTENSIVE DISORDERS OF PREGNANCY

Hypertension in pregnancy wears many faces and is a condition that is not always discernible or well understood. It has been known since the pre-Hippocratic period as a convulsive disorder. In 1596 convulsions of pregnancy were attributed to epilepsy, and not until 1739 were convulsions differentiated from epilepsy and called *eclampsia*. In 1843 Lever discovered that proteinuria occurred with eclampsia in pregnancy and confused it with nephritis. Eclampsia continued to be thought of as a renal disease until the 1940s. In the late 1930s, essential hypertension was recognized in pregnancy, with residual hypertension occurring in the postpartum period. *Preeclampsia* became the term used to designate women with hypertension, proteinuria, and edema but without convulsions. Although they are misnomers, preeclampsia and eclampsia have remained the terms used to refer to the classic triad of hypertension, proteinuria, and edema.

Today, the term *pregnancy-induced hypertension* (PIH) is gaining in popularity, and *PIH* and *preeclampsia* are used interchangeably in this text. PIH, however, is still an inadequate description. In fact, hypertensive disorders of pregnancy encompass many facets that are poorly understood. The term is used to describe women in the following classes:

- Women diagnosed and treated for hypertension prior to pregnancy but who had no known underlying disease
- Women found to have underlying renal or cardiovascular problems
- Women with no prior history who developed hypertension during pregnancy, which resolved in the postpartum period

Incidence

Pregnancy-induced hypertension (PIH) occurs in 5% to 7% of all pregnancies. It is the third leading cause of maternal death in the United States and is a major cause of perinatal morbidity (especially intrauterine growth retardation) and mortality. Hypertensive disorders, including preeclampsia, eclampsia, and postpartum eclampsia, may develop insidiously or dramatically and affect nearly every maternal organ system. Women with these complications of pregnancy require specialized prenatal care as well as expert intrapartal care to optimize maternal and neonatal outcomes.

PIH is characterized by intermittent vasospasm and accompanying hematologic changes, deposition of fibrin and fibrinogen in the vessels, tissue ischemia and hypovolemia due to a shift of fluid from vascular to extravascular spaces, and increased central nervous system irritabil-ity. Although this disorder typically develops antenatally and improves rapidly after delivery, eclampsia may develop during the postpartum period as well.

The incidence of hypertensive disorders in pregnancy in the United States is approximately 6%, but in reality there are wide variations. Geographic, ethnic, and racial factors play a role. Primigravidas are six to eight times more likely to develop PIH than are multiparas. Chronic hypertension is three to four times more prevalent in black than in white women. Additionally, there is a familial predisposition to the development of preeclampsia. In one study, 25% of daughters of mothers who had had preeclampsia developed preeclampsia themselves, whereas only 6% of daughters-in-law developed the disease (Chesley 1981).

Maternal/Fetal Implications

Regardless of the cause, hypertension in pregnancy places the mother and infant at increasing risk as pregnancy progresses. Although there is a low incidence of maternal fatalities, mothers face the risk of eclamptic seizures, cerebral vascular accidents, cardiopulmonary insufficiency, renal shutdown, coma, DIC, and death. For the developing infant, PIH is often associated with intrauterine growth retardation and increased mental retardation in surviving infants. Infant death may result from hypoxia and prematurity.

Intermittent vasospasms seem to be a major underlying alteration that leads to much of the pathophysiology of the disease. Fluid shifting from the vascular system into intracellular spaces results in tissue ischemia as well as hypovolemia. Although the triggering mechanism and the order of progression of the illness are not well understood, its influence on the major systems has been determined from tissue biopsy and other laboratory studies. Despite these major alterations, recovery is usually complete after delivery, with return of normal function to all major systems. Table 19–1 lists pathophysiologic changes observed in major organ systems. Changes basic to all these systems are tissue ischemia, vasospasms, and fibrin/fibrinogen deposits in the vessels' walls.

Depending on the severity of the disease, a variety of symptoms may be observed. However, the disease is defined by the classic triad of hypertension, proteinuria, and edema.

On the basis of studies that demonstrate physiologic changes, a blood pressure reading of 140/90 is deemed to be a hypertensive state for an adult. In fact, blood pressure varies according to race, age, weight, heredity, and other factors. A more accurate assessment of hypertension in pregnancy is achieved if it is defined as an elevation of 30 mmHg systolic and 15 mmHg diastolic pressure from the baseline or prepregnant blood pressure.

The presence of proteinuria is determined from a urine

(text continued on page 511)

NURSING CARE PLAN

The Patient With Mild Pregnancy-Induced Hypertension

Nursing Diagnosis (Patient Problem) and Assessment Data	Nursing Interventions	Rationale
Potential Complication: *pregnancy-induced hypertension*		
Risk factors: • Primigravidity • Multiple pregnancy • Vascular disease • Familial tendency • Severe malnutrition • Hydatidiform mole • Polyhydramnios • Diabetes mellitus • Maternal age <18 or >35	Prenatal assessment includes recording blood pressure to establish a baseline. At each subsequent visit, check the patient's weight and blood pressure, and check for the presence of edema and proteinuria	Assessment enables ongoing evaluation of changes in patient's health. During the second trimester systolic blood pressure decreases by 2–3 mm Hg and diastolic by 5–10 mm Hg because of blood volume expansion. As a result, a rise of blood pressure may be significant even if the nonpregnant 140/90 limit of abnormality is not reached
	Obtain a nutritional history on the first or second visit.	Many pregnant women are at nutritional risk. Early identification of risk and nutritional counseling may help to avoid or decrease problems associated with malnutrition, such as PIH and anemia.

Expected Outcome:

The at-risk patient responds to appropriate prenatal and nutritional care before symptoms develop.

Probable Complication: *pregnancy-induced hypertension*		
• Rising diastolic blood pressure	Alert physician of an increase of 30 mm Hg systolic and a 15 mm Hg diastolic over the baseline	In the presence of other symptoms, this increase is diagnostic for PIH
• Proteinuria	Readings of 1+ or 2+ may be persistent and need to be identified and reported	Early diagnosis/treatment of urinary tract infection or possible kidney damage is important.
• Edema	When dependent edema is not resolved after a night of sleep, the height the edema rises (*e.g.,* sacrum) should be noted	Physiologic edema is difficult to differentiate from generalized edema and must be carefully assessed.
• Hyperreflexia	Hyperreflexia may be elicited and noted.	Hyperreflexia is more significant in conjunction with other positive symptoms. Clonus appears with severe PIH.

(continued)

The Patient With Mild Pregnancy-Induced Hypertension

Nursing Diagnosis (Patient Problem) and Assessment Data	Nursing Interventions	Rationale
• Excessive weight gain	Assess weight gain at each prenatal visit.	The normal weight curve is a 10-lb weight gain at 20 weeks with 0.5-lb gain per week until 40 weeks. In PIH weight gain usually exceeds 30 lb by the third trimester.
• Headache, visual changes	In early PIH warn the patient about these changes and the importance of seeking immediate care.	Blind spots, photophobia, or blurred vision indicate severe PIH

Expected Outcome:

The patient with PIH responds to treatment as evidenced by maintenance of normal blood pressure, weight gain, and no signs of fetal compromise until delivery can be accomplished.

Potential Complication:
compromised placental perfusion

	Assess uterine growth relative to gestational age.	Decreased fetal growth may be suspected when McDonald's measurements are less than expected for gestational age.
		Premature calcification and decreased blood flow to the placenta may result in intrauterine growth retardation and decreased fetal movement when PIH is severe.
	Facilitate nonstress testing, ultrasound, amniocentesis.	Tests assess fetal growth and placental function.
		Amniocentesis can be used to determine fetal lung maturity when delivery is being considered.

Expected Outcome:

The patient with PIH maintains normal uterine growth and demonstrates no signs of compromised fetal status.

Nursing Diagnosis:
knowledge deficit related to self-care for PIH

	Explain to the client any medication ordered. If edema is present, order	When the client is aware of her increasing symptoms and the necessity for

(continued)

NURSING CARE PLAN (continued)

The Patient With Mild Pregnancy-Induced Hypertension

Nursing Diagnosis (Patient Problem) and Assessment Data	Nursing Interventions	Rationale
	bed rest on left side. Teach the client and family about the danger signs of PIH. Determine if family knows how to get emergency service. Teach the family how to provide care. Help the family plan for needed homemaking activities. Identify ways the client may avoid boredom. Consult with the visiting nurse for close supervision.	complete bed rest and continued assessment of fetal health, she will better understand the importance of maintaining bed rest and medication regimen. Additional support may be needed to allow maintenance of bed rest and safe care at home.

Expected Outcome:

The patient verbalizes an understanding of the treatment regimen for PIH and demonstrates ability for appropriate self-care at home with assistance

---

dipstick test of a clean-catch or catheterized specimen. A reading of proteinuria (1+) on two or more occasions should be followed by a 24-hour urine collection so that the total amount of protein can be quantified.

The presence of significant edema is determined both by the amount of edema present in a specific tissue area and by the extent to which edema is found at various body sites. Initially, edema is noted in the most dependent parts of the body, such as the feet and ankles, and extends up to the knees and the sacrum. Hands usually swell at about the same time as feet and ankles, whereas facial and generalized edema are late signs.

Although still described as mild, moderate, or severe, PIH is a progressive condition, as reflected by the symptomatology presented in Table 19–2.

Treatment

Screening for PIH occurs at each prenatal visit. The patient is weighed, blood pressure is recorded, and the urine checked for protein. By establishing a baseline of these values and taking into account expected patterns in pregnancy, the care provider can better assess any subse-

quent change. Without a prepregnant or first-trimester blood pressure reading, it is difficult to assess the meaning of blood pressure changes in the second and third trimesters. It is important to remember that the blood pressure normally decreases in the second trimester (systolic by 2 to 3 mmHg and diastolic by 5 to 10 mmHg) secondary to blood volume expansion. As a result, the patient may have a significant rise in blood pressure without reaching 140/90.

Careful assessment of total and interval weight gain in conjunction with knowledge of the patient's eating habits will help in evaluating the edema associated with rapid weight gain. Examination of the legs and ankles for evidence of dependent edema enables the clinician to grade the degree of edema present. Pressing the skin against a bony part, such as the ankle or tibia, for 30 seconds and then examining the depth of the indentation determines whether the edema is classified as trace, +1, +2, and so on. The hands often become swollen at the same time as the feet or shortly thereafter. Edema of the face is a more ominous sign. The severity of edema can also be judged by whether edema is present in the morning or evening.

Table 19-1   **Pathophysiologic Changes in Preeclampsia/Eclampsia**

Organ	Change
Kidneys	Endothelial cells become swollen
	Amorphous material is deposited in cytoplasm
	Glomerular capillaries become narrow
	Glomerular blood flow diminishes
	Glomerular filtration rate decreases
Liver	Most common lesion is hemorrhagic necrosis
	Vessel compression and extravasation may occur
	Fibrin clots may form, with systemic hypercoagulability.
	There is high risk for disseminated intravascular coagulation
	Hemorrhage under the liver capsule may occur
	Intra-abdominal bleeding may occur, causing an acute surgical emergency
Lungs	Pulmonary edema may occur
	Diffuse hemorrhagic bronchopneumonia may occur
	Heart may be affected, causing impaired cardiac reserve, arrhythmia, and rapid pulse
Placenta	Signs of premature aging may appear
	Tissue degenerates and calcifies
	Thrombosis of arterioles may occur
	Intervillous spaces may become congested

Dependent edema caused by decreased circulatory return from the lower extremities usually results in evening edema. This edema often diminishes when the legs are elevated. The patient should sleep in the supine position to assist circulatory return to the heart. Generalized edema may be indicated by an indentation left on the abdomen from the pressure applied by the fetoscope or by residual indentation after pressing for 30 seconds on the sacrum.

Protein (albumin) molecules are large and usually will not pass through the renal filtration system. Most proteins excreted in the daily output of urine are globulins. Therefore, proteinuria indicates that the kidney has been assaulted in some manner. The cause may be an acute or chronic infection, renal abnormalities, or the arteriospasms of PIH. Trace proteinuria is never an indicator of PIH. If the urine dipstick test shows a trace of protein, contamination from vaginal secretions must be considered and a repeat, clean-catch specimen must be examined. The patient should be questioned about the possible presence of excessive discharge, burning or itching, or change in vaginal odor that would suggest vaginal infection. The urine specimen should be retained for culture, if necessary. The definitive evaluation of the degree of proteinuria is a quantitative analysis of a 24-hour urine collection. Nonpregnant women rarely excrete more than 150 mg of protein per day, whereas normal pregnant women often excrete more. A level of 500 mg (0.5 g) is accepted as the upper limit of normal in pregnancy. When total protein is being determined, analysis for creatinine clearance is also performed on the 24-hour specimen to rule out renal disease as a cause of proteinuria. Urinalysis and culture eliminate the possibility of infection.

Implications for Nursing Care

The purpose of frequent and careful assessment during the perinatal period is the prevention of PIH. The only known "cure" for PIH is delivery. Except in the most severe cases, the patient's laboratory values usually return to normal within 48 hours after delivery. The objective of prenatal care is to detect early indicators of PIH for prompt intervention to forestall further complications and promote health maintenance.

When the patient's blood pressure rises persistently, she is instructed to begin resting on her side for a period of 2 hours in the afternoon, in addition to 8 hours rest at night. Resting in the left lateral position will aid circulatory return to the heart, since in this position the large blood vessels are not constricted by the weight of the enlarged uterus. The patient should refrain from resting on her back to avoid supine hypotensive syndrome. Resting also promotes blood perfusion to the kidneys, increasing urinary output and decreasing edema. Antihypertensive therapy may also be ordered (see Table 19-3).

During World War I, a low incidence of preeclampsia was noted during pregnancy, and led to the belief that a decreased protein intake reduced the incidence of preeclampsia. Pregnant women were advised that weight gain should be restricted to a maximum of 16 to 20 pounds. It is now known that neither of these approaches is valid. In recent years, Dr. Thomas Brewer has written extensively about the importance of good nutrition in reducing the tendency to hypovolemia and hypoperfusion. A shift of protein from the intravascular to the extravascular spaces during pregnancy results in increased edema. Although the mechanisms are poorly understood, they have been related to diet. A nutrient intake that approximates the RDA allowance for pregnancy not only seems beneficial, but also teaches sound nutritional habits to women who are feeding growing families.

Excessive intake of nutrients is *not* recommended. Excessive sodium intake is probably the most common failing of the American diet. With the increase in glomerular filtration rate in pregnancy, the amount of sodium filtered through the kidney is increased. The renin-angiotensin-aldosterone system compensates by retaining sodium in the body. Therefore, the RDA sodium intake during pregnancy is 1100 to 3300 mg/day. Excessive sodium intake over prolonged periods has been identified as a significant factor in the development of hypertension. Studies suggest that if salt intake is kept at low levels, 20% fewer salt-sensitive individuals may develop hypertension in

Table 19-2   **Signs and Symptoms of Pregnancy-Induced Hypertension (PIH)**

Sign	Early PIH	Mild to Moderate PIH	Severe PIH
Blood Pressure	Rising diastolic pressure, especially in second trimester, but still within normal limits	Increase of 30 mmHg in systole and 15 mmHg in diastole over baseline or reading between 140/90 and 160/110	Over 160/110
Proteinuria			
Qualitative, dipstick test	Absent	May still be absent +1 or +2 reading may be sporadic or persistent	+3 to +4 reading persistent
Quantitative, 24-hr analysis	Not indicated	0.5 to 2.5 g total protein lost in 24 hr (variable)	5.0 g or more each 24 hr
Edema	Absent	If present, difficult to differentiate from physiologic edema Present in hands, feet, and ankles	Generalized and noticeable in face; classic facies of coarse features, broad nose, puffy eyes
Reflexes	Unchanged from normal baseline of +1 to +2	May be hyper-reflexion; +3, brisk No clonus	Hyper-reflexion Clonus
Total weight gain	Within normal range, or greater than 2 lb/wk in absence of other signs	2 lb/wk or more Greater than 6 lb/month	2 lb/wk or more Usually total gain over 30 lb in third trimester
Gastric/epigastric function	No problems	Impossible to distinguish from indigestion caused by increasing uterine size	Nausea and vomiting Epigastric pain (classic warning sign of imminent seizure)
Central nervous system function	No signs	No signs	Headache Visual changes: blind spots, photophobia, blurred vision
Renal function	No signs	Proteinuria	Impaired renal function Oliguria (output less than 30 ml/hr)
Placental function	No signs	Decreased blood flow	Decreased blood flow Significant premature calcification found on ultrasound
Fetal well-being	No signs	Decreased fetal growth, established by baseline ultrasound	Intrauterine growth retardation Decreased fetal movement

later life. These facts and recommendations indicate that excessive sodium should be eliminated from the diet.

Increased fluid intake goes hand-in-hand with reduced sodium intake. Adequate fluid intake will help to maintain optimal fluid volume, interact with sodium and the intravascular and extravascular shifts, and aid renal perfusion and filtration. The recommended intake is eight to ten glasses of fluid per day. This quantity of fluid intake is easily recommended but laboriously achieved. Water is preferable because it lacks calories and sodium. But water is boring. To enhance compliance, the nurse may suggest

• Diet soda — no calories but 30 mg sodium
• Iced tea — no sugar added or with sugar substitute
• Lemon-lime seltzer — no calories but 10 mg sodium

When other drinks are recommended they should contain some nutrients if they are caloric. Fruit juices are good.

Avoid fruit-flavored drinks that are high in sugar but lack nutrients. Artificially added vitamin C is not a good substitute for fruit.

When a patient is being monitored for early signs of PIH, a baseline sonogram should be obtained. Then, interval sonograms can be done as indicated to detect intrauterine growth retardation (IUGR). If hypertension persists or the sonogram indicates changes consistent with IUGR, weekly nonstress tests may be performed to assess placental sufficiency (see Chapter 17).

If all of the above recommendations have been followed and the patient with PIH has not improved with increasing bed rest, hospitalization may be necessary. Since the definitive treatment of preeclampsia is delivery, the physician must evaluate the status of the mother and infant to determine the feasibility of delivery. (See Chapter 28 for a discussion of inpatient nursing care of patients with severe PIH.)

Table 19–3   **Drugs That May Be Indicated in Control of PIH in Outpatient Care**

Drug	Dosage	Indications and Adverse Reactions	Nursing Implications
Antihypertensives			
Aldomet (methyldopa)	500 to 1000 mg orally q.i.d.	Drug is indicated in essential hypertension and used for outpatient maintenance. It is also an adrenergic blocker with many systemic side effects. Its safety in pregnancy is not established, but no specific fetal effects are known.	Regular interval readings are needed during period of adjustment. Initial sedative effect is beneficial to maintaining bedrest with PIH. Drug may enhance orthostatic hypotension. Observe for symptoms of mental depression. Tolerance may occur in 2 to 3 wk of therapy, indicated by rise in blood pressure. This must be reported to physician. Compliance tends to be poor because of drug's many side-effects. Encourage patient to keep appointments.
Hydrodiuril (hydrochlorothiazide)	50 to 100 mg orally daily	Drug may be used as first-line therapy for pre-existing hypertension. Usually patient is maintained on previous medications. Because of its diuretic action, drug may be discontinued if moderate or severe PIH develops. There are no known adverse effects to the fetus.	Advise patient to eat potassium-rich foods. Check potassium level with periodic serum electrolytes.
Anticonvulsants/Sedatives			
Valium (diazepam)	5 to 10 mg orally b.i.d.	This mild sedative and CNS depressant aids compliance with complete bedrest when patient is being treated at home. It reduces CNS stimulation with progressing PIH. Since it also depresses fetus, it should be discontinued several days before delivery.	If given within 24 hr of delivery, watch for flattened baseline or other changes on the fetal monitor indicating depression. Report such changes to physician.

CHAPTER SUMMARY

Pregnancy is a normal physiologic process. The family has every right to expect it will remain so. Complications in pregnancy cause the family stress, anxiety, and fear. The health care team expands in relation to the severity of complication. The nurse plays a pivotal role on the health care team by coordinating activities to achieve the care necessary for health maintenance throughout the pregnancy. She plays an advocacy role, serving as the person consistently available to the family and knowledgeable about the care. In this way, she strongly influences the family's childbirth experience.

STUDY QUESTIONS

1. List three clinical findings that may indicate the presence of twins.
2. The most common anemia is recognized by what signs or symptoms?
3. List foods other than meat that are rich sources of iron.
4. A woman is 10 weeks pregnant and comes to the emergency room with brown vaginal spotting. She asks if this means she is "losing the baby"? How will you respond?
5. Define the term *at-risk pregnancy*.

6. List five drugs that are contraindicated during pregnancy and state the adverse effect of each on the mother or fetus.

REFERENCES/BIBLIOGRAPHY

Barrows JJ: Nursing role in management: Blood pressure disturbances. In Lewis SM, Collier IC (eds): Medical – Surgical Nursing: Assessment and Management of Clinical Problems, 2nd ed, p 729. New York, McGraw-Hill, 1987

Bragonier JR, Cushner IM, Hobel CJ: Social and personal factors in the etiology of preterm birth. In Fuchs F, Stubblefield PG (eds): Preterm Birth: Causes, Prevention and Management. New York, Macmillan, 1984

Cagney EN: Nursing care during the treatment of preterm labor. In Fuchs F, Stubblefield PG (eds): Preterm Birth: Causes, Prevention and Management, p 288 – 97. New York, Macmillan, 1984

Chesley LC: Hypertension during gestation. In Iffy L, Kaminetsky HA (eds): Principles and Practice of Obstetrics and Perinatology, Vol 2, p 1268. New York, John Wiley & Sons, 1981

Creasy RK: Preterm labor and delivery. In Creasy RK, Resnik R (eds): Maternal – Fetal Medicine: Principles and Practice, p. 415 – 443. Philadelphia, WB Saunders, 1984

Dyson DC: Fetal surveillance vs labor induction at 42 weeks in post term gestation. J Reprod Med 33(3):262 – 269, 1986

Iams JD, Johnson FF, O'Shaughnessy RW et al: A prospective random trial of home uterine activity monitoring in pregnancies at increased risk of preterm labor. Am J Obstet Gynecol 157(3):638 – 643, 1987

Institute of Medicine: Preventing Low Birthweight. Washington, DC, National Academy Press, 1985

Main DM, Gabbe SG: Risk scoring for preterm labor: Where do we do from here? Am J Obstet Gynecol 157(4):789 – 793, 1987

Kelly JY, Iffy L: Placenta previa. In Iffy L, Kaminetsky HA (eds): Principles and Practice of Obstetrics and Perinatology, Vol 2, p 1105. New York, John Wiley & Sons, 1981

Mannino F: Neonatal complications of postterm gestation. J Reprod Med 33(3):271 – 276, 1988

Mannor SM: Hyperemesis gravidarum. In Iffy L, Kaminetsky HA (eds): Principles and Practice of Obstetrics and Perinatology, Vol 2, p 1155. New York, John Wiley & Sons, 1981

SUGGESTED READINGS

Barnes D, Perez L: An influx of hydatidiform moles. Female Patient 11(1):100 – 104, 1986

Bengman SL, Burns MK: Hypertensive crisis in L & D. AJNurs 88(3):325 – 328, 1988

Byce RL, Stanley FJ, Enkin MW: The role of social support in the prevention of preterm birth. Birth 15(1):19 – 23, 1988

Dilorio C: The management of nausea and vomiting in pregnancy. Nurse Pract 13(5):23 – 28, 1988

Dorfman SF: Ectopic pregnancy. Female Patient 11(2):121 – 129, 1986

Moleti CA: Caring for socially high-risk pregnant women. Am J Matern Child Nurs 13(1):24 – 27, 1988

Neidahardt A: Why me? Second trimester abortion. AJN 86(10):1188 – 1135, 1986

Prevention of perinatal transmission of Hepatitis B virus: Prenatal screening of all pregnant women for Hepatitis B surface antigen. MMWR 37(22):341 – 346, 1988

Snyder DJ: Peer group support for high-risk mothers. MCN 13(2):114 – 117, 1988

Wilson D: An overview of sexually transmittable diseases in the perinatal period. J Nurse Midwif 33(3):115 – 128, 1988

20 medical conditions complicating pregnancy

LEARNING OBJECTIVES

After studying the material in this chapter, the student should be able to

- Describe physiologic changes with specific complications of pregnancy

- Discuss the impact of specified medical conditions on pregnancy and identify the clinical signs of each

- Enumerate social and behavioral factors that may place women at risk for pregnancy complications

- Identify essential adjustments in nursing management based on the assessed condition

- Demonstrate an understanding of the nurse's role in anticipatory guidance and health teaching when pregnancy is at risk

KEY TERMS

Embolism

Glucosuria

Hyperglycemia

Hyperthyroidism

Hypothyroidism

Immunosuppression

Infant of Diabetic Mother (IDM)

Ischemia

Jaundice

Macrosomia

Myocarditis

Polyhydramnios

Sensitized

Thrombosis

Titer

Advancing technology has improved and prolonged the quality of life for those with chronic medical problems. It is not uncommon to see women in whom pregnancy is superimposed on a preexisting medical condition. Some of the medical conditions arise from imbalances or malfunctions of organ systems; some arise from exposure to infectious processes; and others result from social circumstances. At times the pregnancy and the condition interact, causing either the illness and/or pregnancy to deteriorate. Because this interactive effect is variable, it is imperative that the pregnancy be observed closely.

NURSING RESEARCH

Pregnancy Complicated by Chronic Illness

An exploratory study was conducted to examine how a group of chronically ill pregnant women managed their own medical risk factors associated with their pregnancies. Data were collected through four in-depth interviews (two prior to delivery and two subsequent to delivery), and by observations during prenatal visits, in the hospital, and at home.

Data were analyzed using techniques for qualitative data to generate a description of how women managed pregnancy with a superimposed chronic illness. Women described a process of assessing the risks and benefits of medical interventions, balancing these and controlling them through self-care measures. Factors that affected the woman's ability to accomplish this process included: her own knowledge about her illness and the treatment plan, the level of support available to her (such as financial, emotional), the stability of her illness, and the woman's own perceived sense of control over events and situations likely to increase risk.

Implications of this study center on the woman's need for information about her own illness, her pregnancy status, and the risks/benefits of proposed medical management. Women want healthy babies, and will do what they believe to be in their babies' best interest, even if that requires going against medical advice. Thus, establishing a trusting relationship early on with the chronically-ill gravida is essential to promote optimal health status. If such a relationship is established, the woman is more likely to be willing to negotiate with the health care team to reach a compromise beneficial for her and her unborn child.

Corbin J: Women's perceptions and management of a pregnancy complicated by chronic illness. Health Care Women Int 8:317–337, 1987

The nurse is challenged to apply the principles of sound maternity care to the specific patient needs presented by each of these conditions.

Preventive health care is the basis of nursing management. The objective is to guide and support the pregnant woman in achieving or maintaining optimal health for both herself and her fetus. The nurse employs anticipatory guidance and health education directed toward both the illness and the pregnancy. The nurse assumes the role of interpreter in helping the patient understand the "whys and wherefores" of her care. As the nurse has frequent or extended contact with the patient, she is often privy to the patient's concerns, uncertainties, and responses. In this regard, the nurse also assumes the role of a listener who provides both emotional and informative reassurance.

DIABETES MELLITUS

Diabetes mellitus is a chronic familial disease in which inadequate insulin production and/or utilization and faulty metabolism of carbohydrates, fats, and proteins result in hyperglycemia and glycosuria. Long-term systemic effects may result in microvascular and macrovascular changes and neuropathies. The four classic symptoms are polyphagia (increased appetite), polydipsia (increased thirst), polyuria (increased urine volume), and loss of weight and strength. Physiologic changes in metabolism resulting in increased serum glucose levels may exceed the renal threshold and glucosuria may result. When fats are oxidized faster than they are utilized, ketonuria may occur.

Hormonal influences can best be appreciated if they are divided into the first and second half of pregnancy. In the first 20 weeks of pregnancy, increases in estrogen and progesterone induce metabolic alterations causing:

- Hypertrophy of the pancreas with an increase in beta cells, which are the insulin-secreting cells in the Islets of Langerhans
- Increased liver glycogen
- Increased glycogen synthesis
- Suppressed gluconeogenesis
- Increased insulin action at the level of muscle and adipose tissue

As a result of these changes, the action of insulin is facilitated.

During the second half of pregnancy, observed changes in carbohydrate metabolism suggest insulin resistance. Increased levels of HCS (human chorionic somatomammotropin) cause peripheral insulin resistance. Circulating free cortisol overrides the action of estrogen and progesterone. As a result, increased metabolic activity breaks down more complex substances to make greater quantities of simple sugars available. These simple sugars cross the placenta, but maternal insulin does not. The hyperglycemic state stimulates the fetal pancreas to produce insulin and fetal hyperinsulinemia often results. This maternal–fetal dynamic has been identified as the possible etiology for fetal death, macrosomia, and delayed pulmonary development (Gibbons 1982).

Class A diabetes is also referred to as *gestational diabetes*. Gestational diabetes is defined as a state of carbohydrate intolerance with the onset or recognition occurring during pregnancy. This hyperglycemic response may not be restricted to pregnancy, as many women with gestational diabetes will develop overt diabetes in later life. All other classes of diabetes refer to age at onset and duration of overt insulin-dependent diabetes (see Classification of Diabetes in Pregnancy).

Maternal Implications

Before insulin was available, diabetic women were frequently infertile. Of those who conceived, one third died during pregnancy, and few infants survived. With insulin

Classification of Diabetes in Pregnancy

Class A	Patient with abnormal glucose tolerance test with normal fasting blood sugar Controlled with diet alone
Class B	Insulin-treated diabetic Onset after age 20 Duration less than 10 yr No vascular disease or retinopathy
Class C	Insulin-treated diabetic Onset between ages 10 and 20 Duration between 10 and 20 yr No vascular disease or retinopathy
Class D	Insulin-treated diabetic Onset before age 10 Duration more than 20 yr Retinopathy
Class E	Any pregnant diabetic with calcification of the pelvic vasculature
Class F	Any pregnant diabetic with diabetic nephropathy
Class R	Any pregnant diabetic with proliferative retinopathy

Queenan JT (ed): Management of High-Risk Pregnancy. Oradell, NJ, Medical Economics Books, 1980

control, fertility among diabetics equals that of the general population, and maternal health has shown significant improvement. Nevertheless, maternal and fetal complications are still seen today.

Infections are common in diabetic patients. In particular, urinary and vaginal infections are common in pregnancy. Asymptomatic bacteriuria is three times more common in the pregnant diabetic than in the general population, regardless of classification. Therefore, periodic urine culture screening of diabetics is recommended during the prenatal period. Prompt treatment with antibiotic therapy and follow-up culture is recommended if any infection is found.

Although various types of vaginal infections may be noted during pregnancy, *Candida* vaginitis is most frequently found in the diabetic patient. Recurrent *Candida* infections may alert the nurse to screen pregnant women for diabetes. During pregnancy, *Candida* vaginitis may recur, requiring repeated therapy throughout pregnancy.

The incidence of pregnancy-induced hypertension (PIH) is increased among diabetics, probably due to underlying renal disease caused by vasculopathy.

Diabetic ketoacidosis (DKA) occurs more frequently and at a lower blood glucose level during pregnancy. DKA is a serious metabolic aberration that generally occurs due to diminished glucose availability (from inadequate insulin levels) and is accelerated in the presence of infection. Prevention is almost always possible with careful urine testing for ketones, especially when an infectious process is present. Perinatal mortality may be as high as 50%–80% with DKA. Treatment includes intravenous insulin administration, rehydration and provision of glucose once serum levels fall to 200 mg/dl. Bicarbonate may be required to correct acidosis.

Fetal/Neonatal Implications
Problems of a more serious nature include

- Congenital malformations
- Hydramnios (excessive amount of amniotic fluid)
- Macrosomia (large body)
- Unexplained fetal death near term
- Respiratory distress
- Birth injury resulting from macrosomia
- Metabolic abnormalities

Fetal malformations result from hyperglycemia during the period of organogenesis (Lander et al 1967). When glycohemoglobin (HgA_1C) is elevated during the first 8 weeks of fetal development, there is an increased risk of fetal anomaly. With normal blood glucose and glycohemoglobin levels in this early period, fetal anomalies approximate that of the nondiabetic population at 2% to 3%.

Macrosomia is most likely to occur in women who are hyperglycemic and results from induced fetal hyperinsulinemia. Birth injuries are increased when fetal macrosomia occurs. The neonate is at risk for metabolic abnormalities such as hypoglycemia, which is caused by high circulating insulin levels at birth combined with acute glucose withdrawal as the umbilical cord is severed. Other metabolic abnormalities affecting the IDM include hyperbilirubinemia, polycythemia and hypocalcemia (See Chapter 34 for a discussion of nursing care for the IDM).

Hydramnios results from maternal hyperglycemia. If the woman is controlled to a euglycemic state, hydramnios may resolve.

Unexplained fetal death or intrauterine fetal demise (IUFD) is thought to occur as a result of accelerated placental maturation and breakdown. Thus, the fetal respiratory and metabolic needs may "outgrow" placental functioning.

Preconception Counseling for Diabetics

Preconception counseling is an important role for the nurse-educator. For the diabetic, Classes B through R, pregnancy counseling should begin 3 to 6 months before conception. The objective is to achieve euglycemia and thereby reduce the incidence of congenital malformations among infants of diabetic mothers (IDM). Goals during this time are directed toward

- Assessment of maternal vasculopathy
- Achieving strict diabetic control by intensive self blood glucose monitoring, nutritional adjustment, and insulin manipulation
- Providing genetic counseling
- Encouraging emotional and financial preparation for the intensive dual management of diabetes and pregnancy

Glucose monitoring during pregnancy is often more sophisticated and intensive than most patients have used prior to pregnancy. Adjustment to new equipment and frequent testing requires a period of exploration of differences between old methods and new ones. Monitoring periodic glycohemoglobin levels periodically becomes a motivator, when patients see the glycohemoglobin values moving closer to the normal range (Langer et al 1987).

Diabetic patients of long duration may be reluctant to alter their personally adjusted regimen of diet, insulin, and exercise for fear of "losing control" of their diabetes. Time and patience are essential ingredients in providing nursing education during this time. Barrier contraceptives should be used by the couple, until they have adapted to the new self-care regimen and achieved adequate blood glucose control.

Screening

The American Diabetic Association (1985) reports that selective screening based on clinical attributes or past obstetric history has been shown to be inadequate. Therefore, glucose screening for *all* pregnant women is recommended.

Screening is accomplished by determining the serum glucose level. Since gestational diabetes is evident in the insulin-resistant, altered metabolism of the latter half of pregnancy, screening is recommended between 24 and 28 weeks of gestation.

Patients who are at risk for gestational diabetes, such as those with glycosuria, macrosomia, hydramnios or other complications associated with gestational diabetes, should be screened early in pregnancy. If this initial screening is negative, the patient should be rescreened at 24 to 28 weeks' gestation. Currently, the preferred method of testing is the 50-g glucose load test. The patient is given 50 g of a concentrated glucose solution to drink. After an hour, a blood sample is drawn so that the serum glucose level can be determined.

For screening, no prior fasting is needed. Test values in excess of 112 mg/dl for whole blood or 130 mg/dl for plasma are an indication for further testing with the 3-hour oral glucose tolerance test (OGTT).

Before the glucose tolerance test is administered, the patient should be instructed to eat a high-carbohydrate diet (at least 100 g) for 3 days. The glucose values derived from the test may be calculated from either whole blood or plasma, and the range will vary slightly from one laboratory to another.

If two of the following serum glucose levels are exceeded, diabetes is diagnosed:

Fasting	105 mg/dl
1 hour	190 mg/dl
2 hours	165 mg/dl
3 hours	145 mg/dl

Although the urine is routinely checked for glucose at each prenatal visit, urine tests are never considered diagnostic for diabetes. Glucosuria results from alterations in glomerular filtration, with a lowering of the renal threshold for glucose. Urine testing for glucose is a gross screening tool and should be used only as an indication for further investigation.

Management

There are four basic principles to follow when managing the diabetic woman, as shown in the display, opposite. The management of the gestational diabetic and the man-

Principles of Management of Diabetes During Pregnancy

Principle 1: Strict control of maternal blood glucose levels
Principle 2: Prompt detection and treatment of maternal complications
Principle 3: Fetal surveillance, including diagnosis of fetal macrosomia
Principle 4: Avoidance of unnecessary premature delivery

Adapted from Gibbons JM: Diabetes in pregnancy. In Schnatz JD (ed): Diabetes Mellitus: Problems in Management. Menlo Park, CA, Addison-Wesley, 1982

agement of the insulin-dependent diabetic are different. To distinguish these differences clearly, management for each will be discussed separately.

Gestational Diabetes

The prognosis for the gestational diabetic is excellent when close prenatal surveillance is employed. The principles previously outlined in the display are implemented as follows.

Controlling Serum Glucose

Strict control of the serum glucose level is necessary. This may be accomplished through:

- Dietary control
- Regulated physical activity
- Insulin use, if necessary
- Monitoring of serum glucose levels
- Careful control of nausea and vomiting, if present

If nutritional therapy is insufficient to control blood glucose, insulin may become necessary. The most commonly used insulins are combinations of regular and NPH, or regular and Ultralente insulin.

Detecting and Treating Maternal Complications

Prompt detection and treatment of maternal complications protect the health of the mother and infant. The pregnancy should be especially monitored for:

- Asymptomatic bacteriuria
- Ketoacidosis
- Hypertension
- Hydramnios

Approximately one third of gestational diabetics will have significant bacteriuria without the presence of symptoms. Routine screening with clean-catch urine cultures and appropriate health teaching is the best way to prevent urinary tract infections. Even in the absence of symptoms, bacteriuria should be treated promptly.

Diabetics are particularly susceptible to ketoacidosis, since the fetus also uses glucose and amino acids. A bedtime snack and an adequate breakfast are essential to prevention, since ketoacidosis is most likely to occur during long periods of fasting. The presence of ketones in the urine may indicate the need for additional calories or insulin.

Diabetes is one of the many factors known to increase the incidence of PIH, probably because of early vasculopathy and affected renal function. Home blood glucose monitoring may be helpful in the assessment of hypertension. Proteinuria may occur due to nephropathy and thus make the diagnosis of PIH difficult.

Both hydramnios and macrosomia result from the alterations in metabolism associated with the combination of pregnancy and diabetes. Recent studies with strictly controlled diabetics have shown that these changes need not occur. The incidence can be reduced by adherence to Principle 1 — strict control of the serum glucose level.

Implications for Nursing Care

The newly diagnosed pregnant diabetic struggles with the acceptance of a medical problem that threatens the welfare of the unborn infant while demanding rigorous and continuous self-care. The success of this adjustment rests largely with the patient's ability to integrate the requirements of self-care into her usual daily activities. The nurse plays a key role in providing knowledge of the techniques of:

- Dietary adjustment
- Accurate self-glucose monitoring and recordkeeping
- Self-injection with insulin
- Preventing, recognizing, and treating insulin reactions and ketonuria

While a nutritionist is often the health-team member who teaches dietary adjustments, it is the nurse who is responsible for the ongoing assessment of patient compliance. The nurse should be familiar with the specific division of kilocalories for the required 24-hour intake.

In general, the modified carbohydrate diet totals 1800 to 2400 calories per day. The average diet for the pregnant diabetic consists of 20% of the calories from protein, 45% from carbohydrates, and 35% from fat. The diet should be tailored to the patient's usual preferences, as much as possible.

Accurate recordkeeping is necessary for ongoing assessments of adequacy of self-care. Some patients may use reagent strips for self blood glucose monitoring. Preferably, the patient will be using a glucose meter for a more accurate reading of glucose levels. It is well-documented that patients often do not keep a correct and accurate record of their daily glucose values (Langer and Mazze 1987). The nurse should attempt to discern if the blood glucose values are accurate and direct her care to whatever difficulties the patient is encountering.

Insulin-Dependent Diabetes

Pregnancy imposes a substantial burden on the insulin-dependent diabetic and her family. The normal physical and psychologic discomforts of pregnancy are magnified, and prenatal visits, unexpected hospitalizations, frequent testing procedures, and stringent limitations on physical activity require considerable adaptability and cooperation on the part of the patient's support system. Psychologic stress is intensified by the fear of congenital anomalies and intrauterine fetal death (IUFD). Hospitalization requires a sudden separation from the family. Referral to a distant specialized center intensifies stress. Yet, family members are often highly cooperative, even enthusiastic, and do all they can to promote a healthy outcome for mother and infant.

Controlling Serum Glucose

Prenatal visits are primarily for the purpose of achieving *strict control of serum glucose levels.* Insulin and dietary adjustments are based on the self blood glucose monitoring levels. Insulin and calorie needs will vary at different stages of pregnancy. For example, insulin requirements will markedly increase in the second half of pregnancy because the influence of the hormones tends to counteract the effects of insulin. Injections of regular and intermediate-acting insulin are divided into morning and early evening doses. Long-acting insulin may also be used with mealtime doses of regular insulin. Calories are carefully distributed throughout the day to balance the blood glucose. The patient who is noninsulin-dependent (diet-controlled) prior to pregnancy generally requires insulin therapy during pregnancy because of its diabetogenic effects.

Detecting and Treating Maternal Complications

Prompt detection and treatment of maternal complications are essential, since unrecognized or untreated maternal complications will most certainly result in an increased risk to the fetus.

Infections cause a rapid deterioration in the control of the diabetic and the development of DKA. In particular, asymptomatic bacteriuria occurs frequently, and early detection and treatment are important. If untreated, 25% of the cases of asymptomatic bacteriuria will progress to pyelonephritis, a condition associated with preterm labor.

Urine cultures should be obtained routinely. If the bacterial count is greater than 100,000, even asymptomatic patients should be treated vigorously with antibiotics until a repeat urine culture is sterile. Preventive care includes daily prophylactic antibiotics for the remainder of the pregnancy.

Infection predisposes the patient to ketoacidosis, which carries with it a high risk of intrauterine fetal death. If ketonuria is found, further investigation is required, since ketonuria is presumed to be a sign of ketoacidosis until proven otherwise. Patients who have an infection should check their urine at least 3 times daily for ketones.

Monitoring for Fetal Well-Being

Fetal surveillance is important throughout the pregnancy. Observations include evaluation for macrosomia, congenital anomalies, appropriate interval growth, and fetal lung maturity.

For antepartum testing, nonstress or contraction stress testing or biophysical profile may be used and testing generally begins at 32 weeks' gestation. The type of test used and the frequency of monitoring will be determined by the type of diabetes, degree of vasculopathy, previous obstetric history and present maternal status (see Chapter 17 for discussion of assessment of fetal well-being).

Preventing Prematurity

A balance must be struck between the principle of *preventing unnecessary prematurity* and preventing sudden fetal death by early delivery. This survival is most dependent on the maturity of the fetal lungs, which is assessed by testing the amniotic fluid.

The amniotic fluid is tested to determine the L/S ratio and whether PG is present. These tests are used to predict the infant's ability to ventilate once born. If results for both tests are favorable, the incidence of RDS is very slight (usually < 1%).

Implications for Nursing Care

The nurse is the coordinator of care and the advocate for the diabetic patient. As such, her responsibilities are vast and varied and may include:

- Testing the urine specimen for glucosuria and ketonuria.
- Scheduling the patient at intervals for a clean-catch urine specimen for culture
- Scheduling an ultrasound examination at 20 weeks and 32 weeks, unless otherwise indicated
- Providing appropriate laboratory slips for glucose screening

- Reviewing the patient's chart for previous test results and following up on all abnormal results
- Recording blood pressure and, if it is elevated over previous readings, retaking blood pressure
- Instructing the patient in preparation for various tests, including ultrasound, nonstress test, glucose tolerance test, and so on
- Making each visit a time for health teaching appropriate to the trimester of pregnancy, including
    - Understanding of diabetes
    - Self-care techniques
    - Nutrition
    - Support for a healthy pregnancy
    - Clarification of treatment options to assist the patient in making an informed choice
- Teaching the patient self-care techniques, including how to
    - Test blood glucose levels
    - Maintain the diabetic diet
    - Prevent, recognize, and treat hypoglycemia
    - Administer insulin
    - Test urine ketone levels
    - Recognize the symptoms of urinary tract infections
    - Maintain health and hygiene to prevent infections

Care of the diabetic patient is dependent on establishing a balance between nutritional intake, insulin, and daily activity. In pregnancy there is an increase in nutritional requirements, changes in glucose utilization and insulin effectiveness, and varying activity levels from full-time work to bed rest. The potential changeability of the diabetic condition requires the nurse to assess all three components of care.

Dietary Assessment.   The care of the pregnant diabetic requires the attention of a registered dietician (RD) for assessment, diet prescription, and patient teaching. The nurse may assess the following:

- Hour of rising and of retiring
- Eating pattern
- Ethnic influence
- Likes and dislikes
- Usual activities
- Food budget
- Other members of the household
- Who cooks and shops

The nurse should discuss any difficulties in adhering to the diet and seek further consultation with the RD.

Insulin.   The nurse should review the patient's log book, in which the patient records the results of glucose testing. She should note, in particular, if there are consist-

---

The Insulin Infusion Pump

The currently available insulin pumps are approximately the size of a pocket calculator. Most models are motor-driven syringes that run on rechargeable batteries. All pumps infuse only regular insulin through a catheter with a 26–27 gauge needle. The patient places the infusion set in the subcutaneous tissue every 1 to 3 days and tapes it in place. The pumps are set at an appropriate basal rate between 0.5 and 1.5 U/hr that is delivered in miniboluses of about 0.1 units every 10 to 15 minutes around the clock. Twenty or 30 minutes before each meal, the patient delivers an extra dosage (bolus) by pushing a button on the pump. Determination of the extra dose is primarily based on the carbohydrate content of the food. This mode of insulin delivery mimics the function of the normal human pancreas.

Adapted from Frank HJL: Insulin preparations and insulin delivery systems. In Nuwayhid BS, Brinkman CR, Lieb SM (eds): Management of the Diabetic Pregnancy, p 39. New York, Elsevier, 1987

---

ent periods of hyperglycemia or hypoglycemia. Self-blood glucose monitoring is generally performed prior to each meal and at bedtime. The patient may also test blood glucose levels at 3 A.M. periodically.

The nurse should review both the method and insulin dosage prescribed. And finally, the nurse should review the subjective signs and symptoms of hypoglycemia or hyperglycemia noted by the patient and what action was taken.

Activity and Exercise.   The above information should be correlated with any changes in daily activity or exercise. Increased activity may lead to hypoglycemia if planned snacks are not included. Exercise is generally acceptable if the woman is accustomed to it, has no other complications (such as hypertension), and does not become overtired. Exercise should NOT be attempted if blood glucose is in excess of 250 mg/dl.

Psychological Assessment.   The psychological assessment for the newly diagnosed diabetic should include assessment of the family's adjustment. The chronicity of the illness and the regimentation of daily activities require that all members of the family adapt. The nurse may encourage family members to attend prenatal visits and refer families to diabetes classes and support groups as needed.

(text continued on page 526)

NURSING CARE PLAN

The Pregnant Woman at Risk Because of Diabetes Mellitus

Nursing Diagnosis (Patient Problem) and Assessment Data	Nursing Interventions	Rationale
Potential Complication: *gestational diabetes*		
Maternal risk factors: • Gravida more than 25 years old and obese • Family history of diabetes mellitus • Previous pregnancy loss • Previous neonatal death, unexplained stillbirth, anomaly, or premature infant • Previous infant weighing over 4500 g • Previous gestational diabetes • Hydramnios • Glucosuria on two or more visits	Perform glucose urine dipstick test at each prenatal visit. If glucose is identified, determine if the patient ingested sweets before urine collection. Early diabetic screening is needed for women identified at risk. A 50-g glucose load test is ordered. Explain the method of testing. If this initial screen is negative, repeat testing is indicated at 24–28 weeks.	Dipstick test is used as a screening tool but is not diagnostic. Occasional trace amounts of glucose in the urine are common in pregnancy. Lowered renal threshold and high blood sugar level may result in a physiologic glycosuria.
	All patients who have a positive screen should be evaluated by a standard 3 hour glucose tolerance test.	If the screen is positive, > 112 mg/dl (whole blood) > 130 mg/dl (plasma). oral glucose tolerance test should be performed. Two blood glucose values must be abnormal to diagnose diabetes: Serum FBS > 105 1 hour > 195 2 hour > 165 3 hour > 145

Expected Outcome:

The patient in return demonstrates her knowledge of diabetes mellitus and testing by stating significance of diabetes for pregnancy, what symptoms to report, and significance of prompt reporting.

Complication: *gestational diabetes*	Schedule prenatal visits every 2 weeks.	The objective is to achieve strict control of serum glucose level.
	Provide for dietary control by arranging ongoing consultations with a nutritionist.	Gestational diabetes may be controlled through dietary and activity regulation.
	Assess the woman's activities.	Patient activity burns calories. The patient's intake of food must be correlated with activity level.

Expected Outcome:

The patient complies with prenatal visits schedule and demonstrates compliance with self-care.

(continued)

The Pregnant Woman at Risk Because of Diabetes Mellitus

Nursing Diagnosis (Patient Problem) and Assessment Data	Nursing Interventions	Rationale
Potential Complications Related to Gestational Diabetes: *impaired uterine perfusion; fetal macrosomia*	Through symptom analysis and testing, monitor the patient for asymptomatic bacteriuria, ketoacidosis, hypertension, and hydramnios.	The patient is at risk for developing these problems; early identification will allow prompt dietary change or treatment of the problem.
	Teach patient to report signs of infection or pregnancy complication.	
	Plan for nonstress or contraction stress testing.	
	Plan for ultrasound assessment at 20 weeks of gestation.	A baseline ultrasound to compare with the later ultrasound will permit documentation of interval fetal growth and will reveal macrosomia and polyhydramnios.

Expected Outcome:

The patient experiences no complications and demonstrates normal blood glucose levels, a normal pattern of weight gain, uterine growth, and fetal development throughout pregnancy.

Potential Complication:
insulin-dependent diabetes

	Assess serum glucose levels.	Strict control of serum glucose levels is necessary to prevent maternal and fetal complications.
	Explain necessity for frequent prenatal visits.	Insulin dependence increases risk to mother and baby and necessitates increased testing and hospitalization, causing psychological stress to the woman and her family.
	In collaboration with the nutritionist, ensure that insulin and dietary adjustments are made, based on the blood glucose level.	Insulin and dietary needs vary at different stages of pregnancy and require frequent adjustment.
	Ensure that urine cultures are collected monthly.	Infections cause rapid deterioration of diabetic control.
	Collect a clean-catch urine specimen at each prenatal visit to check for ketones (also glucose and protein).	Ketoacidosis in the mother suggests presence of DKA, which places fetus at risk for intrauterine death.
	Measure fundal height to assess for excessive intrauterine fluid.	Hydramnios that is clinically evident may indicate poor blood glucose control.

(continued)

NURSING CARE PLAN (continued)

The Pregnant Woman at Risk Because of Diabetes Mellitus

Nursing Diagnosis (Patient Problem) and Assessment Data	Nursing Interventions	Rationale
	Make arrangements for antepartum testing after 32 weeks. Explain the test, how it will be done, and what it monitors.	Antepartum testing can detect possible difficulties in placental functioning.

Expected Outcome:

The pregnant diabetic remains free of complications, and demonstrates normal blood glucose levels, a normal pattern of weight gain, uterine growth, and fetal development for remainder of pregnancy.

Nursing Diagnosis:
knowledge deficit related to managing diabetes during pregnancy:

	Nursing Interventions	Rationale
	Assess patient's knowledge base, and her ability to: • Perform self blood glucose monitoring • Maintain her diabetic diet. • Self-administer insulin (including mixing insulins). • Prevent, recognize, and treat hypoglycemia. • Assess urinary ketones and prevent diabetic ketoacidosis. • Seek early care for urinary tract or other infections.	Treatment of diabetes is based on self-care. The more the diabetic mother can learn about her illness and its effects on her pregnancy, the better she will be equipped to intervene or seek help with problems as they arise.

Expected Outcome:

The patient demonstrates her understanding of teaching by modifying her diet and balancing her insulin and activity to maintain optimal blood glucose levels throughout pregnancy.

Management in the Third Trimester

Fetal surveillance and preventing unnecessary prematurity are the management principles of the third trimester. The nurse's role continues to be that of educator and advocate. She can help the patient to understand the reason for frequent monitoring, allay fears that arise, and buffer the abrasiveness of technical procedures. At the same time, she is preparing the patient for birth.

Ideally, the patient will have attended prenatal and childbirth preparation classes. But it is the nurse who will realistically prepare the patient for her specific experience. Assuming the diabetes is uncomplicated and under control, the patient may generally anticipate induced labor at 38 weeks following the attainment of mature lung indices to avoid macrosomia and IUFD.

Diabetic women with complications such as pregnancy-induced hypertension, retinopathy, nephropathy, or fetal compromise may require earlier delivery. Approximately 50% of pregnant diabetics have cesarean births.

Close monitoring and control of glucose levels is essential during the intrapartum period. Maternal hyperglycemia may result in fetal hyperinsulinemia with resultant hypoglycemia of the newborn. Glucose levels should be monitored hourly until stable, then every 2 hours. Glucose control may be maintained by the continuous intravenous infusion of regular insulin. Postpartally, the maternal insulin requirements drop rapidly with the decrease in human chorionic somatomammotropin (HCS). After delivery, glucose levels are monitored; however, most patients do not require insulin in the first 24 hours.

INFECTIONS

Infections of the Urinary Tract

The frequency and seriousness of urinary tract infections during pregnancy has been well documented. Dilatation and stasis in the kidney and ureters provide an ideal medium for bacterial growth and the ascent of infections from the bladder to the kidney.

Asymptomatic Bacteriuria

Asymptomatic bacteriuria is a condition in which significant numbers of bacteria are found on urine culture (greater than 100,000 colonies/ml urine) in the absence of symptoms. This condition can progress to pyelonephritis during pregnancy as a result of the following physiologic changes:

* Dilatation and stasis of the kidney and ureters
* Reflux of urine from the bladder to the ureters
* Changes in the composition of the urine, such as, for example, glucosuria, which support bacterial growth

The overall prevalence of bacteriuria in pregnancy ranges from 4% to 13%. Since the condition may occur without the usual symptoms of urinary tract infections, every woman should be screened for bacteriuria during the course of prenatal care.

Symptomatic Urinary Tract Infections

Urinary tract infection is a general term applied to a urinary infection presenting with the classic symptoms of urgency, frequency, and dysuria, often accompanied by increased nocturia and occasionally by hematuria. It may be a lower tract infection, or cystitis, in which the inflammatory process is restricted to the bladder, or there may be upper tract involvement of the ureters and kidneys. The likelihood of renal involvement can be assessed through careful history-taking that specifically notes indications of upper tract involvement. These indications include the following:

* Long-standing symptoms. The longer symptoms have been present, the more likely is upper tract involvement.
* Symptoms of systemic illness, such as fever, malaise, lack of appetite, nausea
* Abdominal or back pain. Ureteral spasms are usually noted anteriorly and laterally and may radiate into the inguinal area. Kidney pain is usually noted at the costal–vertebral angle (CVA) region of the back.

The definitive diagnosis is determined by urine culture showing bacterial growth greater than 100,000 colonies per milliliter of urine. A sensitivity test of the culture growth will identify the most effective antibiotic for therapy. Many antibiotics are contraindicated for use in pregnancy. In general, sulfa-based drugs and ampicillin are effective in treating urinary tract infections when no patient allergies exist.

For women with a history of recurrent urinary tract infections, prophylactic use of antibiotics may be indicated.

Implications for Nursing Care

All women should be screened with a urine culture during the course of prenatal care, and this is often done on the first prenatal visit. In particular, the nurse should note any history of urinary tract infections, recording past symptoms, treatment, number of incidences, renal or x-ray studies, and known causative factors. The nurse should review the signs of urinary tract infections and screen for current symptomatology.

For women with a history of, or current urinary tract infection, the nurse should emphasize health care behaviors to prevent recurrence, such as those outlined in the accompanying Self-Care Teaching display.

SELF-CARE TEACHING

The Patient With Urinary Tract Infection

* Drink eight 8-oz glasses of fluid a day.
* Drink cranberry juice: it may help to acidify the urine.
* Void frequently.
* Void before and after intercourse.
* Take vitamin C 500–1000 mg/day to acidify the urine.
* Wear cotton underpants and practice good hygiene.
* Avoid carbohydrate and sugar binges to reduce the incidence of glucosuria
* Seek immediate treatment for any recurrence of symptoms.

NURSING CARE PLAN

The Woman With Possible Urinary Tract Infection

Nursing Diagnosis (Patient Problem) and Assessment Data	Nursing Interventions	Rationale
Potential Complication: *urinary tract infection*		
• Pain with urination • Urgency • Frequency • Nocturia	Collect a clean-catch urine specimen and send for microscopic examination. Order urine culture and sensitivity tests.	The presence of over five bacteria per high-power field may indicate urinary tract infection.

Expected Outcome:

The pregnant woman continues with self care and an uncomplicated pregnancy as evidenced by normal parameters of pregnancy and routine follow-up care.

Probable Complication: *urinary tract infection*		

• WBCs and protein in urine
• Patient reports fever, chills, flank and/or suprapubic pain
	Seek physician consultation and assessment for medication.
	
	Ask patient about known allergies. Ensure that the following contraindicated drugs are not used:
	
	    Sulfonamides
	    Tetracycline
	    Nitrofurantoin
	
	Take a history that includes
	
	• Onset of symptoms
	• Symptoms of systemic illness
	• Symptoms of pain
		Sulfonamides should not be used in late pregnancy as they may cause neonatal jaundice. They should be avoided in patients with G6PD disease to avoid hemolysis. After 16 weeks of gestation, tetracycline will cause permanent discoloration in fetal deciduous teeth. Late in pregnancy nitrofurantoin may cause neonatal hemolysis and jaundice.
		
		Symptoms experienced over a long period may indicate kidney involvement. Fever, malaise, nausea, lack of appetite, and back, abdominal, and inguinal pain and costovertebral angle tenderness are all indicative of kidney infection. Pregnant women with kidney infection are at risk for premature labor and are generally hospitalized.

Expected Outcome:

The patient returns to asymptomatic status within 24–36 hours of treatment and remains free of infection throughout pregnancy.

(continued)

NURSING CARE PLAN (continued)

The Woman With Possible Urinary Tract Infection

Nursing Diagnosis (Patient Problem) and Assessment Data	Nursing Interventions	Rationale
Nursing Diagnosis: *knowledge deficit related to self-care for urinary tract infection:*	Review prescribed antibiotic regimen. Counsel patient to:	
	• Drink eight, 8-oz glasses of fluid per day.	Flushing out the bladder helps prevent recurrence. Delay encourages bacterial growth and bladder over-distension.
	• Void before and after sexual intercourse.	Urination washes out bacteria.
	• Wear cotton underwear and practice good hygiene.	Keeping the vulva dry discourages bacterial growth.
	• Avoid carbohydrate and sugar binges to reduce glycosuria.	Glycosuria encourages bacteria to grow.
	• Seek immediate treatment if symptoms recur.	Prompt treatment will effect early resolution of symptoms and infection.
	• Take vitamin C 500 mg/day	Acid urine retards infection.
	Instruct patient regarding need for follow-up, routine collection of midstream clean-catch urine samples.	

Expected Outcome:

The patient demonstrates understanding of instruction by stating symptoms of urinary tract infection and importance of reporting symptoms within 24 hours of onset.

As symptoms are often relieved within 48 hours of antibiotic therapy, the nurse should emphasize the importance of completing the full course of therapy. Following completion of therapy, the urine culture is repeated because asymptomatic bacteriuria may persist.

TORCH Infections

The nurse should be aware of the role viruses play in contemporary health problems. They are more virulent than bacteria, more insidious, less responsive to treatment, and more devastating in their sequelae.

TORCH infections (Table 20–1) are often discussed collectively because they have the ability to actively infect the fetus during pregnancy. The name is derived from the first letter of each infectious condition.

T oxoplasmosis
O ther (syphilis, hepatitis, and HIV)
R ubella
C ytomegalovirus
H erpes

These infections may or may not be sexually transmitted. However, they all share the ability to infect the fetus,

Table 20-1   **TORCH Infections**

Infection and Transmission	Maternal Symptoms	Fetal Effects	Nursing Intervention
Toxoplasmosis			
Protozoa transmitted via undercooked meat, cat feces, and transplacentally	Usually asymptomatic or mild and self-limiting symptoms, so most infections are not diagnosed during pregnancy Swollen cervical lymph nodes in some cases Difficult to differentiate from mononucleosis Serologic testing necessary for diagnosis	If disease is acquired during pregnancy, 40% of fetuses will be infected In early pregnancy, increased abortion, stillbirth, IUGR, and severe congenital infection In newborns, jaundice, hepatosplenomegaly, encephalitis Sequelae in surviving infected infants: microcephaly, cerebral calcification, chorioretinitis, mental retardation Newborn may be asymptomatic	Instruct pregnant women about the source of disease Instruct in how to cook meat Instruct to avoid cleaning kitty litter box
Other*			
Syphilis			
Spirochete transmitted via sexual contact and transplacentally	In primary infection, chancre possible in genital area Rash possible on hands and feet Premature labor common Serologic testing required prenatally	Secondary infection with skin rash and purulent nasal discharge CNS damage Hearing loss Mortality 10%-30% if untreated	Include VDRL in laboratory studies on first prenatal visit Review history for past infections and treatment Observe preterm newborns for evidence of a palmar rash and "snuffles"
Hepatitis			
Virus A transmitted via contaminated water, fecal-oral route. B transmitted by sexual contact, contaminated needles, and transplacentally[†]	Fever, headache, abdominal pain, tea-colored urine, jaundice Virus found in all body fluids, including urine, feces, and semen	Symptomatic chronic hepatitis Jaundice at 3-4 months of age Mental retardation possible from high bilirubin levels	Obtain hepatitis B surface antigen screen at first prenatal visit Discuss sexual transmission of disease Make public health referral for evaluation of home environment (many of those affected are drug users) Give HB immune globulin to infants born to women with active HB Schedule follow-up pediatric or public health care for repeat of injection 1 month and 6 months
Rubella			
Virus transmitted via nasopharynx droplet, transplacentally	Usually mild illness Swollen lymph nodes preceding a rash Rash beginning on face, neck, chest, and spreading to abdomen and extremities Joint pain common in adults	In early pregnancy, abortion, stillbirth, gross abnormalities May remain chronically infected for months Classic anomalies: microcephaly, heart defects, cataracts, and deafness	Screen with rubella titer on first prenatal visit If not immune, schedule immunization in immediate postpartum period Isolate infected newborns: virus is shed in saliva and urine

*This category also includes Group B streptococcal infections, chlamydia, varicella zoster, and HIV.
[†]Major effects on fetus relate to hepatitis B.

(continued)

Table 20–1   **TORCH Infections** (continued)

Infections and Transmission	Maternal Symptoms	Fetal Effects	Nursing Intervention
Cytomegalovirus			
Virus transmitted via contact with body fluids, including colostrum, or contact with cervical mucus	Positive antibodies from prior exposure in 50%–60% of pregnant women Usually asymptomatic Tends to be latent but activated with immunosuppression of pregnancy Serologic testing necessary for diagnosis	May be subclinical to severe, including hyperbilirubinemia, hepatosplenomegaly, pneumonitis, and encephalitis Of those with encephalitis, 5% will die, 85% will have CNS abnormalities If symptomatic at birth: SGA, long-term developmental and learning disabilities Early exposure results in classic tetrad: microcephaly, cerebral calcification, severe mental retardation, and chorioretinitis	Isolate infected newborns: virus is shed in saliva and urine No effective treatment known No immunization available
Herpes Simplex, Type I and II			
Virus transmitted via sexual contact, contact with cervical mucus, or transplacentally	Mostly found in adolescents and young adults Primary infection: painful vesicles on labia, vagina, or cervix, with systemic symptoms of fever, headache, malaise, and anorexia Recurrent infection: localized painful lesions — systemic symptoms are rare	In early pregnancy, increase in abortions Later in pregnancy, increase in preterm labor Infected newborn has 60% risk of mortality Severe neurologic sequelae in 50% of infected survivors	Discuss sexual transmission Culture if symptoms persist. Patients in early labor or with ROM who have a recent positive culture or a symptomatic lesion are usually delivered by cesarean Record and report rupture of membranes during labor Culture possibly infected newborn for herpes Isolate and observe for signs of infection

either by crossing the placenta or by way of an ascending infection after rupture of the membranes and cervical dilatation. When the organism crosses the placenta in early pregnancy, the fetus may develop major malformations. If the organism crosses the placenta in the latter half of pregnancy, the infant may be born with active disease. Since the newborn has an immature immunologic system, an ascending infection may become overwhelmingly systemic, causing encephalitis, meningitis, or both. If the infant survives, he or she may suffer severe neurologic impairment.

These conditions are increasing in incidence, are often difficult to detect in the adult, and may not be obvious in the newborn until weeks or months after birth. All of these conditions may be diagnosed by testing for a serum titer level that indicates a past or current infectious process and the formation of antibodies. Currently, only ru-

bella and syphilis are routinely screened for during the prenatal period. Rubella screening has been mandated by law, since the rubella epidemic of the 1960s resulted in the birth of 30,000 children with major malformations.

Greater attention has been given to herpes infections since the marked increase in sexually transmitted herpes in the 1970s. The condition does not affect the development of the fetus, but infants who contract herpes at birth are likely to develop meningoencephalitis with severe neurologic sequelae. Cesarean birth is generally chosen as the method of delivery when a lesion is present and delivery is imminent.

Cytomegalovirus (CMV), a herpes-related virus, was discovered in 1956. The infection is subclinical in adults, but antibody screening reveals that up to 50% show evidence of previous infection. If the mother is infected during pregnancy, the fetus may also become infected. The condition may affect fetal development, causing manifestations similar to toxoplasmosis, which include:

- Microcephaly
- Cerebral calcification
- Mental retardation
- Chorioretinitis of the eye

On the other hand, there may be no evidence of cytomegalovirus at birth, and it may not be diagnosed until neurologic problems develop in the infant. Cytomegalovirus is thought to be a major cause of mental retardation.

Hepatitis

The incidence of hepatitis has risen sharply over the last decade. There are four forms of hepatitis:

- Type A is a relatively benign, self-limiting disease.
- Type B is a more serious form, the incidence of which has increased over the decade.
- Type D can only replicate in the presence of Type B and is more likely to progress to chronic severe liver disease.
- Type Non-A, Non-B is the name given to encompass at least three additional distinct forms of the disease. Clinical manifestations are similar to Type B.

Type A (HA) is commonly known as infectious hepatitis and is primarily transmitted by oral–fecal contamination through water and food sources. The 2-week interval following exposure, but prior to the onset of jaundice, is the period of greatest infectivity. Fecal virus excretion diminishes rapidly after the onset of jaundice. Type A seems not to be transmitted to the fetus unless infection occurs less than 1 week before delivery.

Type B (HB) is transmitted perinatally, parenterally, and sexually. The dramatic rise in incidence is attributed to Southeast Asian immigration, drug abuse, and frequent intercourse with varied sexual partners. Approximately 40% of the Southeast Asian population carries the virus and most acquire the infection at birth or during childhood.

Forty to sixty percent of those infected with hepatitis will become symptomatic. Clinical cases vary in severity from mild to critical. The earliest positive serologic test appears 1 to 2 months after exposure.

American College of Obstetricians and Gynecologists (ACOG) currently recommends routine screening of all pregnant women for HB. Testing for surface antigen is generally done at the first prenatal visit and a positive result usually indicates past infection, although an infection work-up is still indicated. All infants of hepatitis surface antigen-positive women should receive HB immunotherapy within 12 hours of birth to prevent a chronic carrier state.

Implications for Nursing Care

Intrapartally, preventing transmission to the newborn and care providers focuses on avoiding contact with maternal exudate, especially blood. The following precautions should be taken:

- During labor, avoid the use of a scalp electrode. External monitoring should be used.
- Dispose of needles without recapping to avoid self-puncture
- Wear gown, gloves, and protective eyewear in the delivery area
- Handle the newborn with gloves, until the baby has been bathed.
- Delay giving the newborn injections or blood sampling until the baby has been bathed.
- Administer HB immunotherapy within 12 hours following delivery and arrange for follow-up with HBV vaccine and boosters.
- Use universal isolation techniques (see Nursing Alerts, on Universal Precautions, Chapters 23 and 32).

HIV Infection and Acquired Immunodeficiency Syndrome (AIDS)

AIDS results from immunosuppression caused by a retrovirus (T-cell lymphotrophic virus type III) referred to as HIV. HIV can be transmitted by exposure to an infected person's blood, semen, or cervical–vaginal secretions; blood products or contaminated needles; or it can be transmitted transplacentally (Feldblum et al 1988).

This section focuses on HIV infection and AIDS in pregnancy. See Chapter 10 for a full discussion of AIDS as a sexually transmitted disease.

While most people with AIDS are homosexual men, the incidence among women, especially black and hispanic women, is increasing dramatically. Women who are at high risk for exposure to HIV are:

- IV drug users or sexual partners of IV drug users
- Sexual partners of persons with AIDS
- Sexual partners of bisexuals or hemophiliacs
- Women with multiple sexual partners since 1978
- Recipients of blood products between 1979 and 1985
- Donor inseminated women
- Women who have resided in endemic areas of Africa and Haiti (Booth 1988)

Pregnancy is associated with suppression of cell-mediated immunity and increased susceptibility to some infections. The T helper to T suppressor ratio is lowest in the third trimester of pregnancy. Studies suggest that preg-

(text continued on page 535)

NURSING CARE PLAN

The Pregnant HIV-Positive Patient

Nursing Diagnosis (Patient Problem) and Assessment Data	Nursing Interventions	Rationale
Nursing Diagnosis: *potential for infection or transmission of HIV to fetus/infant*		
	Minimize vaginal examinations.	Reduce the risk of transmitting HIV infection to the fetus.
	Minimize fetal blood samples, intrauterine catheters or fetal scalp electrodes. Inform patient that breast-feeding is contraindicated. Educate parents to importance of handwashing and infection prevention for infant.	Research indicates the HIV can be transmitted via the placenta. HIV has been isolated in cervical mucus and in breast milk.

Expected Outcome:

Precautions to minimize transmission potential are followed by staff and family.

Nursing Diagnosis (Patient Problem) and Assessment Data	Nursing Interventions	Rationale
Nursing Diagnosis: *potential for infection or transmission to staff and/or other patients*		
	Provide intrapartal care in single room with private bathroom. Use blood and body fluid precautions.	To protect the health care staff and other patients from infection with HIV and associated opportunistic pathogens.
	Needles must not be bent or recapped after use; needles and other sharps must be discarded immediately in a puncture-resistant waterproof container.	Meticulous care needed in disposal of sharps to prevent needlestick injuries with possible HIV transmission.
	All specimens sent to laboratory must be clearly labelled and placed in an impervious bag for transport. Label "Risk of Infection;" "HIV Precautions."	Protect confidentiality of patient's diagnosis.
	Spillage of body fluids must be saturated with an appropriate disinfectant, left for 30 minutes, then carefully wiped up by nursing staff, using paper towels that are then placed in appropriate containers (indicating "Infection Precautions") and sent for incineration.	

(continued)

The Pregnant HIV-Positive Patient

Nursing Diagnosis (Patient Problem) and Assessment Data	Nursing Interventions	Rationale

Expected Outcome:

Infection precautions are implemented consistently and no "sharps" injuries or body fluid contacts are reported by staff.

Nursing Diagnosis:
fear related to potential transmission of HIV to fetus

| | Acknowledge patient's feelings | Help relieve fears. |
| | Encourage ventilation of feelings; provide emotional support. | Convey support and decrease sense of isolation. |

Expected Outcome:

Patient acknowledges fear of transmission to the baby and is able to express her concerns openly with nursing staff.

Nursing Diagnosis:
fear related to potential worsening of maternal condition

| | Assess available support systems; with patient's consent, call friends or family to mobilize support. | Assist significant others to provide needed support. |
| | Provide information as desired; correct misconceptions, but avoid destroying hope. | |

Expected Outcome:

Patient demonstrates her acceptance of support systems verbalizing her fears with them and stating needs.

Nursing Diagnosis:
anticipatory grieving related to decreasing quality of life and future loss of life and of fetus if pregnancy termination is chosen

| | Acknowledge patient's verbal and nonverbal expressions of grief and anger. | Assist patient in grief process. |
| | Encourage expressions of negative emotions; explore alternative ways of expressing emotions if support persons and family respond by isolating patient. | To assist others to adjust to difficult situation without excessive distancing from patient. |

(continued)

NURSING CARE PLAN (continued)

The Pregnant HIV-Positive Patient

Nursing Diagnosis (Patient Problem) and Assessment Data	Nursing Interventions	Rationale
	If patient is withdrawn, and expresses feelings of helplessness, provide caring physical presence even if patient remains silent. Avoid forcing interaction, but prevent unnecessary isolation.	Adults respond to loss with sadness and grief, and may direct anger inwards, blaming themselves. They may become withdrawn and increasingly unable to initiate interactions. A sign that grief may be resolving in some cases is movement from depression and withdrawal to anger and blaming others for their loss.
	Encourage physical activity.	
	Provide information as patient appears ready for it.	

Expected Outcome:

The patient works through grieving as demonstrated by movement through the steps of the grieving process and by improved interactions with others.

---

nancy increases an infected woman's risk of developing AIDS or ARC (Centers for Disease Control 1985).

Women in high-risk categories should be offered testing early in the prenatal period. ELISA is the commercially prepared product used for initial screening. If the results of the initial ELISA screening test are reactive, the test is repeated. If repeatedly reactive, it is recommended by the CDC that ELISA be followed with the Western Blot test to eliminate any false-positive results. Pregnant women who are reactive to both should have a thorough physical examination, including a CBC with differential. The presence of specific antibody should be considered presumptive evidence of current infection and infectiousness.

If the results are nonreactive, additional testing should be done just prior to delivery. If negative, there is no risk of exposure and the care of mother and infant should follow the normal course.

Pregnant women who test positive must face the difficult issue of continuing or terminating the pregnancy. When it is too late to terminate the pregnancy or she chooses not to, the pregnant woman may experience enormous guilt, fear, and anxiety during the remainder of the pregnancy.

Even though a pregnant woman knows she is infected and is advised that she risks an infected child, she may continue her pregnancy, or choose not to abort an early fetus because she feels well and denies illness. Many other women who receive no prenatal care, and have been unaware of their infection through IV drug use, are diagnosed only at the time of delivery.

Transmission of HIV to the baby may occur

- Through transplacental transfer in pregnancy
- By contact with maternal blood at the time of delivery
- From breast-feeding

Even though a pregnant woman is totally asymptomatic, it has been demonstrated that by the middle of the first trimester, the placenta and fetus can be infected with HIV in asymptomatic seropositive women.

Seventy-five percent of AIDS in children may be attributable to *in utero* transmission of the disease. The prognosis for these infants is disheartening since approximately 60% die within the first year of life. Survival rate for these infants is estimated to be 6 months (Willimas 1986).

HIV positive women should be screened for hepatitis B, cytomegalovirus, and tuberculosis as these conditions are found to be concomitant with AIDS (Shannon 1987). Precautions for the care of the HIV-infected woman during pregnancy and the woman and her fetus/newborn during the intrapartal and postpartal periods are the same as listed in hepatitis B.

Pregnant infected women will require additional medical and psychosocial support during the prenatal period. They may experience:

- A profound sense of isolation
- The need to keep their illness secret, thus depriving themselves of family and community support
- Grief related to termination of pregnancy, if chosen
- Grief related to loss of health, body image, sexuality, and loss of childbearing potential
- Limited sexual expression/may not disclose infection to new sexual partner
- Inability to fulfill parenting responsibilities because of illness or overwhelming depression.
- Guilt about potential transmission to fetus
- Responsibility to plan for surviving children
- Problems finding primary health care sensitive and specific to her needs
- Fear of dying

See the accompanying Nursing Care Plan for the HIV-infected pregnant woman.

SUBSTANCE ABUSE

The fetus is the recipient of food and other substances ingested by the mother. In the case of drugs, the severity and type of adverse effects that result from a given drug depend on a number of factors. These include:

- Size of dose and frequency of ingestion
- Route of administration
- State and stage of the pregnancy
- Maternal health and status of nutrition
- Genetic makeup of the mother and fetus
- Previous obstetric history
- Environmental factors, such as smoking, drugs, and exposure to chemicals and pollutants

The safety of any drug used during pregnancy is difficult to determine, and the effects of many preparations have been incompletely studied.

Alcohol

One of the commonest drug abuse problems in our society is alcoholism. In the United States it affects 1 million women in the childbearing group from 21 to 29 years. Women are drinking more and starting at an earlier age. It is estimated that the incidence of fetal alcohol syndrome is 1 to 2 cases per 1000 live births. Thus, alcohol may be the primary environmental teratogen.

Alcoholic beverages contain not only ethanol (grain alcohol) but many other chemicals, such as congeners, which impart aroma and flavor to the alcohol, and aldehydes (oxidation products). High levels of these drugs are distributed to the organs of the fetus, including the liver, pancreas, kidneys, lungs, thymus, and brain, and as yet little is known about their effects.

Effects of Fetal Alcohol Syndrome on the Infant

Head and Facial Abnormalities

- Eyes: shortened palpebral fissures, ptosis, strabismus, myopia, microphthalmia (abnormally small eye size), tortuosity of the arterial and venous retinal vasculature
- Nose: short and upturned nose, low, broad bridge, hypoplastic philtrum (flat or absent groove above upper lip), and greater than normal distance from upper lip to nose
- Ears: large, low-set ears, rotated posteriorly
- Jaw: underdeveloped upper and lower jawbones

Cardiovascular Abnormalities

- Ventricular septal defect, tetralogy of Fallot, patent ductus arteriosus, great vessel defects

Urogenital Abnormalities

- Hydronephrosis, kidney hypoplasia, renal agenesis (absence of one or both kidneys), undescended testicles, clitoral hypertrophy, labial hypoplasia

Skeletal Deformities

- Microcephaly, hypoplastic nails (defective development), shortened fingers or toes, cervical spinal fusion, clinodactyly (permanent deflection of one or more fingers), aberrant palmar creases, and numerous less common deformities

Central Nervous System Disorders

- Mental retardation, hyperactivity (impulsivity, and difficulty in focusing attention), sleep disturbances, developmental delay, decreased muscle tone, and weak sucking

Growth Deficiency

- IUGR, failure to thrive

Fetal Implications: Fetal Alcohol Syndrome

The term *fetal alcohol syndrome* (FAS) has been applied to a set of problems exhibited by some neonates. These problems, discussed in more detail in Chapter 35, include:

- Prenatal or postnatal growth retardation (below the tenth percentile for body weight, length, or head circumference)
- Characteristic facial anomalies (at least two of the following three):
    Microcephaly (below the third percentile)
    Microphthalmia or short palpebral fissures
    Underdeveloped philtrum (medial groove on the upper lip), thin upper lip, and maxillary hypoplasia
- Central nervous system dysfunction (neurologic abnormality, mental deficiency, developmental delay).

When these three criteria are not met, the Fetal Alcohol Study Group of the Research Society on Alcoholism has proposed that the term *possible fetal alcohol effects* be used to describe the characteristics suspected to be related to alcohol consumption. The number of infants experiencing fetal alcohol effects—4.4 for every 1000 live born infants—is much higher than the number with FAS. It is also recommended that the FAS diagnosis be corroborated with maternal alcoholism because of its close resemblance to fetal hydantoin syndrome.

Precisely how alcohol causes fetal alcohol syndrome is not known. Alcohol appears to enter maternal and fetal circulation at the same rate, but the fetal blood alcohol level remains higher because the immature fetal liver is unable to metabolize it. Some anomalies in infants with fetal alcohol syndrome are clearly the result of disruption during organogenesis. Heavy intake of alcohol during the early weeks of pregnancy may be particularly damaging. The effect of alcohol on fetal brain cell development in the last trimester is also of concern.

Fetal malformations from FAS may be related to the quantity and frequency of alcohol intake during pregnancy. The mother does not have to be an alcoholic for anomalies to occur. Moderate daily drinking or infrequent bouts of high alcohol ingestion, especially during the embryonic period, can cause permanent mental and physical disability. Risk to the fetus increases when the mother takes two or more drinks daily. These include intrauterine growth retardation (IUGR), immature motor activity, increased risk of anomalies, decreased muscle tone, poor sucking, increased rate of stillbirths, and decreased placental weight. Ingestion of five or more drinks at a time on an irregular basis increases the risk of structural brain abnormalities; six or more drinks per day will frequently cause FAS.

Many health care professionals believe that there is no safe level of alcohol consumption during pregnancy. To be perfectly safe, *women should not consume alcohol when pregnant.* The effects of alcohol use in pregnancy are potentially so severe—yet absolutely preventable—that educating pregnant women about them is essential. Nurses who work in prenatal, family planning, or women's clinics are in an excellent position to provide such information.

Marijuana

The dried leaves, stalks, and flowering tops of the plant *Cannabis sativa* are called *marijuana* (or hashish, grass, dagga, kif). This complex substance contains over 400 chemicals. The psychoactive ingredients it contains depend on the soil of the area in which it was grown. The component that provides the "high" is delta-9-tetrahydrocannabinol (THC), 5 to 10 mg of which is sufficient to produce this effect. The flowering top of the plant contains the most concentrated THC and provides the material for hashish. Marijuana contains 1% to 5% THC, whereas hashish oil contains as much as 30% to 90%.

Also contained in marijuana are compounds called cannabinoids, which cause increased heart rate, bronchodilation, reddened conjunctiva, and impaired memory and psychomotor performance. These substances are fat-soluble and accumulated in fatty tissue, including the brain.

SELF-CARE TEACHING

The Patient Who Smokes Marijuana

- Because marijuana interferes with the production of hormones critical for sexual and reproductive development, its use by sexually immature girls and boys carries a particular long-term risk.
- Marijuana also has a very potent inhibitory effect on reproductive hormones in adults. Although these appear to be reversible after discontinuation of drug use, individuals with impaired fertility or sexual function should be particularly cautious about using marijuana.
- The U.S. Surgeon General has warned that use of marijuana during pregnancy may harm the baby's health. Pregnant women and couples trying to conceive should not use it.

From Asch RH, Smith CG: Effects of marijuana on reproduction. Contemp Ob/Gyn October 1982, p. 217. Copyright 1983. Oradell, NJ, Medical Economics Books. Reprinted with permission.

Maternal/Fetal Implications

It has been estimated that approximately 43 million Americans have used marijuana and 16 million are current users. Young adults make up the bulk of users, and young women of reproductive age are becoming increasingly exposed to marijuana. Since use of marijuana is illegal, it has not been well studied. Research has necessarily been limited to effects on rhesus monkeys. Results of some studies show that THC disrupts the reproductive cycle in both men and women, as shown in Table 20–2.

The effect on the newborn of exposure to THC during the critical period of embryonic development is unknown. In studies of mice, fetal death and decreased body weight have resulted from use of marijuana. Decreased uterine blood flow and IUGR may result from THC's interference with estrogen conversion in the placenta. During labor and delivery, mothers who were marijuana users had a higher incidence of meconium problems, more abnormally short or long labors, and more infants who appeared "stoned" and needed resuscitation.

THC has also been detected in the blood of breast-fed mice whose mothers were given the drug. Lactation may also be affected: the amount of milk is reduced as a result of a decrease in mammary gland enzymes necessary for the growth of normal mammary tissue.

The mechanism that causes disruption of the male and female reproductive systems has not yet been determined. It is known that THC and marijuana cause infertility in both sexes, but their effects have been shown to be reversible in mature animals after 63 days of abstinence. It is possible, however, that long-term exposure during the critical adolescent growth period may permanently impair fertility.

Table 20–2   **Reported Action of Marijuana on Reproductive Systems**

Females	Males
Decreases levels of follicle-stimulating hormone (FSH), luteinizing hormone (LH), and prolactin (PRL)	Decreases FSH, LH, and PRL levels
Inhibits ovulation	Decreases testosterone levels (tolerance develops)
Disrupts menstrual cycle (tolerance develops)	Inhibits spermatogenesis and sperm motility
Crosses placenta and may affect fetal growth and development	Alters sperm function
Passes readily into milk	

Asch RH, Smith CG: Effects of marijuana on reproduction. Contemp Ob/Gyn October 1982, p 217. Copyright 1983. Oradell, NJ, Medical Economics Books. Reprinted with permission.

Tobacco

Before the 1920s, very few women smoked. An extravagant advertising campaign convinced women that smoking was fashionable and, since that time, the number of women who smoke has increased significantly. It has been estimated that 40% of women smoke at least occasionally during pregnancy.

In the 1930s and 1940s, research studies involving animals reported that maternal smoking increased fetal heart rate and caused increased resorption of embryos, increased stillbirths, and reduced birth weight. These studies were deemed irrelevant to humans and ignored by the medical establishment. Since that time, much has been learned about the hazards of smoking to the pregnant woman and to the fetus.

Smoking permits rapid absorption of nicotine in the body, 90% being absorbed by the lungs. The nicotine content of the last puff of a cigarette is two to three times greater than that of the first puff. Since nicotine is fat- and water-soluble, it is rapidly distributed throughout body tissues and fluids. The highest concentrations are found in the brain, pituitary, and adrenals.

After smoking just one cigarette, pregnant women have peak blood nicotine levels of 14 to 41 mg/ml. The wide variation reflects the different ways in which cigarettes are smoked. The depth and length of inhalation, the number of inhalations per cigarette, puff pressure, the brand of cigarette, and the amount of the cigarette smoked all affect the nicotine blood level (Abel 1983). Cigarette smoke also contains tar, carbon monoxide, and other substances.

Maternal/Fetal Implications

The commonest effect of maternal smoking on the infant is *reduced birth weight*. This reduction may range from 40 to 430 g, the average reduction being 200 g (7 oz). This effect may result from the high level of carboxyhemoglobin in the fetal circulation as a result of carbon monoxide exposure from the smoke. The amount of oxygen available to the fetus is decreased, causing hypoxia. There is also a close relationship between the number of cigarettes smoked during pregnancy and the infant's weight: the more cigarettes smoked, the lower the birth weight.

At one time, this effect was thought to be a result of the lower weight gain during pregnancy of women who smoke. It was believed that increasing weight gain during pregnancy would help to offset the harmful effects of smoking on the fetus. However, more recent evidence indicates that even when the weight gain and dietary intake of smoking and nonsmoking mothers are similar, infants of smoking mothers still experience a higher rate of IUGR and lower birth weight.

How tobacco smoking inhibits *fetal growth* is not well understood. Some experts theorize that carbon monoxide in the maternal blood crosses the placenta and binds with fetal hemoglobin, thus reducing the effectiveness of fetal oxygen transport. Others suggest that the vasoconstrictive action of nicotine in cigarette smoke reduces utero-placental perfusion. In view of the known health risks of smoking in general and the more specific risks to fetal growth, the nurse should advise the pregnant woman to stop, or at least reduce, her smoking for the duration of pregnancy. Since the risks to the fetus decrease with a decrease in the number of cigarettes smoked per day, cutting down smoking may be helpful.

Spontaneous abortion (SAB) normally occurs in about 20% of recognized pregnancies. Although the statistics are difficult to assess, the average number of SABs in maternal smokers may be as high as 24.5%, as opposed to 7.8% for nonsmokers. The increased rate of spontaneous abortions in smokers has not been fully explained, but it may result from changes in the placenta that render it unable to support the pregnancy.

Increased death rates during delivery and the early neonatal period have been noted in babies of smoking mothers. Women who smoke 11 or more cigarettes a day increase their risk of having a stillborn infant by over 50%.

The risk of sudden infant death (SID) for babies of smokers is twice that for babies of nonsmoking mothers. Disorders of the respiratory system are also higher in children of smokers and are thought to result from impairment of the immune system. There does not appear to be a strong association between maternal smoking and risk of malformations, although an association between smoking in pregnancy and increased incidence of cleft lip and palate has been noted.

Breast milk is also affected by smoking. Nicotine is secreted into the milk and can be detected as long as 7 to 8 hours after the last cigarette. Its concentration in the milk depends on the amount and depth of inhalation, the amount of the cigarette smoked, and the frequency of smoking.

Positive change can occur if the pregnant woman stops smoking during pregnancy. When smoking is stopped by the fourth month, the risks to the baby are minimized and may even be eliminated. With most hazardous substances, the risk to the fetus is greatest during the early first trimester. The effects of smoking, however, are most potent during the latter months of pregnancy, when the central nervous system of the fetus is growing and developing.

Narcotics

Narcotic addiction does not appear to increase the risk of major developmental anomalies in the fetus. It is difficult to assess the effect because compounding factors may include poor prenatal care, exposure to infections with IV drug use, especially hepatitis and HIV, and abuse of other substances (Lake 1987). A major complication of narcotic addiction is neonatal withdrawal. If the pregnant woman continues to use drugs during pregnancy, gradually decreasing the daily intake to a low level by the third trimester will be beneficial to the newborn.

Cocaine

Cocaine use, in the form of snorting, free-basing, or crack, has complicated one in ten pregnancies in major urban areas. The complications of pregnancy arising from the vasoconstriction of cocaine are

- Spontaneous abortion
- Placenta abruptio
- Low birth weight
- Intrauterine growth retardation
- Maternal hypertension

Additionally, cocaine is known to stimulate uterine contractions, which places these patients at very high risk for preterm birth.

Implications for Nursing Care

Caring for the patient with a substance abuse problem presents a difficult challenge in establishing a truthful, trusting relationship. Referral to specialized programs for pregnant women may be necessary to enable safe and effective behavior change. For the addict who presents in labor, the nurse should ascertain the time and amount of the last drug usage, and the frequency and type of drugs usually used. Generally, the patient will be screened to determine which drugs are currently found on blood sampling.

Intrapartally, drug users are difficult to care for in labor. They tolerate pain poorly, and become irritable and belligerent when they begin to withdraw. The nurse is challenged to provide care for the laboring woman while maintaining support and firm direction.

OTHER MEDICAL CONDITIONS

Trauma in Pregnancy

The most frequent cause of death in women under the age of 35 is trauma (Smith and Phelan 1987). The fetus is sometimes the victim as well in automobile accidents, shootings, stabbings, and family violence. Minor trauma is seldom associated with a poor pregnancy outcome. This includes soft-tissue deceleration injuries caused by seat

NURSING RESEARCH

Seat Belt Practices Among Pregnant Women

A study was conducted to examine the seat belt practices of 87 pregnant women. Of these women, nearly half (40) reported using seat belts regularly during pregnancy. However, almost one third of these did not adjust them for maximum protection (for lap-type belts, as low as possible across the hips below the abdomen; shoulder harnesses, across the shoulder, chest, and upper abdomen). Older women and those with more education were more likely to use their seat belts routinely. Only 20 women remembered receiving information about seat belt use during their pregnancies; 48 women would have appreciated receiving more information.

Seat belts have been proven effective in reducing deaths and serious injuries; maternal death is the leading cause of fetal death related to accidents, and seat belts significantly reduce the mother's risk of death or serious injury in an automobile accident. Teaching about seat belt use during pregnancy should be routinely included in prenatal visits and in organized classes for expectant parents. Nurses are in an ideal position to positively influence health promotion behaviors such as seat belt use among pregnant women.

Arneson S, Beltz E, Hahnemann B et al: Automobile seat belt practices of pregnant women. J Obstet Gynecol Neonatal Nurs 15(4):339–344, 1986

belts. ACOG reports that as few as 20% of pregnant women wear seat belts, yet the injuries are likely to be minor in comparison to unbelted passengers (ACOG 1983). Stress fractures are a more frequent injury, now seen in obstetrics with the increase in jogging and aerobic exercise. Several cases of fractures of the pubic bone at delivery have been reported (Moran 1988).

Implications for Nursing Care

Acute accidental traumas may result in emergency room care. However, perinatal units are increasingly updating services to include intensive care capabilities such as invasive hemodynamic monitoring and mechanical ventilation. Table 20–3 lists the ways trauma may be influenced by pregnancy. The nurse needs to direct health education toward patient awareness of these changes as well as toward a consciousness of accident avoidance, as listed in the accompanying Self-Care Teaching display.

Thyroid Conditions

Thyroid conditions, whether hypothyroid or hyperthyroid, are a risk to pregnancy if the patient is untreated. A study of pregnant hypothyroid women showed a stillbirth rate double that found in the general population. On neurologic testing, children of these women were found to have lower scores up to 7 years of age. Hyperthyroid women were found to have low birth weight infants.

Normal thyroid hormone levels affect

- Oxygen consumption
- Growth
- Heat production
- Gluconeogenesis
- Glucose utilization
- Milk production

During pregnancy, renal changes result in increased iodine loss. Physiologic compensation occurs with an increase in the size of the gland and increased hormone production (Berry et al 1987).

Symptoms of changes in thyroid function include the following:

Hyperthyroidism	Hypothyroidism
Weakness	Weakness
Increased appetite	Puffy face
Diarrhea	Hoarseness
Weight loss	Cold intolerance
Heat intolerance	Hair loss
Sweating	Dry skin
Tremors	Brittle nails
Nervousness	Thick tongue
Tachycardia	
Vomiting	

The goal of treatment is to keep the patient's thyroid function normal with a minimum of medication. Regular evaluations of thyroid function are needed to ascertain values for a maintenance dose of medication, which is taken daily. The patient whose thyroid hormone levels return to normal usually feels immediate improvement with increased energy, restful sleep, and stabilized weight gain.

Hyperthyroidism can be treated with any one of the following regimens:

- Antithyroid drug therapy alone
- Antithyroid drug therapy in combination with thyroid hormone therapy

Table 20-3   **Physiologic Adaptations to Pregnancy That Affect Maternal Response to Trauma**

System	Alteration	Clinical Effect
Genitourinary	Uterine enlargement	Predisposes to injury
		Protects bowel
	Bladder becomes intra-abdominal	Predisposes to injury
	Ureteral dilation	Abnormal IVP
Gastrointestinal	Decreased motility	Prolonged gastric emptying; regurgitation/aspiration
	Distended abdomen	Reduces peritoneal signs
Pulmonary	Increased minute ventilation; increased oxygen consumption; reduced functional residual capacity	Predisposes to hypoxemia with apnea
Cardiovascular	Increased cardiac output	
	Aortocaval compression	Supine hypotension
	Increased blood volume	Protects against hemorrhage
	Decreased peripheral resistance	Increased skin temperature
Hematologic	Larger relative increase in plasma volume	Physiologic anemia
	Leukocytosis	

Smith CV, Phelan JP: Trauma in pregnancy. In Clark SL, Phelan JP, Cotton DB (eds): Critical Care Obstetrics, p 387. Oradel, NJ, Medical Economics Books, 1984. Reprinted with permission.

- Antithyroid drug therapy followed by subtotal thyroidectomy in the second trimester and postoperative thyroid hormone therapy.

Methimazole and propylthiouracil are drugs commonly used in treatment. Dosages are reduced in pregnancy because the drugs readily cross the placenta and can induce goiter and even cretinism in the developing fetus. It is important, therefore, that the dosage be sufficient but not excessive. Postpartum patients receiving antithyroid drugs should not breast-feed their infants.

SELF-CARE TEACHING

Avoiding Accidental Trauma

- Always wear a seat belt.
- Be aware of body habitus and changes in center of gravity—avoid climbing and stretching for objects.
- Avoid lifting heavy objects.
- Remove yourself from threatening situations—don't provoke an argument and don't walk alone at night.
- Don't drive if not seated comfortably and in control of the car.
- The best exercise is daily walking in a supportive shoe.

Implications for Nursing Care

While the patient is being treated and a maintenance dosage being established, the nurse should

- Record vital signs every 4 hours
- Observe and record the patient's overt symptoms, since dosage may require adjustment
- Weigh the patient weekly or at the time of each prenatal visit. Weight gain unrelated to pregnancy may be seen several weeks after initiation of therapy.

Heart Disease

Heart function, like that of most organ systems, is altered by pregnancy, and altered findings on physical examination may, in fact, be normal, as shown in the Cardiac Signs and Symptoms in Pregnancy display, page 542. The physiologic changes that produce these altered findings include the following:

- Cardiac volume increase
- Elevation of the diaphragm by the enlarging uterus, displacing the heart to the left and upward
- Lowered blood viscosity and torsion of the great vessels as a result of displacement caused by the enlarging uterus
- Plasma volume increase

NURSING ALERT

Cardiac Signs and Symptoms During Pregnancy

Usually significant
   Diastolic murmur
   Focal pulmonary rales
   Distended neck veins
   Increased cardiac size (chest roentgenogram)
   Dysrhythmias (except sinus tachycardia and paroxysmal atrial tachycardia)

May be normal observation in pregnancy
   Systolic flow murmur
   Slight breathlessness
   Decreased exercise tolerance
   Extracardiac flow murmur (mammary artery)
   Wide splitting of S_1
   Resting tachycardia

Malkasian G, Noller K, Aaro L et al: Miscellaneous medical complications. In Iffy L, Kaminetzky HA (eds): Principles and Practice of Obstetrics and Perinatology, Vol 2. New York, John Wiley & Sons, 1981

New York Heart Association Functional Classification (Modified)

Class I	No limitation of physical activity
Class II	No symptoms at rest
	Minor limitation of physical activity (fatigue, palpitations, minor dyspnea, etc.)
Class III	No symptoms at rest
	Marked limitation of physical activity due to symptoms of cardiac disease
Class IV	Symptoms at rest
	Discomfort increased with any physical activity

Malkasian G, Noller K, Aaro L et al: Miscellaneous medical complications. In Iffy L, Kaminetzky HA (eds): Principles and Practice of Obstetrics and Perinatology, Vol 2. New York, John Wiley & Sons, 1981

- Heart rate increase
- Cardiac output increase
- Red blood cell volume increase
- Accelerated production of red blood cells
- Decrease in total peripheral resistance
- Stagnation of blood in lower extremities
- Blood pressure decrease in first half of pregnancy, followed by rise to prepregnant state or higher

Because of the increased cardiovascular workload, the presence of decompensation can endanger the life of the mother and infant. The subject of heart disease covers a variety of conditions that vary considerably in their severity and impact on pregnancy. Rheumatic heart disease accounts for 65% to 80% of all cardiac disease. Congenital heart disease is the next largest category.

It is not within the scope of this section to discuss specific conditions. Management of the pregnant woman with a cardiac condition is guided by the New York Heart Association classification, shown in the accompanying display, and is based on the presenting symptomatology and the degree of disruption in daily activities. The same management approach is used for Classes I and II. A more aggressive approach is used for Classes III and IV.

The best time to diagnose and treat cardiac disease is prior to pregnancy. When it is discovered during the pregnancy, maternal risk is greater and fetal prognosis worse. In general, women in Classes I and II tolerate pregnancy reasonably well. The outlook is much worse for women in Classes III and IV. Women in Class III have an 80% risk of significant heart failure, and their mortality exceeds 5%. Maternal mortality for women in Class IV is approximately 25%. Generally, these women should be counseled to avoid pregnancy.

If symptomatic with hypertension and edema, the Class II cardiac patient may require management with diuretics, low-salt diet, and bedrest. For the advanced cardiac patient, a variety of drugs may be employed to assist with the increasing cardiac workload. Table 20-4 discusses these drugs as they pertain to pregnancy.

Implications for Nursing Care

The management of pregnant women in Classes I and II encompasses the following:

- Limited strenuous activity
- Adequate rest
- Low-salt diet
- Avoidance of anemia
- Aggressive treatment of infections
- Frequent prenatal visits
- Cardiology consultation
- Monitoring for dysrhythmias

The balance between rest and activity is determined after the patient's symptoms are assessed. An evaluation of the patient's living situation will aid in tailoring activities. For example, the patient who has to climb stairs to

Table 20-4   **Common Maintenance Drugs for the Cardiac Patient**

Drug Name and Type	Dosage	Effects and Adverse Reactions	Nursing Implications
Digoxin (cardiac glycoside)	0.5–1 mg/day digitalizing dose; 0.125–0.5 mg/day, orally, maintenance dose	Increases the force of cardiac contraction and refractory period Decreases conductivity May cause GI disturbances Depletes potassium when given with thiazides No adverse effects reported on fetus	Know high and low limits of pulse rate range outside of which drug should be withheld Take apical pulse for a full minute before administration. Withhold dose if pulse <60 Check cardiac monitor for arrhythmias Withhold drug if GI disturbances are noted Observe for hypokalemia Provide foods high in potassium
Hydrodiuril (thiazide diuretic)	50–100 mg/day	Promotes excretion of water, sodium, and chloride Causes excretion of potassium, biocarbonate, and other ions Lowers peripheral resistance Used as an adjunct in treating edema in congestive heart failure	Weigh patient daily Observe for signs of electrolyte imbalance Review laboratory studies of renal function and electrolytes
Heparin (anti-coagulant)*	10,000 U followed by 5,000–10,000 U every 4–6 hr IV *or* 10,000–20,000 U followed by 8,000–10,000 U t.i.d. SC	Interferes with most aspects of clotting mechanism Prolongs clotting time but does not affect bleeding time Increases risk of hemorrhage Is highly acidic, so imcompatible with most antibiotics Does not cross the placenta	Monitor daily coagulation studies If SC injection, rotate injection sites Check sites for hemorrhage and avoid massage Type and cross-match patient on admission
Quinidine (antiarrhythmic)	0.2–0.3 g t.i.d. or q.i.d., orally	Depresses cardiac excitability, conduction velocity, and contractability Has an anticholinergic action Effect is reduced if hypokalemia is present Sensitivity causes tinnitus, headache, nausea Does not cause uterine contractions No adverse effects reported on fetus	Monitor for arrhythmias Monitor serum electrolytes frequently
Inderal (beta-adrenergic blocker)	Contraindicated during pregnancy, since it may cause premature closing of fetal ductus arteriosus		

*Oral anticoagulants have been known to cause hemorrhage in the fetus, and therefore they are contraindicated in pregnancy

enter the home may spend more time at home than she would if she lived at ground floor level.

The goal of rest periods is to provide the best possible perfusion to the uterus. The patient should be instructed to rest in the left lateral recumbent position to facilitate blood flow through the great vessels. If dependent edema is present, the feet should be raised higher than the level of the heart. The patient should be advised to take a minimum of 8 to 10 hours of sleep per day, with frequent rest periods during the day.

The degree of salt restriction in the diet depends on the severity of the condition. The nurse should provide examples of how best to achieve a low-salt diet while still enjoying food. (Suggestions for Self-Care Teaching are given in the display on page 544.)

Anemia is avoided through sound nutrition, with an emphasis on foods high in iron, and supplemental iron. Routine prenatal assessment of the complete blood count will indicate whether iron intake needs adjustment.

Management for the patient with Class III or IV cardiac problems is directed at avoiding congestive failure and

SELF-CARE TEACHING

The Patient on a Low-Salt Diet

- Begin by eliminating foods coated with salt, such as crackers, chips, and french fries.
- Eliminate canned meats and all luncheon meats.
- All canned tomato products, including ketchup, are high in sodium. Use fresh tomatoes or reduced-sodium products.
- Other canned vegetables are high in sodium as well. Use fresh products as much as possible. Steam vegetables without adding salt.
- Do not salt any foods while cooking: learn to season with herbs and spices.
- Most cheeses are high in sodium, especially processed cheeses. Substitute low-sodium cheeses, such as mozzarella, ricotta, Swiss, cream cheese, and gruyere, which contain less than 150 mg sodium per ounce.

---

pulmonary edema resulting from the increased cardiac workload. The patient may need to be hospitalized for digitalis therapy. When therapy is being initiated, the nurse needs to monitor and assist the patient by

- Providing oxygenation
- Suggesting appropriate guidelines for rest and activity
- Providing emotional support
- Monitoring daily weights
- Providing skin care
- Promoting good nutrition
- Ensuring that constipation is avoided
- Providing medications
- Monitoring digitalis therapy

Once the patient is stabilized and discharged on digitalis, continued monitoring of her cardiac status is carried out during the prenatal period. The patient must maintain stabilization by self-care. Health care teaching by the nurse should include

- Planning a sample menu that includes the recommended sodium and fluid restrictions
- Developing a plan of activities that will avoid dyspnea and fatigue
- Assisting the patient to maintain the medication regimen by
    Teaching the name, dose, frequency, and side effects
    Teaching the use of each medication
    Teaching what symptoms should be reported immediately

Intrapartal and Postpartal Care

Pregnant women with cardiac disease are at risk for a slow onset of congestive heart failure or an acute episode of heart failure with pulmonary edema. This risk is greatest during labor and after the delivery of the placenta. Shifts in fluid balance occurring during this time are

- Delivery of the placenta with contraction of the uterus causing a significant decrease in intravascular space
- Fluid shift from tissues to intravascular space
- Increased cardiac return with decompression of the vena cava by the uterus

Eighty percent of maternal deaths occur under these conditions.

Women with a symptomatic cardiac condition need intensive care during labor. Vital signs are taken every 15 minutes. Signs of impending cardiac failure include respiratory rate above 24 and a pulse rate above 100. Both mother and fetus are under continuous electronic monitoring. Women should be resting in the left lateral recumbent position to facilitate vascular flow. Bearing down efforts should be avoided (Clark 1987).

For Class II and III cardiac patients, immediate postpartal nursing care is directed to hourly monitoring of intake and output. The patient may be assisted in diuresing, with the administration of intravenous Lasix. Pulse and respiratory rate should be monitored, as in labor. In addition to observation for signs of cardiac failure, the patient should be monitored for hemorrhage and thrombophlebitis.

Rest lowers the workload of the heart and is the critical component of self-care. The patient will need support from family and health care team in order to tolerate a restricted pregnancy. It is important for the nurse to listen to the patient's concerns and frustration with prolonged bedrest. The nurse should help the patient anticipate her needs for the immediate postpartum period, if restricted activity is continued (Bosak et al 1987).

Thrombophlebitis

Deep venous thrombosis occurs in about 0.018% to 0.29% of all deliveries (Rutherford and Phelan 1987). The condition is most likely diagnosed in the postpartum period (see Chapter 30 for further discussion). Women are at 3 to 5 times greater risk of thromboembolic disorders if they

- Are delivered by Cesarean birth
- Are older women with high parity
- Are obese
- Are restricted in ambulating
- Have cardiac disease.

Superficial venous thrombosis and varicosities are more commonly seen prenatally. When treated, they rarely present a serious problem (Rutherford et al 1987).

Implications for Nursing Care

The presence of varicosities may be assessed by direct examination of the legs or by patient report of tired, aching legs. Fitting with support stockings can significantly reduce any increased risk of serious complications. In her teaching, the nurse should include the points listed in the accompanying Self-Care Teaching display.

Renal Disease

A study of 30 pregnant women with renal disease found that those with normal renal function tests showed no evidence of deterioration during pregnancy (Klockars et al 1980). This study included women who had glomerulonephritis, pyelonephritis, or polycystic kidney disease. The perinatal mortality in women with impaired renal function resulted from hypertension (PIH), placenta abruptio, and preterm delivery. Women with successful renal transplants who maintain adequate renal function for at least 2 years may deliver term infants without complications.

This discussion of renal disease is limited to insults that have resulted in impaired renal function. The effect of renal disease on pregnancy is in part dependent on the presence of hypertension. In the absence of hypertension, renal disease may not directly affect the mother and fetus. Rather, it increases the risk of other complications developing during pregnancy, such as the following:

* Pregnancy-induced hypertension (PIH)
* Urinary tract infections

SELF-CARE TEACHING

The Patient With Thrombophlebitis

* Rest with legs elevated above the level of the heart.
* Use correct method for putting on support (Jobst) stockings: lie flat with legs elevated and roll on stockings.
* Do not sit with legs crossed.
* Wear loose clothing.
* Do not wear garters or other tight restrictions around the legs.
* If sitting most of day, get up and move around every hour.

* Preterm labor
* Intrauterine growth retardation

In the kidneys, as in other systems, many physiologic changes take place as a result of pregnancy.

* Kidney size increases
* Ureters and kidney pelves dilate, with relaxation of smooth muscles
* Glomerular filtration rate increases
* Renal plasma flow increases
* Growing uterus causes mechanical obstruction

The triad of symptoms indicative of renal disease are the same as those for PIH: hypertension, proteinuria, and edema. Renal function studies will establish a baseline in early pregnancy and will serve as a comparison with later studies, if the patient's condition is worsening clinically. These studies include a complete blood count, electrolyte tests, and serum creatinine and blood urea nitrogen (BUN) tests. Urinary studies include urinalysis, bacteria culture, and a 24-hour collection for protein and creatinine clearance.

The treatment approach is similar to that for PIH:

* More frequent prenatal visits
* Serial ultrasound for interval fetal growth
* Monthly assessment of renal function
* Monthly screening with urine cultures for asymptomatic bacteriuria
* Careful assessment of blood pressure for early detection of hypertensive changes
* Antepartum surveillance beginning at 32 to 34 weeks

Implications for Nursing Care

Assessment of the urine at each prenatal visit will establish a valuable comparative record. The nurse should review the record for the incidence of proteinuria. Trace proteinuria can be expected and is not significant. Proteinuria at the level of +1 to +2 is an indication for further analysis with a 24-hour collection for total protein.

For both the urinalysis and the cultures, an uncontaminated specimen is essential. If efforts to obtain a clean-catch midstream specimen are unsatisfactory, catheterization may be indicated.

Careful assessment of the blood pressure includes

* Reviewing the prepregnant blood pressure and current prenatal readings
* Using the correct cuff size for the size of the patient
* Retaking the blood pressure after the patient has rested on her left side for 10 minutes, if the initial reading shows elevation

The degree and location of edema should be evaluated, reviewing the following points:

- When in the day does the patient notice the swelling? Morning edema may either be renal or PIH related. If edema appears in the evening only, it is probably pregnancy related.

- Where does the patient most notice the edema? Edema of the feet and ankles is probably pregnancy related. Edema of the face or generalized edema is either renal or PIH related.

- Is the edema constant or intermittent? Pregnancy related edema may appear during periods of increased activity, prolonged standing, or warm humid days. Renal induced edema is related to intake of salts, protein, and fluids, as well as renal perfusion and is likely to remain constant.

Preterm labor and intrauterine growth retardation are common complications for women with renal impairment. See sections regarding self-care for preterm labor prevention and third trimester fetal assessment. Women with renal impairment enter pregnancy with *known* risk. The health care team needs to keep her and the family realistically informed of the progress of the pregnancy.

Asthma

Asthma is a condition of intermittent airway obstruction resulting in a restricted capacity to breathe. The condition varies greatly in its severity, ranging from acute attacks requiring hospitalization to a mild chronic form controlled by medication. Only in the most severe form, reflected by altered blood gases, is oxygenation of the fetus affected. Asthma may result in an increased incidence of abortion and preterm labor and, in its most severe form, may be life-threatening to the mother.

SELF-CARE TEACHING

The Patient With Asthma

- Try to identify the factors that aggravate your condition.
- Seek medical care at the onset of an upper respiratory infection.
- Discuss adverse reactions to the medications and any relation to the discomforts of pregnancy with care-provider.
- If the asthma is allergy-related, adjust your diet or environment to reduce the incidence of reactions.
- If the asthma is stress-related, discuss your concerns and request referrals as needed.

Stimuli associated with asthmatic episodes are allergies and stress. Depending on whether the patient is exposed to these stimuli, asthma may or may not present a problem during pregnancy.

Asthma presents with the respiratory symptoms of an expiratory wheeze, dyspnea, and a productive cough of tenacious mucus. A prolonged episode of asthma may result in hypoxemia, hypercarbia, and atelectasis.

The objective of treatment is the relief of symptoms and the reduction of stimuli that may precipitate or aggravate asthma. The treatment is accomplished by the use of various bronchodilators. Depending on symptoms, the drugs and dosage may vary during the course of pregnancy. Since these are often controlled by the patient, the nurse should instruct her on the use of each medication. Table 20–5 lists the drugs most commonly used in the treatment of asthma.

The patient may be concerned about the teratogenic effects of the daily use of medication during pregnancy. These concerns should be explored, since they may affect her compliance in the use of needed medications. To date, no teratogenic effects have been related to the drugs listed in Table 20–5.

Depending on the severity of asthma, the medication regimen follows a progressive pattern:

1. For chronic mild asthma, theophylline compounds may be tried with adrenergic inhalants, as needed.
2. If the above approach is not effective, oral beta-adrenergic agents are added in divided doses.
3. For severe asthma causing interference with daily living, oral steroids are added in addition to the above.
4. If a patient on the above regimen finds that symptoms are not controlled by it, she should report to the Emergency Room for evaluation.

Implications for Nursing Care

Since the interaction between asthma and pregnancy is so variable, the nurse should briefly review the status of the patient's asthma since the last prenatal visit. Approximately 75% of patients will either improve or remain unchanged. The nurse should focus on self-care health teaching that will help the patient to avoid any precipitating or aggravating factors.

CHAPTER SUMMARY

With advances in medical care, women, who in the past would not have conceived, are now able to carry a pregnancy to near term or term. The challenge to the health care team is to maintain the best balance possible between care of the medical condition and care of the preg-

Table 20-5   **Common Maintenance Drugs for the Asthmatic Patient**

Drug	Dosage	Effects and Adverse Reactions	Nursing Implications
Epinephrine 1:1000 solution	0.3 to 0.5 ml SC or IM	Elevates blod pressure Increases heart rate Causes vasoconstriction In pregnancy, has same effect on fetus Not known to be teratogenic Quick acting with short duration	Epinephrine is usually administered in emergency room at onset of attack. Patients become anxious when having diffculty breathing, and anxiety is increased with palpitations. Provide calm reassurance and support oxygen inhalation
Ephedrine, Tedral (contains ephedrine, theophylline, phenobarbital)	25 to 50 mg every 4 to 6 hours orally	Longer-acting agent than epinephrine Causes bronchodilation Causes cerebral agitation (confusion, disorientation, behavioral changes, etc.), unless taken in combined form, as in Tedral	Patient may be maintained on this drug for extended periods Stress need for medical follow-up to determine minimum effective dosage
Isoproterenol (Isuprel), isoetharine (Bronkosol)	No more than two inhalants t.i.d.	Causes bronchodilation Quick-acting, short duration Death has resulted from overuse	Review use pattern with patient Stress use only as needed
Terbutaline (Bricanyl, Brethine)	2.5–5 mg every 6 hours	Causes bronchodilation Frequently causes increased heart rate and tremors. Often causes palpitations, sweating, headache, and cramps in hands and feet. Drug appears to be effective in stopping preterm labor. Maintenance dose is often required until 37 weeks of gestation. Relaxes smooth muscles	Monitor pulse rate Anxiety is increased with palpitations. Provide calm reassurance and support Discuss side-effects and encourage patient compliance

nancy. It often requires the patient and her family to adjust their lifestyle to accommodate the self-care required. In the process, the patient undergoes physiologic changes in her health status and psychosocial changes in her self-identity, infant bonding, family relationships, and possibly her entire social structure. The nurse is challenged to address the full scope of needs in facilitating the patient's and family's access to appropriate health team members and community resources.

STUDY QUESTIONS

1. What are the goals of preconception counseling?
2. A Class II cardiac patient who is pregnant is advised to avoid all strenuous activity. List those activities that you would consider as needing modification.
3. What action would you take if you found a +2 glucose level on a routine urine test during a prenatal visit?
4. Why is the most effective time to screen for diabetes after the 24th week of gestation?
5. Laboring women with significant cardiac disease are at risk for developing what two complications?

6. What are the classic symptoms of a urinary tract infection?
7. The principles for caring for the pregnant patient with renal impairment are similar to those followed in pregnancy-induced hypertension. List these principles.
8. List three sexually transmitted diseases that can be transmitted to the fetus.
9. Give three reasons why hepatitis Type B, and not Type A, is a perinatal concern.
10. List five conditions that put women at risk for exposure to HIV.
11. What complications of pregnancy are women who use cocaine likely to experience?
12. Discuss health teaching points to help women avoid accidental trauma in pregnancy.

REFERENCES/BIBLIOGRAPHY

Abel EJ: Marijuana, Tobacco, Alcohol, and Reproduction. Boca Raton, FL, CRC Press, 1983
Abel EL: Fetal Alcohol Syndrome and Fetal Alcoholic Effects. New York, Plenum Press, 1984

ACOG Committee on Technical Bulletins of the American College of Obstetricians and Gynecologists. Automobile Passenger Restraints for Children and Women, #74. Washington, D.C., American College of Obstetricians and Gynecologists, 1983

American Diabetes Association. Position Statement on Gestational Diabetes Mellitus. Diabetes, 34:123–26, 1985

Berry JL, Swank AB, Gabbe SG: Endocrine considerations in pregnancy: Diabetes mellitus and thyroid disease. In Sonstegard LJ, Kowalski KM, Jennings B (eds): Women's Health: Crisis and Illness in Childbearing, vol 3. New York, Grune & Stratton, Inc. 1987, pp 205–212

Boehme TL: Hepatitis B: The nurse-midwife's role in management and prevention. J Nurse-Midwifery, 30:79–87, 1985

Booth W: CDC paints a picture of HIV infection in U.S. Science 239(4837):253, 1988

Bosak PJ, Larson DM: Cardiac disease and DIC in pregnancy. In Sonstegard LJ, Kowalski KM, Jennings B (eds): Women's Health: Crisis Illness and Childbearing, vol 3. New York, Grune & Stratton, 1987, p 169

Center for Disease Control: Recommendations for assisting in the prevention of perinatal transmission of human T-lymphotropic virus Type III/lymphadenopathy-associated virus and acquired immunodeficiency syndrome. MMWR 34(48):721–32, 1985

Clark SL: Structural cardiac disease in pregnancy. In Clark SL, Phelan JP, Cotton DB (eds): Critical Care Obstetrics. Oradell, NJ, Medical Economics Books, 1987, pp 92–113

DiClemente RJ, Boyer CB, Morales ES: Minorities and AIDS: Knowledge, attitudes, and misconceptions among black and latino adolescents. Am J Public Health 78:55–57, 1988

Feldblum PJ, Fortney JA: Condoms, spermicides, and the transmission of human immunodeficiency virus: A review of the literature. Am J Public Health 78:52–3, 1988

Gibbons JM: Diabetes in pregnancy. In Schnatz JD (ed): Diabetes Mellitus: Problems of Management. Menlo Park, CA, Addison-Wesley Publishing Co, 1982, p 171

Khoury A, Nuwayhid B: Blood glucose control. In Nuwayhid BS, Brinkman III CR, Lieb SM (eds): Management of the Diabetic Pregnancy. New York, Elsevier, 1987, pp 49–59

Klockars M, Saarikoski S, Ikonen E, et al: Pregnancy in patients with renal disease. Acta Med Scand 207:214–18, 1980

Krugman S: Viral hepatitis: 1985 update. Pediatr Rev 7:3–10, 1985

Lake KD: Drugs and pregnancy. In Sonstegard LJ, Kowalski KM, Jennings B (eds): Women's Health and Illness in Childbearing, vol. 3. New York, Grune & Stratton, 1987, p 249

Landon MB, Gabbe SG, Piana R, et al: Neonatal morbidity in pregnancy complicated by diabetes mellitus: Predictive value of maternal glycemic profiles. Am J Obstet Gynecol 156:1089–93, 1987

Langer O, Mazze R: Diabetes in pregnancy: Evaluating self-monitoring performance and glycemic control with memory-based reflective meters. Am J Obstet Gynecol 155:635–41, 1987

MacGregor SN, Keith LG, Chasnoff IJ, et al: Cocaine use during pregnancy: Adverse perinatal outcome. Am J Obstet Gynecol 157:686–90, 1987

Moran JJM: Stress fractures in pregnancy. Am J Obstet Gynecol 158:1274–77, 1988

Nitzan M: Diabetes mellitus. In Schulman JD, Simpson JL (eds): Genetic Disorders in Pregnancy: Maternal Effects of Fetal Outcome. New York, Academic Press, 1981, p 340

Pastorek II, JG, Miller JR, Summers PR: The effect of hepatitis B antigenemia in pregnancy outcome. Am J Obstet Gynecol 158:486–9, 1988

Rutherford SE, Phelan JP: Deep venous thrombosis and pulmonary embolus. In Clark SL, Phelan JP, Cotton DB (eds): Critical Care Obstetrics. Oradell, NJ, Medical Economics Books, 1987, pp 126–134

Shannon M: Acquired Immunodeficiency syndrome (AIDS) Screening. In Star WL, Shannon MT, Sammons LN, et al (eds): Ambulatory Obstetrics: Protocol for Nurse Practitioners/Nurse Midwives. San Francisco, University of California, San Francisco Press, 1987, pp 159–62

Smith CV, Phelan JP: Trauma in pregnancy. In Clark SL, Phelan JP, Cotton DB (eds): Critical Care Obstetrics. Oradell, NJ, Medical Economics Books, 1987, pp 382–89

Willimas A: Public health implications of HIV infection. Nurse Pract 1:8–13, 1986

SUGGESTED READINGS

Alexander L: The pregnant smoker: nursing implications. J Obstet Gynecol Neonatal Nurs 15(3):167, 1987

Arneson S, Beltz E, Hahnemann B et al: Automobile seat belt practices of pregnant women. J Obstet Gynecol Neonatal Nurs 15(4): 339, 1986

Avery P, McKenzie O: Expanding the scope of childbirth education to meet the needs of hospitalized, high risk patients. J Obstet Gynecol Neonatal Nurs 16(6):418, 1987

Gavin JR: Diabetes and exercise. Am J Nursing 88(2):178, 1988

Harris BAA: Pregnancy in the diabetic woman. Part I: Screening and preconception care. Female Patient 10(10):57, 1985

Lipman TH: What causes diabetes? MCN 13(1):40, 1988

Shaw FE, Maynard JE: Hepatitis B: still a concern for you and your patients. Contemp OB/GYN 27(Special issue):27, 1986

Smith J: The dangers of prenatal cocaine use. MCN 13(3):174, 1988

Snyder D: Peer group support for high-risk mothers. MCN 13(2):114, 1988

Van Dorten JP: Pyelonephritis in pregnancy. Female Patient 11(3):100, 1986

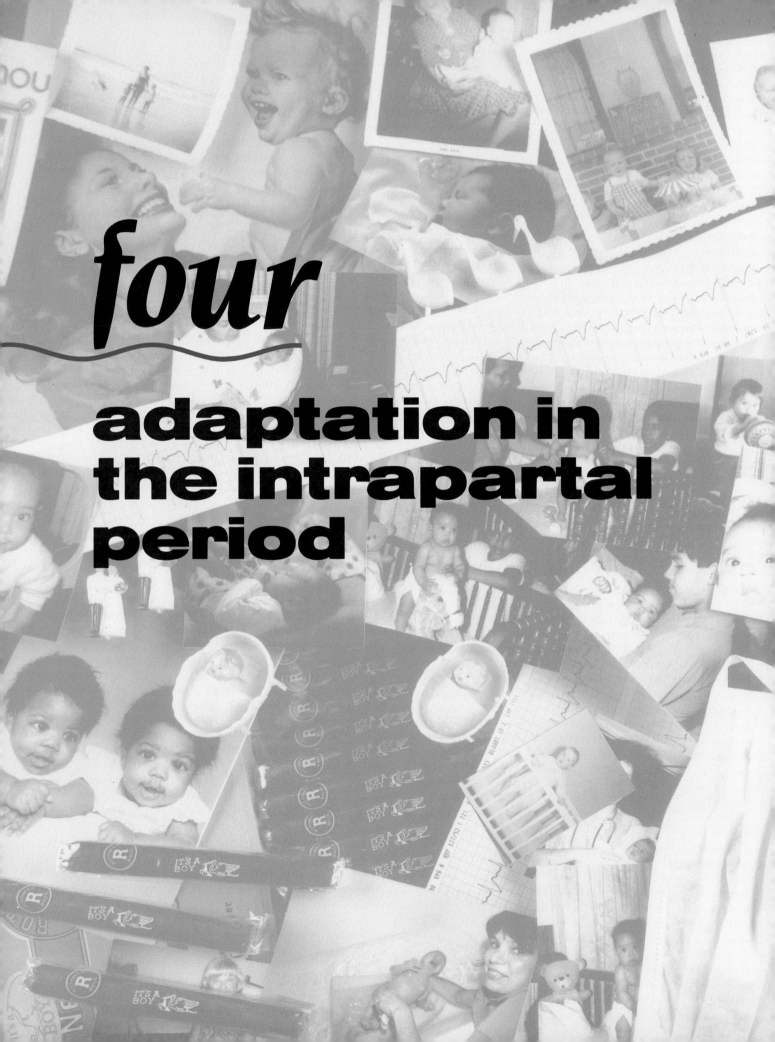

four

adaptation in the intrapartal period

21 preparation for childbirth

LEARNING OBJECTIVES

After studying the material in this chapter, the student should be able to

- Describe the major components included in most forms of childbirth preparation

- Describe commonly used labor coping techniques and explain the underlying theory of their effectiveness

- Explain the key points of appropriate nursing care of laboring patients using specific labor coping techniques

- Describe the documented effects of childbirth education

- Identify organizations involved in childbirth education and the current status of teacher certification in the field

- Discuss nursing roles in childbirth preparation

KEY TERMS

Conditioned response

Effleurage

Hyperventilation

Pain threshold

Pain tolerance

Progressive relaxation

Psychoprophylaxis

Sensate focus

Signal or cleansing breath

Tonus

Visualization

In the early part of the 20th century, birth was seen as an almost inevitable and uncontrollable event in a family's life. In the mid-1960s childbirth in the United States and other industrialized countries underwent a dramatic shift. Childbirth has become an event that many families consciously choose to experience and over which they increasingly want to exert some measure of personal control. Many other aspects of birth have changed as well, including the range of places in which birth occurs, the medical technology available, and customary birth attendants.

Since the maternity nurse is the person primarily responsible for assisting and supporting laboring women and their families, it is important for her to understand some of the history and background of the prepared childbirth movement and to be familiar with a variety of methods of preparing for childbirth so that she can provide safe and supportive care, regardless of the level or type of preparation of her patient.

Providing safe and sensitive care to families during pregnancy and birth, regardless of the pregnant woman's level of preparation, is a major goal of maternity nursing care. However, more and more families are attending childbirth classes and planning to use prepared childbirth techniques during labor. This trend is being extended to a broad range of socioeconomic and cultural groups, and in many communities the majority of expectant mothers and their partners attend some sort of childbirth classes.

The purpose of this chapter is to present information about prepared childbirth so that the nurse can deliver safe and appropriate care to women and families who choose to use these techniques, and to alert the nurse to developments in childbirth education that directly affect nursing practice in the obstetric setting.

SOME HISTORICAL PERSPECTIVES ON PREPARED CHILDBIRTH

One of the most important changes in birth in America has been the shift from home to hospital birth and from traditional birth attendants to physicians. In the United States in 1900, over 90% of births took place in the home, and the usual birth attendant was the so-called granny midwife. By 1940, more than half of all births took place in hospitals and were attended by physicians, either general practitioners or specialists in obstetrics. By 1970, the transition was complete, with more than 95% of births taking place in hospital settings, the vast majority attended by obstetricians.

Introduction of Routine Medical Intervention

As physicians increasingly managed the processes of labor and birth, more and more medical interventions and technology were developed to deal with the problems physicians observed. The use of anesthesia to ease the pain of labor and birth and the use of forceps to facilitate difficult births are examples of early medical interventions. As birth moved into the hospital setting, practices that had developed in other areas of medical care were introduced into obstetrics and became part of routine management. Many practices were borrowed directly from the standard surgical care of the day, such as routine transfer of the patient from one specialized area of the hospital to another (rather than moving medical and nursing staff), vigilance about sterile procedures, preparation procedures (including routine shaving and enemas for women in labor), and delivery of the infant on a specialized table in the delivery room.

Many of these changes were intended to improve outcomes for mothers and infants. However, as hospital practices in birth continued to evolve, some changes were introduced that were clearly not in the best interests of mothers, fathers, or babies. In the early part of the century, a drug known as "twilight sleep" was introduced from Great Britain. Touted as the best anesthesia for childbirth, it was a combination of morphine and scopolamine. Women were not aware of their surroundings with this analgesia and had no memory of the birth. This type of anesthesia became popular among middle- and upper-class women. However, it increased the risk of respiratory depression in the newborn, and the need for more intensive medical support gave further momentum to the trend toward hospitalization for childbirth.

Standard obstetric practice gradually included more use of analgesia. By the 1940s, women were often "snowed" during labor, given morphine or opiate substitutes and general anesthesia for uncomplicated vaginal births. Along with the increased use of analgesia and anesthesia came the need for more intensive medical and nursing care, such as complete bed rest, intravenous fluids, and urinary catheters, as well as the undesirable side-effects of prolonged labors and depressed neonates.

The increased use of medical technology in normal childbirth had other undesirable effects on families. Fathers began to be routinely excluded from participation in the birth; by the 1950s, they were frequently barred from the floor of the hospital on which the labor and delivery room was located and were not allowed to hold their babies or even see them, except through nursery viewing windows at visiting hours. Participation and hospital visits by other family members were practically unheard of (Wertz and Wertz 1977).

Beginnings of the "Natural Childbirth" Movement

In response to the increasing "medicalization" of birth, a grassroots movement began promoting the advantages of "natural childbirth." Dr. Grantly Dick–Read's book *Childbirth Without Fear,* published in the United States in 1944, gained popularity in Great Britain and the United States. Dick–Read stressed that if mothers were educated about the process of birth as a healthy, normal event, their fear would be reduced and so would muscular tension during labor and birth, resulting in less pain. In time, women who had had successful birth experiences following Dick–Read's principles began to organize, sometimes with the support of health care professionals, to offer teaching and support to other women. The International Childbirth Education Association (ICEA) was established in 1960. The ICEA promoted various childbirth preparation programs and is still a major force in childbirth education today.

Shortly after the introduction of Dick–Read's teaching to this country, another school of thought in the area of natural childbirth appeared. The work of Dr. Ferdinand Lamaze, a French obstetrician, became known in the United States, in large part because of the publication in 1959 of *Thank You, Dr. Lamaze* by Marjorie Karmel. Lamaze's notion of "childbirth without pain through the psychoprophylactic method" grew out of the then-new concept of Pavlovian conditioning. This method gained increasing popularity in the United States. Again parents banded together with professionals to organize a nationally recognized teacher-training program and promote this method of birth. Their efforts resulted in the formation of the American Society for Psychoprophylaxis in Obstetrics (ASPO) in 1960.

Shortly thereafter, another view of natural childbirth was presented by an American obstetrician, Robert Bradley, in his 1965 book, *Husband-Coached Childbirth,* which emphasized the use of deep relaxation techniques for labor and the role of the husband as coach. An organization of parents and professionals called the American Academy of Husband-Coached Childbirth evolved to make Bradley's teachings widely available and to prepare teachers.

Some of the distinguishing characteristics of these three methods, as they were first developed, are shown in the accompanying display. Contemporary childbirth education practices are eclectic and combine features of all three methods.

The Struggle to Reform Birth Practices in the United States

Acceptance of the Dick–Read, Lamaze, and Bradley views of childbirth was achieved only after much struggle. The parents, teachers, and health professionals who be-

---

Contributions of Early Developers of Prepared Childbirth

Grantly Dick–Read

- Suggested that education reduces fear of the unknown, thus eliminating the "fear–tension–pain" cycle
- Stressed the importance of muscular relaxation and slow breathing

Ferdinand Lamaze

- Proposed that psychoprophylaxis ("mind prevention") could eliminate or greatly reduce the perception of pain through the formation of new conditioned reflexes in response to uterine contractions
- Developed a technique combining relaxation, concentration and focusing, and complex breathing patterns to decrease the perception of pain

Robert Bradley

- Believed that the father, as the woman's loved one and intimate partner, was the most effective person for labor support
- Proposed that imitation of behaviors observed among other mammals, such as slow breathing, deep relaxation, and reduced responsiveness to external stimuli, would promote comfort during labor

---

lieved in and promoted these methods met considerable resistance from the medical and nursing professions in the 1960s and 1970s. The struggle was so intense that in 1973 a bill was introduced into the House of Representatives (H.R. 1502), which, if it had been passed into law, would have made it mandatory for all hospitals receiving federal funds to permit the father to attend the labor and delivery as long as he had the permission of the mother and physician. Many nurses and physicians who joined parents in this struggle were ostracized; in some cases nurses lost their jobs.

The change was difficult, in part because there was little organized support from within medicine and nursing, and changing a system from the outside is usually difficult. Sasmor (1979) points out that early proponents of natural childbirth (usually childbirth educators) by and large ignored the importance of the labor nurse in parents' experiences of birth. Early efforts to reform birth practices often led to adversarial rather than collaborative relationships between parents and health professionals. This probably delayed the adoption of family-centered obstetric care in many areas of the country and perhaps still hinders its acceptance to some extent.

Nevertheless the natural childbirth movement was successful not only in promoting education and preparation for birth, but also in paving the way for the development of the family-centered or "alternative" birth practices discussed in detail in Chapter 2. Prepared childbirth, as it is more often called now, has gone from being a fashionable practice among educated middle-class couples to being a resource available to and used by a wide variety of parents.

Childbirth Education: A Social Trend

Prepared childbirth is rapidly becoming a standard part of prenatal care in the United States. It is a central part of family-centered maternity care, and the scope of prenatal education has become much broader than simply teaching parents techniques for coping with labor. There is considerable agreement among the major organizations involved in prenatal education about what areas are important to address; the basic components of prenatal education programs are listed in the accompanying display.

In many hospitals, most parents have obtained prenatal education. However, prepared childbirth is still a predominantly middle-class phenomenon and is not easily accessible to members of disadvantaged and minority groups or tailored to their needs. This is clearly reflected in the characteristics of those who choose prepared childbirth. Women who attend childbirth classes are more likely to be primiparous, better educated, more affluent, more knowledgeable about pregnancy and birth, and more likely to have a positive self-concept, favor nontraditional male and female roles, plan to have their husband present at birth, and to breast-feed than are women who do not attend prenatal classes.

Childbirth education has grown from the activities of small groups of largely self-taught childbirth educators scattered across the country to the current programs of several national organizations that provide coordination, teacher training, and certification for childbirth educators. Most communities now have childbirth educators in private practice as well as in hospital-based programs (Fig. 21 – 1). In many communities, parent education programs are sponsored by such organizations as the Ameri-

---

Basic Components of Prenatal Education Programs

The following are basic components of prenatal education programs, according to the *ICEA Position Paper on Planning Comprehensive Maternal and Newborn Services for the Childbearing Year* and NAACOG *Guidelines for Childbirth Education:*

- Human reproduction, including the anatomy, physiology, and psychology of labor, birth, and the postpartum period; signs of pregnancy; normal physical and psychological changes during pregnancy; health maintenance and care during pregnancy; fetal development; signs and stages of labor; postpartum health care
- Basic nutritional needs and their relationship to fetal development
- Self-help techniques and comfort measures for pregnancy, labor, birth, and the postpartum period, including posture, body mechanics, maintenance of muscle tone and physical fitness, control of tension and relaxation, breathing techniques, childbirth and postpartum exercises
- Role and support techniques for the companion in labor and birth
- Social and psychological roles and relationships in the family; sexual roles
- Roles of health care providers in the management of labor, birth, and the postpartum period
- Options in labor and birth procedures and in the birth environment; rooming-in; early discharge; family visitation; home care follow-up
- Rights of the expectant family; responsibilities of the childbearing woman for self care and decision making
- High-risk birth, including indications and procedures for prenatal tests for fetal growth and well-being, electronic fetal monitoring, intravenous fluids, induction and augmentation, analgesia, anesthesia, episiotomy, forceps, and cesarean birth, as well as the risks and benefits associated with them and alternatives where appropriate; parents' participation in the care of a sick newborn
- Preparation for parenting, including the roles of family members, infant care, infant feeding (breast and bottle), child growth and development, child safety, well-baby care, immunizations, family planning, and the couple's sexual relationship; identification of community resource groups dealing with breast-feeding, parenting, cesarean family support, nutritional programs, and physical fitness
- Tour of maternity-newborn unit

Adapted from Young D: Changing Childbirth: Family Birth in the Hospital. Rochester Childbirth Graphics, 1982

EFFECTIVENESS OF PREPARED CHILDBIRTH

Research on the effectiveness of prepared childbirth has been made more difficult in some ways because of the special characteristics of parents who choose to attend prenatal classes and because its popularity has grown rapidly (Beck et al 1980). Are the "effects" of prepared childbirth actually caused by the education and the techniques themselves, or are they a result of the high levels of motivation and education found among parents who attend these classes? In addition, nearly everywhere in the United States, expectant parents have heard claims about the effectiveness of prepared childbirth. Are "effects" achieved because the techniques work, or because parents *expect* them to work? Few studies have been sufficiently well controlled to allow conclusive findings. However, there is agreement about some effects of prepared childbirth.

Documented Effects of Prepared Childbirth

Participation in prepared childbirth classes does contribute to increased knowledge about the functioning of the body in childbearing, and about the course of pregnancy, labor, and birth. Preparation for childbirth appears to lead to more positive attitudes about childbirth in general and to the reduced use of medication during labor and birth. It is not clear whether preparation for childbirth reduces the actual pain experienced or increases the woman's ability to cope with pain. Early in the history of the prepared childbirth movement, proponents claimed that these techniques could produce "painless childbirth" and shorter labors. Contemporary experts do *not* make this claim but stress that the techniques enable the woman to cope more effectively with the stress of labor by reducing anxiety and promoting relaxation.

Unsupported Claims About Prepared Childbirth

The nurse as a health care professional must always be aware that overenthusiastic proponents sometimes exaggerate the benefits of new and innovative developments in health care. For some reason, this seems to be especially common in relation to practices in maternity care. Parents may hear that prepared childbirth classes will "make them better parents," "will increase parent–infant bonding," or "will improve the husband–wife relationship." Any of these might happen to an individual couple during the course of prenatal classes, but there is no evidence to indicate that preparation for parenthood has a long-term effect on marital or parent–infant relationships.

However, many of the original claims about the useful-

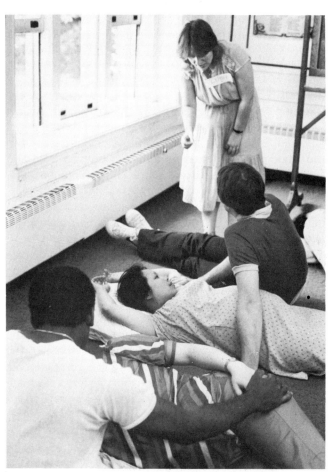

Figure 21–1. A maternity nurse/childbirth educator provides individualized teaching for expectant parents in childbirth preparation classes. (Courtesy of John B. Franklin Maternity Hospital, formerly Booth Maternity Center, Philadelphia)

can Red Cross. Libraries and bookstores hold a wide range of written materials for expectant and new parents. There is a growing trend toward offering a greater variety of classes for expectant and new parents, including early pregnancy classes, father and sibling classes, and support groups for expectant and new parents. Organizations involved in prenatal education have provided leadership in the development of these types of educational programs.

Several organizations, including ASPO/Lamaze and ICEA, have developed teaching-training and certification programs to ensure that childbirth educators have similar knowledge and competencies. Most childbirth educators certified by one of these organizations add the initials CCE (certified childbirth educator), or some variation of that designation after their names. However, childbirth education is not regulated by law, and anyone who chooses to do so can practice as a childbirth educator. The nurse should encourage parents to seek out a childbirth educator who has a good reputation in the community, who works in collaboration with professionals and hospitals, and who is certified by a national organization.

ness of prepared childbirth to help reduce stress by increasing coping during labor have been supported. For this reason, it is important that the nurse understands the theoretical basis for prepared childbirth practices.

THEORETICAL BASIS FOR PREPARED CHILDBIRTH

The major schools of prepared childbirth in the United States evolved separately, and each used a different theory to explain the effectiveness of its techniques. Dick–Read (1959) stressed the importance of giving the mother adequate information prenatally to reduce her fear of the unknown and thus minimize muscle tension. He described a cycle of "fear–tension–pain" in which fear of the unknown intensifies muscular tension, which in turn increases the perception of pain. Thus, the Dick–Read method focuses on relaxing the mind as well as the body.

The Lamaze method, which was developed slightly later, focuses on the idea that pain and uterine contractions are separate phenomena that became linked in the human mind. The Lamaze method is directed toward reducing the negative preconceptions women have about labor through education and the formation of new conditioned reflexes in response to uterine contractions. Selected breathing and active relaxation techniques are practiced until they are accomplished with ease. Early proponents theorized that these practiced responses decreased the perception of pain by blocking impulses to the cerebral cortex. More recently, it has been suggested that pain impulses are blocked in the dorsal horn cells of the spinal cord by varied tactile and pressure stimuli together with selective focusing on breathing and relaxation (the "gate control" theory). The effectiveness of these activities has also been linked to the body's ability to produce its own endogenous analgesics, the endorphins (Nichols and Humenick 1988).

Sasmor (1979), a nurse and childbirth educator, suggests that the effectiveness of all forms of childbirth preparation can be best explained by Selye's stress adaptation theory. Selye proposed that human beings function on three inter-related planes: the physiologic, the psychologic, and the biologic. Any change in one plane results in changes in the other two. An example would be the case of the woman in labor who becomes increasingly fearful (a psychologic change), resulting in the increased secretion of adrenalin (physiologic), which can disrupt the pattern of uterine contractions (biologic).

Viewed from this perspective, childbirth preparation can be seen as a form of stress adaptation, giving the mother mechanisms with which she can cope more effectively with the stresses of labor and birth. First, the woman is given factual information, which reduces the fear of the unknown and contributes to a positive mental attitude about labor and birth. This often results in an increased sense of confidence and control. Second, the woman is taught relaxation exercises to use in response to the sensations of labor. The more the woman concentrates on selective relaxation and on a particular sensate focus, the less she is aware of the painful sensations of labor. In addition, relaxation of muscles not involved in the labor process avoids unnecessary energy drain and fatigue, which can lead to an increased perception of pain. Finally, she is taught to concentrate on and to use deliberate behavior patterns, such as breathing techniques, to alter her perception of pain and reduce it to a manageable level.

Virtually all childbirth preparation methods advocate having a trained support person present during labor. The presence of a support person provides psychologic reassurance, which augments the coping mechanisms available to the mother. Attending to simple comfort measures, providing emotional reassurance, and acting as the spokesperson for the woman in labor are some of the functions of the labor partner, whose role complements that of the nurse. Most often, the labor partner is the mate of the woman in labor, but a friend, her mother, or another relative can also fill this role. The woman may choose to have more than one person available for support.

GOALS AND PRACTICES OF PREPARED CHILDBIRTH

The nurse working in obstetrics must be aware of the goals and practices of prepared childbirth and must be skilled in supporting and supplementing the parents' own efforts in labor and birth.

The overall goals of preparation for childbirth are

- To provide parents with the knowledge and skill they need to cope with the stress of pregnancy, labor, and birth
- To prepare parents to be intelligent consumers of maternity care
- To assist parents in achieving a safe, positive, and rewarding labor and birth experience

The various modes of preparation for childbirth all share these goals.

Observers of childbirth education in the United States have noted that in recent years the distinctions between the schools of prepared childbirth have faded and that many childbirth educators present a more eclectic approach to labor techniques, including the most effective techniques from each method. Since the nurse in the obstetric setting rarely has much contact with expectant parents prior to labor, she must be acquainted with the full range of techniques used to support parents regardless of their mode of preparation. Sasmor (1979) states that all approaches to childbirth education have the following common features:

- Factual information about human reproduction and detailed descriptions of labor and birth
- Techniques for achieving and maintaining relaxation
- Specific learned breathing techniques to be used in response to the sensations of labor

The following section will discuss these last two areas in detail and outline appropriate nursing actions to support the couple using these techniques during labor.

Techniques for Coping With Labor

Most methods of prepared childbirth teach two kinds of techniques for coping with labor, *relaxation techniques* and *learned breathing techniques*.

Relaxation

Relaxation is "a state of low arousal in which such bodily responses as muscle tension, heart rate, breathing rate, and metabolism diminish so as to bring these functions into equilibrium" (Shrock 1988). The stress response, the opposite of relaxation, can interfere with any of the four major physiologic systems — muscular, vascular, hormonal, or neurotransmitter.

Relaxation techniques

Relaxation techniques are designed to help the woman achieve a deep level of relaxation of muscles not directly involved in the work of labor. Uterine contractions use tremendous amounts of energy; avoiding unnecessary muscular tension conserves energy and oxygen reserves needed for the work of labor. Few people are skilled at achieving and maintaining states of mental and physical relaxation, so specific techniques must be learned and practiced in preparation for birth (Fig. 21–2). Techniques for relaxation are most effective when they are selected according to which physiologic system is in disequilibrium; Table 21–1 shows common effects of prolonged stress and lists relaxation techniques with which the nurse should be familiar.

Preparation for childbirth involves many types of relaxation techniques. Some of the most frequently taught are the following:

- *Progressive relaxation:* leads to a state of deep relaxation of the entire body by systematically tensing and releasing muscle groups in a pattern

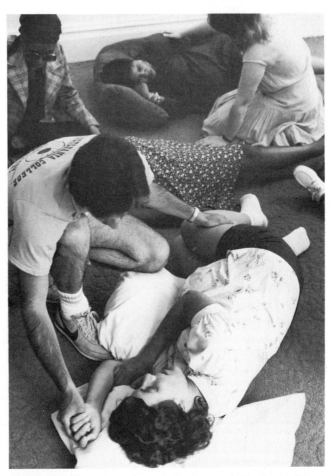

Figure 21–2. The father or support person helps the mother learn to use relaxation techniques in preparation for childbirth. (Courtesy of John B. Franklin Maternity Hospital, formerly Booth Maternity Center, Philadelphia)

- *Neuromuscular dissociation:* teaches the woman to consciously tense and release a particular muscle group while maintaining deep relaxation elsewhere
- *Visualization:* affects a woman's manner of response by combining mental and visual processes to form calming and peaceful images.

Table 21–2 describes these and other types of relaxation techniques and approaches to teaching them. The nurse should be familiar with these in order to help laboring women and their partners to utilize relaxation as a coping technique during labor. This will enable the nurse to assist the woman in achieving and maintaining optimum relaxation and will help the support person to do the same. The nurse's familiarity and comfort with these techniques sometimes makes the difference between adequate and *excellent* supportive nursing care during labor.

Another important point: relaxation training is probably one of the safest, most effective, and most *underuti-

Table 21 – 1   **Effects of Prolonged Stress and Suggested Relaxation Techniques**

Dominant System Affected	Symptoms Produced	Suggested Techniques
Muscular Response Increased muscle tone, which may compress veins and lymphatics, resulting in waste-product accumulation and further increases in muscle tone	Fatigue, increased susceptibility to infection Muscle spasms in the shoulder Low back pain Tension headaches	Neuromuscular relaxation supported by biofeedback or feedback from coach
Vascular System	Increased heart rate and blood pressure Cold extremities Sweaty palms Possibly migraines, angina	Autogenic training with feedback based on hand temperature, using sensation, mood ring, thermometer, or Biodot
Hormonal System Increase in ACTH, adrenalin, norepinephrine and thyroid hormone Decrease in follicle-stimulating hormone	Hypermotility of stomach, intestines Amenorrhea Retardation of immune response Compulsive eating or anorexia	Meditation, including focal points and concentration on breathing patterns Body imagery
Neurotransmitter System Possible excess, deficiency, or alteration of neurotransmitters	Increase in cortical activity, fear, depression Increased use of alcohol, nicotine, and caffeine with higher than average potential for addiction	Systematic desensitization and focus training, in conjunction with other types of relaxation training

Adapted from Humenick S: Teaching relaxation. Childbirth Educ 3(4):48, 1984

lized interventions in nursing. Relaxation can be safely and effectively used in a variety of nursing situations, such as caring for a patient in pain or assisting a patient to relax and sleep. As suggested in Table 21 – 1, relaxation (especially autogenic training) may also be of use in reducing blood pressure and heart rate secondary to high levels of stress and may assist in the control of habits associated with stress, such as smoking and overeating.

Progressive relaxation exercises are not used during actual labor but are taught to enable the woman to achieve a relaxed state easily and release tension when it develops in a particular body part. Neuromuscular dissociation exercises are believed to be useful for simulating the experience of a uterine contraction while keeping other muscles relaxed. Visualization can be used during actual labor and can be an effective means of pain management. It may be used to induce a generalized response similar to that achieved by progressive relaxation, or the goal may be to accomplish a specific physiologic response. During labor, visualizing the opening cervix may help to minimize unproductive tension. At the birth, picturing the baby moving down the birth canal may mobilize the forces needed to deliver the baby. Generalized relaxation responses may come from the suggestion to mentally picture and recall the sensations associated with

pleasant places the patient has been, to build an imagined picture following the verbal suggestions of her partner, or to visualize energy flowing into her body or the diminution of some symbol of pain. Imagery can be effectively used with an untrained woman, if suggestions are simple and within the woman's frame of reference. The nurse's skill in assessing the woman's particular fears and in establishing trust will be particularly valuable. The display on page 560 gives an example of a simple visualization exercise.

Several other techniques that can enhance relaxation are taught in many childbirth classes. The most common of these are the use of a sensate focus (or focal point), gentle massage, counterpressure to the back, and effleurage. The nurse should be able to identify the particular techniques a woman and her support person have been taught and assist in their use. The nurse should also observe the woman's level of relaxation and comfort throughout her labor and be prepared to suggest and teach other techniques that might be useful.

Use of a Sensate Focus

Focused concentration on a particular sensory stimulus can be quite effective in achieving and maintaining a level of deep relaxation. Lamaze teachers typically in-

Table 21–2   **Approaches to Teaching Relaxation Techniques**

Name and Type	Description	Feedback
Progressive relaxation (modifies muscular responses)	Consists of systematically tensing and releasing muscles. Developed by E Jacobson, modified by J Wolpe into a 6-wk approach with home practice.	Primary feedback from awareness of participant, who focuses on sensation of tensing and relaxing each muscle. Either coach or electromyograph can provide further feedback.
Neuromuscular dissociation (modifies muscular responses)	Modifies progressive relaxation by asking the participant to tense some muscles and relax others simultaneously. Introduced in this country by E Bing.	Feedback from coach who checks relaxation and tension. Introduced by Karmel and Bing. Not mentioned by Lamaze or Chabon.
Autogenic training (mental control modifies muscular and autonomic systems responses)	Uses suggestions, such as "my right arm is heavy" or "my left arm is warm." Effects include slowing heart and respiration as well as cooling forehead. Developed by J Schultz and W Luther.	Primary feedback from awareness of participant. Biofeedback equipment, thermometers, etc., may also be used.
Meditation (modifies vascular and neurotransmitter responses)	Is defined by H Benson as dwelling on an object (repeating a sound or gazing at an object) while emptying the mind of all thoughts and distractions in a quiet atmosphere in a comfortable position. Used in transcendental meditation and yoga.	Self-monitoring by participant or feedback from coach on concentration on a focal point or breathing patterns.
Visual imagery	Includes techniques such as visualizing oneself on a warm beach or as a bag of cement or going down a staircase. Often precedes introduction of other kinds of relaxation. May also be used to visualize and potentially affect specific body parts, as in cancer therapy. May be used in desensitization, in which one relaxes while visualizing a potentially threatening situation. Used in labor rehearsals.	
Touching/massage	Has always been a way for one person to calm another. There is evidence of actual transfer of energy through some forms of touching. In childbirth preparation, touching is associated with muscular relaxation (S Kissinger).	Feedback from coach, which includes informing the subject when muscle tension is felt. Advanced coaching needed. Coaches may need first to discern relaxation by moving a limb.
Biofeedback	Uses various devices: Electromyograph: measures neuromuscular tension Thermometer: measures skin temperature at extremities Galvanic skin reflex: records conductivity changes because of the action of sweat glands at the surface of the skin Electroencephalograph: distinguishes alpha, beta, and theta waves in the brain	Feedback from all of these machines in one or more of these forms: visualization of a meter, listening to a sound, or watching a set of flashing lights

Adapted from Humenick S: Teaching relaxation. Childbirth Educ 3(4):48, 1984

struct women to select an external "focal point"—an object, such as a small toy, a picture, or a vase of flowers, on which to focus their eyes during contractions. Other childbirth teachers, especially those using Bradley techniques, encourage women to close their eyes during a contraction and concentrate on the sound of their support person's voice, taped music, or a particular body sensation, such as the touch of the support person's hand. All of these examples operate on the same principle—the idea that deliberate attention to a sensate focus can alter and diminish the perception of pain. For this technique to be effective, consistency and avoidance of interruptions during contractions are important.

Gentle Massage and Counterpressure

Some methods of childbirth preparation encourage the use of gentle massage to enhance the relaxation and comfort of the woman in labor. Several massage tech-

Visualization Exercise for Childbirth Preparation

Go to a quiet, tranquil place where you won't be disturbed. Lie down in a comfortable position with your body well supported with pillows. Close your eyes, inhale slowly as you breathe in fresh oxygen, then exhale completely while you release your body tension. As you continue to inhale oxygen and release tension, your breathing will become slower and more even.

Continue to rest and allow your mind to take you to a very special place where you feel comfortable, safe, and tranquil. Allow yourself to enter this favorite place. Take in the sights, sounds, and smells of this place and allow those feelings to enter your body.

What sounds are you hearing? Pause and listen to all that you can. What scents are you smelling? Pause and enjoy the fragrances. What sights are you seeing? Pause and look around to enjoy all that you are seeing, the vibrant colors, the various shapes and sizes of all that you see.

Note the temperature in this special place, the warmth, the coolness, and allow your body to enjoy all the sensations while feeling comfortable, safe, and secure.

While in this special place, imagine your baby growing in your womb, being comfortable, safe, and secure.

Stay in this special place for a few minutes and enjoy all the good feelings of being there. . . . And now, bringing those good feelings with you, slowly come back to the here-and-now by counting backwards from 5 to 1. Five—move your feet and toes. Four—move your upper body. Three—open your eyes and take a good look around. Two—take a good stretch. One—sit up slowly as you come back to your present surroundings.

niques are shown in Figure 21–3. *Effleurage,* a light, rhythmic, circular stroking of the abdomen with the fingertips, may be soothing to the woman and may complement the use of learned breathing techniques.

Gentle massage of the back and shoulders, using talcum powder or lotion to reduce friction on the skin, can also be comforting to the mother. This can be done in a variety of ways, allowing the woman to decide what is most effective for her. Massage of the legs should be done only lightly and *with caution;* there is a small increased risk of thrombosis in pregnant women, and vigorous massage might dislodge a blood clot, causing embolism.

Firm counterpressure may also be offered as a counterirritant to sensations of internal pressure and pain, particularly in the lower back. Other areas where pressure can exert a calming effect are the pelvis, thighs, feet, shoulders, and hand. The effectiveness and comfort provided by gentle massage and counterpressure during labor must be re-evaluated frequently. The amount of comfort the woman in labor derives from massage may change as her labor proceeds, and a touch that was relaxing early in labor may become intolerable later. For this reason, the nurse and support person should observe the woman's nonverbal behavior closely, assess her comfort level regularly, and make adjustments as necessary. Figure 21–4 shows several ways a labor partner may apply counterpressure or other comfort measures to relieve back pain during labor.

Learned Breathing Techniques

All of the most common childbirth preparation methods include some kind of learned breathing techniques for use in response to contractions in labor. Techniques have evolved slightly differently in each school of childbirth education, and it is common to find slight variations, depending on local practices and instructor preferences. However, the underlying principles in the use of breathing techniques are the same.

First, deliberate and controlled breathing patterns are directly linked to optimum relaxation. The breathing patterns by themselves are not effective in altering pain perception, but must be done in combination with relaxation techniques. Second, particularly in Lamaze preparation, it is the *concentration* on performing complex breathing patterns that alters the perception of pain and helps the woman to accept the sensations of labor and not be overwhelmed by them. Each breathing technique is used according to need, not according to particular stage in labor; if one technique is not effective in helping the woman cope with her contractions at a particular point in labor, another technique (usually a more complex one) should be used. Finally, all commonly used breathing techniques must be done in a way that maintains adequate respiratory function without tiring the woman unnecessarily.

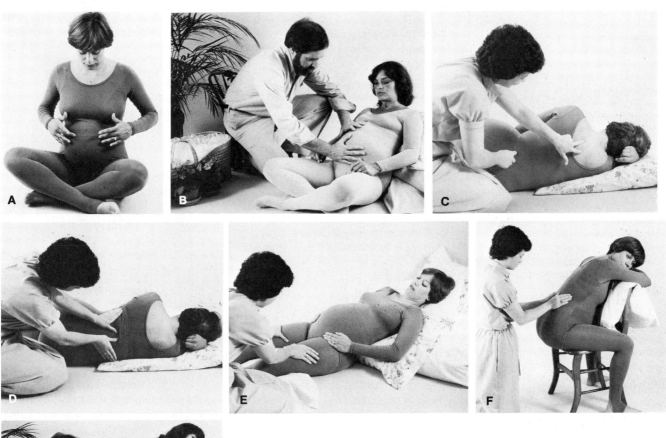

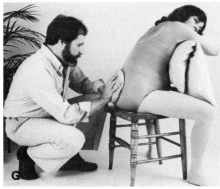

Figure 21-3. Massage techniques for labor. (*A*) Effleurage (light rhythmic stroking) may be soothing for the woman in labor. (*B*) The support person or nurse may also provide this type of massage. (*C*) Back massage may also enhance the laboring woman's relaxation and comfort. Either long downward strokes along the spine or firm thumb strokes (*D*) may be used. (*E*) Gentle thigh massage may relieve cramped or trembling legs and facilitate perineal relaxation. (*F*) Firm pressure on the sacral area of the lower back may assist the woman in coping with back pain. Counterpressure may be applied with the hand, a warm or cold pack (*G*), or a firm object such as a soda can or tennis ball, which can be rolled rhythmically to provide additional countersensation. (Photo: Childbirth Graphics)

Doing the techniques incorrectly can lead to hyperventilation, causing changes in blood chemistry.

The four major breathing techniques commonly used in childbirth preparation are slow paced breathing, modified paced breathing, patterned paced breathing, and expulsion breathing. All techniques should be individualized to promote optimum relaxation and oxygenation. In determining the pace and depth suitable for each person, the nurse should consider the patient's body position, her usual resting respiratory rate, her particular learned style of breathing, and the fetal station. Couples will use a variety of techniques, depending on the type of prenatal education they received, their skill, and the effectiveness of these techniques in maintaining the woman's comfort.

The nurse must be flexible and adjust her care as much as possible to the couple's individual pattern during labor.

Slow Paced Breathing

The technique called "slow paced breathing" in the Lamaze method is also taught as slow abdominal breathing in other methods. It involves breathing at approximately half the normal breathing rate. It can be done through the nose, mouth, or both throughout the duration of a contraction. Slow paced breathing provides the best oxygenation, is calming, and is the least fatiguing of the breathing techniques. To counteract the tendency to habituate to this technique, thereby reducing its effectiveness in altering pain perception, the woman should be

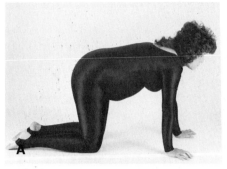
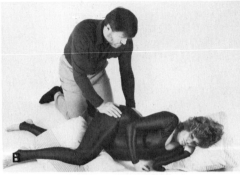
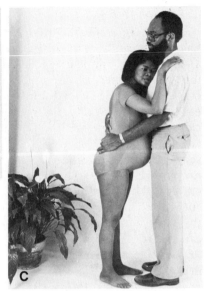

Figure 21–4. Relief of back pain in labor. (*A*) The woman may find that assuming a hands-and-knees position and rocking her pelvis helps to relieve back pain. (*B*) Assisting the woman to find a position of comfort, either with pillows and gentle massage or by ambulation and gentle partner support (*C*), may reduce back pain. (Photo: Childbirth Graphics)

encouraged to vary its use by incorporating a variety of other strategies. Some of these might be counting with each inhalation and exhalation, picturing the breath moving throughout the body, coordinating breathing with the partner's touch, walking or rocking in rhythm to the breath, or chanting a word or phrase with each exhalation.

After delivery of the infant, the woman may use slow paced breathing and relaxation techniques to deal with the discomforts of the early postpartum period.

Modified Paced Breathing

Modified paced breathing is used when slow, rhythmic breathing is no longer effective and a more alert state is needed. It begins with a cleansing breath (a deep inhalation through the nose and exhalation through the mouth) at the beginning of a contraction, shifts to breathing characterized by a slightly accelerated rate and increased use of the intercostal muscles, and ends with a cleansing breath. The rate should not exceed twice the woman's average respiratory rate. The primary considerations in determining rate are adequate oxygenation and the woman's comfort.

If this breathing technique alone is not effective, the strategies mentioned above for use with slow paced breathing or effleurage may be added. Effleurage is done slowly but in rhythm with the breathing. Again, the concentration required for this complex combination helps alter the woman's perception of the pain associated with the contraction.

Preventing Hyperventilation

As the pace of respiration increases, the nurse must remember that if respirations become *deep* and rapid, there is a risk of hyperventilation. Hyperventilation re-

sults in an increased carbon dioxide loss and respiratory alkalosis. Symptoms include lightheadedness and tingling of lips, face, hands, or feet. Hyperventilation can occur, if the woman or labor partner is breathing too rapidly or begins to panic. Should this occur, the nurse should have them breathe into their cupped hands or a paper bag until the symptoms disappear. Measures to restore relaxation, such as verbal reassurance in a quiet, calm manner or a firm touch, should be taken. When the breathing pattern is resumed with the next contraction, respirations should be kept moderate-to-slow in rate. With careful assessment and action, such episodes are usually brief. However, prolonged hyperventilation can eventually cause loss of consciousness, severe maternal respiratory alkalosis, and a resulting decrease in uterine blood flow.

Patterned Paced Breathing

During the last phase of cervical dilatation (7–10 cm) and the beginning of the second stage of labor, often called "transition," the woman may experience the sensations associated with labor most intensely. During this time, she may require a rhythmic breathing pattern to assist her in working with her labor. Patterned paced breathing is a series of 1 to 6 breaths of the same quality as modified paced breathing but interspersed with a soft blow at regular intervals. The rhythmic quality and the need for concentration on a pattern make this technique effective for the most stressful periods of labor. A series of soft blows may be used to counteract the desire to push, if the woman begins to experience it before her cervix is completely dilated, or to slow the descent of the fetal head and avoid a too rapid delivery that might be difficult to control.

Expulsion Breathing

The teaching of techniques for bearing-down efforts has recently undergone a change (Nichols and Humenick 1988). Women may be taught to push with a closed glottis (breathholding) or with an open glottis (exhaling). Conclusive evidence on the advantages and disadvantages of each technique is still lacking. Although pushing with a closed glottis, the traditional method, is taught and encouraged in many labor and delivery settings, there is some controversy about whether, over an extended period of time, it is the safest and most effective method for childbirth. It may cause an increase in intrathoracic pressure, which in turn causes a reduction in venous return to the heart and a fall in cardiac output. This decreased cardiac output may cause reduced placental blood flow. Reduced placental perfusion is known to cause a decrease in available oxygen to the fetus, with resulting fetal hypoxia and acidosis. Proponents of open-glottis pushing assert that forced exhalation of air while pushing ("candle-blowing" or groaning) does not inhibit venous return to the heart and causes the abdominal muscles to contract and press on the uterus, aiding in expulsion of the fetus. (See Chapter 24 for a more detailed discussion of bearing-down efforts during labor.)

IMPLICATIONS FOR NURSING CARE

Individual nurses have played important roles in the evolution of childbirth education in the United States. Many of the first practicing childbirth educators were nurses who became involved in childbirth education through their professional work or their own experiences in childbearing. Collectively, however, nursing has not been highly visible in the field until recently. The Nurses' Association of the American College of Obstetricians and Gynecologists (NAACOG) developed *Guidelines for Childbirth Education,* which outlined the scope of childbirth education and identified competencies that should be expected of childbirth educators. Health education for the childbearing family is central to the practice of obstetric nursing, a view reflected in *Standards of OGN Nursing,* also published by NAACOG (1981).

Nurses are increasingly responsible for the development and implementation of hospital- or clinic-based parent education programs. Some of these programs have been extremely innovative and effective in reaching disadvantaged or minority families and creating a comprehensive approach to parent education (Rising 1982). Nurses were also among the first to develop sibling and grandparent classes, and classes for hearing- or sight-impaired parents to supplement the more traditional types of childbirth education (Baranowski 1983, Perez 1979).

NURSING RESEARCH

Perceptions of the Nurse's Role in Labor and Birth

A study was conducted to examine the role of the labor and delivery room nurse as perceived by expectant mothers trained in the Lamaze method, mothers without Lamaze training, and labor and delivery nurses themselves. The authors hypothesized that the Lamaze-trained mothers would perceive the nurses' role to be more important in terms of physical support, whereas the non-Lamaze-trained mothers would perceive the nurse's role to be more important in terms of emotional support and their expectations of the nurse would be met more easily. However, none of these hypotheses were supported; that is, expectations of the nurse's role in labor and delivery were generally consistent between trained and untrained mothers and the nurses themselves.

The authors suggest that this study underscores the importance of both emotional and physical support for the laboring woman. Care must be individualized, based on the mother's expectations and perceptions; however, it is unwise to make assumptions about the importance of one aspect of nursing support over another, based only on the mother's level of childbirth preparation.

Collins B: The role of the nurse in labor and delivery as perceived by nurses and patients. J Obstet Gynecol Neonatal Nurs 15(5):412–419, 1986

Probably the most important nursing role, however, is the effective and compassionate nursing support of couples during labor in the hospital setting. This is where nurses make a unique contribution to the quality of the childbirth experience. The nurse has a key role in helping parents put into practice what they have learned in prenatal education or in teaching useful techniques to assist unprepared couples in labor and birth. The nurse should never underestimate the extent to which her attitudes, skills, and knowledge contribute to a positive, fulfilling birth experience for families in her care.

The nurse's role in caring for women or couples using prepared childbirth techniques is the same as her role in any other labor situation, except that she is working with a better-informed and prepared patient. Nursing care during labor and birth is discussed in detail in Chapters 23 and 24. However, some aspects of care should be emphasized when the nurse is caring for a woman or a couple using prepared childbirth techniques. These can be broken down into several areas: supporting the support person, providing comfort and reassurance, maintaining relaxation and concentration, and giving information. Although these aspects of nursing care are important for *all* women in labor and their partners, the following section will highlight points of particular importance for couples using prepared childbirth techniques.

Assessment

The nurse in the labor and delivery setting must initially assess the type of childbirth preparation, if any, the parents have had, and what their plans and expectations are in regard to using particular coping techniques. Information such as this is often gathered and recorded as part of the nursing history. In addition, the nurse must assess the woman's responses to the sensations of labor, and gauge the effectiveness of any particular technique in helping her to cope with the stress of labor. The process of this assessment of the patient in labor is detailed in Chapter 24.

Diagnosis

The nurse assesses the woman's responses to labor as well as those of the father and/or support person on an ongoing basis throughout labor, and formulates working nursing diagnoses that help to direct nursing care. Some nursing diagnoses that may be addressed in independently providing labor support for the woman and her support person are

Anxiety related to expectations of "coaching performance" in labor

Altered comfort: Pain associated with uterine contraction

Fatigue related to physical exertion of labor coping techniques

Knowledge deficit related to coping techniques for labor

Fear related to maternal expressions of pain, maternal "panic"

Planning and Implementation

The process of integrating "prepared childbirth techniques" into nursing care is discussed in the chapters on labor and delivery (Chapters 23–24). Some key points related to the diagnoses listed in the previous section are highlighted in those chapters.

FAMILY CONSIDERATION

The "Father" vs the "Coach"

The nurse should be especially careful not to "typecast" the father as the "coach," during labor and birth, for several reasons. First, the coach concept tends to focus attention on the father's role during a relatively brief period on the childbearing cycle — labor and delivery — and detracts attention from other important aspects of father involvement in pregnancy, the growing bond between unborn/newborn and the father, and the emotional preparation necessary for fatherhood. Second, the concept of "father as coach" reinforces stereotypical and sexist gender roles, while it holds both parents to unreasonable expectations. At best, the concept of "coach" reinforces the image of the father as just a prop and deemphasizes him as a unique individual in the process of sharing a challenging life experience with his partner. At worst, it implies that the father should provide direction and should assume responsibility if things go badly during labor and birth, while it discourages the woman's reliance on her own self-knowledge and ability during childbirth.

We should "fire" the coach, and help fathers find their own place in the experience of birth by

- Erasing "coach" from our vocabulary. Try substituting the label "support person," and do not use "father" and "support person" synonymously. The father may provide labor support, but that is not all he does.
- Try to change arbitrary institutional policies that restrict women to one labor-support person, and then encourage parents to consider arranging for additional labor support, regardless of whether the father intends to provide labor support.
- Remind fathers that nursing personnel are responsible for providing support as well as professional care during labor and he does not have to "do it all."

May K: The father's role: Is it time to fire the coach? CBE-Childbirth Educ (Winter): 30–35, 1988

Supporting the Support Person

The nurse must be present to monitor progress, assess maternal–fetal status, and give support to the woman and her support person in their efforts during labor (Fig. 21–5). Usually the support person is the father of the baby. No matter how well prepared he is for his support role, he is *not* in a position to make professional judgments about the progress of labor, nor is he necessarily capable of providing effective emotional and physical support throughout the labor process. The father who

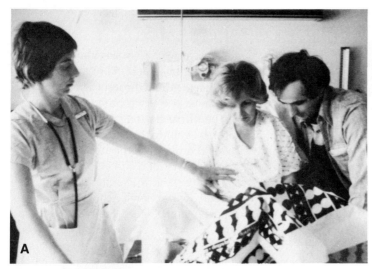

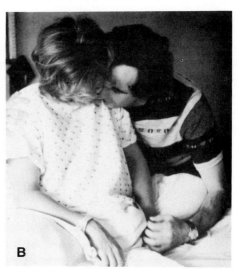

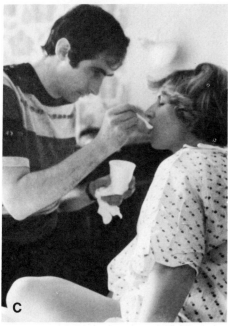

Figure 21–5. Partner support in labor. (*A*) The nurse should assess the support person's adaptation to the labor situation and assist him in his efforts to help his partner. (*B*) The support person, usually the father, may provide valuable emotional support and comfort measures, such as ice chips, massage, or comforting physical contact. (*C*) However, the father may not recognize the laboring woman's needs on his own, and the nurse should suggest and demonstrate comfort measures that the father can then carry out. (Photo: BABES, Inc.)

acts as support person during labor is in a situation that may be extremely stressful and sometimes frightening. As he watches his partner struggle with the difficult, painful work of labor, he may feel as if he is helpless to assist her in a meaningful way. Even when labor is going well, he is intensely concerned about the safety and well-being of his partner and the baby. If the nurse is not working with him closely and supporting his efforts, he is likely to feel anxious and alone. The woman will probably pick up his emotional discomfort, and this cannot help but increase her feelings of vulnerability and fear.

The nurse can assist by giving frequent and appropriate reassurance and feedback about the support person's effectiveness. The nurse should talk to *both* the woman and the support person, not just one or the other. Many

prepared couples have discussed their hopes and expectations in advance so that the support person can "speak for" the woman in labor. The nurse should take note of the support person's view of the situation, and assess the condition of the woman in labor directly; comments or actions that might be seen as discounting the support person's opinion should be avoided.

The nurse should observe whether the support person is comfortable and suggest breaks, reassuring both the woman and the support person that someone will be available to stay with her. It is important that the nurse recognize the *cumulative* effects of stress and fatigue on the support person. Late in labor, the support person's emotional and physical energy may be at a low point, and he or she will need additional encouragement and relief.

If the mother is to be transferred to another room for the birth, the nurse should prepare the support person well in advance to avoid an unsettling last-minute rush. The support person should be told specifically what preparation, such as scrubbing or special attire, is required. The nurse should give clear instructions to the support person about the type of "coaching" needed during the actual delivery and should frequently observe the support person's level of comfort during this time.

Maximizing the support person's effectiveness by providing assistance and encouragement not only benefits the woman in labor but also helps to make the birth experience a positive one for the father. This may indirectly affect his feelings about his spouse and infant and his role as a father.

Providing Comfort and Reassurance

A major aspect of caring for couples using prepared childbirth techniques is providing for their comfort and reassuring them that they are managing well and making progress. The physical presence of a caring nurse, even if no words are spoken, is reassuring. While taking into account a couple's need for privacy and uninterrupted periods, the nurse should avoid leaving couples alone during labor for long, even if they seem to be managing well.

Comfort measures for the woman — ice chips, a cold cloth for her face, propping her with pillows in a comfortable position, back or leg rubs with talcum powder, balm for chapped lips, or a warm shower — may be particularly helpful. The support person may not remember to suggest such measures or may not be aware of them. The nurse can model this behavior for the support person and seek his opinion about what the woman may find comforting.

If prepared childbirth techniques and other comfort measures are not effective, the woman is clearly struggling and in a great deal of pain, and she is still more than 2 hours from expected delivery, the nurse should discuss appropriate analgesia with the woman and her support person. Comments like "you don't need to go all the way" imply failure and should be avoided. Instead, the nurse may point out that other techniques have not helped and explain that the mother's emotional and physical comfort is important for a safe birth. The nurse should assist the woman and her support person in making their own decision about the use of analgesia, within the limits of safety for mother and baby. Parents should be reminded that the desired outcome is a healthy baby and a healthy and happy mother and father, and in some cases analgesia and other types of medical intervention will help achieve that goal.

Maintaining Relaxation and Concentration

The nurse can also intervene to assist the woman and her support person to establish and maintain high levels of relaxation and concentration through the labor process. One way is to make the environment conducive to the work of labor. The nurse should promote a calm and relaxed atmosphere by keeping the activity level and distractions in the labor room to a minimum. Distractions, such as unnecessary conversation late in labor, will drain energy the woman needs. The nurse should encourage rest and sleep between contractions. As labor intensifies, the nurse and support person should keep directions and questions short and relevant. Voices should be low and comforting. Lowering, rather than raising the voice and whispering directly into the woman's ear during the most intense parts of labor may be the most effective way of regaining control during periods of panic. The support person should sit down or get near to the woman's eye level when supporting her through a contraction.

The nurse should attempt to do all necessary procedures between contractions. If a vaginal (internal) examination must be performed during a contraction, the woman may be more comfortable if the examiner's fingers are inserted into the vagina before a contraction and held there, rather than inserted after a contraction has started.

Giving Information

Couples who have attended childbirth education classes are generally knowledgeable about the progress of labor and will expect to be kept informed. The nurse should give the woman and her support person frequent information about the progress of labor, including the degree of dilatation and effacement and descent of the fetal head. If electronic fetal monitoring is used, the nurse should explain the significance of tracings; it is especially important to explain some of the common "nonemergencies" that may arise with monitoring equipment, such as the need to shift the tocodynamometer and the appearance of artifacts on the tracing, and to give hints on how to position cords. This should be done early in labor so that parents are not unnecessarily worried about these common problems.

Supporting the "Unprepared" Woman

The nurse should not assume that all pregnant women want to take prepared childbirth classes or want to use prepared childbirth techniques in their labor. Cultural and family backgrounds strongly affect a woman's expectations about labor and birth. Women from some ethnic groups (Hispanic and some Middle Eastern groups, for example) choose not to attend childbirth classes because it is not customary or acceptable for men to accompany their wives in labor. Some women will moan or scream throughout their labor because this is a culturally acceptable practice for them. Others may find the idea of a labor and birth without anesthesia horrifying and regard the traditional hospital birth with general anesthesia as modern and desirable. In these situations the nurse must explain the risks of unnecessary medication and assist these women in making safe decisions for themselves and their babies. However, the labor and delivery suite is not the place to try to change women's expectations about birth, nor is it appropriate to impose the nurse's value judgments about a "good" labor on these patients.

When the nurse finds herself caring for women and family members who have not taken any kind of prepared childbirth classes and who are not well informed about what to expect in labor and birth, she may, if she has a working knowledge of labor coping techniques, be able to teach some of these techniques on the spot, *if* the woman seems to be interested in learning ways to cope with her labor. Visualization may be particularly effective if the nurse can encourage pleasant imagery with suggestions appropriate to the woman's frame of reference. An "unprepared" support person can be taught to give effective comfort measures, some as simple as hand-holding and loving, reassuring talk.

Evaluation

Evaluating the effectiveness of care directed toward supporting prepared childbirth techniques is probably most often done by collecting information about the family's "satisfaction" with their birth experience. Most often, couples who have made specific plans for childbirth preparation are likely to regard their birth experience more positively if these plans are taken into account to the extent made possible by the health professional.

Of course, most parents recognize that obstetric problems may require medical interventions, which make their birth plan impossible. However, the nurse plays a critical role in explaining how plans can be modified within the demands of a given labor situation, and in assuring that parental wishes are respected to the maximum possible extent. Indeed, the difference between a "satisfying" and "unsatisfying" birth experience for some well-prepared and goal-oriented couples may be the nurse who genuinely listened to their desires and

helped the parents actualize as much of their birth plan as possible. Thus, it is essential the nurse be well-versed in the types of childbirth preparation available to patients and be prepared to individualize her intrapartal nursing care on that basis.

CHAPTER SUMMARY

Preparation for childbirth evolved in response to consumer concerns about the increasing medical control and technologic management of normal labor and birth. Early proponents developed techniques intended to reduce pain perception and increase relaxation during labor and birth. Their goal was to reduce the need for analgesia, anesthesia, and other types of medical intervention in childbirth. Childbirth education attained early popularity among middle-class groups. Specialized educational services have been developed to meet the needs of disadvantaged and other high-risk groups, but more work is needed in this area.

Most types of childbirth education include factual information about the process of labor and birth, specific techniques for achieving and maintaining relaxation, and coping techniques to use in response to the sensations of labor. The nurse must be knowledgeable about the range of techniques taught in childbirth classes in order to act as a resource for parents seeking prenatal education and to provide effective and supportive care to women in labor and their families. Nurses have played an important role in the development of innovative programs of parent education. High-quality and creative parent education during the childbearing year must continue to be a priority of nurses involved in maternity care.

STUDY QUESTIONS

1. List the major components of childbirth preparation as currently practiced in the United States.
2. Identify some commonly taught labor-coping techniques, explain the rationale for their use, and outline supportive nursing actions for couples using these techniques.
3. What are some documented effects of childbirth education? What are some undocumented claims parents might hear about childbirth education? What might the nurse tell parents about the advantages of childbirth education?
4. Discuss childbirth educator practice in the United

States. What are the advantages of teacher certification?

5. Discuss some key nursing contributions to the field of childbirth education.

REFERENCES/BIBLIOGRAPHY

Baranowski E: Childbirth education classes for expectant deaf parents. MCN 8:143, 1983

Beck N, Siegel L: Preparation for childbirth and contemporary research on pain, anxiety, and stress reduction: A review and critique. Psychosom Med 42:429, 1980

Dick–Read G: Childbirth Without Fear. New York, Harper and Row, 1959

NAACOG: Guidelines for Childbirth Education. Chicago, NAACOG, 1981

NAACOG: Standards for OGN nursing. Chicago, NAACOG, 1981

Nichols F, Humenick S: Childbirth Education: Practice, Research, Theory. Philadelphia, WB Saunders, 1988

Rising S, Lindell S: The childbearing, childrearing center: A nursing model. Nurs Clin North Am 17(1):11, 1982

Sasmor J: Childbirth Education: A Nursing Perspective. New York, John Wiley and Sons, 1979

Schrock P: Relaxation. In Nichols F, Humenick S (eds): Childbirth Education: Practice, Research, Theory. Philadelphia, WB Saunders, 1988

Wertz R, Wertz D: Lying In: A History of Childbirth in America. New York, Free Press, 1977

Young D: Changing Childbirth: Family Birth in the Hospital. Rochester, NY, Childbirth Graphics, 1982

SUGGESTED READINGS

Eakin P: The American Way of Birth. Philadelphia, Temple University Press, 1986

Leavitt J: Brought to Bed: Childbearing in America, 1750–1950 New York, Oxford University Press, 1986

Nichols F, Humenick S: Childbirth Education: Practice, Research, Theory. Philadelphia: WB Saunders, 1988

Simkin P: Stress, pain, and catecholamines in labor. Birth 13(4):223–241, 1986

22 the process of labor and birth: maternal and fetal adaptations

LEARNING OBJECTIVES

After studying the material in this chapter, the student should be able to

- Understand the dynamic relationship between the bony pelvis, the fetus, and the pelvic and perineal muscles and ligaments during the process of labor and birth

- Define and describe the stages of labor

- Describe the cardinal movements of the fetus during labor and birth

- Explain the possible causes of onset of labor

- Describe the processes of cervical effacement and dilatation and their significance for progress in labor

- Describe maternal psychophysiologic responses during labor and birth

- Identify signs of labor and distinguish between false and true labor

- Outline maternal physiologic and behavioral adaptations during labor and birth

- Describe fetal physiologic and behavioral adaptations during labor and birth

KEY TERMS

Attitude

Contraction

Crowning

Dilatation

Effacement

Fontanelle

Labor

Lie

Parturient

Presentation

Station

The process of labor and birth is a fairly predictable sequence of events that usually occur in a harmonious fashion and result in a healthy mother and neonate. Many individual and environmental factors affect this process, so that each labor and birth is unique. The course of labor can be prolonged or accelerated, painful or gentle. Labor may require aggressive medical and nursing management or only supportive care.

Nursing care during childbirth can change dramatically in a period of minutes as the woman moves through the stages of labor. To accurately assess the woman's progress through labor and to anticipate and meet her needs, the nurse must have a thorough understanding of the anatomical and physiologic changes that occur during labor and birth. How well the nurse understands this process will determine the appropriateness and effectiveness of the care she can provide.

This chapter reviews these anatomic and physiologic changes and discusses behavioral changes in both the mother and the fetus. Chapters 23 to 28 discuss nursing care for women and their families in normal, moderate-risk, and high-risk labor and birth.

FORCES OF LABOR: PASSAGE, PASSENGER, POWERS, AND PSYCHE

Four factors, commonly known as the "four *P*s," are of critical importance in the process of childbirth: passage, passenger, powers, and psyche. In normal labor, the pelvic anatomy (passage) must be adequate for the individual fetus; the fetus (passenger) must be in an advantageous position; uterine contractions (powers) must be rhythmic, coordinated, and efficient; and maternal efforts (psyche) must be adequate to accomplish the delivery of the fetus. All of these factors interact dynamically with the environment to accomplish spontaneous delivery. An alteration in any one component will require compensation in another. If compensation does not occur, the process of labor will be altered, and active intervention may be required to accomplish delivery. In many cases, the nurse can facilitate the physiologic progress of normal labor by assessing each component and providing nursing support to prevent any drastic alteration of the labor process.

Passage: The Pelvis

The passage is determined by maternal pelvic anatomy: the bony pelvis and the muscles of the pelvic floor and perineum. (See Chapter 5 for the muscular and bony anatomy of the pelvis and Chapter 16 for the classification

and assessment of pelvic types.) Specific pelvic landmarks and measurements are important when considering the complementary relationship between the bony pelvis and the fetus.

Pelvic Planes and Measurements

The pelvis consists of four bones: two innominate bones (formed by the ilium, ischium, and pubis), the sacrum, and the coccyx. The configuration of these bones is of considerable importance when one is measuring the capacity of the pelvis. For obstetric purposes, the pelvis is described as having three planes: the *inlet,* the *midpelvis,* and the *outlet,* as shown in Figure 22–1.

Pelvic Inlet

The *pelvic inlet* is bounded by the sacrum posteriorly, the linea terminalis laterally, and the symphysis pubis anteriorly. The linea terminalis demarcates the true pelvis from the false pelvis. Four diameters of the pelvic inlet are important for measurement purposes: the anteroposterior, the biischial (or transverse), and the two oblique diameters. Of these, the anteroposterior and biischial (Fig. 22–2) are the most important in most cases: oblique diameters generally only assume significance when there is an abnormality in pelvic structure. The shortest anteroposterior diameter of the pelvic inlet is also called the *obstetric conjugate* (Fig. 22–3). It usually measures 10 cm or more. If the obstetric conjugate is narrow, the presenting part may never engage in the bony pelvis. Immediately above the obstetric conjugate is the *true conjugate,* which extends from the top of the symphysis to the tip of the sacral promontory (Fig. 22–4). It is usually a little wider than the obstetric conjugate.

Midpelvis

The plane of the *midpelvis* is bounded anteriorly by the bottom of the symphysis and at the sides by the ischial spines. The midpelvis is of obstetric significance because it normally contains the narrowest portion of the pelvis. The smallest diameter of the pelvis is the interspinous diameter, usually measuring about 10 cm. The shortest anteroposterior diameter at the ischial spines usually measures 11.5 cm. If labor fails to progress after the presenting part is engaged, there may be narrowing in some aspect of the midpelvis.

Pelvic Outlet

The *pelvic outlet* consists of a line drawn between the two ischial tuberosities. This line is a transverse diameter, and 10 cm or more is considered adequate for obstetric purposes. The immobility and position of the sacrococcygeal joint can narrow the anterior-posterior diameter of the outlet if the coccyx is fixed or juts out.

Factors Influencing Progress in Labor and Birth

Maternal Age

Maternal age may affect the progress of normal labor and birth. The very young woman (under 16 years) may have an immature, small pelvis, increasing the risk of cephalopelvic disproportion, and is at increased risk for preeclampsia. The older woman (over 35 years) is more likely to have twins, breech, or occiput posterior presentations, and a longer second stage of labor.

Maternal Weight

Overweight women are at risk for delays or arrests in latent or active phases of labor and for soft tissue dystocia, the slowing of the second stage as a result of excessive weight.

Birth Interval

When the interval since the last birth is less than 1 year, the woman is at risk for a more rapid labor and a smaller infant.

Birth Weight and Gestational Age

Preterm and small fetuses are usually born after a fast labor, whereas large fetuses are generally associated with longer labors, especially longer second-stage labor. Gestational age of less than 37 weeks is associated with a higher rate of malpresentation, which can affect the progress of labor. Gestational age of more than 42 weeks is associated with *macrosomia,* or large body size in the fetus, and a higher risk of birth complications.

Fetal Position

Labor progresses most effectively when the fetus is in a well-flexed vertex position.

Status of Amniotic Sac

Early rupture of the amniotic sac may interfere with the progress of labor because the synthesis in the chorion of prostaglandins, substances that cause uterine contraction, is impaired. There is no evidence that rupture of the amniotic sac shortens labor and some evidence that the fetus may be at higher risk for acidosis when membranes are ruptured before the second stage of labor.

Site of Placental Implantation

High or fundal implantation of the placenta has been shown to be associated with prolonged labor, possibly because of interference with myometrial contractility in the area.

Maternal Position During Labor

Maternal position during labor has been shown to affect uterine activity. Standing or upright positions have been found to be most efficient in dilating the cervix and have been associated with lower incidence of umbilical cord compression and increased maternal comfort. The lateral recumbent position appears to result in less efficient uterine contractions than the upright position. The supine position is associated with more frequent but less efficient contractions.

In addition, the supine position puts the mother at risk for maternal supine hypotensive syndrome, caused by the compression of the inferior vena cava by the heavy gravid uterus. Maternal symptoms of supine hypotension include dizziness, breathlessness, visual changes, and numbness and tingling in the extremities. Uterine arterial circulation may also be impaired by compression of the abdominal aorta by the uterus.

Psychologic Factors

Maternal psychological status has direct effects on the progress of labor. Stress and anxiety stimulate the release of stress hormones called catecholamines, which are known to inhibit uterine activity. Childbirth preparation has been shown to be helpful in reducing stress and anxiety associated with labor and birth and may contribute to more favorable labor progress and outcome.

Medications

The use of narcotic analgesia has been shown to slow down the active phase of labor. Magnesium sulfate, used in the treatment of preeclampsia, has been shown to diminish the frequency and intensity of uterine contractions and also reduces the resting tone of the uterus. There is some controversy about whether regional anesthesia slows the progress of labor and contributes to increased need for oxytocin augmentation and cesarean delivery.

Assessment of Pelvic Capacity

When assessing pelvic capacity, other important landmarks and measurements are considered as well. The curve and length of the *sacrum* determines the posterior capacity of the pelvis in all three planes. The sacrum may be concave, flat, or convex; the latter two characteristics decrease pelvic capacity. The characteristics of the *ischial spines* are also important in assessing pelvic capacity for childbirth. Sharp, encroaching spines greatly decrease the transverse diameter of the midpelvis. The *pubic arch,* or subpubic angle, should be wide and rounded at 90° or more to allow the fetal head to pivot under it. A narrow or acute pubic angle will force the fetal head down onto the

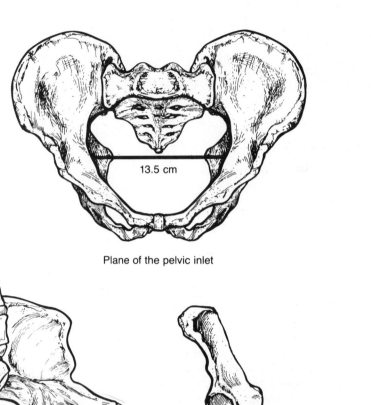

Plane of the pelvic inlet

13.5 cm

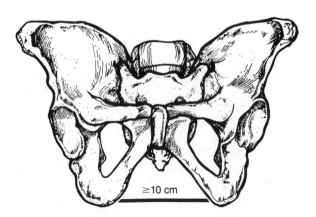

Anteroposterior diameter
of the midpelvis

11.5 cm

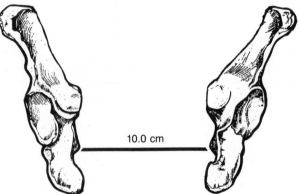

Ischial spines:
Midplane, or plane of least pelvic dimensions—the smallest
diameter of the pelvis

10.0 cm

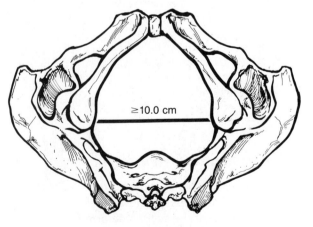

Biischial diameter or the transverse diameter of the outlet

≥10 cm

Inferior view of the outlet. The transverse diameter is the
distance between the inner edges of the ischial tuberosities

≥10.0 cm

Figure 22–1. Planes of the pelvis. Figures give average measurements. (Childbirth Graphics)

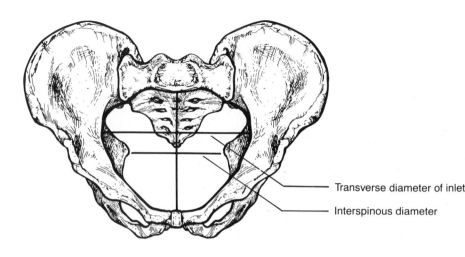

Transverse diameter of inlet

Interspinous diameter

Figure 22–2. The transverse diameter of the pelvic inlet, and interspinous diameter of the midpelvis. (Childbirth Graphics)

perineum and may cause major perineal tears or require an operative delivery.

The physician or nurse midwife will draw conclusions about the capacity of a woman's pelvis for normal childbirth from clinical evaluation of the pelvis (see Chapter 16 for a detailed review of the pelvic examination) as well as estimates of fetal weight and position. A diagnosis of *cephalopelvic disproportion* indicates that the combination of fetal size, fetal position, and pelvic architecture is not favorable for a vaginal delivery and usually leads to a decision for a cesarean delivery. However, unless gross pelvic inadequacies are found, this diagnosis is not safely

made on the basis of clinical evaluation of the pelvis alone for several reasons. First, clinical evaluation of pelvic size and architecture by vaginal examination depends on the skill and experience of the examiner and may be open to subjective error. Second, fetal size is sometimes difficult to estimate accurately without confirmation by sonography. Finally, a fetus that is well positioned or "flexible" may be able to negotiate passage through a tight pelvis, although another fetus of the same size may not.

X-ray pelvimetry is sometimes used to gain information about the shape and inclination of the pelvis, its length and diameters, and the relationship and fit of the fetus to the pelvis. However, there is considerable controversy about the value of pelvimetry. The pelvic capacity and position of the fetus are only two of the many factors that determine obstetric outcome, and the prognosis for a successful vaginal delivery cannot be established on the basis of x-ray pelvimetry alone.

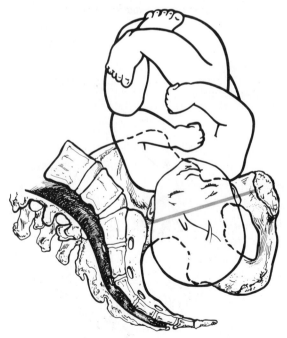

Figure 22–3. Obstetric conjugate. This obstetrically important diameter is the shortest anteroposterior distance between the sacral promontory and the symphysis pubis. (Childbirth Graphics)

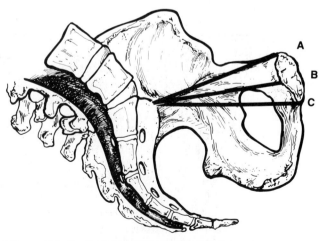

A
B
C

Figure 22–4. Anterior–posterior diameters of the pelvic inlet. (*A*) True conjugate. (*B*) Obstetric conjugate. (*C*) Diagonal conjugate. (Childbirth Graphics)

Computed Tomography (CT) Pelvimetry. Because traditional x-ray pelvimetry has been shown to have limited usefulness in predicting the progress of labor, a new technique, known as CT pelvimetry, is being used in selected settings to evaluate the adequacy of the maternal pelvis. A very low dose of radiation (22 m rad) is absorbed in comparison to conventional x-ray pelvimetry (885 m rad). Its usefulness in assessing pelvic dimensions in breech presentations and in estimating shoulder widths in macrosomic fetuses is also being evaluated (Kitzmiller 1987).

Passenger: The Fetus

The fetus, as passenger, must undergo a series of predictable and synchronized maneuvers to accommodate itself to and descend through the maternal pelvis. The anatomy and placement of the fetal head in the bony pelvis and the movements of the fetus through the pelvis play an important part in the progress of normal labor.

Fetal Head

In labor and birth, the head, or *cranium,* is viewed as the most important part of the fetus. The head is usually the presenting part; is not compressible, as is the softer tissue of the rest of the body; and, along with the shoulders, represents the largest part of the term infant.

Fetal Cranial Anatomy

The fetal cranium is composed of the *occipital bone,* two *parietal bones,* two *temporal bones,* and two *frontal bones* (Fig. 22–5). At birth, these bones are only partially ossified and are joined by tough, membranous connective tissue. This allows some movement of the bones and overlapping under pressure. Thus, the fetal head can adapt somewhat to the maternal pelvis through a process called *molding,* usually without damage to the underlying tissue.

The membranous spaces between the bony plates of the cranium are called *sutures.* Where these sutures intersect, there are wide, membranous spaces called *fontanelles.* The characteristic arrangement of sutures and fontanelles provides a useful way of determining the position of the fetal head in relation to the maternal pelvis. In a vaginal examination during labor, the examiner can feel the sutures and fontanelles through the dilated cervix.

The *sagittal suture* is the most readily felt. It runs in an anterior-posterior direction between the two parietal bones, connecting the anterior and posterior fontanelles. The *frontal suture* is the anterior continuation of the sagittal suture between the two frontal bones. The *coronal sutures,* extending in a transverse direction from the anterior fontanelle, lie between the parietal and frontal bones. At the back of the head, the *lambdoid sutures*

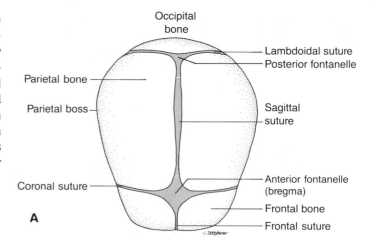

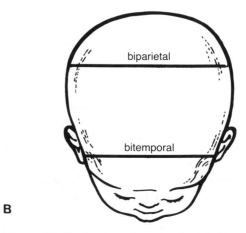

Figure 22–5. Fetal cranium superior. (*A*) Bones. (*B*) Transverse diameters. (Childbirth Graphics)

extend in a transverse direction from the posterior fontanelle, dividing the occipital bone from the parietals.

Other important landmarks of the fetal skull are shown in Figure 22–6. These areas of the cranium are as follows:

- *Occiput:* back of the head formed by the occipital bone
- *Vertex:* top of the head between the two fontanelles
- *Bregma:* front of the head formed by the frontal bone
- *Mentum:* chin
- *Sinciput:* brow
- *Glabella:* elevated area between the orbital ridges
- *Nasion:* root of the nose
- *Parietal eminences* or *bosses:* widest areas on each side of the parietal bones

Diameters of the Fetal Skull

The diameters of the fetal skull are the distances between reference points in the cranium (Fig. 22–7). In general, fetal descent through the maternal pelvis is accomplished by movements that present the smallest fetal

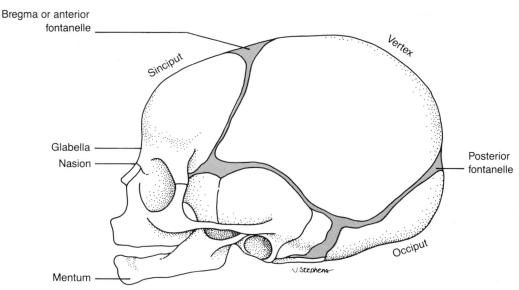

Figure 22-6. Fetal cranium, lateral view. (Childbirth Graphics)

skull diameter. The particular diameter of the fetal skull presented to the maternal pelvis will be determined by how flexed or extended the fetal head is throughout labor. Complete extension or flexion of the fetal head presents the smallest fetal head diameter and facilitates passage of the head through the bony pelvis.

The fetal skull diameter of the greatest obstetric importance is the *biparietal diameter.* This diameter is assessed in ultrasonic measurements of fetal head size. It is the distance between the parietal bosses and represents the largest transverse diameter of the fetal head, averaging 9.25 cm at term. The *suboccipitobregmatic diameter* extends from the lower edge of the occipital bone (near the neck) to the bregma, or forehead. This is the anterior-posterior diameter that presents to the maternal pelvis

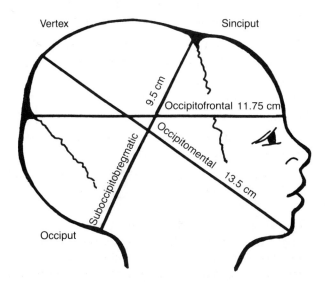

Figure 22-7. Diameters of the fetal skull. (Childbirth Graphics)

when the fetal head is well flexed; it averages 9.5 cm at term. The *occipitofrontal diameter* extends from the external occipital protuberance (back of the head) to the glabella. This diameter presents to the maternal pelvis when the fetal head is neither well flexed nor well extended but straight, in which case the fetus is sometimes said to be in a "military attitude." The *verticomental diameter* extends from the vertex to the mentum and is applied to the pelvis in brow presentations with partial extension of the head. The *submentobregmatic diameter* presents with complete extension of the head, as in face presentations.

Fetopelvic Relationships

Another set of terms is used to describe the relationship of the fetal body to the maternal pelvis. These terms are useful in describing the positioning of the fetus in the pelvis and the level of its descent through the pelvis.

Station

The term *station* refers to the level of the presenting part of the fetus, usually the head, in relation to the ischial spines in the midpelvis, as shown in Figure 22-8. When the presenting part is at the level of the ischial spines, it is said to be at 0 station, or to be *engaged.* Levels above the ischial spines are referred to as *minus stations;* stations of −4 to −1 indicate centimeters above the ischial spines. Levels below the ischial spines are *plus* stations; stations of +1 to +4 indicate centimeters below the level of the spines.

Fetal Lie

The term *fetal lie* refers to the relationship of the long axis of the fetus to the long axis of the mother, as shown in Figure 22-9. A *longitudinal lie,* with the fetal and mater-

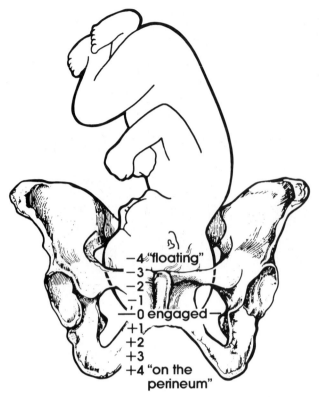

Figure 22–8. Stations of the fetal head. (Childbirth Graphics)

Presentation

The term *presentation* refers to the part of the fetus that enters, or presents to, the maternal pelvis. The major variations in fetal presentation are shown in Figure 22–10. The most common is *cephalic* or vertex presentation, which occurs in 95% of labors. *Breech,* or buttock, presentations occur in approximately 4% of labors. Breech presentations can be further divided into three types:

- *Frank breech:* most common type, characterized by fetal flexion at the thighs and extension at the knees
- *Complete breech:* characterized by fetal flexion at thighs and knees
- *Footling or incomplete breech:* characterized by extension at knees and thighs

Breech presentations are shown in Figure 22–11. The rarest types of presentations are *shoulder* and *face* presentations, and presentations of other body parts.

Depending on the estimated size of the fetus and the progress of labor, some breech presentations can be successfully delivered vaginally. However, many cases of breech presentation and virtually all shoulder and face presentations require cesarean delivery.

Position

The term *position* refers to the relationship of a particular reference point of the presenting part to the maternal pelvis, as shown in Figure 22–12. In vertex presentations, the reference point on the head may be the occiput, the brow, or the chin, depending on whether the head is flexed or extended. In breech presentations, the reference point is the fetal sacrum, and in shoulder presentations, it is the fetal scapula.

In describing fetal position, the maternal pelvis is di-

nal spines parallel, is normal and occurs most often. In *transverse lie,* the fetus is in a horizontal position relative to the maternal spine, whereas an *oblique lie* is at a slight angle off a true transverse lie. Transverse and oblique lies will prevent the fetus from entering the bony pelvis; thus, they eliminate the possibility of a vaginal delivery, unless they convert to a longitudinal lie at the beginning of labor.

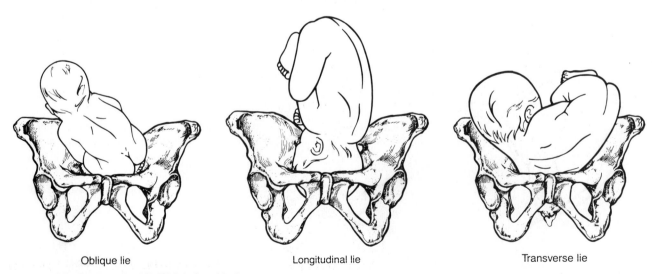

Oblique lie   Longitudinal lie   Transverse lie

Figure 22–9. Fetal lie. (Childbirth Graphics)

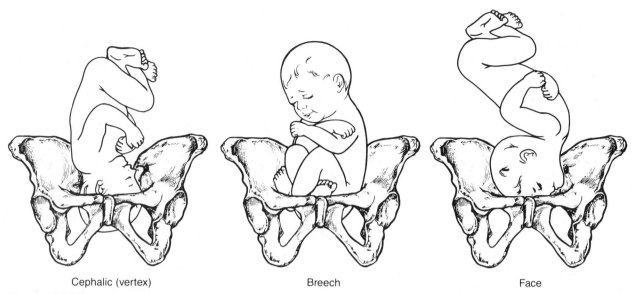

Cephalic (vertex)   Breech   Face

Figure 22-10. Fetal presentations. (Childbirth Graphics)

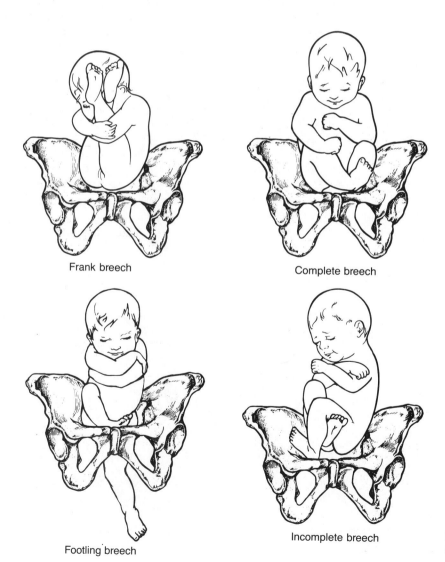

Frank breech   Complete breech

Footling breech   Incomplete breech

Figure 22-11. Types of breech presentations. (Childbirth Graphics)

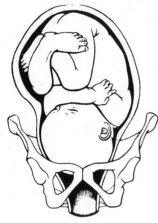

Left occipital posterior

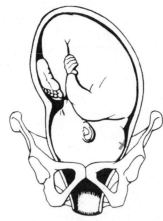

Left occipital transverse

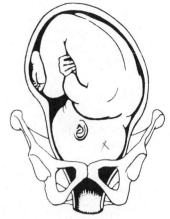

Left occipital anterior

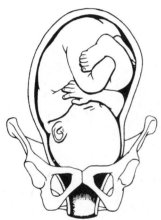

Right occipital posterior

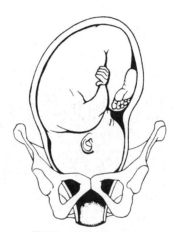

Right occipital transverse

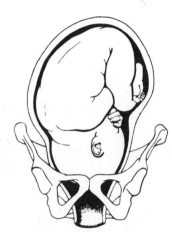

Right occipital anterior

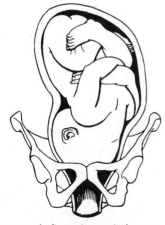

Left mentum anterior

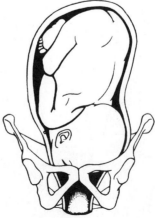

Right mentum posterior

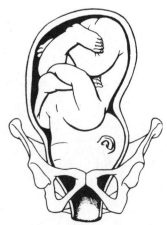

Right mentum anterior

Figure 22–12. Fetal positions. (Childbirth Graphics)

vided into four segments: right and left anterior and right and left posterior. These are labeled according to the mother's perspective, not the examiner's. It may be helpful to visualize the top of the bony pelvis as the face of a clock, with 12 o'clock at the mother's back. Thus, the area from 9 o'clock to 12 corresponds to the right posterior area (the mother's right, the examiner's left); 12 to 3 o'clock corresponds to the left posterior area; and so on. Thus, if the presenting part can be palpated on vaginal examination, the reference point of the presenting part can be identified in terms of its position in the pelvis.

Each fetal position is identified by a standard abbreviation with three elements. The elements appear in the following order: the first indicates whether the presenting part is to the left, to the right, or transverse in the maternal pelvis; the second indicates what the presenting part is; and the third indicates whether it is in the anterior or posterior half of the pelvis (see the accompanying display, Standard Abbreviations Describing Fetal Positions). For example, *left occiput anterior (LOA) position* describes the situation in which the occiput of the fetal head is on the mother's left in the front part of the pelvis. The fetal head usually enters the pelvis during labor in an oblique or transverse position; LOA, LOT, ROA, and ROT are the most common fetal positions encountered during labor. The shape of the pelvic inlet influences fetal position. If the anterior half of the pelvis is narrow, the back of the fetal head may be pushed to the rear so that the shorter bitemporal diameter presents to the narrow forepelvis, resulting in an *occiput posterior* position (Fig. 22–12).

An occiput posterior position usually causes labor to progress more slowly than normal, with accentuated back pain, sometimes called "back labor." Most fetuses in the occiput posterior position during labor spontaneously rotate anteriorly, and delivery proceeds normally. Certain maternal positions, such as kneeling on all fours or lying on the side opposite to the one on which the fetal occiput is detected, may allow gravity to rotate the fetal spine

Standard Abbreviations Describing Fetal Positions
Side of Maternal Pelvis?
L Left
R Right
T Transverse

Presenting Part?
O Occiput
S Sacrum
Sc Scapula
M Mentum

Part of Maternal Pelvis?
A Anterior   T Transverse
P Posterior

toward the anterior position. Approximately 10% of fetuses in occiput posterior positions do not rotate, and the infant is born in a face-to-pubis position; alternatively, the birth attendant may rotate the infant to an anterior position manually or with forceps.

Attitude

The term *attitude* refers to the relationship of fetal parts to each other. The fetus usually assumes a flexed position, in part to accommodate the shape of the uterine cavity. The back is flexed, the chin is placed on the chest, the arms are folded across the chest, and the thighs are drawn up against the abdomen with the knees flexed. The attitude of the head determines which part of the skull is the presenting part, as shown in Figure 22–13. If the

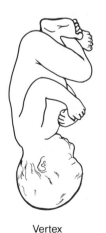
Vertex (Flexion)

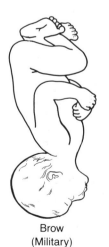
Sinciput (Military)

Brow

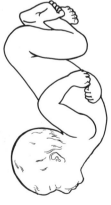
Face (Extension)

Figure 22–13. Fetal attitude. (Childbirth Graphics)

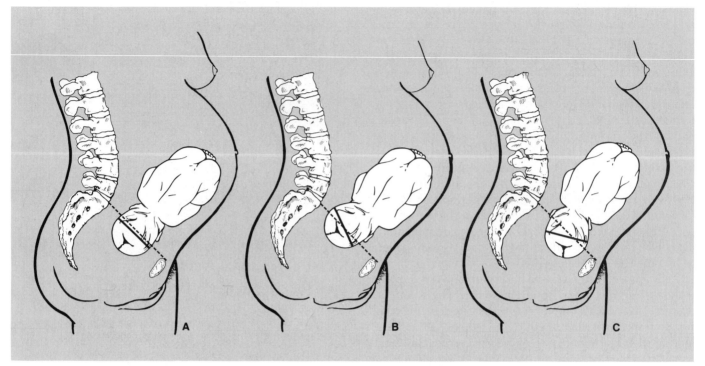

Figure 22–14. (*A*) Synclitism. Position of the fetal head when the sagittal suture is halfway between the sacral promontory and the symphysis pubis. (*B*) Posterior asynclitism. Position of the fetal head when the sagittal suture is closer to the sacral promontory. (*C*) Anterior asynclitism. Position of the fetal head when the sagittal suture is closer to the symphysis pubis. (Childbirth Graphics)

head is flexed, the occiput presents first, and the posterior fontanelle is palpable on vaginal examination. If the head is extended, the brow will present; if the head is hyperextended, the chin will present. If the head is neither flexed nor extended (*i.e.,* the fetus is in the military attitude), the sinciput will present, and the anterior fontanelle will be palpable.

Synclitism and Asynclitism

Synclitism and *asynclitism* refer to the position of the fetal head in relation to the anterior–posterior diameter of the maternal pelvis (Fig. 22–14). *Synclitism* refers to the position of the fetal head when the sagittal suture (which runs from front to back along the top of the head) is halfway between the sacral promontory and the symphysis pubis, so that the planes of the maternal pelvis and the fetal skull are parallel. *Asynclitism* refers to the position of the fetal head when the sagittal suture is closer to the sacral promontory (posterior asynclitism) or the symphysis pubis (anterior asynclitism). These positions occur normally as the fetal head shifts to accommodate the irregular shape of the pelvic cavity. Exaggerated or prolonged asynclitism, however, usually reflects cephalopelvic disproportion.

Cardinal Movements of Labor

The cardinal movements of the fetus during labor have been described in the same way since the 18th century. These movements or mechanisms are a series of passive adjustments of position as the fetus descends through the pelvis during labor (Fig. 22–15). These movements flow smoothly and often overlap as labor progresses; failure to achieve one or more of these adjustments usually indicates a need for some form of obstetric intervention.

Descent. Descent, or the downward movement of the fetus, continues throughout normal labor. Descent is brought about by the pressure of uterine contractions and is aided in the second stage by maternal bearing-down efforts. An upright maternal position in labor allows gravity to aid in the descent of the fetus.

Flexion. Flexion is the natural attitude of the fetus because of the shape of the uterine cavity and, during labor, because of the resistance of the pelvic floor to fetal descent. Flexion is also aided by thickening of the uterine fundus, which decreases the available space; the fetus is forced to flex into a compact, ovoid shape. Flexion of the fetal head is important because, as mentioned before, it

(text continued on page 584)

Internal Rotation

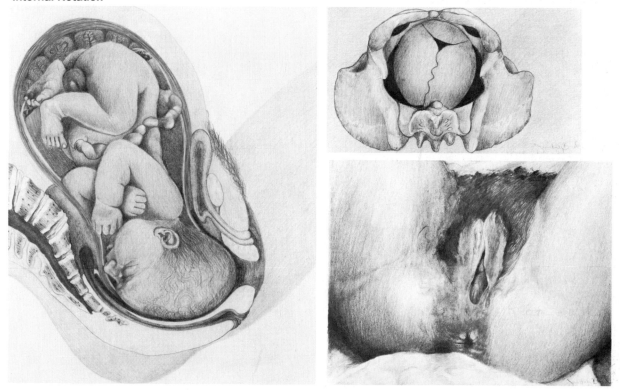

Figure 22–15. Internal rotation occurs as the fetal head enters the bony pelvis in a transverse position and rotates to an anteroposterior position because of pressure from the encroaching ischial spines. The bispinous diameter is too small to admit a normal-sized head in a transverse position. (Childbirth Graphics)

Extension Beginning

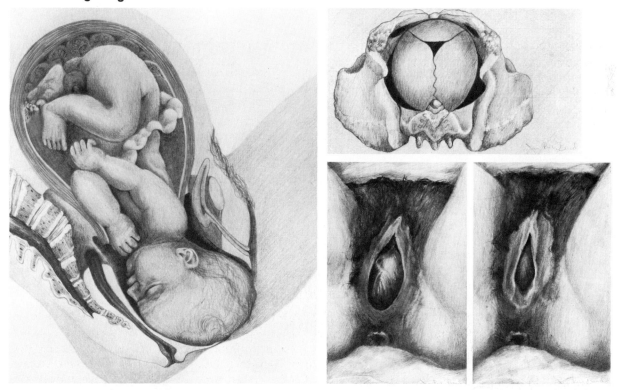

Figure 22–15 *(continued).* Extension occurs when the head reaches the pelvic floor and is deflected anteriorly away from the sacrum. The distention of the perineum becomes apparent. The head can be seen to advance with contractions and bearing down efforts and to retreat between contractions.

Crowning

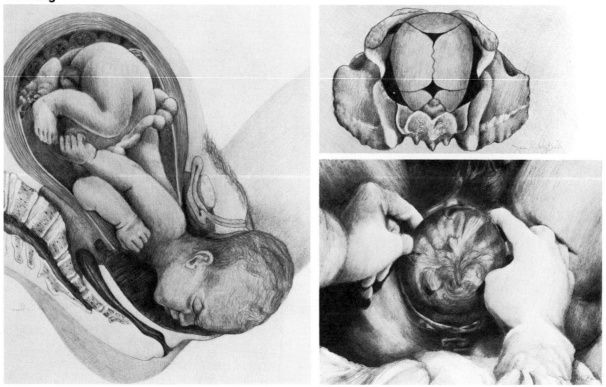

Figure 22–15 *(continued).* Crowning occurs when the head distends the perineum maximally so that the head is fully encircled.

Extension Complete

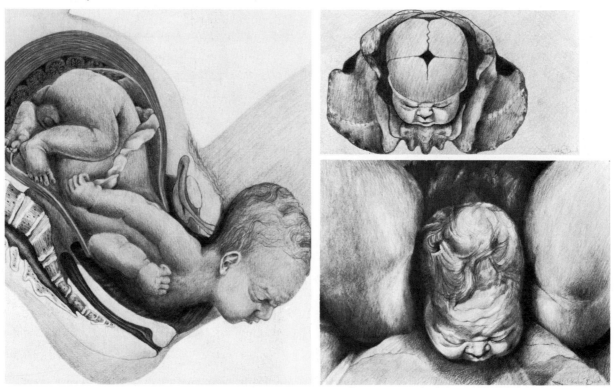

Figure 22–15 *(continued).* As the head emerges the symphysis exerts pressure on the neck. The continued downward pressure from contractions forces the baby's head to pivot under the symphysis.

External Rotation (Restitution)

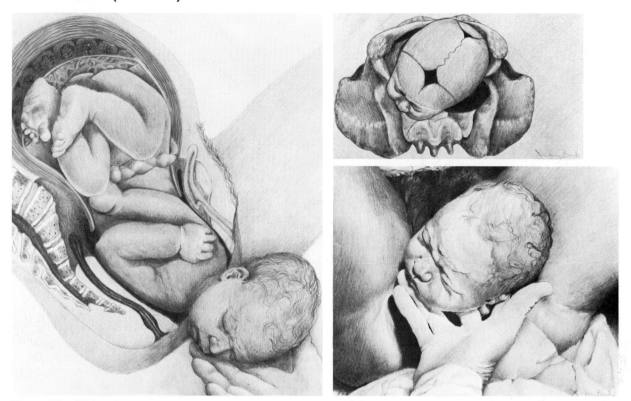

Figure 22–15 *(continued)*. External rotation occurs when the head rotates back to the oblique position in which it entered the pelvis, thus realigning the head, neck, and shoulders.

External Rotation (Shoulder Rotation)

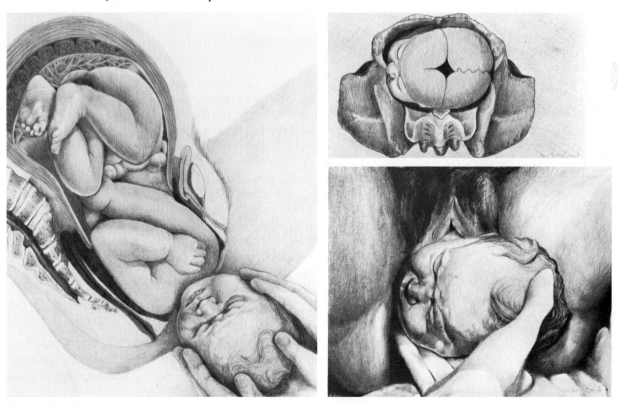

Figure 22–15 *(continued)*. The shoulders are now in an anteroposterior position; the anterior shoulder is born under the symphysis and the posterior shoulder slides over the perineum.

Expulsion

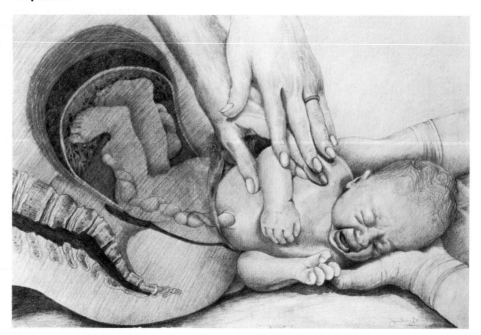

Figure 22–15 *(continued).* Expulsion occurs as the rest of the body is born; because the head and shoulders are the largest part of the neonate, the rest of the body is delivered easily.

causes the smallest fetal head diameter to present to the maternal pelvis. Flexion begins at the pelvic inlet and continues until the head reaches the pelvic floor.

Internal Rotation. Internal rotation must occur, since the fetal head usually enters the pelvis in a transverse or oblique position and must rotate 45° to 90° to an occiput anterior position at the midpelvis to accommodate the narrowest transverse diameters of the pelvis. In most cases, the head rotates to an occiput anterior position because of the shape of the bony pelvis and the downward and forward slope of the pelvic musculature. As mentioned before, some fetuses rotate to an occiput posterior position. Internal rotation usually occurs during the second stage of labor; however, it may occur earlier in multiparas and is sometimes accomplished in one contraction.

Extension. Extension of the fetal head is caused by the continued downward pressure of uterine contractions and the resistance of the pelvic floor to continued descent. Because of the greater length of the sacrum, the face of the fetus in the occiput anterior position has a greater distance to travel than does the occiput. The flexion of the head usually continues until crowning so that the smallest diameter of the fetal head presents and distends the perineum. The neck of the infant then pivots in the subpubic angle and allows the head to extend. As the head extends, the brow, face, and chin move past the sacrum and coccyx and are born over the perineum; at this point, the infant's head is in an occiput anterior position. Extension is said to be complete when the entire head is born.

Restitution. While the head rotates to the anterior position, the shoulders remain in the oblique or transverse position; thus, the infant's neck is slightly twisted. Once the head is delivered, the neck rotates 45° and the head returns to its normal relationship with the shoulders, which may be the original position in which the head entered the pelvis. This is known as *restitution* and usually occurs automatically once the head is delivered.

External Rotation and Expulsion. External rotation sometimes appears to be part of *restitution,* since they often occur together. External rotation of the head an additional 45° occurs along with the internal rotation of the shoulders. As the head extends and is delivered, the shoulders reach the pelvic floor. The shoulders then must rotate to the anterior–posterior diameter of the pelvis. Once the shoulders have rotated, the anterior shoulder is born under the symphysis pubis and the posterior shoulder slides out over the perineum. The head and shoulders are delivered, expulsion occurs as the rest of the infant is born without difficulty through the mother's bearing-down efforts.

Powers: The Uterus in Labor

A major force contributing to the process of labor and birth is the power of uterine contractions. The appropriately timed onset of labor, uterine contractility patterns, and progressive cervical effacement and dilatation must occur in a coordinated fashion in order to bring about fetal descent and birth.

Theories on Causes of Initiation of Labor

A complex interaction of maternal, fetal, and placental factors is responsible for initiating labor; however, the exact mechanism by which labor is initiated is still not well understood. Many theories have been proposed to explain the onset of labor, but none can stand alone as the complete explanation. Additional research will undoubtedly provide answers in the future. The following explanations are among those currently being investigated.

Uterine Stretch Theory.   The uterine stretch theory proposes that labor begins when the uterus is stretched to a certain point. This theory partially explains the early onset of labor in multiple gestations and cases of polyhydramnios (an excess amount of amniotic fluid), but does not help to explain what causes preterm labor.

Pressure Theory.   The pressure theory of labor initiation proposes that the descent of the presenting part stimulates pressure receptors in the lower uterine segment. This in turn causes increased secretion of oxytocin by the maternal posterior pituitary gland. Oxytocin stimulates the myometrium to contract and start labor.

Placental Aging Theory.   The placental aging theory suggests that after 40 weeks of gestation, placental circulation decreases as a result of the degeneration of trophoblastic tissue. This alteration in placental vascularization then causes a disruption in the production of placental hormones or perhaps causes the secretion of a new hormone that causes labor to begin.

Changes in the Estrogen/Progesterone Ratio. During pregnancy, the proper balance between concentrations of estrogen and progesterone allows pregnancy to continue. However, there is some controversy as to whether progesterone levels decrease or remain the same before labor (Nathaniels 1976).

Uterine Contraction

Although much is still to be learned about the mechanisms that trigger labor, the mechanisms of labor itself are better understood. The actual work of labor is accomplished through uterine contractions, which, over a period of hours, open and thin the cervix and facilitate descent of the fetus. Uterine contractions are augmented by the "power" of maternal bearing-down efforts in the second stage.

A *contraction* is a periodic, rhythmic shortening or tightening of the uterine musculature in response to a stimulus. Each contraction has three phases: the *increment,* the period during which the intensity of the contraction increases; the *acme,* the strongest point of the contraction; and the *decrement,* the period of decreasing intensity. The *intervals* between contractions are charac-

terized by a relaxation of the muscle to its normal resting tone or *tonus.* During normal labor, contractions occur 2 to 20 minutes apart, last 15 to 90 seconds, and are of varying intensity depending on the stage of labor. A typical pattern of uterine contraction is shown in Figure 22 – 16.

Contractions serve several purposes in labor: they efface and dilate the cervix; they facilitate the descent and rotation of the fetus; they cause the separation and expulsion of the placenta after birth; and after the expulsion of the placenta, they maintain hemostasis of the uterus by compressing blood vessels. Normal uterine contractions are involuntary, rhythmic, and intermittent. Intervals between contractions allow the uterine muscle to rest and to receive uninterrupted blood circulation.

If contractions are constant (with intervals of less than 30 seconds between contractions) or prolonged (lasting more than 90 seconds), medical evaluation of the patient is necessary. Strong, constant uterine contractions may result in actual rupture of the uterine muscle. Further, vasoconstriction occurs during the contraction because of the pressure of the contracting tissue, dramatically reducing oxygen exchange with the fetus. The interval between contractions allows the flow of oxygenated blood into the intervillous spaces to resume. If intervals between contractions are short, the fetus is at risk for anoxia.

Contractions increase in intensity, frequency, and duration throughout labor because of the mechanical stretching of the cervix. This phenomenon is known as *Ferguson's reflex;* contractions stimulate stretch and pressure receptors in the cervix. These receptors act to stimulate increased oxytocin secretion, which in turn stimulates the uterus to contract more vigorously.

The uterine contraction has been described as having three major characteristics. First, contractions normally start in a pacemaker near the *uterotubal junction* of the fundus at the top of the uterus and radiate downward toward the cervix. This characteristic is called *fundal dominance.* Second, the contraction diminishes in intensity as

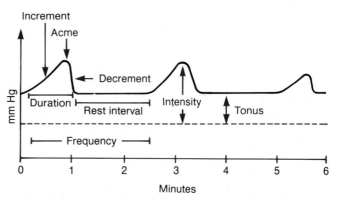

Figure 22 – 16. Characteristic pattern of uterine contraction.

it moves away from the pacemaker, so that contraction of the upper segment of the uterus is stronger than contraction of the lower segment. Third, the duration of the contraction diminishes as it moves away from the pacemaker. Thus, contraction of the upper segment is longer than that of the lower segment. All three of these characteristics must be present to ensure efficient uterine functioning and normal progress in labor. For reasons not completely understood, contractions will sometimes start in another area of the uterine muscle and spread in an uncoordinated fashion through the uterus rather than in this orderly fundus-to-cervix pattern. Contractions of this sort are not efficient and will not contribute to the work of thinning and opening the cervix in labor.

Changes in the Uterus During Labor

The process of labor requires the uterus to change dramatically in shape. These changes reflect two different processes: the development of upper and lower uterine segments, and cervical dilatation and effacement. Both processes facilitate the descent and eventual delivery of the fetus.

Development of the Uterine Segments

As labor contractions proceed, the uterus differentiates into two distinct portions or segments. The *upper segment* is the more active fundal region; it becomes thicker and its muscle fibers become shorter as labor advances. The upper uterine segment contracts, retracts, and forces the fetus to descend and eventually be expelled from the uterus. Contraction of the uterus never totally relaxes during labor, and the muscle becomes fixed at its shorter length to maintain the downward pressure it attains with each contraction. As a result of this contraction and retraction, the upper uterine segment becomes thicker through the first and second stages and tremendously thick after the third stage.

The *lower segment* is much less active. Its muscle fibers relax and stretch, and during labor the lower segment becomes a thin-walled passage for the fetus. The differentiation between the two segments becomes quite marked during labor. The boundary between them is called the *physiologic retraction ring.*

Cervical Effacement and Dilatation

The second major change that occurs in the uterus during labor is the process of cervical effacement and dilatation (Fig. 22–17). *Effacement* is the softening, thinning, and shortening of the cervical canal. During pregnancy, the cervical canal is approximately 2 cm in length. As labor progresses, the cervix is shortened and thinned until it is completely assimilated into the lower uterine segment itself. This change results from the contractions

of the uterus and the pressure of the presenting part and the amniotic sac.

Effacement is evaluated during labor in terms of percentages: 0% indicates no effacement, and 100% indicates complete effacement. Frequently, especially in multiparas, the cervix will be 50% or more effaced by Braxton Hicks contractions before labor begins. After labor begins, effacement and dilatation will occur simultaneously in a multigravida, whereas in the primigravida effacement is usually advanced before dilatation of the os begins.

Dilatation, sometimes known as dilation, is the opening and enlargement of the external cervical os from a few millimeters during pregnancy to 10 cm at complete dilatation in labor. Dilatation is caused by the retraction of the cervix into the lower uterine segment as a result of labor contractions and the pressure of the amniotic sac.

Assessment of cervical effacement and dilatation during labor is accomplished by direct fingertip palpation of the cervix during vaginal examination (Fig. 22–18). It requires practice to develop consistency and accuracy in this assessment, and even among experienced clinicians there may be some small differences in assessments of the same patient.

Psyche: Maternal State of Mind

The woman's state of mind is also a critical aspect in the process of labor and birth. Her perception of the process of birth is influenced by her self-confidence, her patterns of coping with uncertainty and stress, her own attitudes and expectations about labor and birth and those of her family and care-providers, and her response to pain, anxiety, and other alterations in functioning that occur during labor.

A knowledgeable and sensitive nurse can support the woman in making the most positive adaptation to labor possible, given the unique characteristics and course of each labor and birth. Chapters 23 and 24 address in more detail some specific nursing actions to facilitate healthy psychosocial and physiologic adaptation to labor and birth. A few key areas important to an overall understanding of the impact of the psyche on labor and birth will be highlighted here.

Negative Attitudes About Childbirth

Many women see childbirth as a challenge to be met or, more fatalistically, as a brief experience to be endured and forgotten. Other women have much more negative attitudes about childbirth or are extremely fearful of it. These attitudes often affect the progress of labor and birth.

Childbirth as a Threat to Safety. Negative attitudes toward childbirth may arise from the threat it poses to

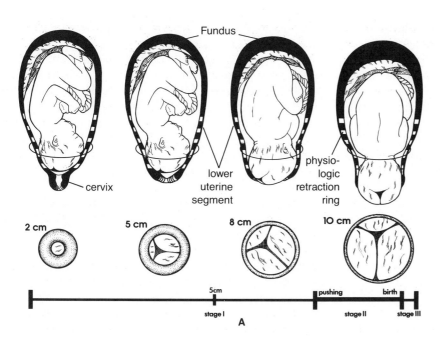

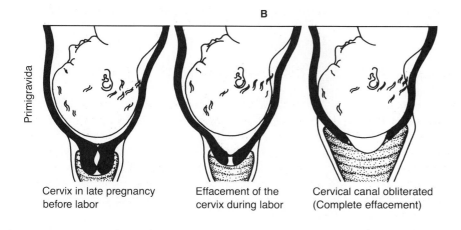

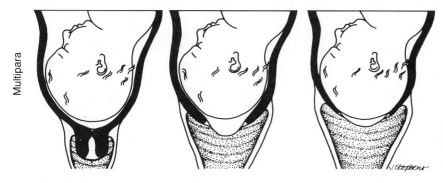

Figure 22–17. (*A*) Cervical effacement and dilatation. (*B*) Comparison of cervical effacement and dilatation in the primigravida and multipara. (Childbirth Graphics)

physical safety—the mother's own and her infant's. These fears are based to some degree on fact, since childbirth entails an element of physical risk that cannot always be anticipated or reduced. They are likely to be intensified by "horror stories" shared and sometimes embellished by other women. If the woman is a primigravida, she fears the unknown. If she has had children before, she may fear a repetition of previous negative experiences or, if earlier births were easy, worry that this one will be difficult. Such attitudes may be hard to change

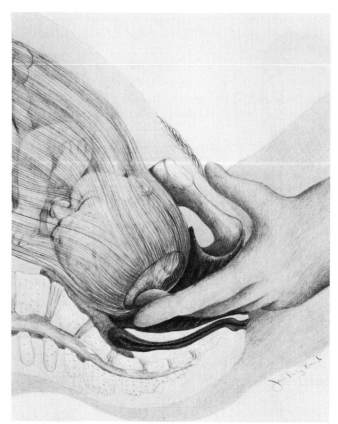

Figure 22–18. Cervical dilatation. The degree of cervical effacement and dilatation is determined by manual examination. The examiner's first and second fingers are placed in the vagina and the cervix is located. The fingers are swept over the cervical margin from one side to the other to determine its approximate dilatation in centimeters and to estimate its effacement. When the cervix is fully dilated its diameter is approximately 10 cm. At the same time, the level of the presenting fetal part in the birth canal (station) is also identified. (Childbirth Graphics)

for two reasons. First, these fears are in part based in reality. Second, friends, family members, and the woman's partner, if he chooses to prepare for and attend the birth, are likely to respond to the dangerous aspect of childbirth and unintentionally reinforce the woman's own fears.

Childbirth as a Threat to Self-Image. Childbirth can also be seen as a significant threat to the woman's self-image. Birth requires giving up control of one's body and one's behavior to a certain degree, which can be quite disturbing to some women. Childbirth also represents a real threat to a woman's body image. In addition, she may view childbirth as the symbol of motherhood, and if she has negative feelings about what motherhood entails, such as loss of physical beauty or sexual attractiveness,

Psychological Factors That Influence The Progress of Labor

Childbirth as a Threat to Safety

Fears about personal safety and safety of fetus generated by:
> Previous experiences with illness and pain
> "Horror stories" shared by other women

Fear of the unknown

Childbirth as a Threat to Self-Image

Vulnerability to loss of control over:
> Bodily functions and privacy
> Verbalizations and behavior

Concerns about body image

Negative attitudes about childbirth and motherhood related to:
> Loss of physical beauty or sexual attractiveness
> Decreased occupational or career potential
> Increased dependency

Unrealistic expectations about childbirth and childrearing

The "Medicalization" of Childbirth

Decreased decision-making power for woman and family

Isolation of birth experience in hospital setting

Illness-oriented health care practices and setting

Lack of respect for the woman and her family shown through:
> Inappropriate use of technical language
> Value judgments about woman's behavior by providers
> Paternalistic practices of providers
> Arbitrary exclusion of support people and family members from participating in childbirth

The Meaning of Pain Experienced During Childbirth

Past experience with pain

Cultural background

Physical status

Psychological status

Progress of labor

Stage of labor

increasing dependency on others, or loss of occupational potential, she is likely to be less positive about birth itself. A woman may also have unrealistic expectations about herself in relation to childbirth and child-rearing and may see herself as having something to prove to herself or others. Such expectations may contribute to negative attitudes toward childbirth.

The "Medicalization" of Childbirth.   Childbirth in Western society is viewed as an "illness" state requiring medical intervention, including hospitalization, medical management, the use of technology, and sometimes surgery to accomplish delivery. At times this trend contributes to a view of the childbearing woman as dependent, passive, and even childlike, with no real role in decision making. More women today reject this passive role, but the view that childbirth is a medical condition requiring treatment, instead of a normal physiologic process, is still prevalent. Labor and birth usually take place in the hospital setting, where the mother and her support person are relatively isolated. This restricts the amount of "second-hand" knowledge women gain about childbirth and reduces the amount of emotional support the laboring woman may have from friends, family, and experienced women.

Although these negative attitudes may have some impact on the woman's psychosocial adaptation to labor, they can usually be assessed and addressed to some extent through effective maternity care. Attendance at childbirth classes and anticipatory guidance during pregnancy may go a long way toward reducing their effects in labor. Yet, as noted before, each labor is unique and, in some ways, unpredictable. Thus, the woman's psychosocial adaptation to labor will depend in large part on her perception of events as they unfold. One of the most important factors affecting her adaptation is her response to labor pain.

Pain in Labor and Birth

Most women anticipate and, in fact, do experience some pain in childbirth. Labor pain is sometimes described as the most intense pain a person may experience, and the pain of labor is often the aspect of childbirth most worrisome to expectant parents. There is undoubtedly a physiologic basis for pain in labor, although the intensity of the pain experienced varies a great deal from one woman to another. Although pain is usually associated with pathology, in the case of childbirth it is due to normal physiologic processes.

Factors Affecting Perception of Pain in Labor.   Dr. Joyce Roberts, a nurse midwife and scientist, notes that a woman's responses to pain in labor are influenced to a great extent by her own history of pain, her cultural background, her psychological and physical state and the interpretation she places on the pain-producing situation (Roberts 1983). The intensity of reported labor pain increases as labor progresses, peaks at transition, and declines during the actual delivery; however, some women report a decrease in pain during the second stage as well.

All of these factors — threats to personal safety and one's self image, the medicalization of childbirth, and the meaning of pain — may arouse anxiety in the woman and

alter the normal course of labor and delivery. Excessive anxiety can alter the woman's perception of labor, intensifying her response to pain and fatigue. A study by a nurse scientist, Dr. Regina Lederman, has shown that high levels of anxiety are related to the secretion of catecholamines, which in turn may inhibit uterine activity and result in less effective uterine contractions and an increased risk of intrapartal complications (Lederman 1978). There is some evidence that preparation for childbirth may reduce anxiety during labor by minimizing the fear of the unknown and allow the woman to interpret the sensations of labor and events in her environment more accurately.

STAGES AND PHASES OF LABOR

Labor is divided into four stages during which cervical effacement, dilatation, and the cardinal movements of the fetus occur.

The First Stage

The first stage of labor begins with the onset of regular contractions and ends with complete dilatation of the cervix (10 cm). The first stage is further divided into two phases: the *latent phase* and the *active phase* (Table 22–1). The early or *latent* phase begins with the initiation of true labor contractions and is completed when the cervix is dilated 3 to 4 cm. It is the longer of the two phases, and in primigravidas it is the period during which the cervix effaces.

Uterine contractions during the latent phase are usually mild. The uterus is easily indented with the fingertips, when it is palpated through a contraction, and exerts a pressure of only 20 to 30 mmHg. Contractions often last only 15 to 30 seconds and are relatively infrequent (occurring as infrequently as every 10 to 20 minutes). Many women complete the latent phase at home in the comfort of familiar surroundings. They are able to ambulate without difficulty, at times even through contractions.

The *active phase* of labor, also called the dilatation phase, begins at 4 to 5 cm dilatation and ends when the woman's cervix is completely dilated. It is subdivided into three periods: (1) the acceleration phase (4 to 5 cm), (2) the phase of maximum slope (5 to 9 cm), and (3) the deceleration phase (9 to 10 cm).

During the acceleration phase, contractions become longer (30 to 45 seconds), stronger (exerting up to 50 mmHg pressure or greater) and occur more frequently (as often as every 3 to 5 minutes). The woman may find it is more difficult to continue walking during contractions and the nurse will note an obvious change in the parturient. Mild cramping sensations and a low, dull backache may give way to perceptions of mild-to-moderate discomfort or pain during contractions.

During the phase of maximum slope (5 to 9 cm), the cervix dilates most rapidly. Uterine contractions continue to increase in frequency (every 2 to 3 minutes), intensity, and duration (45 to 90 seconds). There is often an increase in bloody show. The woman may experience moderate-to-severe discomfort or pain in the latter half of this phase. By 7 cm dilatation, many women wish to sit or recline for periods of time and may find ambulation difficult or impossible at the acme of the contraction.

The interval between 8 and 10 cm is also referred to as the *transition stage*. The laboring woman may experience intense sensations of discomfort or pain, and an urge to bear down as she begins to feel the pressure of the fetal presenting part deep in the pelvis. Nausea, vomiting, increased irritability, and even a sense of panic may occur as she is bombarded with multiple, intense stimuli.

The culmination of the active phase of labor is the deceleration phase (9 to 10 cm). The rate of cervical dilatation slows slightly. A noticeable change in the woman's responses to labor may be noted as she approaches complete dilatation. She may feel more relaxed and perceive less pain or discomfort, or the intensity, frequency, and duration of contractions may peak along with an irresistable urge to push.

The Second Stage

The second stage of labor, or stage of expulsion, begins with complete dilatation of the cervix and ends with the birth of the infant (see Table 22–1). Uterine contractions often decrease in intensity, frequency, and duration for a short period of time. The woman may immediately feel an urge to push, or it may take time for fetal descent to stimulate stretch receptors in the lower pelvis. It may, therefore, be appropriate in some instances to allow the woman a short period of rest, especially after a tumultuous first stage, before initiating bearing-down efforts.

Intra-abdominal pressure is now combined with uterine contractions to expel the fetus. The perineum begins to bulge and flatten out as the presenting part emerges (see Fig. 22–15). Protrusion of the rectal mucous membrane through the anus may also occur. The labia majora and minora begin to separate as the head emerges. With each contraction, a larger portion of the presenting part is visible at the introitus and is referred to as crowning.

The woman may experience intense rectal pressure and a sensation of stretching, tearing, or burning of the perineum as the head is born. With the birth of the head, there is a sudden sense of relief, as well as diminution in pressure and pain. The shoulders and body are then expelled.

Rupture of Membranes.   The membranes may rupture at any time before or during the first stage of labor, but occasionally remain intact until the cervix is completely dilated. The birth attendant will usually artificially rupture the membranes if they have not ruptured during the course of the second stage of labor. This is done so as to visualize the color of the amniotic fluid. If meconium (fetal intestinal contents) has been expelled *in utero*, a special suction technique is required at birth to prevent aspiration of meconium by the neonate as it takes its first breath. (See Chapter 33 for further description of suctioning.)

The Third Stage

The third stage of labor, or the placental stage, begins with the birth of the infant and ends with delivery of the placenta (see Table 22–1). Contractions may cease for several minutes after the infant is born, and with their resumption (usually within 5 minutes), the placenta is delivered in 2 phases: (1) the separation phase and (2) the expulsion phase.

The Separation Phase

With the birth of the neonate, the uterus contracts, becomes smaller and firmer, and often appears to stand up in the maternal abdomen. Within minutes after the infant has been expelled, the uterus becomes a thick muscular sac. The walls of the uterine cavity collapse, eliminating the large cavity that was recently occupied. This sudden decrease in uterine size results in a decreased area for placental attachment and causes the decidua and fetal membranes to fold. The placenta is forced to accommodate to the decreased surface area by buckling off the wall of the uterus in the decidua spongiosa layer. The blood vessels in this central area begin to bleed, and a hematoma forms between the placenta and the remaining decidua. As this retroplacental hematoma enlarges, it forces additional cleavage of the placenta from the uterine wall, as shown in Figure 22–19. Visible maternal bleeding is usually minimal during this process, but there may be a gush or spurt of blood from the vagina, signaling placental separation.

It is believed that separation of the placenta usually begins in the central area, within minutes of delivery. The peripheral areas are more firmly attached. Part of the decidua comes off with the placenta, and a varying amount remains attached to the myometrium to be shed during the next several weeks. The fetal membranes are peeled off the uterine wall by contraction of the myometrium and traction of the separated placenta as it slides down the uterine walls into the lower uterine segment. From there, the placenta may be expelled from the uterus and vagina by increased abdominal pressure due to ma-

Table 22-1   Stages and Phase of Normal Labor and Related Physical Characteristics

| Stage | Phase | Dilatation | Contractions | | | Physical Characteristics |
			Frequency	*Intensity*	*Duration*	
First Stage (0–10 cm)	Latent	0–4 cm	Q. 10–20 min but may occur more often: Q. 5–10 min.	Mild	15–30 sec	Mild "menstrual-like" cramps Low, dull backache Sensation of uterine tightening Expulsion of mucous Light bloody show Diarrhea Possible rupture of membranes Ambulation without difficulty
	Active	4–10 cm				Mild-to-moderate discomfort or pain with UCs
	Acceleration	4–5 cm	Q. 3–5 min	Moderate	30–45 sec	Increased bloody show Possible rupture of membranes Persistent backache with occiput posterior position Ambulation without difficulty
		Maximum Slope 5–9 cm	Q. 2–3 min	Moderate to intense	60–90 sec	Moderate-to-severe discomfort or pain with UCs Increased bloody show Increasing rectal pressure Intermittent urge to push Nausea, vomiting, hiccoughing, leg cramps, diaphoresis Involuntary shaking Periods of amnesia Possible rupture of membranes Ambulation difficult or impossible with UCs
Transition Stage (8–10 cm)	Deceleration	9–10 cm	As frequent as Q. 1–2 min	Moderate to intense	45–90 sec	Moderate to severe discomfort or pain with UCs Increased bloody show Increasing urge to push Increasing rectal pressure Possible rupture of membranes
Second Stage (10 cm to birth of infant)			(May initially decrease in frequency, intensity and duration). As frequent as Q. 1–2 min			Strong urge to push with descent of presenting part Increasing rectal and perineal pressure Desire in some women to assume squatting position Bulging of perineum Prolapse of rectal mucosa Emergence of fetal presenting part—"crowning" Possible rupture of membranes

(continued)

Table 22–1   **Stages and Phase of Normal Labor and Related Physical Characteristics** (continued)

| Stage | Phase | Dilatation | Contractions | | | Physical Characteristics |
			Frequency	*Intensity*	*Duration*	
Third Stage (Birth of infant to birth of placenta)			(Initial cessation of contractions)			Sensation of burning, stretching, or tearing as head is born Perineal anesthesia due to extreme stretching of perineum Mild-to-moderate uterine cramping with re-initiation of UCs Feeling of fullness in vagina as placenta is expelled
Fourth Stage (1–4 hr postbirth)			(Continuous contraction of uterus to prevent bleeding from spiral arteries)			Perineal tenderness Intermittent mild-to-moderate menstrual-like cramps Involuntary shivering in some women (neurogenic response to intensity of labor)

ternal pushing efforts. Other methods of assistance may be needed if the woman is in a recumbent position. If she is in an upright position, gravity will aid expulsion. A commonly used method of assistance in placental delivery involves applying a hand over the uterine fundus and using the uterus as a piston to expel the placenta while applying gentle cord traction at the same time (Fig. 22–20).

Uterine musculature is arranged in three layers: the *outer layer,* which arches over the fundus and extends into the various uterine ligaments; the *inner layer,* which consists of sphincterlike fibers that surround the openings into the uterus, the fallopian tubes, and internal os of the cervix; and the substantial *middle layer,* which forms a dense crisscrossing network of muscle fibers in which are interlaced the many blood vessels of the uterus.

As a result of this structure, the contraction of the middle-layer muscle fibers results in hemostasis of the uterine blood vessels at the placental site. Immediately following placental delivery, the uterine muscle should feel firm, and the fundus should be apparent at or below the umbilicus.

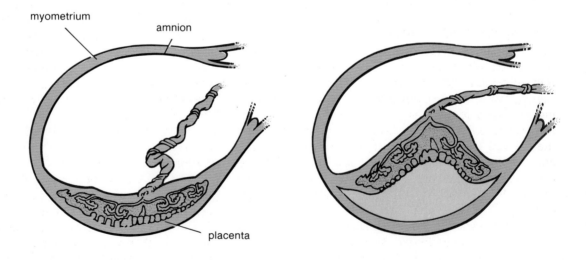

A Placenta attached to uterine wall   **B** Placenta separated from uterine wall

Figure 22–19. Placental separation. (*A*) Placenta attached to uterine wall. (*B*) Placenta separated from uterine wall.

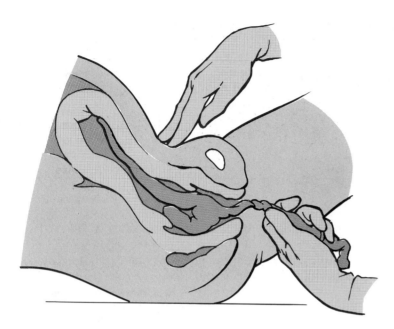

Figure 22–20. Placental delivery.

Normally, third-stage labor lasts from a few minutes to 30 minutes. The incidence of complications increases after 30 minutes.

Placental Separation and Expulsion

The classic signs of placental separation are the following:

- A gush of blood from the vagina
- A change in the size, shape, and consistency of the uterus
- Lengthening of the umbilical cord from the vagina
- Maternal report of a contraction

Mechanisms of Expulsion

There are two mechanisms by which the placenta can be expelled from the uterus. The more common of these is called *Schultze's mechanism.* In Schultze's mechanism, the central region of the placenta separates first. As bleeding from torn vessels continues, a *retroplacental hematoma* is formed, and this further eases the placenta off the uterine wall. The central portion is followed by the peripheral portions. The hematoma and any free bleeding is contained in the trailing membranes as they are inverted behind the placenta. The shiny fetal surface of the placenta appears first at the introitus.

In *Duncan's mechanism,* separation of the placenta occurs first at the periphery. Blood collects between the placenta and the uterine wall and may spurt or gush from the vagina when separation occurs. The placenta descends sideways in this case, and the dull and irregular maternal surface appears first at the introitus. Placental separation by Duncan's mechanism carries a slightly in-

creased risk of retained placental fragments in the uterus after delivery owing to incomplete separation. Thus, when the placenta is delivered by this mechanism, examination of the placenta and assessment of the uterine position, tone and bleeding after delivery must be particularly careful.

Because of the quality of the presenting surface in the two mechanisms, they are often remembered as *shiny Schultze* and *dirty Duncan.*

Duration of Labor

The length of time required to complete the work of childbirth varies according to a number of factors — fetal size and position, strength and pattern of uterine contractions, maternal position and activity, and maternal age and parity, to name a few. However, certain patterns in the duration of each stage and in the course of labor overall help to indicate whether an individual woman's labor is progressing normally.

Perhaps the most comprehensive study of the duration and progress of normal labor and birth was undertaken by Emmanuel Friedman, an obstetrician. He studied a large number of births and examined how long individual stages of labor and the entire course of labor lasted under normal conditions in cases in which outcomes were good (Friedman 1978). The results of his study on the length of stages of labor among primigravidas and multigravidas are shown in Table 22–2. The upper ranges represent the longest time that labor continued and still concluded normally. The characteristically shorter labor of the multigravida can be seen in this table. These results are used widely as guidelines for judging whether the progress of a

Table 22-2   **Lengths of Phases in Normal Labor**

Phase	Primigravidas		Multiparas	
	Average	*Upper Normal*	*Average*	*Upper Normal*
Latent phase	8.6 hr	20.0 hr	5.3 hr	14.0 hr
Active phase	5.8 hr	12.0 hr	2.5 hr	6.0 hr
First stage	13.3 hr	28.5 hr	7.5 hr	20.0 hr
Second stage	57 min	150 min	18 min	50 min
Rate of cervical dilatation in active phase	Under 1.2 cm/hr is abnormal		Under 1.5 cm/hr is abnormal	

particular woman's labor is within normal limits. However, as noted below, these findings may have limitations and must be used cautiously.

The Friedman Curve

These guidelines have been translated into a graphic representation of the progress of labor (Fig. 22–21). The so-called *Friedman curve* is frequently used in labor assessment and may appear in hospital settings in pre-printed labor progress records on which the woman's progress is charted. The nurse should recognize that these guidelines must not be used in isolation but must always be used along with other clinical data, such as fetal heart rate and maternal status, to determine whether more active management of labor is needed.

Further, there is some evidence that the Friedman curve may not always accurately represent the upper safe limits of time in labor. Research on the second stage suggests that it may safely extend to more than 2.5 hours for a primigravida, as long as the fetus appears to be doing well. Also, these guidelines may not accurately reflect patterns of normal labor in unmedicated and ambulating or upright parturients. As research continues, these guidelines may be further revised.

Signs and Symptoms of Labor

Before the onset of labor, certain phenomena may alert the patient to approaching labor.

Braxton Hicks Contractions

Although Braxton Hicks contractions occur throughout pregnancy, these tightenings of the uterine musculature become more noticeable in the last 4 to 6 weeks. Multigravidas often experience more discomfort from them than do primigravidas. Braxton Hicks contractions are usually painless, irregular in frequency and intensity, and they may be unusually long in duration. They are noted as a tightening or pulling sensation low in the abdomen over the pubic bone. These contractions may be helpful in developing the neuromuscular pathways needed for the coordinated contractions of labor. They may also assist in early changes of the cervix before labor begins. A series of Braxton Hicks contractions may be referred to as *false labor.*

Lightening

Lightening refers to the settling or engagement of the presenting part in the maternal pelvis. It usually occurs 2 to 3 weeks before the onset of labor in primigravidas and may not occur in multigravidas until labor begins. Although it is often described as a subjective sensation felt by the woman, lightening may be evident as a decrease in prenatal fundal height near 37 or 38 weeks of gestation. The woman is usually aware of this settling of the baby in the lower uterine segment, which is often described in lay terms as the "baby dropping." She feels increased movement low in the uterus, may experience less difficulty breathing, and observes that her uterus protrudes more. In addition, bladder capacity is further decreased and urination may be frequent. Leg cramps, pedal edema, and pelvic pressure may also increase.

Cervical and Vaginal Changes

Cervical changes, often referred to as "ripening," include softening, effacement (shortening and thinning), and sometimes dilatation. Uterine contractions late in pregnancy begin to pull the cervix upward as the lower uterine segment is formed. This results in the loosening of fibrous connective tissue of the cervix. The cervix becomes softer, shorter, more pliable, and thinner in preparation for dilatation. It may also move from a posterior to an anterior location in the vagina. There may also be increased vaginal discharge due to the increased pelvic congestion in early labor.

Persistent Backache

Relaxin, the placental hormone responsible for relaxation of pelvic ligaments, has maximally affected the sacroiliacs and other pelvic joints by late pregnancy. As a result, strain on the muscles of the lower back is increased. The postural changes associated with pregnancy may add to this problem.

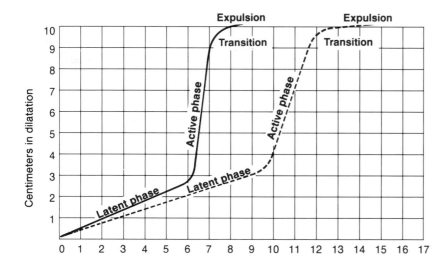

Figure 22–21. Graphic analysis of labor utilizing Friedman's curve. The mean labor duration for primigravidas is shown by the dotted line, and the mean for multigravidas is shown by the solid line.

Weight Loss and Gastrointestinal Upset

As estrogen and progesterone levels change in late pregnancy, electrolyte shifts occur that result in loss of body water. Weight loss of 1 to 3 pounds can occur. Many women also experience diarrhea 1 or 2 days before labor begins; the cause of this is unknown.

Nesting Behavior

A flurry of activity by the pregnant woman is not uncommon in the final days before labor begins. The woman can feel compelled to "have everything ready" for the arrival of the baby. She should take care not to overdo this and begin labor in an exhausted state.

Signs of True Labor

Uterine Contractions.   True labor contractions usually occur at regular intervals. The contractions get closer, increase in duration and intensity, and bring about pro-gressive change in the cervix and descent of the fetus. Women describe true labor contractions as starting in the back and radiating to the front. Activity, such as walking, may increase the intensity of true labor contractions.

Spontaneous Rupture of Membranes (SROM). Rupture of the membranes may occur as a leak or a gush of amniotic fluid. This fluid is usually clear and odorless, although in some cases it may be greenish because of *meconium staining,* or fetal passage of intestinal contents *in utero,* a sign of possible fetal distress. Labor contractions usually start within 8 to 12 hours of spontaneous rupture; if labor does not ensue, more active obstetric management to stimulate labor may be advised because of the increasing risk that infection will ascend into the uterus and threaten the fetus.

Bloody Show.   Bloody show, or blood-tinged vaginal secretions, may occur at the onset of labor or several days beforehand. It is caused by rupture of minute capillaries in the cervix as it softens, dilates, and effaces in preparation for labor.

MATERNAL AND FETAL ADAPTATIONS

Maternal Physiologic Adaptations

In addition to the adaptations that occur in the reproductive system, there are also normal alterations in other body systems, which indicate a healthy adaptation to the process of labor and birth.

Neurologic Adaptations

Neurologic adaptations have not been extensively studied to date. As noted, certain behavioral responses have been noted just prior to the onset of labor, such as

---

Signs and Symptoms of Impending Labor

- Braxton Hicks contractions
- Lightening
- Cervical changes (softening, effacement, and dilation)
- Increased vaginal discharge, in some cases
- Persistent backache
- Weight loss
- Nesting behavior
- Signs of true labor:

  Uterine contractions

  Spontaneous rupture of membranes

  Bloody show

nesting behavior and energy spurts, which may reflect central nervous system adaptations. The neurochemical basis for these alterations in activity are poorly understood. Sleep disturbances have also been noted and have been attributed to frequent fetal movement, Braxton Hicks contractions, need to urinate frequently, and the gravida's inability to assume a comfortable resting position in late gestation. But hormonal changes in pregnancy may, in fact, alter circadian rhythms and the percentage of time spent in REM sleep, contributing to sleep disturbances.

Cardiovascular Adaptations

Cardiac Output.   Cardiac output steadily rises during labor, with a 15% to 20% increase during contractions caused by catecholamine release and the expulsion of blood from the uterine vessels back into the circulatory system. Cardiac output may increase as much as 40% to 50% in the second stage of labor, with expulsive effort and peaks in the third stage at 80% above prelabor levels. This is caused by the loss of the uteroplacental vascular bed and the release of pressure on the vena cava.

Blood Pressure.   Arterial blood pressure increases during labor. The systolic pressure may increase an average of 15 mmHg and diastolic 5 to 10 mmHg. Higher levels may indicate pathology (see Chapter 28). During contractions, the blood pressure may rise temporarily higher with pain sensations, anxiety, and catecholamine release, as well as by compression of the distal aorta and common iliac arteries.

Heart Rate.   The pulse rate increases over time to 100 beats per minute (bpm) or slightly higher by the second stage of labor, with sensations of pain, anxiety, increased activity, and catecholamine release. During the peak of contractions, a reflex bradycardia accompanies the increase in cardiac output and blood pressure. Between contractions, the pulse rate returns to the resting rate, which averages 80 to 90 bpm.

Stroke Volume.   There is also a progressive increase in stroke volume during labor, which peaks at delivery.

Blood Volume.   There is no change in blood volume during normal labor, but the parturient may lose up to 500 ml during delivery. The hypervolemia of pregnancy allows the woman to adapt to the rapid blood loss. Other cardiovascular responses that also aid in the successful adaptation, include elimination of the large uteroplacental vascular bed and fluid shifts from the extravascular compartment back to the circulatory system.

Hematologic Adaptations

Blood coagulation time decreases slightly during labor but plasma fibrinogen levels increase. There is a progressive leukocytosis (an average increase to 15,000 mm³) by the end of the first stage. With heavy exertion, the white cell count may rise to 25,000 to 35,000 mm³.

Pulmonary Adaptations

The respiratory rate increases during labor, and there is an increase in oxygen consumption secondary to the rise in metabolic rate and the work of labor. Some women may hyperventilate during the peak of contractions, but persistent hyperventilation is abnormal.

Biochemical Adaptations

While the maternal pH remains within norms (7.35 to 7.45), a rise in blood lactate and a fall in pH are noted in the late first stage of labor. This metabolic acidosis results from several factors, including increased muscular activity, which produces acid metabolites, and starvation ketosis caused by the catabolism of fat to meet energy requirements.

Renal Adaptations

Increased fluid losses and changes in electrolyte balance during labor result from several significant factors. Polyuria is common with increased cardiac output and a resultant rise in the glomerular filtration rate. Diaphoresis and hyperventilation contribute to insensible water loss. Reduced oral intake of fluids due to nausea, pain sensations, and the administration of analgesia or anesthesia further alter fluid and electrolyte balance. The hypervolemia of pregnancy protects the parturient to some extent, but dehydration, ketonuria, and electrolyte aberrations are observed with prolonged labor, persistent nausea and vomiting, and maternal exhaustion.

Slight proteinuria (trace) is also usually noted in as many as one-third to one-half of women secondary to an increased metabolic rate and muscle breakdown during the work of labor. Greater levels of proteinuria are indicative of pathology (see Chapter 28).

Inability to void and bladder distention are often observed in the laboring woman. A relaxed bladder muscle tone occurs when progesterone levels in pregnancy predispose the parturient to distention. Compression of the urethra and bladder by the uterus and fetus may make it impossible for her to void. Distention may cause a reflex diminution in the forces of labor and can lead to trauma of the bladder mucosa during birth of the infant.

Gastrointestinal Adaptations

Gastrointestinal motility and absorption decrease during labor, as do gastric secretions. Thus, gastric emptying time is prolonged and undigested food may remain in the stomach throughout labor. Nausea and vomiting are not uncommon, especially in the transition stage. Liquids are, however, absorbed rapidly and the parturient experiencing an uncomplicated labor and birth is encouraged to ingest clear fluids, high in glucose, to meet energy requirements. Diarrhea is also observed in some women, particularly as a sign of impending labor.

Metabolic Adaptations

The increased metabolic activity that occurs during labor causes an increased pulse rate, respiratory rate, body temperature, and insensible fluid loss. The slight elevation in body temperature should not exceed 0.5°C to 1.0°C and any increase should be observed closely, as it may be an indication of maternal infection or chorioamnionitis.

Both aerobic and anaerobic carbohydrate metabolism increase during labor secondary to muscle activity and catecholamine release. Blood sugar levels decrease during labor, and the parturient may require fluids with glucose supplementation during prolonged labor, or with persistent nausea and vomiting.

Maternal Behavioral Adaptations

A woman's responses to the pain and physical demands of labor produce systematic changes in behavior and require alterations in her psychologic functioning as labor progresses. Many experienced labor nurses can judge with great accuracy how far cervical change has progressed in the unmedicated laboring woman by observing her behavior and her interaction with the environment. Excitement and anticipation are typical in early labor, and the woman interacts easily with her partner, other support people, and staff. Conversations or other activities readily distract her from attending to her labor, and only the recurring contractions themselves refocus her attention on the process that has begun.

However, as labor becomes well established, the physical sensations become more compelling. As she reaches the midway point of cervical dilatation, the woman must work to cope with contractions. Interactions with others are limited to the work at hand, and only between contractions can her attention be directed away from the sensations she is experiencing. Observers have described this as a process of *ego constriction:* the woman's attention gradually narrows from her normal engagement with the outside world to the world of her labor room.

The nurse may observe a gradual loss of modesty as the work of labor becomes paramount in the woman's mind. A woman who in early labor was concerned about keeping her body covered now may not even notice when she is uncovered; as labor reaches a peak during transition, she may actively remove coverings. The woman in active hard labor gradually becomes less and less able to focus on matters not directly related to her own comfort and safety. As she approaches complete dilatation, the sensations associated with contractions may be almost overwhelming. The woman's attention is totally self-focused. She may fall asleep or close her eyes between contractions and interact little with others, except to respond to directions or ask for help.

Once dilatation is complete, the sensations associated with labor compel her to bear down, and this work of pushing demands her full concentration. However, as she makes progress and delivery becomes imminent, her attention expands to include the soon-to-be born infant. She may watch the crowning and the birth with growing excitement and react with joy at the first sight of the infant. The mother often will then "reconnect" with her support person, especially if it is the father: looking to see his response, sharing tears of joy and laughter with him. Rapidly, the mother's psychological space expands to include both baby and father.

However, this process of behavioral adaptation to labor is influenced by many factors. Obviously, if regional anesthesia is used during labor, this level of psychological adaptation to the physical stress of labor is not necessary. Thus, changes in the woman's behavior may be far less dramatic. If complications arise, the woman is forced not only to cope with labor but also to adjust to a rapidly changing "risk" situation. She may become acutely attuned to interactions around her, looking for information and reassurance. Anxiety, sensory alterations, and the supportive presence of others also affect the woman's psychological adaptation to labor.

Fetal Physiologic Adaptations

In addition to the positional and attitudinal adaptations that occur in the fetus during labor and birth, the following adjustments are made.

Neurologic Adaptations

An intact brain and autonomic nervous system function to regulate fetal heart rate, cardiac output, and blood pressure. The *parasympathetic nervous system* (cardiodecelerator system) and its primary nerve—the vagus nerve—increase in dominance during gestation, and the fetal heart rate gradually slows. During labor, when the vagus nerve is stimulated, for example by compression of the fetal head during contractions, the heart rate will temporarily slow until pressure on the head ceases.

The *sympathetic nervous system* (cardioaccelerator system) has nerve fibers that are widely distributed in heart muscle. When stimulated by the mild hypoxia the fetus experiences during contractions, the heart rate is increased. The parasympathetic and sympathetic nervous systems interplay to control both the fetal heart rate and the variability in the heart rate pattern. The balance between these systems is altered by changes in the intrauterine environment, fetal activity, external stimuli, and changes in maternal or fetal PO_2 or PCO_2 concentrations (Murray 1988).

Cardiovascular Adaptations

Heart Rate.   During labor, the fetal heart rate normally ranges between 120 and 160 bpm. In some term or post-term fetuses, the baseline heart rate ranges between 100 and 120 bpm as a result of neurologic maturity (Murray 1988). With uterine contractions, the increase in uterine tension reduces the flow of oxygenated maternal blood to the intervillous spaces. At approximately 50 mmHg pressure, blood flow ceases, and the fetus must rely on oxygen reserves in the intervillous spaces. If these reserves are exhausted, fetal hypoxemia and tissue hypoxia will occur. Mild hypoxia causes an increase in fetal heart rate, and with moderate to severe hypoxia, the fetal heart rate will slow.

Blood Pressure.   Baroreceptors at the junction of the internal and external carotid arteries and chemoreceptors in the aortic arch, carotid bodies, and brain control fetal blood pressure and heart rate. If fetal blood pressure increases, baroreceptors cause a reflex decrease in cardiac output and blood pressure. This may occur with sudden compression of the fetal umbilical cord. Umbilical arteries are compressed, preventing outflow of fetal blood and increasing systemic blood pressure. Baroreceptors then slow the fetal heart rate and lower the blood pressure.

Chemoreceptors located in the brain are stimulated by adverse changes in fetal pH, PO_2, and PCO_2 and cause an initial increase in fetal heart rate and blood pressure. This initial rise in pressure is a protective mechanism that improves blood flow to the brain. With moderate-to-severe hypoxia, blood is selectively shunted to essential fetal organs (brain, heart, and adrenal glands) and away from the gastrointestinal tract, skeletal muscles, and skin.

Hematologic Adaptations

Oxygen utilization by the fetus is very high during labor. The fetal PO_2 is approximately 30 to 35 mmHg in the carotid artery, and although this is an extremely low oxygen tension, the fetus is able to meet its metabolic demands for oxygen in several ways. Hemoglobin levels are very high (15 to 20 g/dL); the fetal hemoglobin has a greater affinity for oxygen and a greater oxygen carrying capacity than the adult.

Pulmonary Adaptations

The placenta functions as the organ of respiration during intrauterine life. With the onset of labor, small amounts of fetal lung fluid are expelled from fetal airways during passage through the birth canal. This allows for an easier inflow of air when the neonate takes its first breath after birth. Ultrasonic examination of the fetus during labor confirms the continuation of rhythmic fetal breathing movements, which began early in the gestational period.

Gastrointestinal Adaptations

The healthy fetus may pass meconium (intestinal contents) during labor without adverse outcomes. Meconium may be also be swallowed and reabsorbed. However, many studies have reported lower Apgar scores, lower pH values, and higher perinatal morbidity and mortality rates among neonates who pass meconium *in utero*. In instances of moderate-to-severe intrauterine hypoxia, compensatory mechanisms shunt blood from the fetal GI tract, and this action may result in necrosis of intestinal tissue postnatally.

Renal Adaptations

The fetal kidneys produce urine and the fetus may urinate *in utero* during labor without adverse sequelae.

Biochemical Adaptations

Normal fetal pH ranges between 7.25 and 7.35 during labor. An oscillation in fetal pH occurs with uterine activity. Fetal blood pH decreases during contractions by as much as 0.05 pH units. In the period between contractions, excess carbon dioxide and acid metabolites are transported to the intervillous spaces and across the placental membrane. Carbon dioxide diffuses across the placental membrane at a much faster rate than does lactic acid (at least 20 to 30 minutes), thus the fetus can remain acidotic for some time after a hypoxic episode (Murray 1988).

Fetal pH is also influenced by maternal pH. Maternal starvation, increased muscle activity, and catecholamine release will falsely decrease the fetal pH in the absence of hypoxia. Correction of the maternal condition will, in these cases, reverse the lowered fetal pH.

Hormonal Adaptations

If fetal hypoxia occurs, the adrenal medulla releases epinephrine and norepinephrine. These catecholamines act directly on the fetal heart and cardiovascular system to increase blood pressure, heart rate, and the force of myocardial contractility.

Fetal Behavioral Adaptations

Only recently have researchers begun to explore behavioral states in the human fetus during birth. Using ultrasound technology, investigators have identified awake states characterized by mouthing movements (opening or closing of the jaw), eyelid closure and opening, and general body movements (rotation, flexion and extension of extremities). The fetus also exhibits periods of quiet and active sleep, even with increasing intensity of labor and rupture of membranes (Griffin 1985).

CHAPTER SUMMARY

The essential components of childbirth can be summarized as the "four *Ps*": passage, passenger, powers, and psyche. Each of these components involves a complex set of maternal and fetal adjustments. The *passage*, or maternal pelvis, must be adequate in size and shape to accommodate the descent and delivery of the fetus. The *passenger*, or fetus, must negotiate passage through the pelvis by fitting the smallest parts of its body to the narrow diameters of the pelvis. This is accomplished through a series of position changes known as the *cardinal movements of labor*. The *powers*, or uterine contractions, must be coordinated and of sufficient strength and quality to dilate and efface the cervix and, in concert with maternal expulsive efforts, push the fetus down and deliver it. The *psyche*, or maternal adaptation, must allow the woman to cope with the pain and physical demands of labor so that she can maintain physiologic and emotional balance and can actively push the fetus out during the second stage.

The parturient and the fetus undergo major physical and behavioral adaptations during the four stages of labor. During the first stage of labor, the gravida experiences an increasing intensity in physical and psychologic sensations as the cervix dilates and the fetus begins its descent through the birth canal. During the second stage, the physical work of labor reaches its peak as the mother-to-be must literally push the newborn into the world. The fetus is also experiencing drastic changes in pressure, position, and posture, which require complex physiologic adaptations. While the third stage is characterized by relief and elation for the new mother as the placenta is delivered, the fetus is faced with its greatest challenge as it makes the transition to extrauterine life. During the fourth stage, maternal physiologic stability is achieved, but the psychologic adaptation to parenthood is just beginning.

The nurse relies on her knowledge of each of these components to provide information about the progress of labor and to guide nursing care to support maternal adaptation. The following chapter outlines this nursing care.

STUDY QUESTIONS

1. Name and describe the obstetric significance of the three pelvic planes.

2. Identify five maternal factors affecting birth outcome.

3. Define the following terms: fetal lie, presentation, station, position, attitude, and synclitism.

4. What are the cardinal movements of labor? Why does each movement occur?

5. Discuss three current theories regarding the initiation of labor.

6. Describe the process of cervical effacement and dilatation.

7. What are the major stages and phases of labor? What are major defining characteristics of each?

8. Describe the major maternal physiologic and behavioral adaptions, which occur during labor and birth.

9. Describe the major fetal physiologic and behavioral adaptations, which occur during labor and birth.

10. Compare the typical labor pattern of a primigravida with that of a multigravida.

11. What factors are known to influence a woman's perception of labor and her satisfaction with the birth experience?

REFERENCES/BIBLIOGRAPHY

Friedman E: Labor: Clinical Evaluation and Management, 2nd ed. New York, Appleton-Century-Croft, 1978

Griffin RL, Caron RJ, Geijn HV: Behavioral states in the human fetus during labor. Am J Obstet Gynecol 152:828–833, 1985

Gustavii B: Human decidua and uterine contractility. In Fetus and Birth, p 351. CIBA Foundation Symposia No 47. Amsterdam, Excerpta Medica, North-Holland Biomedical Press, 1977

Kitzmiller JL, Mall JC, Gin GD et al: Measurement of fetal shoulder width with computed tomography in diabetic women. Obstet Gynecol 70:941–945, 1987

Lederman R, Lederman E, Work B et al: The relationship of maternal anxiety, plasma catecholamines, and plasma cortisol to progress in labor. Am J Obstet Gynecol 132:495, 1978

Murray M: Antepartal and Intrapartal Fetal Monitoring. Washington, DC, NAACOG, 1988

Roberts J: Factors influencing distress from pain during labor. MCN 6(3):62, 1983

SUGGESTED READINGS

Flanagan TA, Mulchahey KM, Korenbrot CC et al: Management of term breech presentation. Am Obstet Gynecol 156:1492–1502, 1987

McKay S, Roberts J: Second stage labor: What is normal? J Obstet Gynecol Neonatal Nurs 14:101–106, 1985

23 nursing care in normal labor: first stage

LEARNING OBJECTIVES

After studying the materials in this chapter, the student should be able to

- Discuss the application of the nursing process in caring for a woman and her family in active labor

- Identify signs of labor and distinguish between false and true labor

- Outline differences between physiologic and active management of labor

- Explain the technique of timing and palpating uterine contractions

- Describe nonpharmacologic strategies for pain relief in labor

- Outline the standard of nursing care for assessment of the woman in latent and active phase labor

- Describe the advantages and disadvantages of electronic fetal monitoring

KEY TERMS

Active phase of labor

Bloody show

Latent phase of labor

Transition

Childbirth requires little obstetric intervention for most women identified as "low risk;" in these cases, *physiologic management of labor* is appropriate. The primary goal of physiologic labor management is a healthy mother and fetus during the labor process. Physiologic management of labor is based on the following principles:

- Labor is a normal physiologic process in most cases.
- Most childbearing women are healthy and at low risk.
- The healthy fetus benefits from minimal obstetric intervention.
- Medication and other obstetric interventions are unnecessary, unless preferred by parents, for most normal labors.
- Women are more comfortable and less stressed when care emphasizes physiologic management.

If deviations from the normal course of labor appear, more active management may be needed. *Active management of labor* features interventions to promote and improve upon the body's own mechanisms.

For the past 50 years, obstetrics has been moving toward a more active management style. Consumers and professionals have raised questions about this approach and have begun to stress the need for less intervention in normal labor and birth, reserving active intervention for situations in which abnormal progress may increase risks to mother or fetus and for women who are deemed to be at moderate or high risk for complications.

Nursing care of families during labor focuses on maintaining normal physiologic and emotional status of all family members — mother, fetus/newborn, and father or significant others — as they move through the rapid changes of the intrapartal period. The labor nurse individualizes her care according to the family's needs and desires and within the physician's or nurse midwife's framework of obstetric management.

Proper nursing care during the process of labor is essential to ensure the wellbeing and security of the childbearing family. Labor and birth, as a progression of normal physiologic and psychological events, requires expert nursing assessment skills and timely problem identification, intervention, and evaluation on a continuous basis.

This chapter focuses on nursing care during the first stage of labor. Chapter 24 addresses nursing care from the second stage through delivery and the immediate postpartum recovery.

LATENT PHASE

Assessment

Most women will spend a significant portion of latent-phase labor at home. The nurse may have telephone contact with women who require assistance in determining whether symptoms they are experiencing are indications of early labor, or who have been instructed by their careprovider to come to the hospital for evaluation of their symptoms, in order to distinguish between true and false labor.

Distinguishing Between True and False Labor

Occasionally women experiencing uterine contractions are not sure if they are actually in labor. The labor nurse is often called upon to help in making this determination. Distinguishing characteristics of true and false labor are shown in Table 23–1.

Diagnosis

Although diagnosis and planning usually do not begin until the woman is admitted, the following diagnoses may be useful in caring for patients in the early latent phase:

- Altered health maintenance related to labor and birth
- Fear/anxiety related to impending labor and birth

Table 23–1   Distinguishing Between True and False Labor

True Labor	False Labor
Uterine Contractions	
Show regular pattern	Show irregular pattern
Usually become closer together, stronger and longer	Usually vary
Increase in intensity with walking	May stop with walking or position change
Are usually felt in lower back, radiating to lower abdomen	Are usually felt in back, upper fundus
Are not stopped by relaxation techniques such as hot bath, heating pad, alcoholic drink, or sedation	Will eventually stop with relaxation techniques
Cervix	
Softens, effaces, and dilates	May soften; no significant change in dilatation or effacement
Fetus	
Starts descent into pelvis	No noticeable change in position

See the section on Admission to Labor and Delivery for a discussion of potential complications.

Planning and Implementation

The labor nurse may be responsible for making a preliminary determination of whether or not a woman is in labor and should be admitted to the labor unit. If the nurse determines that a patient may be in early labor, she then begins to plan for admission. However, if the nurse determines the woman is experiencing "false labor," she should explain the situation to the couple and review with them the characteristics of true onset of labor. The nurse should reassure the woman that this difficulty is not uncommon, and that she should contact the labor unit or her physician or nurse midwife if she is uncertain about whether or not labor has begun.

Nursing interventions in early labor are primarily aimed at encouraging women to remain at home and prepare themselves for admission to the labor unit. Important goals for nursing intervention are meeting the woman's need for information, promoting effective self-care during early labor, and giving emotional support.

Providing Information and Promoting Self-care

Women are generally excited and happy during this phase. They are likely to be confident and comfortable and can continue their activities at home. The nurse's primary task is likely to be telephone consultation, especially with parents who are unsure whether the woman is actually in labor and who need encouragement to stay home because of their excitement or inexperience. The

SELF-CARE TEACHING POINTS

Early Labor

- Rest, relax, and conserve energy
- Keep your mind occupied with something enjoyable.
- Try comfort measures such as a warm bath, walking, or massage.
- Empty your bladder frequently and eat lightly (unless otherwise directed by your birth attendant).
- Keep taking clear fluids, such as water, juice, or soothing teas.
- Time your contractions, and don't use labor coping techniques (such as breathing techniques) until you really need them to help you stay comfortable.

nurse may wish to review with them the directions to the hospital, the location of the appropriate entrance, what to bring to the hospital, and important information about the admission procedure. Even if parents already have this information, reviewing it quickly may alleviate their worry and increase their confidence about upcoming events.

During the latent phase of early labor, the patient should be encouraged to remain at home where she can relax, complete last-minute preparations, and eat lightly. She should be encouraged to call the labor unit if she has questions about her labor status and to come to the labor unit when contractions become regular or when rupture of membranes occurs. The nurse should assist the woman in making an accurate assessment of whether she is in actual labor.

The nurse should also encourage the woman and her partner to be calm, and to call if they have further questions.

Expected Outcomes:

- The woman utilizes effective comfort and relaxation techniques at home, until a regular labor pattern is established.
- The woman and her support person distinguish between true and false labor as evidenced by coming to the hospital or birthing center when a regular labor pattern is established.

Providing Emotional Support

The nurse should also consider the anticipatory guidance that may be necessary for women and their families. The nurse should include the support person in communications with the family in early labor. If the father is going to be an active participant in the labor, the nurse may want to speak to him to assess how well he is adapting to early labor and the level of support he is giving his partner. It may also be useful to review guidelines about family or support-person participation in labor and birth, if the parents are not already familiar with that information.

Expected Outcome: The support person understands his part in the labor and birth process, as evidenced by his verbal adaptation to labor.

Admission to Labor and Delivery

Usually, families arrive on the labor and delivery unit near the end of the latent-phase labor. The physician, nurse midwife, or labor nurse will decide when admission

Nursing Support During Admission

- Introduce yourself to the patient and her support person(s)
- Communicate your role as a supportive, nurturing, and knowledgeable nurse both verbally and nonverbally; use of touch is important
- Orient the patient and her support person(s) to the surroundings, including how the labor bed works, location of bathroom, call light, towels, tissues, emesis basin, water, ice, and other items useful during labor
- Show approval, consideration, and regard for the patient and support person(s)
- Keep patient and support person(s) informed of progress after pelvic examinations
- Offer comfort measures or medication as appropriate
- Act as liaison between patient and the physician/midwife or nurse

is appropriate, based on the determination that labor has begun. Key components of this assessment focus on the pattern of uterine contractions, cervical status, and the state of amniotic membranes. An important nursing responsibility is to orient the family to the unit, acquaint them with the professionals who will care for them, and promote relaxation while labor status is assessed.

Assessment

Uterine Contraction Patterns

An essential part of the nurse's initial and ongoing assessment in labor is an evaluation of the pattern of uterine contractions. To palpate contractions, the nurse places her fingertips on the mother's abdomen over the uterine fundus. As the contraction begins, tension or tightening of the uterus will be felt in the fingertips, sometimes even before the patient senses the contraction. The nurse's assessment must include *intensity, duration,* and *frequency.*

The *intensity* of the contraction normally will increase and reach a peak and then slowly diminish. Intensity is described as mild, moderate, or strong. With *mild contractions,* the fingertips can indent the abdomen easily (similar to feeling the fleshy cheeks of the face). With *moderate contractions,* the fingertips can indent the fundus only slightly (similar to feeling the chin). With *strong contractions,* the fingertips cannot indent the abdomen (similar to feeling the forehead).

Duration is measured from the beginning to the end of the contraction in seconds. *Frequency* is measured by noting the time in minutes from the beginning of one contraction to the beginning of the next. (Review Figure 22–16 for these characteristics of uterine contractions.)

Determining the Status of Amniotic Membranes

Another important nursing assessment is the determination of whether amniotic membranes are intact or ruptured. If the mother reports having already experienced persistent leaking or a gush of fluid, the nurse should inquire about its color and its odor, if any. If membranes have ruptured, the nurse should note the time of rupture and the color and odor of amniotic fluid.

Normally, amniotic fluid is clear, pale amber, and has a slight fleshy odor. Any unpleasant odor or thick consistency of fluid suggests infection (amnionitis). Greenish fluid suggests recent fetal passage of meconium; yellowish fluid may suggest meconium passage more than 36 hours before rupture of membranes, or possibly fetal hemolytic disease. Wine-colored amniotic fluid indicates the presence of blood and may signal premature separation of the placenta.

Women often may be unsure whether they have experienced rupture of membranes or urinary incontinence caused by the pressure of the uterus on the bladder, a symptom not uncommon in late pregnancy. The labor nurse may use several tests to help establish membrane status.

Nitrazine paper, which is sensitive to *p*H, will turn bright blue when applied to moist vaginal tissue or a perineal pad if membranes are ruptured, indicating the slight alkalinity of amniotic fluid. With urine and vaginal fluid, which are slightly acidic, the yellow color of the strip remains unchanged.

Ferning, the characteristic frondlike pattern of crystallization of amniotic fluid, may be observed by obtaining a swab specimen of vaginal fluid, allowing it to dry on a microscopic slide, and then observing it under magnification. Urine and vaginal discharge will not show this pattern.

Pooling of fluid in the vagina can be observed on sterile speculum examination. The patient may be asked to bear down or cough, which will force amniotic fluid into the vagina, if membranes are ruptured.

None of these tests is an *absolute* indicator of ruptured membranes, but they all are helpful determinants when a woman with a possible slow amniotic membrane leak is being assessed or when membrane status is uncertain. If membranes are ruptured, subsequent vaginal examinations to determine the progress of labor should be kept to a minimum to reduce the risk of infection.

Admission History and Physical Examination

When a woman is admitted to the labor unit, a complete history and physical assessment will be needed. The nurse reviews the patient's history, which should contain the following items:

- Identifying information, such as name, age, gravida, para, LMP, EDC.
- Pregnancy history, including prenatal care, laboratory work, special tests (amniocentesis, sonography). Details of any complications or problems and their treatment. A complete review of the prenatal record is in order, if it is available.
- Past pregnancy history, including number, previous complications, size of infant(s), birth intervals, length of labor, and condition of children (normal, term, or premature, congenital defects, early death [sudden infant death syndrome], etc.).
- Past medical and family history. This can be obtained from the prenatal chart. Drug allergies, previous blood transfusions, and major medical problems should be reconfirmed with the patient.
- Attendance at childbirth preparation classes.

The nurse is responsible for conducting a complete systems assessment of the parturient, regardless of the type of birthing facility she has chosen and whether or not the birth attendant is also present to evaluate patient status. Nursing diagnoses can be made only after the following systems review is completed:

- Assessment of vital signs, including temperature, pulse, respirations
- Assessment of blood pressure in a sitting position and left lateral position
- Gross examination and systems review including:

1. Neurologic
   Deep tendon reflexes and evidence of clonus
   Headache or visual disturbances
   Syncope or convulsions
   Numbness or tingling in extremities or around mouth
2. Cardiovascular
   Heart rate and rhythm
   Skin color and capillary fill-time in nailbeds
   Edema: presence, extent, and location
   Varicosities
3. Hematologic
   Pallor
   Petechiae or ecchymosis
   Bleeding from mucous membranes or venipuncture sites

4. Pulmonary
   Respiratory rate and pattern
   Breath sounds
   Dyspnea, shortness of breath, cough
   Hiccoughs
   Odor of breath (fruity or alcohol)
5. Gastrointestinal
   Nausea, vomiting, diarrhea
   Epigastric distress
   Time of last meal and fluid intake
6. Renal
   Urine specific gravity and pH
   Leukocytes, glucose, protein or blood in urine upon urine dipstick
   Costovertebral (CVA) tenderness
   Urinary frequency or dysuria
7. Genital
   Bloody show or mucus discharge
   Active vaginal bleeding
   Leakage or gush of fluid from vagina (color, odor, and amount)
   Lesions of external genitalia (signs of sexually transmitted disease)
   Redness or edema of external genitalia (signs of vaginitis — Candidiasis)
   Vulvar varicosities
8. Musculoskeletal
   Deformities, fractures, chronic back pain
9. Skin and mucous membranes
   Skin turgor
   Rashes, lesions, lacerations, ecchymosis
   Track marks (substance abuse)
   Nasal discharge, nose bleeds
   Scars (previous surgery)
   Jaundice
   Moistness of mucous membranes
   Dentures

In addition, the nurse should weigh the woman to determine if there has been a sudden weight gain or loss.

The present labor history, including onset of contractions, bloody show, rupture of membranes, fetal movement, frequency, duration, and intensity of contractions is obtained. Finally, a thorough abdominal and pelvic examination is essential. In many settings this assessment is a nursing responsibility. Abdominal examination should include

- General observation of the abdomen for scars, contour, and size
- Abdominal palpation for fetal presentation, lie, position, estimated size, and station (floating or fixed)

ASSESSMENT TOOL

Labor Admission Record

AGE	GRAVIDA	PARA	EDC	WEEKS FROM LMP

UNIT NUMBER

PT. NAME

DATE LMP	LIVE BIRTHS		OTHER TERMINATIONS	
/ /	Living	Dead	< 20 Wk	≥ 20 Wk
BLOOD TYPE	ANTIBODY SCREEN		SEROLOGY	RUBELLA

BIRTHDATE

TIME OF ADMISSION	DATE	TEAM

FEEDING: ○ BREAST ○ BOTTLE   Admitted to Alt. Birth Room: ○ YES ○ NO

LOCATION   DATE

EARLY DISCHARGE: ○ YES   ○ NO

PRIVATE PEDIATRICIAN   ALLERGIES:

Previous Pregnancy Problems: Date Last Live Birth (Mo./Yr.) [/]   Date Last Termination (Mo./Yr.) [/]

Present Pregnancy Problems:

History of Labor: Onset: _____ Character of Contractions _____ Comment: _____

Weight Gain [ ] kg   Prenatal Care: ○ Regular ○ Teen ○ HiRisk ○ Private ○ Other

Month First Prenatal Visit [ ] (1st, 2nd, etc.)   Total Number Visits [ ]

Comment: _____

Phys. Exam: Weight [ ] kg Height [ ] cm Blood Pressure [ ] T [ ] °c R [ ] P [ ]

○ Normal Head & Neck   ○ Abnormal: _____
                                         (Describe)
○ Normal Heart & Lungs   ○ Abnormal: _____
                                         (Describe)
○ Normal Breasts   ○ Abnormal: _____
                                         (Describe)

Abdomen: Presentation [ ]   Position [ ]

FHT [ ]   EFW [ ] g

○ Normal Extremities   ○ Abnormal: _____
                                         (Describe)

○ Normal Reflexes   ○ Abnormal: _____
                                         (Describe)

Vaginal: Dilatation [ ] cm   Station [ ]   Effacement [ ] cm

Pelvimetry: _____

Membranes: ○ Intact ○ Ruptured ○ Spontaneous ○ Artificial   Date/Time [/ /]

Fluid: ○ Clear ○ Light meconium ○ Thick meconium

Laboratory: Hct [ ] %   Urine Protein [ ]   Sugar [ ]

Other: _____

Diagnosis: _____

Proposed Management: _____

_____ M.D. __ __ __ __

_____ Clinical Clerk

_____ M.D. __ __ __ __

NURSING ALERT

HIV Precautions for the Labor and Delivery Nurse

Recently, the Centers for Disease Control (CDC) reported that health care workers have acquired human immuno-deficiency viral infection (HIV) after their unprotected mucous membranes or broken skin were exposed to the body fluids of AIDS patients. The labor and delivery nurse is employed in an environment where there is a high risk of exposure to body fluids, including blood, amniotic fluid, urine, and feces. Emergency situations and sudden changes in patient status occur frequently and the practitioner has limited time to don barriers such as gloves, impermeable cover gowns, goggles, or face shields to prevent direct contact with body fluids.

Universal blood and body-fluid precautions should be used in the care of *all* patients, but the labor and delivery nurse should take added precautions based on the nature of the setting.

- Wear clear glass or prescription-lens eye wear at all times in labor/delivery to prevent unexpected splashes with body fluids (*i.e.*, sudden rupture of membranes, snapping of an umbilical cord during birth).
- Carry a pair of unsterile gloves in a pocket at all times in case of precipitate birth or sudden hemorrhage.
- Wear unsterile gloves whenever assisting birth attendants with vaginal exams, insertion of internal fetal monitor probes, or amniotomies as fluid splashes and contamination of linens are likely to occur.
- Have impermeable barrier gowns in each labor room in case of precipitate delivery or sudden hemorrhage.
- Stock knee-high boots for birth attendants and scrub nurses to wear to prevent contamination of the lower legs during birth.
- Stock face shields for use in surgical or other procedures that generate splashes.
- Institute a policy for placing all used sharps (*i.e.*, suture needles and local anesthesia infusion needles) in *one specified location on the delivery* table so that housekeeping personnel or nurses do not accidentally receive puncture wounds.

- Fundal measurement (to be compared with weeks of gestation and used in assessment of fetal size)
- Assessment of pattern, strength, and duration of contractions
- Auscultation of fetal heart tones (FHTs)
- Observation of any fetal movement

NURSING ALERT

Fetal Assessment Upon Admission of the Woman in Labor

Standards of nursing practice continually change as a result of research, legal imperatives, and consumer demands. While current research suggests that electronic fetal monitoring (EFM) of the low-risk woman provides no beneficial effects over intermittent auscultation, it is now strongly recommended that the fetus be initially evaluated for 20 to 30 min with an external EFM when the parturient is admitted to the birthing unit.

Electronic fetal surveillance yields more precise information regarding variability in the fetal heart rate pattern over time, may identify positive signs of adaptation (accelerations in the heart rate), and nonreassuring signs in fetal status with the onset of labor. If the fetus of the low-risk parturient demonstrates a normal fetal heart rate, rhythm, and pattern of variability during the 20- to 30-min assessment, the EFM may be disconnected and fetal heart rate auscultated intermittently for the remainder of labor.

Pelvic examination should include assessment of

- Cervical effacement and dilatation
- Position of the cervix (anterior, posterior, midposition)
- Fetal station
- Presenting part and position, if possible
- Presence of molding or caput
- Status of fetal membranes
- Pelvic capacity
- Status of perineum

While the comprehensiveness of this nursing assessment is modified if the parturient presents in very active labor or delivery is imminent, it is imperative that as much information be elicited as possible in order to provide her with appropriate supportive or active care.

Laboratory Tests

An evaluation of the patient's *prenatal laboratory tests* should be made, especially the hematocrit (which may reflect anemia), blood type, and Rh tests (which will determine the need for Rh-immune globulin administration in the immediate postpartum period). On admission to the labor unit, hematocrit and urinalysis testing for protein, glucose, and ketones is repeated. Blood samples are collected for typing and cross-matching in case transfusion becomes necessary, and a complete blood count (CBC) is done to establish a baseline for later assessment.

The nurse should review findings of previous laboratory studies and note any pending studies as part of her initial assessment.

The nurse reviews the information provided by the history, physical examination, and laboratory tests to assess the patient's level of obstetric risk. Each maternity unit has explicit risk criteria, which are used in determining the type of obstetric and nursing care given to the woman and her family. An example of criteria used in determining whether a delivery may take place in a birth-

ing room is shown in the accompanying display, Birthing Room Risk Criteria.

Admission to the hospital or birthing center in active labor is a stressful event for most women and their partners. As part of the admission procedure, the nurse should focus on stress reduction for the laboring woman and her support person(s). It is well documented that excessive stress and anxiety is harmful for the mother and fetus (Lederman 1979, Levinson et al 1979). The nurse can play a key role in stress reduction while she

---

Birthing Room Risk Criteria

Factors Precluding Admission to the Birthing Room

Social factors

- Less than three prenatal visits
- Maternal age: primipara over 35 years of age; multipara over 40 years of age*
- Maternal substance abuse

Preexisting Maternal Disease

- Chronic hypertension
- Moderate or severe renal disease
- Heart disease, Class II–IV
- History of toxemia with seizures
- Diabetes
- Anemia (hemoglobin level less than 9.5 g/100 ml)
- Tuberculosis
- Chronic or acute pulmonary problem
- Psychiatric disease requiring major tranquilizer

Previous Obstetric History

- Previous stillbirth of unknown etiology
- Previous Cesarean section
- Rh sensitivity
- Multiparity greater than 5†
- Previous infant with respiratory distress syndrome at same gestation

Factors in Present Pregnancy

- Pregnancy Induced Hypertension
- Gestational age less than 37 wk or more than 42 wk
- Multiple pregnancy
- Abnormal presentation

- Third-trimester bleeding or known placenta previa
- Prolonged rupture of membranes (over 24 hr)
- Evidence of intrauterine growth retardation
- Contracted pelvis on any plane
- Pelvic diseases, such as adnexal mass, uterine malformation, herpes, pelvic tumors, polyhydramnios
- Treatment with reserpine, lithium, or magnesium
- Induction
- Spinal or general anesthesia
- Any other acute or chronic medical or psychiatric illness that would increase risk to mother or infant

Factors Developing After Admission That Require Transfer to Labor and Delivery Unit†

- Hemoglobin level less than 9.5 g/100 ml
- Temperature over 100.4°F (38°C)
- Significant variation in maternal blood pressure from previous recordings
- Amniotic fluid deeply stained with meconium
- Abnormal fetal heart rate pattern
- Prolonged true labor (over 24 hr)
- Prolonged second-stage labor (over 2 hr for primagravida; over 1 hour for multigravida)
- Arrest of labor in active phase
- Significant vaginal bleeding
- Development of any factor that requires continuous electronic fetal monitoring
- Any labor pattern or maternal–fetal complication that the physician, nurse midwife, or nurse believes requires more sophisticated diagnosis or treatment than is available in the birthing room

Relative contraindication: patient may use the birthing room after a period of fetal monitoring in active labor
†*May use the birthing room with an IV during labor*
‡*Should the problem resolve, the woman may be moved back to the birth room*

begins caring for a woman in labor by attention to the details of providing support.

Once the nurse has completed the initial assessment of the woman in labor, the birth attendant is notified of findings. In many instances, the physician or nurse midwife is not present in the birthing unit and a telephone report is made. Critical elements of the report are presented in the accompanying box. The physician or nurse midwife depend on the labor nurse to provide an accurate and complete report in order to make appropriate decisions about subsequent care of the parturient. Written or verbal orders are obtained by the nurse to guide practice. Preprinted standing orders for labor and delivery are frequently used by physicians or midwives to expedite the admission process. An example of standing orders is provided (page 610).

Maternal Physiologic Status

The nurse must be totally cognizant of adaptations that occur during labor and birth and their resultant impact on maternal vital signs. Standards of nursing practice require evaluation of the maternal status at specific time intervals. Table 23–2 lists recommendations for the assessment of vital signs during latent-phase labor. If, at any point in time, aberrations in vital signs are noted, the birth attendant must be notified and more frequent evaluation of the parturient is indicated.

Progress in Labor

Progress in cervical dilatation, effacement, and fetal descent should be charted using a labor progress chart. Vaginal examination should be done on admission, at any change in labor pattern, and to verify full dilatation and effacement when maternal urge to push appears at the beginning of the second stage.

Other parameters of progress in labor that should be evaluated and documented at regular intervals include the presence of bloody show; rupture of membranes; color, amount, and unusual odor of amniotic fluid; nature of contraction pattern; and alterations in behavioral states. Table 23–3 summarizes these signs and recommended standards for frequency of nursing assessment in the latent phase.

Fetal Physiologic Status: Heart Rate

Fetal heart rate (FHR) should remain between 120 and 160 bpm, and may be *auscultated* throughout labor, if the pattern remains within normal limits and no other complications arise.

Both the baseline FHR and the response to contractions should be noted. Baseline FHR is determined by auscultation for 1 full minute between contractions; screening for FHR variations is done by auscultation throughout a contraction and for 30 seconds afterwards.

If FHR is within normal limits, it should be monitored throughout labor as follows:

- Every 30 minutes during the active phase
- Every 15 minutes during the second stage
- Immediately after rupture of membranes
- Immediately after any change in contraction pattern
- After every contraction during second stage
- At maternal request

Report to Attending Physician or Nurse Midwife

When the patient has been admitted and assessed by the nurse, the attending physician or nurse midwife should be notified. A report should be given in an orderly manner to facilitate patient care. The following order of report is suggested:

Identifying data
  Name
  Age
  Gravida, para
  LMP EDC
  Weeks of gestation by dates and by examination
Assessment
Chief complaint or problem (*e.g.,* normal labor, active phase)
Significant prenatal history

Significant medical or obstetric problems
Significant laboratory data
Current vital signs and urinalysis
Other symptoms — edema, hyperreflexia, costovertebral angle tenderness
Results of abdominal evaluation — height of fundus, fetal lie, presentation, position, estimated fetal weight, FHTs, other significant findings
Results of pelvic examination — station, effacement, dilatation, status of fetal membranes, fetal position, other significant findings
Maternal and family responses to labor — emotional status and comfort level as evidenced by self-report and observed behavior

ASSESSMENT TOOL

Standing Orders Form

INSTRUCTIONS
(Doctors write in black ink, nurses in red. Nurse checks orders with the time as she notes them. Doctors and nurses sign their notes. When an order is discontinued, doctor writes "Discontinue, etc." giving date and naming order.
Authorization is given for dispensing by nonproprietary name unless drug order is initiated by the physician opposite the name of the drug.

DATE	TIME

STANDING ORDER—LABOR AND DELIVERY

Admit to Labor and Delivery

Diagnosis:

Allergies:

Activity:

Diet: Clear Liquids

Vital Signs: Maternal—Temperature every 4 hr. (Every 2 hr if R.O.M.)

BP, P+R every 2–4 hr in early labor, and every 1 hr in active stage.

Obtain initial fetal heart rate/uterine contraction tracing for 20 minutes.

Monitoring:

Fetal Heart Rate:

Uterine Activity:

Labs: Urine—Dipstick for glucose/protein/ketones

Blood—Hold clot for blood bank and purple top. Spin hct.

Notify Anesthesia of patient's admission.

Additional Orders:

SIGNATURE _____ M.D. ___ ___ ___
_____ Checked By _____ R.N.   Time: _____

Table 23-2   **Standards of Care for Assessment of Maternal Vital Signs During the First Stage of Labor**

	Latent Phase (0-4 cm)	Active Phase (5-10 cm)
Blood Pressure	Q. 60 min	Q. 60 min
Pulse and Respirations*	Q. 60 min	Q. 60 min
Temperature†	Q. 4 hr	Q. 4 hr

*An increase in pulse or respiratory rate may be the first indication of maternal infection
†When membranes rupture, the temperature is assessed every 2 hr

If FHR is outside the normal range or maternal risk factors are present, auscultation should be done:

- Every 15 minutes during active phase
- Every 5 minutes during second stage

Auscultation may also be replaced by continuous external monitoring for a 20-minute interval to determine the nature of any variation detected on auscultation (NAACOG 1988).

Equipment Used for Intermittent FHR Assessment

The *fetoscope* is a modified stethoscope with a head piece that allows FHR to be heard more clearly by using bone conduction as well as air conduction of sound. Auscultation is inexpensive and noninvasive. The fetoscope must be used with the woman in a supine or semisitting position. The instrument is most effectively used to auscultate during and immediately following a uterine contraction. However, only gross abnormalities can be detected, and if the patient is obese, effectiveness is reduced.

The *Doppler unit (Doptone)* is a portable electronic instrument that is used like a stethoscope. The unit emits ultrasound (high-frequency sound) waves that, when reflected off a moving object, in this case the fetal heart,

NURSING ALERT

Monitoring Maternal Well-being in Labor

If maternal blood pressure is greater than 140/90, or shows 10-15 mmHg elevation over pregnant levels, notify the attending physician or nurse midwife: the elevation may signal developing preeclampsia. If pulse rate is over 100 bpm, or respiration rate is over 20/min, notify the attending physician or nurse midwife: the elevation may signal maternal dehydration, developing infection, or hemorrhage. An elevated pulse rate often is the first sign of impending maternal hemorrhage and precedes any drop in blood pressure following rapid blood loss.

produce echoes. The unit processes these echoes and transmits audible "clicks" to the listener at the rate the fetal heart is beating. The advantages of the Doppler unit are: (1) it is effective when FHR is difficult to hear and (2) it will usually detect the FHR regardless of maternal position.

The *electronic fetal monitor* is a more stationary instrument that allows for intermittent or continuous external monitoring of FHR and of the intensity of uterine contractions through sensors strapped to the mother's abdomen. External electronic fetal monitoring uses an ultrasound transducer to monitor the FHR in the same way as the portable Doppler unit. The electronic fetal monitor usually displays a digital readout of the FHR and produces both amplified sound and a continuous graphic display of the FHR pattern. In addition, the monitor also has a tocodynamometer, which, when positioned on the uterine fundus, records the frequency and intensity of uterine contractions. The advantages of electronic fetal monitoring are that a continuous readout of FHR patterns is provided and FHR can be correlated with uterine activity. Disadvantages are that some limitations are placed on

Table 23-3   **Standards of Care for Assessment of Maternal Progress During the First Stage of Labor**

	Latent Phase (0-4 cm)	Active Phase (5-7 cm)	Transition Phase (8-10 cm)
Contraction Pattern	Q. 30-60 min	Q. 30 min	Q. 15 min
Bloody Show	Q. 60 min	Q. 30 min	Q. 15 min
Amniotic Fluid	Q. 60 min	Q. 30 min	Q. 15 min
Behavior Pattern	Q. 60 min	Q. 30 min	Q. 15 min

Although the parturient should be evaluated *at least* every 15 min, the nurse's continuous presence at the bedside may be indicated because rapid alterations in maternal status occur in the transition period.

NURSING ALERT

Assessment of FHR Pattern

The following FHR patterns detected by auscultation require further, more precise assessment of fetal heart rate pattern:

Baseline Fetal Heart Rate

Tachycardia: FHR of 160 bpm or more for 10 min
Bradycardia: FHR of 80 to 120 bpm for more than 10 min

Periodic Changes

Acceleration: Transitory increase of 15 bpm or more above the baseline. Acceleration is not associated with fetal distress, but when it occurs consistently and uniformly with uterine contractions, it may be a forerunner for more serious patterns.

Deceleration: Transitory decrease of 15 bpm or more below the baseline. Deceleration that occurs with the onset of contractions and in which FHR returns to baseline rate *by the end of the uterine contraction* (early deceleration) is not of clinical concern. All other deceleration patterns require further assessment.

If FHR variations are detected:

- Initiate continuous external electronic monitoring of FHR
- Place the mother in a side-lying position to eliminate possible maternal supine hypotension or positional cord compression
- Alert the physician or nurse midwife as to the nature of the FHR variation, and response to position change
- Administer oxygen by tight face mask at 8–12 liter/min to reduce possible fetal hypoxia
- Explain actions to patient. Explain that more evaluation, and possibly treatment, may be needed

maternal ambulation and position in labor because of the connections to the monitor, and there is a possibility that unnecessary medical intervention may result from observation of questionable FHR patterns that are, in fact, benign or caused by machine failure. (See Monitoring the At-Risk Fetus, Chapter 25, for further discussion.)

Behavioral Adaptation

The nurse's assessment of the emotional status and behavioral adaptation of the woman and her partner or support person completes the data on which nursing care

will be based. The labor nurse notes psychosocial factors likely to affect how the parents will respond to labor, including the following:

- Age, educational level, socioeconomic level
- Overall response to pregnancy
- Previous experience with childbearing
- Cultural background
- Family support and partner status
- Nature of contact with care providers (clinic or private patient? consistent prenatal care? preference for particular provider and birth "options"?)
- Extent and type of preparation for birth and parenthood

Some facilities have nursing history forms that facilitate the collection and recording of this type of information during pregnancy and allow it to be easily communicated to the labor nurse. A sample of such a form is shown in the accompanying Assessment Tool, page 614.

As the labor nurse assists both members of the couple with admission procedures and completes her initial assessment, she asks questions about their feelings and concerns about being in labor and observes nonverbal cues. (Note: throughout this Chapter we refer to the "couple" or "family" and to "mother" and "father" or "partner," reflecting the fact that most women are in a partner relationship with the father of the baby and that a large majority of women are now accompanied to the labor and birth setting by the father. Where this is not the case, the nurse will need to adjust her care accordingly.)

Maternal Responses

The nurse should observe the mother's responses to admission procedures, to her partner or support person, and to the uterine contractions in order to make a preliminary assessment of her emotional status. Is she excited and eager for information? Is she understanding much of what is said and seemingly well-prepared for labor? Does she appear fearful, uncomfortable, and confused by conversations and activities around her?

The nurse should ask the mother how she has been feeling for the last 24 hours before admission: has she been sleeping well or poorly? Has she been unusually active? Does she feel tired now? When did she last eat? Does she feel as though things are "under control" at home? These factors may help the nurse assess the mother's responses to early labor and to plan for possible needs as labor progresses.

The nurse should also observe the mother's interaction with her support person and try to identify how the mother is likely to utilize that support. The presence of supportive others, especially the father, has been shown

Advantages and Disadvantages of Electronic Fetal Monitoring

Advantages	Disadvantages
Reliably identifies healthy fetuses	Reduces maternal mobility in labor
Improves outcome for low birth-weight infants	Monitor belts increase maternal discomfort
Identifies more acidotic fetuses than intermittent auscultation	Monitor belts interfere with effleurage
High-risk infants have significantly improved 5-min Apgar scores	May cause anxiety in woman and labor support person
Allows woman or coach to see contractions and assist woman with breathing	Inexperience with interpretation may lead to unnecessary obstetric interventions and higher cesarean rate
Hearing heart beat may reassure woman	Has limited value between 20 and 30 wk gestation
Avoids need to interrupt woman to auscultate fetal heart rate during contractions	Nurse may spend more time observing monitor than patient

Adapted from Murray M: Antepartal and Intrapartal Fetal monitoring. Washington DC, NAACOG, 1988

to have a positive effect on the mother's perception of her labor, probably by reducing the level of distress and helplessness the woman feels in coping with labor pain. The father's supportive presence, rather than his training or skill at labor support techniques, seems to be the important factor. In several studies and in a variety of low- and high-risk birth situations, women have reported they were more comfortable, less fearful, and perceived their childbirth experience more positively when their partners were present (Cranley et al 1983, Mercer et al 1983). One way the nurse can determine the nature of the couple's relationship is to ask how the couple prepared for labor. Does the mother rely on her partner to assist with labor coping techniques (such as breathing or relaxation) or for reassurance and emotional support? Does she expect little actual support but expects her partner to be present for "the experience"? How the mother seeks out and uses partner support during labor is an important aspect of the nurse's assessment, since the most effective nursing interventions will be tailored to fit that pattern.

For instance, if the mother relies on her partner for emotional support and reassuring presence, the nurse can help the partner by providing information and facilitating close contact. If the mother appears to rely on her partner for labor coaching, the nurse may want to concentrate her activities on additional comfort measures that will enhance his coaching efforts. If the mother appears to expect little direct support from her partner, the nurse must plan to provide that support and to evaluate, as labor progresses, whether drawing him into a more active role will meet both of their needs, or whether both are more comfortable with him in an onlooker role.

Paternal Responses

The nurse should also assess the father's responses to early labor and to the admission procedures along similar lines. Does the father appear confident or unusually anxious? Does he appear to understand conversations and activities around him? Does he seem to have a sense of what to expect? The nurse should engage the father as much as possible in her conversation with the mother; how the father responds will give the nurse valuable cues about his own status and how he sees his role in labor.

Diagnosis

Based on a systematic assessment of maternal/fetal physiologic status and the behavioral adaptation of the patient and her family members, the nurse identifies needs that will direct ongoing care during the latent phase of first-stage labor. The following nursing diagnoses indicate needs of families admitted in latent-phase labor. They may be addressed independently, and priorities are based on such nursing diagnoses.

- Anxiety related to unfamiliar surroundings and pain
- Altered comfort: pain related to uterine contractions
- Anxiety related to prolonged latent-phase labor

Careful monitoring and active nursing management may be required for some women whose early labor does not follow normal patterns. The most common problems of this type are *prolonged latent phase*, or *prodromal labor*, and *premature rupture of membranes*. Patients experienc-

ASSESSMENT TOOL

Obstetric Patient History

GENERAL DATA

A. Name _____ B. Age _____

C. Marital status (circle one)   Married − Living with − Single − Div. − Sep. − Wid.

D. Highest level of educations you have completed (circle one)

    Grammar school − High school − College − Other _____

E. Your occupation _____

F. Partner's occupation _____

GENERAL HEALTH DATA

A. Height _____ B. Usual weight before pregnancy _____

C. Special health problems _____

D. Medications taken regularly _____

E. Allergies _____ F. Special diet _____

G. You wear: Dentures − contacts − glasses − none − other _____

H. Frequency of bowel movements: 1/day − 1 every other day − other _____

I. Usual sleep pattern: 6-8 hrs/night − 8-10 hrs/night − other _____

    Bedtime _____ Usual time of arising _____

CHILDBEARING DATA

A. Number of pregnancies including this one: _____

B. This pregnancy was: planned − unplanned

C. Number of children at home: _____ Ages: _____

D. Pediatrician: Private _____ UCSF _____

E. Childbirth classes attended or plan to attend _____

F. Infant feeding preference: Breast − bottle   Experienced?   yes − no   How long? _____

G. Plans for birth control: Diaphragm − IUD − rhythm − condom/foam −

                        tubal ligation − vasectomy − birth control pills − undecided

H. Past pregnancy experiences: normal − complicated

    If complicated, explain _____

I. Present pregnancy experience: normal − complicated

    If complicated, explain _____

J. How long do you expect to stay after delivery: 24 hrs. − 2 days − 3 days − Family Centered Birthing

    24 hr. rooming-in − other _____

K. What would you like instruction in?   breast-feeding − bottle-feeding − baby bath − baby care −

    postpartum exercises − birth control methods − other _____

L. Expected help at home after baby is born: parents − friends − partner

    other _____

M. If there is any other information about yourself which you feel would assist us in planning your care, please write

    it here: _____

    _____

Thank you − UCSF Nursing Staff

Signature: _____ Date/Time: _____

              (Nurse)

ing these problems are likely to be admitted to the labor unit for observation and obstetric intervention.

The above problems may become complications requiring collaboration with other members of the health care team. The nurse should monitor for complications and notify the physician or nurse-midwife if such problems arise. Premature rupture of membranes may create a potential for infection.

Planning and Implementation

By the 40th week of gestation, most women are eager for the birth of the infant and the concomitant release from the minor discomforts of pregnancy. As the first signs of labor begin, however, anxiety may be aroused by perceived threats to self and the fetus. Perceptions of pain

Routine "PREPS" for Labor and Birth

In some facilities, standard admission care includes a *perineal prep* and an *enema* in early labor. The routine use of both procedures is controversial and is declining in many areas. Some clinicians believe that shaving the perineum facilitates postdelivery repair and improves perineal hygiene in the postpartum period. The routine administration of an enema in early labor is believed by some to stimulate labor and avoids the possibility of expelling bowel contents with consequent embarrassment to the patient during bearing down efforts in second-stage labor.

However, other care providers point out that shaving the perineum may actually increase the risk of infection and does not aid in postdelivery repair. Further, an enema itself is likely to be uncomfortable and embarrassing to the woman in labor and does not ensure that bowel contents will be totally absent by the second stage of labor. Many patients also question the need for perineal shaving and an enema in early labor. The nurse should determine the woman's wishes, verify the attending physician or midwife's directions, and identify contraindications for routine perineal prep and enema before proceeding.

A *complete prep* usually involves shaving all pubic, perineal, and rectal hair, whereas a *mini prep* involves shaving the hair between the level of the clitoris and the rectum. Disposable prep kits include the necessary supplies. The nurse should position the woman comfortably and ensure adequate lighting. The labia and perineum are shaved, with the woman positioned as for a vaginal examination; when this is complete, the woman is helped to the side-lying position to shave the rectal area. The nurse should take care that contaminants from the rectal area do not enter the vaginal area.

Rapid labor progress with imminent delivery is a contraindication for a routine prep and enema, since monitoring maternal and fetal status and preparation for delivery are nursing priorities in these circumstances. A history or presence of vaginal bleeding contraindicates the administration of an enema, since these signs suggest a placental problem, such as placenta previa or placental abruption; in both cases, stimulation of labor must be avoided. Administration of an enema is also contraindicated in the absence of labor and a well-engaged presenting part, since peristalsis and straining caused by the enema may contribute to premature rupture of membranes and umbilical cord prolapse.

LEGAL/ETHICAL ISSUES

Nursing Care of the Homeless or Indigent Childbearing Family

The birth experience for homeless families and those with severely limited resources often occurs in public or charitable hospitals in the United States. The physical setting may not permit privacy or be conducive to gentle birthing. These facilities are frequently affiliated with teaching institutions (medical and nursing schools), and patients may be asked to participate in research or permit assessment and care by students.

The nurse, in this setting, must be particularly vigilant in the role of patient advocate. When women in labor are asked for their permission to perform procedures or to conduct research, it must be determined that language barriers or limited education do not prevent informed consent. The clinician should be familiar with the support services available to assist new families, such as social services and the Women – Infant – Children Supplemental Food Program (WIC). Every effort must be made to respect the patient's rights, and the nurse must be resourceful in manipulating the environment to provide the best childbirth experience possible.

put the woman and her partner at ease. All procedures should be explained before implementation. Admission procedures and orientation to the unit or birthing room should be accomplished, without haste, in the latent phase of labor to minimize the risk of sensory overload. The family should be encouraged to voice concerns and to ask questions as they arise. The woman is made to feel at home in her new surroundings and free to ambulate and take light nourishment and liquids during this early phase of labor. Indigent patients, or those from other cultures, may require special nursing attention as they enter the hospital environment (see accompanying box, above).

Expected Outcome: The woman in labor demonstrates a decrease in anxiety, as evidenced by verbalization of her understanding of interventions and her satisfaction with the emotional support provided by the nurse.

may heighten the anxiety, and knowledge deficits add another dimension to the parturient's fears.

Providing Emotional Support

Nursing interventions are aimed at minimizing anxiety. A warm, supportive, and empathetic demeanor can

Promoting Rest and Comfort

Although uterine contractions are generally mild during latent-phase labor, each woman's perceptions of discomfort will be different. The body area most affected by pain sensations will also vary. Many strategies may be

ASSESSMENT TOOL

Labor and Delivery Nursing Assessment

I. ADMISSION DATA:
   A. Medication taken during pregnancy: _____
   B. Date and time of last dose: _____
   C. Contact with communicable disease: (Circle one)   Rubella   –   Measles
          Hepatitis   –   Mumps   –   Herpes   –   Gonorrhea   –   Other
   D. BP range during pregnancy: _____
   E. Date and time of last meal: _____
   F. Valuables: Yes No   G. Disposition of valuables: sent home – held in safe – to postpartum
   H. Fatigue level: Rested – Tired – Exhausted
   I. Anxiety level: Alert – Excited – Maintains control – Fearful – Anxious – Out of control
   J. Support person present: _____
II. ADMISSION ASSESSMENT: _____

Nurse's
Signature: _____   Date: _____   Time: _____

III. DELIVERY AND PARENTAL–INFANT INTERACTION DATA:
   A. Behavior of infant (Circle appropriate response):
       1. Crying: None – Periodic – Almost continuous
       2. Affect: Difficult to arouse – Dozes – Eyes open – Very alert
   B. Verbal responses of mother (Circle those that apply):
       1. Calls baby by name
       2. Comments on beauty of baby and/or on realistic defects
       3. Talks about baby
       4. Asks husband or nurse if baby is all right
       5. Voices unhappiness over sex of baby
       6. Answers in monosyllables
       7. Complains of difficult labor and delivery
       8. Doesn't talk about baby   10. Calls baby "it"
       9. Requests baby be taken to nursery   11. Uses unhappy or scolding inflection
   C. Nonverbal responses of mother (Circle those that apply):
       1. Looks, reaches out to baby   8. Tenses face, arms
       2. Hugs, kisses baby   9. Turns head from baby
       3. Smiles at baby   10. Unresponsive to partner/nurse
       4. Positive eye contact with partner   11. Doesn't touch baby
       5. Holds hand of partner   12. Doesn't look at baby
       6. Breast feeds baby   13. Pushes baby away
       7. Sleepy, not drug-induced   14. Cries unhappily

IV. ASSESSMENT OF PARENT RESPONSE TO BABY: _____
_____
Did this family meet their expectations of labor and delivery? _____
If no, why not? _____
_____
_____
_____
_____

Signature _____   Date/Time _____
                Nurse

---

employed to alleviate discomfort, and a major responsibility of the labor and delivery nurse is promoting comfort and using nonpharmacologic techniques to minimize pain.

Encouraging early ambulation and rest in an upright position, suggesting a refreshing shower or bath, and recommending massage by the labor coach are activities often employed in early labor to reduce restlessness, discomfort, and anxiety. It may be helpful for the woman to listen to soothing music. Television viewing may be an effective distraction strategy for others. Breathing techniques can be employed, but should not be started too early or maternal exhaustion might occur later. Normalizing the experience for the woman is the key to promoting comfort. For a discussion of pharmacologic measures, see Chapter 27 on Managing Maternal Pain.

Expected Outcome: The woman in labor adjusts to the level of pain by continuing to ambulate, continuing to use effective breathing and relaxation techniques, and by assuming a position of comfort, as evidenced by verbalization of maximum comfort.

Providing Support in Prolonged Latent-Phase Labor

The latent phase of labor is prolonged if it exceeds 20 hours for the primigravida or 14 hours for the multipara. The unripe cervix is the most common cause, especially in primigravidas, since time and continued uterine activity are required for cervical softening, thinning, and effacement. When this is accomplished, the woman's labor will often proceed normally. Other causes for a prolonged, latent phase of labor include

- Abnormal fetal position
- Cephalopelvic disproportion
- Dysfunctional labor
- Administration of sedation or analgesia early in labor

Although prolonged latent phase is not harmful to the fetus, it can cause maternal exhaustion and increased anxiety. Nursing support should include reassurance, encouragement, and information about the nature of the problem; continued comfort measures, such as warm showers, ambulation, rest, and diversion; maintenance of energy and hydration with juices and other clear liquids.

Active nursing management may include encouraging active labor through ambulation and instructing the woman about the possible usefulness of nipple stimulation to increase secretion of oxytocin, which may enhance uterine activity (Curtis et al 1984). The nurse may also consult with the physician or nurse midwife about the use of mild sedatives to promote sleep and avoid maternal exhaustion. (See Chapter 26 on modifying labor pattern.)

Expected Outcomes:

- The woman in labor expresses decrease in anxiety as evidenced by ease in verbalizing her fears or frustrations regarding prolonged labor.
- The woman in labor employs effective relaxation strategies to reduce fatigue, maintains adequate fluid and caloric intake to meet energy needs, and verbalizes her understanding of interventions employed to promote sleep or encourage active labor.

Monitoring For Complications
Potential for Infection Related to Prolonged Rupture of Membranes

The rupture of membranes 1 hour or more before the onset of labor is called *premature rupture of membranes* (PROM). This occurs in 10% to 12% of all pregnancies; of these, nearly a quarter are preterm pregnancies. The cause of premature rupture in term pregnancies is unknown. Spontaneous labor within 48 hours occurs in 50% to 70% of women with premature rupture of membranes. Premature rupture increases perinatal morbidity and mortality slightly; there is an increased risk of infection to mother and infant and a risk of fetal distress due to cord prolapse if a loop of the cord escapes through the cervix with the gushing amniotic fluid. Cord prolapse is more likely to occur when the presenting fetal part is not well engaged in the cervix or does not fill the pelvis, as in presentations other then vertex. Accurate assessment of station of the fetal head is essential to ensure appropriate care of the mother with premature rupture of membranes.

There is currently some controversy about optimal obstetric management of premature rupture in term pregnancies. Some physicians and nurse midwives will watch closely for signs of ascending infection or fetal distress but will wait several days to see if labor begins spontaneously. Others will wait only 6 to 8 hours before initiating steps to bring about delivery.

Nursing intervention will vary to some degree accordingly. Nursing support should include monitoring fetal status, decreasing risk of infection, and providing support for the woman and her family. Fetal status may be assessed by frequent or continuous fetal heart monitoring (see Chapter 25). Infection prevention includes limiting vaginal examinations or procedures to reduce the risk of introducing contaminants, and close monitoring for signs of maternal infection. Vital signs and temperature are recorded every 1 to 2 hours and maternal CBC every 24 hours. Prophylactic antibiotics may be ordered as well.

Active nursing management includes interventions aimed at promoting labor, as described above for prolonged latent phase. In addition, the nurse may be responsible for administering and monitoring oxytocin (Pitocin) by intravenous drip to induce labor. (See Chapter 26 for nursing care during induction and augmentation of labor.)

Expected Outcomes:

- The patient appreciates the danger of infection as evidenced by her use of appropriate perineal hygiene techniques to reduce the risk of infection.

• The patient remains free of signs and symptoms of infection secondary to PROM.

ACTIVE PHASE

The major part of intrapartal nursing care is focused on the active phase of labor. Normally, women are admitted to the labor unit in active labor. The major characteristics of this phase are increased uterine activity with descent of the fetus into the bony pelvis.

Nursing care is focused on monitoring maternal physiologic and behavioral adaptations as well as fetal adjustments during this period of rapid change. Goals of care include assuming self-care activities for the parturient as she moves through active labor, providing appropriate emotional support and comfort measures, and monitoring her for fetal well-being and normal labor progress.

Assessment

Nursing assessment is done throughout labor. If the woman is admitted in active labor, the initial assessment is especially important (Fig. 23–1). The nurse's initial assessment of the physical and emotional status of the woman and of the father or support person lays the foundation for nursing care. The nurse's assessment includes components of the admission assessment as previously described (assessment of labor and membrane status,

review of history and physical examination, abdominal/vaginal examination, review of laboratory tests, and assessment of psychosocial and emotional status).

A sample nursing assessment form used in labor and delivery is shown in the accompanying Assessment Tool. Note that both an admission assessment and an assessment of parent–infant interactions are entered in this form for ease in later communication with nurses responsible for postpartum care.

After completing the initial assessment, the nurse begins the process of assessing the maternal, fetal, and family responses to labor. This ongoing assessment focuses on the following major areas:

• Maternal physiologic status
• Progress of labor
• Fetal physiologic status
• Behavioral adaptations

Maternal Physiologic Status

Maternal vital signs should be assessed throughout labor. Table 23–2 summarizes the standards of nursing care for assessment of maternal vital signs in active labor. The nurse must also evaluate, in a systematic fashion, normal maternal physiologic and behavioral adaptations to establish accurate nursing diagnoses and plan appropriate interventions.

Progress of Labor

With experience, the nurse will be able to determine the extent of cervical change and progress in labor by

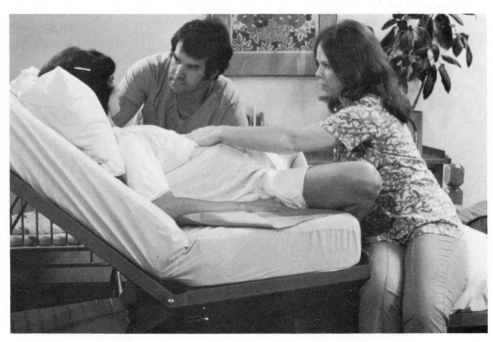

Figure 23–1. The labor nurse assesses the intensity of the woman's contraction by palpation and observes the woman's response to the first stage of labor. (Photo courtesy Hill–Rom)

observing the woman's behavioral cues. The accompanying display lists behavioral clues to the phase of labor.

Pelvic or vaginal examinations during labor are done periodically to evaluate progress in effacement, dilatation, station, status of membranes, and position of the presenting part. Fetal molding and caput are also noted. The frequency with which vaginal examinations are done depends on the patient's condition and on the nurse's and attendant's ability to determine progress in labor by other means, such as behavioral clues, contraction pattern, and change in location of FHTs. If membranes have ruptured, pelvic examinations should be restricted in number because of the possibility of infection. In these circumstances they are usually done only on admission in labor to verify complete dilatation prior to pushing, and to

Behavioral Clues to Labor Phase

Latent Phase

Anticipation
Excitement
Animation, happiness
Relief that labor has started
Some fear and anxiety
Relaxation

Active Phase

Seriousness, growing apprehension
Sense of purpose
Introspection
Fear of being alone, desire for companionship
Change from relaxation to tension
Internal conflict of confidence versus fear
Ill-defined doubts and fears

Transition Phase

Acute sensitivity and irritability
Difficulty in controlling behaviors
Uninhibited behavior
Fatigue, sleepiness
Amnesia
Horror of being left alone but little desire for interaction
Discouragement and fright
Frustration
Pronounced introspection

Many physical symptoms, including leg cramps, shaking and chills, perspiration, hiccoughing, belching, flatulence, nausea and vomiting, heavy bloody show, pulling and stretching sensations low in the pelvis, and severe backache.

NURSING ALERT

Signs of Inadequate Uterine Relaxation

Placental perfusion is decreased during uterine contraction. Healthy fetuses can tolerate this over the course of labor in the following circumstances:

- If the uterus relaxes well between contractions for long enough (more than 30 seconds) to allow normal perfusion between contractions
- If contractions are not unusually long (*i.e.,* last less than 90 sec).

Abnormally long, strong contractions, termed *tetanic contractions,* may follow oxytocin administration to stimulate or augment labor and placental abruption.

If uterine contractions last more than 90 sec or there is 30 sec or less between contractions:

- Stop oxytocin administration
- Change mother to left lateral position
- Administer oxygen by tight face mask at 8–12 liter/min
- Assess fetal heart rate pattern
- Notify physician

check for prolapsed cord when membranes rupture. An examination is also in order before pain medication is administered because sudden progress in labor may be the cause of the increased pain level. The purposes and technique of the vaginal examination during labor are outlined in the display on page 620.

The pattern and intensity of uterine contractions are also noted; the nurse palpates the intensity of contractions at the fundus and assesses the woman's response to her labor.

The progress of labor, as noted by periodic vaginal examinations, is recorded on a labor graph, such as the one shown in the accompanying Assessment Tool, page 621. Such graphs can then be compared to Friedman curves for normal labor, which are discussed in Chapter 22. Other important data, such as quality of contractions and contraction patterns, maternal vital signs, FHR, administration of medications or intravenous fluids, and intake and output, are often charted using a flow chart such as the one shown in the Assessment Tool on page 622.

Fetal Physiologic Status

Evaluation of fetal well-being is done throughout labor. Presentation, position, station, fetal heart rate, and heart rate patterns are all important issues. Presentation, posi-

Vaginal Examination to Assess Progress in Labor

Purpose

Vaginal examinations are performed to assess progress in labor by noting changes in cervical softening, dilatation, and effacement as well as fetal descent. Examinations are done only when necessary and only with aseptic technique.

Vaginal examinations are *contraindicated* if vaginal bleeding is present.

Technique

1. Place the woman comfortably in a supine position with legs flexed and separated. A pillow should be used to support the woman's head. Place a small pillow or rolled towel under the woman's right hip to prevent the heavy uterus from pressing on the vena cava and causing supine hypotension. Explain that the vaginal examination will allow an assessment of progress in labor, and while it may be uncomfortable, should not cause pain.

2. Put on a sterile glove and lubricate the examining hand with antiseptic solution (if status of membranes has yet to be determined, sterile water may be used as a lubricant, since some antiseptic solutions affect nitrazine paper, which is used to detect presence of amniotic fluid). Place the other hand on the mother's abdomen to allow slight downward pressure on the fundus. This applies the presenting part more directly to the cervix and may help in determining fetal position. Introduce the index and middle fingers into the vagina with slight downward pressure; you may pause here briefly to allow the mother to become accustomed to the sensation. Then advance the fingers and rotate the hand so that the thumb rests outside and above the symphysis pubis.

3. Advance the examining hand so that the cervix can be felt. This pressure may be uncomfortable, especially during a contraction. Encourage the woman to use relaxation techniques and reassure her during the examination.

4. Make the following assessments:

   Status of membranes: are they intact? bulging through the cervix?

   Status of cervix: is it soft or firm? how much dilatation? how much effacement?

   Fetal presentation: what is the presenting part? (head, breech, other fetal part?) what is the fetal position? (left/right, anterior/posterior/transverse)

   Fetal station: where is the presenting part in relation to the ischial spines?

   Engagement: is the presenting part well applied to the cervix?

5. Remove the examining hand gently, and explain the findings to the woman and her partner. Dry the perineal area and place clean absorbent pads under the buttocks. Help the woman to a comfortable position.

---

tion, and station are evaluated during maternal pelvic examinations. The presence of fetal molding and caput succedaneum (scalp edema) helps the nurse assess feto-pelvic adaptation during labor.

To evaluate FHT, the fetal back is located and the fetoscope or ultrasonic device is placed over it, because the fetal back is usually where the tones are heard most clearly. This point is called the *point of maximum intensity*. A head piece should be used with the fetoscope, since this device functions partly through bone conduction. When an ultrasonic device is used, it must be directed toward the fetal heart; thus, the nurse may need to alter the orientation of the device on the maternal abdomen to maximize the pickup as fetal position changes in labor. The point of maximum intensity changes as the fetus descends and rotates, usually to locations lower on the abdomen near the midline.

FHTs should be auscultated at the following times:

- On admission, to establish a baseline (see Nursing Alert, page 607)

- At least every 30 minutes during active labor and more frequently if indicated
- Following spontaneous or artificial rupture of the fetal membranes (see Nursing Alert, page 630)
- Following any sudden change in the labor or contraction pattern, such as:
  Tetanic or prolonged contraction
  Precipitous labor
- Following the administration of any medication
- Following any obstetric or medical complication during labor
- Following any obstetric procedure, such as vaginal examination, manual rotation, and so forth
- At the request of the mother

When FHTs are not being continuously recorded with the electronic fetal monitor (see Chapter 25 for electronic fetal monitoring) the fetal stethoscope or ultrasonic device should be placed over the point of maximum intensity midway between contractions. The nurse listens to the FHTs for a full minute to determine the fetal heart rate in

ASSESSMENT TOOL

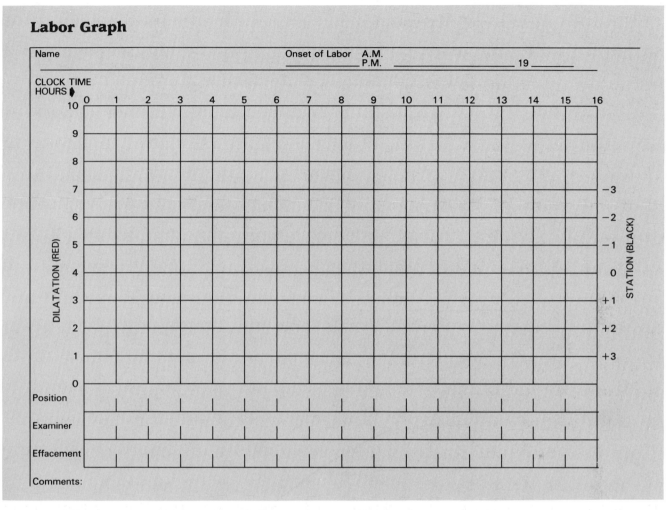

Labor Graph

beats per minute. The usual range is from 120 to 160 bpm. The nurse then listens to the FHTs during the next contraction and for at least 30 seconds following the contraction. Any irregularity should be noted and documented. The nurse should palpate the uterus while listening to determine if FHTs change in relation to the contraction. If changes occur, external electronic monitoring may be indicated to assist in determining the precise nature of the FHT changes (see Chapter 25).

Behavioral Adaptation

The nurse also must assess both the mother's and father's psychosocial responses to active labor on an ongoing basis. The following areas are important parts of the nurse's assessment of both partners as they adapt to the demands of active labor:

- Body posture/movement
- Interaction with partner and staff
- Perceptual status

- Energy/fatigue level
- Responses to disturbing stimuli
- Expressions of discomfort/pain

Each will be discussed in more detail in the following sections.

Maternal Responses

The mother's responses to labor involve physiologic and psychologic adaptation to stress. The nurse should observe her *body movements and posture* for cues of growing fatigue, tension, or pain. If the mother is using relaxation techniques, growing muscular tension should be noted as a sign of increasing stress. However, the nurse should not assume that certain body movements signal an increase in pain. The mother's movements may be calming or soothing by themselves. Cultural patterns play a part in woman's behavior in labor; thrashing and crying out may be expected and do not necessarily indicate a need for immediate nursing intervention. Likewise, quiet, stoic behavior does not always indicate that the woman is

ASSESSMENT TOOL

Obstetric Flow Chart

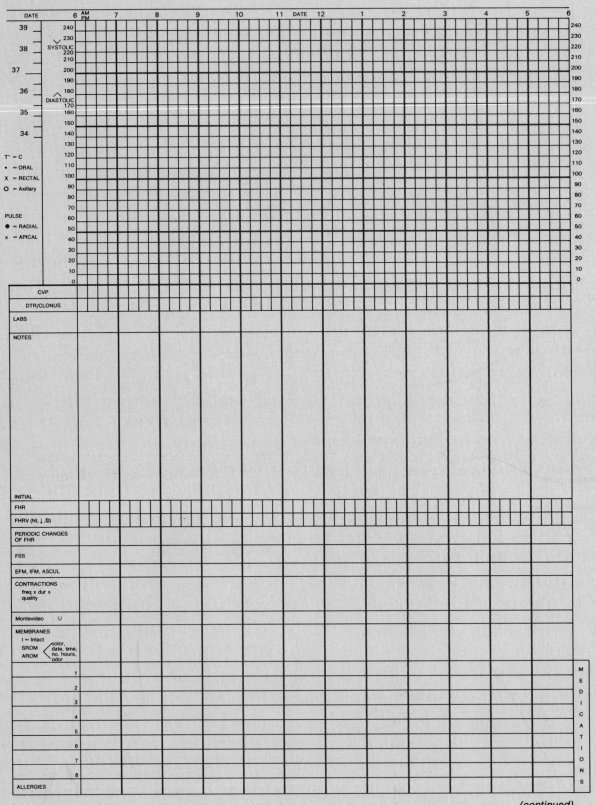

(continued)

ASSESSMENT TOOL (continued)

HOURLY INTAKE	I.V.										
	PO										
	OTHER										
HOURLY OUTPUT	URINE										
	OTHER										
UA	PROT										
	SG										
	GLUCOSE										
	KETONE										
	HEME										
	OTHER										

START TIME	BOTTLE NO.	PARENTERAL SOLUTION & ADDITIVES	TIME CHECKED	AMOUNT ABSORBED	LEFT IN BOTTLE	BLOOD		

INTAKE: I.V. / PO / BLOOD / OTHER / 12° TOTAL

OUTPUT: URINE / EBL / EMESIS / OTHER / 12° TOTAL

WEIGHT

experiencing little discomfort. The nurse should frequently ask the mother about her discomfort and make use of what the mother says as well as of observations of the woman's behavior.

The mother's *interactions* with her partner and staff also give important cues to the progress of labor (Fig. 23–2). The woman's attention and energy normally become much more focused inward as labor progresses, and interaction will become more difficult. This process requires the father and staff to utilize more direct methods of interaction, such as touch and direct short instructions to communicate with the woman in labor. The mother's inward focus will also diminish her *perceptions* outside her physical experience, so that subtle behavioral changes in her partner or information not relating to her own condition may not be taken in. The woman may gradually lose concern about bodily modesty, and remove clothing and bedding as she focuses intensely on coping with labor. However, the woman's perceptual acuity may also increase if she becomes more anxious, and she may respond dramatically to small bits of information, such as an overheard conversation or a slight change in an attendant's facial expression.

The mother's *energy and fatigue level* will shift as labor progresses. This will be most noticeable in the later part of active labor. She will gradually avoid unnecessary activity and will rest or even sleep between contractions. However, she may respond to *disturbing stimuli* with greater irritability—for example, by pushing helping hands away, not permitting painful vaginal examinations or other procedures, attempting to remove monitor or intravenous lines.

The mother's *expressions of discomfort and pain* are a major focus of the nurse's assessment. The nurse should observe for increasing restlessness and muscular tension, signs of rising anxiety, and increasing "clinging" or fearfulness. These signs may indicate that pain is increasing and that more effective comfort measures are needed. Another reason that the nurse should be alert for these signs is that they may signal rapid cervical change and faster progress toward delivery.

The mother's *responses to labor* also reflect how well the actual experience fits with her expectations. For instance, if she expected breathing techniques to reduce her pain and they seem to have little effect, she will likely become increasingly anxious and uncomfortable. If she expected labor to progress quickly and it does not, or if unexpected problems arise, she will likely become dis-

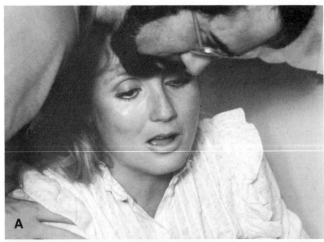
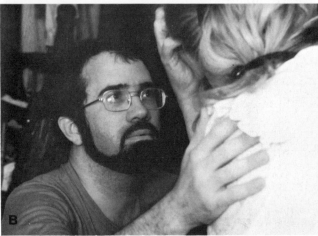

Figure 23-2. The labor nurse should assess how well the mother responds to her partner's support (A), and how well the father is able to interpret his mate's needs as labor progresses (B). (Photo: BABES, Inc.)

couraged and doubt her ability to "make it." This emotional state will decrease her ability to tolerate the demands of labor, at least until she gathers additional energy and support to help her cope. On the other hand, if the sensations and progress of labor are about what she expected, or if she can sense movement toward resolution and relief, she probably will tolerate labor more easily.

Paternal Responses

Paternal responses to their partners' labor show more variability, because the father's responses are based not only on physiologic changes but on the type of involvement he has established (Fig. 23-3). However, regardless of the father's level of involvement in labor, the nurse should remember two important points. First, virtually all fathers with whom the labor nurse will have contact are fearful and concerned about their partner's well-being and the well-being of their baby. Second, no matter how involved they are in the labor process or how well pre-

pared they appear for labor coaching, most fathers feel uncomfortable and unsure of themselves in this situation and are unsettled by some of what they see and hear. The nurse must keep in mind that commonplace events on a labor unit may be mystifying and frightening to a father, and her care should be directed toward reducing the father's fears by providing information and emotional and practical support.

The nurse should observe the father's *body posture* and nonverbal cues. He may stay very close to his partner, actively supporting her through contractions, or he may stay on the periphery, observing. A change in the father's posture or position may signal increasing fatigue or fear and should be further evaluated. The nurse should also observe the actively involved father for signs of muscle fatigue and the strain of bending over or physically supporting his partner and relieve him as necessary.

The father's *interactions* with his partner and staff will depend in large part on the type of involvement he establishes. An actively involved father may need occasional assistance in interpreting his partner's needs as her attention becomes increasingly focused and withdrawn in advanced labor. Sometimes a father will need to be shown how to touch or comfort his partner in a different way. The nurse should not imply that the father is not doing a good job in comforting his partner; this will undermine his confidence and probably raise his anxiety about his ability to carry out his role. Rather, the nurse should point out what she noticed about his partner's response to his comforting, stressing that a woman's responses to labor are not always predictable, and that trial and error may be needed to find the best way of comforting each individual woman.

The father's *perceptions* and his *energy and fatigue level* will change as labor progresses. The nurse should suggest frequent breaks for rest and food and relieve him as needed. Especially during a long or painful labor, the father is likely to become somewhat discouraged and unable to take in events around him. Reassuring him and pointing out tangible signs of progress may help.

The nurse should be especially alert to the father's responses to *disturbing stimuli* and try to limit them as much as possible. Potentially disturbing stimuli include the appearance (grimacing, gradual loss of bodily modesty, bloody vaginal discharge) and sounds (moans or cries) of a woman in labor, as well as the sometimes painful vaginal examinations and dramatic perineal changes late in labor. The nurse should tell the father what to expect as often as possible before it happens, and observe him for signs of increasing discomfort. If the nurse observes that the father is disturbed by these sights, she can encourage him to "take a break" while she stays with his partner, or can move him up toward his partner's head to comfort her, thus limiting his view of some sights that may be distressing to him.

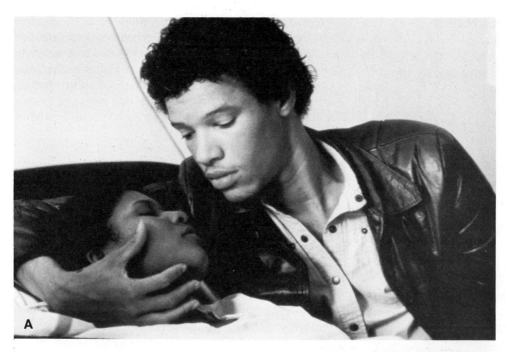

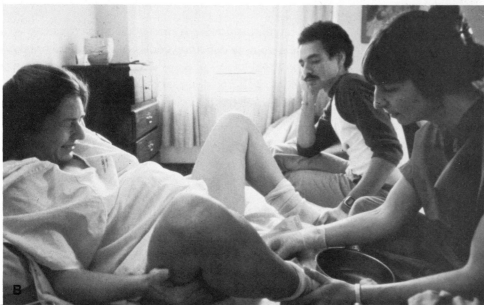

Figure 23–3. The nurse should assess the father's response to labor and his ability and readiness to provide support to his partner. Some men undertake a supportive role with ease *(A)*, whereas others do not *(B)*. This may reflect personality or cultural differences and does not necessarily reflect lack of concern. (Photo: Kathy Sloane)

Responses of Other Family Members

In many birth settings, other family members will be present as support persons, and older children may be present for part of labor. The nurse's responsibility includes monitoring the responses of those persons and supporting them so that their presence does not distract the woman or cause her additional stress. Adolescent mothers in labor are often supported very effectively by their own mothers; in these cases, the nurse should be alert for the grandmother's need for information and explain procedures that may be unfamiliar to her (Fig. 23–4).

Settings in which older siblings are present typically have protocols designed to ensure a positive birth experience for all concerned. Such protocols nearly always require that each child have a support person whose responsibility it is to attend to the child's needs and monitor his or her responses to labor. In addition, the protocols identify the circumstances in which siblings will be excluded from attending labor and birth. The nurse's responsibility in this area is limited to monitoring the sibling's and parent's responses, and identifying situations in which the presence of the child may be over-stressful for the parents or the sibling. In those circumstances, the

FAMILY CONSIDERATIONS

Presence of Siblings at the Birth of the Infant

Some parents wish to have siblings present at the birth of the infant. Many facilities have instituted programs to prepare children for this experience. It is often required that an adult, other than the labor coach or partner, be present to supervise the child. The nurse must, however, also assess the sibling's reaction and be prepared to provide comfort and guidance at any time.

Behavioral responses will vary with the age of the child. The clinician must be alert to subtle cues of discomfort, mild anxiety, or distress, and be prepared to direct the support person if he or she is unable to deal effectively with an upset child. Research to date suggests positive outcomes for the family when a properly prepared sibling participates in the birth experience. However, further study is indicated to distinguish benefits among different age groups and to identify the risks of permitting siblings to be present during childbirth.

Daniels MB: The birth experience for the sibling. Description and evaluation of a program. J Nurse-Midwifery 28(5):21–26, 1988

nurse should discuss her observations with the parents and the child's support person; often it is preferable for children to be present less during labor (because their attention span is limited and because sights and sounds are disturbing to them) but to be invited in shortly before the birth itself, which is usually the most important aspect of sibling participation for children and parents alike.

Diagnosis

The nurse's ongoing assessment of the mother's physiologic and emotional status, of the progress being made, of fetal well-being, and of the father's responses to active labor provide the basis for ongoing care. The following nursing diagnoses may be useful in caring for women and their families in the normal physiologic and behavioral problems of the active phase of labor. These nursing diagnoses may be addressed independently by the nurse and priorities established based on them.

- Altered nutrition: Less than body requirements
- Fluid volume deficit related to decreased oral intake/ abnormal loss
- Altered patterns of urinary elimination
- Anxiety related to perceived threat to self/fetus, impending birth
- Ineffective coping related to fatigue and discomfort of labor

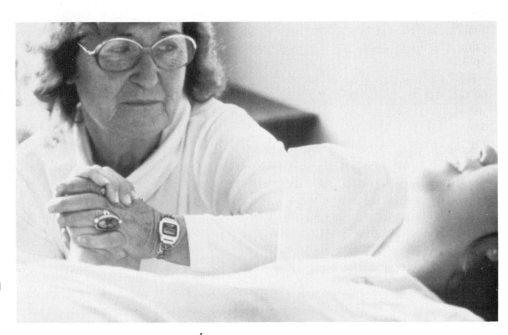

Figure 23–4. Adolescent mothers are often well supported by their own mothers in labor. (Photo: Kathy Sloane)

- Altered comfort: Pain related to contractions or nausea/vomiting
- Impaired physical mobility related to discomfort, pain, or interventions
- Sensory–perceptual alterations
- Self-care deficit: Hygiene related to energy depletion and pain in labor

Complications requiring collaboration with other team members may arise during the active phase. Such potential complications include fetal distress and maternal hyperventilation. Both are discussed at the end of this chapter.

Planning and Implementation

The nurse's assessment and diagnoses may indicate the need for continuing nursing support, if physiologic management of active labor is proving successful, or the need for more active nursing management if variations from normal progress arise.

Promoting Physiologic Adaptation
Promoting Nutrition and Hydration

The practice of using intravenous infusion routinely as a means of providing the laboring woman with fluids, calories, and electrolytes arose in large part because of a rapid increase in the use of general and regional anesthesia for labor and birth in the last 40 years. A patient who receives anesthesia or narcotic analgesia is at risk for vomiting and aspiration of gastric contents. Thus, when these medical interventions were used widely for women in labor, the practice of prohibiting oral intake and providing calories and fluids intravenously became well accepted.

However, more recent research suggests that without the neutralizing effects of food and oral fluids, maternal gastric contents may be more damaging to lung tissue, if aspirated. Further, there is new evidence that gastric emptying time, long thought to be greatly delayed in labor, may in fact be normal in unmedicated women in early labor, and only slightly delayed in active labor. However, gastric emptying time is greatly increased in women who receive narcotic analgesia during labor. Perhaps even more important, general anesthesia (which carries the greatest risk of aspiration) is rarely used except in obstetric emergencies (Broach et al 1988).

For these reasons, increasing numbers of physicians and nurse midwives do not routinely limit oral fluids and food intake during labor, and do not order routine intravenous replacement (Keppler 1988). Normal, healthy women may be permitted to eat lightly in early labor and should stop eating in active labor. Low-residue, simple energy-packed foods, such as toast with honey, crackers, jello, broth, or frozen juice bars, are recommended for early labor. Soothing teas with honey, water, fruit juice, or ginger ale can be taken throughout labor.

However, other providers regard the risk of aspiration as still too high and believe that while routine use of intravenous fluids may not be indicated, oral intake should be restricted. An indwelling intravenous catheter may be inserted and attached to a heparin lock in the event that fluids are needed to treat a specific problem (Douglas 1988).

The nurse must be aware of physician and nurse midwife preferences, as well as established hospital policies regarding oral intake during labor, and advise patients of these policies. When labor does not proceed as expected, if complications arise, or if the woman is unwilling to take oral fluids or vomits frequently, intravenous hydration is indicated.

When intravenous fluids are ordered in labor, the nurse's responsibility includes administration and monitoring. Physiologic solutions, such as Ringer's lactate in 5% dextrose, is often ordered and administered at 100–150 ml/hr. The nurse should guard against fluid overloading, especially when oxytocin or other medications are being administered, and carefully record intake and output. The nurse must be especially careful to monitor urinary output to prevent bladder distension when intravenous therapy is instituted.

Expected Outcome: The woman in labor maintains an adequate caloric intake to meet energy needs and maintains adequate fluid intake to prevent dehydration.

Promoting Bladder Elimination

The bladder should be evaluated frequently to ensure that it is not becoming distended. A full bladder can impede fetal descent, is uncomfortable for the patient, and may become a predisposing cause of postpartum hemorrhage. The bladder can be evaluated when other abdominal assessments are carried out. Catheterization may become necessary, if efforts to keep the bladder empty fail. The possibility of urinary tract infection after catheterization in labor is great, however, so strict aseptic technique should be used.

A small flexible catheter (usually a 14F) should be well lubricated and inserted *between* contractions for the patient's comfort. Output should be recorded, and the patient encouraged to void at least every 2 hours thereafter.

Expected Outcome: The woman in active labor voids 25 to 30 ml/hr voluntarily at least every 2 hours and maintains urine specific gravity below 1.020.

Promoting Behavioral Adaptation

Providing Emotional Support and Promoting Effective Coping

A major nursing responsibility is providing the woman in labor and her partner with psychosocial support as labor progresses. The woman becomes increasingly uncomfortable and fatigued as active labor progresses. Interaction with others becomes more difficult for her, since she is preoccupied with coping with contractions. Gradually, she will be less able to tolerate distractions and interruptions and may begin to doubt her ability to cope with labor. She finds it difficult to relax and needs constant reminders and encouragement.

The nurse should periodically note the woman's changing behavior and tailor intervention to her changing needs. A gentle reassuring touch is an important nursing tool. The nurse may also find that she can assist the woman to maintain her concentration and control by establishing close eye contact or by speaking quietly in her ear during contractions.

The nurse also should assess how the father is coping and provide encouragement and help. No matter how skillful a father appears to be as a labor support person, he is still experiencing a great deal of stress and requires emotional support as well as reassurance about his performance. The nurse should also remember that the father has physical needs and should remind him to take breaks while she remains with the mother. This is especially important during a long or painful labor; the father's ability to support his partner depends to a great extent on his own comfort level. A brief rest, hot food or coffee, or a walk around the block may boost his energy and increase his effectiveness as a labor support.

The nurse should also point out and explain changes in the woman's behaviors as labor progresses. This helps the father to interpret her behavior and adjust his caregiving to her changing needs. This is especially important if the woman rejects his touch or comfort measures; the father is likely to interpret that as rejection of him, rather than as a reflection of the woman's need to reduce the sensory stimulation with which she has to cope.

The nurse should also be careful not to assume the father is able to provide effective labor support. Many men are not accustomed to being in a caretaking role, especially in a situation as foreign to them as a labor unit. Some fathers can provide reassurance and comfort to their partners by their presence, by holding hands, and by giving encouragement, but will not be comfortable or effective in more direct caregiving (see Fig. 23–3). If the father is anxious or uncomfortable in an active role, the nurse should point out how his quiet presence and physical contact help the woman and encourage him to participate in this way. Fathers differ in their abilities and responses to the labor situation, and the nurse can often contribute directly to the woman's comfort by promoting the *father's* comfort.

Emotional support and reassurance from professionals is very important to parents throughout labor. The nurse should reiterate progress in labor, give positive reinforcement, give expert advice when asked, and communicate empathy for the patient and her family. The nurse should be particularly aware of the fact that time is often seen as an enemy during labor.

The longer labor lasts, the more worried parents and professionals become. The nurse should avoid focusing on the passage of time, since parents are often unaware of the amount of time spent in labor, unless the staff reminds them and directs attention to time as a limiting factor. When no serious complications arise, time during labor can be viewed as an ally. With enough passage of time, many problems are solved in labor, without intervention. The nurse's attention should more appropriately be focused on assessing the patient and family and on meeting other needs for comfort, relaxation, and safety.

Expected Outcomes: The woman in active labor verbalizes feelings related to her current emotional state. The woman in active labor utilizes effective coping strategies to enhance feelings of control and well-being and makes appropriate decisions with the input of significant others and the health care team to change problem situations.

Promoting Comfort

Many nursing support measures facilitate the patient's comfort and relaxation throughout labor. Patients will vary in their need for and response to these measures. Careful and thorough nursing assessment and evaluation are needed to meet the individualized needs of each patient and each labor.

Massage.   Various forms of massage, including *effleurage* (light stroking), kneading, and counterpressure, are often soothing to the patient. This tactile stimulation helps with relaxation and pain relief. Effleurage is often used on the lower abdomen, over the lower half of the uterus. It can also be used on the legs or face. Kneading is particularly useful for reducing tension in the neck, shoulders, and back. (Occasionally, this is helpful for the support persons as well!) Massage of the feet can be relaxing for some women. Counterpressure is frequently used over the sacrum or the inner thighs. (See Massage Techniques, Chapter 21.)

Baths and Showers. These nursing measures to promote comfort and relaxation have been underused. Unfortunately, many labor and delivery units do not have bathtubs. Sometimes the staff views labor in the bathroom as undesirable, either because it is inconvenient or because the bathroom is shared with other patients. Ideally, for each woman in labor there should be a private bathroom, including tub and shower. If this is not possible, flexible rules should be established for the use of the bath or shower, including the presence of a support person. The advantages of hydrotherapy include relaxation and pain relief, distraction, and maintenance of the upright position. In a normal labor, these advantages would seem to outweigh any inconveniences incurred by the staff.

A single, long hot bath or shower may be helpful to the patient, or, during a long or very painful labor, several 1- to 2-hour sessions may both be helpful and assist with general cleanliness.

Little is known about the possible risk of ascending infection when bathing with ruptured membranes. Therefore, the patient should use the tub only when membranes are intact. Showers may be taken, regardless of membrane status.

Cold Packs and Hot Compresses. Cold packs and hot compresses can be used to promote relaxation and pain relief, as well as maternal comfort. Cold packs can be made from an ice bag or rubber glove filled with ice. A silica gel cold pack can also be used. Cold packs are particularly helpful over the sacral area. They can be used with counterpressure or alternated with counterpressure when backache is severe. Cool, moist cloths on the forehead, back of the neck, or upper chest can be soothing and refreshing to the perspiring woman. Hot compresses can be made from hot water bottles, or a towel soaked in hot water and wrapped in plastic, or a blue pad. If firm, warm pressure is desired, plastic fluid bottles can be kept in a warming cabinet and can be used against the patient's back. Hot compresses may also be helpful over the sacral area, since some patients prefer hot application over cold for the sacral area. In addition, hot compresses can be soothing when placed on the lower abdomen. This can be alternated with massage. Care must be taken not to harm the patient's skin with excessive heat, since sensation will diminish after repeated applications of heat or cold.

Relaxation and Visualization. Many women will have practiced relaxation exercises prenatally. They will have spent time consciously focusing on the muscles of the body in a relaxed state and on rhythmic breathing to

facilitate relaxation. The nurse should encourage the use of whatever relaxation and breathing methods the patient has been practicing, and assist the father or support person in using those methods. Simple relaxation methods can be taught on the spot to those who have not previously learned them. The nurse can ask the patient to relax specific muscle groups, such as the legs, neck, face, and perineum. Relaxed rhythmic breathing can be encouraged to help "breathe out the tension" with each exhalation. Relaxation allows the woman to focus her mind on her body, thus experiencing the labor as a psychophysical experience. She neither controls the experience nor totally yields to it. The process of labor and birth is very much affected by the degree of integration between the mind and the body. The woman can gain confidence during the labor by recognizing the "wisdom" of her body.

Visualization, or mental picturing of the biophysical events of labor and birth, can also encourage women to work with, rather than resist, the normal physiologic progression of labor and birth.

The nurse may suggest the use of visualization to strengthen the mind-body connection during labor. The nurse can enlist such images as contractions opening the cervix for the baby (rather than being just painful); breathing bringing in healthy, cleansing oxygen to the fetus and getting rid of waste products and tension; blood flow to the placenta and fetus increasing as blood vessels relax; and the baby sliding down the birth canal.

The nurse should communicate in a calm, soothing voice, using touch to assist the woman's concentration. The nurse should also explain these techniques to the father or support person, who may be able to help the woman visualize calm, favorite scenes, or who may have special knowledge about things the woman finds calming (such as having her hair brushed or massage). (See Chapter 21 for further discussion and sample visualization exercise and Chapter 27 on Managing Maternal Pain.)

Ambulation and Position Changes

In some obstetric units, women are encouraged to stay in bed once they are admitted in labor, because of concern about cord prolapse during ambulation. This is a highly unlikely event, even when membranes are ruptured. To evaluate the possible risk of cord prolapse, the woman can be examined vaginally in a standing position to assess how well the fetal head is applied to the cervix. If the head is not well applied, or the presentation is breech, risk of cord prolapse is increased. If the head is well applied, however, ambulation can be encouraged. If membranes rupture during ambulation, the woman should be examined immediately for the presence of prolapsed cord, and the FHR should be auscultated at that time. Most women should be encouraged to move around, walk in the halls, around their room, to the nursery, and so on. Walking

NURSING ALERT

Prolapsed Umbilical Cord

The umbilical cord can become prolapsed at any time in active labor if the presenting part is not well applied to the cervix. However, cord prolapse is most likely to occur at the time of rupture of membranes or shortly thereafter, and in presentations other than vertex.

Precautions:

Auscultate FHR immediately after rupture of membranes and with next contraction. Abrupt and variable decelerations suggest cord compression.

If cord prolapse is suspected:

- Perform gloved vaginal examination.
- If cord is palpable in the vagina, apply two fingers against presenting part with cord in between fingers and press presenting part up into pelvis to relieve pressure on cord. Do not compress cord between fingers.
- Call for help.
- Maintain upward pressure on presenting part.
- Instruct others to assist mother to knee–chest position with hips elevated as high as possible; this allows gravity to pull presenting part off prolapsed cord.
- Instruct others to administer oxygen by mask at 8–12 liter/min and prepare for emergency cesarean delivery.

increases their level of comfort and promotes less frequent, more efficient contractions. The upright position allows the full benefit of gravity in encouraging dilatation and optimizes the fetal position in the birth canal. Arrested labors may be augmented by walking. There are also reports that walking reduces discomfort, including pain from contractions and backache (Roberts et al 1983, Read et al 1983). The slight movements of the joints during walking may facilitate rotation and descent of the fetus.

A laboring woman will be most able, willing, and interested in walking if she is unencumbered by machinery and if she is awake and aware, not drowsy from medication or weakened by anesthesia. Telemetric electronic fetal monitoring may soon be more widely available so that ambulation and continuous monitoring can be done simultaneously.

Position changes during labor can be used to enhance maternal comfort or to correct or prevent problems in labor, as described in the accompanying display. Position change is a simple, harmless tool the nurse or the woman herself can use. Research indicates that women prefer a mixture of positions, including sitting and standing/

walking for most of the first stage and lying down only late in labor (Read et al 1983).

Maternal positioning can be used to prevent or correct malpositions of the fetus. An all-fours or side-lying position combined with the pelvic rock motion may be used to turn an occiput posterior fetus to a more favorable position. Firm abdominal stroking (in the direction that you want the baby to turn) can also be done (Andrews 1981). Prolonged back-lying or semisitting, and even prolonged side-lying, may impede rotation and progress in labor. Frequent position changes appear to be effective in facilitating fetal rotation and descent. Figure 23–5 displays some of the commonly used positions for labor.

Position changes are sometimes helpful in alleviating mild fetal distress, if the distress is due to supine hypotension syndrome or cord compression. Trial and error methods must be used by monitoring FHR in various positions to determine which to avoid and which to encourage in each individual patient.

When backache, often called *back labor,* occurs, it is usually caused by pressure of the presenting part on the sacrum, which refers pain to the lower back. It is particularly acute with a posterior presentation. Positioning can facilitate rotation and promote maternal comfort and relaxation.

Other measures can be used as well, including counterpressure (Fig. 23–6), hot or cold packs, and showers. (See Chapter 21 for relief measures for back labor.)

Expected Outcomes:

- The woman in active labor uses effective nonpharmacologic techniques to enhance comfort and reduce pain, as evidenced by her verbalization of a reduction in discomfort or pain.
- The woman in active labor ambulates in the area and voices her increased comfort as evidenced by less frequent, more effective contractions.

Promoting Optimal Sensory Stimulation

Sensory alterations during labor and birth are due to a combination of factors. A woman's usual daily activities are often disrupted by early labor; thus, she may not have eaten well or slept well for hours or even a day or two before labor begins. The unfamiliar physical environment of the birth setting may contribute to this disruption.

Some degree of sensory overload can be expected during labor because of such physiologic phenomena as uterine contractions, unusual secretions, rupture of membranes, nausea and vomiting, fetal descent, and pelvic pressure. These physical sensations may range from mild and easily tolerable to overwhelming. Routine care also introduces additional sensory input from vaginal ex-

Physiologic Positions for Labor and Birth

Position	Advantages
Standing	Takes advantage of gravity during and between contractions Contractions are less painful and more productive Fetus is well aligned with angle of pelvis May speed labor May increase urge to push in second stage
Standing and leaning forward	Takes advantage of gravity during and between contractions Contractions are often less painful and more productive Fetus is well aligned with angle of pelvis May speed labor Relieves backache May be more restful than standing
Walking	Takes advantage of gravity during and between contractions Contractions are often less painful and more productive Fetus is well aligned with angle of pelvis May speed labor Relieves backache Encourages descent through pelvic mobility
Sitting upright	Good resting position Some gravity advantage Can be used with electronic fetal monitor
Semisitting	Good resting position Some gravity advantage Can be used with electronic fetal monitor Vaginal exams possible Easy position to get into on bed or delivery table
Sitting, leaning forward with support	Good resting position Some gravity advantage Can be used with electronic fetal monitor Relieves backache Good position for back rub
Hands and knees	Helps relieve backache Assists rotation of baby in occiput posterior position Allows for pelvic rocking and body movements Allows for vaginal exams Takes pressure off hemorrhoids
Kneeling, leaning forward with support	Helps relieve backache Assists rotation of baby in occiput posterior position Allows for pelvic rocking Less strain on wrists and hands than hands and knees position

(continued)

Physiologic Positions for Labor and Birth (continued)

Position	Advantages
Side-lying	Very good resting position
	Convenient for many interventions
	Helps lower elevated blood pressure
	Safe if pain medications have been used
	May promote progress of labor when alternated with walking
	Gravity-neutral
	Useful to slow a very rapid second stage
	Takes pressure off hemorrhoids
	Facilitates relaxation between pushing efforts
	Allows posterior sacral movement in second stage
Squatting	May be comfortable and relieve backache
	Takes advantage of gravity
	Widens pelvic outlet to its maximum
	Requires less bearing down effort
	May enhance rotation and descent in a difficult birth
	Helpful if mother does not feel an urge to push
	Allows freedom to shift weight for comfort
Sitting on toilet or commode	May help perineum for effective bearing down
	Takes advantage of gravity
Supported squat	Maximizes diameters of bony pelvis
(mother leaning with back against support person who holds her under the arms and takes all her weight)	Permits relaxation while avoiding stretching of the muscles connected to the pelvis
	Takes advantage of gravity

aminations, use of monitoring devices, laboratory tests, room changes, and personnel changes. Unusual situations that demand quick staff responses, such as instances of fetal distress or other developments requiring emergency procedures, cause very high levels of environmental activity and can contribute to the sensory overload experienced by the woman in labor.

In other instances, if progress is slow, the woman has no support person with her, and continuous nursing support is not possible, she may experience some deprivation of sensory input as a result of her environment (darkened rooms with limited visual interest), limitations on her activity or movement, the unfamiliarity of her surroundings, and lack of distractions from the somatic sensations of labor.

During active-phase labor, the nurse can minimize sensory overload by approaching the woman in labor in an unhurried, gentle manner. All procedures should be explained before they are implemented and time should

be provided for the parturient to prepare herself for pelvic examinations and other necessary interventions. The environment should be conducive to rest and relaxation. Bright overhead lights can be dimmed, and natural light or small table lamps used whenever possible to reduce visual stimuli. The nurse should speak in a low, calm voice and efforts should be made to reduce noise and unnecessary conversations immediately outside of the woman's room. If an electronic fetal monitor is used, the audio output for the fetal heart beat should be reduced as much as possible.

If a support person or coach is not present, the woman in labor will benefit by the nurse's frequent or continuous presence. One of the most frightening experiences for the parturient in active or transition-stage labor is to be left alone. If the woman has neither family nor friends present, the nurse becomes her link to reality. She translates the intense sensations and often overwhelming stimuli into an understandable experience, and reassures

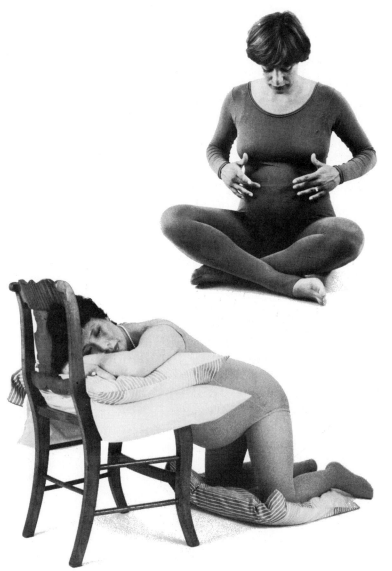
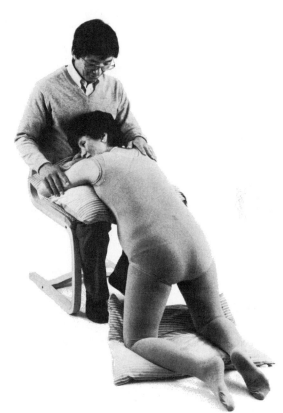

Figure 23–5. Some commonly used physiologic positions for labor. All of these positions avoid compression of the vena cava and resulting maternal hypotension. Many of these positions are ones laboring women will naturally adopt as positions of comfort in labor if movement is not restricted. (Childbirth Graphics)

the woman that she will not be alone during the birth of her infant.

Expected Outcome   The woman in active labor experiences relief from sensory overload, as evidenced by her relaxed and calm response to labor or she verbalizes feeling relaxed and supported.

Supporting Appropriate Self-Care

Supportive care becomes increasingly important as labor progresses. The woman in labor becomes less able to meet her own needs effectively as her attention and energy are directed toward the physical and mental demands of labor. The nurse can assist the mother in main-

taining a sense of control by encouraging her to perform easy self-care measures, such as effleurage, to urinate frequently, and ambulate and rest quietly between contractions.

The nurse can also assist the father or support person in taking on some self-care measures on the woman's behalf. These measures may reflect self-care as much for the father as for the mother, since they give the father a sense of purpose and reward if he sees that they help his partner. The father or support person may be especially able to assist the woman with maintaining the room environment the way the woman prefers it (door open or shut, lights dimmed or bright, music or quiet). Other comfort measures the father can offer are massage, hot or cold packs on the lower back, sips of fluid or ice chips, and

(text continued on page 636)

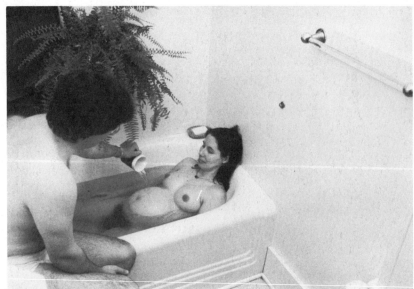

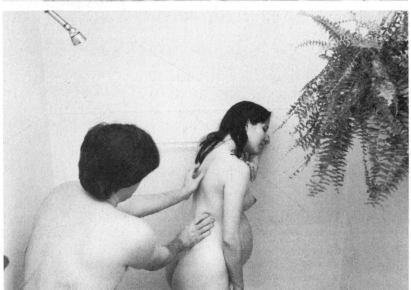

Figure 23–5. (cont.)

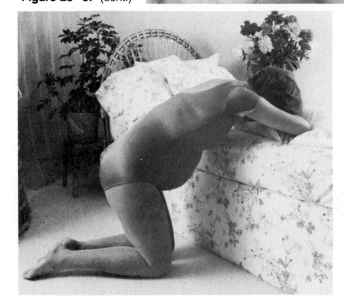

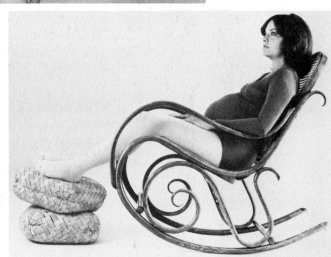

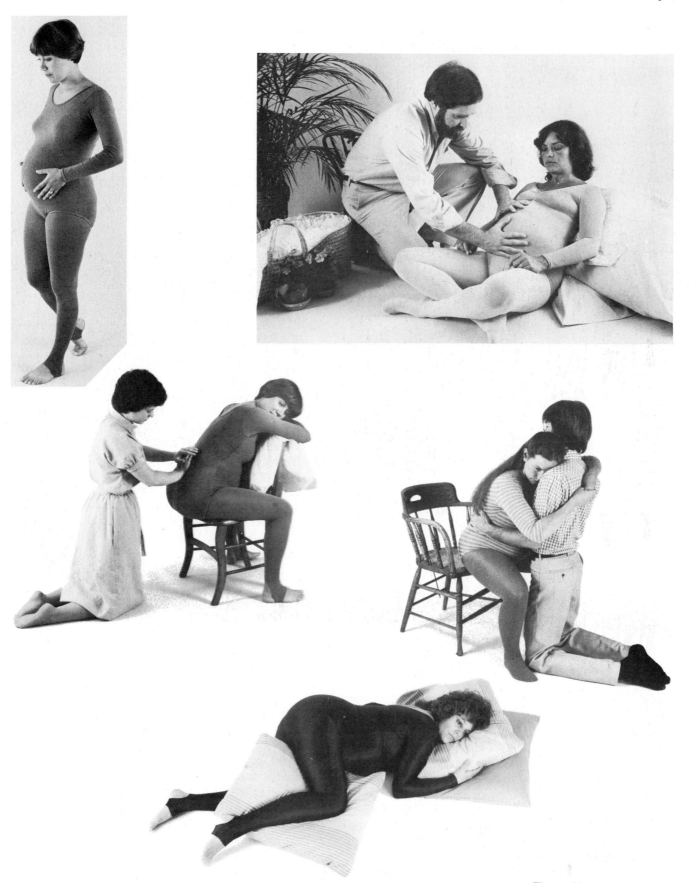

Figure 23–5. (continued)

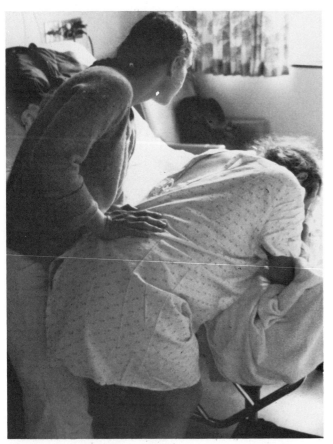

Figure 23–6. The labor nurse provides sacral counterpressure for a woman experiencing back labor. Note how the woman is positioned (standing and leaning forward) to facilitate fetal rotation from posterior to anterior position). (Photo: BABES, Inc.)

NURSING RESEARCH

The Use of Music as a Therapeutic Modality During Labor

Nurses are continuously seeking ways to provide diversion and enhance relaxation in early labor and reduce pain and sensory–perceptual alterations in the active phase. Sammons (1984) examined the effects of music during childbirth. Subjects reported music establishes a favorable mood, humanizes or normalizes the birth environment, and induces relaxation.

Some subjects who chose not to listen to music stated that they did not want to be distracted from relaxation and breathing activities, but the majority stated that they had not thought of it as an option. Further research is definitely indicated to clarify the benefits and disadvantages of music therapy during labor, but clinicians may offer the option to women as it appears that many have not even considered its use during birth.

Sammons LN: The use of music by women during childbirth. J Nurse-Midwifery 29(4):266–270, 1984

comforting physical contact. The father may also help the woman in labor in a warm shower or bath by providing reassuring physical contact and assistance.

One area in which the woman and her partner can exercise effective self-care is in promoting progress in labor. Ambulation and upright positions may encourage progress; the nurse can explain this to the father and guide him in supporting his partner. If the progress of labor continues to be slow, the father may assist the mother with breast or nipple stimulation to promote cervical ripening and labor (Elliott et al 1983). The nurse can explain this option and assist the father or provide privacy for parents as appropriate. In some cases, this technique may help to avoid the need for other measures to stimulate labor, such as artificial rupture of the membranes or oxytocin augmentation of labor: these interventions, while useful for many patients, are not without risk. (See Chapter 26 for further discussion.)

As the parturient's energy resources are depleted, the nurse assumes a larger share of the self-care needs. She will provide perineal care after vaginal exams, with rupture of the membranes, and when bloody show is evident. A sponge bath may be very refreshing at the end of the transition period, before the woman begins the expulsive stage of labor. Attention to mouth care is important, as breathing efforts and decreased oral intake dry the mucous membranes.

Expected Outcome: The woman in active-phase labor implements, or her support person implements, specific self-care measures and verbalizes satisfaction with the comfort and hygiene measures performed by herself or others.

Transition

The last part of active-phase labor is typically called *transition,* reflecting the impending shift from the first stage of labor to the second stage. This phase of labor is often described as the most intense, and it presents the labor nurse with challenging patient needs. Although transition is technically part active-phase labor, because of its unique characteristics, it is described in detail here.

Nursing assessment during the transition phase of labor is directed toward careful monitoring of maternal and fetal status and of the progress of labor. Because of the intensity of this phase, the woman may exhibit marked apprehension, restlessness, and irritability. Her attention is focused only on her situation, and she has difficulty responding to others. She may not wish to be touched or comforted, but cannot cope with labor alone. The woman may appear confused and unable to understand directions. She may feel overwhelmed by the contractions and have little strength to cope with the demands of labor. She may experience panic and beg to be "put to sleep" or for staff to "get the baby out." These characteristic responses may suggest to the nurse that first-stage labor is ending, and the patient may be moving into second-stage labor.

Transition marks an especially demanding phase in the care of the woman in labor and her family. If progress appears to be normal, the nurse begins to plan for imminent delivery—especially for the multipara, who will likely move through this phase in 15 to 20 minutes. The labor nurse should not leave the mother alone at this time and may need other staff assistance for preparations. The father or support person will need to be prepared for the birth; if special clothing is needed, the father should be shown where to change, exactly what clothes are needed and how they are to be worn, and where to wait if the woman is to be transferred immediately. The physician or nurse midwife should be called. If the birth is to occur in the labor bed, any equipment likely to be needed at delivery is collected.

Controlling the Urge to Push

A common variation in normal labor during the transition phase, which may require active nursing management, is a phenomenon called *premature urge to push,* which occurs when the urge to push is felt by the patient in labor before the cervix is completely dilated. Traditional obstetric practice encourages attendants to prevent the woman from pushing until the cervix is completely dilated. The dangers, to mother and fetus, of pushing against an undilated cervix are not well documented, but are thought to include increased fetal head compression, cervical laceration, cervical edema, and a subsequent prolonged labor, and maternal exhaustion as a result of prolonged ineffective pushing.

The urge to push is a reflex action stimulated by descent of the presenting part. The stretch and pressure receptors of the lower uterine segment and vagina are activated as the fetus descends. The obstetric conditions usually accompanying a premature urge to push are advanced labor, cervical dilatation of at least 8 cm, +1 station of descent or more, and moderate-to-strong uterine contractions.

Nursing interventions in caring for the woman with a

premature urge to push during transition focus on assisting her to avoid pushing or bearing down until the cervix is completely dilated. The nurse must explain to the woman why bearing down should be delayed and encourage her to "blow the contractions away" by blowing out short breaths of air through pursed lips during the urge to push with contractions. The nurse can increase the effectiveness of this technique by maintaining close eye contact with the patient and breathing with her. The woman should be helped to a gravity-neutral position, such as the side-lying position, to decrease the intensity of downward pelvic pressure. The nurse may also suggest that the patient visualize the last rim of the cervix being retracted over the baby's head with a strong contraction; this may help her to focus her attention and resist the urge to push.

The nurse should also be alert for signs of progress in labor, since the urge to push may signal rapid movement into the second stage of labor. For this reason, the woman experiencing a premature urge to push should never be left alone.

Promoting Comfort

Nursing care when maternal and fetal status and the progress of labor are normal is directed toward providing comfort and emotional support.

The nurse should assist the woman during transition by providing whatever physical comfort measures are possible and by providing encouragement and a calm presence. If the woman is using relaxation and breathing techniques, the nurse can help the father to keep the mother focused on these activities.

During this time, sacral counterpressure, cool cloths on the forehead, and ice chips may be especially welcome. An emesis basin should be kept on hand; if the woman experiences nausea, deep breaths and moving her to a sitting or semisitting position may help. Table 23–4 reviews common nursing support techniques used during the transition stage.

Managing Sensory Overload

For many women, the potential for sensory overload is greatest during the transition period. The nurse's presence is absolutely essential to support the parturient and her partner through this period of overwhelming sensory stimuli. Profound changes in behavior that frighten the partner may occur. Previously successful coaching techniques may fail to help the gravida, owing to the intensity of the experience.

It may be necessary to speak directly into the woman's ear or maintain close eye contact to prevent her from feeling overwhelmed by her contractions. The nurse should give firm, precise directions when needed, and keep unnecessary conversation to a minimum to allow

Table 23–4   **Nursing Support Measures During Transition**

Common Physiologic Characteristics	Nursing Support Measures
Shaking, chills	Hold extremities; use warm blankets
Perspiration, feeling hot	Use fan; wipe with cool cloth; give ice chips
Restlessness, irritability, increased apprehension	Give encouragement; work on relaxation techniques; avoid behaviors irritating to patient; increase verbal cues for relaxation
Inability to focus; confusion	Give firm but kind instruction; repeat instruction and show understanding; breathe with patient; use eye contact
Increased pain, especially sacral	Apply sacral counterpressure; give other comfort measures
Inability to cope	Give reassurance; maintain physical presence; focus on shortness of phase. Give overwhelming support—"baby is almost here." Take one contraction at a time.
Exhaustion	Facilitate rest and sleep between contractions. Alert patient to beginning of contraction.
Hiccoughing, burping, flatulance	Patient is often embarrassed. Reassure that this is normal.
Nausea and vomiting	Reassure that this is normal and will be over soon; use comfort measures, such as cold cloth to throat; position with head elevated or on left side
Urge to push	Check for complete dilatation. If not complete, try side-lying position and "blowing contractions away."
Carpopedal spasm	Extend patient's leg and flex foot; check for warmth of extremities, provide blanket as needed

the woman to concentrate on coping with each contraction. The woman should be encouraged to rest and sleep, if possible, between contractions. Interruptions should be minimized to allow for quiet, undisturbed rest.

The nurse should explain to the father or support person that the woman's irritable or angry behavior is a normal response to this part of labor. The woman may find certain kinds of contact very irritating, such as touch or conversation. The nurse can explain this and help to reduce those irritating stimuli as much as possible. The nurse may also need to interpret the woman's needs to other staff, based on the observations and knowledge acquired from working with the woman throughout her labor.

Providing Emotional Support

The woman and her support person are more likely to need reassurance and calm guidance at this point in labor than at any other time. The nurse should encourage both parents and commend them frequently on their efforts. Information about labor progress should be given freely when it is likely to be encouraging. The mother can be reminded that the baby will soon be born and that she needs to cope with labor only a little while longer, if that can be said with reasonable certainty. The father may be particularly distressed at his partner's obvious pain, and may need additional encouragement and reassurance. The nurse should anticipate questions and concerns and explain what the father can expect in the next few minutes so that he can adjust more easily to the faster pace of activity.

Expected Outcome: The woman in transition experiences less anxiety and fear, as evidenced by her verbalization of feelings and of satisfaction with their emotional support provided by significant others and the health care team.

Monitoring for Potential Complications

Potential Complication: Fetal Compromise.   The nurse must maintain a close watch on fetal status during the transition phase of labor. Rapid cervical change and fetal descent can sometimes occur at this time. The nurse should never leave a woman in labor alone during this phase and should always investigate, by perineal inspection or vaginal examination, if the mother says birth is imminent. Fetal heart tones should be monitored at the end of each contraction, at this point in labor. Because contractions may be longer and more frequent, with little resting time in between, placental oxygenation is decreased and fetal hypoxia is a possibility.

Potential Complication: Hyperventilation.   Because of the intense physiologic demands and her apprehension, the mother is prone to hyperventilation during this time, especially if she is using shallow, patterned breathing in an effort to cope with her contractions. Hyperventilation results from breathing too fast or too deeply, causing an excess amount of carbon dioxide to be blown off, leading to respiratory alkalosis. Symptoms of hyperventilation include numbness and tingling in the lips, fingers, or toes; dizziness; light-headedness; and confusion. The father or support person may also hyperventilate, either from excitement or from attempting to assist the woman to control her breathing. Treatment for hyperventilation consists of rebreathing exhaled carbon dioxide either from cupped hands around the mouth or from a paper bag.

Expected Outcome: The woman in transition uses effective techniques to cope with intense physical and emotional sensations of transition and verbalizes the rationale for implementing specific medical or nursing interventions.

Evaluation of First-Stage Labor Care

The final step in the nursing process is the systematic comparison of the woman's physical and emotional status with expected outcomes. The nurse carries out a comprehensive assessment of the client so as to make appropriate changes in the nursing diagnoses and implementation of care, if expected outcomes have not been achieved. During latent-phase labor, the evaluation process may be done in an unhurried manner, providing an opportunity to foster the growing nurse–client relationship. During active labor, particularly the transition stage, rapid changes in the parturient's condition require swift reappraisal and timely interventions.

CHAPTER SUMMARY

The first stage of labor is a period of concentrated nursing attention to the changing needs of the mother, the fetus, the father, or the support person. The nurse must systematically assess and diagnose needs as they change through the latent phase to and through active labor. Further, she must implement care and evaluate its effectiveness in meeting patient needs in the context of ongoing change in the patient and in family responses to labor. As the intensity of labor increases during the transition phase, the nurse begins to prepare for the second stage and the dramatic event of delivery.

STUDY QUESTIONS

1. How would you help a women distinguish between true and false labor during a telephone conversation?

2. What information should you give to a woman calling the labor unit, who suspects that her membranes have ruptured? Why is this information important?
3. How would you instruct a father supporting his wife in labor to distinguish between mild, moderate, and strong contractions?
4. Describe the current disagreement among authorities about maternal oral intake during labor. What implications do you see for nursing care?

REFERENCES/BIBLIOGRAPHY

Andrews C: Changing fetal position through maternal posturing. In Raff B (ed): Perinatal Parental Behavior: Nursing Research and Implications for Newborn Health. White Plains, March of Dimes, 1981
Broach J, Newton N: Food and beverages in labor. Part II: The effects of cessation of oral intake during labor. Birth 15(2):88–92, 1988
Cranley M, Hedahl K, Pegg S: Women's perception of vaginal and cesarean deliveries. Nurs Res 32(1):10, 1983
Curtis P, Rimer R: Breast stimulation to enhance labor. Med World News February 27, 1984
Douglas M: The case against a more liberal food and fluid policy in labor. Birth 15(2):93–94, 1988
Elliott J, Flaherty JF: The use of breast stimulation to ripen the cervix in term pregnancies. Am J Obstet Gynecol 145:553, 1983
Keppler A: Use of intravenous fluids during labor. Birth 15(2):75–79, 1988
Lederman R, Lederman E, Work B et al: Relationship of psychologic factors in pregnancy to progress in labor. Nurs Res 28:94, 1979
Levinson G, Schnider S: Catecholamines, the effects of maternal fear and its treatment on uterine function and circulation. Birth Fam J 6:167, 1979
Mercer R, Hackley K, Bostrom A: Relationship between psychosocial and perinatal variables to perception of childbirth. Nurs Res 32(4):201, 1983
NAACOG. Nursing Responsibilities in Implementing Intrapartum Fetal Heart Rate Monitoring. Washington, D.C.: NAACOG, 1988
Read JA, Miller FC, Pauh RH: Randomized clinical trial of ambulation vs. oxytocin for labor enhancement: A preliminary report. Am J Obstet Gynecol 139:669, 1981
Roberts J, Mendez-Bauer C, Wodell D: The effects of maternal position on uterine contractility and efficiency. Birth 10:243, 1983

SUGGESTED READINGS

Chute GE: Expectation and experience in alternative and conventional birth. J Obstet Gynecol Neonatal Nurs 14:61–67, 1985

Hazle NR: Hydration in labor. J Nurse-Midwifery 31(4):171–175, 1986

Hedstrom L, Newton N: Touch in labor: A comparison of cultures and eras. Birth 13(3):181–186, 1986

Kintz D: Nursing support in labor. J Obstet Gynecol Neonatal Nurs 16(2):126–130, 1987

Lupe PJ, Gross TL: Maternal upright posture and mobility in labor: A review. Obstet Gynecol 67(5):727–734, 1986

Mercer RT: Relationship of the birth experience to later mothering behaviors. J Nurse-Midwifery 30(4):204–211, 1985

Phillips CR: Single-room maternity care for maximum cost-efficiency. Perinatol-Neonatol Mar/Apr: 22–31, 1988

Young J, Poppe C: Breast pump stimulation to promote labor. MCN 12(2):124–126, 1987

24 nursing care in normal birth: second-stage labor through recovery

LEARNING OBJECTIVES

After studying the materials in this chapter, the student should be able to

- Discuss the application of the nursing process in caring for a woman and her family during second-stage labor through recovery

- Discuss the types, indications, risks, and benefits of episiotomy

- Assess the placenta, cord, and fetal membranes for normalcy and completeness

- Perform an immediate assessment of the neonate at delivery

- Explain the procedure and rationale for postpartum fundal massage

- Identify maternal and neonatal needs in the first hour after birth

- Discuss family needs and identify advantages of family-centered birth care

KEY TERMS

Apgar score

Caput succedaneum

Cotyledon

Crowning

Episiotomy

Velamentous insertion

This chapter completes the discussion of nursing care for the family experiencing a normal childbirth. The physiologic and behavioral changes of first-stage labor become increasingly dramatic as the process of fetal descent becomes dominant in second-stage labor. Again, in a low-risk case, nursing care centers on enhancing the body's own mechanisms and monitoring maternal/fetal status to detect deviations from normal.

Nursing care of families late in labor and through the birth and early recovery period is exciting and immensely rewarding. The nurse continues to assess maternal, fetal, and family well-being on an ongoing basis, and identifies diagnoses and collaborative problems, which direct her care. Her plan of care is continually revised in light of changing patient needs as labor progresses. In addition, the nurse collaborates with the birth attendant in preparation for and management of the actual delivery of the neonate. Finally, the nurse completes the process of labor and birth care as she assists the family during the immediate postpartum recovery period and prepares them for discharge to postpartum care.

CARE OF THE FAMILY DURING SECOND-STAGE LABOR

The second stage of labor begins with complete dilatation of the cervix and ends with the birth of the infant. This stage can last from 15 minutes to 2 hours or more. During this stage, the fetus descends through the maternal pelvis and the vaginal canal. This descent is caused both by continuing uterine contractions and by the pushing or bearing-down efforts (BDE) of the mother.

The labor nurse provides one-to-one care at this time for the woman in labor, and has much responsibility for support and active nursing management of the patient in the second stage of labor.

Assessment

Nursing assessments in second-stage labor again focus on monitoring maternal and fetal physiologic status, assessing the effectiveness of the mother's bearing-down efforts, and assessing the emotional state of both parents. The nurse should be providing uninterrupted one-to-one care during second-stage labor, so assessments are made on an ongoing basis.

Maternal and Fetal Physiologic Status

The mother's blood pressure, pulse, and respirations are monitored every 5 to 15 minutes throughout the second stage. Effects of fatigue and increased physical activity become apparent in the second stage of labor: flushing, increased perspiration, and muscle weakness and tremors. The mother should be encouraged to void, and the bladder should be assessed for signs of distention, especially if intravenous or oral fluids have been administered during labor.

Fetal heart rate should be auscultated or observed on a monitor tracing between and after each contraction to assess for changes in baseline FHR and variations in response to contractions and maternal bearing-down efforts. In second-stage labor, the FHT usually is best heard over the midline in the lower abdomen as fetal descent progresses (Fig. 24-1).

Progress of Labor: Maternal Bearing-Down Efforts

The nurse should observe the mother's bearing-down efforts and assist her in positioning and pushing efforts that will result in labor progress. The nurse should help the mother into a comfortable position, most often a

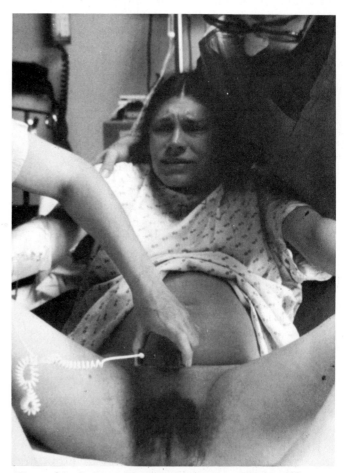

Figure 24-1. Intermittent fetal heart rate monitoring with a Doppler ultrasound device during bearing-down efforts in a low-risk labor. (Photo: BABES, Inc.)

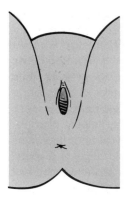 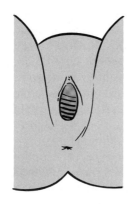 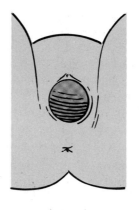 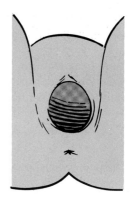

Anteroposterior slit   Oval opening   Circular shape   Crowning

Figure 24–2. Perineal changes in second-stage labor.

semisitting position, with legs well flexed at the hips and arms positioned to pull on handles or bedrails. The mother may also choose to push in a squatting or kneeling position. Whatever position is selected, the woman should use the diaphragm and abdominal muscles to help in bearing down, while keeping other muscle groups as relaxed as possible to decrease fatigue.

Effective bearing-down efforts will result in steady descent of the fetal head, and first flattening, then distention and bulging of the perineum (Fig. 24–2). Once the head is visible at the introitus, the nurse should observe the head advances with bearing-down efforts and retreats slightly between contractions. However, the head should make steady, noticeable progress toward the perineum.

Behavioral Adaptations

Despite the physical demands of labor, the woman may be able to cope more easily with contractions and may be encouraged if progress is apparent. However, if progress is slow or questionable, the woman and her partner are extremely vulnerable and may become fearful and discouraged. This is especially true if the labor is being managed with an eye toward a time limitation for the second stage (usually 2 hours). The nurse can assist by providing encouragement, keeping the parents informed of any progress, and by active nursing management to facilitate the progress of labor.

Maternal Comfort

The parturient experiences multiple foci of discomfort and pain during the second stage of labor. Pain caused by vaginal and perineal distention becomes prominent as the fetus descends into the birth canal. Persistent, intense back pain can also occur, especially with an occiput posterior presentation of the fetal head. The woman may experience painful leg cramps and general muscular achiness

after long hours of labor. Fatigue adds to the general sense of discomfort the gravida experiences during the expulsive stage of labor.

The nurse continues her surveillance of the woman's comfort level and the location, nature, and extent of discomfort or pain. This may require gently questioning the woman, as she may be unable to express herself well by the onset of the second stage due to sensory–perceptual alterations, fatigue, and pain. Body cues can alert the nurse to the location of pain. The parturient may, for example, reach for her lower back with each contraction. The nurse should also assess the general comfort of the partner. Hours of coaching, including physical support of the gravida and massage may exhaust the support person after a long labor.

Diagnosis

Based on these and data obtained from other assessments through the pregnancy and admission, the nurse formulates applicable diagnoses. The following are nursing diagnoses reflecting possible problems that may arise during the second stage of labor and that may be addressed independently.

- Altered comfort: pain related to descent and perineal stretching
- Fear related to impending birth

Complications may arise during the second stage of labor. Such complications are related to bearing-down efforts and include alterations in maternal tissue perfusion, fetal compromise, and perineal injury. The nurse is responsible for monitoring for potential complications.

Planning and Implementation

Nursing interventions during the second stage of labor focus on promoting comfort, providing support, and monitoring for potential complications.

Promoting Comfort

The pain caused by vaginal and perineal stretching as the head begins to crown has been referred to as the "ring of fire." Hot compresses to the perineum, perineal massage, or "ironing the perineum" (massaging and flattening the perineum between a finger inserted over the lower inner aspect of the vagina and the thumb) may help to promote perineal relaxation and tissue flexibility.

The nurse should encourage the mother to consciously relax the perineum and to visualize the perineum thinning out to accommodate the baby. Providing a mirror and helping the mother to see the fetal head as it becomes visible or to touch the fetal head may help her to do this. The mother should be reminded to relax as much as possible between contractions, and to keep her face, neck, and mouth as relaxed as possible during bearing-down efforts. Shortly before birth, the woman may become unable to concentrate. The nurse can assist her by giving repeated and direct instructions on bearing-down efforts and giving encouragement.

Backache caused by fetal descent or an occiput posterior position may be alleviated in several ways. Pelvic rocking and counterpressure on the lower back may ameliorate the discomfort (see Chapter 21). Position changes should be frequent (at least every 15 minutes), and positions selected to promote physiologic bearing-down efforts. Squatting or hands-and-knees positions may be especially comfortable during the second stage. However, the nurse must be aware that the woman will require careful physical support in these positions.

The nurse should continue such comfort measures as supplying cool compresses and ice chips, since the woman typically becomes quite warm from the exertion of second-stage labor. Mouth dryness is especially common because of mouth breathing with bearing-down efforts and because of dehydration. Sucking on large, hard, candy lollipops (not small candies, which may be kept in the mouth and might be aspirated) or frozen juice bars may be especially welcome and provides a source of food energy.

Expected Outcome: The woman in labor verbalizes her understanding of the interventions used to promote comfort and also verbalizes a decrease in

Figure 24–3. The labor nurse provides comfort and encouragement to the laboring woman *(A)*. The father supports his mate in active labor *(B)*. This mother has chosen to labor in a hands-and-knees position. (Photo: BABES, Inc.)

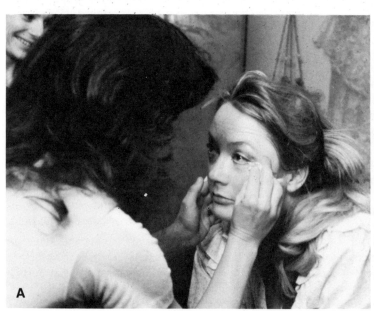

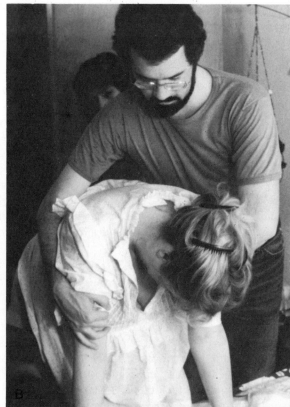

her discomfort or pain. She shows visible signs of relaxation between expulsive efforts.

Providing Support

The nurse should observe the interaction between the woman and her partner and be prepared to model encouragement and support techniques (Fig. 24–3). Support persons may have a tendency to become either overenthusiastic or too nondirective in their coaching efforts during the second stage. The nurse should explain what is needed and demonstrate it to the partner, reassuring him that he is doing well.

The nurse should also begin to prepare the woman and her partner for their first contact with their newborn. This can be done by providing a mirror so the woman can see the fetal head on the perineum and asking the father if he wants to watch the progress that the baby's head makes during pushing.

The nurse should keep the mother and father well informed of progress during this phase and provide encouragement if progress appears slow. Slow progress can be especially demoralizing, and nursing support of the parents' confidence and spirits can be very helpful.

Expected Outcome: The woman in labor and her support person verbalize a decrease in anxiety.

Monitoring for Complications

Complications in the second stage of labor are related to the efforts of bearing down. Alterations in maternal tissue perfusion, fetal compromise, and perineal injury may result if the woman is not monitored continuously.

The nurse remains in constant attendance as the parturient begins bearing-down efforts. A variety of effective positions can be assumed to facilitate effective expulsive efforts. The nurse must assess the appropriateness of the woman's position and the efficacy of efforts to expel the fetus. Figure 24–4 illustrates a variety of commonly used positions for pushing in second-stage labor. If the parturient is uncomfortable with a particular position or efforts appear ineffective in bringing down the presenting part, the nurse should not hesitate to try a different approach.

Traditional Methods of Pushing.   Research has questioned the exclusive use of the lithotomy and other recumbent positions for pushing in the second stage of labor (Roberts 1987, Russell 1982). These positions cause maternal supine hypotension (due to aortal compression by the heavy uterus), which may result in fetal distress. Furthermore, the traditional methods of pushing or bear-

ing-down during the second stage have utilized the Valsalva maneuver. When the mother uses this type of bearing-down effort, she closes the glottis and pushes throughout a contraction, holding her breath as long as possible to build up intrathoracic pressure to assist in expelling the fetus. Hemodynamic changes result. Blood is driven from the pulmonary circulation into the left heart, causing maternal blood pressure to rise. However, as breath-holding continues, the blood pressure begins to fall steadily. The longer the breath is held, the lower the blood pressure may drop. Subsequent breath-holding episodes have a cumulative effect as well. Effects on the mother include exhaustion, cardiovascular strain due to blood pressure changes, and possible tissue damage with the birth. Fetal effects may be even more pronounced. During a Valsalva maneuver of 6 seconds or more, maternal oxygenation is impaired and placental blood flow decreases. This may result in increased fetal blood pH, decreased PO_2, increased PCO_2, and an increased incidence of fetal heart rate abnormalities. Prolonged maternal bearing down may result in fetal hypoxia and acidosis, and in lower Apgar scores for the newborn.

The Valsalva maneuver has also been found to stimulate the maternal sympathetic nervous system and thus increase catecholamine release. This response may decrease uterine activity, adversely affecting progress in labor.

Open-Glottis Pushing.   Recently, an alternative style of pushing has been proposed for use in the second stage. Called "open-glottis" or "gentle" pushing, this style encourages the woman to push in short, 6- to 7-second periods and *only* when she has the urge to do so (not continuously through each contraction), and to push while exhaling slightly, which ensures an open glottis.

When the woman in labor exhales while pushing, cardiovascular changes are not as pronounced. High intrathoracic pressure is not maintained and there is minimal rise and fall in maternal blood pressure. Some suggest that placental blood flow is maintained with this method, and fetal hypoxia and distress is therefore decreased. Research has demonstrated that women who used open-glottis or exhalation pushing may have babies with higher umbilical arterial and venous blood pH and better Apgar scores than babies whose mothers used prolonged breathholding when pushing (Caldeyro–Barcia 1979).

Open-glottis pushing has other benefits as well. It allows for relaxation of the perineum and gentle delivery of the infant's head. It is also a pushing style women naturally adopt when they have not been trained to push in the traditional manner. Roberts and associates described these voluntary, periodic, short bearing-down efforts of women in the second stage and found that progress was adequate and fetal outcome good when prolonged breath-holding was avoided (Roberts 1987).

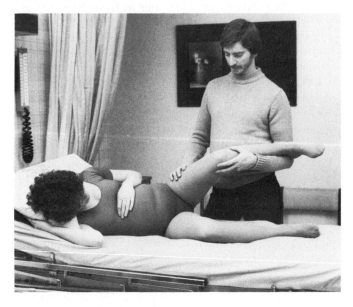

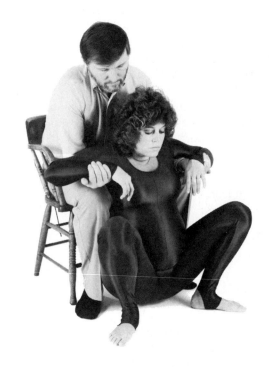

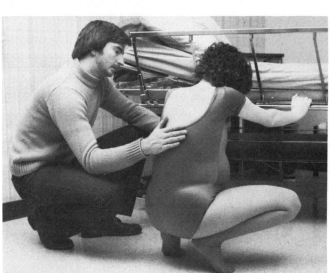

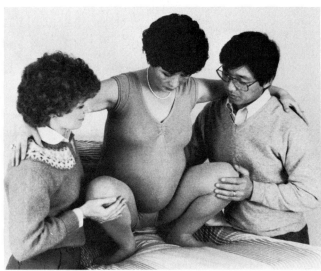

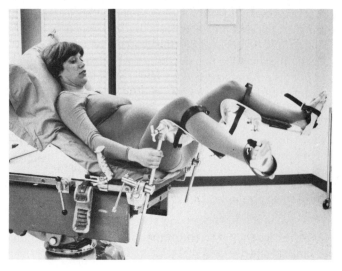

Figure 24–4. Commonly used positions for pushing in second-stage labor. Most of these positions take advantage of gravity to aid bearing-down efforts. Many of these positions are ones laboring women will naturally assume for bearing down, if position choices are not restricted.

The urge-to-push comes and goes, occurring in "surges" three to five times during each contraction. The nurse may feel the surges by palpating the fundus. Increased tension in the uterus is felt for 5 to 7 seconds. If the mother is encouraged to behave spontaneously, her behavior will include short, 5- to 7-second breath-holds during these surges, with time for several breaths in between (Roberts 1987). Grunting or other expiratory sounds may be heard.

Restraint in Pushing. In some instances, uterine contractions are so intense and descent of the fetal head so rapid, that expulsive efforts must be restrained to prevent perineal lacerations. In this case, the woman must be coached to pant or pant-blow through the contractions. Assuming a side-lying position may also help to decrease the urge to push.

Maternal position can be varied during the second stage for the following reasons:

- Promote comfort
- Enhance or slow down fetal descent
- Rotate a malpositioned baby
- Avoid exacerbation of hemorrhoids
- Increase bearing-down sensations
- Protect the perineum from lacerations or episiotomy
- Intervene when fetal distress occurs due to umbilical cord compression or supine hypotension

Expected Outcome:

- The woman in labor uses effective breathing and expulsive techniques.
- The woman in labor assumes positions that facilitate expulsive efforts, maintain placental perfusion, and prevent or alleviate umbilical cord compression.

CARE OF THE FAMILY DURING BIRTH

The atmosphere surrounding birth often appears chaotic, since nursing tasks during this time are varied and urgent, and the birth occurs in a relatively short period of time. The following are nursing priorities immediately prior to and following birth:

- Monitoring maternal and fetal physiologic status
- Preparing supplies and equipment needed for delivery
- Giving emotional support to both the father and woman in labor

- Assisting the mother and father with position changes and viewing the birth
- Supporting the mother's bearing-down efforts and instructing her, as necessary
- Administering medications, including analgesics and oxytocics as ordered
- Performing the initial assessment of the newborn
- Following identification procedures for newborn

Monitoring Maternal and Fetal Physiologic Status

The nurse must continue to monitor maternal vital signs (blood pressure, pulse, and respirations) at 10- to 15-minute intervals during the final moments before birth. The fetal heart rate is also evaluated after each contraction. If electronic fetal monitoring has been employed, and the mother is transferred to a delivery room for the birth, it is imperative the monitor be reapplied, when the mother is positioned on the delivery table, and the fetus continuously monitored until birth.

Preparing for Delivery
Supplies for Asepsis

Infection control guidelines for asepsis during delivery will vary from facility to facility. Sterile technique is used in the conventional hospital delivery room or operating room. Caps, masks, shoe covers, and sterile gowns and gloves are required for personnel, and the father is given a cap, mask, shoe covers, and gown. Once the woman is positioned on the delivery table, a perineal scrub is often done, and the area is draped. A delivery pack of sterile instruments will be opened and laid out for the physician or nurse midwife. This pack contains the instruments used for an episiotomy, for suctioning the neonate, and for clamping and cutting the umbilical cord.

In a labor room or alternative birth center delivery, personnel usually wear clean gowns and sterile gloves for the delivery; masks and caps are usually not worn. A small sterile field may be created by putting a sterile drape under the woman's buttocks just before delivery; a perineal scrub is optional and may be limited to cleansing of only the perineum and anal area. A sterile instrument pack will be opened and laid out. Infection rates have not been shown to be increased in settings using these more relaxed guidelines for asepsis in normal childbirth.

Equipment and Personnel Needed for Delivery

A large quantity of equipment is not necessary for a spontaneous vaginal birth. Essential equipment, usually provided in a standard delivery pack, includes the following items:

- Gloves for the birth attendant
- Sterile drapes

- Gauze sponges for drying the infant's face
- Bulb syringe for suctioning the infant
- Two clamps for the umbilical cord
- Two scissors: one for the cord and one for the episiotomy, if needed
- A large basin for the placenta
- Gauze sponges and ring forceps for inspection of the vagina and perineum

In addition, there is an infant linen pack containing infant blankets, sterile towels for handling the neonate, and a cap. All equipment and linen should be handled with aseptic technique and should be readily available to the birth attendant. An additional light source should be available in case it is needed. A radiant warmer for use during the initial assessment of the neonate and access to resuscitation equipment are important. The nurse should verify that this equipment is present and in working order prior to delivery (Fig. 24–5).

A birth attendant and a labor nurse should be present. When neonatal complications are anticipated, a pediatrician and a nursery nurse are essential and should be called in advance. If additional staff are called, the labor nurse should provide them with a brief summary of the labor and introduce them to the parents.

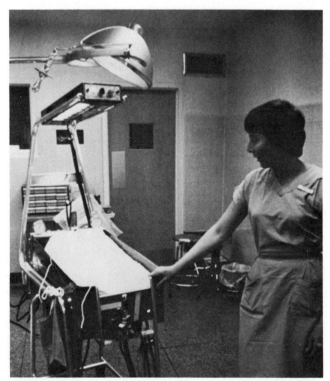

Figure 24–5. The labor nurse checks the radiant heat crib used in a conventional delivery room setting. (Photo: BABES, Inc.)

Transfer to Delivery Room

If the birth is to take place in the delivery room, the primigravida should be transferred by gurney or in the labor bed when the perineum is bulging. The multipara should be transferred at 8 cm of cervical dilatation. If electronic fetal monitoring has been used, this equipment accompanies the patient to the delivery room. To the extent possible, the nurse should leave ample time for a calm transfer, allowing the patient to move between contractions.

Positioning for Delivery

Throughout history, women have preferred the upright position for childbirth. However, in the last 50 years most women in the United States have given birth in the lithotomy, modified lithotomy, or recumbent position. Many reasons have been suggested for these positions including increased use of analgesics and anesthesia, operative delivery, continuous electronic fetal monitoring, episiotomy, and the more active management of delivery by the attendant (Rossi 1986).

Recently, this practice has come into question. The lithotomy position for birth has been linked to increased perineal lacerations and maternal discomfort caused by stretching the leg muscles, torsion on the hip joints, and pressure on the coccyx. Thus, the lithotomy position does not facilitate physiologic labor and birth and can be a disadvantage to the mother and infant. This position is the position of choice only when operative procedures are needed to complete the delivery.

Use of the Lithotomy Position for Birth

Indications

- Operative delivery
- Obstetric procedures
- Episiotomy or laceration repair
- Choice of birth attendant

Technique

1. Place a rolled towel or cushion under the woman's right hip to displace the uterus to the left to alleviate the effects of the supine hypotension syndrome.
2. Dorsiflex the patient's feet, if she experiences leg cramps; pad the stirrups for comfort.
3. Minimize the length of time this position is used.
4. Remove both patient's legs together from the stirrups to avoid trauma to the sacroiliac joints.

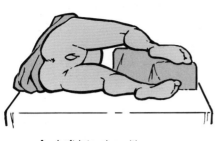

A   Left lateral position

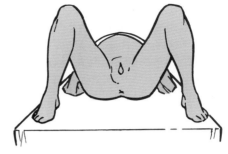

B   Dorsal position

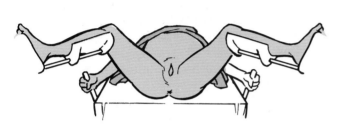

C   Lithotomy position

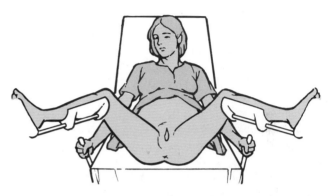

D   Back elevated: semisitting position

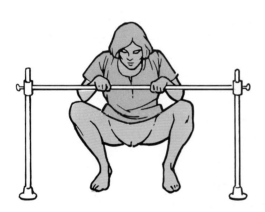

E   Squatting position

Figure 24–6. Positions for delivery. *(A)* Left lateral position. *(B)* Dorsal position. *(C)* Lithotomy position. *(D)* Back elevated and semisitting position. *(E)* Squatting position.

Any delivery position used should allow the bearing-down efforts of the mother to be aided by gravity, promote fetal descent and rotation, and avoid supine hypotension. Descent and rotation are best aided by a position that provides for mobility of the pelvis into a pelvic tilt so that the sacral promontory is pulled away from the uterus, creating larger pelvic diameters in all planes. Radiographic studies have shown an increase of 0.5 to 2.0 cm in pelvic diameters when the mother is in a squatting position (Russell 1982). Figure 24–6 illustrates phys-

iologic positions for delivery. It should be kept in mind that no one position is ideal for second-stage labor. Each must be evaluated according to the particular circumstances.

Positioning the woman properly on the delivery table or bed is an important nursing responsibility. It requires practice and familiarity with the equipment, which may be a birthing chair, a birthing bed, or a conventional delivery table, as shown in Figure 24–7.

If a conventional delivery table is to be used, the

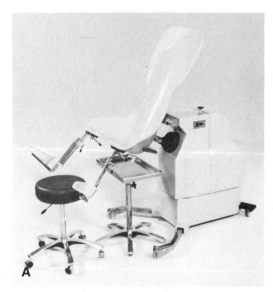

Figure 24–7. To accommodate a range of maternal positions in second-stage labor, birth settings utilize a variety of beds and equipment. *(A)* A modern birthing chair that enables the woman to maintain a semisitting position while still allowing easy access to the perineum.

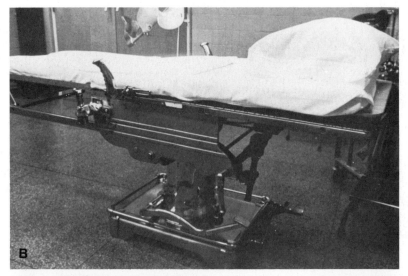

(B) A standard delivery room table in its extended or flat position, which also serves as an operative table if cesarean delivery is needed.

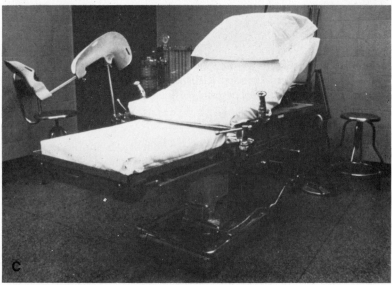

(C) The same table in its "broken" position, ready for use in second-stage labor; this position will support the woman in a semisitting position for delivery. (Photo A courtesy of Century Manufacturing Co., Inc.; B and C, BABES, Inc.)

NURSING RESEARCH

The Effects of The Birthing Chair on Maternal Outcomes in Labor and Delivery

Although many practitioners now question the automatic use of the lithotomy position for birth, few studies have clearly demonstrated that the use of the birth chair is advantageous. Researchers have reported mixed findings. Several studies have demonstrated shortened second-stage labor for multiparas using the chair. Other investigators have found no differences. The effect of the birthing chair on blood loss and perineal swelling is also unclear. Some clinical researchers suggest that the chair should be pivoted to a horizontal position after birth of the infant or significant blood loss can occur with placental separation and from the episiotomy site.

Further study is indicated. Currently practitioners may continue to use the birthing chair, but should observe the perineum closely during second-stage expulsive efforts for signs of edema. They may also consider changing the position of the chair to the horizontal plane immediately after birth, if an episiotomy was performed or significant bleeding occurs.

Shannahan MD, Cottrell BH: Effect of the birth chair on duration of second-stage labor and maternal outcome. Nurs Res 35:364–366, 1986

woman should be positioned in a semisitting position with the head of the table elevated from 30° to 60° or with pillows and partner assistance used to support the woman's back and head as shown in Figure 24–8. The bottom of the delivery table should remain extended until the birth attendant is present.

If stirrups are to be used, the woman's legs should be positioned simultaneously, and both stirrups should be adjusted for the woman's comfort. The nurse should check that excessive pressure is not placed on the calf or popliteal area because this may predispose the woman to thrombophlebitis in the postpartum period. The nurse should never leave a woman unattended, once she is positioned for delivery, and should respect the woman's modesty by covering her as much as possible while preserving an easy view of the perineum. A perineal scrub may be done at this time, followed by sterile draping of the area.

Modern delivery tables allow a variety of positions for delivery, which promotes the woman's comfort and gives the birth attendant a clear view and good access to the perineum. The woman's body should be supported so that she can curl forward and pull on handles with bearing-down efforts, yet relax between contractions.

Maternal position and preparation procedures vary more widely in labor or birthing room deliveries. Birthing beds eliminate the need for transferring the mother to a delivery table, and stirrups are usually not used (Fig. 24–9). Draping is usually not done, and a minimal perineal scrub may be done just before delivery, or may be omitted altogether.

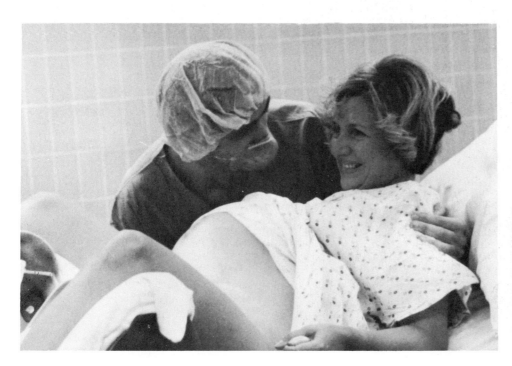

Figure 24–8. Maternal bearing-down efforts in a conventional delivery room. The mother is supported in a semirecumbent position by pillows and by her partner. Her legs are supported by well-padded stirrups; handholds are in place to assist pushing efforts. (Photo: BABES, Inc.)

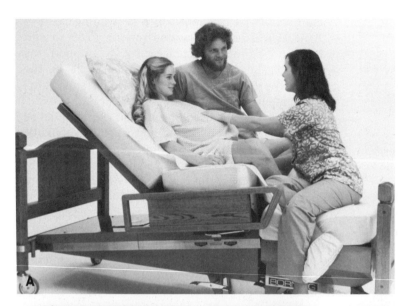

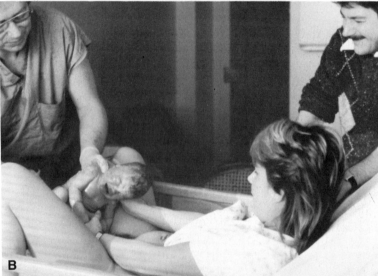

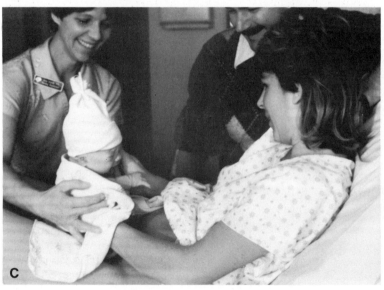

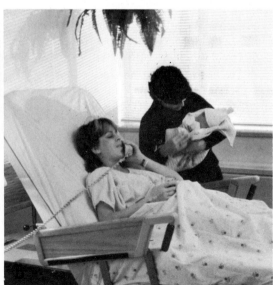

Figure 24–9. The trend toward use of a single room for labor, birth, and postpartum recovery has been made possible by the development of birthing beds that offer a range of positions for labor and birth. *(A)* A birthing bed as used in labor. *(B)* A birthing bed used for delivery in a semisitting position, which allows immediate contact with the newborn *(C)* while still allowing easy access for third-stage labor care. *(D)* The same unit as a postpartum room, allowing the mother to rest comfortably after birth without transfer to another room. The mother will remain in this room until discharge. (Photo courtesy of Hill–Rom)

As the mother pushes, the baby's head will advance, receding between bearing-down efforts until the vaginal opening completely encircles the head. This event is known as "crowning." If the amniotic sac is still intact at this point, the birth attendant will tear it to prevent the neonate from aspirating amniotic fluid with its first respiratory effort. If it appears that the vaginal opening will lacerate before the head is delivered, the birth attendant will administer local anesthesia, either through infiltration of the perineum or by pudendal block, and will perform an episiotomy as shown in Figure 24–10.

Episiotomy

Episiotomy is an incision made from the lower aspect of the vaginal opening into the perineum during the second stage to enlarge the opening to accommodate the fetal head; this is done in an attempt to prevent tearing the underlying muscle and fascia as the head is born. Episiotomy is the second most common surgical procedure performed, excluding cutting of the umbilical cord. Over 65% of vaginal deliveries in the United States include episiotomy. Among primigravidas, the incidence reaches 80%.

The routine use of episiotomy is controversial. Nurse midwifery practice has historically relied on nonsurgical methods of protecting the perineum during the second stage, including perineal massage and the use of alternative maternal positions to enhance perineal stretching while minimizing pressure on the tissue. Physicians may perform episiotomy more often because they have not

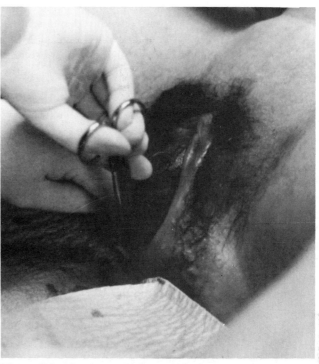

Figure 24–10. The birth attendant performs an episiotomy to facilitate delivery. (Photo: BABES, Inc.)

Benefits and Risks of Episiotomy

Benefits of Episiotomy

The following list reflects general beliefs that are based on observations in clinical practice and are not necessarily documented by clinical research.

- Maternal

  May maintain pelvic floor integrity
  May lower incidence of serious lacerations with delivery of large infant
  Heals more rapidly than a laceration

- Fetal

  Shortens second stage, which may be important with compromised fetus
  May prevent fetal brain damage by reducing pressure on fetal head from pelvic floor; may be important with premature fetus

- Obstetric

  Facilitates obstetric maneuvers, such as forceps delivery, vacuum extraction
  Facilitates delivery of malpresenting or large infants
  Shortens second stage

Risks of Episiotomy

The following risks have been documented in clinical research and practice:

- Severe postepisiotomy pain is estimated to occur in 60% of women
- Risk of infection is increased
- Pain and edema may inhibit urination and defecation after delivery
- Risk of significant blood loss is increased
- Risk of persistent dyspareunia, which may last 6 months or more, is increased

had extensive experience in delivering over an intact perineum. Scientific studies to date have not demonstrated benefits of episiotomy in well-controlled clinical trials, and the risks of episiotomy are not insignificant (Banta 1982).

Types of Episiotomy

There are two major types of episiotomy: the median and the mediolateral, shown in Figure 24–11. Both are usually performed under local anesthesia by the physician or nurse midwife as shown in Figure 24–12. In some cases, the perineum is naturally numbed by stretching and the pressure of the fetal head, and the episiotomy can be performed without anesthesia, if necessary. Infiltration of the perineum itself with lidocaine produces perineal anesthesia both for the episiotomy and for its repair. Injection of lidocaine, using long needle guides, into the vaginal walls near the ischial spines blocks pain impulses through the pudendal nerve and provides anesthesia of the lower two thirds of the vagina and the perineum. This technique, known as *pudendal block,* also provides short-duration anesthesia for delivery and perineal repair. It is safe and effective and has little effect on the fetus. Pudendal block may temporarily blunt the mother's urge to bear down in the second stage.

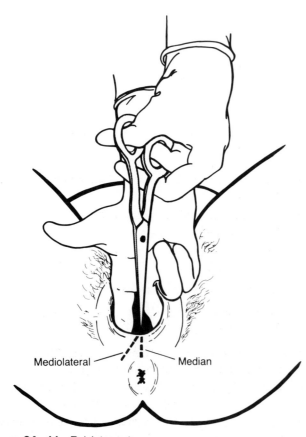

Mediolateral ———   Median

Figure 24–11. Episiotomy types.

Median Incision. The median episiotomy incision is the type most commonly used in the United States. It is reported to be easier to repair, less painful, less disfiguring, and associated with less blood loss and more rapid healing than the mediolateral incision. A disadvantage of the median incision is a higher incidence of extension (tearing beyond the incision) through the anal sphincter into the rectum.

Mediolateral Incision. The mediolateral episiotomy incision is used frequently in Europe and other parts of the world. Its advantages are that it provides more room for obstetric maneuvers and has less tendency to extend into the rectum than the median episiotomy. However, its disadvantages are regarded as significant and account for the rarity of its use in the United States. They include increased difficulty in repairing the incision, longer wound healing time, increased blood loss, greater distortion in perineal configuration, and consequent sexual dysfunction, including persistent dyspareunia.

The decision as to whether an episiotomy is necessary must be made by the birth attendant, with as much participation as possible by the patient. No woman can be guaranteed that episiotomy will not be necessary, since many unexpected events may occur during labor and birth. The nurse can play an important role in minimizing the need for episiotomy during the intrapartal period.

When the patient wishes to avoid episiotomy and the birth attendant is cooperative, the nurse may use the following techniques to maximize the chances that the perineum will remain intact as shown in Figure 24–13.

- Apply hot compresses to the perineum during the second stage of labor to promote relaxation, increased circulation, and increased pliability of the perineal tissues.
- Encourage gentle pushing during the second stage to allow for gradual distention of the perineal tissue.
- Encourage the patient to avoid bearing-down efforts when crowning occurs.
- Use a lubricant to massage the perineum during the second stage.
- Apply an icepack on the clitoral or periurethral area during crowning to reduce the burning and stinging that accompany stretching of the vagina and to enhance perineal relaxation.
- Use maternal positions for delivery that avoid overstretching the perineum, such as the sidelying or semisitting positions. When stirrups are used, position to avoid hyperextension of the legs and extreme perineal stretching.

Some conditions necessitate the use of episiotomy, and the birth attendant is in the best position to deter-

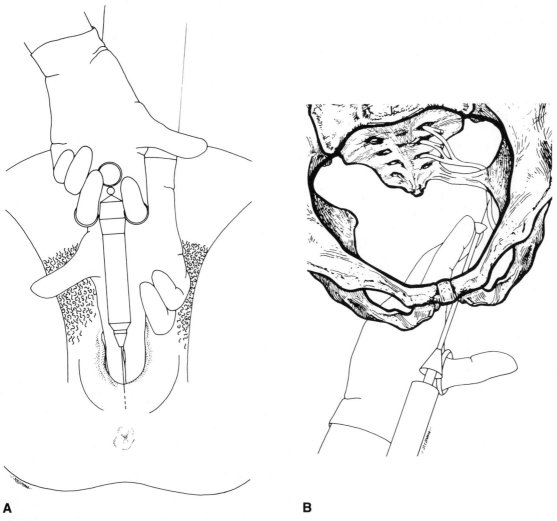

A   **B**

Figure 24–12. Local anesthesia for episiotomy. *(A)* Local infiltration of the perineum. *(B)* Pudendal block. (Childbirth Graphics)

mine the best course of action for the health of mother and infant. The nurse can encourage women to avoid unnecessary episiotomy by using these techniques but should discourage women from focusing on this intervention to the detriment of the rest of the birth experience.

Lacerations of the Perineum and Vaginal Tract

Lacerations of the perineum, the vagina, occasionally the cervix, or, rarely, the body of the uterus may occur during delivery. Cervical or uterine lacerations usually occur in association with difficult deliveries or operative procedures for delivery. Factors associated with lacerations of the perineum and vagina include the following:

- Rapid, precipitous, uncontrolled delivery

- Malpresentations, such as occiput posterior or face presentation
- Use of exaggerated lithotomy position
- Use of perineal anesthesia
- Friable or tense maternal tissue
- Operative delivery
- Inadequate length of episiotomy incision

Lacerations are classified according to the tissues involved, as follows:

- *First degree:* involving the skin or vaginal mucosa but not extending into the muscular layers
- *Second degree:* extending from the skin and vaginal mucosa into the muscles of the perineum
- *Third degree:* extending from the skin, vaginal mucosa, and muscle into the anal sphincter

Delivery of the Neonate

The birth attendant applies gentle pressure on the advancing head to control the delivery and prevent too-rapid expulsion. The other hand supports the perineum and prepares to receive the head as it emerges. The mother is instructed to pant or breathe through her contractions and to bear down only when asked to do so. The nurse should explain that this assists in controlling the birth, and reduces the risk of an over-rapid delivery. The head is usually delivered between contractions.

Once the head is delivered, the birth attendant suctions the mouth and nose and checks for a nuchal cord. This is done by inserting two fingers along the back of the neonate's neck. A nuchal cord (a loop of umbilical cord around the baby's neck) is found in approximately 25% of deliveries and usually causes no difficulty. The loose loop is pulled out and slipped over the baby's head to allow for delivery (Fig. 24–14); the attendant should then feel for a second loop and remove it in the same way. If the loop is too tight to be pulled over the head, it is double-clamped and cut between the clamps.

The birth attendant then holds the head in both hands and applies gentle downward pressure to ease the anterior shoulder under the symphysis. The woman is then asked to push gently to deliver the anterior shoulder; gentle upward pressure is then applied to deliver the pos-

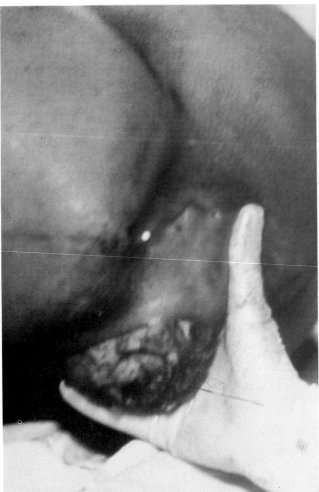

Figure 24–13. Thinned-out perineum. This mother has chosen to deliver in a squatting position; note how the nurse midwife has "ironed out" the perineum to stretch easily and without resistance over the baby's head. (Photo: Kathy Sloane)

- *Fourth degree:* extending through the rectal mucosa into the lumen of the rectum

Other genital lacerations that may result from vaginal delivery include *periurethral tears,* which occur near the urethral meatus, and *periclitoral tears,* which occur near the clitoris. Lacerations may bleed profusely, depending on their location and degree. They are generally repaired in the same way as an episiotomy. (See Labor: Third Stage, later in this chapter.)

The vagina and perineum are routinely examined after delivery for lacerations or extension of an episiotomy. Cervical inspection may not be done routinely because of maternal discomfort, but if cervical bleeding is suspected, inspection will be necessary. It may be done under pudendal block or, less frequently, under light inhalation anesthesia.

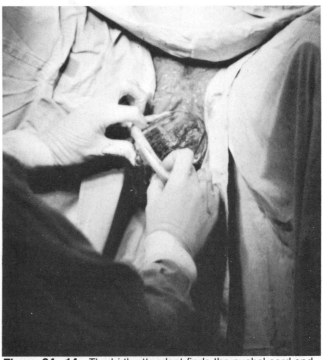

Figure 24–14. The birth attendant finds the nuchal cord and slips the loop over the baby's head. Notice the sterile draping in a delivery room setting. (Photo: BABES, Inc.)

terior shoulder. The rest of the baby slips out easily, once the shoulders are delivered. The nurse should note the time of delivery for recording purposes and for timing 1- and 5-minute Apgar scoring.

The birth attendant typically shows the baby to the parents briefly, then will hold the baby at the level of the introitus in a head-down position to facilitate drainage of mucus and perfusion through the umbilical cord. The

birth attendant will place the newborn in a head-down position, dry it, and assess for adequacy of respiratory effort. If stimulation is necessary, it is administered by rubbing the newborn's back and the soles of the feet briskly until respiratory effort is satisfactory. The newborn is then typically placed skin-to-skin on the mother's abdomen with the head turned to the side and slightly lowered to facilitate the drainage of mucus. This should

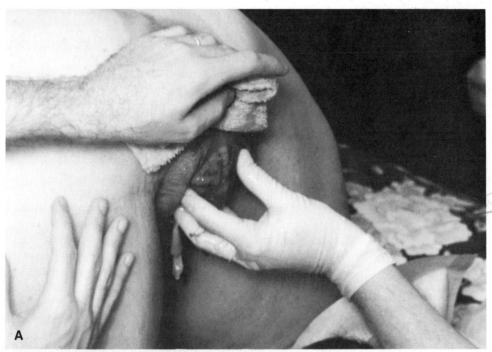

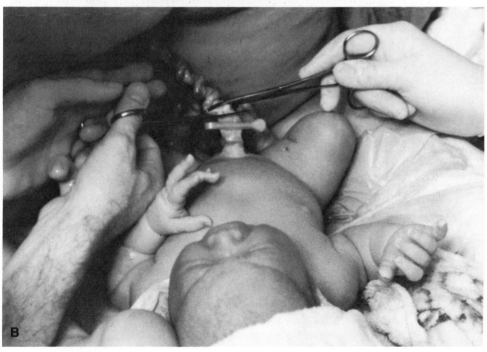

Figure 24–15. This woman has chosen to deliver in a hands-and-knees position. *(A)* The birth attendant controls delivery of the head while the father's hands provide perineal support. *(B)* The baby has been quickly dried and suctioned; the cord has been clamped and the father cuts it. (Photo: BABES, Inc.)

be done without traction on the umbilical cord. The newborn should then be dried and covered for warmth.

When cord pulsation has ceased, two sterile clamps are placed on the cord 2 to 4 inches from the umbilicus, and the cord is cut between the clamps with sterile scissors. Some birth attendants permit the father to cut the cord, under close supervision, as seen in Figure 24 – 15.

The birth attendant then observes for signs of placental separation (slight gush of blood from the vagina, lengthening of cord, rising of rounded uterine fundus palpable through the abdomen). When these signs are observed, the mother is asked to push slightly with a contraction to deliver the placenta. The placenta is received into a basin for later examination.

CARE OF THE FAMILY IN THIRD-STAGE LABOR

The third stage of labor is defined as the period from delivery of the neonate through separation and expulsion of the placenta. This period is usually one of dramatic release and high emotion for the new mother and her partner as they greet the newborn. Nursing responsibilities during this relatively short period of time are many and pressing, such as ongoing assessment of maternal and neonatal status, completion of delivery records, obtaining and labeling laboratory samples, and facilitating early parent – neonate interaction. The nurse must anticipate patient needs during this period as well, such as monitoring for signs of excessive postpartum bleeding, and obtaining any additional instruments or supplies needed by the birth attendant.

Assessment

The birth attendant is responsible for monitoring signs of placental separation and delivery during this stage of labor. Nursing priorities during this period focus on the assessment of neonatal and maternal physiologic status, and early family responses to the newborn.

Neonatal Physiologic Status: Apgar Score

The nurse is responsible for most aspects of the initial assessment of the normal newborn. The birth attendant suctions the nose and mouth and assesses spontaneous onset of respiration. Once respiration is established, additional assessment of the newborn begins, using the Apgar score.

Apgar scores are recorded officially at 1 and 5 minutes after birth. However, initial assessments of the newborn's

condition and necessary steps to support respiration and cardiac function are completed immediately after delivery. Responsibility for designating the Apgar score may be the birth attendant's or the nurse's, depending on standard procedures in the facility.

As soon as the infant is born, the nurse notes the exact time. Assessment of the newborn's transition to extra-uterine life begins immediately, whether the infant is placed under a radiant warmer or on the maternal abdomen. The Apgar scoring system is used to assess heart rate, respiratory effort, muscle tone, reflex irritability, and color. The optimum score is 10, with 2 points being given for each criterion, as shown in Table 24 – 1.

The initial newborn assessment and 1- and 5-minute Apgar scores are generally completed during this time; the normal newborn remains with its parents under the watchful eye of the nurse. The nurse observes the neonate carefully for abnormal skin color (mottling or cyanosis of face and trunk) as well as signs of respiratory difficulty, and monitors thermoregulation in the newborn.

Maternal Physiologic Status

Maternal physiologic status during the third stage of labor is determined primarily through monitoring blood pressure, the process of placental separation and delivery, and blood loss. Maternal blood pressure and pulse should be monitored before and after signs of placental separation are noted. If uterine bleeding is excessive, an increasing pulse rate may be the first sign; any drop in blood pressure caused by bleeding will be temporarily compensated for by the increased systemic volume created by loss of the placental circulation. However, this compensation is only temporary, and hypotension and hypovolemic shock can develop quickly in the newly delivered woman.

Family Responses to the Newborn

The nurse observes and notes the parents' first responses to the newborn. These responses often give clues to the extent to which parents have attached to their infant prenatally and provide information that helps direct ongoing family-centered care.

Parents are often overjoyed with the arrival of the newborn, immediately ask about its gender and its health, and call it by name (Fig. 24 – 16). First-time parents often express wonder and pleasure at the newborn's appearance.

However, behavioral responses vary widely and depend on many factors, including:

- Maternal fatigue level
- Administration of analgesia or anesthesia
- Level of discomfort or pain
- Maternal parity
- Cultural background

Table 24–1   **Apgar Scoring**

Sign	Score*		
	0	1	2
Heart rate	Absent	Slow (below 100)	Over 100
Respiratory rate	Absent	Slow, irregular	Good, crying
Muscle tone	Flaccid	Some flexion of extremities	Active motion
Reflex irritability†	No response	Grimace	Cry
Color	Blue, pale	Body pink, extremities blue	Completely pink

* This method is used for evaluating the immediate postnatal adjustment of the newborn baby. The total score of the five signs if 8 to 10 when the initial adjustment is good. Infants with lower scores require special attention. Scores under 4 indicate that the child is seriously depressed.

† Tested by inserting the tip of a catheter into the nostril.

(Courtesy of Virginia Apgar, M.D., and Smith, Kline & French Laboratories, Philadelphia)

The nurse must be cautious about drawing conclusions regarding the nature of the parent–infant acquaintance process based on initial maternal responses. Many birthing units employ an assessment tool that documents maternal behavioral responses in the immediate postbirth period. The data collected should be viewed only as a beginning evaluation of parent–infant attachment, and this nursing assessment must be placed within the context of the factors listed above.

If family responses to the newborn do not seem to fit the expected norm, additional observation and interaction with the parents will be needed before a conclusive nursing diagnosis can be made. Responses that reflect some difficulty in prenatal attachment or signal the parent–infant relationship may be at risk include an unwillingness to hold or look at the newborn, expressions of displeasure about appearance or sex, and blaming the newborn for a difficult labor and birth. If these responses continue into the postpartum period, there is a possibility that the parent–infant relationship may be at risk.

The third stage of labor passes relatively quickly (5–30 minutes); the nurse is unlikely to establish new nursing diagnoses during this brief period. However, this time is important for beginning the assessment of maternal, neonatal and family adaptation. During this time, the nurse also begins to plan for transfer of the mother and her

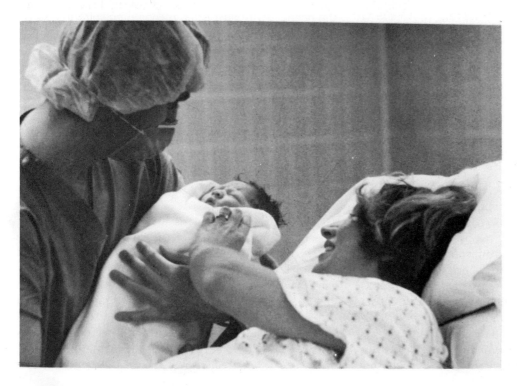

Figure 24–16. Happy parents greet their newborn. (Photo: BABES, Inc.)

family from the delivery room to a recovery room and, if necessary, for the initiation of postpartum care and transfer of the newborn to the admission nursery.

Diagnosis

The following are nursing diagnoses that reflect possible problems that may arise during the third stage of labor and may be addressed independently by the nurse. Priorities in care may be established based on the following:

- Potential ineffective airway clearance (newborn)
- Hypothermia (newborn)
- Altered comfort related to involution of uterus
- Potential altered parenting

Complications requiring collaboration with other health care team members may arise during the third stage of labor. In addition to routine nursing care, the nurse is responsible for monitoring for potential complications. Such complications include postpartum hemorrhage (maternal), need for perineal repair, and cord/placental abnormalities.

Planning and Implementation

The nurse's primary task during the third stage of labor is to monitor maternal and newborn status and support the family unit. The nurse also remains alert to the needs of the birth attendant and provides any required assistance. Nursing interventions center on supporting maternal physiologic status, supporting the newborn's transition to extrauterine life, and supporting the family unit through assistance with interaction and early breast-feeding.

Promoting Newborn Physiologic Adaptation

Initial assessment of the newborn, including 1- and 5-minute Apgar scoring, is usually completed during this period. It is especially important to observe the newborn carefully for signs of respiratory difficulty and to ensure that heat loss is minimized. The newborn should be dried and covered while it is on the mother's abdomen. Mucus should be suctioned from the nares and mouth with a bulb syringe, as needed during this period, and the respiratory effort observed carefully. If the nurse has concerns about the newborn's status, it should be moved to a radiant warmer within sight of the parents, so careful obser-

vation is possible. If the newborn's status is good, a more complete neonatal assessment is usually deferred until after the third stage of labor is completed.

Suctioning and Positioning

The newborn very often has difficulty in getting rid of respiratory secretions. Immediate respiratory support of the newborn is discussed in greater detail in Chapter 33; major points are presented here in summary form. Suctioning with a rubber-bulb syringe or a mechanical suction device will help the newborn to maintain a patent airway. Bulb suctioning is used to clear mucus from nose and mouth. It can be done while the newborn is on the mother's abdomen or in her arms (Fig. 24–17).

Suctioning with a mechanical suction device is done to clear the nasopharynx, to aspirate gastric content, or to check patency of nares or esophagus. This method is more efficient than suctioning with a bulb syringe, and suctions deeper when necessary. It requires placing the newborn in a radiant warmer and positioning it on its back with the neck slightly extended. Deep suctioning should not be done routinely, but only in response to the need of the neonate. Prolonged suctioning may lead to bradycardia and other cardiac arrhythmias as a result of vagal stimulation.

Suctioning must be done as the head is born if respiratory efforts begin, or if amniotic fluid is meconium-stained. In the latter case, thorough suctioning and visualization of the vocal cords is done by the pediatrician or intensive care nursery nurse to prevent aspiration or to determine the extent of meconium aspiration. (Support of the neonate with suspected meconium aspiration is discussed in detail in Chapter 34.)

Positioning the normal, healthy baby immediately after birth should meet the following criteria:

- Allow for maintenance of an airway
- Provide a safe, secure location for the newborn
- Provide for thermoregulation of the newborn
- Allow for frequent assessment by the staff
- Facilitate drainage of secretions
- Facilitate family interaction and bonding

Any number of positions would meet these criteria, depending on the status of the infant. One commonly used position is placement of the infant on the mother's abdomen, skin to skin, with the infant's abdominal surface facing the mother. The infant usually clutches the mother's body and the mother or father can easily place a hand to secure the infant. The baby's head can be turned to the side easily to facilitate drainage of secretions. Warm blankets should be used to cover the infant, or a radiant warmer can be directed over the area. A hat should be

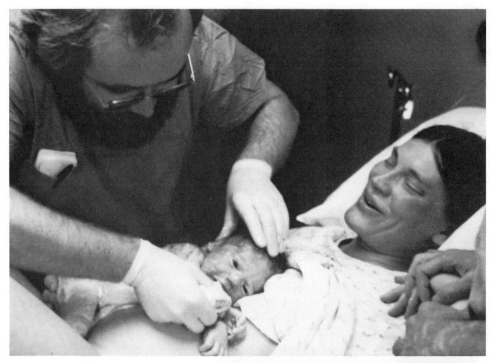

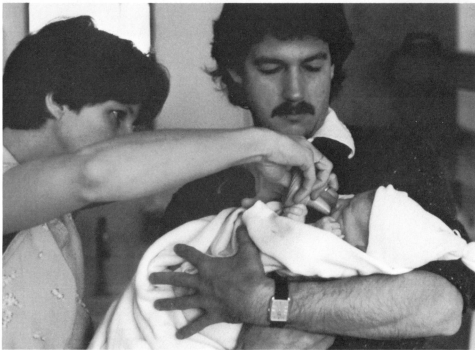

Figure 24–17. Bulb suctioning can be adapted to the delivery scene. *(A)* Conventional delivery room: The baby is placed on the mother's abdomen while the birth attendant continues suctioning. *(B)* Alternative birth center: father holds the baby while the labor nurse uses bulb suctioning. (Photo A: BABES, Inc.; B: Courtesy of Hill–Rom)

placed on the baby as well to prevent heat loss. Assessments of heart rate can be done by palpating the umbilical artery pulsations with a hand under the blankets or by auscultating, if needed or desired. Respiratory effort, reflex irritability, muscle tone, and color can be assessed as well. If there is difficulty in the assessment or a change in the status of the infant, the nurse should reposition the infant. The infant may also be positioned in the radiant warmer immediately after birth to facilitate the attendant's assessment or the performance of necessary procedures.

Expected Outcome: The newborn breathes spontaneously with a minimum of respiratory secretions.

Supporting Thermoregulation

At birth, the newborn's body temperature drops 3.5° to 5.3°F (2°–3°C) because it is no longer protected by the uterus and its body heat is conducted to cold objects that touch the infant's skin or is lost through (1) the evaporation of moisture from wet skin, (2) radiation to a cool environment, or (3) convection to cool air. The heat loss causes an increased need for oxygenation. In addition, the infant responds by vasoconstricting and increasing heat production through nonshivering thermogenesis, using stored brown fat. Hypothermia and resulting cold stress can become life-threatening, if severe or prolonged, as heart and respiratory rates decrease (see Chapter 31 for an in-depth discussion of neonatal thermoregulation).

Body heat can be maintained in the normal newborn by observing the following procedures:

- Providing a warm, draft-free environment for delivery
- Avoiding placing the baby in contact with cold instruments, hands, blankets, and so on
- Drying the baby thoroughly immediately after delivery

- Using radiant heat or skin-to-skin contact and covering the baby with warm blankets
- Placing a hat on the baby to prevent evaporative heat loss from wet hair.

Expected Outcome: Newborn maintains body temperature as measured by axillary body temperature between 36.4° and 37.2°C in the first hour.

Promoting Maternal Physiologic Adaptation

The nurse monitors maternal physiologic status during the third stage of labor primarily by attention to maternal blood loss and blood pressure before and after the placenta is delivered. Maternal blood pressure should be monitored every 5 to 10 minutes during this part of labor. The nurse should watch for signs of placental separation and may need to alert the mother to assist placental deliv-

Figure 24–18. Fundal massage. Two hands are used for fundal massage. One hand anchors the lower uterine segment just above the symphysis. The other gently massages the fundal area. (Childbirth Graphics)

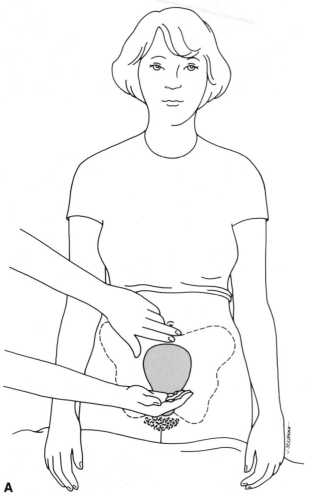

A

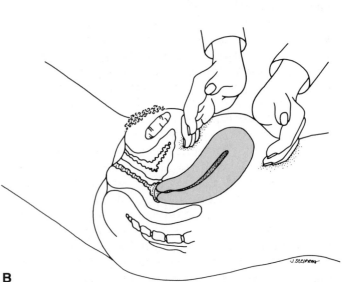

B

ery with bearing-down efforts. Blood pressure should be assessed shortly after the placenta is delivered and at regular intervals thereafter.

Massaging the Uterine Fundus

Massage of the uterine fundus in the immediate post-partum period stimulates the myometrium to contract and promotes hemostasis and the expulsion of clots. The nurse uses two hands for fundal massage: one hand anchors the lower uterine segment just above the symphysis while the other gently massages the fundal area as shown in Figure 24–18. Fundal massage must be done *gently,* with adequate support of the lower segment, because the uterine suspensory ligaments are relaxed after delivery and offer little resistance. Aggressive massage may result in partial or complete uterine prolapse, a serious obstetric complication. Further, fundal massage should be done only when the fundus is not firm, since overstimulation of the myometrium can contribute to muscle fatigue and a tendency toward relaxation.

The nurse should explain why the fundal massage is necessary, and further explain the contractionlike twinges of discomfort the woman will have during involution of the uterus (for further discussion see Chapter 29).

Expected Outcome: Postpartum mother expresses comfort with fundal massage and bleeding is within normal limits with firm uterine tone and normal maternal vital signs.

Promoting Behavioral Adaptation

Promoting Parent–Infant Interaction

If the newborn is placed on the mother's abdomen immediately after delivery, the nurse can encourage the parents to touch the newborn and to assist with drying and wrapping. If early breast-feeding is desired, the nurse should assist the mother into a comfortable position and help her to place the newborn to the breast. The nurse may want to stress that the newborn may be more interested in looking at its parents' faces than in breast-feeding in the first moments after birth (Fig. 24–19). The parents will progressively explore their baby, often unaware of other events around them.

The nurse can also encourage the father to hold the newborn in the first minutes after birth. The nurse should assess the father's physical and emotional state and should not hand the newborn to the father abruptly. Some men, especially first-time fathers, may feel very excited and shaken after birth, and may feel unprepared to handle their newborn immediately. The nurse may ask the father to take a seat at the mother's side before handing the well-wrapped newborn to the father.

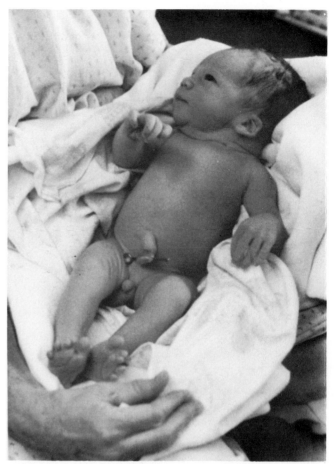

Figure 24–19. After the baby is dried he is returned to his parents. Notice his interest in his mother's face. (Photo: BABES, Inc.)

The period immediately following the birth can be very exciting for parents. When the newborn's condition is normal, the nurse should assist parents with interaction as soon as possible. If the neonatal support measures described in Chapter 33 are necessary to establish effective respiratory effort, the nurse should explain to the parents what is being done and assist parent-newborn interaction at the earliest safe opportunity.

Expected Outcome: Parents and newborn begin interaction characterized by intent face-to-face gazing and parental exploration of the newborn.

Monitoring for Potential Complications

Potential Complication: Postpartum Hemorrhage

Brisk bleeding immediately after deliver is usually caused by uterine atony. Fundal massage, administration of oxytocics, and nipple stimulation may all help to pro-

NURSING ALERT

Signs of Impending Postpartum Hemorrhage

Immediate nursing action is required if any of the following conditions are noted in the first 1 to 2 hr after delivery:

- Two perineal pads are soaked within 30 min (excessive bleeding)
- Mother complains of light-headedness, nausea, or visual disturbances (possible impending hypovolemic shock)
- Mother is anxious, skin color is pale or ashen, skin is clammy and cool (impending hypovolemic shock)
- Pulse and respirations are elevated, blood pressure is unchanged or slightly lowered (impending hypovolemic shock)

If any of the above are noted in the newly delivered woman, the nurse should take the following steps, in this order:

1. Summon help immediately by emergency call light; have care provider notified
2. Check uterine tone, massage fundus gently if not firm, and assess effect on bleeding and presence of clots, if any
3. Elevate patient's legs, lower head of bed to facilitate blood return
4. Increase intravenous infusion, if present, and start O₂ at 7–8 liter/min by mask
5. Start intravenous infusion with 16- to 18-gauge angiocath

---

mote uterine tone and hemostasis. The nurse must be alert for signs of impending postpartum hemorrhage.

If fundal massage and nipple stimulation are not sufficient to keep the uterus well contracted, the nurse must notify the birth attendant, who may order administration of oxytocics.

If bleeding is brisk and the uterus is firm, the placenta should be thoroughly examined for retained placental fragments or membranes, which may be preventing the myometrium from completely contracting. Placental fragments may be retained if uterine force is insufficient to expel the entire placenta; if attempts to remove the placenta manually leave shreds at resistant sites; if there are defects in the decidua; or if oxytocics are administered before there are clear signs of placental separation. Retained placental fragments are removed manually by the physician under sterile conditions. Once this is done, the uterus usually contracts firmly to maintain hemostasis.

Cervical, vaginal, or perineal tears, or an unligated vessel in an episiotomy can also bleed profusely. The repair must be done promptly to prevent further blood loss.

Administration of Oxytocics

Some birth attendants advocate the administration of oxytocics (Pitocin, Syntocin) immediately after delivery to promote uterine contractility and ensure hemostasis. Oxytocics may be given intramuscularly or added to intravenous fluids as the placenta delivers. The usual dose is 10 IU to 30 IU, given intramuscularly or added to 1 liter of fluid and infused over a period of hours. This medication generally is available in ampules containing 10 IU/ml. Oxytocin is usually *not* given in a bolus because doing so can induce hypotension and tachycardia. Intramuscular injection usually causes a transient burning sensation at the injection site.

Ergotrate (Ergonovine), a natural ergot preparation, and methylergonovine (Methergine), a synthetic ergot, may be given intramuscularly to stimulate a sustained tetanic-type contraction to control postpartum hemorrhage. The usual dose is 0.2 mg, given intramuscularly or orally. A single dose is usually sufficient to achieve hemostasis, but it can be repeated in 2 to 4 hours if needed.

These drugs are never administered intravenously or before delivery because they are powerful vasoconstrictors. Ergotrate is slightly more likely to cause elevation in blood pressure in normotensive women than is methylergonovine. Sudden hypertensive crisis and cerebral vascular accident may result with intravenous administration. These drugs are also contraindicated for women with hypertensive disease and for women who have received regional anesthesia because they are at risk for vasomotor instability. Either drug can be used safely in combination with oxytocin.

Measuring Maternal Blood Loss

The estimation of maternal blood loss is important in planning appropriate maternal care in the immediate postpartum period. At delivery, normal blood loss is derived by direct measurement from the placenta basin or other collection containers, and by assessing the amount of blood in drapes, towels, and sponges. On the average, a 300- to 400-ml blood loss can be expected during vaginal delivery with an episiotomy; this blood loss results from bleeding from the placental site. In addition, blood loss can result from any cervical, vaginal, or perineal tears or episiotomy.

The extent of blood loss provides an indication of the woman's relative risk for hypovolemic shock in the immediate postpartum period, as well as of the need for monitoring hemoglobin and hematocrit levels during the woman's postpartum recovery.

Assisting at Perineal Repair

The episiotomy or perineal lacerations are repaired by the birth attendant after the placenta is delivered and when the mother's condition permits. First-degree lacerations that are small (less than 1 cm) and not bleeding are often not repaired, since they will heal well without suturing. Other lacerations are sutured to ensure approximation of the wound edges and to reduce formation of scar tissue.

Perineal repair requires adequate anesthesia, usually through pudendal block or local infiltration of the perineum. Sutures are placed using sterile technique; often the birth attendant will request the nurse to assist with clean gloves and clean sterile drapes under the perineum and on the woman's abdomen. The birth attendant examines the vulva, perineum, and vagina for lacerations, and any extension of the episiotomy. The birth attendant applies direct pressure to bleeding sites using sterile pads; the vaginal incision will tend to bleed most. The birth attendant or the nurse should explain the procedure to the woman, and assess the adequacy of perineal anesthesia as suturing is begun. The vaginal mucosa is sutured first, beginning at the apex and working toward the perineum. Then the perineal muscle layers, the subcutaneous layers, and finally the skin edges are approximated and sutured.

Examination of the Placenta, Membranes, and Umbilical Cord

The nurse or birth attendant should examine the placenta and membranes to determine their completeness and to check for any abnormality. A technique for examining the placenta and membranes follows.

1. With the placenta maternal side down, grasp the membranes and approximate the edges to determine if they are complete.
2. Inspect the fetal side.
   a. Check the location of the insertion of the cord (central, marginal, or velamentous).
   b. Trace blood vessels to the periphery to detect any torn vessels, which might indicate a succenturiate or extra lobe of the placenta.
3. Inspect the maternal surface.
   a. Check the cotyledons to determine if they are all there.
   b. Observe for areas of abruption, infarction, or calcification.
4. Inspect the umbilical cord.
   a. Check the number of blood vessels (two arteries and one vein).
   b. Check the length of the cord (appropriate [50–55 cm], long, or short).
   c. Check for the presence of a true knot, varicosities, or other abnormalities.

The examination of the placenta may also be used as a teaching tool for patients, if they express a desire to see it. The nurse should chart the examination of the placenta, noting particularly any abnormalities, since these may have significance for the newborn.

Common Variations of the Placenta, Membranes, and Cord

Areas of *abruption* may be seen adhering to the maternal surface of the placenta. They appear dark red and clotted and indicate premature separation of the placenta before the third stage is completed. An area of abruption is measured in square centimeters of surface area covered or as a percentage of the total placental area.

An *infarct* may also be located on the maternal side of the placenta. It appears as a dense, sharply defined lesion in various shades of red, yellow, gray, or white. Infarcts are areas of placental necrosis with destruction of the intervillous space. They impair maternal-fetal exchange by decreasing the amount of functioning placental surface. Infarcts may be related to placental aging.

Calcifications, usually scattered randomly on the maternal surface, appear as white or gray dots. Although their significance is uncertain, they are often seen on the placentas of post-term, hypertensive, and diabetic gravidas and gravidas who smoke.

Circumvallate placenta is marked by a ring on the fetal surface, either complete or incomplete. It is significant because the placental vessels terminate at the ring and fold back upon themselves. This greatly reduces the functioning surface area of the placenta. This type of placenta may be related to uteroplacental insufficiency, late abortion, or stillbirth.

The *Battledore placenta* contains a velamentous insertion of the cord along the edge of the placenta. This tenuous attachment of the cord may sometimes be noted after a perfectly normal pregnancy, labor, and birth. However, it may also be related to fetal hemorrhage with cord detachment *in utero;* to small-for-gestational-age growth due to chronic uteroplacental insufficiency; or to fetal distress in labor, especially when the fetus descends and puts traction on the cord.

A *succenturiate lobe* is an aberrant lobe or entire cotyledon connected to the main body of the placenta by blood vessels, but it is anatomically separate. It may be torn off from the main portion of the placenta during separation and expulsion and be left behind, where it may cause postpartum hemorrhage or infection.

The cord occasionally contains two blood vessels (one artery and one vein) instead of the usual three (two arteries and one vein). This finding is associated with an increased possibility of other congenital abnormalities.

NURSING ALERT

Identification Procedures for the Newborn

The nurse is responsible for accurate identification of the newborn before mother and newborn are transferred out of the labor unit. Because prompt and accurate identification was lacking, newborns have been given to the wrong parents in maternity settings. To prevent this, the following procedures can be used:

• Apply matching identification bands showing name and patient record number on both mother and infant; usually two bands are placed on the infant (one wrist and one ankle). Take care to place bands on newborn snugly, since weight loss (5%–10% of birth weight) is common in the first days of life.

• Fingerprint the mother and footprint the newborn.* Take care to clean and dry both surfaces before taking the prints.

• When taking an infant to its mother, address the mother by name, and verify that the mother's band and infant's bands match.

* Not done in all birthing facilities. Very low birthweight infants lack identifying whorls and creases on hands and feet.

Expected Outcome: The postpartum woman remains free of complications as evidenced by a less than 300- to 400-ml blood loss and a normal placenta.

Documenting Intrapartal Care

A major nursing responsibility during the third stage of labor is accurate documentation of intrapartal care. Important details of this documentation include the following:

• Time of delivery of infant and placenta
• 1- and 5-minute Apgar scores
• Any immediate neonatal care required
• Extent and repair of perineal lacerations or episiotomy
• Estimated maternal blood loss
• Medications administered prior, during, and after delivery

• Placement of identification bands on mother and newborn; footprint identification of newborn
• Maternal vital signs

Most institutions have standard forms for documenting intrapartal care; an example is shown in the accompanying Assessment Tool, opposite page.

CARE OF THE FAMILY DURING FOURTH-STAGE LABOR

Although technically it is not part of labor, the immediate postpartum recovery period is sometimes labeled the fourth stage of labor because of its great importance. The first hour after the third stage has been completed is critical to maternal and neonatal recovery and important in the establishment of early family interaction and breast-feeding.

Many facilities that use conventional delivery rooms have a separate postpartum recovery room where mothers and their families are moved after third-stage labor is completed. In others the mother and newborn may recover in the delivery room itself for the first hour, and are then transported to the postpartum unit. Settings with single-unit maternity systems allow the mother and newborn to recover and remain in their room until discharge. Regardless of how immediate postpartum recovery care is arranged, close nursing observation is absolutely essential to ensure optimal maternal and neonatal adaptation and to promote optimal family interaction in the first hour after birth.

Assessment

An essential aspect of postdelivery care is careful assessment of maternal and neonatal status and of family responses to the newborn. These assessments are done frequently through the first hours after birth. Ideally, the nurse who accompanied the family during labor and birth should also provide this one-to-one recovery care.

Maternal Physiologic Status

The nurse should complete a systematic assessment of the mother's physiologic status, her comfort needs, and her needs for interaction, nutrition and hydration, and rest during the first few hours after delivery. Frequent assessments are necessary because changes in maternal status that can result in life-threatening complications—

ASSESSMENT TOOL

Delivery, Third Stage, and Newborn Record

SEROLOGY	TYPE Rh

LABOR

○ SPONTANEOUS ○ NONE
○ AUGMENTED ── ○ MEDICAL AGENT ____
○ INDUCED ── ○ SURGICAL

○ NORMAL   ○ FAILURE OF DESCENT
○ PROLONGED LATENT   ○ TRANSVERSE ARREST
○ ACTIVE PHASE ARREST   ○ PERSISTENT OP
○ SLOW SLOPE ACTIVITY   ○ PROLONGED 2ND STAGE
○ NONE

LABOR ONSET: DATE ___ TIME ___   END OF 1ST STAGE: DATE ___ TIME ___

MONITORING: ○ INTERNAL   ○ EXTERNAL   ○ BOTH   ○ NONE

FETAL SCALP SAMPLING: ○ NO   ○ YES   NUMBER ___   1st STAGE ___ HRS.-MIN.

ANESTHESIA   ○ GENERAL   ○ EPIDURAL   ○ SADDLE-BACK   ○ LOCAL/PUDENDAL   ○ PARACERVICAL   ANESTHESIA TIME ___ HRS.

MEDICATION DURING LAST HOUR OF LABOR:

DELIVERY   POSITION AT DELIVERY: ___   STATION: ___   DATE ___   TIME ___

VAGINAL   ○ VERTEX: ○ SPONTANEOUS   (○ ASSISTED   ○ UNASSISTED)
○ VACUUM EXTRACTOR (○ LOW   ○ MID*)
○ FORCEPS   (○ LOW   ○ MID*)

EPISIOTOMY   ○ BREECH:*   ○ SPONTANEOUS   (○ MAN. ASSIS. ○ EXTRACT   ○ FORCEPS)
○ MEDIAN   ○ MEDIOLATERAL   ○ NONE

2nd STAGE ___ HRS.-MIN.
○ *ROTATE   METHOD
FROM ___   ○ Manual
TO ___   ○ Forceps   ○ Vacuum

LACERATIONS:

ALTERNATIVE BIRTH PROGRAM: LABOR: ○ NO ○ YES   DELIVERY ○ NO ○ YES   POST PARTUM ○ NO ○ YES

LOCATION OF DELIVERY: ○ DR   ○ LABOR ROOM   ○ ABC   ○ OR   ○ Other ____

SECOND STAGE COMPLICATIONS:

CAESAREAN SECTION   ○ LOW TRANSVERSE   ○ LOW VERTICAL   ○ STERILIZATION   OPERATING TIME ___ HRS.
○ CLASSICAL   ○ HYSTERECTOMY   ○ OTHER ____

THIRD STAGE   PLACENTA: ○ EXPRESSED   ○ SPONTANEOUS   ○ REMOVED   DATE ___   TIME ___

UTERUS EXPLORED: ○ NO   ○ YES   COMMENT: ____

EBL ___ ML   PLAC. WT. ___ gm   CORD VESSELS ___   3rd STAGE ___ MIN.

THIRD STAGE COMPLICATIONS: TOTAL LABOR

MEDICATIONS: ___ HRS.-MIN.

INFANT   ○ FEMALE   ○ MALE   WEIGHT ___ gms   SUSTAINED RESPIRATION   ○ <90 SEC.   ○ ≥90 SEC.

RESPIRATION SPONTANEOUS: ○ YES   ○ NO   RESUSCITATED: ○ O₂   ○ MASK   ○ INTUBATION   ○ OTHER ____
NASOGASTRIC TUBE PASSED: ○ LEFT   ○ RIGHT

GASTRIC ASPIRATE: ___ cc   ROM: ___ HRS.

	APGAR SCORE						AMNIOTIC FLUID:
TIME	HEART RATE	RESP. EFF.	MUSCLE TONE	REFLEX	COLOR	TOTAL	○ CLEAR
1 MIN.							○ MECONIUM: INTUBATED: ○ YES ○ NO
5 MIN.							○ CLOUDY

AMNIOTIC FLUID: ○ NOT DONE

ASPIRATE ___ cc
BABY TO: ○ ICN   ○ REGULAR NURSERY

CORD BLOOD
○ YES
○ NO
○ NEWBORN ABNORMALITIES:

ANESTHESIOLOGISTS
_____ MD _ _ _ _
_____ MD _ _ _ _
NURSE: _____ RN

OBSTETRICIANS
_____ MD _ _ _ _
_____ MD _ _ _ _
_____ MD _ _ _ _
D/C/A

(ORIGINAL—OB RECORD;   COPY—NEWBORN RECORD;   PINK—LOG)

most notably excessive bleeding and postpartum hemorrhage — can occur vary rapidly.

The nurse monitors the mother's blood pressure, pulse, respiration, position and tone of the uterus, and the amount and quality of lochia. The mother's temperature should also be taken at least once during this time to check for elevation associated with dehydration or developing infection. Usually, an elevation in temperature within 24 hours of delivery is due to dehydration and will respond to fluid replacement. However, if the membranes ruptured prematurely and the elevation recurs, a developing infection should be suspected.

Uterine Tone and Position.   The nurse assesses uterine tone, height, and position every 15 minutes during the first hour. Usually, uterine tone and the amount of lochia are correlated: if the uterus is firmly contracted, the flow of lochia will be small, whereas if the uterus is large and soft ("boggy"), flow may be moderate to large. The nurse should also note the height and position of the uterus. The fundus should remain at or slightly below the level of the umbilicus on the midline. Enlargement may indicate that the uterus is filling with blood and clots and that a postpartum hemorrhage is imminent. Elevation and deviation of the fundus to one side, usually the right, often indicates that the uterus is being displaced by a full bladder. A full bladder will inhibit uterine contraction and may predispose the woman to postpartum hemorrhage, and steps must be taken promptly to alleviate bladder distention.

Perineum and Lochia.   The nurse should assess the perineum and the amount of lochia every 15 minutes for the first hour. The nurse should observe lochial flow while fundal massage is being done. Lochia will usually flow in a slow, intermittent trickle; a continuous trickle of blood suggests a laceration of the cervix or vagina.

Normally, lochia will be bright red in color and contain a few small clots. Saturation of more than two perineal pads in the first hour or a rapid pooling of blood under the buttocks indicates excessive bleeding and requires further evaluation. If tissue is present in lochia, it should be saved for examination by the birth attendant.

The perineum is assessed frequently for increasing edema, asymmetric edema, bruising, gaping, and bleeding from perineal repair. The nurse should ask the mother if she is experiencing a great deal of perineal pain. Occasionally, a hematoma will form as a result of a broken blood vessel bleeding into the connective tissue underlying skin or mucosa of the vagina and perineum. A hematoma will feel fluctuant and is likely to be extremely painful when touched. The following symptoms of hematoma formation must be reported to the birth attendant promptly:

- Increasing, severe perineal pain
- Asymmetric perineal swelling
- Ecchymosis of the overlying skin or mucosa
- Increased tautness of skin or mucosa
- Complaint of rectal pressure

Neonatal Physiologic Status

Ongoing assessment of the normal newborn in the first hour after delivery is usually the responsibility of the labor and delivery nurse. Many labor and delivery units now provide family-centered recovery care, in which the newborn is screened for abnormalities in the delivery room and, if normal, stays with parents for the first hours after delivery. Other settings request that the newborn be taken away briefly for evaluation in the admission nursery and returned as soon as possible to the parents, while still others request that the newborn spend some time in the admission nursery for observation.

The nurse should be sensitive to parents' wishes in this matter and attempt to maintain early parent–newborn contact within the limits of safe practice in that particular setting (Fig. 24–20). If the newborn is to remain with the mother and father, the nurse must perform regular and systematic assessments of the newborn's physiologic status. The nurse must be alert for potential neonatal problems, which necessitate close observation or admission to the nursery.

Nursing responsibilities in the initial neonatal assessment are discussed in detail in Chapter 31.

Family Responses to the Newborn

The mother and father usually are very joyful during this time and respond with wonder, excitement, and delight to their newborn. This early response can contribute to increased feelings of attraction, and connectedness to the newborn and may lay the groundwork for and facilitate parent–infant attachment. Behaviors thought to signify the beginning of positive parent–infant interaction include:

- Progression of touch from tentative touch with fingertips to more confident touch and enfolding of the infant
- Active reaching for the infant rather than passive receiving
- Active attempts to make and hold eye contact with the infant in the same vertical plane, known as *en face* positioning
- Expressions of approval or satisfaction with infant's sex, weight, condition, appearance, and size

The nurse should observe the nature of the parents' first responses, since they are the basis for the unfolding future relationship with the newborn.

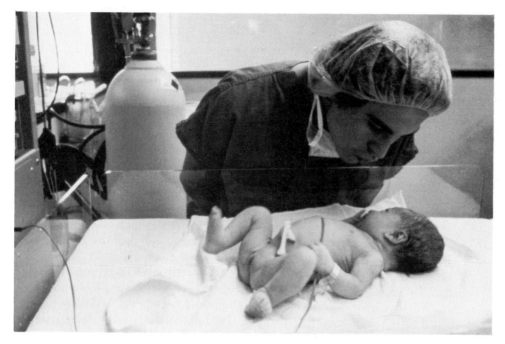

Figure 24-20. This newborn was slightly hypothermic after delivery and was transferred to the admission nursery and put under a radiant heater. The father accompanies the newborn and has an excellent opportunity to explore and interact with his new daughter. (Photo: Kathy Sloane)

Close contact with the newborn in the first hours after birth is very important to many parents. The opportunity to be with the newborn in its first alert phase, which lasts 1 or 2 hours after birth, is precious and should be protected. The nurse will observe that most parents are overwhelmingly positive about their newborns and are eager for close contact and interaction.

However, some parents will seem less eager for interaction or will express concerns or disappointment about the newborn's appearance or sex. This reaction may be the result of a long, painful labor, of unmet expectations for the birth or the newborn, of physical pain and fatigue, of an unwanted pregnancy, or of cultural differences. The nurse should be careful not to assess such interactions as being atypical or worrisome too quickly; close observation and sensitive listening to and acknowledgment of parents' feelings and concerns, and communication of observations to postpartum nursing staff are in order.

The following are nursing diagnoses that may be useful in the care of families during the immediate postpartum period.

- Altered patterns in urinary elimination
- Altered comfort related to perineal trauma, uterine cramping, and "postpartum chill"
- Ineffective airway clearance (neonatal)
- Hypothermia (neonatal)
- Health maintenance: need for parent–neonate interaction

Complications of the immediate postpartum period include possible postpartum maternal hemorrhage and complications of the newborn, such as respiratory problems, hypothermia, and hypoglycemia. Part of the nurse's responsibilities of the fourth stage of labor, then, is monitoring for possible complications.

Diagnosis

Nursing diagnoses during the immediate postpartum recovery period guide the nurse in setting priorities for care in the first hours after birth. More immediate plans for transferring the family to the postpartum unit are made, if necessary. Communication with the postpartum staff, who will be providing care throughout the rest of the hospital stay, will lead to a smooth transition of care.

Planning and Implementation

The period immediately after delivery is often the most rewarding time for the nurse working with a family during childbirth. The woman and her partner have completed the difficult work of labor and birth and now have the opportunity to become acquainted with their newborn. Nursing care for the woman and her family is directed at supporting maternal and neonatal physiologic status, providing for comfort needs, supporting family interaction, and monitoring for possible complications of the mother and newborn. Priorities for care are based on assessment data and nursing diagnoses.

Promoting Maternal Physiologic Adaptation

Promoting Urinary Elimination

If the mother's condition is stable and alert, she may be offered clear liquids; if these are tolerated well, a normal or high-residue diet may be instituted. Both parents may be quite hungry at this point and may welcome a meal.

The mother should be encouraged to empty her bladder as soon as she is able to do so after delivery, whether or not she has the urge to urinate. Because of perineal anesthesia and postdelivery edema, she may not feel the urge to void even when the bladder is distended. Normal postdelivery diuresis and administration of intravenous fluids predispose the woman to bladder distention during this period.

The nurse should help the woman walk to the bathroom and stay with her as she voids to provide any needed assistance and guard against a fall caused by muscle weakness or fainting. The voiding should be measured and entered in intake and output records. Color and amount should be noted as indications of the level of hydration of the patient. If less than 100 ml is voided, the nurse should be alert for the possibility that this represents overflow of urine from an overdistended bladder, and careful continued monitoring of output is required. If the mother has difficulty voiding, measures such as running water, pouring warm water over the perineum, and applying light suprapubic pressure may be helpful. If the bladder is palpable and the woman is unable to void, a straight catheterization is indicated.

Expected Outcome: The woman demonstrates complete emptying of bladder by voiding voluntarily within 6 hours after birth or when her bladder becomes distended.

Promoting Comfort

Perineal edema and ecchymosis commonly occur secondary to birth trauma. Ice packs may be applied to the perineum for the first 24 hours postpartum to reduce pain, swelling, and resulting difficulty with voiding. Chemical ice packs are available, but a sterile glove filled with crushed ice is just as effective. The nurse should explain the purpose of the ice pack. In some cultures, it is considered essential to avoid cold for successful recovery from birth. In this case, use of an ice pack may be objec-

tionable, but the woman's initial concerns may be overcome by the nurse's sensitivity to cultural beliefs and careful teaching regarding the benefits of cold in the reduction of swelling.

If an episiotomy was performed or vaginal lacerations occurred, the woman may begin to experience perineal pain as the effects of the local anesthetic begin to wear off. If the woman has hemorrhoids, they may also contribute to sensations of pain. The application of an ice pack to the perineum during the first 24 hours may reduce pain sensations, but some women may require analgesia such as plain acetaminophen or a combination of acetaminophen and codeine. The nurse can also demonstrate techniques for sitting and getting out of bed, which reduce tension on the episiotomy site.

Fundal massage is likely to be uncomfortable for the mother. The nurse can increase her comfort by instructing her how to do fundal massage, why it is important, and encouraging her to take some responsibility for this aspect of her care. The nurse can also remind her to utilize relaxation techniques to ease this discomfort.

Other nursing actions that will contribute to the general comfort of the new mother include a sponge bath or shower and gentle perineal hygiene.

The new mother may experience shaking and chills in the first hour after delivery. The cause is unknown, but it may be related to an elevated core body temperature with relatively cool skin and extremities, or it may reflect a generalized immune response to fetal cells that entered the maternal circulation at the time of placental separation. The nurse should reassure parents that this is a normal phenomenon, cover the mother with a warmed blanket or two, and offer warm nonstimulating liquids, such as herb tea or soup.

Expected Outcome: The woman practices self-care comfort and pain-relief techniques resulting in decreasing levels of pain and increased maternal mobility.

Promoting Newborn Physiologic Adaptation

As long as the neonate's physiologic status is within normal limits, nursing support remains centered on preventing excessive heat loss and promoting effective airway clearance. The neonate is vulnerable to excessive heat loss in the first 1 to 2 hours after delivery. The nurse should ensure that the neonate is well dried and well covered at all times. A hat should be used to prevent heat loss from the head. The neonate also may need assistance in keeping the upper airway clear of mucus. The presence of excess mucus is signaled by bubbling from the mouth, sneezing, or noisy respiration. Bulb suctioning of the nares and mouth should be done, as needed. (Thermoregulation and airway maintenance are discussed further in Unit V.)

Expected Outcome: The newborn maintains a patent airway and an axillary body temperature between 36.4° and 37.2°C in the first 2 hours after delivery.

Promoting Parent–Newborn Interaction

An important nursing responsibility in the immediate postpartum recovery period is supporting family interaction and parent education. This phase of labor provides an excellent opportunity for parent–newborn interaction for several reasons:

- The newborn is likely to be in a quiet alert state for 1 or 2 hours, will gaze at faces, and will initiate breast-feeding with assistance

- Early contact with the alert newborn provides the parents with cues about its temperament and its needs, which helps them interact with the newborn as an individual

- The mother and father are often excited and eager to interact with the newborn as the reward for their hard work in labor; fatigue, and discomfort may not be significant enough to interfere with this interaction

- Parents may feel a special closeness with each other and with the newborn during this time, and interaction takes on a special significance

The nurse can help in many ways to support family interaction during this special time. Promoting the comfort of both parents' and helping them to become settled for a time will allow them to enjoy this interaction. Assessing the mother's physical comfort, providing food or fluids as appropriate, and providing extra blankets, a clean gown, or clean bedding may be helpful.

The nurse's regular assessments of the newborn's status provide an opportunity for teaching parents about their newborn. Although the nurse should take care not to overwhelm them with information, tips about important aspects of care—such as keeping the newborn warm, checking for excessive mucus, and using the bulb syringe—and the information about the newborn's ability to see, hear, and orient to sounds may be new for first-time parents and will be especially welcome.

Assistance with early breast-feeding is often especially appreciated during this period. The newborn typically will not nurse long and may be more interested in gazing at faces. However, the mother–newborn contact will assist

in maintaining uterine tone and hemostasis and may facilitate early initiation of lactation. The nurse should ensure that the mother is comfortably positioned and can support the newborn at the breast without fatigue or strain; this is easily done by positioning the newborn on the breast and supporting its weight and the mother's arm on pillows to enable the mother to relax as much as possible.

The nurse should also assess how much contact the father wants with the newborn and facilitate father–newborn interaction, as appropriate. Most mothers will ask their partner if he wants to hold the baby, and many fathers do not hesitate to do so. However, some tend to hold back, either because they believe it is "more important" for the mother to hold the newborn, or because they are uncertain about how to hold a new baby. The nurse should provide a comfortable chair, check that the baby is well wrapped, both to prevent heat loss and to provide a more easily handled "bundle," and then hand the newborn to the father. Reassurance, encouragement, and pointing out how the newborn orients toward and seeks out the father's voice may provide powerful reinforcement to a father who is feeling unsure about his role.

Once these things are done, the nurse can ensure that the family has some private time without interruptions. This may require the nurse to reorganize the timing of periodic assessments of maternal and infant status or of the administration of medications. However, this privacy can be very special to the family. The nurse should assure the family that she is nearby in case she is needed and indicate when she will return. Whenever possible, the nurse should defer routine newborn care (for example, the administration of eye medication) until the second or third hour to allow the newborn to remain with the parents in a quiet alert state.

The nurse should provide an opportunity for interaction with other family members, if desired. Many institutions allow for brief visits by other family, especially grandparents and siblings, during this time. Although care is needed to prevent overstimulating the newborn and parents, brief periods of family "togetherness" to greet the newborn can be especially meaningful for many families. It is especially important to be aware of ethnic customs in the postpartum period (Fig. 24–21).

Both parents will likely experience great excitement and will interact with the newborn for a period. This is followed by growing awareness of their fatigue. At this point, both parents should be encouraged to rest (Fig. 24–22). Once made comfortable, the mother will probably sleep intermittently. The nurse should help her find a comfortable position for rest and for breast-feeding as needed. Pillows can be positioned to support the newborn and to support tired limbs. The father should be encouraged to rest or sleep and offered a comfortable place with his family, if possible.

Expected Outcome: Parents demonstrate beginning attachment behaviors as evidenced by holding, smiling at, talking to, seeking eye contact with their newborn and demonstrate an understanding of newborn characteristics as evidenced by positive verbalization of feelings about their newborn.

Monitoring for Complications
Potential Complication: Maternal Postpartum Hemorrhage

Maternal physiologic adaptations during the immediate postpartum period are dramatic and require nursing support, if recovery is to be prompt. Of major importance

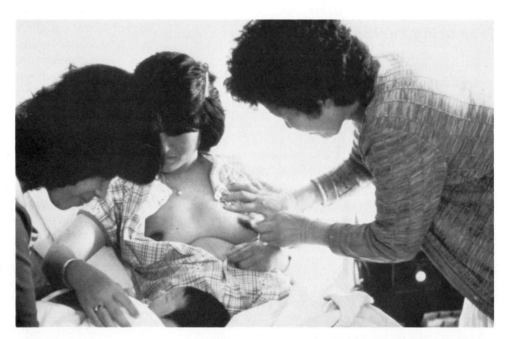

Figure 24–21. Family responses to the newborn are culturally determined in large part. This Asian American mother is being attended by her own mother and her sister. Her mother is bathing her while her sister assumes responsibility for the newborn's care. (Photo: Kathy Sloane)

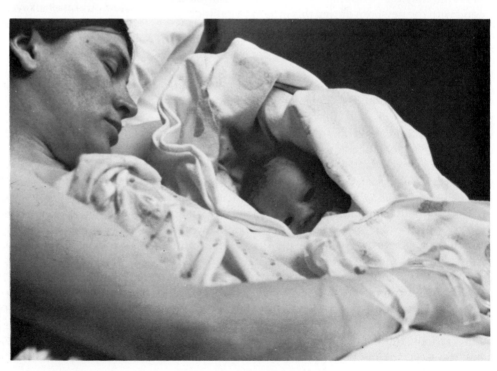

Figure 24–22. Well wrapped and resting with his mother, the baby is contentedly sucking on his hand in a quiet alert state. (Photo: BABES, Inc.)

is nursing intervention to ensure hemostasis and prevent excessive blood loss.

Nursing actions to prevent excessive postpartum bleeding include close monitoring of uterine tone and maternal blood pressure, administration of oxytocics, and maintenance of uterine tone by fundal massage. These were discussed earlier in the chapter and are discussed further in Unit VI.

Expected Outcome: Postpartum mother demonstrates optimum physiologic recovery as evidenced by maintaining uterine tone and normal blood pressure and pulse rate in the first 8 hours after delivery.

Potential Complication: Neonatal Respiratory Problems, Hypothermia, Hypoglycemia

The nurse continues to monitor for these three major complications of the newborn. Airway clearance and thermoregulation were discussed in this chapter and are expanded upon in Unit V. Prevention of hypoglycemia also is discussed in Unit V. In the healthy neonate, early initiation of breast-feeding will also aid in the prevention of hypoglycemia. The newborn should ingest an adequate amount of breast milk or formula to maintain a serum glucose level of 45 mg% or higher and a normal serum calcium of 7.3 to 9.2 mg/dl.

Evaluation of Intrapartal Care

Evaluation of the effectiveness of intrapartal nursing care is challenging. Patient needs are constantly changing, and the time frame in which the nurse must assess, diagnose, plan, and implement care may be very short. Evaluation and modification of the plan of care may become blurred in the constantly shifting picture of patient needs and responses to labor. It is in these situations that the nurse must be knowledgeable about standards of care and parameters of normal and abnormal responses in labor and birth. These provide guidelines against which individual nursing actions can be evaluated.

Nursing care for low-risk families in labor and birth, however, can also be evaluated readily from at least three more general perspectives: promotion of health and appropriate self-care, prevention of complications, and enhancing family satisfaction with the birth experience. In the rapidly changing technologic environment of perinatal health care today, the nurse must work toward these goals as nursing priorities because in so doing, she is assuring individual and family needs will be met.

CONTINUITY OF NURSING CARE INTO THE POSTPARTUM PERIOD

Depending on the setting, the mother and newborn will be transferred to the postpartum unit after 1 or 2 hours. The nurse is responsible for the communication of important information about maternal, newborn, and family status at that time. All nursing care should have been recorded and a verbal report made to the nursing staff responsible for postpartum care. If the newborn is to be admitted to the nursery at this time, a report on the newborn's status is also necessary.

If the nurse is not going to have regular contact with the family during the postpartum period, she may wish to "check in" on the family on an informal basis. The nurse who provides sensitive and expert care during labor and birth often becomes an important person to the mother and father, if only temporarily. Visits from "their" labor nurse are seen as an expression of caring, and give the new mother and father an opportunity to relive their labor experiences and to fill in areas where their recall may not be clear.

A postpartum visit to a family she cared for in labor also gives the nurse a chance to see the full cycle of labor, birth, recovery, and family integration. Caring for a woman and her family in labor is a demanding and rewarding process; often, the results of excellent intrapartal nursing care are best seen in the wonder and excitement of parents as they greet their newborn and as they embark on their life as a new family.

CHAPTER SUMMARY

The nurse plays a major role in supporting the woman and her family during labor, and in protecting maternal, fetal, and family well-being as they adapt to the normal physiologic and psychologic stresses of labor and birth. The needs of the woman and her family change with each phase of labor; nursing care must be continually adjusted to these changing needs. An important aspect of nursing care is attention to the *appropriate* use of technology and obstetric intervention in intrapartal care. Nursing care for women at low risk for complications in the intrapartal period should emphasize providing physical and psychological support, monitoring well-being so that variations from normal status can be identified and treated early, and providing family-centered care that promotes comfort and a positive, healthy beginning for the new family.

STUDY QUESTIONS

1. Describe maternal positions and comfort measures that may be helpful to a woman who is experiencing a slow second stage.
2. What steps should you take in response to a woman who exclaims "My baby is coming!"? Give your rationale.
3. Describe nursing actions that will help to keep the newborn warm immediately after birth.
4. You assess a patient in the first hour after delivery and determine that she has heavy lochial flow. What are the possible causes? What are appropriate nursing interventions? Give your rationale.

REFERENCES/BIBLIOGRAPHY

Banta H, Thackers S: Risks and benefits of episiotomy: A review. Birth 9(1):25, 1982

Caldeyro–Barcia R: The influence of maternal bearing-down efforts during second stage on fetal well-being. Birth Fam J 6:17, 1979

Roberts J: A descriptive analysis of involuntary bearing-down efforts during the expulsive phase of labor. J Obstet Gynecol Neonatal Nurs 16(1):48, 1987

Rossi M: Maternal positions and pushing techniques in a nonprescriptive environment. J Obstet Gynecol Neonatal Nurs 15(3):203, 1986

Russell J: The rationale of primitive delivery positions. Br J Obstet Gynecol 89:712, 1982

SUGGESTED READINGS

Krutsky C: Siblings at birth: Impact on parents. J Nurse Midwifery 30(5):269–276, 1985

Lehrman E: Birth in the left lateral position. J Nurse-Midwifery 30(4):193–197, 1985

Lumley J: Assessing satisfaction with childbirth. Birth 12(3):141–145, 1985

McKay S, Roberts J: Second stage labor: What is normal? J Obstet Gynecol Neonatal Nurs 14(2):101–106, 1985

Romond JL, Baker IT: Squatting in childbirth. J Obstet Gynecol Neonatal Nurs 14:406–411, 1985

Rossi MA, Lindell SG: Maternal positions and pushing techniques in a nonprescriptive environment. J Obstet Gynecol Neonatal Nurs 15:203–208, 1986

Stolte K: A comparison of womens' expectations of labor with the actual event. Birth 14(2):99–103, 1987

25 procedures: monitoring the at-risk fetus

LEARNING OBJECTIVES

After studying the material in this chapter, the student will be able to

- Identify indications for use of electronic fetal monitoring during labor

- Describe advantages and disadvantages of internal and external fetal monitoring

- Describe the key elements of fetal heart rate patterns and their normal range

- Describe the advantages and disadvantages of fetal scalp sampling and fetal scalp stimulation

- Explain the kind of information obtained from fetal scalp sampling and scalp stimulation

KEY TERMS

Amniotomy

Baseline fetal heart rate

Cephalopelvic disproportion

Periodic fetal heart rate changes

Many women have pregnancies that proceed normally and result in spontaneous labor and delivery. These situations require only watchful intrapartal support; little or no obstetric intervention is required to ensure a healthy mother and newborn and a positive experience for the childbearing family. However, a certain proportion of women are known to be at risk for intrapartum complications because of preexisting conditions. Others will encounter unanticipated problems in the intrapartal period after an uneventful pregnancy. Both groups of women then require *active obstetric management,* which includes the use of a variety of techniques designed to lower maternal–fetal risk in the intrapartal period.

Unfortunately, when risk is increased, maternity care tends to become focused more on the medical management of the mother and fetus and less on the emotional needs of the woman. Family-centered care practices may be de-emphasized or withheld entirely, in many cases because of the assumption that such practices would be unsafe or impractical for the moderate-risk or high-risk patient. However, rarely is there clear evidence to support that assumption; more often, restriction of family-centered care to women at increased intrapartal risk is based on a failure of health professionals to question whether family-centered care and active reduction of obstetric risk can coexist. This failure to question traditional modes of care may be depriving families of a valuable source of comfort, since there is convincing evidence that moderate-risk or high-risk patients and their families probably benefit at least as much from family-centered maternity care as do low-risk patients (McKay and Phillips 1984).

Modern maternity care includes a range of procedures designed to reduce intrapartal risk to the mother and fetus/newborn. Each procedure entails specific nursing responsibilities that must be carried out in order to provide safe and sensitive intrapartal care. The nurse in any obstetric setting must be prepared to care for women and their families at increased risk for problems in the intrapartal period in such a way that level of risk is reduced *and* emotional needs are met. Providing high-quality intrapartal care that utilizes advanced medical technology while preserving the important aspects of family-centered care presents a major challenge to nursing.

This is the first of three chapters that highlight procedures intended to reduce maternal and fetal risk in the intrapartal period. Depending on the course of labor and the nature of the actual or potential problem, several of these procedures will be implemented in the course of the patient's intrapartal care. In general, risk-reducing procedures in intrapartal care can be grouped into three major categories:

- Procedures aimed at closer monitoring of fetal status
- Procedures aimed at safe and more effective management of maternal pain

- Procedures that involve modifying the pattern of labor and mode of delivery

This chapter focuses on monitoring the at-risk fetus. The chapters that follow discuss management of maternal pain and procedures that modify the pattern of labor and mode of delivery.

Decisions to implement these types of procedures are made by the physician in consultation with the nurse midwife, the labor nurse, and the family; discussions about risk reduction procedures must always take into account the relative benefits and risks of more active obstetric management. The nurse must be knowledgeable about the nature of each procedure, its indications and contraindications, its relative advantages and disadvantages, and related nursing responsibilities. These aspects of each procedure are discussed here.

MONITORING FETAL STATUS

Fetal distress results from physiologic deprivation that places the fetus at risk when additional demands, such as those of labor and birth, are placed on it. Fetal distress may be either chronic or acute; if untreated, it can lead to fetal and neonatal morbidity and mortality. Even when it is treated promptly, intrauterine fetal distress can result in long-term problems, such as iatrogenic preterm birth, cerebral palsy, epilepsy, and mental retardation.

Chronic fetal distress occurs when the physiologic exchange of nutrients, oxygen, and metabolites from mother to fetus is disrupted over a period of time, often because of systemic maternal problems. These disruptions are often reflected in reduced blood flow to the placenta, abnormalities in placental structure, or deficiency in placental functioning.

Maternal factors that can result in chronic fetal distress include the following:

- Vascular abnormalities associated with maternal hypertension, preeclampsia/eclampsia, diabetes with vascular complications, and pelvic vascular abnormalities
- Inadequate systemic perfusion due to cardiac or pulmonary disease
- Placental abnormalities, such as "aging" in prolonged pregnancy
- Substance abuse

Fetal problems can also result in chronic fetal distress. The most frequent fetal causes of chronic distress are the following:

- Multiple gestation in which there is twin-to-twin transfusion (shared fetoplacental circulation)

- Congenital anomalies or infection
- Rh disease (erythroblastosis fetalis)

Chronic fetal distress is diagnosed by less than adequate uterine growth on the basis of serial antenatal examinations. McDonald's measurements of fundal height and sonography are useful when a slowing of fetal growth is suspected. In addition, during late pregnancy assessment of fetal movement and heart rate changes in response to movement (nonstress testing), discussed in Chapter 17, give indications of fetal physiologic reserves.

Acute fetal distress is often of concern during the intrapartal period. Intrapartal fetal distress is suggested by the following indicators:

- Presence of heavy meconium in amniotic fluid
- Presence of nonreassuring patterns on electronic fetal monitoring (discussed later in this chapter), such as persistent late decelerations, persistent severe variable decelerations, prolonged fetal bradycardia, and absent or decreased beat-to-beat variability

Intrapartal fetal distress is likely when, in addition to any of the above signs, venous blood samples from the fetal scalp reveal increasing acidosis.

When the fetus has been chronically stressed by compromised fetal–maternal exchange, the additional stress of labor compounds fetal risk. The extent to which repetitive uterine contractions contribute to fetal distress depends on the extent of the previous compromise, and when uterine activity is decreased, the distressed fetus will benefit.

The major way to assess fetal risk during the intrapartal period is intensive monitoring of fetal physiologic status. This is primarily done through continuous electronic fetal monitoring and fetal blood sampling.

ELECTRONIC FETAL MONITORING

The electronic fetal monitor (EFM) is a device that provides a graphic display of the fetal heart rate (FHR) and of uterine activity and a digital readout and tracing. Electronic fetal monitoring can be either *external,* which is noninvasive, or *internal,* which requires attachment of an electrode to the presenting fetal part and/or introduction of a pressure-sensing catheter into the uterus. Nursing staff may routinely initiate external EFM; however, initiation of internal EFM generally is done by a physician, nurse midwife, or labor nurse trained by the birthing facility.

Although routine continuous use of EFM is not recommended for low-risk patients in normal labor, there is little disagreement about its value in the moderate- or high-risk obstetric patient. Physicians who advocate continuous monitoring of low-risk women see its usefulness in the early detection of fetal distress and uterine hypotonicity and believe its benefits outweigh its risks.

Perhaps the greatest risk that may result from overreliance on continuous EFM data for labor management is the increased risk of unnecessary obstetric intervention. One study showed a twofold to threefold increase in the cesarean birth rate without an improvement in perinatal outcomes among women who received continuous EFM when compared to those who were assessed by intermittent FHR auscultation (Goodlin 1980). These findings un-

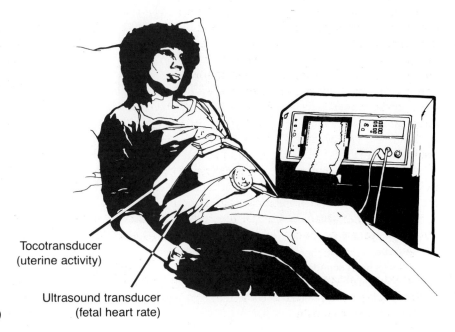

Tocotransducer
(uterine activity)

Ultrasound transducer
(fetal heart rate)

Figure 25–1. External electronic fetal monitoring. The tocotransducer monitors uterine activity. The ultrasound transducer monitors fetal heart rate. (Childbirth Graphics)

derscore the importance of careful FHR auscultation and manual assessment of strength of uterine contractions to verify EFM data before invasive management is instituted. Many settings now use intermittent external EFM for low-risk women in labor — for example, one 20-minute readout strip every 1 to 2 hours — to complement auscultation.

External (Indirect) Monitoring

External EFM relies on ultrasound detection of the FHR, rather than a direct electrocardiogram display, such as that generated by internal monitoring. External EFM is usually used early in labor and may be used on an intermittent or continuous basis. The external monitoring is accomplished by two devices secured by belts to the maternal abdomen and connected to a monitor, as shown in Figure 25–1.

The first of these devices is an *ultrasound transducer,* which detects fetal heart sounds. This device is placed, using a water-soluble conducting gel, on the maternal abdomen at the point of maximum intensity of the fetal heart tones and secured with a snug abdominal belt (Fig. 25–2). Ultrasound waves generated in this device bounce back from organs within the fetus. Information about internal movements (for example, movements of chambers of the fetal heart or of blood in fetal vessels) is then displayed on the monitor by a digital readout, by oscilloscope, and by graphic tracing. This transmission may also reflect movement of blood through a *maternal*

vessel, so abnormally low readings should be checked against the maternal pulse.

The other device used for external EFM is a *tocotransducer,* a pressure-sensing instrument that records relative strength of uterine contractions. As the uterus contracts, pressure is exerted against the tocotransducer and recorded on a graphic display or tracing, as shown in Figure 25–3. This wavelike pattern can be used to record frequency and duration of uterine contractions. Intensity cannot be accurately recorded, since the height of the "wave" depends on the tightness of the belt securing the device to the abdomen. The belt should be secured tightly enough so that the monitor displays an increase in pressure just before or as the patient feels the contraction. This degree of tightness may be annoying to the woman; however, an explanation of why it is needed will usually suffice. When accurate measurement of contraction strength is needed, internal EFM is desirable.

Indications and Contraindications

Indications and contraindications of external EFM are listed in the accompanying display.

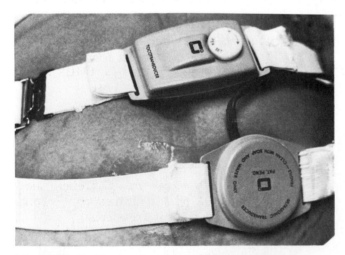

Figure 25–2. The tocotransducer (top) records the pressure of uterine contractions; the ultrasound transducer (bottom) detects fetal heart sounds. Both instruments are secured to the mother's abdomen with belts and are connected to the monitor machine by leads. (Photo: BABES, Inc.)

Indications and Contraindications for External Electronic Fetal Monitoring

Indications

- Variations in fetal heart rate detected by auscultation
- Meconium-stained amniotic fluid
- Induction of labor
- Oxytocin augmentation of labor
- High risk for uteroplacental insufficiency or fetal compromise in patients with:

  Hypertension
  Bleeding
  Preterm or post-term pregnancies
  Intrauterine growth retardation
  Abnormal fetal presentation
  Previous stillbirth
  Diabetes
  Sickle-cell disease
  Hemolytic disease of the fetus

Contraindications

No absolute contraindications

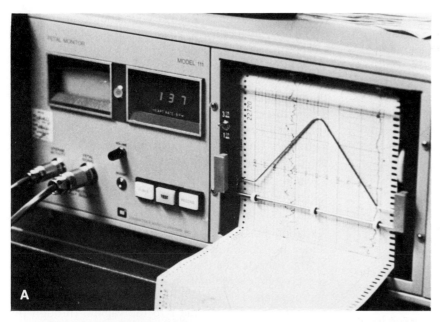

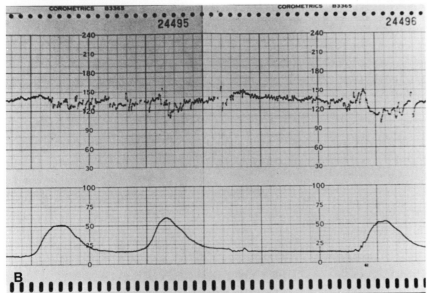

Figure 25–3. The monitor machine *(A)* displays a digital readout of the FHR as well as a continuous graphic tracing of the FHR pattern and contraction pattern on specially marked paper. *(B)* The monitor tracing shows the FHR pattern (top line) in beats per minute. The lower line shows the uterine contraction pattern in mm Hg. This allows observation of changes in FHR patterns in response to uterine activity. (Photo credit: BABES, Inc.)

Advantages and Disadvantages

External EFM is most beneficial as an adjunct to repeated nursing assessments of fetal status and labor pattern by auscultation and palpation. Its *advantages* are that it can be initiated by nursing personnel, it is noninvasive and can be used when membranes are intact and the cervix is undilated, it provides useful information about fetal response to labor, and it may be reassuring and helpful to the woman as she copes with her labor.

Its *disadvantages* include its tendency to limit maternal ambulation and position change and its relative lack of accuracy in recording FHR and uterine contraction strength. Ultrasound transmission may record *artifact*

sounds, including maternal bowel or cardiac sounds, and may be affected by fetal or maternal movement. Belts must be frequently repositioned, and external EFM does not give an accurate measurement of uterine contraction strength, even when the belts are applied carefully. Accuracy of external EFM is further limited by maternal obesity, polyhydramnios, or a very active fetus.

Implications for Nursing Care

The laboring woman being externally monitored should be encouraged to find a comfortable position and to move around the room within the limits of the cord lengths that are attached to the monitor. This attachment may inhibit ambulation, and the nurse should help the woman and her partner to maintain a comfortable level of activity. Both the ultrasound transducer and the toco-transducer will require frequent checking and repositioning if the patient is mobile. However, the advantages of ambulation and frequent position changes, described in Chapter 24, outweigh any inconvenience this may cause. This should be explained to the woman and her partner because some women will limit their movement to avoid "bothering" the nurse to reposition the belts.

While preparing and placing the external monitoring devices, the nurse should instruct the woman and her partner about the function of each device and how it should be positioned. The nurse should also explain what information the monitor provides, how that information can be used to time uterine contractions, and how the volume of the monitor may be adjusted to hear the fetal heart tones. The nurse should point out that attending to the monitor is helpful for some parents, and distracting for others, and should encourage the couple not to focus on the monitor if they do not want to. The nurse should explain that position changes, fetal movement, electronic interference, maternal sounds, ambulation, and occasional disconnection of leads will affect the "readout"; parents should not be automatically alarmed by such a change but should alert the nurse.

Internal (Direct) Monitoring

Internal EFM provides the most precise assessment of FHR and uterine contractility pattern. Fetal heart rates are directly monitored by recording electrical impulses through an electrode attached to the presenting fetal part. Strength of uterine contractions is monitored through a pressure-sensing catheter placed inside the uterus (Fig. 25–4). Because of its invasiveness, internal EFM is used most often when accuracy of information about fetal response to labor or uterine contractility is essential.

Internal monitoring requires access to the fetus and the uterine cavity. The cervix must be dilated to at least 1 cm, and membranes must be ruptured artificially if spontaneous rupture has not occurred. In addition, the presenting part must be engaged and accessible through the cervix.

Internal Spiral Electrode

The internal monitoring devices (that is, the fetal scalp electrode and the uterine pressure catheter) are applied under aseptic conditions in the following manner.

The vulva is cleansed with an antiseptic agent, and a sterile vaginal examination is done to verify the nature and position of the presenting part. A spiral electrode is inserted through a guide into the vagina, through the cervix, and applied to the presenting part, usually the head (Fig. 25–5). This is accomplished by gently twisting the electrode so that it slips beneath the skin of the presenting part. Extreme care must be taken to avoid placing the electrode in such vulnerable body parts as the fontanelles, eyes, or genitals. When the electrode is in place, the guide tube is removed, and wires attached to the presenting part extend through the vagina to the outside. The ends of the wires are attached to a plate secured to the mother's thigh and connected to a cord leading to the monitor, as shown in Figure 25–5. With the internal monitor in place, the mother can change positions more freely and with greater comfort than with the external monitor. Occasionally the electrode becomes dislodged and must be replaced. Ordinarily the electrode remains in place until delivery.

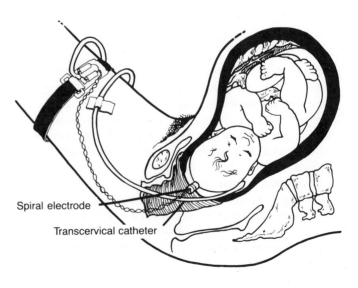

Spiral electrode

Transcervical catheter

Figure 25–4. Internal electronic fetal monitoring. (Childbirth Graphics)

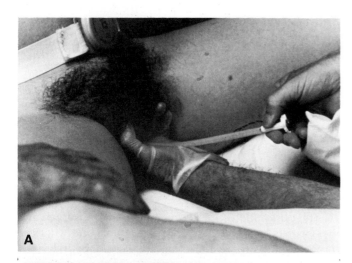

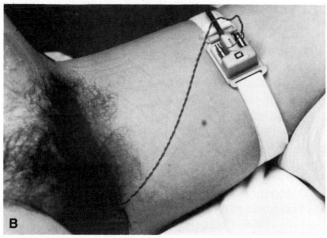

Figure 25–5. Placement of the fetal scalp electrode is done through a guide inserted into the vagina *(A)* and advanced through the cervix to the presenting part. Once the electrode has been attached, the lead is secured to a leg plate on the mother's thigh and connected by a cord to the monitor *(B).* (Photo: BABES, Inc.)

Intrauterine Pressure Catheter

Accurate measurement of uterine contraction strength is made possible by insertion of an intrauterine pressure catheter (IUPC). There are currently two types of catheter available. A hollow, fluid-filled, plastic catheter was the first to be developed. It is threaded through a guide up into the uterus and advanced until a mark on the catheter reaches the introitus. The catheter that extends from the vagina is connected to a strain gauge and then to the monitor.

When intrauterine pressure is exerted on the catheter tip during contractions, it is transmitted via the water-filled catheter, across the transducer diaphragm, to the strain gauge. This mechanical energy is then converted to electrical energy, amplified, and recorded on the monitor paper.

When the fluid-filled catheter is used, sterile water WITHOUT preservative must be used. Saline can corrode the stainless steel diaphragm and preservatives have been linked to morbidity and mortality in very low birth weight fetuses (Murray 1988). For accurate readings of intrauterine pressure, the strain gauge should be positioned at approximately the same level as the catheter tip. The transducer must be calibrated to atmospheric pressure after catheter insertion and every time the patient changes position. Occasionally the catheter tip becomes clogged with blood or meconium and must be flushed to ensure accurate measurements.

Recently a precalibrated, solid, pressure catheter has been introduced. A computer chip located in the tip measures intrauterine pressure. No fluid is used and once the catheter is calibrated and inserted, no further calibration can be done. Both catheters generate a similar uterine pressure tracing.

The intrauterine pressure catheter measures the resting tonus of the uterus as well as the strength of contractions and records this on a tracing calibrated to reflect pressure in mm Hg. This uterine pressure tracing is recorded simultaneously with the FHR. Accuracy of the measurement of uterine contraction strength can be checked by palpating a contraction and comparing this with the monitor tracing. A rise of 25 mm Hg over the resting tonus should correspond to a mild contraction, 50 mm Hg to a moderate contraction, and 70 mm Hg or more to a strong contraction. Patency of the catheter can be checked by asking the woman to cough or apply fundal pressure and observing the tracing for a corresponding rise in intrauterine pressure (Malinowski 1983).

Many birth attendants now use intrauterine pressure monitoring only when assessment of intensity and frequency of uterine contractions is particularly important —for example, during administration of intravenous oxytocin.

Indications and Contraindications

Internal EFM provides the most accurate information about fetal response to labor and uterine contraction patterns, but because of its invasiveness, it is used less frequently than external EFM. Indications and contraindications for internal EFM are listed in the accompanying display, page 682.

Advantages and Disadvantages

Because of its invasiveness and potential risks, the disadvantages of internal EFM outweigh its advantages for routine use. However, when accurate information about a potentially compromised fetus is essential, internal EFM provides information about fetal status, allowing a margin of safety otherwise not possible.

Indications and Contraindications for Internal Electronic Fetal Monitoring

Indications

- Variations in fetal heart rate detected by auscultation
- Meconium-stained amniotic fluid
- Induction of labor
- Oxytocin augmentation of labor
- High risk for uteroplacental insufficiency or fetal compromise (see Indications for External Fetal Monitoring, earlier in the chapter)
- Need for precise determination of FHR pattern, as when abnormality is suspected on the basis of external monitoring
- Failure to progress in labor with suspected uterine dystocia
- Trial of labor for possible vaginal delivery after previous cesarean birth

Contraindications

- Closed cervix
- Presenting part high in the pelvis
- Presenting part that cannot be identified with accuracy
- Presenting part such that application of the electrode would be to the fetal face, fontanelles, or scrotum

Internal EFM has the following advantages:

- It provides beat-by-beat assessment of the fetal heart rate.
- It provides information on uterine contractility when palpation is difficult (because of obesity or presence of fibroids) or when assessment of uterine contractility must be continuous, such as during vaginal delivery after previous cesarean birth or during oxytocin infusion.
- Maternal or fetal position changes do not affect continuous recording of contractions.

Internal EFM has the following disadvantages:

- Before it can be used, membranes must be ruptured, the fetus must have descended, and the cervix must be dilated to at least 1 cm.
- Skilled personnel are needed to apply the equipment and maintain it in operation.
- Fetal scalp abscess or laceration of the scalp or other body part may result from insertion of the spiral electrode.
- There is a risk of infection to the mother.

- There is a risk of perforation of the uterus by the intra-uterine catheter.
- Maternal movement is restricted.
- The incidence of cesarean birth is increased.
- Maternal stress can be induced by early amniotomy.
- There can be trauma to the fetal head because of lack of the amniotic fluid cushion to protect its head.
- There can be a loss of attention to the laboring mother when the focus of attention is on the monitor.

Implications for Nursing Care

The nurse should carefully explain to the woman and her partner why internal EFM is desirable and what the procedure involves, answering any questions they may have. Many will have initial reservations about the procedure, and justifiably so, since it is not risk-free. However, when maternal or fetal conditions make internal monitoring desirable, the woman will probably accept its use without hesitation if she feels her infant is in jeopardy.

The nurse must be aware that close attention to the monitor and its readings may result in decreased attention and concern for the mother's emotional well-being and comfort. The partner should be alerted to the possibility of fixating on the machine to the detriment of the attention needed to support his laboring spouse.

Nursing care should include encouraging the woman to change position frequently, using the baby's heartbeat and uterine contraction patterns to assist with relaxation techniques, and decreasing parental anxiety by explaining that variations in the recording of information on the graphic readout may be artifacts (Fig. 25–6).

Some women welcome EFM because it reassures them and helps them to anticipate contractions. However, the irritation caused by the enforced immobility, loss of control, and loss of privacy may be exacerbated if the monitor receives the attention she desperately needs. Nurses should be particularly sensitive to the needs of women with EFM and remember that clinical skills in palpation of contractions and auscultation of fetal heart rate are crucial to verify EFM findings when caring for laboring women.

Ambulatory Telemetry

A recent innovation in internal EFM is the use of ambulatory telemetry. A radio transmitter attached to a standard scalp electrode and intrauterine pressure catheter transmits information about the fetal heart rate and uterine contractions from an ambulating woman in labor to a central display screen and printer. Although not yet in common use, this telemetry system appears to promote maternal mobility, convenience, and comfort while maintaining the advantages of internal EFM.

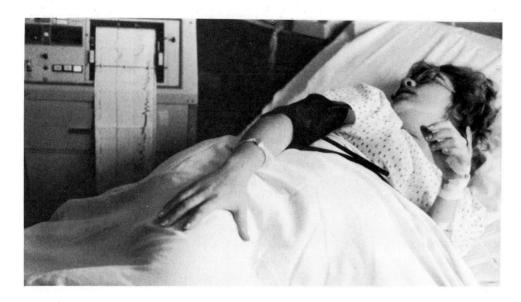

Figure 25–6. The nurse must be sensitive to the parents' responses to electronic fetal monitoring during labor and intervene to provide information and support as needed.

Interpretation of Fetal Heart Rate Patterns

During each uterine contraction there is a transient reduction in maternal blood flow through the placenta. Under normal circumstances placental function and per-

NURSING ALERT

Suspected FHR Abnormalities

- Observe EFM recording strip and identify nature of abnormality.
- Check that monitor straps and lines are properly secured and connected.
- Explain actions and provide reassurance to woman and partner.
- Alert physician or nurse midwife.
- Change mother to lateral position to decrease supine hypotension and correct for possible cord compression.
- If maternal hypotension persists, elevate legs and initiate IV fluids.
- If IV is in place, increase rate of maintenance IV infusion.
- If severe variable decelerations are present, assess for prolapsed compressed cord. If cord is prolapsed, move mother to knee-chest position to relieve pressure on cord; prepare for emergency cesarean delivery. (See Chapter 30, Nursing Alert: Prolapsed Umbilical Cord.)
- Administer oxygen by face mask at 8–12 liter/min.
- Discontinue oxytocin infusion to decrease uterine activity and promote placental perfusion.

fusion provide a "fetal reserve" ensuring that stress to the fetus during labor is minimal. Labor has been described as a stress test for the fetus, who becomes handicapped when certain conditions exist, including the following:

- Placental abnormality
- Maternal disease, such as diabetes, pregnancy-induced hypertension (which produces early placental aging), or decreased perfusion
- Maternal hypotension
- Supine hypotensive syndrome
- Fetal disease, such as erythroblastosis fetalis
- Cord compression
- Analgesic drugs or anesthesia

Assessment of the fetal heart rate by fetoscope during labor, especially if restricted only to the interval between contractions, is not effective for detecting subtle changes in FHR pattern. As discussed, use of continuous EFM is indicated for high-risk fetal labors and when suspicious fluctuations of FHR are detected by fetoscope. Continuous monitoring provides an accurate reading of fetal response to the stress of uterine contractions.

Assessment and interpretation of FHR patterns is a major nursing responsibility in intrapartal care. Interpretation of FHR patterns involves evaluation of both *baseline FHR* and, more important, *periodic FHR changes* that appear in response to uterine contraction.

Baseline FHR

Baseline FHR is determined by the range of the FHR in a 10-minute period in the absence of, or between, contractions. The normal baseline FHR is 120 to 160 beats per minute (bpm). This rate is influenced by the integrity of the autonomic nervous system of the fetus and may be also affected by such factors as prematurity, fetal hypoxia, medications, or maternal fever. If the FHR increases or decreases and remains at this new level for a 10-minute period during labor, this is referred to as a *baseline change,* and a new baseline is established.

The nurse should note that many EFM machines may display double counts or half counts of FHRs that are at the extreme ends of the recording range. If the FHR is 70 or below, the monitor may double the rate and display it as 140 or less, while a FHR of 180 or more may be displayed as 90 or more. This underscores an extremely important point: the nurse should never rely exclusively on machine data for assessment of her patient's status. EFM must *always* be complemented by periodic auscultation of FHR and palpation of uterine contractions.

Fetal Bradycardia

Bradycardia exists when the baseline FHR is below 120 bpm for 10 minutes or more. Bradycardia is described in degrees from moderate to marked. Moderate bradycardia is said to exist if the FHR is between 100 bpm and 119 bpm. This rate is not caused by fetal distress but is a benign change thought to be caused by a vagal response to head compression during labor. Vagal response, due to stimulation of the vagus or 10th cranial nerve, is characterized by parasympathetic nervous system activity, notably slowing of the heart. Marked bradycardia is said to exist if the FHR is less than 100 bpm. This rate is associated with progressive fetal acidosis due to hypoxia and is considered ominous, especially if accompanied by periodic FHR changes. Causes of fetal bradycardia are listed in Table 25–1.

Fetal Tachycardia

Tachycardia is said to exist if the baseline FHR is over 160 bpm for a period longer than 10 minutes. Tachycardia is described as moderate or marked. Moderate tachycar-

dia is said to exist if the FHR is between 161 bpm and 180 bpm. This rate is associated with mild or progressive hypoxia. Marked tachycardia exists if the FHR is over 180 bpm. This rate is considered an ominous sign when associated with periodic FHR changes or minimal baseline variability. Fetal tachycardia may be caused by the factors listed in Table 25–1.

Baseline Variability

Variability in the FHR is a sign of interaction between the fetal sympathetic and parasympathetic nervous systems. Good FHR variability consists of two aspects: cyclic variations of 5 to 15 bpm every 2 to 5 minutes, also called *long-term variability,* and *beat-to-beat variability,* which is continuous fluctuation of 2 to 3 bpm at the baseline. Because of the subtle nature of these changes, variability can *only* be assessed by *internal* continuous electronic fetal monitoring. External EFM produces an average FHR and does not provide information about true variability.

Beat-to-beat variability is described as either present, decreased, or absent. Long-term variability is described in the following degrees:

Absent variability	0–2 bpm
Minimal variability	3–5 bpm
Average variability	6–10 bpm
Moderate variability	11–25 bpm
Marked variability	>26 bpm

Fetal heart rate variability has become one of the most important indicators in the clinical assessment of fetal well-being. Marked variability follows catecholamine release or sympathoadrenal activity in response to mild fetal hypoxia. It is observed most often in association with excessive uterine activity, especially during second stage labor. Reducing uterine activity or temporarily reducing pushing efforts will improve placental gas exchange and may improve this pattern (Murray 1988).

Table 25–1   Causes of Baseline Changes in Fetal Heart Rate

Fetal Bradycardia	Fetal Tachycardia	Reduction in FHR Variability
Fetal hypoxia	Prematurity	Deep fetal sleep (should persist only 20–30 min)
Maternal drugs (anesthetics, oxytocics)	Mild hypoxia resulting in increased cardiac rate to compensate for oxygen debt	Prematurity
Maternal hypotension	Tocolytic agents given to mother to treat preterm labor	Congenital anomalies
Prolonged cord compression	Maternal fever, which increases maternal metabolic levels, and increases fetal oxygen needs	Parasympathetic blocking agents (phenothiazines, atropine)
Congenital fetal cardiac lesion	Maternal anemia or hyperthyroidism	Maternal analgesics
	Administration of phenothiazines or other atropine-like drugs, which interrupt vagal response in fetus	Fetal hypoxia
	Fetal activity	
	Fetal infection	

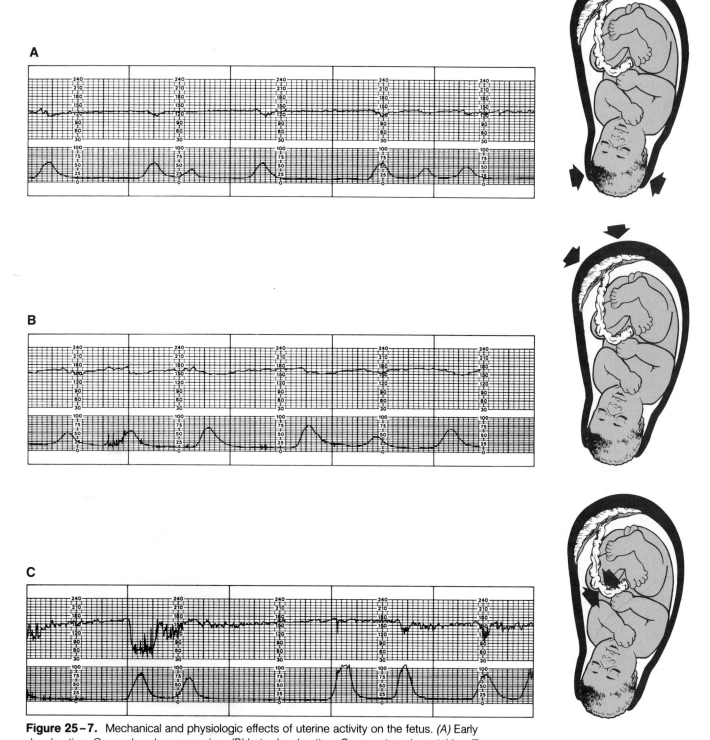

Figure 25 – 7. Mechanical and physiologic effects of uterine activity on the fetus. *(A)* Early deceleration. Cause: head compression. *(B)* Late deceleration. Cause: uteroplacental insufficiency. *(C)* Variable deceleration. Cause: umbilical cord compression. (All fetal line art from Childbirth Graphics. Tracings from Parer JT, Puttler OL Jr, Freeman RK. In Freeman RK (ed): A Clinical Approach to Fetal Monitoring, San Leandro, CA, Berkeley Bio-Engineering, 1974)

Decreasing variability is an indicator of developing fetal distress, and persistent minimal or absent variability is considered an ominous pattern suggesting profound fetal compromise. Some possible causes of reduction in FHR variability are listed in Table 25–1.

Sinusoidal FHR Pattern

The sinusoidal FHR pattern is an unusual pattern that shows uniform wavelike long-term variability of 5 to 15 bpm every 3 to 5 minutes, minimal or absent beat-to-beat variability, and absence of specific responses to uterine contractions. The clinical significance of this pattern is controversial. It has been attributed to severe fetal distress, severe fetal anemia, and maternal medication during labor; however, its causes and its implications for fetal well-being are still unclear.

Periodic Changes in Fetal Heart Rate

Periodic FHR changes are fluctuations from the baseline rate that are associated with uterine contractions. An increase in the baseline associated with a contraction is called an *acceleration* and a decrease is called a *deceleration*. These periodic FHR changes (Fig. 25–7) are thought

Table 25–2   **Patterns of Deceleration Observed on EFM and Appropriate Nursing Care**

Type	Cause	Characteristics	Clinical Significance	Intervention
Early Deceleration	Vagal stimulation from head compression	Onset of deceleration at onset of contraction Ends before contraction ends Uniform wave shape reflects shape of contraction Nadir within normal limits at peak of contraction	Usually innocuous, reassuring pattern May be prevented by avoiding early rupture of membranes	Observe FHR closely to distinguish this from other ominous patterns.
Late Deceleration	Uteroplacental insufficiency due to decreased blood flow during uterine contraction subsequent to: Hypotension (induced by supine position or anesthesia) PIH Tetanic or hypertonic contraction Abruptio placentae Postmaturity	Onset of deceleration at the peak of contraction Ends after contraction ends Uniform wave shape reflects shape of contraction Nadir near end of contraction Tends to occur with every contraction Depth of deceleration does not reflect degree of fetal insult; variability and baseline must also be evaluated.	Ominous sign indicating fetal distress Possible need for cesarean delivery Possible need for fetal scalp *p*H Severe fetal acidosis if baseline variability is lost	Change maternal position to left side, right side, or Trendelenburg to alleviate pattern. Administer O_2 by mask at 8–12 liter/min. Discontinue oxytocin. Increase IV fluids if hypotension is due to regional anesthesia. Notify physician. Prepare for prompt delivery.
Variable Deceleration	Umbilical cord compression against fetal bony part, short or knotted cord, possible prolapse	Deceleration unrelated to contractions Wave forms differ in shape from contraction and from each other. Decelerations usually markedly altered by maternal position change or external manipulation of fetus	Possible severe fetal compromise if decelerations worsen, are prolonged, or are repetitive Possible need for fetal scalp *p*H Possible diminishing fetal reserve if bradycardia is prolonged following deceleration	Change mother to side-lying position. Initiate external manipulation of fetus. Place mother in knee-chest position if deceleration is uncorrected by change to side-lying position. Administer O_2 by face mask. Perform vaginal exam to rule out cord prolapse. Prepare for intra-amniotic saline infusion.

to be related to mechanical and physiologic effects of uterine activity on the fetus.

Accelerations

An acceleration is an abrupt increase of the fetal heart rate that usually lasts less than 10 minutes and is associated with fetal movement. Accelerations are a result of an increase in beta-adrenergic sympathetic nervous system activity and are a reassuring indication of an intact nervous system. They may occur at any time during labor. Repetitive, uniform accelerations with each contraction may occur as an initial response to mild hypoxia that accompanies umbilical vein compression.

Decelerations

A deceleration is an abrupt decrease in the fetal heart rate that usually lasts less than 10 minutes and may be associated with hypoxemia and fetal distress. Decelerations are classified according to their timing in relation to uterine contraction and their shape or waveform as *early, late,* or *variable.* These three major types of decelerations, their causes, characteristics, and clinical significance and the appropriate nursing interventions are summarized in Table 25–2.

Dysrhythmias

Dysrhythmias are irregularities in the fetal heart rhythm. They may be caused by a disturbance in the myocardial cells' ability to form and discharge electrical impulses, resulting in ectopic or premature beats, tachycardia, or bradycardia. Disturbances in conductivity of impulses also occur, leading to heart block. Drugs, acidosis, hypoxia, electrolyte imbalances and cardiac anomalies may precipitate altered rhythms. Many dysrhythmias are benign and require no treatment. It is important to listen to the fetal heart rate with a fetoscope before applying the external EFM in order to detect dysrhythmias and to differentiate them from artifact on the monitor printout.

Implications for Nursing Care

Electronic fetal monitoring has dramatically affected nursing responsibilities in the care of laboring women and their families, especially those who are regarded as being at increased risk in the intrapartal period. The nurse must be knowledgeable about the appropriate use of intermittent and continuous EFM, and must be able to recognize and interpret patterns of FHR change, to report them accurately, and to initiate measures to enhance fetal well-being as needed. In addition, the nurse must be able to rely on learned assessment skills rather than relying exclusively on machinery and must be able to provide sensitive and safe nursing care to the woman and her family despite the potential intrusion of this technology.

Evaluating Findings on EFM Tracings

The nurse must have a systematic approach to evaluating findings on EFM tracings. In assessing FHR patterns, the nurse should first consider the *validity* of the recorded data. Are patterns clear, or does the tracing contain many artifacts and a great deal of "noise"? Are all leads connected? Does the recorded FHR correspond with that noted on auscultation? If not, the EFM may be picking up the maternal pulse or may be halving or doubling the actual FHR. Is the monitor recording the onset and end of uterine contractions simultaneously with the patient's sensation and her own palpation? If not, it is impossible to distinguish between early and late decelerations, a critically important difference. If recordings of uterine contractions are faulty, the pressure catheter may have become dislodged, or the monitor may need to be adjusted or recalibrated.

Events that may have affected the FHR or uterine contraction pattern and other information that aids interpretation must be noted directly on the tracing strip itself. The following types of information are typically recorded on the tracing strip:

- Findings of vaginal examination for progress of labor (station, cervical change, fetal position)
- Spontaneous or artificial ROM
- Maternal vital signs and position changes
- Administration of oxygen or medications
- Changes in maternal status, such as emesis, hiccuping, bearing-down efforts
- Changes from external to internal monitoring
- Adjustments to monitor or leads or any recalibration

If the data are judged to be valid, the nurse then evaluates the tracing for baseline and periodic changes and assesses the quality of the uterine contraction pattern. Data on the tracing are compared with data collected through auscultation, palpation, and observation. Any deviations from normal patterns should be carefully examined and described, and a tentative interpretation of the FHR pattern should be made.

Discriminating Between Reassuring and Nonreassuring FHR Patterns

Once a tentative interpretation of the FHR pattern is made, the nurse must be able to determine whether it is a reassuring or a nonreassuring FHR pattern. Examples of both types are listed in the display on page 688. Reassuring patterns are those associated with fetal well-being and positive outcomes. Nonreassuring, or "warning," patterns suggest decreasing fetal capacity to cope with the stress of labor and may signal frank fetal distress. Ominous FHR patterns are those known to be associated with rapidly developing fetal distress and markedly increased fetal risk.

Fetal Heart Rate Patterns

Reassuring Patterns

Reassuring patterns are those with normal baseline FHR and average variability with

- Mild variable decelerations (less than 30 seconds in duration, with rapid return to baseline)
- Early decelerations (concurrent "mirror image" decrease with contraction)
- Accelerations without other changes

Nonreassuring Patterns (Warning Signs)

- Moderate tachycardia (> 160 bpm)
- Decrease in baseline variability
- Progressive increase or decrease in baseline FHR
- Intermittent late decelerations with good variability

Ominous Patterns

- Persistent late decelerations, especially with decreasing variability
- Variable decelerations with loss of variability, tachycardia, or late return to baseline
- Absence of variability
- Severe bradycardia

The nurse must identify the nature of the change and report nonreassuring or ominous findings to the physician or nurse midwife. Usually, further careful evaluation of maternal and fetal status is then undertaken before decisions about management are made. However, the nurse should be prepared for additional obstetric interventions, such as fetal blood sampling or cesarean delivery.

Since nonreassuring patterns reflect decreasing fetal physiologic reserve to cope with uterine contractions, nursing interventions are directed at maximizing uteroplacental perfusion, providing support and reassurance to the woman and her partner, and preparing for additional obstetric intervention, as necessary. The nurse must notify the physician or nurse midwife immediately and take the following actions to maximize uteroplacental perfusion:

- Position the mother on either the left or right side to reduce the possibility of cord compression and supine hypotension
- Discontinue oxytocin infusion, if there is one, to avoid overstimulation of the uterine muscle and resulting decreased perfusion
- Administer oxygen by face mask at 8–12 liter/minute to increase oxygenation

NURSING ALERT

Administration of Oxygen with Nonreassuring or Ominous Fetal Heart Rate Patterns

If signs of fetal distress occur, a major nursing responsibility is to attempt improvement in fetal oxygen concentrations. Oxygen (100% concentration) should be administered by tight face mask at rates of at least 8 to 10 liters per minute. If maternal, placental, and fetal circulation is not severely compromised, fetal oxygen levels should improve in 1 to 6 minutes.

In the past some facilities used nasal cannulas to deliver oxygen. However, many women in labor breathe through their mouths, especially during contractions, and inspiration of room air (20.9% O_2) will decrease oxygen concentrations to 40% or less, depending upon the woman's breathing pattern. Furthermore, the recommended maximum rate at which oxygen can be delivered by nasal cannula is only 6 liters per minute.

NURSING ALERT

Intrauterine Amnioinfusion

When oligohydramnios is diagnosed or in the event of premature rupture of membranes, the fetus is at increased risk of umbilical cord compression during fetal movement and during contractions. A new technique, intrauterine amnioinfusion, is being utilized in selected medical centers. When severe variable decelerations persist after maternal position changes and oxygen administration have been implemented, amnioinfusion may be attempted.

A hollow intrauterine pressure catheter (IUPC) is inserted into the uterus, and warmed sterile saline is infused at 60 to 100 ml/hour after an initial loading dose of 600 ml/hour for the first hour. Continuous fetal monitoring is required. Potential complications of the procedure include overdistention of the uterus and increased uterine resting tonus. The infusion is therefore stopped every 30 minutes to record resting tone between contractions. Frequent linen protector changes (Chux pads) will be required to maintain patient comfort.

Murray M: Antepartal and Intrapartal Fetal Monitoring. Washington, DC, NAACOG, 1988

- Reassure and support the mother to decrease detrimental effects of fear on uterine blood flow
- Start IV fluids or increase rate of administration
- Prepare for possible intrauterine amnioinfusion

Reassuring and supporting the mother and her partner is a primary nursing responsibility. The nurse should explain the need for the actions outlined above and encourage the couple to ask questions. The nurse should stay with the family, offering encouragement and acknowledging their concerns; use of gentle touch can be very reassuring and quieting to the mother. Providing a calm atmosphere and an explanation of the situation and allowing parents to remain together as much as possible will help them cope with this unwanted turn of events.

If, after further evaluation of fetal status, the FHR is still considered ominous, the physician may decide that prompt delivery is needed. Usually delivery is accomplished by cesarean section; occasionally forceps or vacuum extraction is used if progress well into the second stage has been made. Nursing responsibilities in these situations are discussed later in Chapter 26.

FETAL BLOOD SAMPLING

Fetal hypoxia and the resulting acidosis may be signaled by abnormal FHR patterns. However, at times FHR patterns are inconclusive, and the physician may need additional information to decide whether emergency delivery, usually by cesarean, is needed. If hypoxia is prolonged, the fetus becomes increasingly acidotic and the blood pH decreases. If acidosis is pronounced and uncorrected, fetal well-being is seriously threatened.

Information about fetal blood chemistry can be obtained by fetal blood sampling. A sample can be drawn from the presenting part (usually the scalp) and analyzed to determine pH, oxygen, and carbon dioxide levels. This information can then be used to corroborate or clarify

FHR information. To obtain a fetal blood sample, a cone-shaped endoscope is inserted into the vagina, through the cervix, and is pressed against the presenting part, as shown in Figure 25-8. The scalp is swabbed clean and pricked with a small blade. Fetal blood is collected in a capillary tube and sent immediately to the clinical laboratory for determination of pH and blood gas levels. For this reason, fetal blood sampling is done largely in centers where findings can be interpreted within 10 to 15 minutes; a longer wait for results renders the findings of little value.

While awaiting results of the fetal blood sample, the physician applies compression through one or two uterine contractions to ensure hemostasis and observes the scalp site during a third contraction to verify that there is no bleeding. Even if none is seen, however, continued observation of vaginal discharge is indicated. If there is bloody show following fetal blood sampling, the scalp site should be visualized again to determine if bleeding has resumed. This is important, since any blood loss in a compromised fetus can be disastrous.

Fetal blood pH values are interpreted as follows:

Normal pH (7.25-7.35): No intervention needed; continue to monitor.

Borderline pH (7.2-7.25): Evaluate second sample in 15 to 30 minutes to check for downward trend; continue to monitor.

Acidotic pH (7.2 or less on two consecutive measurements): Severely compromised fetus; immediate forceps or cesarean delivery is necessary.

Indications and Contraindications

Fetal scalp sampling requires access to the fetal presenting part through ruptured membranes and a cervix that is 2 to 3 cm dilated. Access to immediate laboratory analysis and ability to initiate emergency delivery is also necessary. Sampling is done when FHR patterns are

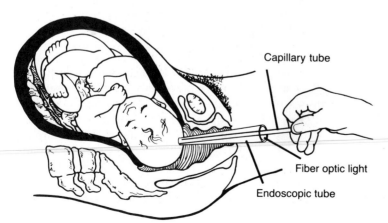

Capillary tube

Fiber optic light

Endoscopic tube

Figure 25-8. Fetal blood sampling to verify fetal distress readings on electronic fetal monitor. (Childbirth Graphics)

inconclusive and potentially worrisome and when additional information about fetal status will make a difference in a decision to delay or expedite delivery. Thus, fetal blood sampling is contraindicated in an obstetric emergency, such as cord prolapse or vaginal bleeding, or when FHR patterns are ominous; in these situations, emergency delivery is indicated.

Advantages and Disadvantages

A major advantage of fetal blood sampling is that it gives direct information about fetal physiologic status that may be used to avoid unnecessary obstetric intervention as well as to initiate emergency procedures when needed. Fetal blood sampling can corroborate and clarify inconclusive FHR findings. However, the procedure also has its disadvantages. Fetal blood sampling requires considerable skill; it is a difficult procedure even under optimal conditions. Further, high-quality and immediately accessible laboratory support is necessary to yield accurate findings that can be used to manage obstetric care. Fetal blood sampling only provides intermittent data, and findings can be influenced by examiner skill and maternal physiologic status. Scalp samples may not accurately reflect pH and blood gas levels in the central circulation, especially if the head is well applied to the cervix and labor is well advanced. Finally, the incision site makes the fetus vulnerable to hemorrhage and subsequent infection.

RELATED RESEARCH

Fetal Scalp Stimulation to Assess Fetal Well-Being

If nonreassuring fetal heart rate patterns persist and a practitioner is not immediately available to perform fetal scalp sampling, a new technique has been suggested to assist in evaluation of fetal well-being. Brisk digital stimulation of the fetal scalp through the dilated cervix is accomplished by the examiner's gloved fingers. Immediate fetal heart rate accelerations in response to stimulation are indicative of a well-oxygenated brain and fetal reserve and have been associated with a scalp pH of greater than 7.19. Fetal scalp stimulation is easy to learn, requires no special technology, and may reduce the number of scalp sampling procedures performed. It also provides the clinician with objective data regarding fetal well-being.

Harvey CJ: Fetal scalp stimulation: Enhancing the interpretation of fetal monitor tracings. J Perinat Neonatal Nurs 1(1):13–21, 1987

Fetal scalp stimulation (see accompanying display) may be appropriate in many cases of suspected fetal distress, and is gaining popularity as an alternative to fetal blood sampling.

Implications for Nursing Care

The nurse must be prepared for problems arising during labor that call for immediate recognition and decisive action. Problems arising suddenly during labor that cause suspicion about fetal status, especially confusing FHR patterns that have ominous aspects, may indicate a need for immediate fetal blood sampling. The procedure demands prompt action and is alarming to the mother and her partner. The nurse's primary tasks are the following:

- To describe the procedure and provide emotional support to the couple that is appropriate, considering the time restraints
- To gather the necessary equipment and assist with the procedure, using strict aseptic technique (During this time the nurse should inform the woman of what is happening and what she can do to help expedite the procedure.)
- While awaiting the pH results, to optimize maternal and fetal status by providing oxygen; by discontinuing any oxytocin infusion (with the physician's permission) to decrease the intensity and frequency of uterine contractions and increase uterine blood flow; by alternating maternal position from the left to the right side to attempt relief of possible cord compression and relieve compression of great vessels
- When the fetal pH is less than 7.20, to prepare the patient for delivery by forceps or cesarean birth, depending on the stage of cervical dilatation
- To interpret the fetal pH results to the couple, to offer support in the event of an emergency delivery, and to stay with the couple as much as possible to keep them apprised of rapidly changing events (Perez 1981)

CHAPTER SUMMARY

The nurse providing care for families during labor must be knowledgeable about procedures used for monitoring fetal status. Electronic fetal monitoring and fetal blood sampling are techniques that enable the clinician to identify the condition of fetal distress and to institute treatment before fetal compromise becomes severe. Nursing responsibilities include recognizing patients for whom these procedures are likely to be beneficial and implementing these procedures safely. Interpretation of fetal

(text continued on page 694)

NURSING CARE PLAN

The Fetus in Distress During Labor

Nursing Diagnosis (Patient Problem) and Assessment Data	Nursing Interventions	Rationale
Potential Complication: *fetal distress* *Risk factors:* • Vaginal bleeding • Diabetes • Pregnancy-induced hypertension • Hypertension • Prematurity • Postmaturity • Multiple pregnancy • Prolonged labor • Meconium-stained amniotic fluid • Maternal infection • Oxytocin induction/augmentation • IUGR • Substance abuse	Apply external EFM for 20 min on admission of all women in labor. Observe and record FHR carefully by intermittent auscultation *during and after contractions* or by continuous electron fetal monitoring. Initiate continuous external EFM. Observe for changes in FHR. Support maternal and fetal physiologic well-being: Provide adequate hydration. Avoid supine hypotension syndrome. Provide comfort measures to minimize need for analgesics.	This establishes baseline FHR information and immediately identifies nonreassuring patterns, if present. Auscultation by skilled nursing staff using fetoscope is acceptable for assessing fetal status in low-risk gravidas. Significance of variations in FHR pattern is often determined by its relationship to contraction pattern. In high-risk cases continuous electronic fetal monitoring is usually preferred because accuracy is greater and monitoring is constant. Fetal stress in labor can be reduced by maximizing uterine blood flow and increasing fetal oxygenation.

Expected Outcome:

Mother delivers healthy newborn by a modified mode of delivery and both maintain physiologic status in appropriate ranges.

Nursing Diagnosis:
fear related to changes in fetal heart rate and labor management

	Explain need for interventions while performing them. Reassure patient/support person.	Parents are sensitive to changes in care-giver reactions. Providing information and support will reduce fear and support coping.

Expected Outcome:

Parents address their fears by voicing them and asking questions concerning procedures and outcomes.

Probable Complication:
umbilical cord compression

• *Variable decelerations*, evidenced by variable shape with sharp drop in FHR and rapid recovery. Decelera-	Observe FHR pattern for continued episodes increasing in severity with decreasing variability.	Mild variable decelerations are usually benign and caused by transient umbilical cord occlusion. Repeated

(continued)

The Fetus in Distress During Labor

Nursing Diagnosis (Patient Problem) and Assessment Data	Nursing Interventions	Rationale
tions can be unrelated to contraction pattern, occasionally severe and prolonged, and associated with rising baseline FHR and decreased variability.	Change mother's position. Administer oxygen at 8–10 liter/min by mask.	stress will diminish fetal oxygen reserve. Position change will often correct pattern by ending cord occlusion. Severe variable decelerations can result in fetal acidosis, loss of baseline variability, and fetal compromise. Correcting cause and replenishing oxygen supply will increase fetal tolerance.
• If severe (FHR < 90 bpm) or recurrent with diminished variability in baseline	Notify physician. Prepare for internal fetal scalp electrode placement, fetal blood pH sampling, and expeditious delivery. Prepare for possible intrauterine amnioinfusion. (See Nursing Alert, this chapter.)	Further evaluation is needed in cases of severe distress. When possible, fetus is delivered. Infusion of fluid may relieve cord compression.

Expected Outcome:

Mother delivers newborn who stabilizes with appropriate respiratory support in first hour after birth.

Probable Complication:
 fetal hypoxia

• Late decelerations evidenced by uniform deceleration that begins midpoint of contraction and recovers well after contraction ends.	Reassure patient. Turn patient on side. Administer oxygen at 8–10 liter/min by mask. Notify physician immediately. Start IV. Take maternal vital signs; correct hypotension if present. Stop or change mother's pushing technique. Discontinue oxytocin. If pattern is determined by auscultation, apply EFM, prepare for application of internal scalp electrode, sampling of fetal blood pH. Monitor carefully, watching for baseline variability, continued decelerations, prolonged fetal bradycardia.	Late decelerations, regardless of magnitude, are *always an ominous sign of fetal hypoxia,* due to uteroplacental insufficiency. Fetal hypoxia and acidosis can result in death. Immediate action is needed to remove cause of hypotension, prolonged breath-holding with contractions, oxytocin-induced hypertoxic uterine contractions. Interventions are aimed at increasing fetal oxygenation. Baseline variability can be assessed only by internal EFM. Fetal pH will determine severity of hypoxia. A subsequent decrease in baseline variability, increase in severity of deceleration, or bradycardia indicate marked fetal hypoxia and acidosis, which could result in death.

(continued)

NURSING CARE PLAN   (continued)

The Fetus in Distress During Labor

Nursing Diagnosis (Patient Problem) and Assessment Data	Nursing Interventions	Rationale
	Be prepared for expeditious vaginal or cesarean delivery. (Type and crossmatch blood).	Worsening of fetal condition may necessitate rapid forceps or emergency cesarean delivery.
	Explain significance of FHR pattern to patient, inform her of possible intervention as fetal condition warrants.	Minor late decelerations are significant but not always obvious. Patient must be informed about condition to prepare her for any intervention, provide support and reassurance, and promote confidence.
• Prolonged, marked deceleration or bradycardia, evidenced by FHR below 90 bpm for longer than 1 min.	Take same actions as for late decelerations.	Marked bradycardia may be due to transient cord compression, placental insufficiency, sudden, rapid progress in labor causing isolated fetal vagal response to head compression.
	Perform vaginal examination.	Vaginal exam will rule out rapid progress or cord prolapse.
• Loss of FHR baseline variability Absent (0–2 bpm)	Check time of last dose of narcotic analgesic.	Narcotics cross placenta, causing depression and transient loss of baseline variability in FHR.
	Review EFM strip for periodic changes in variability.	Decreased variability may be due to fetus's sleep/rest cycle. Should not last longer than 15–20 min.
	Check gestational age.	Premature fetus (under 32 weeks) has immature nervous control mechanism.
	Suspect and react for chronic hypoxia if there have been recent episodes of variable or late decelerations or bradycardia.	Chronic hypoxia leads to fetal acidosis and loss of baseline variability.
• Marked variability >25 bpm	Observe for excess uterine activity and • Stop oxytocics • Reduce pushing efforts • Administer tocolytics • Administer oxygen 8–10 liter/min by mask	Marked variability is response to mild hypoxia and is usually due to increased uterine activity.
• Tachycardia Moderate: 160–180 bpm Severe: 180–200 bpm	Assess maternal temperature.	Maternal infection (chorioamnionitis) is most common cause of fetal tachycardia.
	Confirm fetal heart rate by fetoscope or doppler.	Tachycardia may be due to fetal dysrhythmias. EFM may double slow fetal heart rate.
	Stop oxytocin administration.	Tachycardia may be response to mild fetal hypoxia. Reducing uterine activity may improve placental perfusion.

(continued)

NURSING CARE PLAN (continued)

The Fetus in Distress During Labor

Nursing Diagnosis (Patient Problem) and Assessment Data	Nursing Interventions	Rationale
	Administer oxygen 8–10 liter/min by mask.	Tachycardia is often response to hypoxia.
	Perform vaginal exam.	Tachycardia may result from occult or partial prolapse of umbilical cord.
	Check maternal record for history of hyperthyroidism	Maternal hyperthyroidism may cause fetal tachycardia

Expected Outcome:

Mother delivers newborn who has a one-minute Apgar score of greater than 4 and stabilizes within 24 hours with appropriate respiratory support and specialized neonatal care.

---

heart rate patterns and data from fetal blood sampling has become an essential element of high-risk intrapartal care and requires the nurse to maintain up-to-date skills in order to maintain safe standards of practice.

STUDY QUESTIONS

1. Discuss the nursing actions that should be taken when a deceleration of the fetal heart rate is noted on the monitor strip.
2. Explain the cause and significance of an early deceleration as if you were doing so to a laboring woman.
3. What would you tell a woman who refused electronic fetal monitoring when meconium-stained fluid was the indication?
4. Which fetal heart rate deceleration patterns suggest fetal distress? Why? What patterns are considered reassuring, nonreassuring, and ominous? Why?
5. What is the purpose of fetal scalp sampling? What are normal and abnormal findings?

REFERENCES/BIBLIOGRAPHY

Goodlin R: Low risk obstetric care for low risk mothers. Lancet 10:1017, May 10, 1980

Malinowski J: Nursing Care of the Labor Patient, 2nd ed. Philadelphia, FA Davis, 1983

McKay S, Phillips C: Family-Centered Maternity Care. Rockville, MD, Aspen Systems Corporation, 1984

Murray M: Antepartal and Intrapartal Fetal Monitoring. Washington, DC, NAACOG, 1988

SUGGESTED READINGS

Gilfix MG: Electronic fetal monitoring: Physician liability and informed consent. Am J Law Med 10(1):31–90, 1984

Hager D, Pauly TH: Fetal tachycardia as an indicator of maternal and neonatal morbidity. Obstet Gynecol 66:191–194, 1985

Herbert W, Stuart NN, Butler LS: Electronic fetal heart rate monitoring and intrauterine fetal demise. J Obstet Gynecol Neonatal Nurs 16:249–252, 1987

26 procedures: modifying labor patterns and mode of delivery

LEARNING OBJECTIVES

After studying the material in this chapter, the student should be able to

- Distinguish between induction and augmentation of labor and identify the common modes of each

- Discuss nursing responsibilities during and after amniotomy

- Discuss major precautions to be considered when infusing oxytocin

- Identify indications for and precautions taken during forceps applications

- List indications for cesarean birth

- Discuss nursing responsibilities in caring for the woman and her family before, during, and after cesarean birth

- Discuss the importance of emotional and family-centered support for the woman experiencing cesarean birth

- Identify contraindications and necessary precautions for a trial of labor and vaginal birth after cesarean delivery

KEY TERMS

Augmentation of labor

Cord prolapse

Malpresentation

Meconium

Meconium staining

Oxytocic

Tetanic contraction

Version

Providing care for the woman at increased risk in the intrapartal period requires the nurse to be vigilant in meeting the emotional as well as the physiological needs of the woman and her family. To allow for the safest, most satisfying birth experience possible, the nurse must be able to balance a technological approach to care with intensive emotional support.

For patients requiring interventions designed to modify a less than optimal labor pattern or mode of delivery, nursing care is focused on maintaining optimal maternal and fetal physiological status and providing emotional and physical support while obstetric procedures are initiated. The nurse must be knowledgeable about obstetric procedures and the indications and contraindications of these procedures and must be able to identify both reassuring and worrisome maternal and fetal responses to these procedures.

MODIFYING THE LABOR PATTERN

Maternal–fetal risk in the intrapartal period can be reduced by modifying the pattern of labor, either by induction of labor or by stimulation of labor. *Induction of labor* is typically used when either maternal or fetal status would be improved by delivery but there is no need for cesarean delivery. The most common mode of labor induction is through intravenous infusion of pitocin. *Augmentation (or stimulation) of labor* may be done when the labor pattern is not optimally efficient or effective. Some physiologic techniques for labor stimulation, such as ambulation, maternal position change, and nipple stimulation were discussed in Chapter 23. Labor may also be augmented through oxytocin infusion or through amniotomy. The following section discusses these procedures, their risks and benefits, and implications for nursing care.

Induction of Labor

Induction of labor refers to the deliberate initiation of uterine contractions before they start spontaneously. Induction of labor is a long-standing practice in obstetrics, but it is not without its critics. Induction of labor entails some maternal and fetal risk, and expert medical and nursing care is required to ensure optimal maternal and fetal outcomes. However, induction of labor can also be a lifesaving measure when medical indications for the procedure exist and when the procedure is done safely.

Indications and Contraindications

A specific obstetric indication must be present for an induction to be termed medically indicated. Some of the more common obstetric indications for the induction of labor are listed in the display on the opposite page.

When no medical condition indicates the need to initiate labor, an induction is called *elective* and is performed for the convenience of the physician or patient. Elective inductions are discouraged in many centers because of the increased maternal risk and the danger of delivering a preterm infant. The risks associated with induction must be carefully weighed against the need for the procedure.

Contraindications to induction of labor exist when there are medical reasons to avoid or delay onset of labor or to avoid vaginal delivery. Contraindications to induction of labor can be classified as maternal or fetal in nature.

Advantages and Disadvantages

In addition to resolving the medical condition for which induction is indicated, labor induction offers other advantages in the care of the woman at increased intrapartal risk. These advantages include the following:

- The opportunity for physical and emotional preparation for labor and delivery
- A decreased anesthetic risk, since the patient can be kept NPO and well hydrated
- Adjustment of timing can allow for physician attendance and suitable nursing staff levels

However, disadvantages to induction of labor also exist and include the following:

- Induction may adversely affect the course of labor.
- Induction carries risks to the fetus, including prematurity and fetal distress due to increased uterine activity.
- Induction carries risks to the mother, including prolonged labor, cervical laceration, uterine rupture, and postpartum hemorrhage.
- A failed induction produces emotional and physical stress and is costly in staff time and actual expense.

Assessment of Maternal–Fetal Readiness for Labor

Before induction of labor is considered, the physiologic readiness of both the mother and fetus for delivery must be evaluated. Several factors must be considered in evaluating maternal–fetal readiness for labor.

Fetal readiness or maturity must be well established before induction is attempted; otherwise, there is a risk of delivering a preterm infant, with all the associated risks. A careful maternal history must be taken and verified with the pattern of uterine growth to establish the estimated due date. If there is a question about fetal maturity, other tests should be performed. Amniocentesis may be necessary to obtain an amniotic fluid sample to test for an acceptable L/S ratio and the presence of phosphatidylglycerol (PG), indicating sufficient fetal lung maturity for

Indications and Contraindications to Induction

Indications

- Pregnancy-induced hypertension: This condition may progressively worsen unless resolved by delivery of the fetus.
- Maternal diabetes, classes B-R: Induction and delivery of the fetus 2 to 3 weeks before the EDC may be indicated to prevent fetal demise from placental insufficiency, especially if the diabetes is not well controlled during pregnancy.
- Premature rupture of membranes: Induction may be indicated to prevent uterine infection when membranes have been ruptured 24 hours or more.
- Rh isoimmunization: A rising Rh antibody titer in later pregnancy may indicate maternal sensitization and the need for prompt delivery to prevent erythroblastosis fetalis.
- Postmaturity (more than 42 weeks of gestation): Placental insufficiency and fetal compromise may result from prolonged pregnancy.
- Intrauterine fetal demise: If fetal death has been diagnosed but labor does not ensue, induction may be indicated to reduce maternal risk of disseminated

intravascular coagulation and unwarranted emotional distress.
- Chorioamnionitis

Contraindications

Maternal

- Previous uterine scar or trauma
- Abnormalities of the uterus, vagina, or pelvis
- Placental abnormalities (previa or suspected abruption)
- Herpesvirus Type II in genital tract
- Grand multiparity
- Overdistention of uterus (from multiple gestation, polyhydramnios)
- Invasive cervical carcinoma

Fetal

- Abnormal fetal lie (transverse, breech)
- Low birth weight or preterm fetus
- Fetal distress shown by EFM
- Positive (abnormal) contraction stress test

safe delivery. In addition, ultrasound evaluation may be needed to obtain measurement of the fetal biparietal diameter to assist in estimation of fetal maturity. (See Chapter 17.)

Maternal readiness for induction refers to cervical status and the position of the fetus. Changes normally occur in late pregnancy that prepare or "ripen" the cervix for labor. These changes include a soft consistency, some degree of effacement or shortening, an anterior or centered position relative to the axis of the vagina, and slight dilatation.

A score known as the Bishop score is used to predict cervical favorability for successful induction of labor. This

score assesses cervical dilatation, effacement, consistency, and position as well as fetal station, as shown in Table 26–1. Each factor is assigned a score from 0 to 3, and a total score is calculated. The higher the total score, the higher the likelihood of a successful induction; scores of 6 or more suggest a high probability (95%) of successful induction (Boehm, Davidson, and Barrett 1981).

Other factors that must be considered when readiness for induction is being assessed include open discussion of the indications, relative risks, and probability of success of the induction procedure with the woman and her partner and the provision of information about what the procedure entails and what the parents can expect.

Table 26–1   **Bishop Score for Assessing Readiness for Induction**

Factor	Assigned Value			
	0	**1**	**2**	**3**
Cervical dilatation	0	1–2 cm	3–4 cm	5 cm or more
Cervical effacement	0%–30%	40%–50%	60%–70%	80% or more
Fetal station	−3	−2	−1, 0	+1, +2
Cervical consistency	Firm	Moderate	Soft	
Cervical position	Posterior	Midposition	Anterior	

Adapted from Bishop EH: Pelvic scoring for elective induction. Obstet Gynecol 24:266, 1964

Methods for Ripening the Cervix for Labor

If induction is being considered and the cervix is not favorable for induction, several methods of ripening it may be attempted.

Laminaria Tents. Laminaria tents are stems of round, smooth seaweed that have been dried and sterilized and that readily absorb water. One or more of these laminaria tents may be placed into the cervical canal. Moisture is absorbed and causes the tents to swell; most of this swelling occurs in the first 6 hours after placement. This causes the cervix to become softened and dilated, often to 2 to 3 cm overnight, in preparation for a scheduled morning induction. Maximal cervical effect with laminaria is achieved in 24 hours, whereupon they should be removed.

Prostaglandin E₂. Prostaglandin E_2 in suppositories or cervical gel is being used outside the United States for cervical ripening and induction of labor but is not yet approved for other than experimental use in this country. Prostaglandins are known to have two direct physiologic actions on the labor process: ripening of the cervix and oxytocic stimulation of uterine contraction. Application of a prostaglandin suppository into the vaginal vault or application of gel to the cervix will produce cervical change within 48 hours. In clinical trials many women report mild uterine contractions or backache shortly after administration. Side-effects appear to occur rarely; however, uterine hypertonus, shivering, backache, vomiting, and diarrhea have been reported (Nager, Thomas, and Moore 1987; Glazer and Hulme 1987). Continuous fetal monitoring is required for at least 1 hour after the placement of the gel. If underlying high-risk conditions exist, the woman may remain on the monitor until delivery. A major benefit of the drug appears to be a reduction in the cesarean birthrate due to failed induction when the Bishop score is low. Further evaluations of the drug's safety and effectiveness will be needed before general use in labor induction will be approved.

Stripping of Amniotic Membranes. In the past, stripping of the amniotic membranes from the wall of the lower uterine segment near the cervix was a common method of cervical ripening and labor induction. This was done manually during vaginal examination. However, the risks of rupturing the membranes prematurely and causing prolapse of the cord with a high presenting part and of injuring a low-lying placenta and the discomfort of the procedure have led to a decline in its use.

Once maternal–fetal readiness for labor has been established, induction can safely be considered. By far the most commonly used procedures for induction of labor are amniotomy and intravenous infusion of oxytocin.

Amniotomy

Amniotomy is the artificial rupture of the membranes (AROM), performed by inserting a sterile instrument, usually an Amnihook, into the vaginal canal during vaginal examination and puncturing the amniotic sac, as shown in Figure 26–1. This method of labor induction is thought to be effective because it promotes descent of the presenting part, and mechanical irritation from the presenting part on the parous cervix initiates contractions of the uterus.

The amount of amniotic fluid lost after amniotomy varies and depends upon the amount of fluid contained in the amniotic sac. Descent of the fetal head against the cervix effectively forms a block against further fluid loss and bulging of the membranes. Fluid will continue to leak slowly from the vagina throughout labor. Fluid may be clear or cloudy and is usually odorless. Meconium will turn the fluid greenish or yellowish in color and indicates that the fetus has passed bowel contents. Occasionally, placental abruption will be suspected when an AROM reveals blood-stained fluid, and foul-smelling fluid may indicate infection within the uterus.

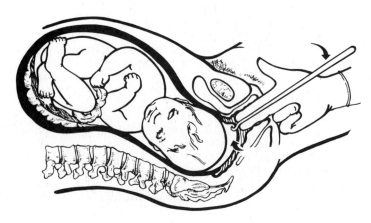

Figure 26–1. Amniotomy (artificial rupture of the membranes). (Childbirth Graphics)

Advantages and Disadvantages

Amniotomy is not without risk to the mother and fetus. It has been associated with increased risk for infection, fetal head compression, and cord prolapse (Gabbe 1976). Amniotomy also removes the protective cushion of the amniotic sac over the fetal head and exposes the presenting part to increased pressure as it is forced against the pelvis and maternal tissues (Baumgarten 1976). Amniotomy may shorten the length of labor, although studies in this area have been conflicting. In fact, no evidence exists to confirm that shorter labors are beneficial to the mother or fetus, and some authors suggest it may even be harmful to the fetus by increasing the risk of acidosis and head trauma.

One advantage of amniotomy is that the use of mechanical means to rupture the membranes avoids the systemic effects of pharmacologic intervention. Amniotomy is also necessary for internal EFM and essential when close monitoring of fetal status is necessary. When fetal hypoxia and acidosis, uterine hyperstimulation, or other high-risk factors are suspected, the benefits of direct fetal monitoring outweigh the risks. For instance, an early amniotomy may reveal meconium-stained fluid, thus allowing early intervention to avert more serious problems.

Indications and Contraindications

Indications and contraindications for amniotomy for induction of labor are given in the accompanying display.

Implications for Nursing Care

The nurse must be aware of the patient's status and of any medical contraindications for amniotomy that may be present. Prior to the procedure, the nurse should assess the woman's condition. When there is evidence that places the merit or safety of an amniotomy in question, the nurse should discuss the findings and rationale with the physician or nurse midwife attending the patient. Circumstances can change in a short time, especially when an induction has been previously planned but the patient has not recently been examined.

When preparing for an amniotomy the nurse should:

- Explain the procedure to the patient, telling her she will experience no more discomfort than with the usual vaginal examination and that she will feel "warm and wet" from the amniotic fluid as it drains
- Assemble the required equipment, which includes an Amnihook, sterile gloves, lubricant, linens, and Doptone
- Help the patient to assume the correct position on her back with her knees flexed and dropped apart
- Monitor the fetal heart tones just before and during the procedure

After the amniotomy the nurse should:

- Assess the fetal heart tones
- Observe and note on the chart the color, amount, and odor of the fluid, recording time of amniotomy and cervical status on EFM graph, if used
- Explain to the patient and her partner the results of the procedure and what is to be expected: onset of uterine contractions, more intense contractions, leakage of fluid
- Change bed linens for the patient's comfort
- Monitor the patient's temperature every 2 hours to assess for possible infection

After the amniotomy, labor usually begins within 4 to 8 hours. When labor has not been established by this time, intravenous oxytocin should be initiated.

Intravenous Oxytocin Infusion

Endogenous oxytocin is released from the posterior lobe of the pituitary gland and stimulates contraction of the uterus. As pregnancy nears term, the uterus becomes sensitive to minute amounts of oxytocin. Synthetic oxytocics, such as Pitocin, when given intravenously, will also act on the uterine muscle, stimulating contraction. Oxytocin also has pronounced cardiovascular and renal effects. Cardiac output and stroke volume are increased, and a significant rise in baseline maternal blood pressure can be noted in some cases. If oxytocin is given in an intravenous bolus, profound hypotension and tachycardia may result. Urinary output decreases significantly because of the drug's antidiuretic effect (Malinowski 1983).

Oxytocin is the most efficient and frequently used drug for induction of labor; it is also used to augment labor

---

Indications and Contraindications to Amniotomy for Induction of Labor

Indications

- Contraindications to use of oxytocin infusion
- Desire for direct fetal monitoring

Contraindications

- High or unengaged presenting part (−2 stations or above)
- Unknown presenting part or abnormal presentation such as transverse lie or breech
- Uncertain EDC
- Placenta previa
- Herpesvirus Type II present in vaginal tract

already in progress (See Augmentation of Labor, later in this chapter). It is a powerful drug, and the patient must be carefully assessed prior to and throughout oxytocin administration.

Advantages and Disadvantages

Advantages of oxytocin use for induction of labor include its efficiency and effectiveness in initiating and stimulating labor, its lack of direct action on the fetus, and its predictability of action. Disadvantages of oxytocin use include the risk of abnormally strong or *tetanic* uterine contractions and the risk of uterine overstimulation, which may result in fetal distress and, in rare cases, uterine rupture. Use of oxytocin has also been associated with increased incidence of preterm deliveries and cesarean deliveries. Safe oxytocin induction requires capability for direct EFM and intrauterine pressure monitoring, physical presence of the physician, and one-to-one expert labor nursing.

Indications and Contraindications

Indications for use of oxytocin to induce labor include all of the general indications for induction, such as threats to maternal–fetal well-being and need to expedite deliv-ery. Indications and contraindications for oxytocin use include those listed in the accompanying display.

The FDA has banned the use of oxytocin for elective inductions and recommends it only for medically indicated inductions.

Implications for Nursing Care

The nurse is responsible for preparing the intravenous solution, assessing the patient before and during administration, and evaluating fetal and uterine response patterns to the medication.

An initial responsibility of the nurse is careful assessment of the patient who is a candidate for oxytocin infusion. The nurse must ensure that there are no contraindications to the drug before the infusion is started. Although the patient will previously have been screened by the physician, the nurse is usually the primary care provider during the infusion and must be aware of all the data relating to the patient.

Most hospitals have detailed policies and procedures concerning the amount, rate, and interval of use of oxy-

LEGAL/ETHICAL ISSUES

Indications and Contraindications to Oxytocin Infusion

Indications

- Pregnancy-induced hypertension
- Maternal diabetes, classes B-R, especially if diabetes is not well controlled during pregnancy
- Premature rupture of membranes
- Rh isoimmunization
- Postmaturity (more than 42 weeks of gestation): placental insufficiency and fetal compromise may result from prolonged pregnancy
- Intrauterine fetal demise

Contraindications

- Cephalopelvic disproportion (CPD)
- Abnormal fetal presentation (transverse, breech)
- Placental abnormalities (placenta previa, suspected abruption)
- Documented fetal distress
- Prematurity (unless maternal or fetal condition warrants delivery)
- Predisposition to uterine rupture (previous uterine scar; multiple gestation or other overdistention of the uterus, such as polyhydramnios, grand multiparity, history of uterine trauma, infection)

Ensuring Patient Safety During Induction of Labor

Induction of labor is based on a benefit–risk ratio for the patient and her fetus. Because risks are inherent in the administration of intravenous oxytocin, it is essential that the labor and delivery unit have a carefully delineated policy and procedure guiding nursing actions that is in accordance with state practice acts. The level and educational preparation of the nurse performing the induction should also be identified in the written protocol and commensurate with the complexity of the procedure.

Institutional policies must allow nurses the flexibility to refuse administration of oxytocin if any question regarding indications arises, the situation is beyond the nurse's expertise, or conditions in the labor unit make it impossible for the nurse to monitor the patient with the frequency required for the provision of safe care. Many resources indicate that the patient being induced should be observed continuously. It is not only appropriate but necessary at times to stop an induction in progress when nursing personnel are not available to assess the maternal–fetal responses to oxytocin infusion. In this case, the physician should be notified immediately.

OGN Nursing Practice Resource: The Nurse's Role in the Induction/Augmentation of Labor. Washington, DC, NAACOG, 1988

tocin infusion. Before initiating an infusion, the policy should be reviewed.

Oxytocin is *always* administered intravenously when used for induction or stimulation of labor. Use of an infusion pump is REQUIRED because it offers precise control of the medication dose. An intravenous piggyback setup is used. The main intravenous line is started with a large-bore needle (usually 16- or 18-gauge) and connected to 1,000 ml of a physiologic electrolyte solution. To a second liter of solution, 10 units (10,000 mU) oxytocin are added (the dose depends on the facility's policy). The piggyback line delivering the medication is connected at the most proximal location to the vein, usually at the needle connection into the hub at the point of insertion. This arrangement allows immediate discontinuation of the oxytocin when necessary, with no residual oxytocin solution remaining in the main IV infusion.

The current standard of care requires a physician to be present in the facility at all times during an oxytocin infusion in order to intervene in a timely manner if complications arise during the induction procedure. The nurse is responsible for notifying the physician before starting the infusion. Since nursing supervision is mandatory and the patient must never be left unattended, adequate staffing should be ensured before infusion is begun. Electronic fetal monitoring is also required, and a 30-minute baseline of fetal heart rate is obtained for comparison if problems arise later. Internal EFM is preferable because FHR and contraction intensity are measured more accurately.

Oxytocin infusion is started at 0.5 to 1.0 mU/min, using a standard infusion guide to calculate flow rate, as shown in Table 26–2. This amount is gradually increased by 1 to 2 mU at every 30- to 60-minute interval until an *optimal uterine response* is achieved: contractions at a frequency of 2 to 3 minutes, with duration of 45 to 60 seconds and moderate to strong (60–70 mm Hg) intensity with at least a 30- to 45-second rest period between contractions (OGN Nursing Practice Resource 1988). To assess uterine contractions, the nurse should palpate the fundus and observe the EFM tracing for intrauterine pressure and FHR response every 15 to 30 minutes. Administration of oxytocin should also be recorded on the EFM tracing itself. In addition, maternal vital signs must be recorded every 15 to 30 minutes. Intake and output recording should be initiated because of the drug's potential antidiuretic effect.

Approximately 15 minutes of infusion is needed to achieve steady blood levels and optimal uterine response. However, sensitivity of the uterine muscle to oxytocin can not be predicted with accuracy. Additional administration of the medication will continue to affect the myometrium after optimal uterine contraction has begun. Hyperstimulation of the uterus may result in *hypertonicity* or tetanic contractions, which are prolonged over 70 seconds. *Tumultuous labor,* or violent, agitated labor, may also result.

Table 26–2 Oxytocin Administration Flow Rate Guide*

Dosage in mU/min	Flow Rate ml/hr
0.5	3
1.0	6
2.0	12
3.0	18
4.0	24
5.0	30
6.0	36
7.0	42
8.0	48
9.0	54
10.0	60
12.0	72
14.0	84
16.0	96
18.0	108
20.0[†]	120

* This guide is for use in administration of oxytocin using intravenous pump that delivers 20 gtt/ml. Infusion solution is 10 units of oxytocin in 1000 ml of intravenous fluid (or 5 units in 500 ml).
[†] If desired contraction pattern is not achieved with dosage of 20.0 mU/minute, consult with physician and obtain order for increased dosage, if appropriate.
Marshall C: The art of induction/augmentation of labor. J Obstet Gynecol Neonatal Nurs 14(1):22, 1985

Hyperstimulation may result in the following sequelae:

- Fetal distress due to impaired uteroplacental perfusion
- Abruption of the placenta
- Amniotic fluid embolism
- Lacerations of the cervix and uterine rupture
- Neonatal trauma

If signs of uterine hypertonicity are observed, the nurse should discontinue the oxytocin infusion immediately and notify the physician. Tocolytics (drugs that inhibit uterine contraction) may be administered to decrease uterine activity. Maternal plasma concentration of oxytocin falls rapidly after the infusion is discontinued, since its circulating half-life is 3 to 4 minutes. After evaluation of the patient's status, the physician may elect to lower the dose of oxytocin, infuse it at a slower rate, or select another method of induction.

Once optimal uterine activity is established, the nurse will need to assess the woman's progress in labor, how she and her partner are responding to the labor, and her comfort level. The nurse should be alert to individual and family needs for support and avoid the tendency to become focused too much on the procedure at hand. Oxytocin administration may be associated with increased maternal pain and fatigue. The nurse should evaluate the need for analgesia, avoiding administration too early

(text continued on page 706)

NURSING CARE PLAN

The Patient Receiving Oxytocin Therapy for Induction/Augmentation of Labor

Nursing Diagnosis (Patient Problem) and Assessment Data	Nursing Interventions	Rationale
Nursing Diagnosis: *potential for injury: trauma related to inappropriate treatment*		
Adequate indications for oxytocin therapy: • For induction: toxemia, diabetes, Rh-sensitization, postmaturity, positive OCT (CST) • For augmentation: arrest of active labor, hypotonic uterine contractions, premature rupture of membranes, irregular or ineffectual labor pattern	Perform vaginal examination for effacement, dilatation, station, presenting part. Assess fundal height. Perform Leopold's maneuvers for presentation, lie, estimated fetal weight. Compare physical findings with prenatal record for verification of gestational age.	The nurse is ultimately responsible for verifying indications, gestation, labor status, and fetal status before initiating oxytocin therapy. The FDA and American College of Obstetricians and Gynecologists *do not* recognize elective inductions for the convenience of patient or physician as appropriate or safe.
Contraindications to oxytocin therapy: • Prematurity (without overriding medical indication). • Uteroplacental insufficiency • Placenta previa • Cephalopelvic disproportion • Previous cesarean section • Overdistension of uterus (*i.e.,* multiple pregnancy) • Grand multiparity, polyhydramnios • Unknown or abnormal fetal lie	Screen patient for contraindications. If contraindication exists: • Recheck information. • Notify physician about findings that contraindicate oxytocin infusion. • Notify nursing supervisor if order to begin infusion appears questionable and is not changed by attending physician. • Thoroughly document relative contraindications with medical justification in patient's chart. If no contraindications exist: • Proceed with preparations. • Explain procedure and anticipated response to patient. • Initiate internal or external electronic fetal monitoring. • Start main IV using an 18 or a 20 gauge needle. • Prepare appropriate mixture oxytocin/IV solution (10–20 IU oxytocin to 1000 ml Lactated Ringer's). Piggyback oxytocin to	The nurse is responsible for knowing all indications and contraindications for any procedures or drug he or she administers. The nurse's responsibility is to *protect the patient* in cases of uncertain practice. Appropriate channels of authority should be followed if an order is questioned. Use of oxytocin infusion is responsible for greatest number of lawsuits involving obstetric practice. Contractions may peak more rapidly and last longer than spontaneous labor. Oxytocin infusion is stressful to fetus. Monitoring of resting tone of uterus is of utmost importance. Large gauge needle is used in case transfusion is needed later. If adverse response to oxytocin occurs, discontinuing infusion assures that no oxytocin remains in IV line if it is connected at proximal point.

(continued)

The Patient Receiving Oxytocin Therapy for Induction/Augmentation of Labor

Nursing Diagnosis (Patient Problem) and Assessment Data	Nursing Interventions	Rationale
	main IV line at most proximal junction to patient. Flow rate is controlled by IV infusion pump.	
	• Notify in-hospital physician of plan to initiate oxytocin infusion.	A physician must be in the hospital during oxytocin infusion.
	• Begin infusion according to protocol (1 to 2 mU/min).	*Patient should never be left unattended during oxytocin infusion* because of danger of fetal distress or hyperstimulation.
	• *Stay with patient.*	
	• Increase dose according to protocol every 30–60 min until desired labor pattern is established. Contractions should be 2–3 min apart, 45–60 sec long and moderate to strong (50 to 75 mm Hg by internal uterine pressure catheter).	
	• Document accurately.	
	• Monitor vital signs, and FHR every 15 minutes. Assess contractions by palpation. If fetal distress or hypertonicity of uterus occur, discontinue infusion immediately; notify physician.	Palpation of contractions is most important indicator of strength. Fetal monitor should never replace "hands on" assessment by the nurse.

Expected Outcome:

Mother proceeds through normal labor following oxytocin therapy without complications and delivers a healthy newborn by vaginal delivery.

Probable Complication:
fetal distress

• Tachycardia	Monitor and record vital signs and FHR every 15 to 30 minutes.	Oxytocin may cause peripheral vasodilation initially, resulting in hypotensive response, decreased uteroplacental perfusion, and fetal distress.
• Bradycardia		
• Decreasing variability		
• Prolonged deceleration		
• Late decelerations	Monitor FHR for normal range of 120 to 160 bpm. If there is loss of variability, late decelerations, or persistent bradycardia (< 120 bpm):	Baseline fetal heart rate should not change significantly with oxytocin infusion. However, frequent contractions of increased strength will stress fetus markedly if uteroplacental insufficiency exists. This is manifested by decreased variability, late decelerations, and bradycardia. O_2 will increase maternal oxygen supply available to the fetus.
• Severe variable decelerations (See Nursing Care Plan: The Fetus in Distress During Labor, Chap. 25.)	• Discontinue oxytocin infusion immediately.	
	• Administer O_2 by mask at 8 to 12 liter/min.	

(continued)

The Patient Receiving Oxytocin Therapy for Induction/Augmentation of Labor

Nursing Diagnosis (Patient Problem) and Assessment Data	Nursing Interventions	Rationale
	• Notify physician.	Notify physician whenever a change in maternal or fetal status occurs.
	• Reposition patient to left side or opposite side.	Repositioning increases placental perfusion.
	• Initiate internal fetal monitoring.	Internal fetal monitoring is more accurate for assessing fetal status. It is the only mechanism for assessing FHR variability.
	• Perform vaginal examination.	Sudden fetal distress may be result of rapid labor progress, descent of fetus or cord prolapse.

Expected Outcome:

Fetus maintains normal activity and heart rate during oxytocin infusion, and mother delivers healthy newborn by vaginal or cesarean delivery.

Nursing Diagnosis:
possible fluid volume excess

Signs of fluid retention: • Bounding pulse • Decreased urine output • Peripheral edema • Sacral edema • Increasing blood pressure • CNS signs (*i.e.,* lethargy, confusion, convulsions) of cerebral edema • Shortness of breath, rales	Monitor intake and output. Monitor amount of oxytocin being infused over course of induction/augmentation.	Slow administration of oxytocin over a prolonged period can result in water intoxication.

Expected Outcome:

Woman in labor maintains normal intake and output with appropriate vital signs during oxytocin induction.

Possible Complication:
maternal hypotension

	• Position patient on side.	A supine position often results in vena caval compression and hypotension, decreased uterine perfusion, and fetal distress.

(continued)

NURSING CARE PLAN (continued)

The Patient Receiving Oxytocin Therapy for Induction/Augmentation of Labor

Nursing Diagnosis (Patient Problem) and Assessment Data	Nursing Interventions	Rationale

Expected Outcome:

The woman in labor maintains normal vital signs during oxytocin therapy without indications of fetal distress.

Probable Complication:
uterine hypertonicity, tetanic contraction

• Contractions >75 mm Hg, >90 seconds duration, or closer than 2 minutes	• Discontinue infusion immediately. • Check maternal vital signs, response. • Assess fetal status. • Notify physician. • Prepare to administer tocolytics as ordered.	Serum half-life of oxytocin is 2 to 3 minutes, thus stopping infusion will diminish uterine activity rapidly. Hypersensitivity is unpredictable and must be carefully monitored. Tocolytics decrease uterine activity.

Expected Outcome:

Laboring woman maintains appropriate level of uterine activity or returns to appropriate level for stage of labor following cessation of infusion.

Potential Complication:
inadequate uterine response

• Absent or weak contractions • Absence of cervical change	Check IV mixture to be sure oxytocin was added, follow IV line for patency and connection. Increase IV flow rate according to protocol; notify physician if maximum rate is achieved.	Error in mixture, IV set up, or faulty connection is often responsible for poor uterine response. Simultaneous administration of magnesium sulfate or epidural anesthesia will inhibit oxytocin effectiveness. Unripe cervix of unready uterus (few oxytocin receptors) will also diminish response. Approximately 20 minutes of infusion at a given dose is needed to achieve steady blood levels. Infusion should be discontinued after 8 to 12 hours and may be restarted next day.
	Observe patient response to contractions. Palpate contractions for quality, duration, relaxation. Perform vaginal exam for labor progress.	What appears to be a "failed" induction or augmentation may be actually promoting labor progress. Patient responses vary and may be misjudged.

(continued)

NURSING CARE PLAN (continued)

The Patient Receiving Oxytocin Therapy for Induction/Augmentation of Labor

Nursing Diagnosis (Patient Problem) and Assessment Data	Nursing Interventions	Rationale

Expected Outcome:

The woman receiving oxytocin induction therapy demonstrates strong contractions of appropriate duration within 8 to 10 hours of beginning the therapy.

Nursing Diagnosis:
potential for injury: trauma related to rapid labor/delivery

Signs of impending birth: • Frequent, strong contractions • Increased bloody show • Urge to push • Rectal pressure • Perineal bulging	Never leave patient unattended. Monitor contractile pattern and patient response for signs of impending delivery. Assess labor progress frequently. Rely on assessment of contractions, response, recent exams to monitor labor. Discontinue oxytocin infusion and notify physician if there is rapid dilatation or delivery is imminent.	Patient must be observed closely for tumultuous labor/precipitate delivery. Patient response may be first indication of impending delivery. Vaginal exam is most accurate assessment of labor progress. Due to the risk of infection, frequent examinations are undesirable. In the event of sudden rapid labor or delivery, the nurse is responsible for discontinuing infusion to prevent such further complications as lacerations, fetal distress, retained placenta, postpartum hemorrhage.

Expected Outcome:

The woman undergoing oxytocin infusion returns to a normal uterine activity pattern and progresses through labor and delivery without oxytocin-induced complications.

(which may prolong labor) and too late (which may produce neonatal depression at delivery). In addition, the woman may make rapid progress in cervical change and fetal descent during oxytocin administration; vaginal examination is indicated when the contraction pattern is optimal and if there is an increase in maternal pain. If the patient is a multigravida, more frequent vaginal examinations may be in order, since she may make more rapid labor progress.

Prolonged infusion of oxytocin may result in hypertension accompanied by a frontal headache, and water intoxication, with symptoms of shortness of breath, rales on chest auscultation, or convulsions. Strict monitoring of vital signs and intake/output is necessary throughout the entire infusion procedure. When labor is not established within 8 to 12 hours, the oxytocin infusion should be discontinued. Depending on the physician's evaluation of the patient's status, the main intravenous line may be kept open and the infusion restarted the following day. Daily or *serial* attempts to induce labor with oxytocin infusions may be indicated. If serial induction fails, cesarean delivery may be indicated.

NURSING RESEARCH

Nonpharmacologic Methods to Stimulate Labor

In an effort to reduce invasive interventions during childbirth, breast stimulation has been suggested as an alternative method to intravenous oxytocin infusion to stimulate labor. Nipple stimulation is known to cause oxytocin release from the posterior pituitary gland, resulting in uterine contractions. Recent studies have evaluated the effectiveness of two breast stimulation techniques in promoting an effective labor pattern: manual rolling of the nipple and use of an electric breast pump. Benefits of breast stimulation may include avoidance of pain related to an IV insertion, elimination of the risk of water intoxication secondary to an intravenous oxytocin infusion, increased patient control during the labor process, and early milk production for the breast-feeding client. Possible adverse effects that may limit the usefulness of this method are uterine hyperstimulation, fetal distress, nipple soreness, and milk production and engorgement in bottle-feeding clients. If breast stimulation is ordered by the physician or midwife, the nurse must carefully instruct the woman in the appropriate technique (see accompanying display), closely monitor uterine and fetal responses to the procedure and be prepared to administer tocolytics, as ordered, if uterine hyperstimulation occurs.

Recommended Technique for Manual Breast Stimulation: Labor Initiation/ Augmentation

- Collect baseline FHR and contraction pattern data for 10 minutes before beginning procedure.
- Instruct patient to roll or tug one nipple under her clothing for a 10-minute period or until the first subsequent contraction.
- Upon contraction, stop stimulation immediately and evaluate quality of contraction and FHR.
- If FHR response and contraction quality are within normal limits, continue nipple rolling for additional 10 minutes or until next subsequent contraction and reevaluate.
- Observe closely for uterine hyperstimulation and adverse FHR response and discontinue breast stimulation if FHR response and exaggerated uterine activity occur (deceleration during any contraction that lasts more than 90 seconds or occurs more frequently than every 2 minutes).

Moenning R, Hill W: A randomized study comparing two methods of performing the breast stimulation stress test. J Obstet Gynecol Neonatal Nurs 6(4):253, 1987

Suggested Procedure for Use of Breast Pump Stimulation

- Obtain an electric breast pump and instruct patient to apply moderate suction on her right breast for 10 minutes and then repeat procedure on left breast.
- Discontinue pumping for 10 minutes; observe FHR and contraction pattern closely for change.
- Repeat the above cycle five times, evaluating closely for uterine hyperstimulation and FHR deceleration (described above). If no positive changes in labor pattern result, discontinue procedure.

Poppe C, Young J: Breast pump stimulation to promote labor. MCN 12:124–126, 1987

Augmentation (Stimulation) of Labor

Augmentation or *stimulation of labor* refers to the process of promoting more effective uterine contractions when labor has already begun but is dysfunctional or has stopped. The most commonly used methods of labor augmentation are also methods for induction of labor: amniotomy, intravenous oxytocin infusion, and nipple and breast stimulation to increase endogenous oxytocin secretion. (Breast stimulation is highlighted in the accompanying displays.) Nursing care of patients receiving these methods of augmentation of labor is identical to that required when these methods are used for labor induction.

As is true of labor induction, amniotomy is not as predictable or effective a stimulator of labor as oxytocin induction. Further, there is some criticism of the practice of amniotomy for labor stimulation, since, as previously mentioned, it may lead to increased incidence of fetal head trauma and increases the risk of cord compression and prolapse and of cesarean delivery.

MODIFYING THE MODE OF DELIVERY

Maternal and fetal risk in the intrapartal period may also be reduced by modifying the mode of delivery. Common obstetric interventions that modify mode of delivery include *version,* a procedure that can convert malpresentation of the fetus; *forceps and vacuum extraction,* procedures that shorten the second stage and facilitate delivery of the fetus; *cesarean birth,* or operative abdominal delivery, which may reduce certain risks posed by vaginal delivery and also allows prompt emergency delivery when either the mother or fetus is in danger; and *trial of labor and vaginal birth after previous cesarean,* which may be attempted to reduce the risks attendant on a repeat cesarean birth.

Version

Version is the manipulation of the fetus to obtain a more favorable position for delivery. *External version* refers to manipulation of the fetus through the maternal abdominal wall, usually to convert a breech presentation to vertex or a persistent transverse lie into a longitudinal presentation. This procedure is usually done at around 37 weeks of gestation; however, it can also be done in early labor.

Advantages and Disadvantages

Many physicians do not attempt this procedure and will advise delivery by cesarean for a persistent malpresentation because of the risk of antepartum hemorrhage, premature rupture of membranes, preterm labor, or fetal death. Others suggest that external version, when done under optimal conditions, can reduce the risks associated with malpresentation and eliminate the need for a consequent cesarean delivery. External version may be attempted after intravenous administration of a tocolytic agent to enhance uterine relaxation. Even if conversion of a malpresentation is successful using this procedure, the fetus may later spontaneously return to the previous position.

Internal podalic version or direct manual manipulation of the fetus inside the uterus was done in the past to convert malpresentation of a second twin. However, internal version poses significant risk to the fetus and is now done only in extreme emergencies, such as profound fetal distress with a prolapsed cord or the need for immediate delivery of a second twin when there is not enough time for cesarean delivery. In this procedure, the physician reaches up into the uterine cavity, grasps the feet of the fetus, and draws them through the cervix, and delivers the fetus as in a breech presentation. This procedure is extremely rare in contemporary obstetric practice.

Indications and Contraindications

Indications for external version are listed in the accompanying display. Contraindications include the absence of any of the requirements listed. External version may stimulate uterine activity and puts mechanical stress on the uterus, membranes, and placenta; thus, the other contraindications in the display apply.

Requirements and Contraindications for External Version
Requirements

External version may be attempted if a breech or transverse presentation is diagnosed, and the following conditions exist:

- Ultrasound evaluation has been done to localize the placenta and rule out multiple gestation.
- The presenting part is not engaged in the pelvis.
- The maternal abdominal wall is thin, permitting accurate palpation of fetal position.
- The uterus is not irritable (prone to contraction with manipulation).
- There is enough amniotic fluid to allow easy movement of the fetus.
- Manipulation can be done without anesthesia, to avoid application of undue force.

Contraindications

- Absence of any of the above conditions
- Previous uterine trauma or surgery
- Any condition that would prohibit a vaginal delivery
- Evidence of third-trimester bleeding or a low-lying placenta

Implications for Nursing Care

Nursing responsibilities after version focus on close monitoring of maternal–fetal status for signs of impending hemorrhage or fetal compromise. Maternal blood pressure should be monitored every 5 minutes throughout the procedure, and continuous FHR monitoring should be in place. The procedure should be discontinued if abnormalities in the FHR appear. Assessment of maternal blood pressure and FHR should be continued during the first 30 minutes following the procedure. If version is done in the intrapartal period, the mother should be monitored closely for signs of postpartum uterine atony and developing hemorrhage secondary to uterine trauma.

Forceps Application

Obstetric *forceps* are curved metal tongs used to facilitate the birth of the baby's head by providing traction and rotation, as shown in Figure 26–2. Blades of the forceps are specially shaped to fit the fetal head and the maternal pelvis; both the blades and the shanks of the forceps are curved to provide the best traction angle for various situa-

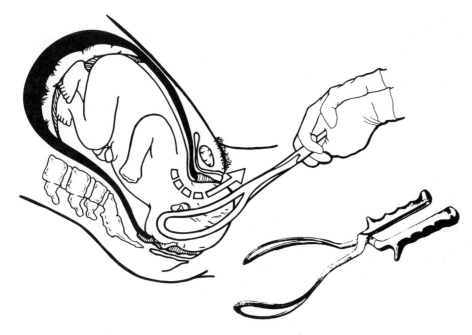

Figure 26-2. Forceps delivery. (Childbirth Graphics)

tions. The incidence of forceps applications will vary according to the facility, the type of analgesia and anesthesia used for labor, customary maternal position for labor and delivery, and the skill and experience of the birth attendant.

Traction is needed when the mother is unable to push the infant out of the vagina spontaneously due to a tight fetopelvic fit, diminished urge to push, or decreased effectiveness of bearing-down efforts as a result of anesthesia, analgesia, fatigue, or improper positioning. In addition, traction may be needed to achieve a rapid delivery if maternal status is compromised or if fetal distress is detected late in the second stage. Preterm infants may also be delivered using forceps to shorten the second stage and protect their vulnerable heads from the prolonged pressure of labor. *Rotation* of the infant by forceps may be done if the fetus presents in a persistent transverse or posterior position and maternal position changes have not been successful in achieving spontaneous rotation.

There are three types of forceps applications. *Low or outlet forceps applications* are done when the fetal head is visible on the perineum; forceps are used in this way primarily to guide and control the delivery of the head. *Midforceps applications* are those in which the head is at the level of the ischial spines and engaged; midforceps deliveries are difficult, and current obstetric management may be replacing midforceps applications with cesarean delivery. *High forceps applications* are those in which forceps are applied through the cervix before the head is engaged in the bony pelvis. Because of the high risk of severe maternal and fetal injury, this practice is no longer used and has been virtually replaced by cesarean delivery.

A *failed forceps delivery* is one in which application was attempted but delivery could not be achieved; cesarean birth is then indicated.

Indications and Contraindications

Indications for forceps application include those conditions that require a shortened second-stage labor: when mother or fetus is in jeopardy or when assistance with maternal bearing-down is needed. The following conditions must exist for a safe forceps delivery:

- Complete dilatation of the cervix and ruptured membranes
- Knowledge of fetal position
- Diagnosed vertex, breech, or face (mentum anterior) presentation
- Absence of cephalopelvic disproportion, sacral or pelvic outlet abnormalities
- Adequate regional or general anesthesia
- Empty maternal bladder to avoid trauma

Without these conditions forceps delivery is unsafe, and cesarean birth is likely indicated.

Advantages and Disadvantages

Advantages of forceps applications include possible avoidance of cesarean delivery when vaginal birth can be safely achieved with mechanical assistance, protection of the preterm fetus's vulnerable head during the second stage, and avoidance of maternal exhaustion from prolonged pushing.

Disadvantages of forceps applications center on

Obstetric Forceps

Obstetric forceps are designed to facilitate delivery of the fetal head. They have blades that are either solid or fenestrated (with an opening), shanks, and handles. The blades are curved to fit the fetal head and the curve of the maternal pelvis. They are designed for specific obstetric purposes; the most commonly used types are described below.

Simpson's forceps (similar to DeLee forceps) are used for low or outlet forceps applications. Note the shanks are well separated near the handle to allow an episiotomy incision to be made after the forceps have been applied.

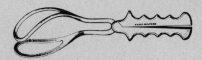

Tucker-McLean forceps are used for low forceps applications and with preterm infants. The solid blades allow easier application and removal, and lessen the potential for soft-tissue or head trauma.

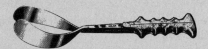

Piper forceps are specifically designed for delivery of the after-coming head in breech deliveries. The shanks are curved down, so that the blades can be higher than the handles when applied to the fetal skull. This allows for easier traction in a breech delivery.

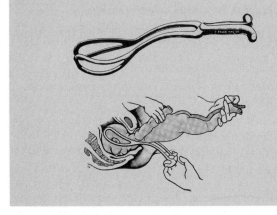

trauma to maternal tissue and the fetal head during delivery. These effects may include:

- Lacerations of the vagina and cervix
- Extension of an episiotomy into the rectum
- Rupture of the uterus
- Increased risk of uterine atony and excessive bleeding
- Increased risk of infection

- Fracture of the coccyx and bladder trauma
- Potential trauma and bruising of neonate's head

Implications for Nursing Care

The decision for a forceps delivery is made by the physician or the nurse midwife. The nurse must be prepared to locate the appropriate type of forceps when requested. Forceps are placed one at a time on either side of the fetal head, while frequent checks are made to ensure proper positioning and avoidance of trauma to the fetal head or maternal tissues. An episiotomy may be made after placement of the forceps. Delivery of the infant is achieved by gentle traction on the forceps handles until full crowning is evident, after which they are removed. When crowning has taken place, the mother then can usually provide the final push to deliver the head and rest of the body.

The nurse must support the mother if she is awake, explaining what is being done and how she can assist in the prompt delivery of her infant. Maternal comfort level should be observed closely; forceps applications should involve sensations of pressure, but adequate regional anesthesia should be established so that no pain results. Inhalation anesthesia may also be used to achieve adequate maternal relaxation for some forceps applications.

The nurse should monitor the FHR closely during application and traction. Fetal bradycardia may be observed as a result of head compression and is transient. Midforceps applications are more dangerous to the fetus, and pediatric assistance should be available, since intensive neonatal support may be necessary. The neonate delivered with forceps should be carefully examined for cerebral trauma or nerve damage (see Chapter 33).

The nurse must be alert for possible sequelae of forceps deliveries. The mother should be observed carefully for excessive bleeding, severe perineal bruising and pain, difficulty in voiding, and cervical or vaginal lacerations.

Vacuum Extraction

Vacuum extraction is accomplished by use of a specialized vacuum extractor, which has a caplike suction device that can be applied to the fetal head to facilitate extraction, as shown in Figure 26–3. Once the suction cup is applied, it is connected with sterile tubing to the suction machine. Suction is initiated at 0.2 kg/cm², and gradually increased in equal increments to a maximum of 0.8 kg/cm². The negative pressure that is achieved pulls the fetal scalp tissue into the suction cup. Fluid accumulates in the subcutaneous tissue of the scalp and it becomes edematous, forming a caput which fits snugly into the cavity of the vacuum cup. This allows traction forces to be applied to the head (Galvan and Broekhuizen 1987). Once the appropriate level of negative pressure is reached, the physician applies traction during uterine contractions

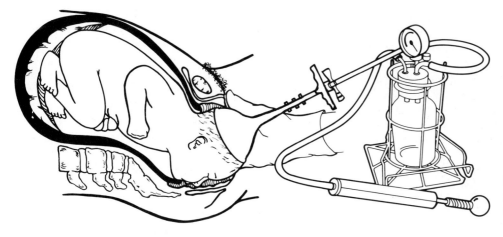

Figure 26-3. Vacuum extractor with suction cup applied to scalp. (Childbirth Graphics)

until descent of the fetal head can be achieved. The suction device should be kept in place no longer than 20 to 30 minutes, and slippage or "pull off" should be avoided because it can cause trauma to fetal scalp or maternal tissue. Caution should be taken to avoid placing the suction device over a previous scalp electrode or blood sampling site, if possible.

Indications and Contraindications

Indications for use of vacuum extraction are similar to those for forceps application. In addition, vacuum extraction can be safely used through a partially dilated cervix to shorten first-stage labor in some cases. Contraindications include profound fetal or maternal distress requiring rapid delivery, evidence of cephalopelvic disproportion, or face or breech presentation.

Advantages and Disadvantages

Vacuum extraction has the following advantages over forceps applications:

- Less trauma to bladder and vaginal tissue
- Lower risk of perineal tearing
- Easier application when the presenting part fits snugly in the birth canal
- Less risk of excessive pressure on fetal head
- No routine need for anesthesia

Disadvantages include the fact that vacuum extraction cannot assist in an emergency where rapid delivery is needed and usually cannot actively achieve rotation of the presenting part, although sometimes spontaneous rotation occurs when traction is applied. Other disadvantages include:

- Risk of fetal scalp bruising, avulsion, and other cerebral trauma from excessive suction or prolonged use (greater than 30 minutes)
- Increased incidence of cephalhematoma

Implications for Nursing Care

Nursing responsibilities during vacuum extraction include informing the mother and support person about the procedure, continued monitoring of maternal and fetal status, and assisting the birth attendant with the procedure. The FHR should be auscultated every 5 minutes if electronic monitoring has not been established, and the nurse should be prepared for forceps application and neonatal resuscitation if prompt delivery is necessary.

During vacuum extraction, the nurse may need to help the physician by connecting the sterile tubing to the suction machine and starting the suction. The nurse may need to release the suction quickly if the cap slips off in order to avoid trauma to maternal tissue. When delivery is achieved, the neonate must be assessed at birth and observed throughout the immediate postpartum period for signs of cerebral trauma secondary to vacuum extraction. A *caput succedaneum* (localized swelling) at the suction cap site is normal and will resolve within 24 hours.

Cesarean Birth

Cesarean birth is an operative procedure in which the fetus is delivered through a surgical incision in the maternal abdominal wall and uterus, as shown in Figure 26-4. The term *cesarean* comes from the Latin root, *caedere,* to cut. Previously called C-section and considered major surgery, the preferred term for the procedure is now *cesarean birth* or *cesarean delivery*. This terminology deemphasizes the operative procedure and stresses the birth experience. Such deliveries may be planned (elective) or arise from an unanticipated problem (emergency).

Currently the incidence of cesarean birth is 15% to 20% of all births in the United States, up from the 4% rate of the late 1960s. This increase may be partly due to the widespread use of electronic fetal monitoring and the resulting concern for fetal well-being during labor, the increased safety of anesthesia and operative care, and the increas-

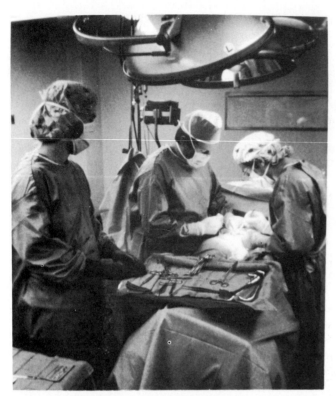

Figure 26–4. Cesarean birth, once a measure of last resort, is now relatively safe and, in many cases, a life-saving procedure. Nevertheless, it is major surgery and is not without risk to both mother and newborn. (Photo: BABES, Inc.)

ing numbers of moderate-risk and high-risk pregnancies being carried to term. In addition, breech presentations are more commonly managed now by cesarean delivery than in the past, and this accounts for some of the recent increase in cesarean rates.

However, there is increasing concern that cesarean deliveries are being performed for maternal or fetal conditions that may not actually require operative delivery. The NIH Consensus Development Statement on Cesarean Childbirth (1980) reports an extensive review of available data on cesarean delivery and perinatal outcomes by an interdisciplinary task force of professionals involved in birth care. This report indicates that for conditions other than frank obstetric emergency, cesarean delivery may not significantly improve maternal and neonatal outcomes.

For example, there is no convincing evidence to support the routine use of cesarean delivery for uncomplicated breech presentations, yet this is standard practice in many facilities. Critics note that this reflects in part the nature of medical training: a physician who receives obstetric training in a setting where certain obstetric conditions tend to be treated by surgical intervention has little opportunity to learn other, equally safe modes. That phy-

sician will then tend to use more intervention than another who observed vaginal breech deliveries and who learned the safe limits of that practice. Further, some critics point out that often when fetal distress is diagnosed and a decision for cesarean birth is made, a healthy newborn with no signs of intrauterine stress is subsequently delivered.

Certainly, the increased rate of cesarean birth is controversial, in large part because cesarean birth is not without significant maternal and neonatal risk. Cesarean birth constitutes major surgery; maternal morbidity is two to four times higher for cesarean than for vaginal deliveries. Wound infections, endometritis, and urinary tract infections are associated with cesarean delivery. Therefore, the need for cesarean delivery in individual clinical cases must be carefully evaluated. Large-scale research on the actual benefits and risks of cesarean delivery to both mother and neonate is still needed.

The increased use of cesarean birth is also controversial because family-centered care is often denied to women and their families when an operative delivery is needed, even if the need is not of an emergency nature. Fathers and support persons are often excluded from the delivery room if a cesarean is required, despite growing evidence that their presence increases the mother's emotional comfort and may contribute to easier postnatal adaptation.

Objections raised to the father's presence at cesarean delivery include the argument that this will increase infection rates, that the sights and sounds of the surgery will be overwhelming to the father, and that malpractice litigation will become more likely if complications arise and he is witness to the care that is rendered. Others argue that if the cesarean is done under general anesthesia, the father cannot support his partner emotionally and therefore has no role in the delivery room. In fact, the opposite appears to be true; infection rates and malpractice cases have not increased in centers allowing fathers to attend cesarean birth, and many parents experience the opportunity to share the birth as a special event. Some fathers whose partners experienced emergency cesareans under general anesthesia were grateful for the opportunity to stay with their partners and to "welcome the baby" for their wives (May and Sollid 1984).

Finally, cesarean birth has been shown to have negative emotional consequences for some women. Certainly an unplanned cesarean birth for a couple planning a shared family-oriented birth is a loss, and some women experience emotional upset after an unanticipated cesarean delivery. They may feel acute disappointment, guilt, and a sense of having failed. These feelings, in addition to the longer postcesarean recovery period, may predispose a woman to difficulty in her adjustment to early motherhood.

Thus, it is important for health professionals to regard cesarean birth as *childbirth* as well as a necessary operative procedure. Women and their families already experience fear and are at increased physical and emotional risk when a cesarean birth is being contemplated. The technology of obstetric care has improved to reduce risk and increase the chances of a good physical outcome for mother and newborn; the remaining challenge to health professionals is to promote family-centered care within the context of cesarean birth.

Cesarean births were, even as late as 1940, procedures of last resort. Now cesarean births are commonplace events in any maternity setting; even emergency cesarean procedures may not be especially noteworthy in many high-risk settings. In many facilities, the labor nurse is responsible for assisting with patient preparation for cesarean delivery, but the procedure itself takes place in the operating room. In other settings, cesarean deliveries are done in the obstetric unit, and the labor nurse assists with all phases of the birth.

Anesthesia for Cesarean Birth

The selection of anesthesia for cesarean birth depends on maternal status and medical history, fetal status, whether the need for prompt delivery is urgent, and whether the operative procedure can be done in the obstetric unit. Regional (either spinal or epidural block) as well as general anesthesia are commonly used for cesarean delivery (see Managing Maternal Pain, Chapter 27). In many settings, general anesthesia is used only in emergency situations where there is insufficient time for administration of regional anesthesia.

Family-centered care is facilitated by use of regional anesthesia, since the mother is alert during the birth and in many cases the father or support person may be present (Fig. 26–5). Many institutions exclude fathers or support people from attending cesarean delivery when general anesthesia is used, on the assumption that the intubation procedure would be unduly upsetting to observers and that because the mother is unconscious, she requires no emotional support during the operative pro-

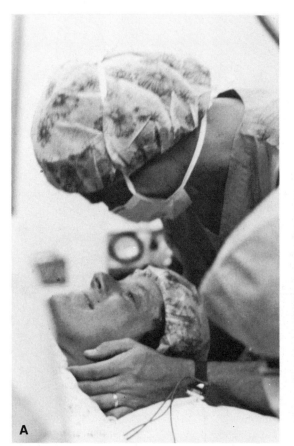
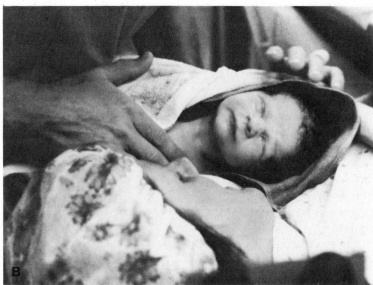

Figure 26–5. *(A)* The father's presence during cesarean birth can be important to both parents and can lead to an increase in their satisfaction with the birth experience. *(B)* Regional anesthesia for cesarean birth permits the mother to be alert and to see her newborn only moments after birth. When circumstances permit, this facilitates parent–newborn interaction and family-centered care. (Photo: BABES, Inc.)

cedure. In addition, when general anesthesia is used, most settings require transfer of the mother to a post-anesthesia recovery unit, during which time she is usually separated from her partner and newborn. In contrast, when regional anesthesia is used, the mother can usually be safely recovered in the obstetric unit.

Types of Cesarean Birth

There are two major types of cesarean deliveries: low-segment and classic. The most commonly used is the low-segment procedure.

In the low-segment delivery, the skin incision is made horizontally. This is called a *Pfannenstiel incision* or, more popularly, the "bikini" cut (Fig. 26–6). The cut is made transversely on the skin at the level of the mons pubis and a horizontal incision is made in the lower segment of the uterus. Since the skin incision is low it is later hidden by pubic hair; thus its name, *bikini cut*. Blood loss is minimal, fewer postdelivery complications occur, and the incision

is easy to repair. A major advantage is that there is less chance of rupture from the uterine scar in future pregnancies. Its major drawback is that the procedure takes longer to perform and thus is not useful in an emergency. Because of the anatomical features of the area, there is limited stretch to the incision and limited space in which to work. This limitation can be alleviated by use of a low-segment vertical incision in the uterus, which has the advantages of the low-segment transverse incision but which can be extended into a classic midline incision, if more room is needed.

Advantages of the low-segment cesarean include the following:

* Less postoperative abdominal distention
* Minimal blood loss since the lower uterine segment is thin compared to the body of the uterus
* Decreased chance of uterine weakening and scar rupture because the tissue of the lower uterine segment is less contractile than the body of the uterus

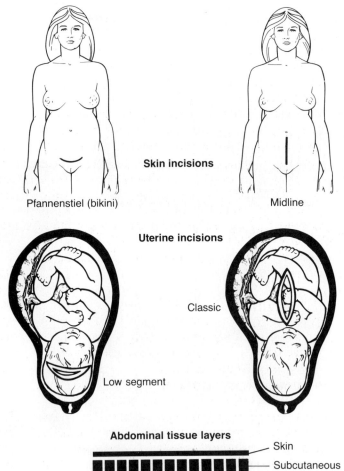

Figure 26–6. Cesarean birth incisions. (Childbirth Graphics)

In a classic cesarean delivery, a vertical midline incision is made in the skin and also into the wall of the *body* of the uterus (Fig. 26–6). This incision is preferable when there are abdominal adhesions from previous surgery and when the fetus is in a transverse lie, because it permits easier access to the fetus for delivery. This type of cesarean is also commonly used in an emergency delivery because more rapid access to the fetus is possible. However, blood loss is increased because large vessels in the myometrium are cut. Further, the uterine musculature is weakened by a midline incision, and there is a greater chance of rupture of the uterine scar in subsequent pregnancies and labor.

Rarely, a cesarean hysterectomy is performed in which the uterus is removed with delivery of the fetus. This is radical surgery reserved for frank obstetric emergencies, including unremitting uterine hemorrhage, placenta accreta (abnormal placental adherence to the uterine wall; see Chapter 28), uterine rupture, or fulminating uterine infection.

The term *primary cesarean* refers to the woman's first cesarean delivery. The term *elective repeat cesarean* refers to a subsequent cesarean that is performed in the absence of a specific indication for operative delivery when either the physician or the woman is unwilling to attempt a vaginal delivery. In the past, a previous cesarean delivery was considered a relative contraindication for subsequent labor and vaginal delivery, even if the cause of the previous cesarean was nonrepeating (such as cord prolapse or breech presentation). This was primarily because of concern about uterine scar rupture during the stress of labor. Although the precise incidence was not known, uterine rupture was thought to be a frank obstetric emergency with high maternal and fetal risk. However, as discussed later in this chapter, the risk of uterine rupture seems to have been overestimated; trial of labor and vaginal birth after cesarean (VBAC) is increasingly regarded as a safe and appropriate mode of obstetric management for selected patients.

Indications and Contraindications

The primary goal of a cesarean delivery is the preservation of the life and well-being of both mother and fetus. A variety of conditions indicate the need for a cesarean birth. A discussion of each follows.

Cephalopelvic disproportion is the most common cause of a cesarean delivery and indicates a spatial inadequacy of the maternal pelvis in relation to the fetal head, which impedes the fetus from negotiating the pelvic canal.

Malpresentation of the fetus exists when the fetus is in a transverse (sideways) or breech (buttocks or feet first) position. Vaginal delivery is potentially dangerous for the mother and fetus when these fetal positions exist. Although vaginal delivery of a fetus in the breech position may be uncomplicated, when the fetal head becomes

---

Indications and Contraindications for Cesarean Delivery

Indications

- Cephalopelvic disproportion
- Malpresentation of the fetus
- Uterine dysfunction
- Previous cesarean delivery
- Soft-tissue dystocia
- Pregnancy-induced hypertension
- Herpesvirus infection of genital tract
- Maternal diabetes
- Maternal complications
- Placental insufficiency
- High-risk obstetric factors: placenta previa, placental abruption, umbilical cord prolapse, fetal distress, previous fetal death or damage, prolonged rupture of membranes with intrapartal infection

Contraindications

- Presence of dead or nonviable fetus

---

obstructed at the vaginal opening, the problem is serious. This problem occurs in breech delivery because the chin, rather than the molded caput, presents at the vaginal opening, making delivery of the head extremely difficult. For this reason some obstetricians feel that all breech presentations should be delivered by cesarean to protect the infant's well-being. Controversy surrounds this practice, but evidence is growing that breech vaginal birth is a safe alternative to cesarean when careful screening and monitoring are used.

Uterine dysfunction describes inefficient or uncoordinated uterine contractions, inability of the cervix to dilate, and prolonged labor. Uterine dysfunction may also be associated with cephalopelvic disproportion or fetal malpresentation. Failure of labor to progress is evidenced by lack of cervical dilatation and fetal descent.

Previous cesarean delivery places the mother at greater risk for uterine rupture. When a previous cesarean incision is subjected to the stress of labor and risk of uterine rupture, planned cesarean births are frequently advised. This trend may be decreasing as more women who experienced previous surgical delivery desire trial labor and vaginal birth. With the increased use of the low-segment incision for cesarean birth, trial labor and vaginal birth has been found to be safer than previously believed. This issue is discussed later in the chapter.

Soft tissue dystocia may be caused by previous surgery or injury to the tissue of the reproductive tract and may result in cervical rigidity, stenosis of the vagina, or scars in the genital tract. During a vaginal birth, hemorrhage or severe lacerations may occur in the previously damaged tissue; thus a cesarean may be required.

Complications of pregnancy, such as pregnancy-induced hypertension (PIH), that are marked by hypertension, edema, and proteinuria may require delivery of the fetus before term to prevent severe maternal compromise.

Unsuccessful induction of labor may occur when the cervix is unripe or unresponsive to oxytocin. In these circumstances cesarean delivery may be required.

Herpes virus infection of the genital tract indicates the need for cesarean delivery. When herpes lesions in the birth canal are actively shedding virus at the time of delivery, as many as 50% of the infants will become infected. During labor and vaginal birth the fetus may become contaminated through the eyes, scalp, skin, umbilical cord, and upper respiratory tract. Congenital herpes may cause long-term disability or death of the infant. In an attempt to avoid infant infection, cesarean delivery is done when the membranes are intact. When the membranes have been ruptured for more than 12 hours, the infant has already been exposed to infection and vaginal delivery is indicated.

Maternal diabetes may lead to a fetus that is larger than average, making vaginal delivery more difficult. Risk of developing PIH is also greater in the diabetic mother. Both of these conditions may require delivery before term although, with careful follow-up and ongoing assessment of maternal diabetic status and fetal well-being, need for early delivery can be eliminated in most cases.

Maternal complications, including cardiac disease, hypertension, Rh incompatibility, uterine anomaly, or previous vaginal repair, may be relative indications for cesarean delivery.

Placental insufficiency, which results from the aging of the placenta in postterm pregnancy, may also suggest the need for an operative delivery. The aging placenta functions less efficiently in supplying the metabolic needs of the fetus. When prenatal testing of the postterm fetus reveals it to be in jeopardy and induction is not feasible, cesarean delivery is performed.

Other high-risk obstetric factors signal the need for immediate cesarean delivery. These factors include placenta previa, placental abruption, umbilical cord prolapse, fetal distress, previous fetal death or damage, and prolonged rupture of membranes with intrapartal infection.

Contraindications for cesarean delivery include the presence of a dead fetus or an immature fetus that could not survive outside the uterine environment. In these situations, the maternal risk of operative delivery is not justified.

Advantages and Disadvantages

Advantages of cesarean birth include the ability to deliver a fetus rapidly when fetal or maternal well-being is threatened, when this threat would be increased by continuing labor, or when a vaginal delivery presents maternal or fetal risk. Although cesarean birth is generally thought to improve maternal and neonatal outcomes, current rates of cesarean delivery (about 1 in 5 births) appear to be higher than would be dictated strictly by considerations of maternal or fetal risk.

Disadvantages of cesarean birth center on the fact that cesarean delivery is major abdominal surgery. Maternal mortality and morbidity are increased over that of vaginal delivery. Surgical complications, such as hemorrhage, anesthetic reactions, injury to pelvic or abdominal organs, and infection, may result.

Implications for Nursing Care

Nursing responsibilities in the care of the woman and her family when cesarean delivery is anticipated combine aspects of surgical and maternity care. In addition, some aspects of nursing care will vary depending on whether the procedure is elective, unanticipated, or under emergency conditions. If the procedure is elective, the couple can be prepared for it either through individual preoperative teaching or through scheduled cesarean classes.

If the need for cesarean birth was not anticipated, the nurse should help the parents to participate in decision making. At times, the need for cesarean delivery is communicated to parents as if there is urgency for delivery when in fact it will make little difference if they take time to consider their decision. The clinician should explain the facts about the labor situation, explain alternative approaches, and discuss the probable consequences of those approaches. The parents should then be given time to consider and to give consent or not, as they choose. If parents feel they have been consulted and have some control over what happens to them, they are likely to respond favorably and perceive their birth experience more positively than if they feel the decision was made for them.

If there is no urgency for delivery, the nurse should still have ample time for explaining to the parents what they should expect during and after the birth. The nurse should allow time for parents to express concerns and encourage them to ask any questions they may have. Whenever possible, the nurse should also allow them some private moments alone to reach out to and support each other. Under emergency conditions, the nurse must assist the parents to adjust as best they can to rapidly changing events. In these circumstances, the nurse will have many pressing tasks in preparation for the procedure. However, providing clear explanations and emotional support to the parents remains an essential element of nursing care.

The nurse should recognize that even when the need for delivery is not urgent, cesarean birth constitutes a risk; parents have fears about pain, physical mutilation of the woman's body, and possible complications or death for the mother or newborn. The parents should be made aware that these fears are to be expected and that the nurse is there to support and assist them. The nurse must also keep in mind that, even in emergency situations, the woman or her partner must be given adequate information and must give informed permission for administration of anesthesia and operative delivery.

Depending on the indication for the cesarean, nursing care will continue up to the transfer to the delivery room. Assessments of maternal vital signs, labor status, and fetal heart rate may be done more frequently. The nurse should also assess the parents' emotional response to the at-risk labor situation and evaluate the kind of information and support they need.

Preoperative Teaching

The nurse should explain the sequence of events leading up to the delivery and what can be expected during postanesthesia recovery. As physical preparations are made, the nurse should explain each procedure, why it is needed, and what sensations the mother may feel. If the father is present, the nurse should explain how he can support his partner during these preparations. The type of anesthesia likely to be used should be explained in terms of what the woman will feel, how long it will last, and what after-effects it may have.

The nurse should explain that if regional anesthesia is used, the mother will be awake during the procedure, that she may feel some abdominal pressure and pulling during the delivery, and that she will be unable to move her legs because of the anesthesia. Specific procedures, such as the use of an electrocoagulation machine to ligate blood vessels (the machine makes a characteristic noise and emits an odor) or the routine sponge count, should be explained to parents so they are not surprised and worried.

If circumstances permit, the nurse should also explain postanesthesia recovery routines and when mother and newborn are likely to be transferred to the postpartum unit. The mother should understand that she will have some pain from the incision and that analgesia will be offered as needed. Preoperative teaching about the importance of early ambulation, coughing, and deep breathing in the postoperative period can be done at this time. The nurse should explain that while these activities will cause discomfort at first, they are essential to reduce the risk of postoperative complications, such as respiratory infection and thromboembolism, and will shorten her recovery time.

Providing Emotional and Family-Centered Support

The nurse should always try to appreciate the effect that an at-risk labor and cesarean delivery may have on the emotional state of the woman and her partner. When possible, parents should be given time alone to gather their strength and take in information and events. Anxiety, tension, and fear are appropriate responses, and they may be expressed through anger, withdrawal, crying, and agitation. The nurse should assess how the woman and her partner are coping with their apprehension and offer support as needed.

The nurse should also facilitate a family-centered approach to the cesarean delivery. If the parents desire it, the father should be permitted to attend the birth; the nurse should explain his role and who will assist him and describe events briefly. If the father cannot or chooses not to be present, the nurse should keep the parents together as long as possible to promote maternal comfort and to allow the father to remain involved. Many women are especially afraid of the administration of regional anesthetic. If the anesthesiologist approves, the father's presence during that procedure may be helpful and reassuring to the woman. If the father is present for the cesarean birth, the nurse must help him obtain suitable operating room attire and explain his role in the delivery room.

The father typically is seated at the mother's head during cesarean delivery. From this position he can touch and converse with the woman, and the anesthesiologist or circulating nurse can provide any needed assistance. Both the mother's and father's view of the surgical field is blocked by a screen; however, the father may stand or look around the screen as he wishes. If the father is to be present at a delivery under general anesthesia, he is usually seated off to the side of the room where he can see the delivery from a slight distance. When he is present, the father is often the first person to hold the newborn after it is stabilized. If the father cannot or chooses not to be present, the nurse can encourage him to stay nearby and perhaps observe through the delivery room window if there are staff who can remain with him and provide reassurance and information. The father can also be encouraged to carry the newborn to the nursery. It is a *nursing* responsibility to keep the father well informed about the status of mother and newborn before, during, and immediately after the operative procedure.

Preoperative Preparation of the Patient

The nurse preparing the precesarean patient should do the following (see Figure 26-7):

(text continued on page 720)

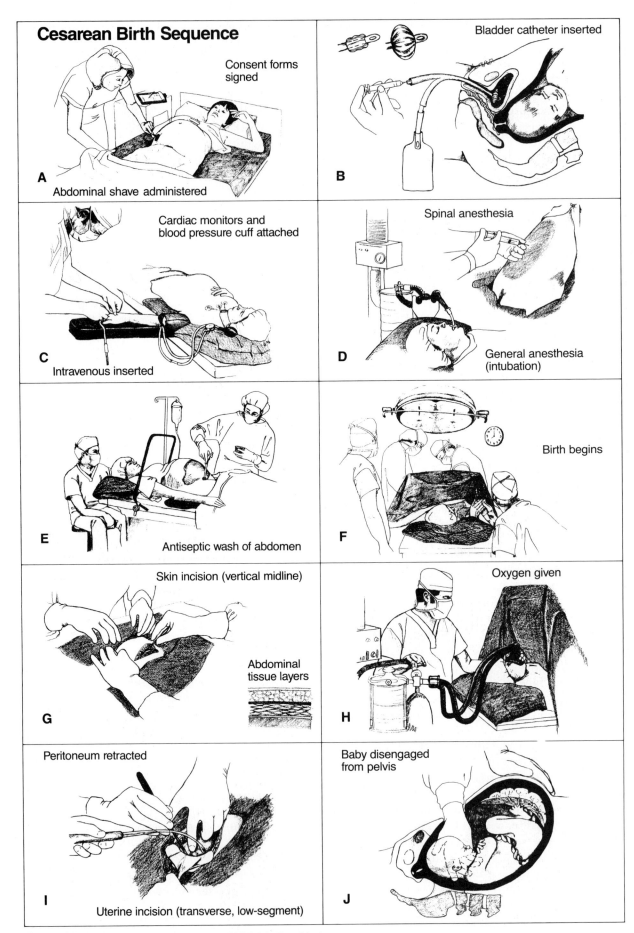

Cesarean Birth Sequence

A Consent forms signed / Abdominal shave administered

B Bladder catheter inserted

C Cardiac monitors and blood pressure cuff attached / Intravenous inserted

D Spinal anesthesia / General anesthesia (intubation)

E Antiseptic wash of abdomen

F Birth begins

G Skin incision (vertical midline) / Abdominal tissue layers

H Oxygen given

I Peritoneum retracted / Uterine incision (transverse, low-segment)

J Baby disengaged from pelvis

Figure 26–7. Steps in cesarean birth. (Childbirth Graphics)

718

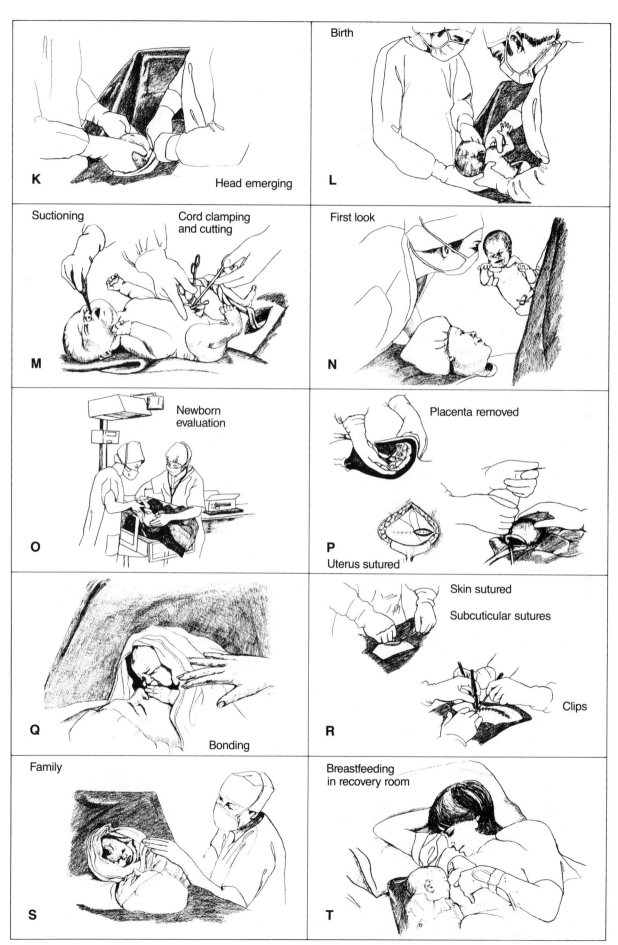

K   Head emerging

Birth

L

Suctioning   Cord clamping and cutting

M

First look

N

Newborn evaluation

O

Placenta removed

P

Uterus sutured

Bonding

Q

Skin sutured

Subcuticular sutures

Clips

R

Family

S

Breastfeeding in recovery room

T

Figure 26–7. *(continued)*

719

- Shave the abdominal area beginning just below the breasts and including the pubic region (Fig. 26 – 7A).

- Insert an indwelling urinary catheter to dependent drainage to prevent bladder distention during delivery (Fig. 26 – 7B).

- Obtain preoperative laboratory tests, including complete blood count (CBC), electrolytes, clotting studies, and type and crossmatch, necessary when ordering units of blood replacement.

- Insert an intravenous line or assess the patency of an existing line to ensure an open route for administration of medications, fluids, and blood (Fig. 26 – 7C). The bore of the needle must be large enough (18 or 16 gauge) for the administration of blood replacement. Infusion of antibiotics may be ordered in the event of prolonged rupture of the membranes and possible ensuing infection. The mother should be kept NPO.

- Help the father or support person with preparations to attend the delivery room or keep him well informed about preparations and patient status.

- Ensure that patient identification is correct. It is also helpful to prepare the baby's identification before delivery and affix it to the front of the mother's chart.

- Administer a nonparticulate antacid 15 minutes before induction of anesthesia. In the event of aspiration during anesthesia induction, the stomach contents will have been neutralized, which helps to prevent aspiration pneumonitis.

- Attend the anesthetist when anesthesia is administered (Fig. 26 – 7D).

- Scrub the entire operative field with antiseptic solution (Fig. 26 – 7E).

- Notify other members of the health care team that the delivery is imminent: pediatrician, intensive care nursery staff, and anesthesia staff. Notify the blood bank when blood replacement is needed.

Intraoperative Care

Functions of the labor nurse during cesarean delivery begin with assisting the mother onto the operating table. She should be positioned comfortably to reduce the risk of muscle strain during the birth. The fetal heart rate is monitored to assess for fetal hypoxia from possible supine hypotensive syndrome, which could occur as a result of the mother lying on her back. If hypotension does occur, the operating table is tilted slightly to one side to relieve pressure of the uterus on the vena cava and maintain optimal circulation to the placenta.

The nurse verifies that the suction and cautery machines are functioning correctly, assists with gowning and gloving of the physicians, and performs an initial sponge count with the scrub nurse and physician. An important function of the nurse is the timing and documentation of

NURSING RESEARCH

Initial Maternal – Infant Interaction in Cesarean Delivered Mothers

The initial mother – infant acquaintance experience for women who have given birth vaginally has been studied in depth. This early pattern of maternal touch is also used by clinicians as a measure of maternal – infant attachment. However, little research regarding early maternal handling has been conducted among women who have given birth by cesarean delivery.

Tulman (1986) recently observed and compared cesarean-delivered mothers and women who gave birth vaginally. Neither group differed in the pattern of initial touch, although the cesarean subjects handled their infants significantly less, were willing to delay seeing the infants, and allowed fathers a more active role in interactions with the newborn. Further study is indicated before clinicians can begin to develop assessment tools appropriate for evaluating maternal – infant interactions after cesarean birth. Nurses should be cautious about interpreting findings regarding the bonding phenomenon if using tools developed for vaginally-delivered women.

Tulman LJ: Initial handling of newborn infants by vaginally and cesarean-delivered mothers. Nurs Res 35(5):296 – 300, 1986

events. This includes the time of the initial incision, the exact time of delivery of the infant, and the time at which the procedure is completed. The nurse stands by to give support to the mother and father, if he is present, and to assist in any way needed by the surgical team. Steps in the cesarean birth sequence are shown in Figure 26 – 7F to L).

The labor nurse may also be needed by the pediatrician to assist with care of the neonate. Help may be required with suctioning of the infant; administering oxygen when necessary; clamping the umbilical cord; evaluating the newborn; injecting intramuscular vitamin K, which enhances clotting, into the infant's anterior thigh (lateral aspect); and verifying the identity of the infant (Fig. 26 – 7M,O).

When the infant has been assessed and is stabilized, it is given to the parents to hold. Nursing support of the family at this time may help to alleviate some of the feeling they may have of being "cheated" out of a family-centered birth (Fig. 26 – 7N,Q,S).

If the newborn is compromised, cardiopulmonary support and resuscitation efforts are begun. The labor nurse assists, as needed, and provides information and support to the parents.

(text continued on page 726)

NURSING CARE PLAN

The Postoperative Cesarean Birth Patient

Nursing Diagnosis (Patient Problem) and Assessment Data	Nursing Interventions	Rationale
Potential Complication: *hemorrhage*		
Risk factors: • Prolonged labor • Difficult operative delivery • Uterine atony	Check vital signs every 5 min until stable then: every 15 min. for 1 hr; every 1–2 hr for 8 hrs.	Vital signs may vary in response to anesthesia or impending hemorrhage.
	Monitor for signs and symptoms of shock: • Thirst • Increased pulse and respiratory rate • Hypotension • Narrowed pulse pressure • Anxiety • Air hunger, dyspnea • Confusion, decreased level of consciousness • Skin cool, clammy, pale • Decreased urine output • Decreasing Hgb, Hct • Abnormal blood gas values ($\downarrow pH$, $\downarrow PaO_2$)	Hemorrhage can occur rapidly in immediate postpartum period, especially following operative delivery.
	Check uterine fundus and its state of contraction every 15 min for 1 hr, more often if indicated.	Fundal massage contracts uterus and decreases bleeding.
	Massage fundus carefully and gently.	Uterus is painful.
	Monitor dressing for amount of bleeding.	Blood loss must be checked.
	Check perineal pads every 15 min 1 hr postop, then every hr for 4 hr or until stable.	Assessment of amount and color of lochia will indicate appropriate uterine involution of possible postpartum hemorrhage.
	Outline area of bleeding on dressing, marking it with date and time every 4 hr for the first 24 hr postop.	To enable comparison of amount of bleeding from previous check.
	Administer oxytocin IV as ordered.	Oxytocin causes uterus to contract to control bleeding.

Expected Outcome:

The mother progresses toward recovery without postsurgical or postbirth complications as evidenced by appropriate vital signs, and contracted uterus and appropriate amount of lochia in first 5 days postbirth.

(continued)

The Postoperative Cesarean Birth Patient

Nursing Diagnosis (Patient Problem) and Assessment Data	Nursing Interventions	Rationale
Nursing Diagnosis: *potential for ineffective airway clearance related to anesthesia/analgesia* *potential for ineffective breathing pattern related to acute pain*	Suction mouth and throat until patient is responsive. Position patient on side to promote mucus drainage. Turn patient frequently. Assist patient to cough every 2 hr for 24 hr. Splint incision while patient coughs, and teach patient to do so. Assess every 8 hr • Decreased depth of respiration • Decreased breath sounds, rales	Respiratory obstruction or aspiration by drainage of mucus must be prevented. Coughing aerates lungs and helps prevent respiratory infection. Splinting decreases incisional pain.

Expected Outcome:

The mother progresses toward recovery without postsurgical respiratory complications as evidenced by appropriate vital signs in first 5 days after birth.

Nursing Diagnosis: *altered comfort: acute incisional pain*		
• Patient complains of incisional pain • Restlessness • Reluctance to move or hold newborn	Assess vital signs before administering pain medication. Confirm that medication is not contraindicated in breast-feeding mothers. Administer analgesic as needed, and prior to ambulation, or handling infant. Provide other comfort measures for pain due to the incision, gas, or uterine cramping such as back rub or massage, heat, positioning, incision splinting.	Blood pressure is often decreased by administration of pain medication. Most medications ingested by the mother are passed into the breast milk. Administration of pain medication before the pain is severe increases medication effectiveness and decreases patient anxiety.

Expected Outcome:

The mother recovering from cesarean birth responds to analgesia and is comfortable as evidenced by verbalization of comfort, more relaxed countenance, relaxation in holding newborn, and stabilizing vital signs.

(continued)

NURSING CARE PLAN   (continued)

The Postoperative Cesarean Birth Patient

Nursing Diagnosis (Patient Problem) and Assessment Data	Nursing Interventions	Rationale
Nursing Diagnosis: *anxiety related to separation from family members*		
	Provide for presence of father or support person and newborn as soon as possible in recovery period.	Parents need opportunity to reassure each other of well-being of family unit, and share acquaintance with the newborn.

Expected Outcome:

Support person participates in birth experience (when permitted/desired) and mother, support person, and newborn share time together in the immediate postcesarean recovery period.

Nursing Diagnosis: *possible altered patterns in urinary elimination*		
• Bladder distention on palpation • Uterine atony • Uterus displaced to side and rising above umbilicus	Check patency of indwelling catheter to dependent drainage.	
	Monitor adequate intake and output.	Bladder distention must be prevented to decrease risk of hemorrhage, ascending urinary tract infection.
	Remove catheter as ordered. Check ability of patient to void, and adequacy of the amount. Assist patient to bathroom. Keep water running in the sink. Pour warm water over the patient's vulva.	This assists spontaneous voiding, avoiding catheterization.

Expected Outcome:

Mother maintains appropriate intake and output and ability to void within 12 hours of delivery.

Nursing Diagnosis: *potential fluid volume deficit related to decreased oral intake*		
	Monitor intake and output. Monitor for signs of dehydration: • Dry skin and mucous membranes • Poor skin turgor • Concentrated urine • Hemoconcentration • Decreased urine output	These signs indicate inadequate fluid intake or abnormal loss.

(continued)

NURSING CARE PLAN (continued)

The Postoperative Cesarean Birth Patient

Nursing Diagnosis (Patient Problem) and Assessment Data	Nursing Interventions	Rationale
	• Increased serum sodium	
	• Thirst	
	• Weakness/lethargy	
	Assess for nausea/vomiting; administer antiemetic as needed.	
	Maintain IV until adequate oral intake established.	

Expected Outcome:

The mother maintains optimal fluid volume balance as evidenced by normal vital signs and urine concentration.

Nursing Diagnosis:
potential fluid volume excess related to IV therapy

	Monitor intake and output, signs of fluid overload:	Patients are often hydrated prior to administration of regional anesthesia and thus may be at risk for subsequent overhydration in immediate postpartum period.
	• Increasing blood pressure	
	• Sacral puffiness	
	• Pitting edema	
	• Fluid intake greater than fluid output	

Expected Outcome:

The mother maintains optimal fluid volume balance as evidenced by normal vital signs and urine output.

Nursing Diagnosis:
probable altered bowel elimination: constipation or postoperative ileus secondary to anesthesia, decreased oral intake, immobility

• Absence of bowel sounds	Auscultate bowel sounds and monitor passage of flatus.	Bowel sounds will be absent immediately postop due to anesthesia, but will return progressively during the following 3 to 5 days.
• Increasing abdominal girth and tension		
• Absence of flatus	Advance progressively to clear liquids, full liquids, regular diet.	Gradual progression of diet from liquids to solids decreases risk for development of paralytic ileus.
• Anorexia, nausea, vomiting		
• Absence of bowel movement	Avoid ice chips.	Overuse tends to reduce intestinal peristalsis.
	Encourage progressive ambulation starting within 24 hr postop. Offer	Initial ambulation will be painful.

(continued)

NURSING CARE PLAN (continued)

The Postoperative Cesarean Birth Patient

Nursing Diagnosis (Patient Problem) and Assessment Data	Nursing Interventions	Rationale
	pain medication prior to ambulation and remain with patient.	
	Explain rationale and importance of early ambulation to the patient.	Ambulation improves bowel function, general circulation; prevents thrombophlebitis; increases aeration of lungs.
	Administer stool softener as ordered, and encourage increased fluid intake.	Normal bowel function must be present before discharge.

Expected Outcome:

Mother returns to normal bowel elimination as evidenced by normal bowel sounds within 3 to 5 days and normal stools by discharge.

Possible Complication:
anemia

• Pallor	Check hematocrit and hemoglobin 8 hr after delivery and the first postop day.	Check identifies possible iron deficiency anemia due to blood loss.
• Tachycardia		
• Orthostatic hypotension	Assess laboratory values: Hgb <10.5 gm, Hct $<30\%$; assess for symptoms of dizziness, lightheadedness, fainting.	Depending on severity of anemia, the patient may need infusion of blood products.
• Vertigo, syncope		
• Moderate to severe blood loss at delivery		

Expected Outcome:

Mother responds to treatment for anemia as demonstrated by Hgb > 10.5 gm upon discharge.

Nursing Diagnosis:
potential for infection: urinary tract infection related to retention, catheterization, bladder trauma during surgery

	Monitor for increased pulse, respiratory rate.	These are nonspecific early signs of infection.
	Check for symptoms of burning with urination, frequency, urgency.	These symptoms may indicate bladder infection.
	Collect urine culture.	Bacterial colonies $>100,000$ indicate bladder infection.
	Assess incision for swelling, drainage, warmth.	These are indicative of wound infection
	Assess for foul-smelling lochia.	Indication of endometritis.
	Notify physician and assist with culture as needed. Administer antibiotic as ordered.	

(continued)

NURSING CARE PLAN (continued)

The Postoperative Cesarean Birth Patient

Nursing Diagnosis (Patient Problem) and Assessment Data	Nursing Interventions	Rationale

Expected Outcome:

Mother progresses toward recovery without complications as evidenced by normal vital signs, appropriate wound healing, and normal lochia upon discharge.

Nursing Diagnosis:
potential altered parenting

• Lack of verbalization of interest in infant	Encourage family interaction as soon as possible.	Anesthesia or discomfort might delay interaction.
• No desire to see, hold, care for infant	Provide the parents early with information about their baby.	New parents have educational needs that are often forgotten because of the mother's physical needs.
	Provide infant and self-care instruction.	
• Verbalization of anger at infant for surgical birth	Encourage discussion of feelings about the cesarean birth and the mother's self-image.	Cesarean birth may cause some to feel inadequate as a woman and mother.
	Attend to maternal needs for comfort, rest, nutrition, and emotional support.	Unmet maternal needs may inhibit acquaintance process.

Expected Outcome:

Parents demonstrate beginning of attachment and parenting as evidenced by interest in reviewing cesarean birth with nurse, discussing care procedures, and participating in return demonstrations in care of the newborn.

After delivery of the infant the placenta will be delivered manually (Fig. 26–7P,R). The anesthesiologist is responsible for administering intravenous oxytocin to the mother, as ordered, at delivery of the placenta.

Lastly, a final sponge count is taken and recorded. A dressing is applied to the incision and the mother is assisted onto the gurney and transferred to the recovery unit.

Immediate Postcesarean Care

Immediate postcesarean care of the woman and her family is similar in many ways to nursing care after a vaginal birth (see Nursing Care Plan). If possible, the family should be kept together in the recovery area and time provided for interaction and closeness (Fig. 26–7T).

The woman's physiologic needs include those of the newly delivered mother as well as those of a postsurgical patient. The tone and position of the uterus must be assessed every 15 minutes for uterine atony, and monitor-

ing of maternal vital signs is important to rule out impending hemorrhage. Palpation of the fundus must be done gently to avoid direct pressure on the incision line. Lochia is assessed as in the vaginally delivered mother. In addition, the abdominal dressing must be checked periodically to ensure that the incision is dry and intact.

Intravenous fluids will be continued for 24 to 48 hours, so accurate intake and output records must be maintained. Blood-tinged urine from an indwelling catheter suggests surgical trauma to the bladder and should be reported to the physician. Dietary intake is generally limited to clear liquids until bowel sounds are heard and then advanced as tolerated to a regular diet.

If the woman received a regional anesthetic, her postoperative care must include assistance with positioning until she has adequate sensation in her legs for movement in bed. The nurse must assess return of sensation and level of anesthesia every 15 minutes until sensation has completely returned. If a general anesthetic is used, the mother is usually recovered in a postanesthesia unit until her condition is stabilized, and then she is transferred to the postpartum unit. As soon as she is fully awake, she should be permitted to see her partner and her newborn, if possible. When possible, the father should be encouraged to bring the newborn to the mother and give her information about it to promote the sense of a shared experience. Nursing care for this mother also must include special attention to coughing and deep breathing in the immediate postoperative period to prevent congestion and risk of infection.

It is especially important for the nurse to spend time in the postpartum period with the mother who delivers by cesarean birth to allow her to talk over her birth experience, to express any feelings of loss or inadequacy, and to be reassured that she did the best she could under difficult circumstances. Both parents may have a need to "relive" the experience by telling it to others in detail; this should be encouraged as a way of working through what may have been an unsettling experience. The mother may also have gaps in her memory of events; these should be filled in as much as possible by the partner or the nurse to facilitate integration of the birth experience. The nurse should encourage as positive a view of the experience as possible and help the family focus on their newborn and on moving into parenthood. If the newborn's condition is uncertain, the family will need additional nursing attention and support in the early postpartum period.

Trial of Labor/Vaginal Birth After Cesarean Delivery

At one time, women who had had previous cesarean births were routinely advised to have repeat cesareans, even if the cause of the previous cesarean was nonrepeating. Fear of uterine rupture during a subsequent labor prevented physicians from considering trial of labor and vaginal birth after cesarean (VBAC) as a safe mode of delivery, since the uterine musculature was believed to be significantly weakened.

However, more recent research suggests that the risks of VBAC may have been overestimated, and the trend toward trial of labor appears to be increasing. Reasons for current VBAC include consumer pressure to avoid operative delivery, cost increases, and maternal and neonatal risks of elective repeat cesarean, which may be greater than careful management of a trial of labor and VBAC.

Indications and Contraindications

Indications for VBAC center on the patient's desire to avoid a repeat cesarean, and on factors that suggest that maternal–fetal risk can be managed, including those listed in the accompanying display. Contraindications include any of the usual contraindications for vaginal delivery as well as those listed in the display.

Advantages and Disadvantages

As noted before, advantages of VBAC include the fact that it may reduce maternal and neonatal risk in selected patients, that it reduces financial costs and length of hospital stay, and that the woman and her partner may view a vaginal delivery as highly desirable. Disadvantages include the small risk of uterine rupture and the need for an emergency cesarean, the need for more intensive monitoring during labor, and the possibility that parents will focus too much on the goal of a vaginal delivery and be greatly disappointed if that turns out to be impossible.

Implications for Nursing Care

Nursing management and care of the patient undergoing trial of labor and VBAC are similar to those for other at-risk patients in labor. Close monitoring of uterine contraction patterns and fetal status is necessary; many facilities require the use of internal monitoring. The nurse must be alert to signs that labor is not progressing normally (arrest of progress, fetal distress, signs of uncoordinated uterine activity). Signs that suggest uterine scar weakening or rupture include maternal report of a "tearing" sensation, abrupt cessation of labor, and developing signs of maternal hypovolemic shock. If observed, these signs must be reported immediately, and an emergency cesarean must be considered likely.

Requirements and Contraindications for Vaginal Birth After Cesarean

Requirements

- Only one previous uterine incision, preferably low-segment incision
- No repeating cause for previous cesarean
- Capability for internal monitoring during labor, with availability of emergency surgical facilities
- Constant physician attendance during labor

Contraindications

- Any contraindications for vaginal delivery
- More than one previous uterine incision
- Previous classic (vertical) uterine incision (considered by some to be a relative, not an absolute, contraindication)
- Malpresentation or possible cephalopelvic disproportion
- Lack of capability for continuous monitoring and emergency operative delivery if necessary

CHAPTER SUMMARY

Labor and birth usually proceed normally without the need for obstetric intervention. However, when the woman or the fetus is seen to be at increased intrapartal risk, various interventions are used to reduce that risk. The nurse plays an important role in identifying women who are at increased risk as they begin the labor process as well as those who develop problems in the intrapartal period.

For both of these groups of women, modern obstetrics offers a range of techniques designed to reduce the risk to mother and fetus/newborn posed by the process of labor and birth. These risk-reduction techniques include monitoring fetal status intensively, managing maternal pain, modifying labor patterns, and modifying the mode of delivery. Each of these modes of risk reduction includes a number of obstetric interventions that can help ensure a positive birth outcome for many women and their newborns. Each obstetric intervention increases the need for expert nursing support in the intrapartal period.

The nurse is responsible for the careful monitoring of women requiring obstetric interventions in the intrapartal period to determine if responses are within normal limits. The nurse must also recognize that with every application of obstetric technology comes the potential for *increased* maternal and fetal risk. The nurse must act to reduce this additional risk through careful monitoring, expert intervention, and understanding of appropriate circumstances for applying that technology.

Finally, the nurse must strive to balance an increasingly technological approach to labor care with an increasingly caring and human emphasis, for women at increased risk in labor and birth need this type of care, perhaps even more than "normal, low-risk" women. To achieve this balance, the nurse must be able to integrate technology and intensive intervention into her care so that it *supplements* her professional hands-on assessment of patient status rather than substituting for it. The nurse must be capable of providing family-centered support for these women and their families in spite of the increased level of medical and nursing intervention required in their care. In this way, nursing makes a significant contribution to the safety and well-being of the woman and her fetus/newborn and to the emotional well-being of the family as a whole.

STUDY QUESTIONS

1. Why is amniotomy not recommended by some health professionals?
2. What are the nurse's responsibilities in the administration of oxytocin for the induction or augmentation of labor?
3. List and define five common indications for cesarean delivery.
4. What preoperative preparation, teaching, and emotional support would you offer a woman before cesarean delivery?
5. You are caring for a patient in labor who delivered her last child by cesarean section. Describe special aspects of your care based on her obstetric history.
6. What should be included in the nursing care of the postoperative cesarean patient?
7. Under what conditions are forceps used during delivery?
8. What is the purpose of the vacuum extraction delivery?

REFERENCES/BIBLIOGRAPHY

Baumgarten K: Advantages and disadvantages of low amniotomy. J Perinat Med 4:2, 1976

Boehm FH, Davidson KK, Barrett JJ: The effect of electronic fetal monitoring on the incidence of cesarean section. Am J Obstet Gynecol 140:295–298, 1981

Gabbe S: Umbilical cord compression associated with amniotomy: Laboratory observation. Am J Obstet Gynecol 125:353, 1976

Galvan FJ, Broekhuizen FF: Obstetric vacuum extraction. J Obstet Gynecol Neonatal Nurs 16:242–248, 1987

Glazer G, Hulme A: Prostaglandin gel for cervical ripening. MCN 12:28–31, 1987

Malinowski J: Nursing Care of the Labor Patient, 2nd ed. Philadelphia, FA Davis, 1983

May K, Sollid D: Unanticipated cesarean birth: From the father's perspective. Birth 11(2):87, 1984

Nager CW, Thomas CK, Moore TR: Cervical ripening and labor outcome with preinduction intracervical prostaglandin E$_2$ (Prepidil) Gel. J Perinatol VII(3):189–193, 1987

National Institute of Health: Cesarean Birth Task Force: Consensus Development Statement on Cesarean Birth. Washington, DC, U.S. Department of Health and Human Services, 1980

OGN Nursing Practice Resource: The Nurse's Role in the Induction/Augmentation of Labor. Washington, DC, NAACOG, 1988

SUGGESTED READINGS

Fortier JC: The relationship of vaginal and cesarean births to father–infant attachment. J Obstet Gynecol Neonatal Nurs 17:128–134, 1988

Leach L, Sproule V: Meeting the challenge of cesarean births. J Obstet Gynecol Neonatal Nurs 13:191–195, 1984

Marshall C: The art of induction/augmentation of labor. J Obstet Gynecol Neonatal Nurs 14:22–28, 1985

27
procedures: managing maternal pain

LEARNING OBJECTIVES

After studying the materials in this chapter, the student should be able to

- Discuss the causes of pain in childbirth

- Outline the adverse effects of pain

- Describe the behavioral cues of pain in the parturient during labor and birth

- Discuss nonpharmacological nursing measures employed to control and relieve pain during the intrapartum period

- Identify the most common types of obstetric analgesia and anesthesia

- List advantages and disadvantages of obstetric analgesia and anesthesia

- Describe nursing responsibilities during the administration of analgesia or anesthesia

- List major complications of obstetric analgesia and anesthesia

KEY TERMS

Anesthesia

General anesthesia

Local anesthesia

Regional anesthesia

Each woman experiences the physical sensations of labor differently. For some, uterine contractions, the process of cervical dilatation and effacement, and fetal descent will create feelings of "discomfort" that range from mild to intense or severe. Others will describe labor and birth in terms of "pain." Labor nurses also differ philosophically in how to describe the sensations evoked by labor and childbirth. Many nurses have been educated to avoid the use of the word "pain" in relation to contractions or have been taught that parturition need not be painful when women are adequately prepared. But few would deny that pain is experienced by the majority of women who labor and give birth, even though it varies widely in nature, extent, and location.

The aim of this chapter is to review the causes of discomfort or pain experienced in labor and discuss both nonpharmacologic techniques and pharmacologic methods employed to control these sensations. Nursing responsibilities in reducing discomfort and pain and in the administration of obstetric analgesia and anesthesia are outlined in detail. Because nonpharmacologic techniques for pain control have been discussed in Chapters 23 and 24, the emphasis in this section will be on pharmacologic modes of pain relief.

PAIN AND DISCOMFORT DURING LABOR AND BIRTH

A crucial role of the nurse during labor and birth entails promotion of comfort and control of pain. The labor nurse engages in an ongoing assessment of the woman's level of comfort and perceptions of pain in order to identify the progress of labor and signs and symptoms of obstetric complications. Decisions about maternal comfort needs are based on observation of the parturient's behavioral cues, assessment of progress in labor, and maternal–fetal status. Planning and implementation of appropriate nursing interventions to control pain are based upon expert knowledge regarding comfort measures and pain relief techniques available today.

Many women have been told that childbirth is the most painful experience they will ever have, and they fully expect to suffer through labor and birth. Others have had previous labors in which their pain was not manageable by prepared childbirth techniques; such women approach labor with a realistic worry that they will not be able to tolerate that level of pain again. Other women may be shocked by a painful, difficult labor when their previous labors were more easily tolerated. Still others will develop problems in the intrapartal period that require active obstetric intervention that cannot be done without adequate maternal anesthesia.

Pain during labor may be related to a variety of physiologic factors (Fig. 27–1), including:

- Cervical stretching during dilatation
- Distention of the lower uterine segment
- Stretching of the uterine ligaments
- Traction on the peritoneum
- Pressure on the bladder and urethra
- Uterine hypoxia
- Pressure on the nerve ganglia around the uterus and vagina
- Maternal parity

Pain in the first stage of labor is due mostly to cervical stretching. Pain impulses are transmitted via sensory pathways that accompany the sympathetic nerves and pass through the spinal nerve to enter the spinal cord. Pain during this stage is usually felt in the lower abdomen and the skin over the lower lumbar spine and upper sacrum. With intense pain, sensations may also be felt above and below these areas, that is, in the upper thighs and the umbilical region.

Pain in the second stage of labor is caused primarily by the distention of the vagina and the perineum with fetal descent. Pain impulses from these areas are transmitted via the sensory fibers of the pudendal nerves, which enter the posterior roots of the second, third, and fourth sacral nerves.

Extreme maternal distress from pain in childbirth itself can constitute a risk factor affecting both maternal and fetal status. Maternal distress from pain can result in an increase in cardiac output and blood pressure. Maternal distress also causes maternal oxygen consumption to increase markedly; when hyperventilation is present, hypocarbia (excessive CO_2 loss) can result in decreased uterine and cerebral blood flow. Stress can result in increased secretion of epinephrine, which may in turn cause vasoconstriction and fetal hypoxia. Distress from pain exacerbates apprehension and muscular tension. This muscular tension increases the metabolic demands on the mother, contributing to acidosis, which may also affect fetal metabolic balance. Finally, muscular tension may result in reflex tightening of the pelvic floor, thus impeding descent and delivery of the fetus (Perez 1981).

The sensation of acute pain may also have immediate and long-term psychological effects on the parturient. A woman who has previously been able to perform breathing and relaxation exercises during contractions and is suddenly unable to do so may become discouraged, frightened, or even panicky. She may experience a loss of self-esteem and confidence in her ability to maintain control of her physical and emotional responses. If the psychological need to remain in control is a strong aspect of the personality, the loss of control can be devastating.

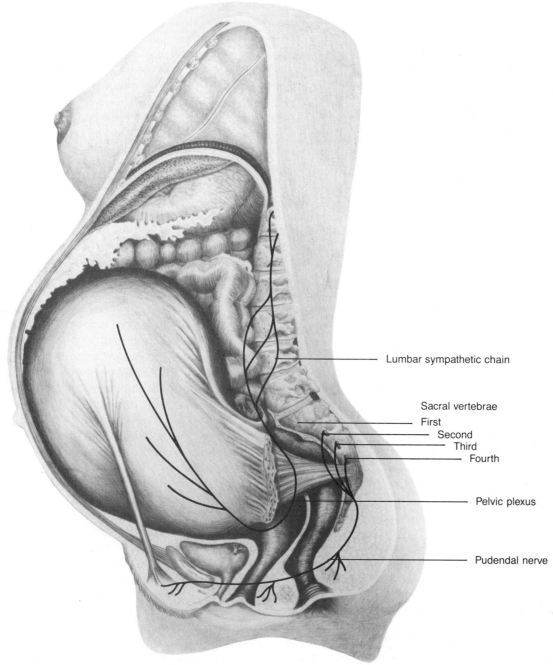

Figure 27-1. Pain sources and pathways. The pain of vaginal delivery primarily originates in the lower genital tract, and painful stimuli from this region are transmitted through the pudendal nerve. Peripheral branches of this nerve provide sensory stimulation to the perineum and anus and to parts of the vulva and clitoris. Sensory fibers of the pudendal nerve originate from the ventral branches of the second, third, and fourth sacral nerves. (Courtesy of Maternity Center Association, New York)

Acute pain that lasts many hours leads to fatigue, distortions in perceptions of time, physical boundaries, and even reality. The woman may be unable to remember parts of her labor experience, or the memories may be grossly distorted. After birth of the infant, the woman may express anger toward the infant, viewing the newborn as the cause of the extreme distress experienced during childbirth. The fear of recurring pain in subsequent labors may diminish sexual responsiveness and hesitancy to become pregnant again.

Managing Maternal Pain

A persistent problem in pain management during labor is that pain itself is not observable. The nurse must rely on observations of behavior or the woman's own reports. The intensity of pain and the distress caused by that pain are not always congruent; that is, although such behavior as restlessness, crying out, rapid breathing, and certain body movements indicates distress, the pain may be mild or quite severe, depending on the factors noted previously. For instance, such behavior is more common in laboring women during the second stage than during the first, but many women actually experience less pain in the second stage.

Assessment of an individual woman's response to labor and the need for physical comfort or analgesia requires sensitivity and experience. The nurse must be knowledgeable about how such factors as fatigue, anxiety and fear, readiness for birth and parenthood, fetal position and presentation, and quality of the labor itself may exacerbate maternal pain.

NURSING RESEARCH

Differences in Perceptions of Pain in Primigravidas and Multigravidas

Pain has been described as a multidimensional, subjective experience of discomfort composed of both sensory and affective components. Very few investigators have explored the differences in the experience of pain between primigravidas and multigravidas. Recently, Johansson and associates (1988) systematically described the dimensions of pain during labor in these two groups of women.

The sensory component of pain was more severe than the affective dimension in both groups. Primigravidas reported more intense sensory pain during the first stage of labor and more affective pain in all stages of childbirth, even though they received more analgesia. The authors note that nonpharmacologic methods for pain relief may be useful for reducing the affective component of pain but that analgesia was more effective for lowering sensory pain intensity. While formulating an individualized care plan for pain control, clinicians should bear in mind that primigravidas may in general experience greater pain and require more intensive emotional and pharmacologic support during labor and birth.

Johansson FG, Fridh G, Norvell KT: Progression of labor pain in primiparas and multiparas. Nurs Res 37(2):86–89, 1988

In order to promote comfort and reduce pain, the nurse must ascertain the nature, degree, and location of discomfort or pain. Assessment begins with admission to the labor unit and may in part help to distinguish between true and false labor (Chapter 23). Determining the location of pain may alert the nurse to fetal presentation and position, stage of labor, and the presence of complications. For instance, low, persistent backache is associated with occiput posterior position, intense rectal pressure may herald the onset of the second stage of labor, and intense abdominal tenderness may indicate intrauterine infection or abruptio placentae.

The nurse should ask the woman to describe the pain; where it is most intense, whether it radiates, and if it is persistent or intermittent in nature. Has the parturient attempted to relieve the pain? What measures has she taken and have her attempts been successful? When did the pain begin? When did it change in intensity? The nurse should also discuss the woman's preparations, if any, for relief of discomfort and pain in labor. Did she attend childbirth preparation classes? What are her plans and desires for pain control and relief during labor? If she is a multipara, what has she experienced in previous pregnancies and what pain control methods were utilized? Finally, were these measures successful, and were there any complications related to their use?

Implementing nonpharmacologic nursing measures (described in Chapter 23) to relieve pain is a major nursing responsibility, outlined in the accompanying Nursing Care Plan. The nurse must work closely with the woman and her support person to promote comfort and control pain sensations and must be familiar with commonly used methods of relaxation and pain relief taught in childbirth education classes. Supporting the woman's efforts to "stay on top," "flow with," "go with," or "avoid fighting" the sensations with which she is bombarded during labor, through use of specific techniques, is crucial. If, however, coping strategies fail to control or relieve pain, the skilled labor nurse should not hesitate to suggest alternative actions or methods.

The nurse should encourage women not to regard the goal of "natural childbirth" as so important that they suffer through a miserable labor experience or refuse medication that may actually improve labor progress and hasten safe delivery of a healthy newborn. On the other hand, a woman experiencing a difficult time during transition may respond positively to intensive support and encouragement and find she can cope without analgesia once she is fully dilated and can push. The nurse's goal is to support the parturient who needs help and encouragement and who wishes to avoid medication during labor. But the woman must be made to feel comfortable asking for pharmacologic pain relief if she needs it. If comfort measures and relaxation techniques are not successful in

(text continued on page 736)

NURSING CARE PLAN

The Mother Experiencing Pain Associated With Uncomplicated Labor and Birth

Nursing Diagnosis (Patient Problem) and Assessment Data	Nursing Interventions	Rationale
Nursing Diagnosis: *anxiety related to unfamiliar situation of labor; fear related to labor pain*		
• Verbalizes fear • Verbalizes fear of pain • Restlessness • Inability to follow requests or coaching • Facial or body tension • Pallor • Tremulousness	Explain procedures before initiating them. Encourage the patient to tell you which comfort measures she prefers.	Having advance warning allows the patient to prepare mentally for the event and promotes her feeling of control and mastery of labor. It decreases anxiety and thus decreases pain.
	Reassure the patient that anxiety and fear are normal.	Patient understanding of the normalcy of the response will lessen the compounding and contagious effect of anxiety. Anxiety interferes with coping mechanisms for pain.
	Explain routine care procedures before initiating them, including vital signs, FHR auscultation, electronic fetal monitoring, vaginal exams and so on.	Routine care may be misinterpreted by the patient as unusual or as cause for alarm if she is not informed, thus increasing anxiety.
	Encourage partner participation and support.	The partner will sense the necessity for a calm environment and take the initiative to minimize anxiety. The partner is often successful in minimizing fears.
	Establish good rapport with patient and family. • Remain with the patient • Listen to expressions of fear/anxiety. • Give positive reinforcement, praise. • Use reassuring touch.	Good rapport demonstrates a genuine care and concern for the patient. Staying with the patient, using touch, and listening to fears will lessen anxiety and increase the patient's ability to cope with the procedures and pain of labor.
	Provide or encourage distraction and attention focusing on conversation, music, television, reading, cards, games, touch.	Perceived intensity of pain is greater when the pain is the focus of attention. Preoccupation with an unrelated activity lessens pain perception.

Expected Outcome:

The woman in labor verbalizes fears and concerns and demonstrates less anxiety by cooperating with pain distraction and relaxation methods.

Nursing Diagnosis:
fatigue related to disrupted sleep

	Encourage rest.	Fatigue and exhaustion exaggerate pain by lowering resistance, energy, control, and coping mechanisms.

(continued)

The Mother Experiencing Pain Associated With Uncomplicated Labor and Birth

Nursing Diagnosis (Patient Problem) and Assessment Data	Nursing Interventions	Rationale

Expected Outcome:

The woman in early labor conserves physical and emotional energy by resting between contractions and verbalizing her feelings of relaxation.

Nursing Diagnosis:
altered comfort: acute pain

Behavioral responses: • Hand clenching • Facial grimacing • Restlessness • Crying • Tremulousness • Inability to speak during contractions • Inability to follow directions • Screaming • Irritability	Ask the patient where she feels the pain. Alleviate secondary causes where possible • Encourage voiding or catheterize the patient if a full bladder is the cause. • Reposition if backache or general achiness is the cause. • Dorsiflex foot if leg cramping is the cause. Encourage the use of, or teach, breathing techniques for labor; suggest a change to more complex breathing pattern. Encourage a position change every 20–30 min to walking, side-lying, or sitting upright position. Encourage ambulation according to protocol for active labor/ruptured membranes.	Laboring mothers often confuse normal indicators of bodily discomfort, such as voiding urge, with the pain of labor. Alleviating secondary causes of pain will often make labor tolerable with usual coping mechanisms. Teaching breathing patterns to patients with no previous childbirth class will discourage breath-holding. Breath-holding decreases O_2, causing increased lactic acid and subsequent pain from uterine contractions. Laboring mothers often maintain one position, fearing that movement will increase pain. Position changes at least every 20 min will decrease stiffness, tension, and pressure soreness, and promote labor progress. Upright position and ambulation increases comfort and shortens labor for some women. Hospital policy may vary.
Physiologic responses: • Increase in pulse, respiration, blood pressure, muscle tension • Physical response: restlessness, grimacing, clutching or grasping with hands, biting lips, rocking, reaching for painful area • Verbal response: groaning, grunting, or cursing: asking about labor length, next examination, or last medication; irritability; screaming	Provide or encourage the coach to provide substitute stimulation, such as stroking, back massage or rubbing, patting, rocking, effleurage. Apply heat or cold to back or forehead or as desired. Promote general comfort by providing ice chips, popsicles, and fluids; warm blankets and clean, dry bed linens; pillow positioning for body support; comfortable room temperature and lighting.	Cutaneous stimulation serves as a distraction and stimulates afferent nerve fibers, blocking pain sensation. Heat helps to relax tense muscles and soothe painful areas. A cool washcloth to the forehead or an ice pack to the back is often used for comfort and the numbing effect of ice. General comfort affects the patient's overall perception of pain and tolerance of labor. Constant attention to minor aspects of comfort avoids exaggeration of pain perception.

(continued)

NURSING CARE PLAN (continued)

The Mother Experiencing Pain Associated With Uncomplicated Labor and Birth

Nursing Diagnosis (Patient Problem) and Assessment Data	Nursing Interventions	Rationale
	Encourage the support person, or significant other to participate in the support of the laboring woman.	The labor support person will probably know most about the patient's tolerance, preferences, and coping mechanisms. This knowledge is vital to the nurse assisting in labor–pain management.
	Discuss and offer pain management options (see Table 27-2).	Ideally, pain management plans should be discussed early in labor to determine expectations and plan care. When this is not possible, the patient should be informed briefly of side-effects and anticipated results.

Expected Outcome:

Laboring woman experiences some relief from labor contractions as a result of comfort measures as evidenced by verbalization of increased comfort and cooperation in providing self-care.

Nursing Diagnosis:
altered comfort: acute pain related to "back labor"

• Complains of extreme back pain. • Inability to remain in one position	Encourage patient to avoid lying on her back. Suggest changing position to side-lying, sitting, all fours, squatting standing, ambulation. Change positions frequently.	Back labor is commonly associated with occiput posterior fetal positions. Supine position hinders rotation of fetus.
	Encourage pelvic rock exercise while side-lying on side opposite baby's back.	Side-lying on side opposite baby's back uses gravity to promote spontaneous rotation of fetus. Pelvic rock exercise relieves backache and jostles the fetus to encourage rotation.
	Provide or encourage the support person to provide firm lower back massage or counterpressure with mother on side (firm pressure on sacrum with heel of one hand while pulling upper hip toward you with other hand) during contractions. Provide comfort measures specific to low back pain: • Support body parts with pillow. • Place a small rolled towel or pillow in small of back. • Apply heat or a cold pack to lower back.	Provides some pain relief by distraction and blocking pain sensation and by promoting general comfort.

(continued)

The Mother Experiencing Pain Associated With Uncomplicated Labor and Birth

Nursing Diagnosis (Patient Problem) and Assessment Data	Nursing Interventions	Rationale
	Provide medication as needed.	Patients often report that usual coping mechanisms, such as breathing techniques, distraction, etc., are not helpful in back labor because of persistent pain between contractions.
	Keep patient informed of contraction onset, peak, and end. Provide support and encouragement.	Constant back pain may hinder patient's perception of contraction frequency and duration.

Expected Outcome:

Laboring woman experiences relief from back labor as a result of comfort measures and/or requested analgesia/anesthesia, as evidenced by verbalization of increased comfort and her increased perception of contraction frequency and duration.

helping the parturient cope with labor pain, the nurse or the birth attendant may suggest pharmacologic pain relief. Both *analgesia,* or the absence or decreased awareness of pain without loss of consciousness, and *anesthesia,* the partial or complete loss of sensation with or without loss of consciousness, may be used in intrapartal care.

There are several major pharmacologic methods of pain relief in common use for childbirth. *Parenteral analgesia,* which includes the use of narcotics, ataractics, and sedatives, is also used commonly to provide quick, effective, and easily administered pain relief during labor. *Conduction anesthesia,* which includes pudendal, epidural, and spinal anesthesia, utilizes anesthetic agents to provide pain relief by blocking sensory nerve impulses from a specific area of the body. *Inhalation anesthesia* may also be used in intrapartal care to provide brief periods of relief, to allow rapid induction of deep anesthesia to permit emergency operative procedures, or to allow operative procedures in situations where conduction anesthesia cannot be used. This section focuses on obstetric analgesia and obstetric anesthesia that are often the methods of choice in situations of increased maternal or fetal risk.

OBSTETRIC ANALGESIA

Obstetric analgesia includes the use of analgesics, sedative-hypnotics, ataractics, tranquilizers, and amnesics (Table 27 – 1).

Analgesics

Analgesics are naturally occurring or synthetic narcotic drugs that provide highly effective pain relief as well as some sedation, decrease in anxiety, euphoria, and antispasmodic action. Maternal side-effects include nausea and vomiting, especially with intravenous administration, mild respiratory depression, and transient mental impairment. Commonly used analgesics in labor are meperidine hydrochloride (Demerol), and morphine sulfate.

These systemic drugs cross the placental barrier readily. Because fetal liver and renal functioning is immature, drugs are metabolized slowly, and fetal blood levels remain high for longer periods than do maternal blood levels. Depressive effects on the neonate are greatest when delivery occurs 2 to 3 hours after intramuscular administration. For this reason, administration of these

Table 27–1   **Drugs Used for Analgesia in Labor**

Drug	Dosage/Route	Maternal Side-Effects	Fetal/Newborn Side-Effects	Nursing Implications
Analgesics				
Morphine sulfate	8–15 mg IM or 1–2 mg IV; peak effect in 60 min after IM and 15–20 min after IV administration with duration 4–6 hr	CNS depression, especially respiratory; nausea/vomiting; possible decrease in uterine activity early in labor	CNS depression; peak effect 2 hr after IM administration	Not commonly used in labor. *Do not* administer if maternal respiratory rate is below 12/min or other signs of CNS depression are present. Avoid administration 1–3 hr before delivery. Prepare to administer narcotic antagonist to neonate if depression is evident.
Meperidine hydrochloride (Demerol)	50–100 mg IM or 25–50 mg IV; peak effect in 40–60 min after IM and 5–10 min after IV administration with duration 3–4 hr	CNS depression, especially respiratory; nausea/vomiting; mild oxytocic effect after initial decrease in contractility; hypotension; drowsiness, blurred vision	Neonatal hypotonia; lethargy up to 72 hr after delivery	Most commonly used narcotic drug for labor. Administered in active phase of labor, preferably at least 2 hr before delivery to minimize CNS depression in newborn. IV is most common administration route because onset is quicker.
Barbiturates				
Sodium secobarbital (Seconal) Sodium pentobarbital (Nembutal) Sodium phenobarbital (Luminal)	100 mg IM or orally	Reduced tension, release of inhibitions; lethargy, hypotension, decreased sensory perception; restlessness in presence of pain or as idiosyncratic reaction in some patients	CNS depression; neonatal hypotonia; delay in establishment of feeding	Used to induce sedation during latent phase labor. *Note:* there is no available antagonist; avoid use in active labor.
Ataractics				
Promazine (Sparine)	25–50 mg IM or IV	Potentiates narcotic effects; antiemetic. Use with analgesic; may produce pseudohypnotic effect.	Potentiates CNS depression	Monitor closely; institute standard safety measures for medicated patients (side rails, bed rest, frequent checking).
Promethazine (Phenergan)	25–50 mg IM or IV	As for promazine	As for promazine	As for promazine
Hydroxyzine (Vistaril, Atarax)	25–50 mg IM or IV	As for promazine	As for promazine	Spasmodic eye or neck movements suggest extrapyramidal effect of phenothiazine; alert care provider.
Diazepam (Valium)	2–10 mg IM or IV	As for promazine	As for promazine	As for hydroxyzine; painful when administered IV

agents within 3 hours of anticipated delivery should be avoided.

If narcotics are administered in labor, the nurse must monitor maternal respiratory rate carefully. Narcotic antagonists, such as nalorphine (Nalline), or naloxone (Narcan) must be on hand to counteract narcotic-induced respiratory depression either in the mother or in the neonate at birth. Narcotic antagonists to reduce narcotic-induced neonatal depression may be administered to the mother intramuscularly 5 to 15 minutes before delivery or to the neonate immediately after birth through intramuscular or intravenous injection of a dilute solution of the medication into the umbilical artery.

Subtle effects on neonatal functioning may be present

NURSING ALERT

Administration of Narcotic Antagonists Before Impending Birth

In some cases, labor progresses more rapidly than expected after administration of a narcotic analgesic. In this case, a decision may be made to administer a narcotic antagonist before delivery of the infant to prevent neonatal narcosis. Extreme caution should be taken, however, when the parturient is known or suspected to be physically dependent on opioids. In such cases an abrupt and complete reversal of narcotic effects may precipitate acute withdrawal syndrome in the gravida. The woman may experience central nervous system, cardiovascular, and gastrointestinal aberrations, including seizures, hypotension, cardiac dysrhythmias, nausea, vomiting, diarrhea, and epigastric distress. It may be advisable in cases of known or suspected opioid dependence to alert pediatric staff and have neonatal Narcan available for use immediately after birth.

in the first 24 hours of life after administration of these medications in labor, regardless of whether antagonists were administered. These effects, which include decreased alertness and responsiveness to stimulation and decreased consolability, may persist for several days.

Sedative-hypnotics

Sedative-hypnotics do not relieve pain but induce relaxation and sleep. They may be used to potentiate the effects of analgesics or to promote rest and sleep when the mother is very apprehensive or becoming exhausted in the latent phase of labor. Among drugs in this class, barbiturates are most commonly used in intrapartal care, including secobarbital sodium (Seconal), pentobarbital sodium (Nembutal), and phenobarbital (Luminal). Usual dose for all of these drugs in 100 mg by mouth or intramuscularly, once the woman is in labor, to obtain satisfactory sedation. Thiopental sodium (Pentothal), a ultra-short-acting drug administered intravenously, is used for rapid induction of anesthesia for operative procedures.

Barbiturates cause maternal sedation and relaxation; side effects may include restlessness (especially when used alone in the presence of moderate to severe pain), hypotension, vertigo, lethargy, and nausea and vomiting. These drugs (with the exception of IV thiopental) should not be used during active labor because of rapid transfer across the placenta, long-lasting effects in the newborn, and the lack of an antagonist to reverse these effects. Effects in the newborn include CNS depression, pro-

longed drowsiness, and delayed establishment of feeding (poor sucking reflex and lower sucking pressure, resulting in decreased intake).

Ataractics

Ataractics (or tranquilizers) are a class of drugs that do not by themselves relieve pain but that decrease apprehension and anxiety and reduce the nausea sometimes produced by analgesics. They potentiate the action of sedatives and analgesics, thereby reducing the dosage needed to produce desired effects. Two groups of ataractics are commonly used in intrapartal care: phenothiazines, including promazine (Sparine) and promethazine (Phenergan) and benzodiazepines, including hydroxyzine (Vistaril, Atarax).

Ataractics may cause maternal hypotension with resultant decreased fetoplacental circulation, drowsiness, and vertigo. Drugs in the phenothiazine group can cause adverse maternal reactions that mimic symptoms of meningitis, including spasmodic eye movements, neck stiffness and spasm, and arching of the neck and back. Both types of ataractics cross the placenta readily, and metabolites can be found in the newborn's system for at least 7 days. Effects on the fetus may include tachycardia and loss of normal beat-to-beat variability on fetal heart monitoring. Effects extending into the neonatal period may include hypotonia, hypothermia, and generalized drowsiness, including reluctance to feed in the first days.

Amnesics

Amnesics are drugs that induce loss of memory. Scopolamine, a drug with sedative and tranquilizing effects, is also referred to as an amnesic because it produces near-total or complete loss of memory of events during its peak action. This drug was commonly used in intrapartal care in the past. It is rarely, if ever, used in contemporary practice because of several undesirable effects.

Scopolamine often produced disorientation, marked delirium, hallucinations, and agitation in laboring women, sometimes necessitating additional sedation or even restraint to minimize agitation and the risk of injury to the mother. Due to the amnesic action of the drug, mothers remembered only fragments of their labor, if anything; usually they believed that they slept through their entire labor and delivery. Psychological effects were also troubling. Women sometimes doubted that their infants were "really theirs" and had difficulty integrating the birth experience into their lives since they remembered none of it. In addition, the repeated doses of scopolamine, usually in combination with meperidine, resulted in a significant amount of physiologic depression in the newborn.

Implications for Nursing Care

The decision to administer analgesia should be a collaborative decision involving the woman in labor and the nurse or birth attendant. The nurse is often given a standing order for analgesia and is expected to evaluate the parturient's responses to labor and determine if and when it should be implemented. The risks and benefits of using pharmacologic agents must be weighed carefully. Maternal and fetal status, expected time frame before delivery, maternal desires regarding the use of analgesia, and the presence of any complications will influence the decision to administer analgesia.

At times the woman in labor will request analgesia. In other situations the nurse may suggest to the parturient that analgesia is indicated. The nurse must conduct an ongoing assessment of the woman's success in controlling pain. If sudden changes in the woman's behavioral and verbal responses suggest an increased pain level, the nurse should examine her to evaluate the progress of labor. Any decision regarding the use of an analgesic is predicated on this vaginal exam. If birth is anticipated within several hours, the risk of neonatal narcosis may preclude the use of analgesia.

If the parturient is opposed to and has refused the use of analgesics in the presence of severe pain, the nurse must remain in close attendance to assess maternal and fetal physiologic responses. As noted, pain can have adverse effects on the parturient and fetus. The birth attendant should be informed and included in further discussions with the parturient regarding pain relief options. If systemic analgesia is refused because of the placental transfer of the agent to the fetus, the parturient may be less opposed to regional or conduction anesthesia.

Nursing care for the patient receiving intrapartal analgesia is described in the Nursing Care Plan, page 740. After administration of the analgesic, the nurse assesses the parturient at frequent intervals (at least every 15 minutes for the first two hours) to evaluate the effectiveness of the drug and to identify idiosyncratic or allergic reactions, side-effects, or other adverse maternal or fetal responses. If the woman continues to experience the same level or greater intensity of pain after peak action of the analgesic is reached, she should be reexamined to determine if further cervical dilatation has occurred. Rapid progress in dilatation and fetal descent often occurs when analgesia is given in active labor. The nurse should be alert for signs of second-stage labor as the patient may be sedated and unaware of the impending birth.

Once the woman in labor receives analgesia, it is advisable to apply an external fetal monitor and tocodynamometer (if intermittent auscultation has been previously used). This permits ongoing assessment of fetal status without disturbing the woman every 15 minutes to auscultate the fetal heart rate. It is common for the sedated woman to sleep until the contraction reaches its acme and then to awake confused and unable to use the relaxation and breathing pattern employed earlier. Using the monitor also allows the labor coach to alert the woman as each contraction begins so that she is not startled or overwhelmed.

The nurse must recognize that none of the medications commonly in use provide completely safe and effective analgesia for the laboring woman. The choice of analgesia in labor must always be made in light of possible adverse effects on the mother, the progress of labor, and the fetus. However, when used wisely, parenteral analgesia can be safe and beneficial to the mother and present little risk to the healthy fetus and newborn.

Administration of these medications and monitoring of their effects during labor are nursing responsibilities (Table 27–2). The nurse must be knowledgeable about the patient's condition, the condition of the fetus, and the safe use of each medication in intrapartal care. The following nursing implications relate to the administration of *any* of these medications to the woman in labor:

- Administration during labor is typically by intramuscular or intravenous route. Dosages are kept to the smallest effective dose so that duration of effect can be better predicted and deleterious effects minimized.
- Intramuscular administration should be done with a needle that is long enough to ensure that the medication is placed in muscle rather than subcutaneous fat, since muscle provides optimal absorption.
- Intravenous administration should be done slowly at a rate of 1 ml/min or less to avoid a too-rapid physiologic response to the drug. Intravenous medication may also be administered at the beginning of a contraction to decrease the amount of medication transferred to the fetus, since placental circulation is markedly decreased during uterine contraction.
- Maternal vital signs, FHR, and cervical status should be assessed and recorded prior to administration. Vital signs and FHR should be checked again 10 to 15 minutes after intramuscular administration and 3 to 5 minutes after intravenous administration to assess possible effects.
- Effects of any parenteral agent will be intensified and potentially more dangerous in the premature or sick fetus or newborn.
- Routine precautions for administration of these medications should be taken: verification of drug and dosage, checking for maternal allergies, raising of side rails, and close monitoring of patient status.
- Positive suggestion will potentiate the effects of analgesics administered to laboring women.

(text continued on page 744)

NURSING CARE PLAN

The Woman Receiving Analgesia During Labor

Nursing Diagnosis (Patient Problem) and Assessment Data	Nursing Interventions	Rationale
Nursing Diagnosis: *altered comfort: pain related to uterine contractions*		

• Restlessness, inability to use self-care techniques in coping with contractions
• Patient requests analgesia
• Contraindication to analgesia:
  Allergy
  Impending birth
  Fetal distress
  Maternal emergency (obstetric or medical)
	Examine patient to determine dilatation of cervix.	Administration of analgesia in latent phase may cause contractions and progress of labor to cease. Administration of analgesia in transition stage may cause neonatal respiratory depression.

Expected Outcome:

Woman responds favorably, as indicated by less restlessness, verbalization of less pain, and ability to relax and rest between contractions within 15 to 20 minutes of administration.

Nursing Diagnosis: *fear related to use of analgesia*		
• Patient uninformed about analgesic choices	Explain type of analgesia to be used, how administered, side-effects, and how patient will feel.	Explanation allows patient to provide informed consent and prepares both her and partner for what to expect when drug administered.

Expected Outcome:

Patient understands use of analgesia, as evidenced by diminished apprehension and ability to give informed consent.

Nursing Diagnosis: *self-concept disturbance related to perceived need for analgesia*		
• Patient verbalizes disappointment, shame, sense of failure or discouragement because she requests analgesia. • Support person "refuses" to "allow" mother to have analgesia.	Reassure patient that analgesia is safe option for pain. Provide information regarding analgesics in nonjudgmental manner. Reassure support person that mother's desires will be respected; encourage joint decision making. Focus support person's attention on maternal responses to contractions and her comfort/fatigue level.	Patient may feel she has failed test of labor. Patient is sensitive to nursing attitudes regarding responses in labor. Fathers or support persons may feel compelled to "protect" patient against "unnecessary" intervention. By focusing on goal (optimum maternal comfort and safety), nurse can deemphasize feelings of "failure" with use of analgesia.

(continued)

NURSING CARE PLAN (continued)

The Woman Receiving Analgesia During Labor

Nursing Diagnosis (Patient Problem) and Assessment Data	Nursing Interventions	Rationale

Expected Outcome:

The patient and support person state that pain relief is needed and, when analgesia has been administered, is achieved, as evidenced by fact that the patient and support person are able to relax and rest between contractions.

Nursing Diagnosis:
potential fluid volume deficit related to decreased oral intake or abnormal loss

	Monitor intake and output. Start IV if nausea or vomiting persists or patient unable to take p.o. fluids or frozen juice bars as source of fluid and calories.	Analgesic sedation results in decreased oral intake and may cause nausea and vomiting. Dehydration can prolong labor and ketosis has adverse fetal effects.

Expected Outcome:

Laboring woman maintains fluid balance through oral intake or IV, as evidenced by adequate urinary output.

Nursing Diagnosis:
potential for injury: fall related to sensory–motor deficit

• Patient unable to move legs or ambulate with confidence • Patient complains of sensory changes in extremities	Place side rails in up position. Instruct patient to remain in bed and call for nurse if needs to void. Place call button within reach.	Analgesia may impair sensation, diminish judgment, and cause vertigo and hypotension.

Expected Outcome:

Woman who has received analgesia understands instructions concerning falls and remaining in bed, as evidenced by compliance during remainder of labor.

Potential Complication:
maternal hypotension related to analgesia

• Patient complains of "lightheadedness" • Increased pulse, decreased BP from previous baseline	Place patient in left lateral recumbent position. Assess BP, pulse and respirations 5 min after IV administration of analgesic and 15 min after IM administration. When IV analgesic given, administer no faster than 1 ml/min.	Prevents supine hypotension and maximizes uteroplacental perfusion. To alert nurse to hypotension or respiratory depression. IV medication has more immediate and pronounced effect on blood pressure

(continued)

The Woman Receiving Analgesia During Labor

Nursing Diagnosis (Patient Problem) and Assessment Data	Nursing Interventions	Rationale

Expected Outcome:

Woman who has received analgesia remains free of maternal hypotension, as evidenced by normal blood pressure and pulse within 15 minutes of administration.

Potential Complication:
fetal distress, decreased placental perfusion related to maternal hypotension

• Nonreassuring FHR pattern, *i.e.*, Late decelerations Decreased variability Pseudosinusoidal pattern	Maintain patient in left lateral recumbent position during and after administration of analgesic.	To improve uteroplacental perfusion. Analgesics can cause maternal hypotension with resultant impaired placental perfusion and fetal hypoxia.
	Begin IV administration with initiation of UC. Give slowly through several UCs.	Administration of IV analgesia with contraction decreases amount of drug transferred to fetus.
	Place external EFM and toco before administration of analgesic if intermittent monitoring done before.	Analgesia causes temporary decreased FHR variability. Placing the toco allows nurse or coach to note onset of each contraction in order to coach patient. EFM allows ongoing evaluation of fetal status without disturbing patient while sedated.

Expected Outcome:

Patient continues in progression of labor and fetus experiences no adverse side-effects as evidenced by normal FHR patterns throughout labor.

Nursing Diagnosis:
altered thought processes related to analgesia

• Patient loses orientation to time, progress of labor, and contraction pattern.	Reorient patient with each assessment. Offer verbal reassurance of progress, fetal well-being.	Orient and reassure patient regarding progress of labor and fetal status.
	Alert patient as the contraction begins to allow initiation of appropriate breathing pattern.	Patient may wake only at acme of contraction and be unable to continue effective breathing pattern unless alerted early.

(continued)

NURSING CARE PLAN (continued)

The Woman Receiving Analgesia During Labor

Nursing Diagnosis (Patient Problem) and Assessment Data	Nursing Interventions	Rationale

Expected Outcome:

Patient understands nursing care as demonstrated by her verbalization regarding labor progress and her compliance with breathing instructions.

Nursing Diagnosis:
potential altered urinary pattern: retention related to analgesia

• Patient unable to void	Have patient void before administering analgesic.	Analgesia can cause urinary retention.
• Bladder distention noted on palpation	Offer bedpan at least every 2 hours while patient is sedated.	Sedation can blunt perceptions of full bladder.

Expected Outcome:

Patient responds to nursing instruction and care as evidenced by voiding when reminded every 2 hours.

Nursing Diagnosis:
potential for injury: precipitous delivery

• Increased bloody show	Assess vital signs at least every 15 to 30 min after analgesia administration and assess for signs of rapid labor.	Analgesia may result in rapid progress of labor while patient is sedated and unable to verbalize sensations of impending birth.
• Involuntary grunting or pushing with contractions		
• Urge to defecate		
• Passage of stool		

Expected Outcome:

Patient continues with normal progression of labor as evidenced by appropriate vital signs and normal, spontaneous delivery.

Table 27–2   Time Sequence for Nursing Support and Administration of Analgesics/Anesthetics During Labor

Early Labor (1–3 cm dilatation)	Active Labor (4–7 cm dilatation)	Transition (8 cm–complete)	Second Stage (pushing)	Birth
Provide nursing support and promote self-care, using the following: Breathing techniques, Back massage, Effleurage/stroking, Application of heat or cold, Position changes, ambulation, Praise, encouragement, Anticipatory teaching	Provide nursing support and promote self-care, using the following: Breathing techniques, Back massage, Effleurage/stroking, Application of heat or cold, Position changes, ambulation, Praise, encouragement, Anticipatory teaching	Provide nursing support and promote self-care, using the following: Breathing techniques, Back massage, Effleurage/stroking, Application of heat or cold, Position changes, ambulation, Praise, encouragement, Anticipatory teaching	Provide nursing support and promote self-care, using the following: Breathing techniques, Back massage, Effleurage/stroking, Application of heat or cold, Position changes, ambulation, Praise, encouragement, Anticipatory teaching	
	Caution patient against hyperventilation. Encourage patient to change breathing techniques.	Instruct patient to blow out if she feels urge to push. Do not leave patient alone.	Assist patient with pushing technique. Assist with positioning if spinal or epidural anesthetic has been given.	
Sedatives may be provided (Seconal, Nembutal, Restoril, Dalmane).	Analgesics may be provided (Demerol, Stadol, Fentanyl).	Analgesic administration may be repeated if >2 hr before expected delivery.	Local or pudendal anesthesia may be provided.	Narcotic antagonist may be provided.
	Epidural anesthesia may be provided.	Epidural anesthesia may be provided. Spinal anesthesia may be provided; Check for bladder distention.	Epidural anesthesia may be provided.	Epidural anesthesia may be provided.

FAMILY CONSIDERATIONS

When the Woman Receives Analgesia or Anesthesia During Labor

When a husband, partner, family member, or close friend has been working intensively with the parturient during childbirth as the labor coach and pharmacologic pain relief is requested, the coaching role may suddenly and drastically change. These labor coaches may feel lost or unable to identify what other roles they may fulfill. On the other hand, if labor has been prolonged and intensely painful, they may be exhausted and relieved when freed from the responsibility of coach. The nurse should be alert to the needs of the labor coach once analgesia or anesthesia has been requested. They may be able to support and encourage the woman during administration of the drug or be required to withdraw temporarily because of hospital policies or their own fears centering on the procedure. Even when analgesia or anesthesia is employed, there is a place for active participation of the labor coach although the role may change. The couple should not be allowed to feel they have failed if pharmacologic methods are requested.

OBSTETRIC ANESTHESIA IN LABOR

Systemic analgesia may be suitable for normal labor, but it may be contraindicated in some situations, such as with a premature or compromised fetus, adverse maternal drug reactions, or when delivery is expected within 1 or 2 hours. Thus, many circumstances may result in a need for more active medical and nursing management of pain through the use of *obstetric anesthesia*.

This section discusses commonly used methods of obstetric anesthesia, including regional and general anesthesia. Perineal and pudendal block, as they are commonly used in low-risk labors, are discussed in Chapter 24. The major types of anesthesia in each group are described, the relative risks and benefits are discussed, and specific nursing responsibilities in caring for patients requiring obstetric anesthesia are identified.

Regional Anesthesia

Regional anesthesia is a term referring to techniques that provide pain relief to a region of the body by directly affecting nerve impulse transmission; this class of anesthetic techniques, sometimes called *conduction anesthesia,* includes *subarachnoid* or *spinal block, epidural block, paracervical block,* and *pudendal block.* In all cases, these blocks produce analgesia and anesthesia by having the anesthetic agent injected in a location where it can stabilize the cell membrane of nervous tissue, thus preventing transmission of sensory impulses. Each block is characterized by a different injection site, which in turn enables different patterns of anesthesia, as discussed later in this section. Spinal and epidural blocks are often referred to as types of *spinal anesthesia* because they involve infiltration into the spinal region. Figure 27–2 shows pertinent spinal anatomy and the infiltration sites for regional anesthesia.

Agents Used in Regional Anesthesia

Several local anesthetic agents are used in regional anesthesia, depending on the type of infiltration and the level of anesthesia desired. There are two major classes of these drugs: *ester-linked anesthetics,* such as procaine (Novocaine), chloroprocaine (Nesacaine), and tetracaine (Pontocaine); and *amide-linked anesthetics,* such as lidocaine (Xylocaine), mepivacaine (Carbocaine), and bupivacaine (Marcaine). These groups are metabolized differently in the body and vary in their duration of action and particularly in their effects on the fetus.

Ester-linked agents are metabolized by plasma cholinesterase in maternal serum and are relatively short acting, do not readily cross into fetal circulation, and may require repeated dosages to achieve satisfactory anesthesia. Amide-linked agents are metabolized by liver enzymes, are longer acting, and are often favored for use in obstetrics for this reason; however, these agents cross the placenta readily and are not easily metabolized by the immature fetal liver, so fetal effects are prolonged (Perez 1981).

Currently, the efficacy and safety of the administration of narcotics, such as morphine and Fentanyl, into the epidural space is being clinically evaluated in the United States. There are opiate receptors found in the spinal column, and intraspinal narcotics may play a role in pain relief during labor and birth. Findings of studies to date have been conflicting. While maternal and fetal cardiovascular, neurologic, and respiratory disturbances are rare, delayed maternal respiratory depression and apnea have been reported, and vomiting and itching (particularly the mouth, face and eyes) are common side-effects. Depression on neurobehavioral examinations also occurred in some infants whose mothers received epidural morphine during labor (Hughes 1982).

More promising is the use of morphine (Duramorph PF) and Fentanyl in combination with lidocaine for cesarean birth. After delivery of the neonate, the narcotic is added to the epidural catheter. Several studies report improved maternal comfort during the latter part of surgery.

More significantly, for the first postoperative day, the need for additional parenteral pain relief may be reduced, allowing the mother greater mobility and alertness for ambulation and interaction with the neonate (Preston et al 1988).

Nursing care of the patient who has received an intraspinal narcotic includes monitoring of respirations every 10 to 15 minutes for the first hour and every 30 minutes for the remaining 24 hours. Delayed respiratory depression with gradual onset has been noted. Narcotic antagonists, such as naloxone hydrochloride (Narcan), are administered to counteract respiratory depression, and antipuritics may be given for severe itching, which occurs in a small number of patients. Further research will undoubtedly be conducted before widespread administration of intraspinal narcotics occurs in obstetrics.

Advantages and Disadvantages

Regional anesthesia for labor and birth has gained popularity in recent years. Advantages of regional anesthesia for labor and birth are that dangers of general anesthesia, particularly aspiration of gastric contents, can be avoided and that the mother can be alert for the birth. Other advantages include the following:

- Pain relief is complete in the area affected by the regional block.
- Doses can be administered repeatedly through use of a catheter for administration of epidural blocks.
- Fetal effects are minimal with spinal and epidural blocks if maternal blood pressure is maintained.

Disadvantages of regional anesthesia include the following:

- Administration requires specialized skill and cannot be done by nursing personnel.
- Anesthetic failures (no effect or only partial effect) can occur.
- Regional anesthesia may be contraindicated or impossible because of spinal abnormality or previous spinal surgery.

In addition, administration of spinal and epidural blocks too early in labor can reduce uterine contractility; however, this can be avoided by delaying administration until the active phase of labor and by avoiding maternal hypotension. Administration of spinal and epidural blocks too early in labor can also create a need for oxytocin augmentation and forceps applications because these blocks reduce the mother's reflex urge to bear down; thus, her bearing-down efforts in the second stage may be less effective.

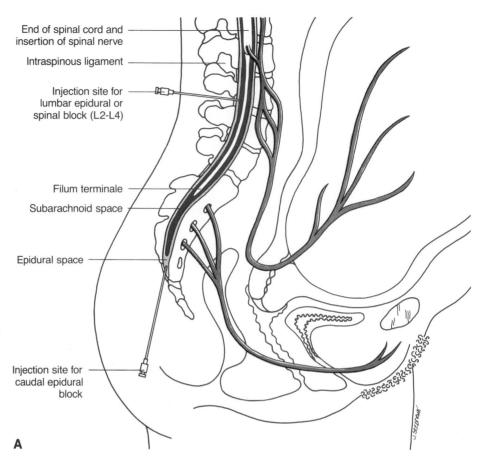

End of spinal cord and
insertion of spinal nerve

Intraspinous ligament

Injection site for
lumbar epidural or
spinal block (L2-L4)

Filum terminale

Subarachnoid space

Epidural space

Injection site for
caudal epidural
block

Figure 27–2. Regional anesthesia. *(A)* Schematic diagram of spinal anatomy. *(B)* Sensation points for determining level of spinal anesthesia. Absence of sensation to cold touch using an alcohol wipe at the midline should be evident 15 minutes after administration. (Childbirth Graphics)

A

Adverse Reactions to Regional Anesthesia

Adverse maternal reactions can occur to any of these types of regional anesthesia; although they are rare, these adverse reactions demand prompt nursing intervention. The most frequent adverse maternal reactions with any type of regional anesthesia are *maternal hypotension* and *allergic or toxic reaction* to the drug itself. A rare but alarming problem is respiratory paralysis resulting from a high spinal block. A less alarming response, but still distressing to the patient, is *partial or total anesthetic failure.* These reactions and appropriate nursing actions are discussed below.

Maternal Hypotension.   Maternal hypotension may follow administration of any regional anesthetic although it is more common after spinal or epidural anesthesia. It is caused by the sympathetic blocking action of the drug and the resulting loss of peripheral vascular resistance and may be compounded by compression of the vena cava if the mother is supine.

The nurse should monitor maternal blood pressure and pulse every 2 to 3 minutes for 20 minutes after injection of the anesthetic and every 10 to 15 minutes thereafter. Steps to prevent maternal hypotension include

- Avoiding compression of the vena cava by using the side-lying position to displace the uterus to the left
- Maintaining adequate maternal hydration with intravenous fluid

A sudden bout of nausea may be an early sign of developing hypotension. Any decrease in systolic pressure should be considered a possible early sign. The nurse should take the following steps if maternal blood pressure is decreasing:

- Place the mother in left side-lying position to relieve pressure on the vena cava and elevate legs to promote venous return.
- Administer oxygen at 8 to 12 liter/min by face mask.
- Increase flow rate of intravenous fluid.
- Have someone else notify the physician of the situation.
- Remain with the patient and provide reassurance.
- Observe FHR pattern for changes.

If these measures are not effective, an intravenous injection of 5 to 25 mg of ephedrine may be ordered to elevate blood pressure.

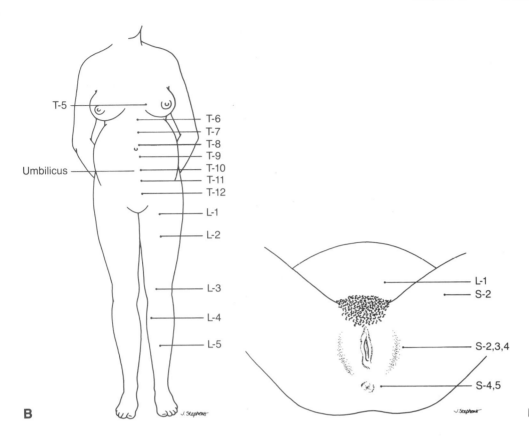

T-5

T-6
T-7
T-8
T-9
Umbilicus — T-10
T-11
T-12

L-1

L-2

L-3

L-4

L-5

L-1
S-2

S-2,3,4

S-4,5

B

Figure 27–2. (continued)

Respiratory Paralysis. Respiratory paralysis can result from spinal block at T-4 or above. This may occur following accidental penetration and injection of the dura with an epidural dose of anesthetic agent. Signs of respiratory paralysis include rapidly developing apnea and hypotension; if it is not corrected, cardiac arrest will result. The nurse should note the patient's comfort level and respiratory status carefully after the block has been administered and the patient has been positioned, especially if anesthesia for cesarean delivery is being attempted. If hypotension develops accompanied by respiratory distress and apnea, the physician is alerted immediately and the nurse takes emergency steps to maintain maternal cardiopulmonary status. Treatment includes the steps for correcting hypotension listed previously; in addition, respiratory effort must be supported, and endotracheal intubation and assisted ventilation may be necessary until the effects of the block have worn off.

Allergic or Toxic Reaction. Both allergic and toxic reactions may occur in response to anesthetic agents. Allergic reactions include urticaria, laryngeal edema, and bronchospasm; this type of reaction is treated by intravenous injection of an antihistamine, usually diphenhydramine. Toxic reactions may also occur when high circulating levels of the drug are introduced, either by inadvertent intravascular injection or by rapid absorption. Although these reactions are *rare,* the nurse must note early signs and notify the physician immediately. The following are signs of drug toxicity in order of increasing severity:

- Lightheadedness, vertigo
- Slurred speech, metallic taste in the mouth, loud ringing in ears
- Numbness of tongue and mouth
- Muscle twitching
- Loss of consciousness
- Sudden cardiovascular collapse
- Generalized convulsions

Treatment of toxic reactions includes administration of oxygen and intravenous or intramuscular injection of drugs to counteract convulsions. Administration of a short-acting barbiturate may be ordered to prevent convulsions. If convulsions are present, intravenous or intramuscular injection of 40 to 60 mg of succinylcholine will be ordered; this controls muscular spasm and allows endotracheal intubation for a patent airway. Once this has been accomplished, assisted ventilation will be initiated, and intravenous fluids and vasopressors will be administered rapidly to support cardiovascular function (Pritchard and Williams 1985).

Toxic reactions in the neonate may also occur, characterized by alterations in CNS functioning, seizures, bradycardia, hypotonia, and apnea. Treatment of newborn anesthetic toxicity includes inducing prompt diuresis with intravenous fluids, supporting respiratory and metabolic status, and using barbiturates or diazepam to control seizures.

Partial or Total Anesthetic Failure.   Occasionally, regional anesthesia will be only partially established or will fail to provide adequate pain relief. There are various causes for this. Malabsorption of the agent may occur because of decreased vascularity in the injection area, dehydration, and poor maternal physical condition. Spinal abnormalities or inaccurate placement of the injection may result in anesthetic failure. In many cases, a partial block can be increased by injection of additional medication; in other cases, however, maternal pain relief remains inadequate, and other procedures, such as systemic or general anesthesia, may be necessary.

Implications for Nursing Care

Patients receiving regional anesthesia for labor and birth are at slightly increased risk simply by virtue of the procedure itself. Nursing care for patients before, during, and after administration of regional anesthesia is extremely important to ensure the safety of the mother and the fetus. The following general functions are of primary concern to the nurse caring for patients receiving any type of regional anesthetic:

- Assisting the attendant with the procedure by preparing the patient and her partner and assisting with positioning of the patient and with the procedure itself, as needed
- Providing support and reassurance for the patient and her partner
- Monitoring maternal and fetal physiologic responses to the anesthesia, observing closely for adverse reactions
- Monitoring for maternal urinary retention resulting from decreased bladder sensation
- Monitoring the pattern of labor for changes resulting from the anesthetic
- Assessing maternal comfort level and monitoring for return of sensation
- Initiating emergency measures in the event of adverse maternal or fetal responses

These nursing responsibilities apply to care of patients receiving any type of regional anesthesia. The following section discusses each type in more detail, and specific nursing care is outlined.

Types of Regional Anesthesia

All of the four major types of regional anesthesia are used in intrapartal care. *Pudendal block* involves infiltration of anesthetic into the perineum near the pudendal nerve and is used to anesthetize the perineum. This type of block, commonly used during normal second-stage labor, is discussed in Chapter 24. The remaining types of regional anesthesia, *paracervical block, spinal block,* and *epidural block* are discussed here.

Paracervical Block

The paracervical block provides anesthesia to the uterus and thus is used to relieve pain of first-stage labor. The anesthetic agent (usually procaine or tetracaine) is injected into the lateral vaginal fornices on either side of the cervix, as shown in Figure 27-3. The patient is usually placed in the lithotomy position, and the injection is done

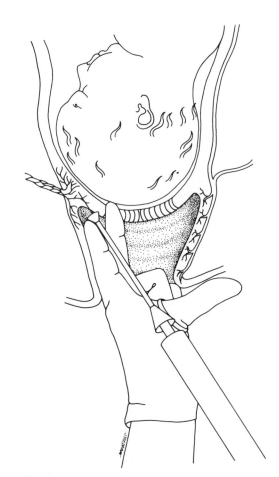

Figure 27-3. Paracervical block is accomplished by injection of local anesthetic into the mucosa in the lateral vaginal fornices by use of a needle guide. Injection of anesthetic agent is kept shallow at a depth of 3 mm to 5 mm to avoid over-rapid absorption of the agent and accidental fetal injection. (Childbirth Graphics)

through a special needle guide 2 to 3 mm into the mucosa in the vicinity of the uterine plexus. Prior to injection, the needle must be aspirated to ensure that the drug is not being injected into a blood vessel, since this can cause a toxic reaction. The standard dose is 5 to 10 ml of low-concentration anesthetic agent on each side of the cervix. Once the injection is completed, the woman should be returned to a side-lying position and, for reasons to be explained shortly, *continuous FHR monitoring* should be implemented for at least 30 minutes after the injection.

Paracervical block relieves uterine pain but anesthesia does not extend to the lower vagina or the perineum, so additional anesthesia (such as pudendal block or local infiltration of the perineum) may be needed for second-stage labor. A paracervical block is administered in active labor, typically at 5 to 6 cm dilatation in a primigravida and 4 cm to 5 cm in a multigravida. It can be administered only while the cervix is still palpable. Anesthetic effect is nearly immediate and lasts 45 to 60 minutes.

Advantages and Disadvantages.

Advantages of a paracervical block include the following:

- The injection is a relatively simple procedure.
- It provides good to excellent anesthesia for pain of uterine contractions and cervical dilatation.
- Maternal side effects are rare.

However, there are some disadvantages to this procedure. A major disadvantage of paracervical block is the fairly high incidence (25%–85%) of fetal bradycardia following administration. This bradycardia is usually transient, appearing within 2 to 10 minutes after injection and lasting 10 to 30 minutes (Perez 1981). There may also be loss of baseline variability and occasional late decelerations before the preblock FHR is reestablished. Fetal bradycardia after paracervical injection is thought to be a result of local vasoconstriction caused by rapid absorption of the drug into the uterine circulation; others suggest that it is a result of cardiac depression caused by transfer of the agent across the placenta to the fetus.

Thus, continuous FHR monitoring before the procedure to establish a baseline FHR and after the procedure to detect bradycardia is considered essential for safe paracervical block. Because of the high incidence of fetal bradycardia, use of paracervical block is *contraindicated* for patients whose fetuses may be compromised or premature or in whom there is evidence of placental insufficiency (Cohen and Friedman 1983). Other disadvantages of paracervical block include the following:

- It is contraindicated when there is evidence of vaginal infection because of the risk of endometritis. (Insertion of a needle into the mucosa when infection is present may spread pathogens into underlying tissue and the uteroplacental circulation.)
- There may be transient decrease in uterine activity for 20 to 30 minutes after injection.
- There is a small but present risk of maternal toxic reaction to the drug due to intravascular injection or rapid absorption (Perez 1981).
- There is a small risk of injecting anesthetic directly into the fetus, which will result in toxicity and, possibly, fetal death.

Implications for Nursing Care.

Nursing responsibilities in caring for a patient receiving a paracervical block include monitoring maternal and fetal physiologic response to the anesthetic and maintaining maternal physiologic functioning once anesthesia has been achieved. The nurse must observe the FHR closely for evidence of bradycardia; if bradycardia is detected, the mother is kept in a side-lying position, and oxygen is administered. If FHR abnormalities persist longer than 30 minutes, the fetus should be considered potentially distressed and the nurse should prepare for fetal blood sampling and emergency delivery. If the fetus is delivered within 30 minutes of the block and before the normal FHR is reestablished, the nurse should be prepared for assistance with a possible acidotic neonate with lowered Apgar scores (Perez 1981).

Maternal blood pressure and pulse should be assessed every 5 to 10 minutes and when there is any change in maternal status; the nurse should carefully observe for early signs of developing toxic response and hypotension in the first 15 minutes after administration. Although these responses are rare, they do occur.

Epidural (Lumbar and Caudal) Block

Epidural blocks can provide excellent anesthesia throughout active and second-stage labor. They can be administered at any point in active labor, but are customarily administered at 4 to 6 cm of cervical dilatation. Anesthesia is achieved by injecting the anesthetic agent into the epidural space outside the dura (Fig. 27–4). The injection may be in the lumbar region at L-2 to L-4 or in the caudal region through the sacral hiatus at S-4. Epidural blocks typically produce blockade from T-10 to S-5, providing complete anesthesia from umbilicus to mid-thigh. They can be extended upward for cesarean delivery by administering larger doses to blockade from T-8 to S-1.

Repeated injection of anesthetic through a plastic catheter inserted in the epidural space and taped securely to the patient's back provides pain relief throughout active labor. The level of anesthesia can be extended from a limited block for active labor to a complete pelvic block for the second stage and delivery. Additional injections or "topping up" can be performed when pain returns.

Procedure for Lumbar and Caudal Epidural Block

Lumbar Epidural Block

1. The patient is positioned on her left side with shoulders aligned and legs slightly flexed. Spinal flexion is not recommended, since it stretches the dura and increases the possibility of puncture and inadvertent spinal block. A sitting position may be necessary for patients when the lumbar interspaces are small.

2. The nurse verifies patency of the intravenous infusion and provides reassurance and support to the patient.

3. The lower back is scrubbed with antiseptic solution and draped for asepsis.

4. A skin wheal is raised by intradermal injection of local anesthetic at the proposed injection site.

5. A short 18-gauge beveled needle is introduced into an interspace between L-2 and L-4 and advanced to the ligamentum flavum. This landmark is noted by resistance to injected fluid or air: injected substance will rebound back into the syringe.

6. The needle is then advanced another millimeter into the peridural space; this is noted by loss of resistance to injected air or fluid. The syringe is aspirated for cerebrospinal fluid or blood. If cerebrospinal fluid or blood is aspirated, the needle is withdrawn and insertion is attempted at another site.

7. A test dose of anesthetic agent is injected. Signs of inadvertent spinal anesthesia (onset of anesthesia after the test dose) are monitored for 5 minutes. The nurse begins assessment of maternal blood pressure, pulse, and respiration every 1 to 2 minutes at this point.

8. If the test dose produces warmth and tingling in lower extremities, but no anesthesia, the needle is judged to be properly placed in the peridural space, and the appropriate amount of anesthetic agent is administered.

If continuous lumbar anesthesia is desired, steps 1 to 6 above are followed by these steps:

7. A plastic catheter is threaded through the needle into the peridural space and advanced 3–5 cm beyond the needle tip. The needle is then removed. (Note: the catheter should not be retracted through the needle because the soft catheter may be shredded or broken off in the peridural space.) Transient hyperesthesia (increased cutaneous sensitivity) may occur in the back, leg, or hip if the catheter touches a nerve in the peridural space.

8. A test dose is administered and is monitored as in steps 7 and 8 above.

9. The catheter is closed off and taped in place, allowing for additional injections by the anesthetist or physician (not the labor nurse), as needed.

Caudal Epidural Block

1. The patient is positioned in a side-lying position and supported by the nurse.

2. The lower back and coccygeal area are scrubbed with antiseptic solution and draped for asepsis.

3. A skin wheal is raised by intradermal injection of local anesthetic over the area of the sacral hiatus of the last sacral vertebra (S-4). With a longer needle the anesthetic solution is injected more deeply into the fascia over the sacral hiatus.

4. An 18-gauge needle is directed toward the sacral hiatus and through the sacrococcygeal membrane and inserted approximately 3 cm into the caudal canal. The syringe should be aspirated; if cerebrospinal fluid or blood is found, the procedure should be discontinued because of the risk of incorrect needle placement into maternal soft tissue or the fetal head.

5. A test dose of anesthetic is administered; the nurse monitors maternal vital signs for signs of spinal block. If no signs are noted after 5 minutes, the caudal dose is administered by the physician or anesthetist.

If continuous caudal anesthesia is desired, steps 1 to 4 above are followed by this step:

5. A plastic catheter is advanced through the needle for a distance of 5 cm, and the needle is withdrawn. The catheter is taped securely in place. A test dose is administered as above. If no adverse signs are noted after 5 minutes, the caudal dose is administered. The catheter is then closed off, and the nurse continues close monitoring of maternal blood pressure, pulse, respiration, and anesthetic level. Additional doses of anesthetic may be administered as needed by the physician or anesthetist.

Continuous epidural block has become the most common type of epidural block. The end of the plastic epidural catheter is attached to a continuous infusion pump and the anesthetic agent is delivered to the patient intravenously at a set rate. This eliminates the need for repeated "topping up" as the anesthetic is metabolized and excreted and pain returns.

A double-catheter approach using both a lumbar and a sacral catheter also can provide flexible and highly effective anesthesia throughout active labor and delivery.

Lumbar epidural blocks are administered with the patient in a sitting or side-lying position. Flexion of the back is not desirable, since it reduces the peridural space and stretches the dura, making it more susceptible to punc-

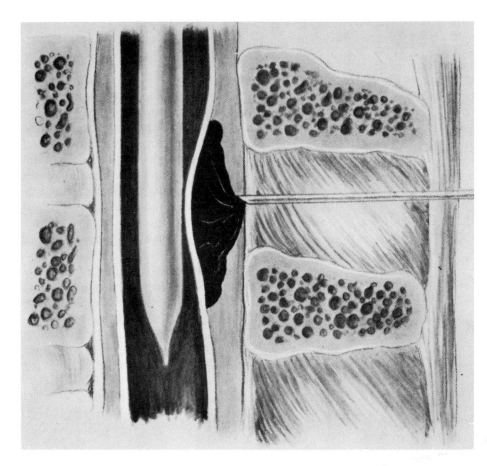

Figure 27–4. Epidural injection is accomplished by introducing a needle through the intraspinous ligament just through the ligamentum flavum into the peridural (epidural) space. The dura protecting the subarachnoid space is pushed away from the needle by the force of the injection. (Moore DC: Regional Block, 4th ed. Springfield, IL, Charles C Thomas, 1967)

ture. Injection is made in an interspace between L-2 and L-4. The procedure is outlined in the accompanying display. First the syringe is aspirated to verify that the needle is correctly placed: puncture of a vessel will yield blood, and aspiration of cerebrospinal fluid indicates the dura has been punctured. In either case the needle is withdrawn and another injection is attempted. If aspiration for blood and fluid is negative, a test dose of anesthetic is injected. If the patient experiences warmth and tingling of the legs with the test dose without paralysis or sensory impairment, the needle has been properly positioned in the epidural space and injection of the full dose can proceed. If continuous administration is desired, a catheter is inserted into the epidural space and a full anesthetic dose is administered and repeated as necessary.

Caudal epidural blocks are administered with the patient in a side-lying position. The fourth sacral vertebra has a U-shaped opening protected by a thin fibrous membrane; this opening is called the sacral hiatus and is the route through which a needle can be advanced into the lowest part of the epidural space. There is less risk of puncturing the dura with a caudal insertion than with a lumbar insertion. However, correct placement of the needle in the sacral hiatus is essential, since incorrect placement may result in puncture of the maternal rectum or of the fetal head, a potentially lethal accident. For this rea-

son, caudal blocks should not be attempted when the presenting part is on the pelvic floor. Correct placement is determined by aspiration and administration of a test dose as with a lumbar insertion. Again, a continuous caudal epidural block can be achieved by insertion of a plastic catheter for administration of repeated doses.

Early signs (Perez 1981) of a successful caudal block include

- Rapid perineal anesthesia
- Loss of anal sphincter reflex
- Loss of urge to push (if previously present)
- Numbness and tingling of toes
- Warmth and dryness of feet

Analgesia will extend upward to the abdomen. Larger doses of anesthetic, compared to doses needed with a lumbar block, are needed to extend a caudal block up to T-8. For this reason, the patient should be monitored carefully for possible accidental spinal block and for toxic reactions, as described in the previous section on adverse reactions to regional anesthesia.

Advantages and Disadvantages. *Advantages of epidural block* include excellent and flexible anesthesia for labor and delivery with little or no identifiable effect on the fetus. In some cases, fetal status may even improve after

NURSING RESEARCH

Maternal Perceptions of Self-Esteem After Childbirth with Epidural Anesthesia

It has been suggested that women who do not experience the physical sensations of birth due to administration of anesthesia may relate differently to the newborn and suffer from feelings of diminished self-esteem. Slavazza and associates (1985) examined the differences in ratings of self-esteem among primiparas who received a variety of analgesics and anesthetics in labor and those who received none. No significant group differences were found in self-esteem, maternal perceptions about the infant, or feelings about the childbirth experience at the time of delivery.

Interestingly, women who had received epidurals described their infants in more positive terms. The authors suggest that the pain relief afforded by the epidural may have led to less fatigue and greater ability to interact with the infant and thus contributed to the more positive feeling. Parturients who received parenteral analgesia were least satisfied with their mode of pain relief. Clinicians should discuss pain relief options with women (preferably early in labor) and help them to understand the possible outcomes of pharmacologic intervention on the birth experience (fatigue, possible decreased mental awareness, absence of sensation of pain and pressure and so forth).

Slavazza KL, Mercer RT, Marut JS, Shnider SM: Anesthesia, analgesia for vaginal childbirth. J Obstet Gynecol Neonatal Nurs 14:321–329, 1985

tress, and in patients with marked hypotension, neurologic disease, or signs of infection at the proposed injection site (Pritchard 1985).

Implications for Nursing Care.   Nursing responsibilities in providing care for a woman receiving an epidural block center on adequately prehydrating the patient with intravenous solutions, assisting her into position for insertion of the catheter, closely monitoring maternal and fetal physiologic status, and providing emotional and physical comfort and support during and after the procedure. The patient is provided information about the epidural by the anesthesiologist and must give informed consent. However, the nurse may need to answer additional questions and explain what the woman and her partner may expect.

A crucial activity prior to placement of the epidural catheter is adequate prehydration of the patient. Epidural anesthesia results in sympathetic block and vasodilatation of the lower extremities and can result in profound hypotension. An intravenous line should be started using a 16- or 18-gauge needle, and a bolus of 500 to 1000 ml of intravenous fluid is administered before initiation of the procedure.

The nurse assists the patient into position and explains the need to avoid movement. The nurse monitors both fetal heart rate and uterine activity and alerts the anesthe-

NURSING ALERT

Pre-hydration Precautions

Women receiving epidural or spinal blocks during childbirth are normally prehydrated with 500 ml to a liter of intravenous fluid prior to the procedure in order to prevent hypotension. Hypotension is a common side-effect of conduction anesthetics, secondary to sympathetic blockade and concomitant vasodilation of the lower extremities. Recent research suggests that the rapid infusion of 5% dextrose in water can have a deleterious effect on fetal acid–base balance. Fetal hyperglycemia, metabolic acidosis, and neonatal hypoglycemia have been associated with a glucose solution bolus. The use of a balanced physiologic solution, such as Ringer's lactate or Plasma-lyte, is recommended for prehydration before administration of conduction anesthesia and for rapid intravenous infusion in cases of maternal hypotension and dehydration.

Philipson EH, Kalhan SC, Riha MM, Pimentel R: Effects of maternal glucose infusion on fetal acid–base status in human pregnancy. Am J Obstet Gynecol 157:866–873, 1987

epidural block because of increased uterine blood flow and decreased pelvic resistance during second-stage labor. *Disadvantages of epidural block* include the risk of maternal hypotension, toxic response to the anesthetic, and disruption of normal labor pattern. Larger doses of anesthetic are required for epidural blocks than for spinal anesthesia. Accidental puncture and injection of an epidural dose of anesthetic into the dura, especially with lumbar epidural block, will result in inadvertent high spinal block, and resultant respiratory paralysis.

In addition, onset of pain relief with epidural block is slower than with spinal anesthesia. If labor proceeds rapidly or if the block is administered late in the first stage, anesthesia may not be established in time for the second stage and delivery. Administration of epidural block also requires considerable skill. Ineffective anesthesia may result from improper placement or irregular nerve pathways.

Epidural blocks are contraindicated in acute fetal dis-

LEGAL/ETHICAL CONSIDERATIONS

Fetal Monitoring During Administration of An Epidural or Spinal Anesthesia

If the decision is made to administer an epidural or spinal anesthetic during childbirth, the nurse has specific responsibilities regarding fetal monitoring during the procedure. Recent changes in standards of practice have occurred as the result of litigation. Currently, the *nurse* assumes primary responsibility for assessing the fetal response during administration of anesthesia. An electronic fetal monitor or doppler must be employed *continuously* during the procedure.

Frequently, the external tocodynamometer belt must be removed during epidural or spinal administration. If the nurse is unable to continuously assess uterine activity, oxytocin infusions should be discontinued during the procedure. The nurse should manually palpate the uterus or ask the patient to inform her of each contraction in order to time their frequency and duration. The anesthesiologist should be notified immediately if fetal bradycardia or prolonged decelerations occur. The procedure should be stopped and measures should be instituted to oxygenate the fetus, improve uteroplacental perfusion, and reduce uterine activity. The birth attendant should examine the patient to rule out prolapsed cord or imminent birth.

siologist to onset of contractions so that the block can be administered between them. Continuous fetal monitoring by EFM or doppler is essential to evaluate fetal response to the epidural block. In order to facilitate frequent assessment of maternal vital signs, it is useful to use an electronic blood pressure monitor that automatically takes the blood pressure and pulse at preset intervals.

A test dose of anesthetic with epinephrine is infused to determine proper placement of the catheter. The nurse monitors the pulse rate during this procedure. If a sudden rise in the pulse rate occurs, inadvertent spinal block may have occurred. If all vital signs remain stable, anesthesia is injected and the catheter taped in place. The blood pressure is monitored every 2 to 3 minutes for the first 20 to 30 minutes and every 5 to 10 minutes thereafter.

The nurse notes the parturient's comfort level, evaluates level of anesthesia using an alcohol wipe (see Figure 27–2B), evaluates mental status (confusion, lethargy, or light-headedness may indicate hypotension), and checks for early signs of adverse reaction to the anesthetic. (These are discussed in the next section.) Care must be taken in positioning the woman to avoid injury to the

lower extremities, since sensory and motor function is diminished or lost. The left lateral position with the head of the bed slightly elevated will promote uteroplacental perfusion and patient comfort.

Bladder distention is a common problem during labor when epidural anesthesia is administered because the block eliminates bladder sensation to some extent. The problem is exacerbated by the administration of large volumes of intravenous fluids to prevent hypotension.

The nurse must monitor intake and output carefully and observe and palpate for bladder distention at least every 30 minutes. The patient can be placed on a bedpan (walking is impossible with an epidural block due to loss of motor function), and some women will be able to void. If the patient is unable to empty her bladder, the birth attendant may decide to place a urinary drainage catheter in the bladder. This prevents the need for repeated cathe-

LEGAL/ETHICAL CONSIDERATIONS

Nursing Responsibilities in the Delivery Room After Administration of Conduction Anesthesia

In many cases the woman receives an epidural or spinal anesthetic in the delivery room just prior to birth of the infant. Nursing malpractice cases frequently result from inadequate supervision of the patient during the interval between administration of anesthesia and birth. The nurse must take specific steps to insure the safety and well-being of both mother and fetus until vaginal or cesarean birth:

- Continuous electronic fetal monitoring and assessment of uterine activity is required.
- Uterine displacement should be effected to prevent compression of the vena cava.
- Extreme caution must be exercised to prevent nerve and tissue damage resulting from pressure on or torsion of legs.
- Care must be taken to restrain the lower limbs to prevent them from falling off the narrow delivery table.
- Care must be taken to prevent patient falls from the narrow delivery table, especially if it is tilted to facilitate uterine displacement.

The patient should NEVER be left unattended in the delivery room. The legs should be positioned in correct anatomical alignment, and stirrups should be padded. Leg restraints should not constrict blood flow. The fetal monitor should not be removed until birth of the infant in the case of vaginal delivery or until abdominal prep is begun in the case of cesarean birth.

terization of the bladder when birth is not anticipated for some time.

Comfort measures such as position changes, frequent replacement of linen protectors as they become soiled, and perineal care are important. Because of the possibility of adverse effects with epidural anesthesia, the patient is usually given nothing by mouth or clear liquids only, once the epidural block is administered. Oral hygiene should be offered as needed to promote comfort and prevent dryness of the mucous membranes.

Because the patient will no longer feel uterine contractions, the nurse must evaluate their frequency, intensity, and duration by palpation and should apply the tocodynamometer to assist in this assessment. The woman will need assistance to bear down effectively during the second stage of labor because, as noted, sensation from the lower body is diminished or eliminated. If the patient is moved to a delivery room, a roller is usually needed to transfer her from the labor bed to delivery table. After birth of the infant, the nurse must make certain that ambulation is not attempted until full motor and sensory function of the lower extremities is regained.

Spinal (Subarachnoid) Block

Spinal block involves introduction of an anesthetic agent into cerebrospinal fluid in the subarachnoid space. Spinal block can be used to provide anesthesia for vaginal delivery or for cesarean delivery by varying the level of sensation loss. Spinal block is usually effective for 1 to 2 hours and so is used primarily at the end of the first stage of labor and for delivery.

The *level of anesthesia* is described both as it relates to the specific location in the spinal column at which impulses are blocked and as it relates to the corresponding loss of sensation. A *saddle block* is achieved by blockade from level S-1 to S-4, with loss of sensation in the perineum, lower pelvis, and inner thighs; uterine contractions will still be felt, and pain with delivery will not be completely eliminated. A *low spinal block* for vaginal delivery requires blockage up to level T-10, with loss of sensation from the umbilicus to the toes. There is loss of sensation of uterine contractions and complete pain relief for delivery. A spinal block for cesarean delivery requires blockage up to the level of T-6, producing complete anesthesia from the nipple line to the toes.

The level of anesthesia is determined by altering the amount of medication injected and by the patient's position after injection, because the anesthetic agent is hyperbaric (heavier than the cerebrospinal fluid). The injection is usually done at L-2 to L-5 for any spinal block, as shown in Figure 27–5. The block is usually administered with the woman in a sitting position or a side-lying position with the head slightly elevated. The patient is asked to place her chin on her chest and arch her back forward

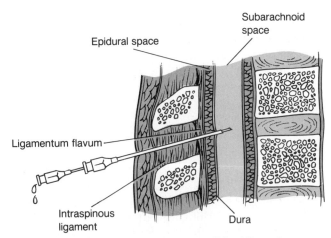

Figure 27–5. Spinal injection is accomplished through a double-needle technique, in which a larger needle is introduced up to the ligamentum flavum, and a smaller needle is used for the injection into the subarachnoid space to minimize the puncture size.

Procedure for Spinal Block

1. The patient is positioned in a sitting or side-lying position and supported by the nurse; the nurse verifies that the intravenous infusion is patent and provides reassurance throughout the procedure.

2. The lower back is scrubbed with an antiseptic solution and draped for asepsis.

3. A skin wheal is raised at the L-3–4 interspace by intradermal injection of local anesthetic.

4. The patient is assisted to curve her back and neck forward, with arms between knees, and is supported in this position by the nurse.

5. A 20- or 21-gauge needle is introduced into the wheal and advanced into the interspinous ligament, the ligamentum flavum, and the epidural space.

6. A smaller-gauge needle (No. 25 or No. 26) is then inserted into the larger needle and advanced through the dura into the subarachnoid space. The presence of spinal fluid in the needle hub verifies that placement is correct.

7. Appropriate amount of anesthetic is injected slowly, and both needles are removed.

8. The nurse assists the patient into the desired position (supine for anesthesia for cesarean birth, sitting for anesthesia for vaginal delivery) for 3 to 5 minutes and begins monitoring blood pressure, respiration, and pulse every 1 to 2 minutes for the first 10 minutes after administration.

9. The nurse observes for signs of toxic reaction or respiratory difficulty, which signals possible respiratory paralysis.

to widen the intervertebral space. (See the accompanying display on spinal block procedure.)

The woman's position within the first 3 to 5 minutes after injection and the amount of medication injected will determine the level at which the anesthetic will act on neural tissue. Injection during bearing-down efforts, coughing, straining, or vomiting must be avoided, since these actions compress the subarachnoid space and force the anesthetic agent to a higher level than desired. If a saddle block or low spinal block for vaginal delivery is desired, the woman is generally kept in a sitting position for 5 minutes to allow time for the anesthetic to become bound to neural tissue. If a higher block for cesarean delivery is needed, more medication is injected and the woman may be asked to move to a supine position immediately after injection. After 5 minutes, maternal position or actions will have little effect on the level of anesthesia produced.

Advantages and Disadvantages.   Advantages of spinal block for intrapartal anesthesia include the following:

- It provides excellent anesthesia for delivery and fourth-stage labor.
- There is little or no direct effect on the fetus if maternal blood pressure is maintained.

Disadvantages of spinal block center on complications that may arise, including maternal hypotension and related fetal compromise; disruption of the normal pattern of labor with decreased effectiveness of bearing-down efforts; possible total or "high" spinal block, which interferes with respiration; postspinal headache; and increased risk of urinary retention in the immediate postpartum period. Each of these will be discussed in detail.

Maternal hypotension may result quickly after administration of the block; it is caused by vasodilation due to blocking of sympathetic nervous system impulses. A severe drop in maternal blood pressure reduces uterine blood flow and can compromise fetal status. This drop can be reduced by ensuring that the patient is well hydrated with intravenous fluids (500–1000 ml) before the block is administered and that supine hypotension syndrome is avoided. Nursing intervention for maternal hypotension is discussed later in this section.

Disruption of normal labor pattern can occur if spinal block is administered before the cervix is fully dilated. If labor is disrupted, oxytocin augmentation may be needed. Further, the block eliminates the woman's reflex urge to push with contractions, so forceps applications are more common among women receiving spinal blocks (Pritchard and Williams 1985).

Total or "high" spinal block (anesthesia level at T-4 or above) with respiratory paralysis may result from a larger than needed dose of anesthetic or upward spread of the agent. Signs of total spinal block are rapidly developing apnea and hypotension and eventual cardiac arrest. (Nursing interventions are discussed in the earlier section on adverse reactions to regional anesthesia.)

Postspinal headache is thought to be caused by leakage of cerebrospinal fluid from the puncture site; when the woman sits or stands, the reduced amount of fluid allows traction on pain-sensitive central nervous system structures. Headache is typically worse upon standing or sitting and is lessened upon bed rest. It usually begins on the second postpartum day, and persists for several days. The incidence of postspinal headache appears to be reduced if a small-gauge (25- or 26-gauge) needle is used for injection and multiple punctures are avoided. There is no convincing evidence that keeping the patient at bed rest for 12 to 24 hours after anesthesia will prevent postspinal headache. Treatment usually includes bed rest, adequate hydration (by IV fluids if necessary), and administration of analgesics. Severe headaches are sometimes treated quite successfully by use of a *homologous blood patch:* about 10 ml of the woman's blood is drawn and immediately injected into the epidural space at the site of the previous puncture; this blood forms a clot and seals the leak (Pritchard and Williams 1985).

Urinary retention, a common problem in the postpartum period, is exacerbated by spinal block in the intrapartal period because intravenous fluids are routinely administered before the anesthesia and the block eliminates bladder sensation. The woman should be monitored closely for urinary retention and catheterized as needed, since this predisposes her to postpartum hemorrhage and later urinary tract infection.

Contraindications for spinal block include maternal hypotension or any factors that predispose to it (suspected hemorrhage, hypovolemia), neurologic disease, coagulation disorders or anticoagulation therapy, infection at the proposed injection site, or acute fetal distress. Because spinal block will produce a rapid and dramatic fall in blood pressure in patients with hypertension, maternal hypertension may be considered a relative contraindication (Pritchard and Williams 1985).

Implications for Nursing Care.   Nursing responsibilities in providing care for a woman receiving a spinal block center on assisting the patient during administration of the block, closely monitoring maternal physiologic status, and promoting comfort and safety. The patient must receive an explanation about the procedure and give consent; usually this is taken care of by the anesthesiologist. However, the nurse may need to answer additional questions and explain what the patient and her partner should expect.

The nurse assists the patient into position for the administration, explains the need to avoid movement, and supports the patient physically. The nurse also alerts the physician to onset of contractions so that the block can be administered between them. The nurse should recognize that spinal procedures are frightening to most patients and should provide emotional support and comforting touch during this time.

Once the patient has remained in the position necessary to establish desired anesthetic level for 5 minutes, the nurse begins monitoring maternal blood pressure every 2 to 3 minutes for 20 minutes, and every 5 to 10 minutes thereafter. The nurse checks the woman's mental state and comfort level frequently for early signs of adverse reactions to the anesthetic. Care must be taken in positioning the woman for delivery to avoid injury to the lower extremities, since self-protective pain sensation will be lost.

The nurse will need to assist the woman to bear down effectively with uterine contractions during the second stage, because sensation from the lower body is diminished or eliminated by the block. In addition, the nurse must take special care in assisting the woman to move after delivery, since some motor paralysis is common. The transfer should be slow and careful to avoid strain to the patient. The nurse must ensure that the patient does not attempt ambulation until full sensation has been regained.

General Anesthesia

General anesthesia, defined as pharmacologic intervention that results in progressive CNS depression with eventual loss of bodily sensation and consciousness, was routinely used in the 1950s and 1960s to manage maternal pain during labor and birth. However, this method of anesthesia is no longer widely used in normal intrapartal care because of the significant maternal and fetal risk it presents and because other modes of anesthesia now provide safer alternatives. However, general anesthesia is still appropriately used in circumstances where regional anesthesia cannot be used and effective maternal pain relief is essential.

The term *general anesthesia* is usually used in obstetrics to refer to inhalation anesthesia, or pain relief through administration of a gaseous agent mixed with oxygen and inhaled until loss of consciousness occurs. Inhalation agents may also be used intermittently for analgesia during labor through inhalers that women can use themselves with close supervision.

General anesthesia may also include the use of intravenous anesthesia—intravenous injection of an agent, usually a short-acting barbiturate, such as pentothal sodium, for pain relief. Intravenous anesthesia provides rapid induction and prompt recovery but is difficult to control and may cause such untoward side effects as ma-

ternal bronchospasm and respiratory arrest. For these reasons, intravenous anesthesia is rarely used alone in modern obstetric care. However, intravenous agents may be used in combination with inhalation anesthetics (see section below on combination or "balanced" anesthesia) to provide appropriate pain relief for women in the intrapartal period.

Agents Used in General Anesthesia

Agents used in general anesthesia include gas anesthetics and induction agents, usually intravenous agents used to assist in the rapid induction of anesthesia. Some gas anesthetics can be self-administered by the patient with the use of an inhaler, a specialized mask that permits the patient to inhale the agent at the beginning of each contraction before pain is felt and to remove (or drop) the mask when anesthesia is sufficient. Inhaler masks should not be held in place for the mother by *anyone* but a skilled anesthetist or anesthesiologist because of the risk of rapid induction of deeper anesthesia and loss of consciousness.

Nitrous Oxide.   Nitrous oxide produces analgesia and alteration of consciousness but not true anesthesia. It provides rapid, pleasant induction without interfering with maternal physiologic status at low dose concentrations (40% nitrous oxide, 60% oxygen). It can be administered by face mask or inhaler and should be given in combination with oxygen in concentrations no higher than 70% to avoid maternal hypoxia. Nitrous oxide has few side effects and is often used both for analgesia in second-stage labor and for induction of anesthesia in combination with other agents (Pritchard and Williams 1985).

Methoxyflurane (Penthrane).   Methoxyflurane can be administered by inhaler for analgesia or in combination with other agents for anesthesia. It provides pleasant but somewhat slower induction and recovery than other gas agents. This agent also is associated with uterine relaxation and increased blood loss in the postpartum period, and for this reason use is typically restricted to low doses for relatively short periods (Pritchard and Williams 1985).

Ketamine.   Ketamine is an intravenous induction agent that produces analgesia, amnesia, and a sleep-like state with some CNS stimulation; it can be used as an induction agent for and in combination with inhalation anesthesia. Ketamine causes an increase in maternal blood pressure and pulse rate. Thus it is useful in situations where maternal hypotension is a concern and is *contraindicated* when the patient is hypertensive. This agent causes minimal respiratory depression; it crosses the placenta readily but does not appear to produce fetal depression in typical doses. Problems with this agent include confusion, delirium, and hallucinations during emergence from anesthesia (Cohen and Friedman 1983).

Pentothal Sodium. Pentothal sodium (thiopental) is an ultrashort-acting barbiturate that produces CNS depression and loss of consciousness within 30 seconds of administration. Its rapid action, its low potential for causing nausea and vomiting, and the prompt recovery time make it useful for induction in obstetric anesthesia. However, it does not produce anesthesia until doses are high enough to cause profound CNS depression; thus pentothal is rarely used alone, being normally used with gas anesthetic agents.

Combination or "Balanced" Anesthesia. Combination anesthesia refers to the use of intravenous induction agents and inhalation anesthesia in combination to achieve a "light" plane of maternal anesthesia that can be rapidly administered but that avoids the risks of maternal–fetal depression caused by deeper anesthesia. Combination anesthesia is especially common for cesarean birth. This practice typically includes induction with an agent such as pentothal sodium followed by administration of an nitrous oxide–oxygen mix to maintain anesthesia. A skeletal muscle relaxant, such as succinylcholine, is then injected intravenously to facilitate endotracheal intubation for the operative procedure, and light inhalation anesthesia is maintained until no longer needed.

Indications and Contraindications

Indications for general anesthesia for delivery are primarily conditions that require considerable uterine and pelvic relaxation (such as difficult forceps applications, breech deliveries, or the presence of tetanic contractions) with prompt effective maternal anesthesia. General anesthesia is often used in emergency vaginal deliveries and emergency cesarean deliveries for fetal distress. General anesthesia is regarded as the anesthetic of choice in the presence of maternal hemorrhage, since regional anesthesia can compound maternal hypotension. Contraindications to general anesthesia include situations where the fetus is already compromised and, because of the possible depressant effect on the fetus/newborn, where delivery cannot be anticipated within minutes of anesthetic administration.

Advantages and Disadvantages

Advantages of general anesthesia include the fact that it produces significant overall muscle relaxation, which is useful in difficult forceps extractions and in breech and cesarean deliveries. This property is also beneficial when the mother has severe preeclampsia or eclampsia, since the muscle relaxation reduces the likelihood of convulsions. General anesthesia can also be rapidly administered and is ideal for emergency situations where delivery must be immediate and maternal pain relief is essential.

Disadvantages of general anesthesia for use in the intrapartal period include the following:

- Delivery must occur within 5 to 7 minutes after administration because inhalation anesthetics rapidly cross the placenta and will cause hypoxia and respiratory depression in the neonate.
- The risk of maternal aspiration of gastric contents with resulting life-threatening pulmonary complications is considerable.
- A skilled anesthetist or anesthesiologist is required for safe administration.
- Immediate postpartum recovery is more difficult, and there is nausea and vomiting and increased risk of uterine atony and postpartum hemorrhage.
- The mother is not alert for the birth and the father is usually excluded from the delivery room.

Several of these points will be discussed in detail.

Respiratory Depression in the Fetus/Neonate. Most general anesthetics rapidly cross the placenta and enter fetal circulation within 2 minutes of administration. The degree of fetal CNS depression from anesthetic agents is proportional to the depth and duration of maternal anesthesia. In circumstances where the fetus is already compromised by hypoxia or prematurity, the depressive effects of anesthesia are additive, and vigorous neonatal resuscitation may be needed at birth (see Chapter 33). The long-term effects of maternal anesthesia on neonatal status are not clearly understood. Effects of general anesthesia are similar to those of other medications but more pronounced; these include decreased response to stimuli, decreased rooting and sucking reflexes, hypotonia and irritability (Perez 1981).

Vomiting and Aspiration During General Anesthesia. Deaths related to anesthesia may account for as much as one half of maternal mortality; the most common cause of anesthesia-related death is pneumonia or chemical pneumonitis resulting from aspiration of gastric contents (Pritchard and Williams 1985). General anesthesia reduces or eliminates the laryngeal and cough reflexes and often induces vomiting. Vomiting is especially likely during emergence from general anesthesia and if fundal pressure is applied to assist with the delivery.

In addition, the laboring woman is at increased risk for aspiration because gastric emptying time may be reduced during labor; she is likely to have particulate food matter in her stomach even hours after eating. Further, the *p*H of gastric acid is lower in pregnancy and secretion of acid may be increased. Aspiration of particulate food matter typically leads to acute respiratory obstruction and aspiration pneumonia. Aspiration of even small amounts (less than 25 ml) of gastric acid is highly destructive to lung tissue and may lead to aspiration pneumonitis or Mendelson's syndrome (adult respiratory distress syndrome).

Vomiting and aspiration during general anesthesia may be silent and unnoticed unless the patient is being closely monitored. Early signs of aspiration pneumonitis are restlessness and agitation, increased respiratory rate, and tachycardia, cyanosis, and shock. Immediate treatment includes positioning the patient on her right side with head down at a 30-degree angle to facilitate airway clearance; endotracheal intubation with assisted ventilation and, possibly, a tracheostomy during the acute phase; systemic corticosteroids to limit the inflammatory reaction; and antibiotics to limit infection.

Measures to prevent aspiration during general anesthesia in the intrapartal period typically include the following:

- Administration of oral antacids (15–20 ml every 2 hours throughout labor and 30–50 ml within an hour prior to administration of general anesthesia)
- Maintenance of NPO status (with ice chips) for laboring women considered likely to require general anesthesia
- Smooth induction of anesthesia followed by prompt endotracheal intubation; intubation should be maintained until the woman is fully awake and has regained cough and laryngeal reflexes to protect her airway
- Application of cricoid pressure (downward pressure on the cricoid cartilage to compress the esophagus, preventing aspiration) during intubation and extubation and when vomiting has occurred

Increased Risk for Postpartum Hemorrhage. Another common problem related to general anesthesia in the intrapartum period is uterine atony and increased risk of postpartum hemorrhage. Most anesthetic gases used for general anesthesia produce profound uterine relaxation, which prevents good contraction and hemostasis. Treatment includes close monitoring of vaginal bleeding and continuous oxytocin infusion begun immediately after the delivery to maintain uterine tone until hemorrhage is no longer considered likely (Pritchard and Williams 1985).

Implications for Nursing Care

Nursing responsibilities for care of the woman receiving general anesthesia for delivery include assisting the anesthetist, as needed, during the procedure. The nurse must be prepared to assist in emergencies such as acute respiratory obstruction. The nurse must be familiar with the location and use of emergency equipment and procedures needed for support of cardiopulmonary status and must be prepared to assist the anesthetist in cardiopulmonary resuscitation efforts.

Nursing care during postanesthesia recovery is of special importance and, in most obstetric settings, the woman will be transferred to a postanesthesia unit. More intensive nursing care is required to avoid postanesthetic respiratory complications, to monitor for uterine atony and potential hemorrhage, and to monitor cardiopulmonary status until anesthetic effects have worn off. The reader is referred to a nursing text on surgical nursing for a fuller discussion of postoperative nursing care.

CHAPTER SUMMARY

A major goal of nursing care during childbirth is the provision of comfort and the control of pain. The nurse employs the nursing process to meet these objectives. From admission through birth and the postpartum period, the nurse assesses the patient's level of discomfort, establishes appropriate nursing diagnoses, and plans effective strategies to manage pain. The quality of the childbirth experience is in large part determined by the nature and extent of discomfort perceived by the patient and the modes of pain relief employed to control it. The woman, her support person, the nurse, and birth attendant are members of a team who must work together to promote comfort and reduce painful sensations in the woman to acceptable levels.

Uncontrolled pain has deleterious effects for both the parturient and her fetus. When comfort measures fail to provide adequate pain control or when complications require such immediate intervention as cesarean birth, pharmacologic methods may be employed. The safety and efficacy of analgesia and anesthesia depend in large part upon the expertise of the clinician. The labor nurse must also have a comprehensive knowledge regarding the drugs and techniques commonly used in childbirth.

Finally, women will differ in their expectations regarding pain during labor and birth, preparations to manage this discomfort, and desire for specific types of pain relief. The nurse must recognize this and individualize the plan of care for the laboring patient by ascertaining the parturient's expectations, goals, and plan for pain management. This approach will enhance the woman's chances of having a safe, meaningful, and satisfying childbirth experience.

STUDY QUESTIONS

1. What are the major sources of discomfort and pain during labor and birth?
2. Describe physiological and psychological effects of pain.

3. Outline major nonpharmacologic methods of pain management during labor.

4. What are the nurse's primary responsibilities when administering analgesia during labor?

5. Why is it inadvisable to administer analgesia during transition-stage labor?

6. What are common forms of conduction anesthesia?

7. What are the nurse's primary responsibilities when epidural or spinal block are administered?

8. What are the major advantages and disadvantages of regional anesthesia?

9. What are the nurse's responsibilities after administration of regional anesthesia prior to cesarean birth?

10. What are common adverse effects of epidural and spinal block?

11. What are the advantages and disadvantages of general anesthesia?

REFERENCES/BIBLIOGRAPHY

Cohen W, Friedman E: Management of labor. Baltimore, University Park Press, 1983

Hughes SC: Intraspinal narcotics in obstetrics. Clin Perinatol 9(1):167–174, 1982

Perez R: Protocols for Nursing Practice. St. Louis, CV Mosby, 1981

Preston PG, Rosen MA, Hughes SC, Glosten B et al: Epidural anesthesia with Fentanyl and Lidocaine for cesarean section: maternal effects and neonatal outcomes. Anesthesiology 68:938–943, 1988

Pritchard J, Williams P: Williams' Obstetrics, 17th ed. New York, Appleton-Century-Crofts, 1985

SUGGESTED READINGS

Carmichael FJ, Rolbin SH, Hew EM: Epidural morphine for analgesia after cesarean section. Can Anaesth Soc J 29(4):359–363, 1982

Geden EA, Beck NC, Anderson JS, Kennish ME et al: Effects of cognitive and pharmacologic strategies on analogued labor pain. Nur Res 35:301–306, 1986

Gibbs RF (ed): Legal Perspectives on Anesthesia. Georgetown, CT, McMahon Publishing, 1984

Hodnett ED, Abel SM: Person–environment interaction as a determinant of labor length variables. Health Care for Women International 7:341–356, 1986

Nicholls ET, Corke BC, Ostheimer GW: Epidural anesthesia for the woman in labor. Am J Nurs 81:1826–1830, 1981

Paterson GM, McQuay HJ, Bullingham RES, Moore RA: Intradural morphine and diamorphine. Anesthesia 39:113–117, 1984

Taylor AG: Duration of pain condition and physical pathology as determinants of nurses' assessments of patients in pain. Nurs Res 33:331–335, 1984

Worthington EL: Labor room and laboratory: A clinical validation of the cold pressor as a means of testing preparation for childbirth strategies. J Psychosom Res 26:223–230, 1982

28 nursing care of the at-risk family in the intrapartal period

LEARNING OBJECTIVES

After studying the material in this chapter, the student should be able to

- Discuss the importance of a family-centered approach to high-risk intrapartal care and ways it can be implemented

- Identify factors that affect how women and their families respond to intrapartal complications

- Identify common causes of third trimester bleeding and outline nursing care for each condition

- Discuss maternal risks that result from abnormal placental adherence and outline appropriate nursing care

- Discuss appropriate nursing care for the patient with premature rupture of membranes

- Identify the risks to mother and fetus of umbilical cord prolapse and outline the emergency interventions needed

- Describe ways in which intrapartal medical and nursing management must be adapted to meet the needs of the mother with preexisting hypertension or diabetes

- Describe the etiology and emergency medical and nursing man-

agement of the major physiologic threats posed by shock and disseminated intravascular coagulation

- Discuss the causes, maternal and fetal risks, and medical and nursing management of preterm labor

- Discuss the nursing implications of grief and loss for families experiencing complications of labor and birth

- Discuss intrauterine fetal demise, its causes, diagnosis, and medical and nursing management

KEY TERMS

Acetylcholine

Bicornuate uterus

Central venous pressure (CVP) monitoring

Chorioamnionitis

Chorionic plate

Cor pulmonale

Ecchymosis

Endotoxin

Exsanguination

Extrinsic coagulation factors

Fetal dystocia

Fetal membranes

Fibrinogen

Goiter

Hypotonic uterus

Petechiae

Podalic version

Retraction ring

Scotoma

Septum

Thromboplastin

Vasa praevia

Velamentous insertion

Usually labor and birth progress with few problems, and outcomes for mother, newborn, and family are generally positive. However, when complications arise in the intrapartal period, they develop rapidly and may have devastating effects on maternal and fetal/newborn well-being. Care providers must identify the nature of the problem and intervene to reduce or limit detrimental effects on mother and infant. The woman must continue to deal with the process of labor and cope with a new set of sensations, fears, procedures, and instructions. The family is thrust into a situation for which they may not be well prepared and over which they have little control. What was expected to be a normal labor and birth becomes a threatening situation in which outcomes are not predictable and even survival seems uncertain.

This chapter first discusses the context of high-risk intrapartal care and intrapartal complications as a family crisis. Family responses to intrapartal crisis are reviewed, with emphasis on the concepts of uncertainty, risk, grief, and loss. The remainder of the chapter focuses on major complications that may arise in the intrapartal period. These complications can be classified in a variety of ways. In this chapter they are divided into the following categories:

Complications primarily involving the placenta, membranes, umbilical cord, and fetus

Complications of fetal descent

Complications involving maternal physiologic systems

Complications involving uterine function

Complications involving the reproductive tract

Specific obstetric complications are described, including etiologic or predisposing factors, maternal and fetal/neonatal implications, treatment and nursing responsibilities.

The nurse plays a central role in identifying and caring for families with complications in the intrapartal period. The quality of nursing care delivered to those families can make the difference between a happy outcome and a tragic one.

FAMILY RESPONSES TO MAJOR INTRAPARTAL COMPLICATIONS

The Nature of High-Risk Intrapartal Care

Providing intrapartal care for women and families experiencing complications is a complex process. First and foremost is the need to identify the nature of the problem promptly and to initiate appropriate medical and nursing care. This alone is a challenge to providers, since the

FAMILY CONSIDERATIONS

Impact of a High-Risk Labor and Birth Experience on Family Functioning

Medical and nursing attention is appropriately focused on the medical or obstetric emergency of the woman in labor. However, the entire family (partner and children) may suffer negative physical and psychological outcomes when the anticipated birth experience is altered by maternal or fetal complications. The father must often assume physical and emotional responsibility for other children and carry both the psychological and financial burdens which arise when the well-being of the woman or fetus is placed in jeopardy.

As a consequence, normal patterns of family coping may be inadequate or inappropriate. Research indicates higher rates of family dysfunction, divorce, and even physical illness in family members following childbirth emergencies. Health care providers must attempt to support family members as they struggle to adapt during the period of crisis. Hospital support services should be recruited to assist the partner. Other nurses not providing direct care to the woman may be in the best position to offer information, guidance, and support. Social and financial services and spiritual counseling referrals should be made, when appropriate.

problem may present as a life-threatening emergency demanding immediate intervention or the problem itself may be difficult to diagnose. Some intrapartal complications may occur suddenly and unpredictably and be true emergencies requiring immediate intervention to ensure maternal and fetal survival. Others may be anticipated because of preexisting maternal or fetal conditions or may progress more slowly so that care can be provided in a less pressured way.

Problems that can be anticipated because of maternal or fetal conditions or that can be stabilized and corrected without emergency measures increasingly are managed in facilities designed to accommodate the high-risk intrapartal patient. However, care providers in any maternity setting must be prepared to deal with rapidly developing complications and obstetric emergencies, since by their very nature these problems usually cannot be predicted.

Regardless of the setting in which care is managed, all care providers must recognize that intrapartal complications involve significant physiologic and emotional risk. Physiologic risk to mother and fetus/newborn should be the focus of initial care. Changes in the mother's physiologic status nearly always adversely affect the fetus. In addition many fetal problems during labor also entail some risk to maternal status, which then increases fetal risk in a spiraling effect. The term "maternal–fetal unit" may be used to express this physiologic interrelatedness.

However, it is important to recognize that once complications have arisen, *all* members of the family must be considered to be "at risk." Both parents are under considerable emotional strain; both mother and father are likely to be fearful for their unborn child's life, even when the identified threat may not be that extreme. The nurse must always remember that although professionals may recognize that there are degrees of risk and margins of safety with any complication, parents usually do not have the knowledge to allow them to make those distinctions. Thus, parents may interpret signs of increasing concern about fetal well-being as indications of a "life-threatening" complication, even when the risk is quite manageable.

When intrapartal complications arise, the mother also usually recognizes that there is some threat to her own well-being, even if only from the emergency treatment required. The father must come to grips with the vulnerability of both his partner and his unborn child. Both parents are likely to feel that they are not prepared to deal with this unanticipated crisis, especially if the usual sources of support are not immediately available to them. Thus, in addition to coping with the usual aspects of childbirth, the family must face a crisis situation over which they may feel they have no control and that involves the potential for devastating loss.

This potential for loss means that the woman and her partner need emotional support and a family-centered approach to care. These may be even more important for families experiencing problems in the intrapartal period than for those whose birth is problem-free. Even if intensive intrapartal treatment for physiologic problems is successful, if emotional needs are not met, the woman and her family may be so stressed that maternal physiologic status is threatened further and long-term individual and family adaptation is compromised. This underscores the need for comprehensive nursing care that emphasizes both the emotional and the physiologic well-being of all family members.

Childbirth or Medical Emergency?

When problems develop in the intrapartal period, it is sometimes difficult to determine whether the situation is a medical emergency or simply a childbirth with complications. In truth, the situation is sometimes both. Some complications are immediately life-threatening and must be managed as emergencies. All efforts must then be directed at interventions to meet the immediate physiologic threat, and supportive care for the family must be deferred until the situation is "stabilized."

However, true emergencies are relatively rare, and

NURSING RESEARCH

The Meaning of Emergency Cesarean Birth For Medically Indigent Women

When a decision is made to perform an emergency cesarean birth due to fetal distress or maternal complications, the values, expectations, and socioeconomic and educational level of the woman in labor appear to influence her view of the experience. Recently, Sandelowski and Bustamante (1986) challenged the assumption that all women who undergo sudden, unexpected emergency cesarean birth with little time for preparation or explanation suffer negative psychological outcomes.

The findings of this study indicate that some women, classified as "medically indigent" and giving birth in public hospitals, may not experience acute disappointment when unable to deliver vaginally. These women emphasized the positive outcomes rather than the process of birth. The investigators suggest that life experiences condition many of the women to surrender control and to avoid anticipating a specific type of birth experience. Further research is essential to identify the variety of responses to technologic interventions during labor and birth and develop appropriate nursing interventions.

Sandelowski M, Bustamante R: Cesarean birth outside of the natural childbirth culture. Res Nurs Health 9:81–88, 1986

many intrapartal complications can be managed effectively with a more deliberate approach to care. One potential problem for care providers is failing to make that distinction in their interactions with patients and their families. Staff may have a tendency to interact with all patients experiencing problems in an intensive, crisis-oriented way. This can decrease the quality of maternity care for women and families experiencing complications in childbirth by leading to ineffective provision of emotional and family-centered support.

Lack of this support may not have immediate visible effects, and some providers may consider it unimportant compared with treatment of physiologic problems. However, parents' emotional responses to the birth experience have been shown to substantially affect the quality of later family life and parenting. Divorce, separation, and family violence occur more frequently among families who experience difficulties in childbearing. Thus, the nurse must remember that interventions during an intrapartal crisis must take into account both short-term and long-term effects and emotional well-being as well as physiologic safety. Many family-centered practices can be incorporated into the care of high-risk families with little reorganization of routine practices, if the nurse is committed to doing so.

Specialization and Regionalization in Perinatal Care

Regionalized perinatal care, established in the late 1960s to provide access to specialized neonatal intensive care units while avoiding duplication of services, has until recently placed much emphasis on neonatal care. Facilities are classified according to the level of neonatal care that can be safely given, ranging from low-risk care to high-risk or "tertiary" level care (see Chapter 34 for a fuller discussion of levels of neonatal care). In the past, complications in the intrapartal period were managed in the local facility, and the sick or compromised neonate was then transported to a tertiary center for care.

However, advances in the understanding and treatment of maternal and fetal physiologic status have resulted in an increasing focus on high-risk intrapartal care. This has given rise to the practice of "maternal transport," or transfer of the woman who is at high risk in the intrapartal period (or, more often, whose fetus is at risk) to a center where a high level of obstetric and neonatal expertise is available. Usually maternal transport is avoided if delivery is judged to be imminent, to preclude the possibility of an out-of-hospital delivery. Some critics question whether the advantages of maternal transport outweigh the hardships involved in removing the mother from her own community for delivery. However, maternal transport has been found to be advantageous in conditions, such as preterm labor, where the mother is the best "incubator" for transport.

The most common indication for maternal transport is a high predicted risk to the neonate, with the need for immediate intensive care. Indications for maternal transport are listed in the accompanying display. Of these, preterm labor is the most common, accounting for almost half of all maternal transports. It is not unusual for a patient to have more than one indication for maternal transport.

The increasing specialization in perinatal care has im-

plications for the delivery of nursing care in the intrapartal period. Some tertiary care settings have established high-risk antenatal and intrapartal units in which medical and nursing staff are experienced in caring for families with complications during childbirth. This has allowed the integration of family-centered practices into high-risk care, since staff are comfortable with individualizing care to meet family needs even in moderate-risk and high-risk situations. Regionalization has also created a need for nurse-staffed maternal transport teams, as well as nursing roles for outreach education and coordination.

Factors Affecting Family Responses

Maternal and fetal complications that arise during the intrapartal period require family members to adapt to unexpected and rapidly changing events and cause a sudden increase in stress. The intrapartal period is one of heightened emotions and stress even under normal conditions. When problems arise, the woman and her partner will be more anxious and fearful. Furthermore, most women and their families have not dealt with such situations before and will feel as if everything is out of their control. This can be viewed as a family crisis, and the degree to which family members can adapt to and cope with this increased stress level will determine how well they will function as a family in the intrapartal and immediate postpartum periods.

Intrapartal complications present a distinct threat of individual and family loss, and the greater the perceived threat, the greater the stress under which the woman and her partner are operating. First, parents are likely to respond with tension-releasing behaviors, such as crying, pacing, or other repetitive physical activity. Parents are then likely to respond with their own characteristic ways of coping with intense emotional distress, such as denying the threat, seeking additional information so as to understand the threat, limiting the amount of information they must deal with, or projecting feelings of guilt through anger directed at staff.

The intensity of this response is determined in large part by how apparent the problem is to the parents and what kind of changes in maternal and fetal status have occurred shortly before and immediately after the problem has been identified, the level of uncertainty about maternal or fetal status and outcomes, and the effectiveness with which the family has adapted to crises in the past. The nurse must understand how these factors affect the responses of the woman and her partner in order to provide appropriate nursing care. The nurse plays an essential role in supporting the woman and her partner when intrapartal problems arise. More specific nursing interventions for providing emotional support are discussed later in this chapter.

Conditions Indicating the Need for Maternal Transport

- Preterm labor
- Severe preeclampsia
- Third-trimester bleeding
- Maternal diseases, including diabetes, hypertension, Rh sensitization, drug abuse
- Multiple gestation

The family's expectations about the intrapartal period will affect their responses to intrapartal complications. If the woman was told she was at increased risk for intrapartal problems, she and her partner are likely to be more prepared and better able to adjust to the situation. Women initially seen to be at low risk may experience more shock and disbelief and may need additional time to accept and cope with the news.

The nature of changes in maternal and fetal status will also have an effect on how the woman and her family respond to intrapartal complications. Changes in maternal and fetal status can be sudden, dramatic, and clearly indicative of an emergency or they may be gradual and subtle, apparent only to skilled professionals. When the threat to maternal and fetal status is obvious to the woman and her partner, they may be better able to adjust to the situation and understand the need for prompt action. However, if signs of developing problems are not obvious to the woman and her partner, they may be confused or suspicious about the need for more active intervention. In such cases the nature of the problem must be clearly explained, and the couple must be included in discussions and decision making about treatment, if at all possible. They should be given the opportunity to ask questions and discuss the situation quietly with each other before treatment plans are implemented.

Another factor that affects how parents respond to intrapartal complications is the level of uncertainty about maternal and fetal risk and expected outcomes. As their anxiety increases, parents may be distressed at the inability of physicians or nurses to predict maternal and fetal outcomes with absolute certainty. Professionals recognize that even in uncomplicated situations there are unknowns; most parents will also recognize this fact under normal conditions. However, when the well-being of mother and fetus/newborn is at stake, parents are likely to respond with fear, impatience, or even anger at what they may interpret as indecisiveness or evasion. Such responses are a result of their fear and are not directed at the professionals personally. In these situations the nurse must assist the parents to obtain and understand whatever information they need and must maintain supportive and calm contact with them.

The woman and her partner will respond in different ways to intrapartal threat because of their different perspectives on the situation. The nurse must be careful to provide assistance and support to both partners if possible or, if it is not, to arrange for partner support to be given by another staff member.

Maternal Responses.   The mother's response to intrapartal threat will be determined in part by how far labor has progressed and by her physical and emotional condition at that point. Her level of physical and emotional fatigue, pain, and fear will affect her response to news of potential or actual complications. As discussed in Chapter 23, the woman usually undergoes a process of psychological withdrawal as labor progresses and as she increasingly directs her energy toward coping with the sensations and demands of labor. If problems arise early in labor, she may be able to take in and understand explanations and comply with requests for her cooperation in the treatment. However, if problems arise later in labor, her focus will be on the present moment and on meeting her bodily and security needs; she may be unable to communicate effectively with others or to comply with their requests, and she may respond with panic.

Paternal Responses.   The father's response to intrapartal complications will also be affected by the level of his participation in the labor process, by his own physical and emotional state, and by his ability to cope with feelings of impotence in the face of this threat to his family. If the problem develops late in labor after many hours of labor support, his emotional and physical reserves will be depleted and he may respond much more emotionally than he would otherwise. The father may also feel that he has somehow failed to protect his partner. He may need to remain close to her and may respond with anger and fear if hospital policy or the situation requires separation (May and Sollid 1984).

COMMON ELEMENTS IN THE CARE OF THE FAMILY WITH MAJOR INTRAPARTAL COMPLICATIONS

No maternity care situation requires more skilled and experienced nursing than the care of the patient with intrapartal complications. Although active obstetric intervention is usually necessary, the quality of ongoing nursing assessment and intervention also greatly influences the eventual results of treatment.

In most settings, patients developing problems in the intrapartal period will be cared for in conventional labor and delivery units (as opposed to birthing rooms) and will require continuous nursing care throughout the intrapartal period. Depending on the nature of the problem, the woman may be kept in the intrapartal unit for longer than is usual for low-risk patients, or she may be transferred to another facility where more intensive neonatal care is available. The challenge to nursing staff is to reduce the stress of hospitalization as far as possible and to provide continuity and coordination of care.

Obstetric and perinatal care for patients with intrapartal complications is focused on reducing maternal and fetal risk. Major ways of managing maternal and fetal risk are discussed in Chapters 25–27.

LEGAL/ETHICAL CONSIDERATIONS

Court-Ordered Interventions and the Nurse

Today, the nurse working in labor and delivery is confronted with unprecedented legal and ethical dilemmas. In the past several years the courts have intervened and overridden the woman's right to self-determination during birth. The courts have ordered obstetrical intervention when the parturient has refused certain procedures deemed necessary by physicians for the well-being of the fetus (including blood transfusion and cesarean delivery). In a recent case both mother and infant died after a court-ordered cesarean birth.

The moral and ethical dilemma facing nurses in these instances is: for whom does the nurse become an advocate — the mother or fetus? What are the clinician's responsibilities and options if she is asked to assist in a court-ordered procedure, such as cesarean delivery, to which the parturient objects? Can the nurse refuse to participate in the procedure? A precedent has been set with therapeutic abortions: nurses may refuse to assist with the termination of pregnancy. Currently, the clinician is advised to discuss the situation carefully with her nurse-manager and the risk-management department and to bring the issue before the ethics committee for review if a court-ordered intervention is anticipated.

Aumann GM: New chances, new choices: Problems with perinatal technology. J Perinat Neonatal Nurs 1(3):1–9, 1988

The nurse can systematically approach the care of patients with intrapartal complications by considering what risk reduction procedures are likely to be needed, given the nature of the problem:

- What type of maternal and fetal monitoring is necessary?
- How can maternal pain be safely managed?
- Will it be necessary to modify (speed up, control, or slow down) the pattern of labor?
- Will it be necessary to modify the mode of delivery to promote maternal and fetal/neonatal safety?
- Are there any legal–ethical dilemmas?

When complications develop in the intrapartal period, the nursing care given must be adapted to the particular needs of the high-risk patient and her family. The specific types of nursing assessments and interventions will vary with the nature of the complication. Overall goals for nursing care of the woman with intrapartal complications include an emphasis on early detection and treatment of intrapartal problems, careful assessment of maternal and fetal status, and efficient implementation of appropriate obstetric care.

Assessment

Assessment is perhaps the most important nursing function in caring for patients with actual or potential intrapartal complications. The nurse is responsible for identifying early signs of maternal or fetal complications and for assessing family responses to labor and to the crisis situation if complications develop. Many potential problems can be anticipated by reviewing information in the patient's prenatal record and the patient's current status and labor progress. Once a problem has been identified and treatment implemented, the nurse is also responsible for continually assessing maternal and fetal physiologic status and responses to treatment.

The nurse must also assess the woman's emotional status and that of her partner, since high levels of fear and distress can have detrimental effects on maternal and fetal physiologic status. Assessing family responses to the situation not only allows the nurse to plan and implement appropriate family-centered care, but also can identify family strengths and coping patterns. Preliminary information of this nature may well be useful in planning ongoing nursing care in the postpartum period.

Diagnosis

When there are complications in the intrapartal period, patients and their families are likely to present with more than one physiologic problem and more than one nursing problem. A variety of nursing diagnoses may be applicable. The following are selected nursing diagnoses that reflect possible problems that may arise in intrapartal nursing care of families experiencing major complications:

- Altered patterns of urinary elimination
- Altered cardiac output
- Altered respiratory function: impaired gas exchange
- Altered tissue perfusion
- Knowledge deficit related to procedures and interventions
- Fear/anxiety related to complications and procedures
- Altered comfort: acute pain

- Ineffective family coping
- Anticipatory grieving
- Self-concept disturbance
- Spiritual distress

The major portion of this chapter discusses collaborative care provided to the at-risk intrapartal family. Potential complications include hemorrhage, infection, and shock. Monitoring for the complications is an integral part of nursing care in this period.

Planning and Implementation

The time available for specifying nursing diagnoses and planning for nursing care is shortened when major intrapartal complications occur. Diagnosis, planning, and implementation of that plan of care may appear to be almost simultaneous as maternal and fetal status changes and steps are taken to limit and reduce risk.

The nurse must be knowledgeable about commonly used risk reduction procedures, as discussed in Chapters 25 through 27, because many of these procedures are used in the management of maternal and fetal complications arising in the intrapartal period. The student may wish to refer to these chapters from time to time to review that material and focus on implications for the nursing care of patients with specific intrapartal problems.

Common nursing interventions for high-risk intrapartal patients and their families tend to cluster in the following categories:

- Monitoring and supporting maternal and fetal physiologic status
- Providing anticipatory guidance to the woman and her partner
- Providing family-centered support
- Coordinating patient care efforts

Monitoring and Supporting Maternal and Fetal Physiologic Status

Patients at increased intrapartal risk require intensive monitoring and support of maternal and fetal physiologic status. The nurse is responsible for regular and frequent monitoring of maternal vital signs and the progress of labor. Electronic fetal monitoring will be continuous, and internal monitoring is usually established at the earliest opportunity. The nurse must be familiar with the immediate procedures taken to support maternal and fetal physiologic status in emergency situations, including the altering of maternal position and the administration of

oxygen. (These are discussed in the Nursing Alert displays in Chapters 23 and 24.)

The nurse is also responsible for implementing medical care, as ordered, and monitoring maternal and fetal responses to treatments. Typically, patients with intrapartal complications will require intravenous fluid administration with careful attention to fluid balance, IV or intramuscular (IM) administration of medications, and preparation for necessary procedures. The types of treatments appropriate for particular intrapartal complications and their nursing implications are discussed in detail later in this chapter.

Expected Outcome: The laboring woman and her fetus maintain normal physiologic status and deviations that arise are identified and corrected promptly.

Providing Anticipatory Guidance

An important nursing responsibility is providing anticipatory guidance to the woman and her partner about what they can expect to happen in the intrapartal and postpartum period. The nurse should collaborate in this effort with the physician or nurse midwife so that information given to the parents is accurate and consistent. Such information helps the parents adjust to rapidly changing events, usually reduces their anxiety, and allows them to prepare themselves emotionally and physically.

The nurse must also evaluate how much information is useful and helpful to the woman and her partner and when it should be given. In stressful situations most people can take in some information about present and immediate future events if it is presented simply and calmly. However, some people function better with more information, whereas others cope with stressful events by avoiding information and decision making and relying instead on others.

Expected Outcome: The at-risk couple understands procedures to be performed as indicated by their questions and their restatement of information given them.

Providing Family-Centered Support

The nurse must provide support to the woman and her partner when complications arise, not only to reduce their anxiety and provide comfort but also to bolster the partner so that he can provide as much emotional comfort as possible to his mate. The nurse should also implement family-centered care as much as the circumstances allow. This requires the nurse to *individualize* care for the high-risk intrapartal patient rather than planning care based on medical diagnosis alone. For example, the nurse may consider whether the father should be present for the delivery, even under unusual conditions, and may wish to discuss this with the physician. Will the parents feel more secure together? Perhaps more important, can the father provide needed emotional and physical support for the mother without experiencing undue strain himself and without creating additional demands on staff attention that cannot be accommodated? In the case of a compromised neonate, can the parents be given the opportunity to see and touch their newborn briefly before transfer to the nursery?

Before considering such questions, the nurse must understand the family's desires and needs, the limits of safe intrapartal practice for this particular patient, and the constraints of the setting. Certainly, these family-centered concerns are secondary to the need for immediate physiologic support and physical safety for mother and fetus/newborn. However, as mentioned before, frank emergencies in intrapartal care are relatively rare, and many high-risk situations lend themselves to creative implementation of family-centered care.

Even in emergencies, concern for the family requires that an effort be made to keep the woman and her partner informed and supported, and this is almost exclusively a nursing responsibility. Parents should *never* be left alone to await procedures or information, even if that requires additional nursing assistance in unexpected emergencies, such as with cesarean deliveries. The benefit of integrating family-centered practices into high-risk intrapartal care is that it increases the likelihood that the family will perceive their birth experience positively, which in turn will promote favorable adaptation in the postpartum period.

Expected Outcome: Couple experiences decreased fear/anxiety and increased comfort as evidenced by verbal expressions of appreciation for support, and increased utilization of coping techniques.

Coordinating Patient Care Efforts

An important area of nursing intervention is coordinating the efforts of the professionals involved in high-risk intrapartal care. Most often this involves arranging for and following up on diagnostic and laboratory tests, arranging for assistance, and communicating with staff about the patient's condition and anticipated needs. Usually coordi-

nation involves intensive care nursery or pediatric staff and postpartum unit staff. This coordination requires the nurse to have accurate and current information about the patient's needs and to be able to communicate clearly with others about the patient's condition.

COMPLICATIONS INVOLVING PLACENTA, MEMBRANES, CORD, AND FETUS

Complications involving the placenta, membranes, cord, and fetus usually place the fetus at some risk and may also increase maternal risk in the intrapartal period. Several common intrapartal complications pose direct threats to fetal well-being, such as fetal distress, umbilical cord prolapse, or other abnormalities, malpresentations, and malpositions. Other, less frequent intrapartal problems are related to multiple gestation, macrosomia (large fetal body size), or hydrocephalus (enlarged fetal head), which may prevent a normal descent into the bony pelvis and vaginal delivery. Premature rupture of membranes or

---

Intrapartal Complications Involving the Placenta, Membranes, Cord, and Fetus

Placental Problems

- Placenta previa
- Abruptio placentae
- Placenta accreta, percreta, and increta
- Placental infarction
- Retained placental fragments

Membrane and Cord Problems

- Premature rupture of membranes
- Chorioamnionitis
- Imbalance of amniotic fluid
- Umbilical cord prolapse
- Congenital absence of the umbilical artery
- Marginal insertion of the umbilical cord
- Velamentous insertion and vasa previa
- Abnormal umbilical cord length

Fetal Problems

- Multiple gestation
- Post-term gestation and postmature fetus
- Fetal anomalies

abnormalities in amniotic fluid also affect the management of labor and birth care. Placental problems, such as placenta previa and placental abruption, directly threaten fetal oxygenation and present a risk of maternal hemorrhage. Fetal demise may occur before or during labor and will affect the course of labor and birth.

Clearly, maternal and fetal status are so intertwined that classifying complications according to maternal or fetal origin requires oversimplification. However, for the purposes of discussion, the following section focuses on problems especially involving the fetus and those originating in the placenta, membranes, or cord.

Placental Problems

The placenta is the life support system of the fetus. Weighing about a pound and measuring about 6 inches in diameter, it allows the transport of oxygen and nourishment as well as the transfer into the fetal circulation of antibodies, metabolites, hormones, and other substances in the maternal bloodstream. Research on placental physiology began in the 1950s; since that time this research has yielded important information about basic cell biology and the functions of hormones and hormone receptor sites in the body. This research has also yielded valuable information about abnormalities in pregnancy. A small percentage of placentas studied after delivery contain evidence of intrauterine or genetic problems. In addition, when fetal death has occurred without apparent reason, the placenta may give clues to the cause through evidence of infection, systemic disease, or genetic abnormalities.

Normal pregnancy and the survival of the fetus require adequate placental functioning, which allows exchange of oxygen, nutrients, and other substances from the maternal circulation and metabolites from the fetal circulation. Normal fetal development depends on the presence of mature and functional vascular channels on both the maternal and the fetal side of the placenta. When placental functioning is disrupted and problems develop in the intrapartal period, often abnormalities are evident either in the placement of the placenta in the uterus or in the tissue structure on the maternal side.

Some placental problems, such as placenta previa and abruptio placentae, are often considered complications of *pregnancy* because they may become evident with the onset of third-trimester bleeding in the absence of labor. Chapter 19 presents a discussion of antenatal management of these two problems; the following section focuses only on intrapartal implications for the nursing care of patients with placental problems.

Placenta Previa

Placenta previa occurs when implantation of the blastocyst takes place in the lower uterine segment and the placenta grows to cover the internal cervical os partially or completely. This condition is frequently revealed by painless third-trimester bleeding. Bleeding results from partial separation of the placenta, often caused by cervical dilatation or effacement; since this bleeding originates from the placenta rather than the endometrium, it cannot be effectively stopped until the placenta has completely separated and the uterus is emptied.

Placenta previa may be classified as follows according to the anticipated position of the placenta at full dilatation of the cervix: *total,* in which the placenta completely obstructs the os; *partial,* in which the amount of the os covered by the placenta a full dilatation is expressed in percentages; *marginal,* in which the edge of the placenta borders on the os; and *low-lying,* in which the placenta can be palpated near the internal margin of the os (see Fig. 19–3).

Etiologic and Predisposing Factors. The precise cause of placenta previa is unknown. Factors thought to be possible causes include late fertilization of the egg and delayed implantation; maternal disease may contribute as well. Predisposing factors also include multiparity; advanced maternal age; previous uterine scarring, such as from previous endometritis; multiple gestation; and increased placental size.

Maternal Implications. The first episode of bleeding in placenta previa is rarely serious; subsequent bleeding episodes may place the mother at risk for severe hemorrhage, embolism, and risks associated with emergency operative delivery. Another risk associated with placenta previa is endometritis, if pathogens gain access to the bleeding site. Other maternal risks are those associated with cesarean delivery, which is the method of delivery typically used.

The existence of placenta previa is often diagnosed before admission to labor and delivery. However, the presenting symptom may be painless, bright-red vaginal bleeding with a soft uterus and the presenting part floating above the symphysis pubis. Maternal pain may signify that labor has started or that abruptio placentae is also present. Diagnosis is often made by visualization of the placenta and the bleeding site through ultrasonography or by direct visualization of the placenta on speculum examination. Manual examination should *never* be performed on a patient presenting with vaginal bleeding unless staff are prepared for *immediate* emergency intervention with a "double setup," meaning blood has been crossmatched, and equipment and staff can accomplish either vaginal or cesarean delivery if profuse hemorrhage results from the examination (see the accompanying display, page 770).

Patients with placenta previa are at increased risk for postpartum hemorrhage as well, since vessels in the less contractile lower uterine segment are not effectively com-

NURSING ALERT

Management of Third-Trimester Bleeding

In the presence of third-trimester bleeding, the nurse *never* performs a vaginal or rectal examination or takes any action that would stimulate uterine activity. Digital examination of the cervical os when placenta previa is present can cause additional placental separation or tear the placenta itself, causing severe hemorrhage, extreme risk to the fetus, and possibly the death of mother or fetus. Until placental location can be established with ultrasonography, no manual examinations should be done. Stimulation of the uterus may result in strong contractions, causing cervical change, sudden placental separation, and rapid hemorrhage.

In some cases of marginal or low-lying placenta previa, the physician may elect to perform vaginal examination with a "double setup." This refers to examination in an operating/delivery room where immediate operative delivery can be initiated if hemorrhage occurs. However, this practice is becoming much less common as ultrasonography has enabled accurate, noninvasive diagnosis. A double setup requires the following:

- IV line in place with IV catheter large enough for administration of blood (16- or 18-gauge)
- Two units of blood crossmatched and on hand
- Equipment and supplies for both vaginal and cesarean delivery set up
- Anesthetist, physician, and scrub nurse present and prepared for surgery
- Pediatric support staff on hand for neonate

pressed. Significant postpartum bleeding can occur even when the fundus is well contracted. If bleeding cannot be controlled with oxytocics, ligation of uterine vessels or hysterectomy may be necessary.

Fetal/Neonatal Implications. Hemorrhage requires early cesarean delivery regardless of fetal maturity, and prematurity accounts for 60% of the fetal deaths associated with placenta previa. Fetal death related to placenta previa may also result from intrauterine asphyxia or fetal hemorrhage, which may result from tearing of the placenta during cesarean delivery or from a vaginal examination that injures fetal vessels. When placental tearing occurs, the amount of fetal blood lost is directly proportional to the time that elapses between placental trauma and the clamping of the umbilical cord with delivery of the fetus. The incidence of congenital abnormalities is increased when placenta previa is present, for reasons not fully understood. In addition, placenta previa encourages

malposition and malpresentation and often prevents engagement of the presenting part.

Treatment. Treatment of placenta previa during the intrapartum period centers on monitoring bleeding, preventing hemorrhage, and replacing blood when necessary to prevent shock. If bleeding has been controlled prior to 38 weeks, an elective cesarean birth can be planned when fetal maturity is assured.

If the parturient presents to labor with active bleeding that cannot be stopped through the use of bed rest and tocolytics, an emergency cesarean birth will be performed immediately.

Once the gestational age can be confirmed at 36 weeks or more, delivery can be safely planned. In many settings, cesarean delivery is the method of choice. Some physicians may choose to proceed with vaginal delivery when the previa is partial at 30% or less. Labor may be induced with amniotomy to promote descent of the presenting part, which applies pressure to the bleeding site (tamponade) and may decrease blood loss. Careful pitocin induction of labor is begun if the presenting part is low, the presentation normal, and the cervix favorable.

Implications for Nursing Care

Nursing responsibilities in providing care for a patient with possible or diagnosed placenta previa during the intrapartum period center on promptly evaluating maternal and fetal physiologic status and minimizing blood loss until delivery can be accomplished through the administration of tocolytics, which reduce uterine activity. The nurse initiates an intravenous infusion using a 16- or 18-gauge needle, which can accommodate the rapid infusion of blood. Emotional support is ongoing and occurs in conjunction with other nursing activities. (See Nursing Care Plan: The Patient with Third-Trimester Vaginal Bleeding.)

Abruptio Placentae

Abruptio placentae, also called premature separation of the placenta, is the sudden separation of a normally implanted placenta (Fig. 28–1). The incidence is estimated at 1 in every 250 pregnancies. The severity of this complication depends on the amount of bleeding and the size of the blood clot that forms on the maternal placental surface. Hemorrhage may be apparent (presence of vaginal bleeding) or concealed. On laparotomy the uterus may also be observed to have large areas of hemorrhage in the musculature itself. This condition is known as *Couvelaire uterus.*

Etiologic and Predisposing Factors. The exact cause of abruptio placentae is unknown. Researchers have noted that the incidence has decreased as obstetric

(text continued on page 774)

NURSING CARE PLAN

The Patient With Third-Trimester Vaginal Bleeding

Nursing Diagnosis (Patient Problem) and Assessment Data	Nursing Interventions	Rationale
Potential Complication: ***third-trimester bleeding*** *Risk factors:* • Uterine anomalies • Multiparity • Pregnancy-induced hypertension • Previous cesarean delivery • Renal or vascular disease • Trauma to abdomen • Previous third-trimester bleed • Large placenta	Closely observe women at risk during the course of labor, and delivery for onset of bleeding.	Third-trimester bleeding episodes are often sudden, acute, and alarming. They are always considered potentially life threatening to mother and fetus. Anticipation and awareness of increased risk will prompt appropriate nursing diagnosis and intervention

Expected Outcome:

Patient proceeds through normal pregnancy and labor as evidenced by no vaginal bleeding.

Probable Complication: ***third-trimester bleeding*** Careful admission history and description of bleeding are needed: *Time of occurrence:* Note related activity, last intercourse *Pain:* absence or presence; duration; quality; type (sharp, dull, stabbing) *Bleeding:* Amount (described in teaspoon, cups, extent of soaking through clothes, perineal pads, etc.); avoid describing bleeding in term of min/moderate/large); color (described as bright red, dark red, brown, pink, watery, etc.); clots (presence or absence) *Contractions:* Presence/absence; frequency (polysystole); duration (continuous or intermittent) *Resting tone:* elevated/normal *fetal activity:* Reported hyperactivity, diminished activity	Perform physical examination: • *No vaginal examination* should be done. • Carefully palpate uterus. • Observe for active bleeding from introitus. Facilitate strict bed rest. Check vital signs every 15 min.	Vaginal exams should never be done on a woman admitted with undiagnosed third-trimester bleeding, since bleeding may be due to placenta previa, which must be confirmed or ruled out by ultrasound or differential diagnosis. Uterus may feel rigid if placental abruption is present. Increasing fundal height may indicate concealed abruption. Color, amount, and duration of bleeding aid in differential diagnosis and identification of the severity (except in placental abruption) and urgency of the situation Activity may aggravate bleeding and increase oxygen consumption The bleeding woman is predisposed to shock due to blood loss. A pulse and respiratory rate elevated above baseline may indicate continued concealed bleeding.

(continued)

NURSING CARE PLAN

The Patient With Third-Trimester Vaginal Bleeding (continued)

Nursing Diagnosis (Patient Problem) and Assessment Data	Nursing Interventions	Rationale
Signs of fetal distress: • Tachycardia • Bradycardia • Prolonged decelerations • Late decelerations • Decreasing or absent variability.	Administer tocolytics as ordered. Maintain continuous fetal monitoring. Observe for signs of fetal distres Start IV with large needle to allow blood administration.	Uterine activity can exacerbate hemorrhage Fetal distress may be the first indicator of maternal hypovolemia or shock and may assist in the diagnosis of abruptio placentae. Care plan may be directed by the presence or absence of fetal distress. To permit fluid replacement, administration of blood (when necessary), and ready access to venous system in case of emergency.

Expected Outcome:

Patient maintains maternal and fetal physiologic status as demonstrated by normal vital signs, fetal activity, and a firm uterus.

Nursing Diagnosis:
fear related to bleeding episode and perinatal risk

• Restlessness • Crying • Facial tension • Body tension • Tremulousness	Provide support and encouragement to mother and family. Explain possible causes while performing initial assessment. Reassure patient while awaiting diagnosis. Do not leave patient unattended. Observe for signs of acute fear/panic.	Third-trimester bleeding is extremely alarming and anxiety-provoking for patient and family. A better verbal history can be obtained if patient is aware of significant factors, and can participate in diagnosis. In all cases of third-trimester bleeding, an apparently stable patient may become critical at any moment. A new bleeding episode, gradual or sudden fetal distress, or shock may necessitate immediate action.

Expected Outcome:

Mother and support person strengthen each other, through nursing support, as evidenced by relaxed expressions and body language and comfort in discussing concerns.

Probable Complication:
placenta previa

• Painless bright red vaginal bleeding • Scanty initial bleeding episode,	• Prepare for possible ultrasound and amniocentesis.	Localization of the placenta via ultrasound is often the safest way to

(continued)

NURSING CARE PLAN

The Patient With Third-Trimester Vaginal Bleeding (continued)

Nursing Diagnosis (Patient Problem) and Assessment Data	Nursing Interventions	Rationale
which subsides spontaneously, but recurs with activity • Uterus soft, relaxes between contractions if labor has begun • Stable fetal heart rate (FHR), unless profuse hemorrhage/shock occurs • Unengaged presenting part, abnormal lie	• Prepare for vaginal examination with double set-up (for emergency cesarean delivery). • Prepare for immediate cesarean delivery • Provide anticipatory cesarean delivery teaching. • Prepare for immediate cesarean delivery if bleeding episodes are recurrent or profuse.	rule out or confirm placenta previa. A skilled ultrasound technician will occasionally be able to locate an area of placental infarct or blood pooling behind the placenta, indicating abruption. With hemorrhage, prompt delivery is indicated to minimize future blood loss and risk to mother and fetus. If vaginal delivery is attempted in cases of marginal placenta previa, vaginal examination or rupture of membranes may initiate a hemorrhage, necessitating immediate cesarean delivery. In case of total previa, immediate cesarean delivery is warranted. Cesarean delivery is performed in cases of total placenta previa and in cases of hemorrhage with marginal previa, regardless of gestational age.

Expected Outcome:

Mother returns to normal physiologic status following cesarean delivery. Newborn adapts to normal physiologic status following cesarean delivery at 36 weeks gestation or more.

Probable Complication:
placental abruption

• Dark red vaginal bleeding • Uterine irritability • Uterine tenderness, continuous pain, sustained contraction • Rigid, boardlike abdomen with sharp abdominal pain • Presence of fetal distress • Enlarging abdomen	• Prepare for labor augmentation via amniotomy or oxytocin infusion • Prepare for immediate cesarean delivery if fetal distress occurs during labor or bleeding continues.	Tocolytic agents to arrest labor are contraindicated in abruptio placentae because of the dangers of fetal distress, hypotensive effects, and hypovolemia. The fetus is considered at danger of complete abruption and death if the pregnancy continues. The amount of external bleeding bears little relation to the severity or extent of abruption.

Expected Outcome:

Mother delivers normal newborn and both return to normal physiologic status postbirth.

(continued)

NURSING CARE PLAN

The Patient With Third-Trimester Vaginal Bleeding (continued)

Nursing Diagnosis (Patient Problem) and Assessment Data	Nursing Interventions	Rationale
Potential Complication: *coagulopathy*		
Observe for signs: • Petechiae • Ecchymosis • Continued bleeding from venipunctures • Hematuria	Facilitate lab tests: • CBC • Type and crossmatch • Blood coagulation studies: fibrinogen level, clotting time, prothrombin time (DIC screen) • APT test	Immediate results from lab tests will assist determination of blood loss, hypovolemia, and urgency of replacement. Disseminated intravascular coagulopathy (DIC) occasionally occurs in conjunction with abruptio placentae because of release of thromboplastin into maternal blood supply, causing numerous tiny clots.

Expected Outcome

Patient maintains normal blood coagulation profile.

Probable Complication: *coagulopathy*		
• Profuse bleeding • Shock • Profound fetal distress	• Prepare for immediate cesarean delivery. • Insert foley catheter and monitor intake and output. • Facilitate DIC screen (coagulation studies). • Administer oxygen 8–12/min by mask. • Place patient in Trendelenburg position. • Facilitate immediate blood replacement.	Disseminated intravascular coagulopathy (DIC) occurs as a result of damage to the uterine wall and retroplacental clotting, which releases large amounts of thromboplastin into the blood supply. Oxygen and Trendelenburg position assist maternal and fetal responses to sudden hypovolemia.

Expected Outcome:

Patient returns to normal physiologic status following oxygen administration, blood replacement, and prompt delivery.

management of pregnancy-induced hypertension (PIH) and cardiovascular disease has improved. However, evidence of any relationship between maternal disease and placental abruption is still considered tentative and somewhat controversial. Cigarette smoking may have detrimental effects on the vascularity of the placental bed, which may lead to necrosis of the uterine decidua. Placental abruption has also been shown to have some association with cocaine use. Other predisposing factors for placental abruption may include external trauma, high

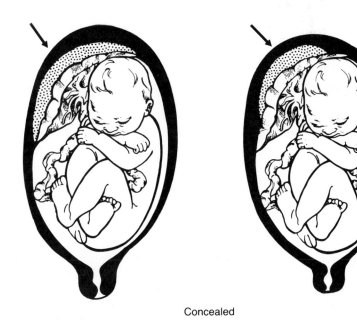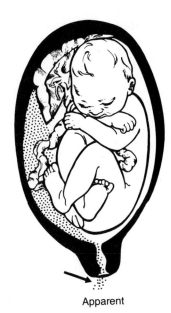

Concealed

Apparent

Figure 28-1. Abruptio placentae. Hemorrhage may be concealed or apparent by vaginal bleeding. (Childbirth Graphics.)

NURSING ALERT

Signs and Symptoms of Abruptio Placentae

When hemorrhage is apparent:

- Bright red or dark, clotted vaginal bleeding
- Uterine irritability with poor relaxation between contractions

When hemorrhage is concealed:

- No vaginal bleeding
- Sudden extreme uterine or abdominal pain
- Rapid increase in uterine size with rigidity
- Signs of acute fetal distress; absence of fetal heart tones

Other clinical signs:

- Hypovolemia and shock secondary to hemorrhage
- Disseminated intravascular coagulation because clotting factors are used in formation of the retroplacental clot

parity, overdistention of the uterus, and history of previous pregnancy loss (abruption recurs in 10% to 25% of cases) (Perrin and Sanders 1984).

Maternal Implications. Women with placental abruption who are most at risk for serious complications are those who have concealed bleeding, are nulliparous, are not in labor and have a closed cervix, and have been diagnosed after some delay. Maternal mortality, estimated to be between 0.5% and 5.0%, results from hemorrhage and cardiac or renal failure. When placental separation is minimal and prompt obstetric diagnosis and treatment are available, mortality is estimated to be between 0.5% and 1.0%. Other potential maternal complications of placental abruption include disseminated intravascular coagulation, renal failure, and postpartum hemorrhage.

Fetal/Neonatal Implications. Prospects for fetal survival are dismal when placental abruption occurs; perinatal mortality associated with this complication ranges from 50% to 80%. In half of the cases where maternal blood transfusion is urgently needed, the fetus is likely to die. In part this is because abruption can occur quickly, before intervention is possible. Among women presenting with signs of placental abruption, 20% will have no detectable fetal heart tones and another 20% will have fetuses showing fetal distress. Of the neonates that do survive, many suffer increased morbidity from effects of hypoxia, birth trauma, and prematurity (Pritchard and MacDonald 1985).

Treatment. Treatment consists of restoration and maintenance of maternal physiologic status, close monitoring of fetal status, and immediate delivery. IV fluid or blood replacement is initiated to counteract hypovolemic shock; central venous pressure monitoring may be instituted to accurately assess maternal hemodynamic status. Fetal status is monitored continuously, and immediate cesarean delivery (or vaginal delivery if the presenting part is low and bleeding is not severe) is indicated.

Implications for Nursing Care

Nursing responsibilities in the care of a patient with suspected or diagnosed abruptio placentae center on early identification of clinical signs, support of maternal physiologic status, monitoring of fetal status, and assistance with prompt delivery. (See Nursing Care Plan: The Patient with Third-Trimester Vaginal Bleeding.)

Placenta Accreta, Percreta, and Increta

Placenta accreta, percreta, and increta are anomalies representing progressively more severe degrees of abnormal placental adherence to the underlying uterine wall (Fig. 28–2). *Placenta accreta* occurs when placental tissue is contiguous with and adherent to the myometrium. *Placenta percreta* occurs when placental tissue—

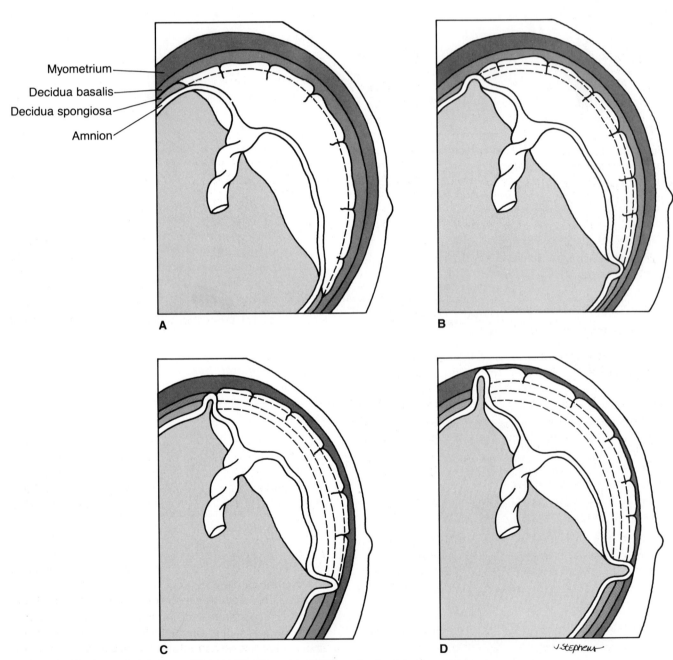

Figure 28–2. Normal and abnormal placental adherence. *(A)* Normal adherence to endometrium. *(B)* Placenta accreta: placental tissue is adherent to myometrium. *(C)* Placenta increta: placenta has penetrated uterine muscle. *(D)* Placenta percreta: placenta has penetrated uterine wall. (Childbirth Graphics)

specifically, the chorionic villi—invades the myometrium. *Placenta increta* occurs when the villi penetrate the full depth of the uterine wall. These conditions are extremely rare; estimated incidence is 1 in 7000 deliveries (Pritchard and MacDonald 1985).

Abnormal placental adherence cannot be diagnosed until delivery, when spontaneous separation does not occur. Attempts to remove an abnormally adherent placenta manually can result in uterine rupture and severe maternal hemorrhage. Third-trimester bleeding with these conditions may occur as a result of a coincident placenta previa.

Etiologic and Predisposing Factors. Placenta accreta, percreta, and increta are believed to result from failure of the decidua (lining of the uterus during pregnancy) to develop in the placental bed, thus allowing placental tissue to have direct contact with the myometrium. The specific cause for this is unknown. Predisposing factors associated with abnormal placental adherence are those that tend to denude or distort the endometrium (lining of nonpregnant uterus) and contribute to abnormal placental implantation, including the following:

* Uterine scarring from previous cesarean delivery
* History of uterine curettage
* Previous manual removal of the placenta
* Previous uterine sepsis
* Presence or surgical removal of uterine leiomyomas (myomectomy)
* Uterine malformation

Maternal Implications. The presence of placenta accreta, percreta, and increta contributes substantially to maternal morbidity, and mortality may be as high as 10%. Approximately one third of emergency postpartum hysterectomies are performed as a result of abnormal attachments of the placenta. Diagnosis is not possible before delivery, since an adherent or penetrating placenta resembles placental tissue that is partially attached. When zealous attempts are made to remove an adherent or penetrating placenta, uterine rupture, hemorrhage, and possibly exsanguination may result.

Fetal/Neonatal Implications. In placenta accreta, percreta, and increta, the placenta functions normally despite its abnormal adherence. In the absence of a concurrent problem, such as placenta previa, the fetus is generally not affected in any way.

Treatment. When minor degrees of placenta accreta exist, adhering tissue may be removed by curettage (scraping), usually without further problems. However, hemorrhage or uterine trauma resulting from attempts to remove invasive placentas constitutes a true emergency, and immediate measures are needed to prevent hemor-

rhagic shock and limit further blood loss. (See Shock, later in this chapter.) An emergency laparotomy will be performed. If the placenta has invaded the lower uterine segment, which is richly supplied with blood vessels, hysterectomy is performed to save the patient from overwhelming hemorrhage. Placental invasion in other areas of the uterus causes less blood loss but may still require hysterectomy. In rare cases most placental tissue can be removed and bleeding can be adequately controlled so that hysterectomy is not required. Subsequent pregnancies can result but with an increased risk of placental abnormality.

Implications for Nursing Care

The nurse caring for a patient with possible or diagnosed abnormal placental adherence must focus on monitoring maternal physiologic status and preparing the patient for surgery. If bleeding is not severe and the mother's condition is stable, uterine exploration and curettage may be attempted; the nurse should provide support, monitor adequacy of maternal analgesia, and be prepared to institute emergency measures should hemorrhage occur. If bleeding is severe, the nurse must be ready to institute emergency measures for hemorrhagic shock and to prepare the patient for immediate surgery. Since hysterectomy is a distinct possibility, informed consent must be obtained from the patient and her partner, if at all possible; the necessity for such surgery must be fully explained and provisions made for contact with a member of the clergy, if the mother desires it and time permits.

PLACENTAL INFARCTION

Placental infarction occurs when the blood supply to an area of the placenta is blocked and tissue necrosis results. Placental infarctions appear most commonly on the maternal surface as circular areas ranging from dark red to yellow white in color. Placental infarctions are most often associated with vascular disease of the uteroplacental unit secondary to maternal hypertension. In the presence of preeclampsia, nearly 33% of placentas will contain infarctions; this increases to 60% in the presence of severe eclampsia (Hibbard 1987).

Infarctions are commonly found at the margin of full-term normal placentas; when restricted to this area, they pose no significant threat to the fetus (Perrin and Sanders 1984). However, when infarctions occur centrally in the placenta, the entire organ may become underperfused. As the infarcted area becomes necrotic, fetal circulation is reduced, because blood flow through the placental villi decreases. However, if the circulation through the rest of the organ is sufficient, a fetus may survive when as much as 20% to 30% of the placenta is infarcted.

Maternal and Fetal/Neonatal Implications. Placental infarcts have no clinical effects on maternal status. Fetal circulation may not be immediately affected by placental infarction. Blood will continue to flow through the ischemic villi for some time, but its capacity for metabolic exchange is limited; affected areas eventually become fibrotic. Small marginal areas of infarction have no effect on fetal status. If infarctions occur centrally and compromise the blood supply to the fetus, growth retardation or even death may result.

Treatment. Placental infarctions cannot be treated *per se*. However, early and comprehensive treatment of underlying maternal disease during pregnancy can decrease the severity and incidence of placental infarcts.

Implications for Nursing Care

The nurse is frequently responsible for examination of the placenta after delivery. When infarctions or other abnormalities are noted, the nurse should bring this to the birth attendant's attention. In most cases such findings have no clinical significance. Rarely, intrauterine growth retardation is diagnosed antenatally, and on delivery the cause may appear to be placental infarction. The nurse should provide appropriate explanations and emotional support for the couple anticipating the birth of a mature but growth-retarded infant. The nurse should also ensure that the parents' need for information is met, through consultation with the pediatrician or neonatologist.

RETAINED PLACENTAL FRAGMENTS

Placental fragments may remain in the uterus and adhere to the uterine wall after the rest of the placenta has separated and been delivered. Often this occurs when overvigorous attempts to hasten placental delivery have occurred and an already contracted uterus has been kneaded. This interferes with the normal physiologic process of placental detachment and may result in fragmentation of the placenta. The diagnosis of retained placental fragments may be made immediately on inspection of the placenta if portions of tissue are missing. However, most often, retained placental fragments are suspected when late postpartum hemorrhage or continued bleeding occurs.

Maternal Implications. Consequences to the mother of retained placental fragments may include steady early (first 24 hours after birth) postpartum bleeding in the presence of a well-contracted uterus, but more

often there is late postpartum hemorrhage (after the first 24 hours). Retained placental fragments may also be suspected if bleeding resumes 1 to 2 weeks after delivery, if the uterus fails to involute normally, or if signs of endometritis develop. (See Chapter 30 for further discussion.) Removal of retained placental fragments is often done during the routine postpartum hospitalization. If diagnosis is delayed, rehospitalization may be necessary. If bleeding is excessive, blood replacement will be required.

Treatment. If retained placental fragments are suspected, the physician will explore the uterine cavity with surgical instruments and remove any placental fragments by curettage. If bleeding has been excessive, blood replacement may be necessary, and if signs of endometritis appear, antibiotic therapy will be initiated.

Implications for Nursing Care

As mentioned before, the nurse is often responsible for examination of the placenta after delivery. If any areas of tissue appear to be missing, the nurse must bring this to the birth attendant's attention. The nurse is also responsible for monitoring the amount and pattern of the patient's postpartum bleeding for signs of retained placental fragments.

Membrane, Amniotic Fluid, and Cord Problems

Complications in the intrapartal period can arise from mechanical or structural problems with amniotic membranes or the umbilical cord or may involve the amniotic fluid itself.

Premature Rupture of the Membranes

Premature rupture of the membranes (PROM) is defined as the rupture of the chorion and amnion 1 hour or more before the onset of labor. With PROM, amniotic fluid leaks from the vagina in the absence of contractions. PROM, especially if prolonged, presents risks for both mother and fetus. There is an increased risk of the intrauterine infection known as *chorioamnionitis,* the fetal protection from trauma provided by the amniotic fluid is lost, and if labor does not begin within 12 to 24 hours, there are the risks associated with obstetric intervention (such as induction of labor or cesarean delivery). The period between rupture of membranes and the onset of labor is called the *latent period*. When this latent period is short (less than 24 hours), the risk of infection is low. However, when the latent period is longer than 24 hours, the risk of infection increases. The signs of chorioamnionitis are shown in the accompanying display. However, some patients do not develop infection, even when the latent period is prolonged; individual risk factors such

NURSING ALERT

Signs and Symptoms of Chorioamnionitis*

- Fetal tachycardia
- Maternal tachycardia and fever
- Malodorous amniotic fluid
- Uterine tenderness

* In order of occurrence and increasing seriousness

as socioeconomic status, nutritional status, and the quality of intrapartal management appear to influence infection rate. In addition, some patients may develop a leak high in the uterine cavity, which may cause slow leakage of fluid throughout gestation but usually does not result in infection.

When PROM occurs at term, risks to mother and fetus are lessened for several reasons. First, most women will begin spontaneous labor within 24 to 48 hours of rupture. In addition, labor can be induced more readily at term, if necessary, and the fetus is mature. PROM occurs in approximately 6% to 10% of term pregnancies. Incidence of PROM rises to 15% among women who experience preterm deliveries, and 30% of neonates born after PROM are low birth weight infants (Danforth 1986).

Etiologic and Predisposing Factors.   The precise cause of PROM is unknown, and specific predisposing factors have not been identified. However, PROM is known to be associated with malpresentations, possible weak areas in the amnion and chorion, subclinical infection, and, possibly, incompetent cervix.

Maternal Implications.   Maternal sepsis subsequent to PROM is usually not serious and can be treated effectively with antibiotic therapy. There is an increased likelihood of more active obstetric intervention, including induction of labor and cesarean delivery.

Fetal/Neonatal Implications.   The significance of PROM to the fetus is that a basic and effective defense mechanism is lost. This is reflected in the fact that the leading cause of fetal death associated with PROM is infection. Approximately 7% of term neonates and 25% of preterm neonates do not survive when chorioamnionitis is present (Creasy 1984). Perinatal mortality from all causes related to PROM is estimated to be 3% to 11%. Fetal outcome depends on the following factors:

- *Size* — infants weighing less than 2500 g do not fare as well as larger infants.

- *Position* — breech positions are associated with more trauma, especially among preterm infants.
- *Presence of infection* — infection increases fetal and neonatal risk.
- *Presence of cord prolapse* — prolapse increases the risk of fetal hypoxia.

Preterm fetuses are at increased risk when PROM occurs because of the dangers of preterm birth and its associated problems, the danger of mechanical trauma (abnormal lie is more common among preterm infants), and the increased probability of cord prolapse and entanglement.

Treatment.   The obstetric management of PROM is based on the assessment of the risks to mother and fetus. *Active management* of PROM involves induction of labor or cesarean delivery if labor does not begin within 24 hours. *Expectant* or *conservative management* involves careful observation without intervention unless signs of amnionitis or fetal distress are seen. When the risk of morbidity associated with PROM is greater than that associated with pregnancy termination, active management is indicated. When risk associated with terminating the pregnancy is considerable, as is the case with prematurity, conservative management is indicated (Creasy and Resnik 1984).

In *management of PROM at 34 weeks of gestation or less,* the risks associated with delivery, such as respiratory distress syndrome (RDS), are considered high. When no signs of fetal infection or distress following PROM are evident, watchful waiting is continued as long as possible. In this case, the use of corticosteroids to speed fetal lung maturation is contraindicated, since they inhibit the normal inflammatory response to infection and increase susceptibility to pathogenic organisms.

At *34 to 36 weeks of gestation,* the risk of RDS is still considerable. However, it is known that fetal lungs mature more rapidly than normal in the presence of stress, such as that imposed by PROM, thereby reducing the risk slightly. In pregnancies at this stage, therefore, induction of labor or delivery may be delayed up to 24 hours to allow for increased lung maturity.

At *36 weeks or more,* there are few complications associated with preterm delivery. Prolongation of the latent period increases the risk of infection, so induction of labor and prompt delivery may be indicated.

In *management of PROM with signs of advanced infection,* such as fever, tachycardia, leukocytosis, purulent vaginal discharge, and sepsis shown by positive blood cultures, delivery of the infant is the first priority, since, regardless of its age, the fetus will have a better chance of survival outside the infected environment of the uterus. In such cases, the mother will be given antibiotics and labor induction will be attempted (the risk of cesarean delivery is increased when the uterus is infected). If induction is unsuccessful, cesarean delivery is necessary.

Prophylactic administration of antibiotics has been tried in order to prevent maternal infection when PROM has occurred. Some findings suggest that there is a decrease in postpartum maternal infection, but perinatal mortality does not appear to be decreased by this practice (Creasy and Resnick 1984).

Implications for Nursing Care

Nursing responsibilities in the care of women experiencing PROM center on minimizing the risk of infection and promoting optimal maternal and fetal status until delivery can be safely achieved. The nurse should instruct pregnant women to contact their care provider if they have persistent leaking or a gush of fluid from the vagina. Patients should be counseled not to douche, have intercourse, take a tub bath, or insert anything into the vagina until the status of the membranes has been evaluated by the care provider, and they should understand the importance of these precautions in minimizing the risk of infection.

The nurse must also take steps to minimize infection while caring for the patient who has suspected or diagnosed PROM. Vaginal examinations should be kept to a minimum. Early and accurate evaluation of membrane status through sterile speculum examination and Nitrazine testing (see Chapter 23) is necessary before appropriate care can be initiated. Admission orders may also include obtaining smear specimens from the vagina and rectum to test for the presence of beta-hemolytic streptococci; presence of this organism increases the risk to the fetus and may be regarded as an indication for prompt delivery.

If evidence of leaking amniotic fluid is found, the nurse must begin close assessment for signs of developing infection. The patient's temperature, pulse, and respiration rate should be assessed on admission and hourly. The color, amount, and odor of fluid from the vagina should be noted. The patient should be checked for signs of uterine tenderness daily and when any other sign of infection is present. Maternal CBC may be ordered every 24 hours to identify early systemic responses to infection. Intermittent or continuous external fetal heart rate monitoring may be initiated, especially if the fetus is premature. When the fetal head is not engaged, the patient may be maintained on bed rest to prevent cord prolapse should additional rupture and loss of fluid occur. If the fetus is judged to be mature, or if risk to mother or fetus is increasing, oxytocin induction of labor may be initiated (see Chapter 26).

If the pregnancy is at term, the nurse should inform the patient that the chances are excellent that spontaneous labor will begin and should encourage the patient and her partner to begin preparing themselves for labor and birth.

If labor does not ensue, or if the fetus is judged to be preterm or at high risk for infection, the nurse should explain the treatment that is likely to be needed and what the couple may experience.

Chorioamnionitis

Chorioamnionitis (sometimes referred to as amnionitis, intrapartal infection, or intra-amniotic infection) involves infection of the chorion, amnion, amniotic fluid, and fetus. During normal pregnancy, the fetus and membranes are protected from infection ascending from the vagina by the mucous plug in the cervix, the intact amniotic membranes, and the normal antibacterial activity of the amniotic fluid. Once protection from these mechanisms is lost, as occurs with PROM, the risk of infection increases, only slightly within the first 24 hours, but exponentially thereafter.

Chorioamnionitis becomes clinically evident in 0.5% to 1.0% of pregnancies, although some researchers report incidences as high as 25% of patients with PROM and speculate that the incidence is probably much higher in economically disadvantaged populations (Creasy and Resnick 1984). Although chorioamnionitis occurs most commonly after rupture of fetal membranes, it may also occur when membranes are intact. Routes of infection are shown in Figure 28–3.

Infection begins when the membranes exposed to the dilating cervix become inflamed. The membranes become stretched and subject to decreased blood supply and may become weakened, thus becoming vulnerable to infection. In blood-borne infections, growth of pathogens begins in the intervillous space; organisms then migrate through the chorion into the amniotic sac. Symptoms worsen rapidly.

Women developing chorioamnionitis usually have early symptoms that are nonspecific. More serious symptoms include elevation of the pulse to over 100 bpm and temperature elevations of 102°F (38.9°C) or above. Dehydration and urinary tract or other infections may be associated with the same symptoms, and these disorders must be ruled out before an early diagnosis of amnionitis is possible. Later symptoms of amnionitis include malodorous amniotic fluid and increasing uterine tenderness and irritability.

Etiologic and Predisposing Factors. Chorioamnionitis may be caused by bacteria or fungi from ascending infections, by viruses, or, less frequently, by bacteria, protozoa, and parasitic organisms in blood-borne infections. The organism most commonly isolated as the cause of amnionitis is *Escherichia coli,* a normal inhabitant of the bowel. Beta-hemolytic streptococci may also be found and may predispose the patient to preterm labor. Anaerobic bacteria should be suspected if foul-smelling amniotic fluid is present. When amniotic fluid is meconium-

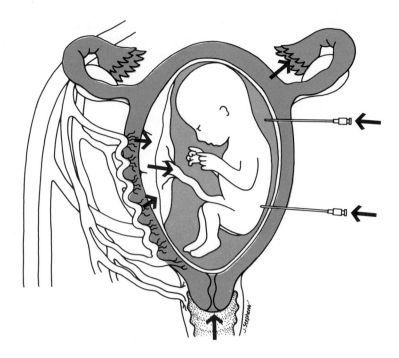

Figure 28–3. Routes of intrauterine infection. Chorioamnionitis can result from contamination as a result of amniocentesis, ascending vaginal microorganisms, or maternal systemic infection through the placenta or the pelvic organs themselves. (Childbirth Graphics)

stained, propagation of pathogenic organisms is greatly enhanced.

Sexual intercourse late in pregnancy has been implicated in the increased incidence and severity of amniotic infections in recent years. Some researchers suggest that sexual activity close to term may cause as much as a fourfold increase in fetal and maternal mortality. Coitus and orgasm late in pregnancy may induce early labor due to maternal oxytocin secretion and the introduction of seminal fluid (containing prostaglandins) into the vagina; infection may then result secondary to membrane rupture. The alkalinity of seminal fluid may also increase the incidence of infection, since a more alkaline environment is more hospitable to microorganisms. (The normal acidity of the vagina provides some protection against infectious organisms.)

Poor maternal nutrition also appears to be an important factor in chorioamnionitis. Malnourished pregnant women are at greater risk for contracting infection because their immune systems are less efficient. Zinc, an element contained in amniotic fluid, confers antibacterial properties; when maternal zinc levels are deficient, defenses against amnionitis are decreased (Perrin and Sanders 1984).

In addition to PROM, sexual intercourse, and poor nutritional status, other factors that predispose the laboring woman to amnionitis include the following:

- Repeated vaginal or rectal examinations
- Internal fetal monitoring
- Presence of vaginitis or cervicitis
- Previous cervical cerclage
- Low socioeconomic status

Diagnosis of chorioamnionitis is often made prenatally solely on the basis of the number and severity of maternal symptoms and the presence of fetal tachycardia (when other causes have been ruled out). Amniocentesis may be used to provide a specimen of amniotic fluid for culture, but this is not always helpful in establishing a diagnosis. Definitive diagnosis is usually retrospective after delivery. Smears of the chorion and amnion, fetal gastric contents, frozen sections of the umbilical cord, and fetal ear canal fluid can all be examined, and cultures can be done to isolate the offending organism or organisms.

Maternal Implications. Chorioamnionitis influences the mode and outcome of delivery. Cesarean deliveries are up to three times as common when infection is present. In addition, there is an increased risk of a range of postpartum complications, including septicemia, pelvic peritonitis, abscess formation, and septic thrombophlebitis. If the infection is unresponsive to antibiotic therapy, hysterectomy may be necessary to remove the source of the infection.

Fetal/Neonatal Implications. The neonate exposed to intrauterine infection is at high risk for sepsis. Infected amniotic fluid in the fetal lungs may result in pneumonia in the neonatal period. Introduction of infected fluid through the eustachian tube into the middle ear may cause otitis media and other septic complications. Early subtle signs of infection in the neonate (discussed further in Chapter 33) include changes in color, muscle tone, feeding, and activity; impaired thermoregulation; apnea; abdominal distention; and jaundice. If diagnosis is delayed, these *ominous* signs may be noted:

- Respiratory grunting, dyspnea, and cyanosis
- Arrhythmias
- Hepatosplenomegaly
- Petechiae
- Seizure activity
- Bulging fontanelles

If treatment is unsuccessful, death may follow.

Treatment.   Some aspects of treatment of amnionitis remain controversial; however, there is agreement that treatment must include delivery of the infant and antibiotic therapy for the mother and possibly the neonate. Unresolved are issues related to the timing of antibiotic therapy and preferred route of delivery. When vaginal delivery is planned, labor and delivery are managed in ways similar to those already described for patients with PROM. Little information is available on complications of cesarean delivery in the presence of uterine infection; operative delivery in this situation is criticized by many as unnecessarily risky for the mother, since preexisting infection increases the likelihood of difficulties in wound healing and other complications following surgery.

There is some disagreement about the appropriate timing of antibiotic therapy as well. Some physicians recommend initiating antibiotic therapy immediately after diagnosis to limit maternal infection and increase protection to the fetus. Others recommend delaying antibiotics until after delivery so that cultures can be obtained from the neonate and therapy can be initiated if needed. However, there is apparent agreement that antibiotics administered during labor will not cross the placenta in sufficient amounts to prevent neonatal infection (Hibbard 1987).

Implications for Nursing Care

Intrapartal nursing care of the patient with chorioamnionitis, in addition to ongoing care for the laboring woman and her family, includes close observation of maternal and fetal status in relation to the stress of infection, administration of antibiotic therapy, as prescribed, and planning for care of a neonate at risk for infection.

Maternal temperature, pulse, and respiration should be monitored every hour when the membranes have ruptured or when greenish, malodorous amniotic fluid or uterine tenderness suggests intrauterine infection. Signs of maternal sepsis (high, spiking fever and increased pulse and respiration rate) must be noted and reported immediately. Intake and output are monitored carefully, and IV fluids are usually initiated, both to ensure adequate hydration and to permit administration of antibiotics. Oxytocin induction or augmentation may be initiated to hasten delivery.

When chorioamnionitis is suspected, the neonate must be regarded as at extremely high risk for infection.

The nurse should make provisions for pediatric support staff to be present at delivery. Upon delivery, cultures of the neonate's ear, nose, and gastric contents are taken; prophylactic antibiotic therapy may be initiated. Signs of sepsis may be present in the neonate at birth or may develop later in the postnatal period. The neonate at risk for sepsis is monitored carefully in the first hours (see Chapter 34). Mother and neonate may require isolation care depending on the nature of the infection and hospital policy.

Imbalance of Amniotic Fluid

Infection is not the only complication involving the intrauterine environment. Problems may arise if too much amniotic fluid accumulates, a condition known as *hydramnios* or *polyhydramnios,* or if too little fluid is present, a condition known as *oligohydramnios.* Amniotic fluid serves several functions. These include

- Protecting the fetus from injury from outside forces
- Maintaining intrauterine temperature
- Allowing free movement
- Minimizing adherence to the amniotic membrane

The volume of amniotic fluid increases as pregnancy progresses, peaking at approximately 980 ml at 34 weeks and then decreasing to approximately 830 ml at term and 550 ml by 41 to 42 weeks. Amniotic fluid is constantly being exchanged, at the rate of 3 to 4 liter/hour at term. The fetus plays an important role in maintaining amniotic fluid volume balance. Close to term, the fetus swallows between 400 and 500 ml amniotic fluid per day (approximately the amount of liquid consumed by the newborn infant) and micturates an equal volume, thus maintaining a steady volume. Interference with either fetal intake or fetal output causes gross alterations in amniotic fluid volume.

Polyhydramnios

Polyhydramnios is the excessive accumulation of amniotic fluid in the amniotic sac; amounts may reach levels of 2000 to 5000 ml or more. This accumulation may be gradual (chronic) or acute, occurring over a period of days to 2 weeks. Polyhydramnios is estimated to occur in 1.5% of all pregnancies (Pritchard and MacDonald 1985). Polyhydramnios has been associated with an increased incidence of fetal abnormalities, many of which can be detected by amniocentesis or by ultrasonography.

Etiologic and Predisposing Factors.   The etiology of polyhydramnios is unclear. While an imbalance between fetal swallowing and micturition may be responsible, evidence is not always conclusive, and in some cases a disruption in water transport in and out of the amniotic cavity may be responsible (Danforth 1986).

Maternal Implications.   Polyhydramnios is usually detected around the seventh month of pregnancy. As increasing amounts of fluid accumulate within the uterus, it becomes more difficult to palpate fetal position and to hear fetal heart tones. Uterine size increases beyond the normal growth curve.

When polyhydramnios is severe (an estimated amniotic fluid volume of more than 5 liters), the mother experiences abdominal discomfort, dyspnea, generalized edema, and difficulty in mobility. The uterine muscle becomes overstretched; this may contribute to later intrapartal uterine dysfunction and increased risk of postpartum hemorrhage due to uterine atony. A small but significant risk of amniotic fluid embolus (see discussion of embolus later in chapter) at the time of birth exists.

When polyhydramnios is detected, evaluation of fetal status to rule out the presence of anomalies will be a high priority. Even if antenatal evidence suggests that the fetus is normal, the intrapartal period is likely to be quite stressful for the mother and her partner until the condition of their infant has been verified.

Fetal/Neonatal Implications.   With the increased risk of fetal anomalies associated with polyhydramnios comes increased risk of fetal or neonatal death secondary to severe anomalies incompatible with life. In the presence of polyhydramnios, approximately 60% of surviving infants will be normal, and the remaining 40% will display some congenital abnormalities. The most commonly associated congenital problems include the following:

- Upper gastrointestinal abnormalities, such as esophageal atresia (absence or closure of the esophagus), duodenal atresia (absence or closure of the duodenum), and esophageal pressure from tumor formation
- Anencephaly (congenital absence of brain and spinal cord)
- Hydrops (erythroblastosis) fetalis
- Hydrocephalus (abnormal accumulation of cerebrospinal fluid within the ventricles of the fetal brain)
- Neural tube defects, including meningocele and spina bifida

Other fetal risks related to polyhydramnios reflect the increased risk of preterm labor and PROM with cord prolapse due to the forceful escape of amniotic fluid. If polyhydramnios is secondary to maternal diabetes, Rh disease, or multiple gestation, these conditions also increase the risk to the fetus or neonate.

Treatment.   Mild or moderate polyhydramnios may not cause significant distress to the mother, and no treatment may be needed. However, because of the increased risk of prolapsed umbilical cord with rupture of membranes, the parturient may be taken to the delivery room and the membranes may be "needled" to allow slow, controlled release of amniotic fluid before spontaneous rupture occurs. The procedure is performed in the delivery room in case sudden rupture of the membranes with resultant prolapse of the umbilical cord does occur.

Implications for Nursing Care.   Intrapartal nursing care for the patient with polyhydramnios focuses on providing comfort measures to relieve maternal distress, emotional support, and information and anticipatory guidance about fetal status and the progress of labor. If antenatal diagnosis of fetal anomalies has been made, the nurse must provide sensitive emotional support of the mother and her partner throughout the labor process. The nurse must also be alert for the increased possibility of cord prolapse with rupture of membranes and maintain close observation of fetal heart tones throughout labor. Ambulation of the woman with polyhydramnios may be contraindicated because of the risk of prolapsed umbilical cord with spontaneous rupture of the membranes.

Oligohydramnios

Oligohydramnios is a rare condition in which the quantity of amniotic fluid is abnormally small. Its precise causes are as yet unknown. Oligohydramnios can occur in postterm pregnancies or when there is a chronic leakage of amniotic fluid. Other conditions associated with or predisposing to oligohydramnios include placental insufficiency and fetal anomalies, especially renal abnormalities.

Renal abnormalities are implicated when oligohydramnios is present, since fetal urination *in utero* plays an important part in amniotic fluid balance; such abnormalities are usually incompatible with life. Renal abnormalities, especially renal agenesis, are likely when amnion nodosum (nodules on the surface of the amnion) is found (Perrin and Sanders 1984). Potter's syndrome, a constellation of fetal abnormalities, including renal agenesis, pulmonary hypoplasia, a flattened facial appearance, deformed and low-set ears with a small mandible, deformed hands, and nuchal webbing, may also be found in the presence of oligohydramnios. This condition occurs in 1 in 4000 births and is more common in males. One third of affected infants are stillborn, and the remainder die within 48 hours of delivery.

Maternal Implications.   In cases of oligohydramnios, the uterine fundus is usually small for gestational age, and the fetal outline may be easily felt through the abdominal wall. Labor may begin before term and is often dysfunctional. Progress may be slow, and the mother may experience severe discomfort, which may in part explain old wives' tales about the difficulty of "dry births."

Fetal/Neonatal Implications. When little amniotic fluid is present, the space in the uterus decreases because its walls are not distended by fluid. The fetus may assume a flexed and cramped attitude. Chronic cord compression may result in intrauterine growth retardation, meconium staining, and fetal hypoxia. At birth, surviving infants appear wizened and have coarse skin; skeletal deformities acquired as a result of the fetus's cramped position may be apparent.

Treatment. Some facilities may attempt an intrauterine amnioinfusion to relieve pressure on the umbilical cord if severe variable decelerations occur (see Nursing Alert, Chapter 25, for discussion of the procedure). Fetal distress may require cesarean delivery in advance of onset of labor.

Implications for Nursing Care. Intrapartal care of the patient with oligohydramnios requires the nurse to provide comfort measures to relieve extreme maternal discomfort during labor, to monitor fetal status closely to identify signs of distress, and to give sensitive emotional support to the mother and her partner if serious fetal anomalies have already been diagnosed.

Umbilical Cord Prolapse

Prolapse of the umbilical cord is a serious intrapartal complication, occurring in approximately 1 out of 200 pregnancies. When a loop of umbilical cord is positioned alongside or in front of the presenting part, it may become compressed between the fetus and the mother's cervix or pelvis. If the fetal presenting part does not completely occlude the pelvic inlet, this loop may be carried down into the vagina by escaping amniotic fluid when membranes rupture. As the presenting part settles down into the pelvis, this prolapsed loop will be compressed and fetoplacental perfusion will be compromised or cut off entirely.

Three types of umbilical cord prolapse have been identified. The classification depends on the position of the cord in relation to the presenting part, as shown in Figure 28–4:

- *Occult prolapse*—the cord lies over the presenting part; membranes are either intact or ruptured, but the cord cannot be palpated on vaginal examination.
- *Forelying prolapse*—the cord precedes the presenting part and is contained within intact membranes; the cord may be palpable through the membranes.
- *Complete prolapse*—membranes are ruptured and the cord drops through the cervix into the vagina; the cord can be palpated on vaginal examination and may be visible at the introitus.

Etiologic and Predisposing Factors. Many obstetrical variables can cause cord prolapse. Common predisposing factors include the following:

- Abnormal fetal position—that is, breech, shoulder, face, brow, or transverse position
- Multiple gestation—prematurity, polyhydramnios, and abnormal fetal position may interfere with descent of the presenting part. Risk of prolapsed cord is 6 times greater in multiple-gestation than in single-gestation pregnancies.
- Premature rupture of membranes prior to engagement of the presenting part
- Fetopelvic disproportion, low-lying placenta, or other conditions that interfere with fetal descent
- Abnormally long umbilical cord

Cord prolapse may also be a result of obstetric intervention, such as amniotomy performed in the presence of a malposition or high presenting part, or obstetric maneuvers, such as manual rotation or flexion of the fetal head, that may disengage the presenting part and allow the cord to slip through.

Maternal Implications. Cord prolapse in the intrapartal period produces an emergency situation in which swift action is needed to save the fetus. Immediate delivery will be attempted, either by cesarean delivery or by forceps application. The mother will be at increased risk for complications related to these emergency interventions, including trauma to the birth canal with rapid forceps extraction, uterine atony resulting from anesthesia, risk of excessive blood loss from operative delivery, and infection (Danforth 1986).

Fetal/Neonatal Implications. Perinatal morbidity and mortality are increased when cord prolapse occurs. The single most critical factor in fetal survival is the interval between the actual prolapse and delivery. When delivery is accomplished within 15 to 30 minutes, fetal survival is approximately 70% to 75%; however, if delivery is delayed more than 1 hour, fetal loss may exceed 50%. Infants who survive may develop later complications related to prematurity, birth trauma, meconium aspiration, and hypoxia; the prognosis is especially guarded for premature infants when meconium staining is noted or when the cord pulse is weak.

Treatment. When prolapsed cord is diagnosed, rapid action is needed to preserve fetal well-being. The goal of obstetric management is to deliver the infant as soon as possible. Vaginal delivery with forceps application may be considered if the cervix is fully dilated, the presenting part is engaged and no malpresentation exists, and pelvic size is normal. If these criteria are not met, however, cesarean delivery is indicated to avoid the further risks of traumatic vaginal delivery.

While preparations for delivery are being made, pressure on the prolapsed cord must be relieved. The fetal presenting part is elevated from the cord with direct man-

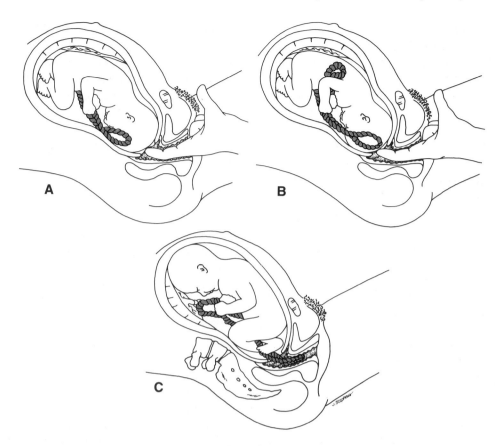

Figure 28-4. Umbilical cord prolapse. *(A)* Occult prolapse and compression of cord by fetal head. *(B)* Forelying cord palpable in cervical os. *(C)* Complete cord prolapse with breech presentation. (Childbirth Graphics)

ual pressure. The patient may be placed in the Trendelenburg, knee-chest, or Sims position to prevent further prolapse and to relieve pressure on the presenting part. However, if fetal demise has occurred (as often happens when prolapse occurs outside the hospital setting and is undetected for some time), emergency surgical intervention is unnecessary and labor should be allowed to proceed (Danforth 1986).

Implications for Nursing Care

The nurse must identify patients who may be at increased risk for cord prolapse and monitor fetal status carefully. When membranes rupture, the nurse should immediately auscultate fetal heart tones for one full minute following the rupture and also during the next uterine contraction to identify signs of acute fetal distress associated with cord compression. In addition, vaginal examination should be done to determine whether the presenting part is engaged and the cord has prolapsed.

If the nurse identifies possible or actual cord prolapse, she must initiate the following emergency measures (review Nursing Alert — Prolapsed Umbilical Cord, Chapter 23). Firm manual pressure should be applied to the presenting part to elevate it and relieve pressure from the cord. The nurse must take care not to further compress the cord itself. However, cord pulsations should be assessed constantly, since they provide direct evidence of

patency and fetal status. Under no circumstances should the hand be removed or the upward pressure released until delivery can be accomplished. No attempts are made to replace the cord into the uterus. Staff must be mobilized for the immediate birth of the infant, in most cases by cesarean delivery. Oxygen and IV fluids will be administered to the mother to increase placental perfusion and reduce hypoxia.

The nurse is also responsible for providing emotional support and reassurance to the mother and her partner. This situation is extremely frightening for both parents, and every effort should be made to provide information and assistance before, during, and after the delivery.

Congenital Absence of the Umbilical Artery

Although umbilical cord prolapse is the most worrisome complication involving the cord, increased intrapartal risk to the fetus/neonate can result from structural abnormalities of the cord and unusual cord length. Normally, the umbilical cord contains two umbilical arteries and one vein. However, single umbilical arteries are observed in 0.2% to 1.0% of pregnancies; the incidence is higher among American Caucasians than among blacks, and more common among infants of diabetic mothers (Perrin and Sanders 1984). The etiology of this condition is unknown. There are no immediate maternal implications.

The condition itself cannot be treated, although the associated problems discussed below may require treatment.

Fetal/Neonatal Implications. The presence of a single umbilical artery may predispose the fetus/neonate to low birth weight. This condition is also associated with a higher incidence of other congenital anomalies. Anomalies may appear in any body system and are evident in as many as 25% to 50% of infants with single umbilical arteries. Other common congenital problems include renal anomalies, tracheoesophageal fistulas, and central nervous system lesions.

Treatment. Treatment of the condition itself is not possible. However, neonates with a single umbilical artery acquire careful screening for other physical anomalies, and attention to possible low birth weight is needed.

Implications for Nursing Care

Nursing responsibilities include accurately identifying congenital absence of the umbilical artery upon inspection of the umbilical cord at delivery, explaining the problem to the parents in collaboration with the physician, and providing them with information and support as further screening for congenital anomalies is undertaken. An interesting finding of recent research indicates that the absence of the normal helix or twist in the umbilical cord may be associated with the presence of only one umbilical artery (Lacro, Jones, and Benirschke 1987).

Marginal Insertion (Battledore Placenta)

Insertion of the umbilical cord at the margin of the placenta rather than centrally may be observed upon inspection of the placenta immediately after delivery. This condition is believed to have no clinical significance.

Velamentous Insertion and Vasa Previa

As mentioned before, the normal umbilical cord contains three blood vessels — two umbilical arteries and one umbilical vein. The cord normally is inserted into the central area of the fetal surface of the placenta. *Velamentous insertion* is characterized by separation of the vessels, which travel over the placental surface for some distance, protected only by the amnion, before entering the placental surface as shown in Figure 28–5. The unprotected vessels may rupture at any time but are particularly vulnerable during labor and delivery, when tears in the amnion may cause fetal exsanguination. Velamentous insertion is more common with multiple gestation and is associated with increased incidence of fetal anomalies. An associated condition called *vasa previa* occurs when the umbilical vessels traverse the cervical os in front of the fetus; fortunately, this condition is quite rare, occurring in fewer than 0.2% of all pregnancies.

Velamentous insertion is usually asymptomatic and may not be diagnosed until the placenta is examined after delivery. However, blood-stained amniotic fluid or small amounts of vaginal bleeding may suggest that fetal hemorrhage has occurred. Vasa previa may be diagnosed by vaginal examination; upon assessment of the cervical os, the examiner may feel a vessel pulsating synchronously with the fetal heart rate in the membranes in front of the presenting part.

When amniotomy is accompanied by an excessive show of blood, the physician or nurse midwife may collect a small amount to be assessed for the presence of fetal cells using the Apt test. The purpose of this test is to differentiate between maternal and fetal blood. Blood is collected in a test tube to which water and potassium hydroxide are added; maternal hemoglobin will denature and turn brown, but fetal hemoglobin will remain pink. Blood identified as fetal in origin is evidence of fetal hemorrhage, and emergency cesarean delivery is necessary.

Etiologic and Predisposing Factors. The precise etiology of these placental abnormalities is unknown, but they are believed to be determined by the angle at which the zygote comes in contact with the myometrium at the time of implantation.

Fetal/Neonatal Implications. As long as the unprotected vessels do not cross the site of amniotic sac rupture, velamentous insertion presents no hazards for the fetus, and most deliveries are without incident. When the condition is discovered, the neonate should be screened carefully for the presence of congenital anomalies. Vasa previa places the fetus at considerable risk; if tears in fetal vessels occur, risk of fetal demise due to exanguination is 60% to 70%.

Treatment. Velamentous insertion requires no treatment unless evidence of fetal hemorrhage exists; emergency cesarean delivery is then indicated. Vasa previa presents an increased risk of fetal hemorrhage as labor progresses; the mother is kept on bed rest, and extremely close external monitoring of fetal heart tones is required. Cesarean delivery may be indicated if the physician believes the risk of hemorrhage is great; any evidence of fetal bleeding or change in fetal heart rate requires emergency cesarean delivery.

Implications for Nursing Care

The nurse must recognize intrapartal signs of placental abnormality, such as pulsating vessels at the cervical os and bloodstained amniotic fluid, and alert the physician at once. Close monitoring of fetal heart tones is essential; any changes in fetal heart rate or incidents of vaginal bleeding must be immediately evaluated to rule out fetal hemorrhage. Stimulation or augmentation of labor is contraindicated for these patients.

The mother will be maintained on bed rest and will

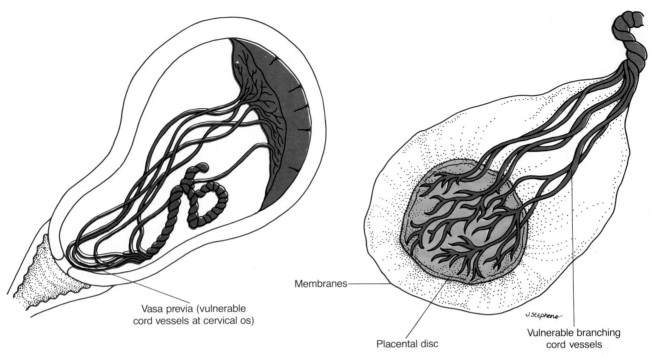

Figure 28–5. Vasa previa and velamentous cord insertion. (Childbirth Graphics)

require an IV line to facilitate emergency obstetric management, should it be needed. In collaboration with the physician, the nurse should explain the situation to the patient and her partner and prepare them for the possibility of a cesarean delivery. Preparations for an emergency delivery — staff, including neonatal intensive care unit staff, supplies, and equipment — should be made in case one is needed.

Abnormal Umbilical Cord Length

The average length of the umbilical cord at term is 54 to 61 cm. In general, larger infants are observed to have longer cords. However, there is considerable variation in individual cord lengths at term and at different points in gestation. An abnormally short cord is defined as one under 32 cm at term, approximately the minimum length necessary to permit a normal vertex delivery. Short cords, using this standard, may be observed in 1% of all deliveries. A cord in excess of 100 cm is considered abnormally long; such cords are found in 0.5% of all births. Causes and predisposing factors for variations in cord length are unknown. Abnormal umbilical cord length has no implications for maternal status intrapartally.

Fetal/Neonatal Implications. Although many neonates with short umbilical cords are delivered without ill effect, asphyxia at delivery is sometimes attributed to excessive traction on a short cord as the fetus descends. Although this happens rarely, a short umbilical cord may also be at risk for rupture during second-stage labor,

presenting the danger of fetal bleeding and hypoxia. An abnormally long cord is susceptible to knotting or entanglement *in utero,* especially around the fetal neck, and to prolapse after membrane rupture, and long cords may limit the efficiency of fetal–placental perfusion.

When chronic mechanical stress (through knots or compression) impedes fetal–placental circulation *in utero,* the fetus may be chronically denied adequate perfusion of oxygen, metabolites, and nutrients; this may result in intrauterine growth retardation (IUGR), a condition placing the neonate at risk for a variety of problems. Acute mechanical stress, such as compression from cord prolapse, a tight nuchal cord, or rupture, presents the danger of rapidly developing fetal hypoxia and death if not discovered promptly.

Implications for Nursing Care

Nursing responsibilities in the intrapartal period center on identifying changes in fetal heart rate that may be associated with cord compression (see Chapter 25) and assisting the birth attendant, as necessary, in the event of a short or nuchal cord at time of delivery. In the event of cord problems, the nurse must be prepared to initiate procedures to support the neonate who has experienced acute or chronic hypoxia (see Chapter 33).

Fetal Problems

A variety of fetal problems may have particular significance in the intrapartal period, increasing either maternal or fetal risk. A major concern is *fetal distress,* already discussed in Chapter 25. Other problems include fetal anomalies that influence the course of labor and birth itself, multiple gestation, which poses additional risks to fetal well-being in the intrapartal period, and intrauterine fetal demise, which affects not only the physiologic but also the psychological process of labor and birth.

Multiple Gestation

Antenatal care of mothers with twin gestations is discussed fully in Chapter 19. This section focuses on the intrapartal assessment and management of labor and delivery in multiple gestation.

During the early intrapartal period, the physician and the family should discuss and decide on the appropriate method of delivery, either vaginal or cesarean. Many problems in delivery with multiple gestation can be prevented when care is planned early, and fetal outcomes may be substantially improved. Occasionally, birth attendants may be surprised by "undiagnosed twins" in the intrapartal period; such events are rare and should be avoided by careful antenatal assessment. However, preterm labor sometimes denies care providers the opportunity for accurate diagnosis of the second fetus.

In order to make early decisions about the appropriate mode of delivery in a twin pregnancy, gestational age and fetal positions must be confirmed. Gestational age must be verified in order to prevent preterm delivery, if possible. Dating from the last menstrual period may be difficult and should be corroborated by other evidence. However, prenatal uterine growth in twin pregnancies is not helpful in establishing gestational age because of the rapid enlargement of the uterus.

Early baseline ultrasound determinations at 12 to 18 weeks provide the most accurate information on gestational age, but these may not have been performed if multiple gestation was not suspected early in pregnancy. Unfortunately, ultrasound determinations of gestational age are less accurate late in pregnancy, and a wider range of possible ages is generated. This is a problem if there is no earlier ultrasound report with which to compare late pregnancy findings. However, ultrasonography will identify the placental site—important information, since placenta previa is more common in multiple gestation—and will give useful information about fetal presentations.

A fetogram, or x-ray film of the uterine contents, may also be used to assess twin gestation and presentation. This may be done to corroborate late pregnancy ultrasound findings and to avoid errors that can result from the variability of fetal positions and crowding. Twins may assume a variety of positions approaching term, including vertex-vertex, vertex-breech, breech-breech, and transverse (Fig. 28–6). These positions are more accu-

rately detected by fetogram. Further, fetograms may detect anomalies not visualized on ultrasound.

Factors Affecting Mode of Delivery. Several circumstances dictate the need for a cesarean delivery to ensure optimal fetal outcomes. First, cesarean delivery may be chosen when fetuses are under 34 weeks of gestation and delivery is imminent or indicated because of maternal condition. Cesarean delivery may be chosen to avoid fetal hypoxia and trauma associated with a preterm vaginal birth, especially if the fetuses are not in vertex presentation. Monoamniotic twins (those sharing a single amniotic sac) have a perinatal mortality rate of over 50% primarily because of cord accidents such as prolapse and entanglement; cesarean delivery may be selected to avoid these problems. Finally, cesarean delivery may be indicated in a term pregnancy when the first twin is in a transverse lie or breech presentation. Cesarean delivery can avoid the possibility of hyperextension of the first fetal head, interlocking twins, cord prolapse, or trauma resulting from vaginal delivery.

If a cesarean delivery is planned, the physician will make decisions regarding the type of anesthesia and abdominal and uterine wall incisions prior to surgery. The abdominal incision may be vertical to allow ample room for manipulation of abnormal presentations. The uterine incision may be low transverse unless fetal positions are difficult to verify, in which case a vertical incision may be used.

If a vaginal delivery is planned, certain precautions are needed. The delivery room must be prepared for immediate cesarean delivery—with any additional staff needed on hand—until the twins are successfully delivered. Anesthesia and analgesia must be carefully administered to avoid depression of the infants. Maternal discomfort may be managed by regional and local anesthesia. Continuous electronic fetal monitoring (EFM) is essential and must be maintained until delivery of the second twin. If the second twin is in a transverse position and does not change position in response to external uterine pressure, cesarean delivery is then indicated. Internal podalic version is never justified (see Chapter 26), because of extreme risk to mother and fetus. Attempts to deliver twins in the presence of dystocia may result in severe trauma and the death of one or both twins.

Maternal Implications. Although the mother carrying a twin pregnancy usually experiences a higher risk of morbidity than one with a singleton pregnancy, mortality is only slightly higher. There is an increased risk of abnormal fetal presentations resulting in cesarean delivery. Premature labor, PROM, and an extended period of labor are common. Polyhydramnios and placenta previa are observed more often in twin pregnancies. Risk for postpartum hemorrhage is increased fivefold because of

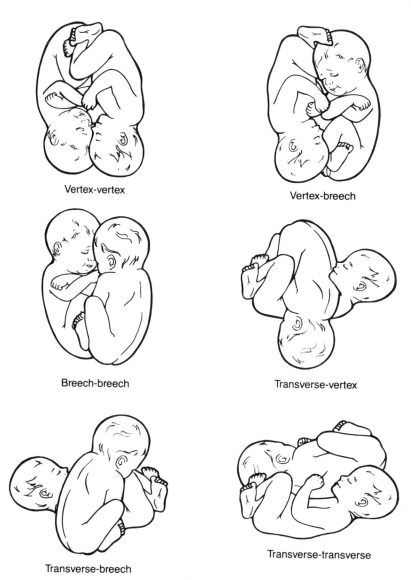

Vertex-vertex

Vertex-breech

Breech-breech

Transverse-vertex

Transverse-breech

Transverse-transverse

Figure 28–6. Twin presentations.

distention of the uterine muscle and subsequent atony. Febrile complications are also five times greater among mothers of twins when compared with mothers with singleton deliveries (Arias and Holcomb 1984).

Fetal/Neonatal Implications. Fetal complications in the intrapartal period are numerous and are responsible for the majority of perinatal deaths in multiple gestation. Complications associated with preterm delivery, especially when the fetuses weigh less than 2000 g, account for most of these losses. PROM with preterm labor resulting in delivery is a significant problem with multiple gestation: this occurs in 25% of twin pregnancies, 50% of triplet pregnancies, and 75% of quadruplet pregnancies (Benson 1987).

The complexities of descent and delivery when more than one fetus is present also account for increased fetal risk. Fetuses may be in abnormal positions that disrupt circulation of one fetus, requiring immediate cesarean delivery. Cord prolapse is more common than with singleton pregnancies. Further, separation of the placenta sometimes occurs before delivery of the second twin, which may cause its death.

Implications for Nursing Care

As mentioned before, twin gestations are usually diagnosed well before the mother is admitted to labor and delivery. However, patients experiencing preterm labor may have undiagnosed twins. The nurse should evaluate the fundal height on her initial assessment; if it is large for gestational age, and if many small parts are palpable, making it difficult to determine fetal position, the nurse should auscultate for two separate heart tones. If two heart tones are found, the physician should be notified immediately. The nurse should establish external fetal heart tone monitoring for each fetus; if possible, the presenting twin may be directly monitored.

The nurse is usually responsible for alerting the delivery team, including neonatal support staff, to prepare for small and possibly compromised infants. A neonatal team and a separate set of equipment and supplies should be available for each baby. Preparations are made for an emergency cesarean delivery, if needed, including having blood typed and crossmatched and a surgical team on hand.

Immediately after the first twin is delivered, the umbilical cord is clamped. A vaginal examination is done to rule out cord prolapse and determine the position of the second twin. If the second amniotic sac is still intact, it is gently pierced with a fine spinal needle to allow for slow descent of the second twin into the pelvis and to prevent cord prolapse. The nurse must monitor the second twin's heart rate continuously throughout this procedure.

Unless some other threatening condition exists, there is no need for prompt delivery of the second twin. Labor may progress as long as both fetus and mother are stable. A dilute solution of Pitocin may be started to stimulate effective contractions if uterine inertia occurs. When the second twin in delivered, the cord is clamped in such a way as to differentiate the umbilical cords for subsequent examination. The nurse is responsible for ensuring accurate identification of the infants, especially if they are born in rapid sequence. A second nurse is needed to receive the second twin while the first nurse cares for the first twin and the mother.

Immediate postpartum care includes careful monitoring of maternal bleeding because of the increased risk of postpartum hemorrhage due to the overdistended uterus and large placental site. Pitocin administration may be needed to decrease maternal blood loss.

The mother and father may be exhausted and overwhelmed by the interaction with two babies. The nurse should provide support and comfort measures, deferring extended contact with the babies until the parents are more comfortable. Parents may also need additional social support, and plans for public health or social work referral or contact with community support groups can be made at this time.

Three or More Fetuses

Problems associated with multiple gestation increase with three or more fetuses. Although they are rare, the widespread use of ovulation-inducing drugs in the management of infertility has increased the number of multiple births. The incidence of multiple gestation among women given gonadotropins is estimated to be 20%. Of this group, 75% are twin gestations and 25% are triplet or higher-number gestations. Among women treated with clomiphene, the incidence of multiple gestation is approximately 10% (Arias and Holcomb 1984).

Cesarean delivery is preferred for these infants because of the increased risks of cord prolapse, hemorrhage from the separating placenta during delivery, malpresentations, and higher mortality risk to the last-delivered fetus. In cases of three or more fetuses, delivery often occurs early, because of either preterm labor or diagnosed fetal distress.

Post-Term Gestation and the Postmature Fetus

Post-term pregnancy is defined as a gestational period greater than 42 weeks. Approximately 6%–12% of births occur after 42 weeks gestation but fewer than 1% after 44 weeks. Placental aging, which occurs after 38 weeks gestation, results in placental infarcts and the deposition of fibrin materials on the surface of the chorionic villi. These changes result in reduced provision of nutrients to the fetus and impaired gas exchange. The fetus is at risk for hypoxia, acidosis, and starvation, with depletion of glycogen stores and fat deposits.

Etiologic and Predisposing Factors.   The causes of post-term pregnancy are not clearly understood. A combination of the presence of inhibitory factors, such as progesterone, and absence of stimulatory factors, such as the release of oxytocin and prostaglandins, may operate to prolong the pregnancy. Maternal conditions associated with post-term gestation are presented in the accompanying box.

When the pregnancy extends beyond 40 weeks, the health care provider must attempt to confirm the gestational age by reviewing the prenatal history (*i.e.*, LMP, pregnancy confirmation date, uterine sizing, recognition of first fetal movement, and ultrasonographic dating). The woman should be examined for signs of post-term pregnancy, which include:

Maternal And Fetal Factors Associated With Post-Term Pregnancy

- Multiparity
- Previous history of post-term pregnancy
- Maternal age (<25 years and >35 years)
- Congenital anomalies (anencephaly, hydrocephaly and osteogenesis imperfecta)
- Occiput posterior position*
- Short umbilical cord*

* Prevents stimulation of cervix and lower uterine segment by presenting part

- Maternal weight loss greater than 3 pounds per week in late pregnancy
- Decrease in volume of amniotic fluid and placental aging, determined by ultrasound
- Evidence of advanced calcification of the fetal skeleton, determined by palpation of an excessively hard, bony head

Maternal Implications. The primary maternal complications are psychological in nature. The gravida frequently becomes frustrated and impatient when the pregnancy continues beyond the expected date of confinement, particularly when friends and relatives question her about when she is going to deliver. Feelings of inadequacy and failure may emerge. Fatigue and physical discomforts of late pregnancy are pronounced and may contribute to depression. Anxiety is aroused by concerns for the fetus, particularly when the health care team begins testing to determine fetal well-being. A second implication of prolonged pregnancy is the increased risk of cesarean section, since many practitioners attempt induction of labor after 42 weeks even in the presence of an unfavorable cervix.

Fetal/Neonatal Implications. The reduction of nutrients and oxygen *in utero* place the fetus at risk for hypoxia and asphyxia. The stress of labor can result in acute fetal distress. Other fetal risks include an increased incidence of umbilical cord compression and hypoxia secondary to oligohydramnios, and failure of fetal descent due to advanced calcification of the fetal skull and lack of cephalic molding.

As a result of intestinal and anal sphincter maturation, the post-term fetus may pass meconium *in utero* in response to hypoxia. With severe asphyxia, the fetus gasps, drawing meconium into the airways and alveoli. At birth the neonate suffers from meconium aspiration syndrome (discussed in Chapter 34). While intubation and aspiration of meconium at birth has reduced perinatal morbidity and mortality, a small percentage of infants still succumb to this pulmonary insult. Permanent neurologic damage as a result of intrauterine asphyxia is another complication of post-term gestation.

Treatment. Once post-term gestation is strongly suspected or confirmed, a series of tests is performed to assess fetal well-being, including biophysical profile, nonstress testing, amniocentesis or amnioscopy to detect the presence of meconium, and recording fetal movement (kick counts). Many practitioners will schedule the woman for induction of labor after the 42nd week, even when signs of fetal well-being are present, particularly if the Bishop score indicates that the cervix is conducive to induction. Expectant management is acceptable with frequent ongoing assessment of fetal well-being, including weekly contraction stress testing.

Clinical trials are now being conducted in the United States to evaluate the safety and effectiveness of prostaglandin E_2 gel for effacement or ripening of the cervix prior to induction of labor. Presently, the cesarean birth rate is high if the induction is attempted when the Bishop score is less than 3. However, recent research suggests that with severe oligohydramnios, the patient should be delivered as soon as possible, regardless of other parameters of well-being, because of the risk of sudden fetal death due to cord compression accidents (Vintzileos et al. 1987).

Implications for Nursing Care

Whether the woman presents for induction of labor or is experiencing spontaneous contractions, nursing care of the parturient with a post-term pregnancy focuses on optimizing uteroplacental perfusion and oxygenation of the fetus. Continuous electronic EFM is indicated, and the patient is maintained in the left lateral recumbent position to improve placental perfusion.

Oxygen is administered at 8 to 10 liter/min by mask if a nonreassuring fetal heart rate pattern is identified. Amniotomy may be performed when possible to attach a fetal scalp electrode and to examine the amniotic fluid for the presence of meconium. The amniotic fluid is evaluated periodically for signs of meconium staining. Fetal scalp sampling may be performed, and the nurse assists the birth attendant and prepares and supports the woman through the procedure.

The nursery should be notified of the impending birth of a postmature infant. Pediatric staff or a health care professional skilled in intubation and aspiration of meconium should be present at the birth to care for the infant (see Chapter 33 for discussion). The nurse should be prepared for sudden fetal decompensation and the need for an emergency cesarean birth, particularly when thick, particulate meconium is evident and administration of oxygen does not improve nonreassuring or ominous fetal heart rate patterns.

Fetal Anomalies Affecting Labor and Birth

Unexpected fetal anomalies may cause difficult labor and delivery, trauma to the fetus, or even fetal—and, rarely, maternal—death. Most often these anomalies are associated with unusual body size or shape; fetal conditions that may cause dystocia include macrosomia, hydrocephalus, fetal tumors, and conjoined twins.

Macrosomia

Macrosomia is defined as a fetal birth weight greater than 4000 g. This condition occurs in approximately 5% of all births. Macrosomia is often associated with poorly controlled maternal diabetes. However, other factors can be responsible, such as genetic predisposition for large babies, maternal obesity, or other metabolic diseases.

Maternal Implications. When the maternal pelvis is sufficiently large, birth of a large infant presents no problem. However, when the maternal pelvis is of only average size, an oversized fetal head cannot accommodate to the pelvis. Cephalopelvic disproportion may cause distention of the myometrium, resulting in uterine inertia and requiring cesarean delivery. This condition also places the mother at increased risk for perineal trauma, uterine rupture, and postpartum hemorrhage.

Fetal/Neonatal Implications. Serious risk to the fetus may result if the maternal pelvis is assumed to be adequate, fetal size is underestimated, and oxytocin augmentation is initiated to stimulate labor. Uterine contractions become regular and strong, forcing the fetal head against the unyielding bony pelvis. Cerebral trauma, neurological damage, hypoxia, and asphyxia may result, with tragic long-term consequences even if cesarean delivery is ultimately performed.

Hydrocephalus

Hydrocephalus is a condition in which an excessive amount of cerebrospinal fluid accumulates within the fetal cranium, causing an abnormally large, softened fetal skull. The enlarged fetal head causes marked cephalopelvic disproportion (Fig. 28–7). Its cause is unknown; it may be genetically linked. Women who have had a previous hydrocephalic infant have a 2% to 5% risk of recurrence.

Hydrocephalus may be suspected when there has been rapid uterine growth in the last trimester, accompanied by hydramnios and/or failure of the fetal head to engage. Ultrasound assessment of the fetal cranium can allow for definitive diagnosis by measurement of the intraventricular width after the second trimester. When hydrocephalus is present, the fetal head may be palpable as a large symmetrical mass over the pubis or in the fundus. Hydramnios may be identified by the tenseness of the uterine wall, which makes palpation of the rest of the fetal outline difficult or impossible. Pelvic examination when the cervix is dilated may reveal abnormally widely separated fetal skull sutures; however, the softness of the skull may sometimes lead to an incorrect diagnosis of breech presentation.

Maternal Implications. The mother may have had a difficult last trimester, with dyspnea, back and abdominal pain, and nausea and vomiting from the pressure of excessive amniotic fluid. If vaginal delivery is attempted as a result of failure to identify the enlarged fetal head, the mother is at risk for dystocia and uterine rupture.

Fetal/Neonatal Implications. Depending on the severity of the fluid accumulation, the damage to the fetal brain, and the availability of early obstetric intervention, the fetus may survive the intrapartal period. However, when the condition is not diagnosed prior to delivery, the risk of traumatic delivery markedly lowers the chances of fetal survival.

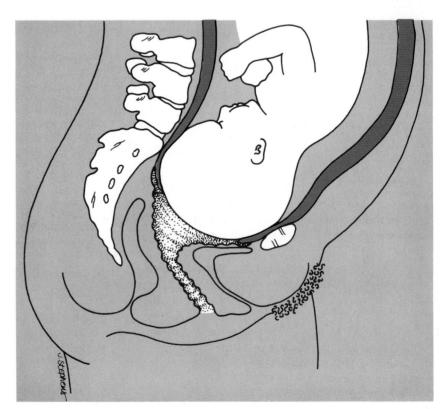

Figure 28–7. Severe dystocia resulting from hydrocephalus. Note the disparity between the fetal head size and diameter of the pelvis between the symphysis and sacrum.

Treatment. Antenatal treatment for hydrocephalus is not widely available, but recent advances in fetal surgery permit surgical treatment in some cases. A ventriculoamniotic shunt has been developed that will allow for release of fluid from the fetal cranium, thus preventing brain damage from excessive pressure; this treatment, however, is still in its experimental stages.

Anencephaly

Anencephaly is a condition in which the fetal cerebrum and cranium fail to develop. The appearance of the fetus, sometimes referred to as an anencephalic "monster," is characteristic: the face is prominent, with protruding eyes, and the cranial vault is absent. This condition is incompatible with life; its cause is unknown. Anencephaly is commonly accompanied by polyhydramnios. The diagnosis can be confirmed by sonography, and, like other neural tube defects, anencephaly may be detected early with amniocentesis.

Maternal Implications. Anencephaly is the most common cause of gross polyhydramnios, a condition requiring amniocentesis. Anencephalic pregnancies tend to be prolonged, especially if polyhydramnios is not present. Further, induction of labor once the diagnosis is made is often difficult, since the uterus may not be responsive to oxytocin induction. Slow aspiration of amniotic fluid in combination with serial induction may be necessary to initiate labor (Pritchard and MacDonald 1985).

Implications for Nursing Care. When labor complications are the result of fetal deformities that may jeopardize the fetus's survival, the nurse's responsibilities center on giving physical and emotional support to the woman and her partner, meeting comfort needs, and providing information sensitively. The nurse must also help the parents to acknowledge their loss so that grieving may begin (see Nursing Care Plan and the section on fetal demise later in this chapter).

Other Fetal Anomalies Affecting Delivery

Unusual tumors may cause enlargement of the fetal abdomen or neck, or strictures of the urethral valve may cause profound distention of the fetal bladder, causing enlargements that interfere with vaginal delivery. In addition, conjoined (Siamese) twins may result in dystocia. These conditions may not be diagnosed until the intrapartal period, when labor fails to progress. In other cases, diagnosis may have been made antenatally.

These conditions are generally not amenable to treatment, and cesarean delivery is often chosen. In some cases, fluid-filled tumors of the fetal abdomen may be reduced by insertion of a needle through the maternal abdomen to drain off fluid and reduce the size of the fetal abdomen. However, this procedure presents an obvious risk of trauma to the fetus. Procedures done even though

the risk of fetal demise is considered high in order to facilitate delivery and preserve maternal well-being are called *destructive* procedures; these are increasingly rare as cesarean deliveries are done more frequently.

COMPLICATIONS INVOLVING FETAL DESCENT: DYSTOCIA

Dystocia literally means difficult labor. Other synonyms include *prolonged* or *abnormal labor* and *uterine inertia*. Many factors contribute to the quality of labor; three factors, however, are of primary importance in determining whether progress toward delivery is made:

- Fetal size and presentation and ability of the fetal head to mold in the pelvis
- Ability of the uterus to contract efficiently
- Pelvic size and internal shape

Problems in any of these areas can cause dystocia, and thus three types of dystocia can be identified: fetal, uterine, and pelvic. These factors may in fact operate in combination, and labor outcome depends on the interaction of fetal, uterine, and pelvic factors in achieving fetal descent. (The student may wish to review Chapter 22 for a full discussion of the process of labor and birth; in this chapter uterine and pelvic factors are discussed specifically in terms of conditions contributing to intrapartal complications.)

Complications Involving Fetal Descent: Dystocia

Fetal Factors

- Unusually large fetus
- Fetal anomaly
- Malpresentations and malpositions

Uterine Factors

- Hypotonic labor
- Hypertonic labor
- Precipitous labor
- Prolonged labor

Pelvic Factors

- Inlet contracture
- Midpelvis contracture
- Outlet contracture

Fetal Factors in Dystocia

Fetal dystocia can result when the fetus has assumed an abnormal position or presentation, is unusually large, or has an anomaly that prevents descent into the bony pelvis. The latter two problems are discussed under Fetal Problems in this chapter. Malpresentations and malpositions, however, are more frequent causes of fetal dystocia. Malpresentations usually reduce the efficiency of labor. For instance, the presenting part cannot adapt to the bony pelvis and exert pressure against the cervix, thus aiding in further dilatation and effacement. The quality and frequency of uterine contractions may decrease, prolonging labor.

Malpresentations also increase the likelihood of PROM, with its attendant maternal and fetal risks. If labor continues when fetal descent is impossible, the integrity of the uterine muscle may be threatened. Pathologic retraction rings may result from excessive retraction of the upper uterine segment with overdistention and thinning of the lower uterine segment. The efficiency of uterine contractions further decreases until the risk of uterine rupture and fetal distress becomes marked as a result of prolonged labor. The following sections discuss malpresentations and their implications for mother and fetus during labor.

Malpresentations and Malpositions

Fetal position (discussed in detail in Chapter 22) refers to the relationship of the fetal skull to the maternal pelvis. Fetal position may contribute to dystocia if the fetus is in a persistent occiput posterior position. More frequently, however, fetal dystocia is related to such malpresentations as breech, brow, face, and shoulder presentation, and shoulder dystocia (see Figs. 22–10, 22–11, and 22–12).

Breech Presentation

Breech presentations are a common cause of dystocia and in many settings are a major cause for cesarean delivery (see Fig. 22–11). Breech presentations are commonly found in the second trimester but are usually spontaneously converted to vertex as the fetus turns to a head-down position before labor begins. Approximately 3% to 4% of singleton deliveries are breech presentations; the incidence is increased in multiple gestation. Breech presentations also appear to correlate with fetal weight, decreasing as fetal weight increases. Breech presentations occur in about 20% of deliveries when fetal weight is 1000 g, decreasing to 12% at 1500 g and less than 5% when fetal weight is 3000 g or more. Breech presentations are classified in the accompanying display.

Breech presentation is usually diagnosed antenatally by abdominal palpation in conjunction with bimanual ex-

---

Classifications of Breech Presentations

- *Frank breech* (65% of breech presentations) — the fetal thighs are flexed at the hips, the legs are extended, and the feet are extended close to the face.
- *Incomplete or footling breech* (25% of breech presentations) — one or both thighs are not flexed, so that one or both feet lie below the buttocks, and a knee or foot is actually the presenting part.
- *Complete breech* (10% of breech presentations) — the fetal thighs are flexed at the hips, and the knees are flexed.

---

amination. The vertex is palpable as a hard, round object in the fundus and is ballotable (*i.e.,* it can be moved independently of the rest of the body). The wider sacrum is palpated in the lower portion of the pelvis, and fetal heart tones are auscultated above the umbilicus. Internal examination when the presenting part is engaged may reveal the soft breech, legs and feet, or the absence of fontanelles. The genitalia of the fetus may be identifiable. When breech presentation is diagnosed, further assessment by radiologic or ultrasound examination may be indicated to confirm fetal position and presentation, localize the placenta, assess fetal head and pelvic size, and identify possible fetal anomalies (Creasy and Resnik 1984).

Dystocia is associated with breech presentation because the larger and less compressible head enters the pelvis and delivers last. For this reason, problems during the second stage are more likely, and in some settings few breech presentations are delivered vaginally. However, there are conditions under which vaginal breech delivery is acceptable (see the display, opposite page).

Maternal Implications. Some increased maternal risk results from breech presentations, even if vaginal delivery is eventually successful. Since the fetal body does not conform well to the lower uterine segment, or to the bony pelvis, the membranes may rupture prematurely, producing increased risk of cord prolapse or infection. Labor may be prolonged and inefficient, since the head cannot assist in cervical or soft tissue dilatation. Forceful delivery of the fetus through a tight pelvis with poor soft tissue dilatation prior to the descent of the head may cause lower uterine segment, cervical, vaginal, or perineal lacerations, especially if forceps application is needed to hasten delivery of the head. Women who require cesarean delivery because of breech presentation are exposed to the additional risks associated with operative intervention.

Vaginal versus Cesarean Delivery in Breech Presentations

All the following criteria should be present for vaginal delivery:

- Frank or complete breech without hyperextension of the fetal head
- Fetal weight estimated at less than 3500 g
- Adequate pelvic size
- Gestational age of 36 to 42 weeks
- Birth attendant experienced in vaginal breech deliveries, and pediatric support available in the event of neonatal problems

Cesarean delivery is preferable under the following circumstances:

- Absence of labor when fetal status requires delivery
- Premature fetus whose condition requires minimal stress in delivery
- Previous history of perinatal death or of a child with residual birth trauma

Fetal/Neonatal Implications. Much of the increased morbidity and mortality associated with breech delivery actually comes from related conditions, such as preterm birth, congenital malformations, PROM, or placental problems (Arias and Holcomb 1984). Factors directly related to breech delivery include prolapse of the umbilical cord, entrapment of the fetal head, and trauma during vaginal delivery, primarily trauma to the after-coming head, which results in central nervous system injuries such as the following:

- Vertebral and medullary injury in infants with hyperextended heads
- Separation of the occipital bone and subdural hemorrhage resulting from pressure on the fetal cranium
- Erb's palsy (facial nerve paralysis)
- Central nervous system damage resulting from hypoxia in delayed delivery

Other types of fetal trauma include muscle damage, bone fracture, and aspiration of amniotic fluid. The last is particularly troublesome, since amniotic fluid is more frequently stained with meconium in breech presentations and so the risk of meconium aspiration may be higher.

Treatment.   When breech presentation is diagnosed early in labor, the decision about the appropriate mode of delivery must be made. When time is needed to assess the fetus, its position, and the adequacy of the maternal pelvis during labor, a tocolytic agent may be administered to slow down or stop labor temporarily. Assessment of the fetus includes ultrasound or radiologic examination to assess fetal weight, whether the fetal head is hyperextended, and the type of presentation. The adequacy of the maternal pelvis may also be determined by x-ray pelvimetry or computed tomography. After these fetal and maternal factors have been considered, the decision for route of delivery is made, as shown in Figure 28–8.

Implications for Nursing Care. Although most breech presentations are diagnosed prenatally, the nurse may sometimes discover an undiagnosed breech presentation in the course of her intrapartal patient assessment. The nurse should notify the birth attendant immediately, since this information may affect the plan of care, especially in settings where vaginal breech deliveries are rare and cesarean delivery is the usual practice. In these cases, the nurse should be prepared to answer the parents' questions and to provide support and reassurance, as needed.

The nurse should be prepared for prompt action if there are difficulties during the delivery of the after-coming head. The fetus should be monitored continuously for evidence of compromise, either from cord prolapse or from cord compression during the second stage. In some cases the nurse must be ready to assist with forceps application and occasionally with emergency measures, such as general anesthesia or cesarean birth, if complications threaten fetal well-being.

Occiput Posterior Position

In the occiput posterior position, the fetal occiput and small posterior fontanelle are located in the posterior segment of the maternal pelvis and the brow and face are in the anterior segment. The occiput posterior position occurs in 15% to 30% of labors; the exact incidence is unknown because most fetuses spontaneously rotate to an occiput anterior position during labor. A right occiput posterior position is five times more common than left occiput posterior.

The position is diagnosed through abdominal assessment and pelvic examination. During abdominal assessment the fetal back is not outlined well, while the fetal small parts are easily felt. FHTs may best be heard in the maternal flank, far from the midline. Occasionally, when the fetus is in occiput posterior position, the contour of the maternal abdomen assumes an hourglass shape that can give the impression of a full bladder. Vaginal examination reveals the position. The fontanelles are at about the same level in the pelvis because of the typical military attitude assumed by the fetus in the occiput posterior presentation.

Etiologic and Predisposing Factors. Factors relating to occiput posterior position include pelvic architecture in which posterior sagittal diameters are larger

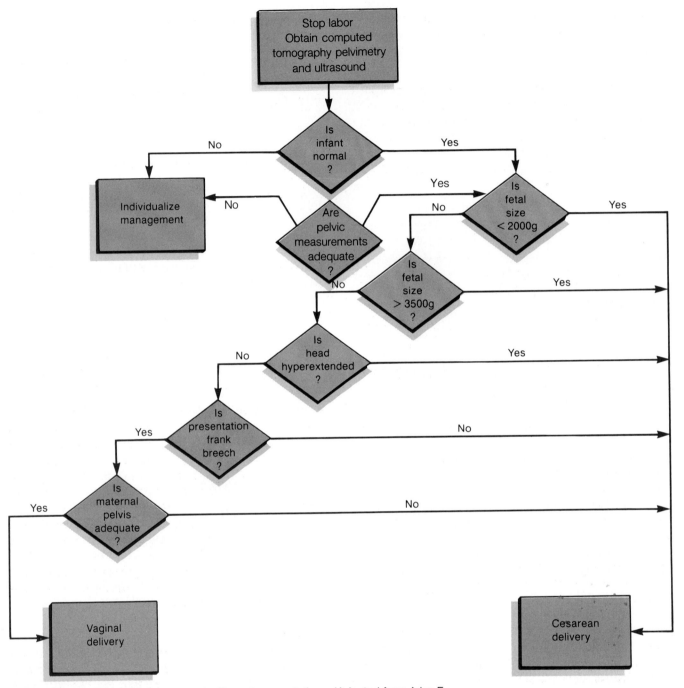

Figure 28–8. Intrapartal management of breech presentations. (Adapted from Arias F, Holcomb W: Abnormal fetal presentations and positions during labor. In Arias F: High-Risk Pregnancy and Delivery, pp 324–325. St Louis, CV Mosby, 1984)

(android and anthropoid pelves) and cephalopelvic disproportion.

Maternal Implications. When the fetus is in occiput posterior position, cervical dilatation and fetal descent are often slow, since the fetal head may not apply even pressure to the cervix. If the malposition is persistent, the fetal head cannot completely flex to present a smaller diameter to the pelvic outlet. Labor may be prolonged significantly.

The parturient may experience excessive backache (back labor) and coupling of uterine contractions. Fatigue, dehydration, and frustration may occur and the patient may become exhausted and anxious. Ketosis may develop with prolonged labor and maternal exhaustion and dehydration and poses a physiologic risk to both mother and fetus.

Fetal/Neonatal Implications. Several complications may occur when the fetus is in a persistent occiput posterior position. If attempts at manual or forceps rotation of the occiput occur, the fetus is at risk for umbilical cord accidents (torsion or compression). The use of forceps may result in ecchymosis or lacerations of the face, facial nerve damage, and, in rare cases, intracranial injury.

Treatment. Many times the fetus in the occiput posterior presentation rotates spontaneously during labor. Having the woman lie on the side of the occiput or in a knee-chest position may facilitate this. Occasionally, spontaneous delivery of the fetus in posterior presentation occurs. The birth attendant may attempt a manual rotation to the occiput anterior position with subsequent forceps delivery. In the case of a low midpelvic arrest with an anthropoid pelvis, an instrument rotation using Kielland's forceps may also be attempted. If manual and or instrument attempts fail, cesarean section is indicated.

Implications for Nursing Care. Once persistent occiput posterior presentation has been diagnosed or is suspected, the nurse may initiate intervention to facilitate rotation and descent of the fetus. She should encourage the woman to use positions for labor that facilitate fetal rotation, including squatting, knee-chest, hands-and-knees, standing and leaning forward, and side-lying on the side opposite the fetal back (which allows gravity to accomplish rotation to anterior position). With the woman in the hands-and-knees position, the nurse may try firm stroking of the maternal abdomen from the same side as the fetal back toward the midline; pelvic rocking movements may assist this technique (review Chapters 21 and 23 on relief of back pain).

Because dehydration and exhaustion can occur with prolonged labor, the nurse should monitor intake and output carefully, encourage adequate fluid and calorie intake, assess the urine for the presence of ketones, and measure its specific gravity. Frequent reassurance of the parturient is essential to prevent frustration and discouragement. The fetal heart rate should be monitored closely for deviations from the norm.

Brow Presentation

Brow presentation occurs when the fetus is in a head-down position with the head straight or slightly extended so that the brow and orbital ridges are the presenting part of the skull, thus presenting the largest skull diameter, the occipitomental, to the pelvic inlet. Frequently, brow presentations convert to face or vertex presentations upon descent into the bony pelvis (Arias and Holcomb 1984).

Etiologic and Predisposing Factors. Brow presentations are thought to be caused by conditions that allow the fetal body to sag forward, resulting in straightening and extension of the neck. Brow presentations are more common in multiparous women or primiparas with small fetuses.

Maternal Implications. If the maternal pelvis is adequate and conversion to a face or vertex presentation occurs, labor may proceed normally. Vaginal delivery with a persistent brow presentation usually results in perineal and vaginal lacerations.

Fetal/Neonatal Implications. Risks to the fetus in brow presentation are similar to those in face presentations: increased danger of trauma to the head, neck, and larynx and of damage to the central nervous system. Trauma may also result from forceps application.

Treatment. Intervention is not needed in cases of brow presentation if the maternal pelvis is adequate and labor is progressing. In the presence of arrested labor or fetal distress, cesarean delivery is indicated.

Implications for Nursing Care. Nursing responsibilities in caring for a patient with a brow presentation include close monitoring of the progress of labor and fetal status throughout labor. The nurse should explain the problem to the parents and assist them in coping with what may be a prolonged and difficult labor. The nurse should also be prepared for the possible need for forceps application and emergency cesarean delivery if fetal status is compromised. If the presentation converts to a face presentation during descent, the nurse should be prepared to explain to the parents the cause and expected duration of any facial swelling and bruising in the neonate and to provide reassurance as needed.

Face Presentation

Face presentation occurs when the fetus is in a head-down position, but with the head hyperextended so that the face is the presenting part (see Fig. 22–10). Face presentation is rare, occurring in 0.2% of deliveries and is more common among multiparous women (Arias and Holcomb 1984).

Etiologic and Predisposing Factors. Face presentations are thought to be the result of brow presentations in which the fetal head has become hyperextended. Thus, any factor that favors extension of the head while preventing its flexion may lead to a face presentation, including:

• Small pelvis
• Large infant

- Congenital goiter or anencephaly (rare)
- Weakness of the maternal abdominal wall, which allows the fetal torso to sag forward, causing straightening of the neck
- Preterm labor

Maternal Implications.   Vaginal delivery may occur in up to 80% of face presentations if the maternal pelvis is adequate and the chin (mentum) is anterior. In mentum posterior positions the chin often becomes arrested against the maternal sacrum. Since no further extension of the fetal head is possible, labor is arrested. Cesarean delivery is often indicated in this instance. However, if labor is progressing well and the fetus is in an anterior position, attempts to manually rotate the fetus to an occiput position should be avoided, and labor should be supported as long as progress continues. Labor may be prolonged, since the face is not as effective in dilating the cervix as is the fetal head. Descent may be more painful, and there is an increased risk of trauma to the genital tract.

Fetal/Neonatal Implications.   When the maternal pelvis is adequate and the fetus is anterior, fetal distress is uncommon. Fetal membranes usually rupture early in labor, and the face becomes swollen, misshapen, and bruised from the pressure against the cervix and throughout descent. The neonate's facial appearance upon delivery may be disturbing to the parents; however, swelling gradually resolves over several days. The molding of the fetal head may be pronounced, with the forehead and occiput protruding. Rarely, prolonged pressure on the infant's hyoid bone during labor may cause edema of the larynx, causing transient respiratory difficulty and requiring close nursing observation throughout the first 24 hours of life.

Treatment.   No treatment for face presentation is needed, unless arrest of progress or fetal distress occurs; in this event, cesarean delivery is indicated.

Implications for Nursing Care.   The nurse should closely monitor the progress of labor and fetal status and be prepared to offer support and provide information to the mother and her partner as they cope with what may be a difficult and prolonged labor. The nurse should also be prepared for the need for emergency delivery and resuscitation efforts if the infant is compromised. However, if vaginal delivery is successful or if a cesarean delivery is needed after considerable time in labor, the nurse should prepare the patients for the infant's facial appearance and, in conjunction with the attending pediatrician, should provide reassurance about the infant's normalcy and the expected resolution of facial swelling and bruising in 3 to 5 days.

Shoulder Presentation (Transverse Lie)

Shoulder presentation is rare, and occurs in 0.3% of singleton births; it is more common among second twins and when fetal weight exceeds 4000 g. Shoulder presentation occurs when the fetus's long axis is perpendicular to the maternal axis in a transverse lie. Inspection of the maternal abdomen shows unusual wideness from side to side, decreased fundal height, and no discernible fetal parts in the fundus (see Fig. 22–9). The head and breech may be palpable on opposite sides of the abdomen. With rupture of membranes, the fetal shoulder dips into the pelvis; an arm may prolapse into the vagina. Attempts to rotate the infant to a more favorable position are generally unsuccessful and may present significant risks of vaginal lacerations and lower uterine segment rupture.

Etiologic and Predisposing Factors.   Factors that predispose to shoulder presentation include the following:

- Multiparity and lax abdominal musculature
- Preterm labor
- Conditions that inhibit normal engagement and descent, such as low-lying placenta, placenta previa, inlet contracture
- Macrosomia

Maternal Implications.   Labor can be dysfunctional, and pathologic retraction rings and even uterine rupture can result if no treatment for shoulder presentation is initiated. When transverse lie is persistent, vaginal delivery is impossible.

Fetal/Neonatal Implications.   There is an increased risk of cord prolapse with a transverse lie as well as the risk of prolapse of the arm into the cervix and vagina. Persistent transverse lie requires cesarean delivery.

Treatment.   When labor is established, treatment for shoulder presentation is cesarean delivery, particularly with a term live fetus. When the fetus is very preterm (<24 weeks) and nonviable (600 g or less), or in the case of IUFD, vaginal delivery may be attempted to avoid the risks associated with cesarean birth.

Shoulder Dystocia

Shoulder dystocia occurs during second-stage labor when the fetal head is born but the shoulders are too broad to rotate and be delivered between the symphysis pubis and the sacrum. This may delay delivery of the body and poses significant risk of fetal asphyxia if the umbilical cord has been brought down and is compressed between the fetal body and the bony pelvis.

Etiologic and Predisposing Factors.   The most common causes of shoulder dystocia are macrosomia and a tight or contracted pelvic outlet.

Maternal and Fetal/Neonatal Implications. If shoulder dystocia occurs, there is increased risk of vaginal or perineal trauma as the birth attendant attempts various maneuvers to facilitate delivery. Risk to the fetus is increased, from asphyxia caused by prolonged cord compression, from overstretching of the neck, and from clavicle fractures sustained during emergency measures to complete delivery. This difficult second stage carries the possibility of cervical nerve damage in the neonate, and the newborn must be observed and assessed carefully for signs of neurologic damage.

Treatment. Shoulder dystocia can be prevented in many cases by careful assessment of fetal size. However, since most estimation errors occur at either end of the range of fetal size — that is, for very small and macrosomic fetuses — other signs that may indicate increased risk for shoulder dystocia must be observed. When a fetus estimated to be large arrests in the midpelvis, vacuum or forceps extractions must be viewed as increasing the potential risk of shoulder dystocia. If shoulder dystocia occurs, the birth attendant may request assistance with manual attempts to extract the fetus. The nurse may be asked to assist in applying suprapubic pressure in an attempt to deliver the shoulder under the symphysis. In extreme cases where delivery cannot be accomplished otherwise, the physician may find it necessary to fracture the infant's clavicles.

Implications for Nursing Care. An important nursing responsibility is the monitoring of labor progress. If fetal descent is slow and difficult, especially when the fetus is estimated to be large, the nurse should be alert for any arrest of progress of the fetal head or shoulders at the symphysis and prepared to assist the birth attendant, as requested. The neonate must be promptly assessed for injuries related to delivery, especially fracture of the clavicle.

Uterine Factors in Dystocia

Uterine dystocia exists when contractions of the uterine muscle are not adequate to dilate the cervix and facilitate the descent of the fetus. Approximately 5% of all labors are complicated by uterine dystocia, most often among primiparas. Uterine dystocia is classified as either *primary,* meaning that uterine contraction patterns appear to be abnormal from their onset, or *secondary,* meaning that a normal labor pattern has become abnormal.

As discussed in Chapter 22, normal uterine contractions begin in a pacemaker site, usually one of the two uterine cornua. From here, electrical impulses sweep down and across the uterus, stimulating a coordinated muscle contraction. As this wave moves away from the pacemaker, the duration and intensity of the contraction decrease so that the contraction is longer and stronger in the fundus than in the less contractile lower uterine segment. Thus, the fundus dominates uterine activity, which permits cervical dilatation and effacement and facilitates the descent of the fetus (Oxorn 1985).

Pathologic Retraction Rings

One sign of dystocia, particularly in prolonged and obstructed labor, is the development of *pathologic retraction rings* in the uterus, also known as *annular uterine strictures.* A pathologic retraction ring is differentiated from a physiologic retraction ring, which is a ridge on the inner surface of the uterus marking the boundary between the contractile upper uterine segment and the passive, distensible lower segment. *Physiologic retraction rings* are normal findings and have little significance for maternal or infant status, except that the lower uterine segment becomes quite thin and vulnerable to trauma.

Pathologic retraction rings, on the other hand, frequently reflect dystocia and are usually associated with the need for cesarean delivery. Pathologic retraction rings are of two types, Bandl's rings and constriction rings (Fig. 28–9 and Table 28–1). The most common type, *Bandl's ring,* begins as a physiologic retraction ring. With prolonged obstructed labor, continuing uterine contractions result in *overretraction* of the upper segment and *overdistention* of the lower segment. With each contraction the ring widens and the lower uterine segment becomes thinner and more distended. Formation of such a ring is considered a sign of impending uterine rupture. The mother may feel pain in the abdomen; the retraction ring is usually palpable only when the abdominal wall is thin. A Bandl's ring may actually impede labor further, since part of the fetus can become trapped above the ring. Cesarean delivery is usually required.

A *constriction ring* occurs when a ring-shaped portion of the uterine musculature becomes tetanic. Constriction rings can occur at any level, but the most common location is 7 to 8 cm above the level of the cervix. This ring prevents fetal descent, and the fetus may become entrapped; thus, a constriction ring is the *cause* rather than the *result* of arrested fetal descent. The ring may be palpable abdominally and causes severe abdominal pain; however, constriction rings do not predispose to uterine rupture. Analgesia and/or anesthesia may relax the constriction; if so, vaginal delivery may be possible as long as fetal status is good and labor progresses well (Oxorn 1985).

Dysfunctional Labor Patterns

Uterine dystocia may be reflected in several different labor patterns, hypotonic labor, hypertonic labor, precipitous labor, and prolonged labor. These patterns are also referred to as dysfunctional labor patterns (Fig. 28–10).

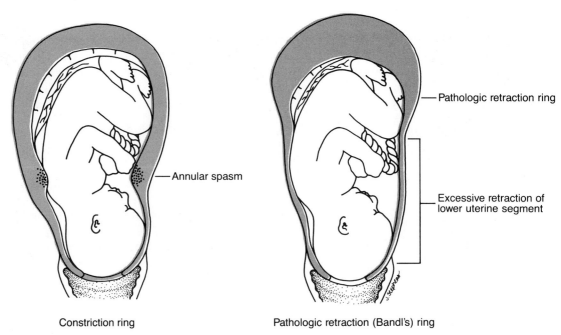

Constriction ring   Pathologic retraction (Bandl's) ring

Figure 28–9. Constriction rings and retraction rings in dystocia. (Childbirth Graphics)

Table 28–1   **Differential Diagnosis of Constriction Ring and Bandl's Ring**

Constriction Ring	Bandl's Ring
Ring is localized area of spastic myometrium.	Ring is formed by excessive retraction of upper segment.
Ring may occur in any part of the uterus.	Ring is always at junction of upper and lower segments.
Muscle at the ring is thicker than above or below it.	Myometrium is much thicker above than below the ring.
Uterus below the ring is neither thin nor distended.	Wall below is thin and overdistended.
Uterus never ruptures.	If uncorrected, uterus may rupture.
Uterus above ring is relaxed and not tender.	Uterus above ring is hard.
Round ligaments are not tense.	Round ligaments are tense and stand out.
Ring may occur in any stage of labor.	Ring usually occurs late in the second stage.
Position of the ring does not change.	The ring gradually rises in the abdomen.
Presenting part is not driven down.	Presenting part is jammed into the pelvis.
Fetus may be wholly or mainly above the ring.	Part of the fetus must be below the ring.
Patient's general condition is good.	Patient's general condition is poor.
Uterine action is inefficient.	Uterine action is efficient or overefficient.
Polarity is abnormal.	Polarity is normal.
Ring results in obstructed labor.	Ring is caused by an obstruction.

From Oxnorn H: Human Labor and Birth, 5th ed. New York, Appleton-Century-Crofts, 1985

Hypotonic Labor

In hypotonic uterine dysfunction, contractions may exhibit a normal pattern in early labor, but then a pattern of infrequent contractions with poor intensity and low resting tone (less than 8 mm Hg on EFM) develops. This pattern is characterized by marked slowing or arrest of cervical dilatation and fetal descent. This pattern may develop in early labor, but is more often seen in the active phase.

Etiologic and Predisposing Factors. Hypotonic labor patterns may result from overstretching of the uterus, administration of sedation in early labor, or varying degrees of cephalopelvic disproportion.

Maternal Implications. Contractions are seldom painful in hypotonic labor. Labor of this kind, however, increases the risk of prolonged labor and PROM, with its attendant problems. There is also the possibility that the

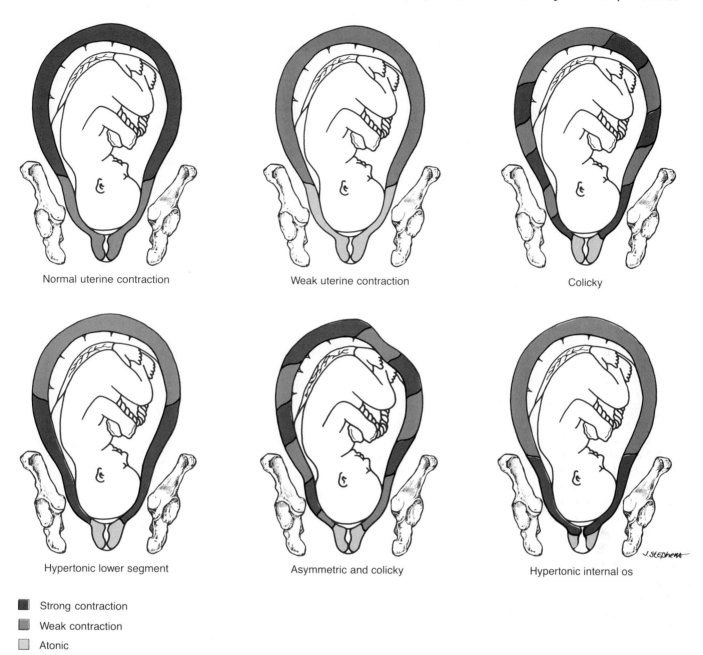

Normal uterine contraction

Weak uterine contraction

Colicky

Hypertonic lower segment

Asymmetric and colicky

Hypertonic internal os

■ Strong contraction

▨ Weak contraction

□ Atonic

Figure 28–10. Normal and dysfunctional uterine contraction. (Childbirth Graphics)

patient will become discouraged or frightened at the lack of noticeable progress and that her mental state will adversely affect her response to labor. She is also at increased risk for uterine atony and associated hemorrhage in the postpartum period.

Fetal/Neonatal Implications. If the fetus is otherwise in good condition, hypotonic labor usually does not cause adverse effects. However, fetal distress can be seen late in hypotonic labor, and subsequent neonatal sepsis may result; the latter is particularly associated with early signs of intrauterine infection.

Treatment. Appropriate treatment first requires that cephalopelvic disproportion, malpresentation, and obstruction due to pelvic or uterine abnormalities be ruled out. When these factors are absent, failure to progress can be assumed to be due to uterine dysfunction. Administration of IV oxytocin to augment labor is usually indicated. Thus, close monitoring of maternal and fetal status and subsequent progress in labor is essential (see Chapter 26).

Implications for Nursing Care. Nursing responsibilities in the care of a patient experiencing hypotonic labor center on close monitoring of labor progress and maternal–fetal status and promotion of effective labor through medical and nursing intervention. The nurse is often the first to identify hypotonic labor by careful analysis of labor progress; she should call this to the attention of the birth attendant with documentation of the contraction pattern and the slowing or arrest of fetal descent in comparison with a normal labor curve (see Chapters 22 and 23). The nurse should also evaluate whether maternal anxiety, sedation, or dehydration might play a role in hypotonic labor and whether comfort measures, ambulation, a change in position, or hydration and rest might facilitate effective uterine contractions. IV fluids may be ordered; the nurse must monitor intake and output and prevent bladder distention. Signs of infection should be watched for, especially if membranes are ruptured; amniotomy may be used as a means of augmenting labor. If oxytocin administration is ordered, the nurse has a major responsibility in monitoring its effects, as discussed in Chapter 26.

Hypertonic Labor

Hypertonic labor occurs when fundal dominance of the contraction pattern is disrupted, often because two or more pacemakers are stimulating contractions. In such cases contractions are usually more frequent but are of only moderate intensity. However, the general resting tone of the uterus is increased, and the uterine muscle does not relax sufficiently between contractions to allow optimal perfusion of the muscle itself. Thus, the woman experiences increased pain with contractions due to the anoxic condition of the uterine muscle. Although contractions are of moderate intensity, frequent, and long, because fundal dominance is lacking, they are not effective in dilating the cervix; thus, little or no progress in labor is seen. Hypertonic labor most often occurs in early labor and, if uncorrected, may develop into prolonged labor.

Maternal Implications. The woman experiencing hypertonic labor quickly becomes exhausted and discouraged, since she is making little progress and must cope with painful contractions far earlier in labor than is typical. In addition, if this condition persists, her physiologic reserves will be depleted, leading to dehydration, acute fatigue, and increasing anxiety.

Fetal/Neonatal Implications. Hypertonicity of the uterus may decrease placental perfusion and place the fetus at risk for uteroplacental insufficiency and subsequent fetal distress. This may develop early and fairly rapidly, since fetal reserves are taxed by prolonged uterine contractions. Excessive pressure on the fetal head also contributes to excessive molding and to caput succedaneum and cephalhematoma formation.

Treatment. Treatment is aimed at stopping this incoordinate labor pattern and promoting more effective uterine contractions. This may be accomplished by encouraging relaxation and sleep through comfort measures and sedation. Often after a period of rest, the patient will awaken to a more normal labor pattern. Rehydration by IV or oral fluids may also be beneficial. If this pattern persists into prolonged labor, the physician may elect amniotomy or oxytocin administration to establish more effective uterine contractions.

Implications for Nursing Care. With uterine hypertonicity, continuous monitoring of maternal and fetal status is especially important. Fetal heart rate patterns should be carefully evaluated for early signs of fetal distress. The nurse must also monitor uterine tone for tetanic contractions or development of a pathologic retraction ring (as discussed above), since both conditions markedly increase the risk of uterine rupture. Because of the physiologic demands on the mother, adequate hydration is important; the nurse must closely monitor intake and output and observe for the presence of ketonuria, a reflection of inadequate energy and fluid balance. The nurse must also face the challenge of finding effective comfort measures and assisting the woman and her partner in coping with this unanticipated and difficult labor experience.

Precipitous Labor

Precipitous labor lasts less than 3 hours before spontaneous delivery. It should be differentiated from *precipitous delivery,* a term applied to an unexpected and often unattended delivery.

Etiologic and Predisposing Factors. The most common cause for precipitous labor is abnormally low resistance of maternal tissue, which allows the fetus to pass easily through the pelvis. In some cases precipitous labor results from a pattern of abnormally strong and frequent uterine contractions, which may achieve an amplitude of 70 mm Hg; in other cases this labor pattern is caused only by an unusually rapid sequence of uterine contractions of moderate intensity. Rarely does precipitous labor result from an absence of pain or unawareness of the progress of labor on the mother's part (Pritchard and MacDonald 1985).

Factors that predispose a woman to precipitous labor include the following:

- Multiparity
- Large bony pelvis
- Soft, pliable genital tissue
- Small fetus in normal vertex position
- Previous precipitous labor
- Cocaine abuse

Maternal Implications. When the cervix is effaced and dilated and the maternal tissues are pliable, serious maternal complications rarely occur as a result of precipitous labor, despite past assertions that such dangers existed. However, maternal risk is substantially increased if precipitous labor occurs when the cervix is long and firm, contractions are vigorous, and maternal tissues are firm and resistant to stretching. These conditions place the mother at high risk for uterine rupture and lacerations of the genital tract; and the risk of amniotic fluid embolism is increased as well. Postpartum maternal risk is increased as well, since vigorous uterine activity may predispose the woman to postpartum uterine atony and hemorrhage (Pritchard and MacDonald 1985).

Fetal/Neonatal Implications. If there is minimal resistance to fetal descent and delivery and if the fetus experiences adequate placental circulation despite the vigorous uterine activity, few fetal complications will result from precipitous labor. However, if the fetus is chronically stressed, its condition may further deteriorate during an abnormally brisk labor, since perfusion is reduced by uterine hypermotility. If there is bony or soft tissue resistance to descent and delivery, trauma to the fetal head may occur. There is also increased risk of neonatal aspiration and hypothermia if the precipitous labor results in an unattended delivery where assistance is not readily available.

Implications for Nursing Care. In the labor and delivery setting, a woman may present who is in advanced labor and exhibiting rapid progress toward delivery. The nurse must be prepared to evaluate the woman's labor status, alert the birth attendant and other staff, as needed, and attend the delivery, if necessary. The nurse immediately assesses the woman's labor pattern, stage of cervical dilatation and effacement, and fetal station and presentation. Fetal heart tones should be auscultated at once and monitored for signs of apparent fetal distress.

Out-of-Hospital Delivery

The nurse may find herself caring for a woman who unexpectedly delivers at home, in a car, or out-of-doors. Major objectives are as follows:

- To support maternal and neonatal physiologic status by:
  Establishing effective respiratory effort in the neonate
  Minimizing maternal blood loss
  Preventing neonatal hypothermia
- To support maternal–newborn interaction by:
  Keeping mother and newborn together
  Promoting early breastfeeding
  Reassuring mother about newborn's status
- To secure appropriate obstetric care as soon as possible without leaving mother and newborn

The nurse's actions are similar to those required in a precipitous birth. However, *cleanliness* and *prevention of*

hypothermia are major concerns. Clean soft cloths can be used to dry the newborn's face, nose, and mouth and to wrap the newborn's head for warmth. The umbilical cord can be tied with *clean* cloth ties and cut with a clean or boiled blade, new razor, or scissors if hospital care is unlikely within an hour or two. If hospital care can be obtained within that time, the cord can be tied off but left intact to avoid the risk of infection from the cutting instrument. The placenta should be wrapped up and kept close to the newborn, avoiding traction on the cord. Clean cloths should be kept under the mother's buttocks, *not* against the perineum.

Hypothermia must be prevented by ensuring a consistent heat source for the newborn and mother. The newborn should be placed skin-to-skin against the mother in a position that allows for breast-feeding. The mother and newborn should be wrapped together in whatever clean materials are available, taking care not to obstruct the newborn's breathing. The newborn should be carefully dried, especially the head, since greatest heat loss will occur from that surface. A hat or head wrap should be fashioned from clean cloth and well secured; the newborn's feet also should be well covered.

Utmost care must be taken to conserve body heat in extreme conditions. Once the pair are well wrapped, covers should be disturbed as little as possible, thus conserving body heat. If the birth occurred out-of-doors, a tent, vehicle, or other shelter may be the warmest place for mother and infant. Building two or three fires around the pair can provide additional warmth. Clean newspapers or plastic bags are good insulators and can be placed under and over the pair, followed by blankets, coats, or sleeping bags. The nurse's own body can provide additional body heat to prevent neonatal hypothermia, if necessary.

The nurse should remain with the mother and newborn until help arrives and, if possible, should accompany the mother to a location where obstetric care can be provided. The nurse must be sure that the infant is clearly identified (either by a note pinned to wrapping or by being with the mother at all times) during the transfer. The nurse should then provide a report to the attending care provider about the circumstances of the birth, to allow appropriate and continuous care for mother and newborn.

Prolonged Labor

Prolonged labor is labor that lasts longer than 24 hours without spontaneous delivery. This problem arises in approximately 1% to 7% of laboring women; however, acceptable obstetric practice requires evaluation of the labor pattern and treatment of causes of prolonged labor prior to 24 hours. In most cases the first stage is prolonged; either the latent or the active phase may be longer than normal. As discussed in more detail in Chapter 22, the latent phase normally lasts no longer than 20 hours in a primigravida and 14 hours in a multipara. The active phase of labor normally lasts from 5.8 hours to 12.0 hours in the primigravida and 2.5 to 6.0 hours in the multigravida; however, the speed of cervical dilatation is the most important factor to consider in the active phase. Dilatation of less than 1.2 cm/hr is considered dysfunctional.

Prolongation of the active phase of labor is further divided into two categories: primary dysfunctional labor and secondary arrest of dilatation. Primary dysfunctional labor occurs when there is steady progress but at a rate slower than normal. Approximately 60% of women experiencing primary dysfunctional labor will go on to deliver vaginally without assistance; the remainder may require forceps application or cesarean delivery, many for subsequent secondary arrest of dilatation. Patients experiencing secondary arrest of dilatation are those who have no cervical dilatation for 2 hours in the presence of adequate uterine contractions.

Etiologic and Predisposing Factors.   One of the major causes of prolonged labor is myometrial dysfunction. During the latent phase this may be caused by an unripe cervix (*i.e.*, one that is long, firm, and closed); uterine contractions must work to overcome the passive resistance of the lower uterine segment and cervix. This process is impeded because the cervix must first be softened and thinned. During the active phase of labor, prolongation tends to be caused by factors that impede cervical dilatation through a lack of pressure by the presenting part, such as fetopelvic disproportion, fetal malposition, PROM, and excessive use of anesthesia or sedation, which decreases uterine motility (Danforth 1986). When these factors have been ruled out, prolonged labor, especially secondary arrest of dilatation, may be caused by myometrial fatigue and excessive maternal discomfort and anxiety.

Maternal Implications.   Prolonged labor places the mother at increased risk for uterine atony and lacerations, resulting in hemorrhage, infection, exhaustion, and severe stress from coping with a difficult labor without noticeable progress toward delivery. The woman and her partner are likely to become increasingly discouraged, especially if additional obstetric intervention, such as forceps application or cesarean delivery, is being considered.

Fetal/Neonatal Implications.   Risk of fetal morbidity and mortality increases as the length of labor increases. This risk comes primarily from the potential for fetal asphyxia as a result of reduced uteroplacental perfusion, infection, and cord prolapse when the presenting part has not engaged. Pressure on the fetal head from the bony pelvis or maternal tissue may cause soft tissue damage and, occasionally, cerebral trauma. Risk of head trauma is also posed by the possibility of forceps application, especially if fetal or maternal condition suddenly requires prompt delivery.

Treatment.   Treatment depends largely on the type of prolonged labor and its cause. Management of prolonged latent phase labor depends on cervical status. If the cervix is ripe, normal labor is likely to ensue with stimulation; nipple stimulation, amniotomy, and oxytocin augmentation may be initiated as discussed in Chapter 26. If the cervix is unripe, the patient may be given comfort measures, fluids, and sedation to promote rest. If dysfunctional labor continues after these measures, amniotomy and oxytocin are then indicated. In the case of secondary arrest of dilatation, again treatment depends on the cause of this dysfunctional labor pattern. If cephalopelvic disproportion is suspected, cesarean delivery is indicated. If it is not suspected, amniotomy may result in progress to a vaginal delivery. If no progress is made in a reasonable time (2 hours), cesarean delivery is then indicated.

Implications for Nursing Care.   The nurse plays an indispensable role in the safe and humane care of women experiencing prolonged labor. Nursing responsibilities include close monitoring of maternal and fetal status for the adverse effects of protracted labor, including signs of fetal distress, infection, and an increasing risk of uterine rupture. The nurse administers and evaluates the effects of medications, such as analgesics, sedatives, and oxytocin. Providing comfort measures and emotional support to the woman and her partner is a major nursing function. Table 28 – 2 describes nursing interventions and rationale for these strategies in caring for women experiencing arrest of labor.

Pelvic Factors in Dystocia

Pelvic dystocia is caused by pelvic contractures or abnormalities in the size or shape of the maternal pelvis. In cases of pelvic dystocia, the fetus is normal but labor and delivery are complicated because of problems in the size and shape of the bony pelvis. As discussed in Chapter 16, there are four types of pelves. The normal configuration, present in 50% of all women, is the gynecoid pelvis. When a normal fetus is present, dystocia in these women is rarely caused by pelvic factors. Other factors, however, such as abnormal fetal presentation or size, may contribute to dystocia. A normal or average pelvis may be too small to permit the descent of a large or malpositioned fetus. Uterine contractions that would otherwise be effective may be inadequate to cause fetal descent if the fetopelvic fit is tight.

The major planes of the bony pelvis are the inlet, the midplane, and the outlet. When the diameter or shape of any of these planes is abnormal, the pelvis is said to be

Table 28–2   **Nursing Interventions for Arrest of Labor**

Causes of Arrest of Descent	Nursing Interventions	Rationale
Cephalopelvic Disproportion		
Maternal Factors		
Inadequate pelvic diameters	Facilitate maternal squatting position.	To increase pelvic diameters
Soft-tissue dystocia	Facilitate maternal upright position; hands and knees or supported squat. Remind patient to relax perineum.	To make use of gravity; relax perineal tissues
Excessive analgesia or anesthesia (especially regional)	Encourage more active bearing-down efforts. Allow medication to wear off. Use maternal upright positions, as tolerated.	To offset decrease in urge to push caused by medication. To make use of gravity
Inadequate pushing	Briefly review physiology of second stage. Use maternal upright position. Hydrate and rest patient. Encourage more active pushing.	To offset possible lack of information. To make use of gravity. To avoid exhaustion and dehydration
Fetal Factors		
Occiput posterior or transverse arrest	Use upright positions; leaning forward, hands, and knees, or side-lying on the side opposite the back of the fetus.	To facilitate rotation to occiput anterior position
Deflexed head, brow, or face presentation	Use upright positions, especially squatting.	To make use of gravity to encourage flexion
Maternal Dehydration and Exhaustion		
	Rehydrate patient with oral or IV fluid. Encourage rest in side-lying position for 20 minutes.	To restore fluid, electrolyte, and glucose levels
Inadequate Contractions		
Maternal stress	Reduce stress. Provide quiet, peaceful, supportive environment.	Maternal stress releases catecholamines that decrease uterine activity and blood flow.
Excessive analgesia/anesthesia	Avoid by using other comfort measures. Use nipple stimulation. Allow medication to wear off. Use upright positions, as tolerated.	Contractions are increased by oxytocin release with nipple stimulation.

contracted. When more than one diameter is contracted, the risk of obstetric problems in labor and delivery is significantly greater than when only one diameter is affected (Pritchard and MacDonald 1985). These planes can be precisely measured only by computed tomography (CT scan) or ultrasonography; however, as discussed in Chapter 16, clinical assessment of the maternal pelvis is routinely done prenatally by bimanual examination.

Any pelvic contracture predisposes the patient to cephalopelvic disproportion and malposition and malpresentation. Variations in the shape of the pelvis result largely from genetic factors dictating the size and conformation of the skeleton. Since treatment and nursing responsibilities are similar regardless of the type of pelvic contracture, these areas are discussed at the end of this section.

Inlet Contracture

The pelvic inlet, known also as the *superior strait,* is considered to be contracted when its anteroposterior (AP) diameter is 10 cm or less, or when its transverse diameter is less than 12 cm. When the measurements of the inlet are smaller than normal, engagement of the presenting part may be difficult. This may result in malpresentations, particularly breech presentations, since the smaller breech may engage; descent of the fetal head is difficult or impossible.

Maternal Implications.   Labor is likely to be prolonged and ineffective, since the presenting part cannot descend and apply pressure to the cervix; cervical dilatation is often slow and incomplete. PROM is common, since the force of uterine activity is exerted on the membranes rather than on the fetal presenting part. If labor continues, risk of pathologic retraction rings and uterine rupture increases.

Fetal/Neonatal Implications.   Inlet contracture increases the risk of perinatal mortality, in part because of the higher percentage of malpositions and malpresentations. Since descent is impeded and the fetal presenting part does not occlude the cervix, the risk of cord prolapse with rupture of membranes is increased. If the fetal head is applied against the bony pelvis for long periods, there is greater danger of soft tissue trauma, excessive molding, and skull fracture and intracranial hemorrhage.

Midpelvis Contracture

The midpelvis (midplane, or plane of least dimensions) is at the level of the ischial spines. As the fetus enters the midplane, three important diameters must be successfully negotiated before it can descend to the pelvic outlet (see Chapter 22 for fuller discussion and diagrams). Contractures are present if any of the following conditions exist:

- The interspinous or transverse diameter is less than 10.9 cm.
- The anteroposterior diameter measured from the inferior border of the symphysis pubis to the juncture of the sacral vertebra (S4-5) is less than 11.5 cm.
- The posterior sagittal diameter between the sacrum and the interspinous diameter is less than 4.5 cm.

Accurate measurement of these diameters requires pelvimetry. However, when large jutting ischial spines and a generally small pelvis are found on clinical examination, contracture of the midpelvis is probable.

Maternal Implications. Contractures of the midpelvis predispose to transverse arrest of the head. If the contracture is marginal, uterine contractions may move the head past it without intervention. If this does not occur, however, cesarean delivery or, rarely, midforceps application to bring the head past the point of the contracture is needed. Since midforceps applications can result in significant trauma to maternal tissue and to the fetal skull, cesarean delivery is often chosen, unless descent is sufficient to permit safe forceps or vacuum extraction.

Fetal/Neonatal Implications. A midpelvis contracture may prevent anterior rotation of the fetal head, turning it into the hollow of the sacrum and thus impeding its downward progress. As with other contractures, if labor is prolonged, excessive pressure on the fetal head may result in soft tissue or skull trauma.

Outlet Contracture

The pelvic outlet is considered to be contracted when the interischial tuberous diameter is less than 8 cm. This condition commonly occurs in conjunction with other pelvic contractures.

Maternal Implications. If descent of the fetal head is protracted and forceps application is difficult, necrosis of maternal soft tissue may result, leading to the formation of fistulas in the vaginal walls. The risk of vaginal hematoma formation may also be increased.

Fetal/Neonatal Implications. Extreme molding and caput succedaneum formation may make it appear that the head has descended lower into the birth canal than it actually has, thus increasing the chances that a difficult low forceps application will be needed to bring the fetal head past the contracture.

Treatment. Treatment for a laboring woman with a suspected pelvic contracture includes close monitoring of labor progress and continuous monitoring of fetal status. Since the exact extent of pelvic contracture and its effect on fetal descent cannot always be accurately predicted, the physician may suggest that the patient have a trial of labor with Pitocin administration to see whether uterine activity might be sufficient to cause fetal descent and eventual delivery. However, trial of labor is justified only if progressive dilatation, effacement, and fetal descent are occurring and maternal and fetal status remains good. If trial of labor is unsuccessful and forceps application is considered unsafe, cesarean delivery is indicated.

Implications for Nursing Care

The nurse must be alert for indications of pelvic contractures. When caring for a nullipara, the nurse must recognize that the pelvis is "untested" and contractures may be present; a multipara who is carrying a normal-sized fetus without evidence of malpresentation and has had previous uncomplicated vaginal deliveries may be considered to be at less risk. Regardless of the patient's obstetric history, however, the nurse must look for any notations about pelvic adequacy on the prenatal chart as well as for signs of delayed engagement of the fetal presenting part, slow cervical dilatation and effacement, and a developing pattern of prolonged labor. Since the nurse often has primary responsibility for monitoring and documenting labor progress, she must alert the birth attendant to deviations that may suggest pelvic contractures and resulting cephalopelvic disproportion.

If a trial of labor is initiated, the nurse is responsible for

Complications Involving Maternal Physiologic Systems
Preexisting Maternal Conditions
- Pregnancy-induced hypertension (PIH)
- Diabetes mellitus

Emergent Maternal Conditions
- Shock
- Disseminated intravascular coagulation (DIC)
- Amniotic fluid embolism

administering and monitoring the Pitocin drip as well as carefully observing maternal and fetal responses, as described in Chapter 26. The nurse must also pay special attention to the comfort and emotional needs of the woman and her partner, as they are experiencing a more difficult and frightening course of labor than they may have anticipated. The nurse must keep the parents informed about the progress of labor and the status of the fetus and be prepared to explain any obstetric interventions that may be needed if labor does not progress.

COMPLICATIONS INVOLVING MATERNAL PHYSIOLOGIC SYSTEMS

Some complications of the intrapartal period involve more than one maternal physiologic system. These arise either because of preexisting maternal conditions, such as diabetes or pregnancy-induced hypertension, or because of emergent problems, such as shock or disseminated intravascular coagulation. Nursing care of patients with these conditions requires expert assessment skills, close monitoring to ensure early detection of signs of complications, interventions to support maternal and fetal physiologic status, and an understanding of the maternal and fetal implications of these conditions.

Preexisting Maternal Conditions: Potential Intrapartal Problems

Preexisting maternal conditions, such as chronic diseases or complications of pregnancy itself, present special intrapartal problems. The nurse plays a key role in providing the specialized intrapartal care these patients require. The following section discusses intrapartal care of patients with diabetes and pregnancy-induced hypertension. (For the prenatal management of these patients, see Chapters 19 and 20.)

Nursing Implications in Intrapartal Care of Patients With Preexisting Maternal Diseases

Hypertensive Cardiovascular Disease

Intrapartal management is similar to that for PIH. If placental function is compromised, early delivery may be necessary. Close monitoring of maternal blood pressure is needed throughout labor to detect possible PIH superimposed on already elevated blood pressure. Spinal anesthesia may be avoided because of the risk of abrupt hypotension and fetal compromise.

Cardiac Disease

About 1% of all pregnant women suffer from preexisting cardiac disease. Patients are usually hospitalized before delivery, with earlier hospitalization in more severe cases. Vaginal delivery is preferable to cesarean delivery if no other complications arise. It is important, however, to minimize maternal anxiety and pain because of their detrimental effects on maternal cardiorespiratory status. Systemic analgesia and pudendal block are customary for vaginal birth. Continuous epidural block may be used, but constant vigilance regarding maternal blood pressure is required to avoid maternal hypotension, which can be fatal to some cardiac patients.

Pulse, respirations, and blood pressure should be monitored every 15 minutes through first-stage labor, and every 5 to 10 minutes through second-stage labor. Increasing pulse (over 100 bpm) and respiratory rate (over 24 per minute) may signal developing cardiac embarrassment. The patient should be maintained on bed rest in the early postpartum period until cardiac function is fully recovered; cardiac decompensation may occur up to 7 days after delivery because of mobilization of extravascular fluid and resulting cardiac overload. Stress and energy expenditure during this time must be minimized.

Hyperthyroidism

There is an increased incidence of preterm labor and birth with hyperthyroidism. Intrapartal management is not unusual, except for closer monitoring of blood and electrolyte values. A cord blood sample should be tested for free T_4 to determine the thyroid status of the neonate.

HIV Infection and Acquired Immune Deficiency Syndrome (AIDS)

HIV infection and acquired immune deficiency syndrome has been reported among pregnant women whose partners had the disease or were in high-risk groups and among women who have received artificial insemination with donor sperm. Intrapartal management requires vigilance to decrease the risk of infection, since the mother's immune system is compromised. To avoid spreading of HIV, health care providers should take the following precautions: scrupulous handwashing, avoidance of accidental needle sticks, gown and glove precautions when in contact with bodily fluids and excretions, and the use of masks if the patient is coughing or has pneumocystosis. The patient's cytomegalovirus titer may be elevated. The probability of transmission to the fetus/newborn is estimated to be as high as 50% to 90%.

Pregnancy-Induced Hypertension

Pregnancy-induced hypertension (PIH) may be mild or severe (see Chapter 19 for a discussion of antepartal management of PIH). The classic triad of symptoms resulting from physiologic changes associated with PIH are the following:

- Hypertension, defined as blood pressure of 140/90, or an increase in systolic pressure of 30 mm Hg over nonpregnant levels, or an increase in diastolic pressure of 15 mm Hg above nonpregnant levels
- Sudden weight gain of more than 2 pounds per week in conjunction with fluid retention and increasing generalized edema
- Proteinuria—0.5 g/liter in 24 hours, or a reading of +1 or +2 on dipstick; usually the last symptom to occur

Eclampsia, a serious obstetric emergency, represents a worsening of preexistent preeclampsia. It usually occurs near term. Symptoms of eclampsia include those of severe preeclampsia and the cardinal signs of clonic-tonic seizures, coma, and hypertensive crisis. Prodromal symptoms—that is, those that signal an impending convulsion—include epigastric or upper right quadrant pain associated with hyperreflexia. The patient exhibiting such signs is seriously ill and must be admitted for immediate emergency care. Other signs that characterize eclampsia are shown in the accompanying display.

Hyperreflexia is a reflection of increased central ner-

NURSING ALERT

Signs and Symptoms of Eclampsia

Symptoms of impending eclampsia:

- Severe headache (due to cerebral edema)
- Visual disturbances, drowsiness, listlessness (due to cerebral edema)
- Vomiting (due to cerebral edema)
- Epigastric pain (an ominous sign caused by the stretching of the liver capsule)

Signs characterizing eclampsia:

- Seizures
- Blood pressure of 160/110 mm Hg (or increases of 60/30 mm Hg over nonpregnant or early pregnant levels)
- Proteinuria: 5 g/24 hr
- Oliguria: 500 ml/24 hr or less
- Hyperreflexia (4+ or sustained clonus)
- Pulmonary edema or cyanosis

vous system irritability, as is seizure activity; it may be caused by cerebral edema and ischemia. The accompanying display reviews the procedure for evaluating deep tendon reflexes (DTRs) and ankle clonus.

Convulsions and hypertensive crises associated with eclampsia may appear before, during, or after labor or in the early postpartum period. During the eclamptic hypertensive crisis, the pulse rate increases dramatically, and blood pressure may reach 200 mm Hg systolic with hyperpyrexia of 103°F to 104°F. Seizure activity is described as similar to that associated with grand mal epilepsy. A typical convulsion may last for 15 to 20 seconds and begins with facial twitching and rolling of the eyes. The muscles of the entire body quickly become rigidly contracted; the face is distorted; the eyes protrude; the arms are flexed; and the hands are clenched. Fixation of the diaphragm occurs and respiration ceases.

After 20 seconds of this tonic contraction, clonic contractions begin with violent opening and closing of the eyes and jaws and contraction and relaxation of the extremities. The patient will thrash about and will need protection to avoid injury. She may also bite her tongue at this time.

When the seizure ends, the patient will take a long, labored breath, after which stertorous and gradually more normal respiration resumes. Coma ensues, and consciousness is gradually regained over a number of hours. Once begun, convulsions usually recur unless treatment is initiated.

Etiologic and Predisposing Factors. As discussed in Chapter 19, the precise cause of PIH is not well understood; however, certain factors are associated with increased risk of this disorder, including

- Nulliparity (especially in teenagers)
- Preexisting hypertensive disease or diabetes
- Family history of PIH or other hypertensive disorders
- Pregnancies with a superabundance of trophoblasts and chorionic villi, such as multiple gestation and hydatidiform mole
- Fetal hydrops
- Malnutrition

In multiparous patients, PIH rarely occurs in the absence of one or more of these factors.

Maternal Implications. The major maternal risks of PIH are those associated with eclampsia and its associated hypertensive and central nervous system abnormalities. Death from preeclampsia itself is relatively rare, whereas maternal mortality among eclamptic patients is estimated to be 10% to 15% (Pritchard and MacDonald 1985). The most frequent causes of maternal death associated with eclampsia are congestive heart failure and intracranial hemorrhage. Hypertensive crises predispose the

Hyperreflexia

Hyperreflexia is determined by deep tendon reflexes (DTRs) on a 0 to 4+ scale:

0   No response

1+   Low normal or somewhat diminished

2+   Normal, average

3+   Above average briskness

4+   Very brisk, hyperactive; also associated with clonus
       (a series of convulsive ankle movements that occur
       when the foot is dorsiflexed)

Assessing Deep Tendon Reflexes and Clonus

Hyperreflexia reflects increased central nervous system irritability. Intrapartal patients with preeclampsia or eclampsia should be frequently evaluated for increasingly brisk DTRs, as this finding suggests worsening of their condition and the possibility of seizure activity. In assessing DTRs, begin with the arms and move to the legs, comparing reflex responses on left and right sides. Note and record any asymmetry. Place the limb to be tested in a relaxed, semiflexed position; a brisk tap places additional tension on the respective tendon and elicits the reflex response.

If in doubt about whether an assessment represents a change in the patient's reflex response, consult with other nurses who have assessed the patient and, if possible, collaborate in another assessment to see whether different results reflect an actual change in status or different evaluations by two nurses.

Biceps Reflex

1. Palpate for the tendon of the biceps brachii muscle in the bend of the elbow and place your thumb over it.

2. Tap your thumb briskly with the pointed end of the reflex hammer and note the reflex movement of the biceps muscle and flexion of the lower arm.

Quadriceps Reflex

1. Position the patient's legs so they are slightly flexed.

2. Supporting the leg under the knee with one arm, palpate the patellar tendon just below the patella and strike it briskly with the pointed end of the reflex hammer, noting the reflex extension of the lower leg.

Ankle Clonus

1. If DTRs are increased, assess for ankle clonus. Position the patient so the knee is slightly flexed.

2. Support the leg under the knee with one arm. With the other hand, grasp the foot, dorsiflex it quickly, and maintain this position. Observe for the rhythmic, repetitive jerks or beats of clonus and chart the number of beats.

---

woman to cerebrovascular accident, coma, and retinal injury. The risk of placental abruption, hemorrhage, and disseminated intravascular coagulation (DIC) is increased. Eclamptic crises necessitate emergency interventions and increase the risk of maternal death from cardiopulmonary arrest. However, with early detection and treatment, these problems can largely be prevented. With appropriate care, most patients improve markedly within 48 hours, and rapid improvement is typical after delivery.

Fetal/Neonatal Implications. The major risk to the fetus is placental insufficiency and ischemia related to vasoconstriction. Placental ischemia may trigger a series of pathologic processes resulting in placental infarction, degeneration, and reduced functioning. The placenta is increasingly prone to abruption, and fetoplacental perfusion is compromised to the point where it may fail to meet the nutritional, metabolic, and oxygen needs of the fetus.

If the fetus is further stressed by drugs, uterine activity, maternal hemorrhage, or hypertensive crisis, its physiologic reserves may be depleted and fetal distress may ensue. If the fetus is preterm or growth retarded, it is at serious risk. Continuous monitoring of the fetal heart rate is essential. Scalp sampling or stimulation to verify fetal status may also be done.

Treatment. Treatment will differ according to the severity of the patient's condition. The preeclamptic or eclamptic patient should be admitted to a labor room supplied with equipment for the management of obstetric emergencies and eclampsia, as listed in the display on page 810.

The patient is kept on strict bed rest. She should be maintained in a lateral recumbent position to increase uteroplacental perfusion, disperse accumulated fluid through systemic circulation, and increase kidney function and excretion of excess fluids. Blood pressure, pulse, respirations, level of consciousness, and reflex irritability are assessed every 15 to 30 minutes or more frequently depending on the patient's condition. Urine intake and output are monitored and a bladder catheter may be inserted to facilitate evaluation of urine output if kidney function is compromised. The urine is tested for proteinuria periodically. Laboratory tests, including platelet

NURSING ALERT

Equipment Used in the Intrapartal Care of the Preeclamptic/Eclamptic Patient

The following equipment is needed for monitoring and intervening in problems associated with preeclampsia. It must be readily accessible to the nurse caring for a preeclamptic or eclamptic patient and should be kept at the bedside for at least 48 hours after delivery. When patients are started on $MgSO_4$, IV therapy should be continued 12 to 24 hours after delivery regardless of the time of the initial loading dose.

Proteinuria

- Dipsticks for testing urine
- Indwelling urinary catheter and collection bag

Hypertension

- Functioning blood pressure cuff
- Apresoline: two vials, 20 mg/ml

Edema

- Graduated container for accurate measurement of urinary output
- Urometer for evaluating specific gravity of urine
- IV flow monitor or metriset/minidrip IV setup to permit accurate administration of small amounts of fluids
- Extra IV poles and 20-gauge needles with tubing for piggyback lines

- Pillows for positioning patient on left side to increase renal flow

Seizures

- Equipment needed for seizure precautions
- Reflex hammer
- $MgSO_4$: multidose vial
- 3-ml syringes with 20-gauge needles for administration of $MgSo_4$
- Patent IV line with Volutrol to allow piggyback administration of $MgSO_4$, essential in case $MgSO_4$ is discontinued immediately because of toxicity and antidote (calcium gluconate or calcium chloride) must be administered via the main IV line
- Valium: 10-mg single-dose vial for administration by IV push
- Adult nasal airway (nasal trumpet): allows for suctioning and oxygen administration; *preferable to padded tongue blade or oral airway* (avoids risk of trauma upon insertion)*
- Suction tubing and connection tubing
- Non-rebreather oxygen mask and functioning O_2
- Functional emergency call light
- Tourniquet for use in obtaining blood sample for arterial blood gases if seizure or respiratory depression occurs
- Calcium gluconate and calcium chloride: 10% in 10 ml = 1 g IV as antidote for $MgSO_4$ toxicity

Adapted from OB Nursing Procedure, University of California, San Francisco
* Snyder M: A Guide to Neurologic and Neurosurgical Nursing, p 280. New York, John Wiley & Sons, 1983

---

counts to monitor coagulation factors, and urinalysis, blood chemistry tests, and creatinine clearance tests are ordered to evaluate liver and kidney function.

In order to optimize the intrauterine environment, oxygen is administered at 8 to 12 liters/minute by tight face mask and the patient is maintained in the left lateral recumbent position to improve uteroplacental perfusion. Continuous fetal monitoring is initiated immediately upon admission, and an electronic scalp electrode is applied as soon as it is feasible. If fetal condition is compromised (indicated by evidence of fetal distress obtained through electronic monitoring of the fetal heart rate or fetal blood sampling), immediate cesarean delivery may be necessary.

Magnesium sulfate is a neuromuscular sedative that decreases the amount of acetylcholine produced by motor nerves and thus effectively blocks neuromuscular transmission. Administration of magnesium sulfate by IV infusion can prevent seizures and permit stabilization of maternal status so that delivery can be accomplished as soon as possible. (See Table 28–3 for dosage and administration.)

Side-effects of magnesium sulfate include the following:

- Increased sodium retention — additional doses should not be administered unless urinary output can be maintained at 25 ml/hour; magnesium sulfate is excreted by the kidneys, and toxicity can result if urinary output is low.

Table 28-3   **Drugs That May Be Indicated in Control of Severe PIH/Eclampsia**

Drug	Dosage	Indications and Adverse Reactions	Nursing Implications
Magnesium sulfate	Initial Dose: 2–4 g MgSO$_4$(USP) as 10% IV solution injected slowly over 15–30 min period Maintenance Dose: 20 g MgSO$_4$ in 1000 ml 5% dextrose in H$_2$O usually 2 g/hr, depending on reflexes, respirations, urinary output, etc.	Drug decreases acetylcholine for neuromuscular transmission. It has a mild hypotensive effect and inhibits uterine contractions. Excessive magnesium in the newborn may cause lethargy and depressed respirations.	If deep tendon reflexes (knee jerk) are depressed, stop drug and call physician. If serum magnesium is above 7 mEq/liter, stop drug. Calcium gluconate is antidote and should be kept at the bedside. Watch for respiratory depression. Rate should be 12 bpm or more. Continue all nursing precautions for the severely preeclamptic patient.
Diuretics Lasix (Furosemide)	40 mg IV (slow push)	Drug is reserved for treatment of pulmonary edema resulting from eclamptic seizures. Caution: it may conceal the degree of hypovolemia and oliguria present. It is usually given after delivery.	See section on nursing management of the eclamptic patient. Monitor CVP line. Maintain intravenous infusion and medications. Monitor hourly urinary output.
Hydrodiuril (hydrochlorothiazide)	Although a diuretic, drug is never used in pregnancy to relieve edema of PIH. It may be used to treat preexisting hypertension.		

- Respiratory paralysis — administration must be withheld or discontinued if respiratory rate is less than 12 or if DTRs are absent; otherwise toxicity may result.

Early signs of magnesium sulfate toxicity include diminished reflexes, hypotension, and muscle flaccidity; later signs include central nervous system depression, especially absence of *patellar reflex,* respiratory paralysis, decreased renal function, and circulatory collapse. Thus, the nurse must determine that DTRs are present, that urinary output is at least 25 ml/hr, and that respiration rate is at least 12 per minute before repeated doses of magnesium sulfate are administered. The antidote for magnesium sulfate toxicity is IV administration of 1 g calcium gluconate or calcium chloride.

Intrapartal care of the eclamptic patient includes the measures listed above; in addition, care involves controlling convulsions, preventing further seizures, and facilitating delivery. During eclamptic seizures and immediately after, efforts are focused on maintaining the airway and stabilizing blood pressure.

Respiratory care of the eclamptic patient is important for two reasons. First, the patient is restricted to bed rest and thus suffers the usual hazards of immobility, including increasing risk of pneumonia. This risk is potentiated by the depressant effect of magnesium sulfate therapy on respiration. Further, if hypertensive crisis or seizures occur, a clear airway and unhampered ventilation become especially important. If the patient is unable to clear secretions from the mouth and throat satisfactorily, suctioning is necessary. Administration of oxygen by mask is usually initiated. Endotracheal intubation or tracheostomy are rare unless tongue biting has occurred or pulmonary edema has developed. In the latter case, the patient is seriously ill and is often transferred to an intensive care unit.

Antihypertensive therapy is indicated only in cases of severe hypertension when the risk of cerebrovascular accident is high. Hydralazine may be used to counteract the generalized vasospasm associated with eclampsia and also to enhance renal flow. However, since a rapid lowering of blood pressure may impair placental perfusion and jeopardize the fetus, close monitoring of maternal blood pressure is essential when using this drug.

Regulation of circulatory volume is another aspect of the management of eclampsia. Hypovolemia is characteristic of eclampsia, and thus the patient requires IV fluid replacement. However, since the vascular bed is constricted as a result of generalized vasospasm, a central venous pressure (CVP) line may be necessary to provide accurate measurement of circulatory volume and to prevent circulatory overload. In severely ill patients, placement of an additional arterial line allows readings of arterial pressure, blood gases, and *p*H necessary for aggressive management.

Once the infant is delivered and the products of conception have been removed from the uterus, patients usually undergo rapid recovery from PIH. Within 8 to 48 hours the following improvements may be noted:

- Stable blood pressure within a normal range while the magnesium sulfate infusion is being maintained
- Urinary output of 60 ml/hour or greater
- Normal deep tendon reflexes with no clonus
- Gradually subsiding levels of proteinuria
- Improved mental status

Implications for Nursing Care

Nursing responsibilities in providing intrapartal care for the patient with PIH focus on careful assessment of maternal and fetal status and ongoing monitoring for changes in that status, support of optimal physiologic status until delivery can be achieved, and emotional support for the patient and her family. The nurse's initial assessment must include a review of the patient's prenatal record to obtain information about the progression of symptoms, baseline weight, DTRs, blood pressure, and proteinuria levels as well as recent changes in fetal activity.

The nurse's initial physical assessment should include blood pressure readings in supine and left lateral positions. These should be done between contractions to eliminate possible effects of pain and anxiety on blood pressure. The patient's weight and level of edema should be noted and compared with the most recent prenatal levels. Changes in these indicators since the last prenatal evaluation should be reported to the physician immediately. DTRs should be evaluated. The presence of hyperreflexia in a woman who has not previously experienced this symptom is an indication that her condition is worsening and should be immediately reported to the physician.

If the nurse's assessment suggests that the patient's condition is unstable on admission, she must stay with the patient, summon help, alert the physician, monitor vital signs, and observe for prodromal signs of eclampsia, which include severe headache, visual disturbance, epigastric pain, or vomiting.

During labor and birth the nurse should be in constant attendance at the woman's bedside. Blood pressure, pulse, and respirations must be assessed every 15 to 30 minutes. The use of an electronic blood pressure monitor

is a useful assessment tool. Reflexes, urinary output, degree of edema, proteinuria, and signs of coagulopathy (petechiae, ecchymosis, oozing of venipunctures and hematuria) are evaluated at least once an hour. Breath sounds should be evaluated, since pulmonary edema is a complication of severe preeclampsia and eclampsia.

The room should be kept quiet and stimulation (including procedures) minimized, since central nervous system irritability may trigger seizures. The patient ingests nothing by mouth and is kept on strict bed rest. Visitors may be permitted on a limited basis; the nurse must explain to them the need for a calm, quiet environment. The patient should never be left without a nurse in attendance.

If seizures occur, the nurse's first concern is maintaining a patent airway and protecting the patient from injury. The patient should be turned on her side to decrease the risk of aspiration should vomiting occur. The nurse should immediately call for emergency assistance and prepare oxygen and suction for use. Past nursing practice for eclamptic patients has included attempts to insert a padded tongue blade ("bite stick") or plastic airway into the mouth at the first sign of seizure activity to prevent tongue biting and allow access for suctioning. However, current emergency management of seizures avoids oral insertion of any object. Instead, a nasal airway (nasopharyngeal airway or nasal trumpet) should be kept at the bedside and inserted by medical or nursing staff during a seizure. The nasal airway must be well lubricated with water-soluble lubricant before insertion. Right and left nasal airways can be distinguished by the pharyngeal end opening, which should face the midline. Once in place, connection tubing can be used for suctioning or for oxygen administration.

Insertion of a nasal airway is preferable to use of a bite stick or oral airway for several reasons. This type of airway is easily inserted into a naris and extends to a point just behind the base of the tongue above the epiglottis, immediately providing a clear airway for oxygen administration and allowing for suctioning, if needed. Use of a nasal airway also prevents possible mouth trauma and dislodging of teeth from a difficult oral insertion during a seizure.

Oxygen should be administered at 8 to 12 liters/minute by mask during the convulsion to maximize fetal oxygenation. To reduce the continued stress on mother and fetus, delivery should quickly follow control of seizures and maternal hypertension. Labor is usually induced, and vaginal delivery under pudendal block can be planned if maternal condition and fetal condition allow. If either is deteriorating, cesarean delivery is indicated.

A major nursing responsibility is attending to the comfort and physical needs of the patient during this enforced inactivity and providing emotional support to the woman and her family. The patient may benefit from quiet visits
(text continued on page 814)

NURSING CARE PLAN

The Patient With Moderate to Severe Pregnancy-Induced Hypertension

Nursing Diagnosis (Patient Problem) and Assessment Data	Nursing Interventions	Rationale
Probable Complication: *moderate to severe PIH*		
• Gestation >20 weeks	Monitor BP, pulse, respirations, reflexes and FHR every 30 min or as indicated.	Maintenance measures and close monitoring assure early identification of change in patient status.
• Hypertension >140/90 or increase of 30/15 over baseline		
• Edema, 3–4+	Monitor hourly intake and output; assess for proteinuria, edema.	Decreased urinary output is a result of poor kidney functioning.
• Proteinuria 72+	Maintain bed rest, lateral position.	To increase uterine and renal perfusion.
	Administer MgSO₄ or other antihypertensives as ordered. Monitor for adverse effects: Check reflexes; if 1 or 0, consult physician. Check respirations; if less than 12, notify physician. If urinary output is less than 30 ml/hr, notify physician	Objective is to reduce blood pressure until the fetus is mature enough to be delivered. Resolution of PIH occurs with delivery. Signs of an overdose of magnesium sulfate are decreased respirations and depressed reflexes.
	Keep calcium gluconate at bedside.	Calcium gluconate is antagonist for MgSO₄ toxicity.
	Never leave the client unattended.	

Expected Outcome:

Patient returns to normal physiologic status, as result of therapy, as evidenced by normal vital signs and balanced intake/output within 24 hours.

Possible Complication: *eclampsia*		
• Epigastric distress	If convulsion occurs, maintain patent airway, give magnesium sulfate as indicated, place the client on her side, protect by padding side rails. After convulsion, maintain intravenous fluids, nothing by mouth.	Epigastric distress or nausea with or without vomiting may indicate a convulsion is impending.
• Nausea and/or vomiting		
• BP >160/110		
	Monitor fetal status, and administer O₂ 8–12 liters/min.	To maintain adequate fetal oxygenation and identify signs of fetal distress.
	Prepare for delivery.	Treatment for severe PIH is delivery of the infant. After delivery the patient undergoes rapid recovery in 8–48 hr with continued care.

Expected Outcome:

The patient with severe PIH experiences no complications associated with drug therapy and returns to normal physiological status within 8 to 48 hours of delivery.

(continued)

NURSING CARE PLAN (continued)

The Patient With Moderate to Severe Pregnancy-Induced Hypertension

Nursing Diagnosis (Patient Problem) and Assessment Data	Nursing Interventions	Rationale
Nursing Diagnosis: *fear related to increased perinatal risk*		
• Expressed fear or signs of dysfunctional anticipatory grief	Provide emotional support.	Support and acceptance of fear as a normal reaction will increase patient's ability to cope.
Expected Outcome:		
Patient accepts fear as normal reaction and responds by cooperating with staff providing her care.		
Nursing Diagnosis: *ineffective family coping*		
• Inability to visit or participate in maternal care	Keep family informed about patient status.	To maintain and support family coping with stressful event.
Expected Outcome:		
Family maintains contact with patient, and both patient and family utilize nursing staff as a source of support during hospitalization.		

from her partner or other family members; some patients rest more easily when family members are present. The nurse must also remember the strain on family members during this time; every effort should be made to reassure them, to allow for close interaction and mutual support, and to create as normal a birth environment as possible.

Diabetes Mellitus

Pregnancy has a profound effect on the diabetic woman and on her prenatal care, as discussed in Chapter 20. Maternal diabetes also affects intrapartal care and may affect both maternal and neonatal outcomes. In the past many diabetic women experienced complicated labors and unexpected third-trimester fetal death. However, current prenatal and intrapartal management of the diabetic patient, including careful regulation of blood glucose and more frequent prenatal visits to monitor maternal and fetal status, has lowered maternal morbidity and improved the chances for good neonatal outcomes.

Diabetics in the Class A (diet-controlled) category, which includes gestational diabetics, have a good chance

of carrying a fetus to term and experiencing an uncomplicated labor and delivery. The prognosis for insulin-dependent diabetics (Class C through F) depends in large part on the degree of diabetic control throughout pregnancy. Pregnant Class B to F diabetic patients should be delivered in a setting with a skilled intrapartal unit staff and a neonatal intensive care unit.

The infant of a diabetic mother (IDM) requires expert neonatal care, since the neonate is at increased risk for macrosomia, hyperinsulinemia, and associated hypoglycemia, hypocalcemia, respiratory distress syndrome and congenital anomalies (see Chapter 34 for nursing care of the IDM).

Maternal Implications. The diabetic mother will be carefully monitored throughout the intrapartal period. Optimal diabetic control is a major goal. Since the mother may be at high risk for preeclampsia, vascular problems, and infection associated with diabetes, early detection of these complications is especially important. Special precautions are needed to ensure maternal and fetal well-being in the intrapartal period, as discussed in the following paragraphs.

Fetal/Neonatal Implications.   The fetus of the diabetic mother is at risk for cardiac and gastrointestinal anomalies, thought to result from altered maternal blood glucose levels in very early pregnancy. The fetus of a diabetic mother is at risk in the last trimester of pregnancy and the intrapartal period, primarily because of decreased uteroplacental perfusion associated with diabetic vascular changes, and resulting fetal hypoxia. However, losses from intrauterine fetal demise (IUFD) are decreasing in number as more careful antenatal monitoring of fetal status, better timing of delivery, and more accurate methods of diabetic control are possible.

The infant of a diabetic mother (IDM) is often macrosomic as a result of maternal hyperglycemia. Birth trauma is more common with macrosomic infants, with effects such as facial palsy, fracture of the humerus and clavicle, bruising, and cephalhematoma. However, not all IDMs are macrosomic; in mothers with Class C to F diabetes, intrauterine growth retardation, low birth weight, and associated problems may also result, although less frequently. Asphyxia, with Apgar scores of less than 7 at 1 minute, is more common in IDMs than in other infants, and respiratory distress syndrome is 5 times more common. The IDM is also at increased risk for hyperbilirubinemia, neuromuscular irritability, and hypoglycemia in the neonatal period. Care of the IDM is discussed in Chapter 34.

Routine preterm delivery of the IDM, regardless of maternal or fetal status, was practiced in the past; however, iatrogenic preterm delivery was eventually shown to present considerable risk to neonatal well-being. Current obstetric practice requires the physician to weigh the increased risk of fetal demise after 37 weeks of gestation among poorly controlled Class C to F diabetic mothers against the risks associated with preterm delivery, taking into consideration assessed fetal status and the quality of past and current diabetic control. If control has been good, no maternal complications develop, and the fetus appears to be uncompromised (as indicated by biophysical profile and nonstress testing), delivery may be delayed on a day-to-day basis until fetal maturity is ensured.

Induction of labor for these patients may be planned when the fetal lungs are mature, if evidence of decreased placental perfusion is present. Conditions indicating the choice of induction of labor or cesarean delivery are listed in the accompanying display.

Intrapartal care of the diabetic patient is dictated in large part by the nature of her disease and the degree of diabetic control during pregnancy.

When blood glucose has been well controlled and no complications arise, the diabetic mother may anticipate a vaginal delivery, with close monitoring of maternal and fetal status throughout labor. If the fetus is not thought to be large (less than 4000 g) and the pelvis is adequate, the physician may await onset of spontaneous labor and plan

---

Delivery of the Infant of a Diabetic Mother

Indications for Induction of Labor

- Pregnancy of 40 weeks or more of gestation
- Fetal macrosomia, with or without hydramnios
- Severe preeclampsia
- Decreasing fetal movement by kick count, or other abnormal indicators of fetal status

Indications for Cesarean Delivery

- Fetal malpresentation, especially breech (because of the risk of macrosomia and dystocia)
- Previous cesarean birth
- Cephalopelvic disproportion
- Long history of infertility
- Worsening complications associated with diabetes

---

for a vaginal delivery. If labor does not begin spontaneously after 38 weeks, nonstress testing may begin (Arias and Holcomb 1984). Obstetric intervention, such as oxytocin induction of labor or cesarean delivery, may be advised sooner for these women than for their nondiabetic counterparts because of the increased risk of macrosomia and cephalopelvic disproportion.

Continuous IV administration of insulin in a dextrose and water solution is initiated to provide optimal diabetic control. Blood glucose levels are monitored hourly, and insulin infusion is adjusted as needed to maintain normal levels (70–110 ml/dl). This reduces not only the risk of maternal problems with glucose regulation during labor and delivery but also the risk of severe neonatal hyperinsulinism, since maternal blood glucose is well regulated before delivery.

Labor may be induced, and if good progress is being made without evidence of maternal or fetal problems, a vaginal delivery will be planned. However, in the presence of suspected cephalopelvic disproportion, developing fetal distress, or maternal problems, such as preeclampsia, cesarean delivery is indicated. After delivery of the placenta, the insulin/glucose infusion is discontinued, and a normal diabetic regimen is established, based on the blood glucose levels in the first postpartum days.

Implications for Nursing Care

Intrapartal care of the diabetic mother requires close monitoring of maternal and fetal status throughout labor. The nurse is responsible for monitoring maternal insulin requirements during continuous insulin/glucose infusion. Hourly blood samples will be necessary. Since the laboratory costs of hourly blood glucose determinations can be considerable, the nurse may suggest that the patient's own glucometer be used. The nurse must have precise orders for adjusting the patient's insulin dosage according to blood glucose determinations. IV infusion of a prescribed dose of insulin in a dextrose in water solution is prepared. Because insulin binds to glass and plastic, 500 ml of normal saline with 50 units of insulin should be run through the tubing to coat it and ensure delivery of accurate insulin dosage in the subsequent administration. The continuous infusion must be administered using an infusion pump.

The nurse must monitor maternal and fetal status carefully, since uteroplacental perfusion may be decreased and premature placental aging may be present. Direct EFM is essential; the nurse must monitor for FHR changes (late decelerations, decreased variability) as well as for signs of placental abruption. The nurse should regularly explain fetal heart rate findings to the parents, since the mother and her partner are likely to be aware of the increased risk to the fetus. The nurse should also be prepared for the need for cesarean delivery and neonatal support if problems arise.

Emergent Maternal Conditions

Shock and disseminated intravascular coagulation (DIC) may develop during the intrapartal period. These maternal conditions involve several physiologic systems and pose a severe threat to both mother and fetus. These are true emergency situations, and though rare, they require immediate diagnosis and treatment to prevent maternal or fetal/neonatal death. The following sections discuss these conditions and a third intrapartal emergency, amniotic fluid embolism, which characteristically presents with both of these problems in the intrapartal patient.

Shock

Shock is the body's response to life-threatening physiologic conditions. A variety of mechanisms are employed to protect the functioning of vital organs. However, the response itself can become a threat to survival and, in extreme cases, can be reversed only through aggressive therapy, often including cardiopulmonary resuscitation.

There are four types of shock: hypovolemic, septic, cardiogenic, and neurogenic. In pregnancy and especially in the intrapartal period, hypovolemic and septic shock are most common. The following section discusses these types of shock, which are summarized in the accompanying display. Signs and symptoms of hypovolemic and septic shock appear in the display on the opposite page.

Hypovolemic Shock.   When large amounts of blood are lost, the body compensates by maintaining blood

Classification of Shock Associated With Obstetrics

1. Hypovolemic shock
    Hemorrhagic shock; associated with

    *   Ectopic pregnancy
    *   Placenta previa, abruptio placentae
    *   Uterine rupture
    *   Postpartum or postabortion hemorrhage
    *   Obstetric surgery

    Fluid loss shock; associated with excessive vomiting
    Supine hypotensive syndrome; associated with compression of the inferior vena cava by the weight of the pregnant uterus

2. Septic shock (endotoxic shock); associated with

    *   Prenatal or postpartum infection
    *   Septic abortion
    *   Chorioamnionitis
    *   Pyelonephritis
    *   Postpartum systemic infection

3. Cardiogenic shock
    Failure of left ventricular filling associated with

    *   Cardiac tamponade associated with coagulation defects
    *   Pulmonary embolism
    *   Thrombophlebitis

4. Neurogenic shock

    Chemical injury; associated with aspiration of gastrointestinal contents
    Drug toxicity; associated with spinal anesthesia
    Inversion of the uterus with vasomotor collapse
    Electrolyte imbalance; associated with hyponatremia

Adapted from Cavanaugh D, Woods RE, O'Connor TCE et al: Obstetric Emergencies, 3rd ed. Philadelphia, Harper & Row, 1982

pressure to minimize the adverse effects of decreased perfusion on tissues. At first, increased respiratory efforts help to maintain venous flow to the heart. Generalized vasoconstriction resulting from catecholamine release from the adrenals ensures that blood pressure and blood flow to essential organs (such as brain, kidneys, heart muscle, and lungs) are temporarily maintained.

This compensatory mechanism is effective until 20% to 25% of circulating blood volume is lost; when this level is surpassed, shock becomes severe. Cardiac output may

NURSING ALERT

Signs and Symptoms of Shock	
Signs	**Symptoms**
Hypovolemic Shock	
Tachycardia	Weak, thready pulse
Hypotension	Anxiety, restlessness
Decreased perfusion	Cool, clammy skin; pallor; blanching of nail beds; flat neck
Oliguria (<50 ml/hr); urine sodium	veins; peripheral cyanosis
= 80 mEq/liter	
Septic Shock	
Tachycardia	Hyperdynamic pulse, palpitations
Hypotension	Faintness, dizziness
Tachypnea, respiratory alkalosis	Anxiety, apprehension, disorientation, stupor
Cerebral ischemia	
Polyuria; urine sodium = 10 mEq/liter	

fall as much as 50%. The body's ability to supply oxygen is overcome, and the continued reduction in cell oxygenation results in an accumulation of lactic acid. Acidosis ensues, and vasodilation in arterioles results in pooling of blood. Perfusion of vital organs is compromised. Renal blood flow is reduced, and urinary output decreases. Massive electrolyte changes occur, and oxygenation of all tissues is compromised. Ultimately, if shock is not reversed, swelling of lung tissue leads to adult respiratory distress syndrome, profound metabolic acidosis, and death. Once adequate perfusion to the brain stops, brain damage and "brain death" occur within 5 minutes (Creasy and Resnik 1984).

Septic Shock. The precipitating factor in septic shock is usually endotoxin from pathologic gram-negative organisms. The incidence of gram-negative sepsis among hospitalized patients has been increasing in recent years, and mortality averages 50% in documented cases. The early phase of septic shock may be referred to as "warm," being characterized by normal or increased cardiac output and warm, dry skin. These symptoms may be easily overlooked, and even by the time they appear, oxygen consumption is already considerably reduced as a result of impaired cellular metabolism. When septic shock is not recognized in this early phase and fluid replacement is not instituted, hypovolemic shock results, and the "cold" phase of septic shock begins. Severe cellular damage from the effects of endotoxins causes malfunction of the vascular system; blood pressure falls dramatically, causing markedly reduced tissue perfusion. At this point severe shock is present, with the associated problems of profound metabolic acidosis. Adult respiratory distress syndrome and death may result.

Etiologic and Predisposing Factors. The most common causes of hypovolemic shock in the intrapartal period are placental accidents, uterine rupture, uterine atony, and severe lacerations of the genital tract. Hypovolemic shock may also be triggered by hemorrhage associated with DIC. Obstetric patients who are at particular risk for septic shock are those with infections resulting from septic abortions, chorioamnionitis, pyelonephritis, and septic pelvic thrombophlebitis.

Maternal Implications. Hypovolemic or septic shock in the intrapartal period poses a direct threat to maternal survival. Symptoms can develop rapidly, producing the need for emergency interventions, including blood and fluid replacement, cesarean delivery, and cardiopulmonary resuscitation. The mother is generally aware of the seriousness of the situation as her condition deteriorates. She may well be cognizant of her surroundings and events taking place, even if she cannot communicate verbally with staff. She may experience fear for her own survival as well as for her fetus if delivery has not been accomplished.

One consequence of severe hemorrhagic shock and DIC is *postdelivery anterior pituitary necrosis,* also known as *Sheehan's syndrome.* This constellation of symptoms, reflecting partial or total loss of endocrine functions, including thyroid, adrenocortical, and gonadal insufficiency, affects a small percentage of patients who survive profound hemorrhagic shock and DIC. The exact etiology of this syndrome is unknown. The symptoms, which include lactation failure, amenorrhea, breast atrophy, genital atrophy, and loss of pubic and axillary hair, suggest varying degrees of anterior pituitary damage and the resulting impaired secretion of its trophic hormones. Treatment, which includes hormonal replacement, is supportive, and the prognosis depends on the degree of damage sustained.

Fetal/Neonatal Implications. The fetus is directly threatened by maternal shock, primarily because utero-placental perfusion is compromised. The fetal response is similar to the mother's. Hypoxemia and acidosis cause bradycardia, vasospasm, and shunting of blood to vital organs. As the maternal condition worsens and these compensatory mechanisms can no longer function, brain damage and fetal death occur.

Treatment. Treatment of maternal shock in the intrapartal period is symptomatic and must be immediate. The patient is placed in a side-lying or supine position with right hip elevated to improve venous return and increase uterine perfusion. The Trendelenburg position is not recommended for a pregnant patient because of the additional risk of supine hypotension. A patent airway must be maintained and oxygen administered at 8 to 12 liter/minute.

Rapid fluid replacement with 5% dextrose in water with 0.20 or 0.45 normal saline should be initiated; however, fluid overload is a concern. The fluid drip rate should be decreased if signs of pulmonary congestion (moist respiratory sounds, dyspnea) develop. A central venous pressure line may be inserted to provide accurate measurement of venous return and adequacy of fluid replacement; an open IV line with a large-bore cannula should be established to allow for blood replacement, if needed. An indwelling urinary catheter is inserted to allow for accurate monitoring of urinary output; 50 ml/hour or more indicates adequate renal perfusion. Output of less than 30 ml/hour indicates continued vasospasm and is not a reassuring sign, reflecting either worsening shock or inadequate fluid replacement.

Maternal pulse, respirations, and blood pressure must be checked and recorded every 2 to 5 minutes; observations of skin color, temperature, and level of consciousness must be recorded as well. Fetal heart tones are monitored constantly for signs of developing distress. Since shock may be complicated by DIC, bruising and signs of bleeding from puncture sites, nose, or gums indicate the need for immediate blood-clotting studies.

The order of priorities in the management of shock is shown in the accompanying display.

Implications for Nursing Care

A primary nursing responsibility is early detection of hemorrhage and signs of impending shock. Tachycardia may be the first sign, followed by hypotension. The nurse must stay with the patient, alert other staff, and take quick action to intervene if, on the basis of these signs, she suspects impending shock. While waiting for assistance, she should position the patient as noted previously,

NURSING ALERT

The ORDER of Priorities in Managing the Patient in Shock

O   OXYGENATE
   Assure an airway
   8–10 liters/min by closed mask, nasal catheter, or endotracheal tube

R   RESTORE CIRCULATING VOLUME
   One or more IV lines
   Initially crystalloids or colloids
   Where possible, blood for blood, but remember clotting factors
   Initial monitoring by central venous pressure

D   DRUG THERAPY
   Avoid vasopressors, as a general rule
   Digitalize if in cardiac failure
   Specific drugs for condition

E   EVALUATE
   Response to therapy
   Basic cause
   Fetal condition, if appropriate

R   REMEDY THE BASIC PROBLEM
   Surgery, if appropriate
   Specific antibiotics, if organism identified

From Cavanaugh D, Marsden DE: In Quilligan EJ (ed): Current Therapy in Obstetrics and Gynecology, 2nd ed. Philadelphia, WB Saunders, 1983

begin oxygen administration, and prepare suction equipment for use. Close monitoring of vital signs and fetal heart rate and assistance with emergency therapeutic measures are primary nursing responsibilities. The nurse must be alert to the need for additional staff support, such as a resuscitation team or neonatal support team, in case an emergency delivery is necessary.

If the partner, other family member, or a support person is present, the nurse should quickly explain the situation, assist him or her to a waiting area, and make an effort to obtain another staff member to keep the family informed and as comfortable as can be expected under the circumstances. The nurse must also recognize that the patient may be cognizant of events although unable to communicate; an effort to explain procedures and provide reassurance should be made without disruption of emergency measures.

Often maternal shock requires immediate delivery to

increase the chances of fetal survival. Thus, the patient may require preparation for emergency cesarean delivery. If maternal condition is not stabilizing and maternal blood loss can be more easily corrected by surgical intervention, this procedure may be lifesaving for both mother and fetus/newborn.

Disseminated Intravascular Coagulation (DIC)

DIC may occur as a result of physiologic insult in late pregnancy or the intrapartal period. This condition is characterized by generation of increased prothrombin, platelets, and other coagulation factors, which cause widespread formation of thrombi throughout the microvasculature. Eventually, the body's clotting factors are expended, and severe hemorrhage begins.

In normal pregnancy the levels of certain clotting factors are increased, which may in fact help prevent exsanguination at birth (Ratnoff 1984). The most significant increase is a 50% increase in fibrinogen concentration over the nonpregnant state, believed to be related to the normally high levels of estrogen during pregnancy. Platelet count and prothrombin levels are not increased in normal pregnancy. However, insults such as placental bleeding, IUFD, and sepsis predispose the pregnant patient to DIC. DIC may develop insidiously during pregnancy or suddenly.

Thrombocytopenia, decreasing fibrinogen, and prolonged prothrombin time are early signs of developing coagulopathy, and baseline laboratory studies should be obtained on women thought to be at risk for DIC. Maternal symptoms include bleeding from puncture sites and gums or other unusual bleeding, such as hematuria, tachycardia, diaphoresis, increasing anxiety and restlessness, and the presence of hemorrhagic areas in the skin (ecchymosis). Platelet count and fibrinogen decrease; prothrombin and partial thromboplastin time (PTT) increase. A tentative diagnosis of DIC can be made when coagulation studies are reported.

Etiologic and Predisposing Factors. A pathologic event, such as IUFD or placental bleeding, activates normal clotting mechanisms and, if clotting factors are depleted, can initiate DIC. Such pathologic events may include the following:

- Septic shock
- Placental or profuse uterine bleeding
- Release of fetal thromboplastin after IUFD
- Amniotic fluid embolism
- Formation of thrombi in kidney, liver, or cerebral vessels secondary to preeclampsia and eclampsia

Maternal Implications. Upon diagnosis of DIC, immediate intensive care is necessary. Often the mother is moved to an intensive care unit, with obstetric staff providing assistance in monitoring fetal status. The mother is extremely ill and will require extensive medical intervention to correct coagulopathy. She may be aware of the seriousness of the situation and is likely to be fearful for her own life and that of her fetus.

Fetal/Neonatal Implications. Fetal/neonatal risk is increased not by DIC itself, but by other maternal physiologic problems, such as sepsis, acidosis, and hypotension. The major risk facing the fetus/neonate is that of hypoxia. In catastrophic situations where maternal status is deteriorating rapidly, emergency cesarean delivery may be necessary to save the life of the fetus.

Treatment. Treatment of DIC must include treatment of the causative factor as well as replacement of maternal coagulation factors and support of physiologic functioning. The first 2 hours of care are critical to survival, and vital signs and renal output must be supported. Treatment of the causative factor usually involves delivery of the fetus, removal of the placenta, and stabilization of maternal condition.

Except when amniotic fluid embolism is the causative factor, evacuation of the uterine contents usually eliminates the cause of DIC. Vaginal delivery is preferable if maternal condition permits. Surgical procedures such as episiotomy and cesarean delivery place more stress on hemostatic mechanisms; however, many patients are too ill for continued labor and vaginal delivery, and in such cases cesarean delivery is indicated.

Replacement of depleted coagulation factors is usually accomplished by whole blood infusion (donor fresh at 6–12 hours). Other blood components may also be used, as shown in Table 28–4. Heparin may be administered by continuous pump infusion to control coagulation.

Renal failure is a serious consequence of DIC; urinary output must be carefully monitored and output maintained at 30 to 50 ml/hour. When blood components are rapidly available and used early, kidney function is usually adequately maintained.

Implications for Nursing Care

An important nursing responsibility is early detection of DIC in the intrapartal patient. The nurse should assess the patient's history for possible predisposing factors. If the patient is identified as at risk, emergency equipment for blood administration and blood components should be readily available.

The nurse must recognize signs of unusual bleeding and notify the physician immediately if bleeding occurs from IV puncture sites, gums, or nose or if there is unusual vaginal bleeding or hematuria. The nurse should alert other staff for assistance, stay with the patient, and apply direct pressure to bleeding puncture sites until bleeding stops. Vital signs and fetal heart rate must be

Table 28–4   **Component Replacement**

Factor	Volume (ml)*	Supplies
Platelet concentrate	40–60	Increased count of viable platelets—by 25,000–35,000
Cryoprecipitate	30–50	Fibrinogen Factors VIII, XIII (3–10 times the equivalent volume of plasma)
Fresh-frozen plasma	200	All factors except platelets; 1 g fibrinogen
Packed RBC	200	Hematocrit 60% to 65%
Fibrinogen†	300	Increased fibrinogen (1–2 g)

From Lavery JP: Component replacement. Contemp Ob/Gyn 95:105, 1982
* Depends on local blood bank service.
† Not available in the United States.

monitored frequently. If the patient exhibits signs of anxiety or agitation, restraints or padded rails are needed to prevent bruising.

The nurse should expedite the process of obtaining laboratory studies and altering the blood bank of the possible need for coagulation factors and other blood components. An IV line with large-bore needle for blood administration and an indwelling urinary catheter will be needed. The nurse should be prepared to assist with placement of a central venous pressure catheter in case one is needed. Oxygen administration by mask should be initiated and the patient placed in a side-lying position to prevent maternal hypotension and fetal hypoxia.

The nurse must also recognize that the woman may well be cognizant of the seriousness of the situation and experience fear for herself and her fetus. The nurse must provide as much emotional support as possible, given the emergency situation; brief explanations of necessary procedures can be given without interrupting the flow of care. Other staff can be mobilized to stay with family members, keeping them informed and providing emotional support.

Amniotic Fluid Embolism

Amniotic fluid embolism is a rare obstetric catastrophe and has been called the most unpredictable and unpreventable cause of maternal death. Its incidence has been reported as ranging from 1 in 8,000 to 1 in 80,000 births (Killan 1985). It is characterized in most cases by rapid and simultaneous onset of shock and DIC. Few women survive amniotic fluid embolism. In the past, this diagnosis could not be confirmed until autopsy, and if the mother survived, the diagnosis was questioned; current diagnostic techniques suggest that survival is possible.

An amniotic fluid embolism occurs when a large amount of amniotic fluid gains access to the central maternal circulation (Fig. 28–11). Multiple emboli form in the pulmonary capillaries, resulting in rapid onset of respiratory distress and shock. Signs and symptoms of amniotic fluid embolism are shown in the accompanying display, opposite page.

Etiologic and Predisposing Factors. Amniotic fluid embolism typically occurs in the intrapartal period. There is considerable speculation about the mechanism involved. One theory suggests that a leak of fluid may occur when a tear in the amnion and chorion allows fluid to enter the chorionic plate; under pressure from the contracting uterus, the fluid is forced into the maternal circulation. It is also postulated that amniotic fluid may enter the maternal circulation through a laceration in the cervix or uterus.

The following have been identified as predisposing factors for amniotic fluid embolism; however, these must be considered speculative, since causation of the condition itself is not well understood.

- High parity
- Advanced maternal age
- Short or tumultuous labor
- Oxytocin augmentation
- Intrauterine fetal death
- Abruptio placentae

The underlying pathology of this condition is not yet well understood. With the onset of symptoms come rapid cardiopulmonary collapse and DIC. This is the only instance in which the agent that triggers defibrination and resulting DIC has been clearly identified; amniotic fluid and mucus found in it contain thromboplastin-like material that activates coagulation.

Events leading to cardiopulmonary collapse are initial pulmonary hypertension, cor pulmonale (acute right heart strain and failure), reduced left atrial pressure, reduced carbon dioxide and systemic hypotension. The

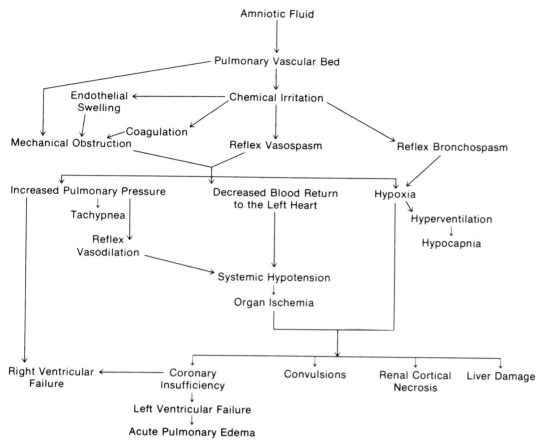

Figure 28–11. Sequence of events leading to cardiopulmonary complications of amniotic fluid embolism. (Abouleish E: Pain Control in Obstetrics. Philadelphia, JB Lippincott, 1977)

NURSING ALERT

Signs and Symptoms of Amniotic Fluid Embolism

Premonitory Symptoms

- Shaking chill and diaphoresis
- Increasing restlessness and anxiety
- Chest pain
- Coughing with frothy pink sputum
- Vomiting
- Seizures

Cardinal Symptoms

- Rapidly developing dyspnea, tachypnea, and cyanosis
- Hemorrhage
- Shock out of proportion to blood loss
- Coma

cause of the initial pulmonary hypertension is not fully understood. It may result from obstruction of the capillary bed by debris (fetal squamous epithelium, lanugo, mucus, and meconium) in the amniotic fluid; the presence of this material in pulmonary vessels at autopsy confirms the diagnosis of amniotic fluid embolism.

Maternal Implications. Approximately 25% of women diagnosed with amniotic fluid embolism die within 1 hour of the onset of symptoms. Mortality for all cases is estimated to be more than 80%; the interval between onset of symptoms and death ranges from 1 to 32 hours. Coagulation failure occurs in up to 50% of patients within 1 hour of onset; significant hemorrhage usually results. Among women surviving the initial crisis, uncontrollable uterine hemorrhage may begin within minutes or hours.

Fetal/Neonatal Implications. The fetus is at profound risk because of the rapid deterioration of maternal status, and immediate delivery is essential. Fetal heart rate is continuously monitored until delivery can be accomplished. Forceps application and emergency vaginal delivery may be possible if labor has progressed sufficiently; otherwise, emergency cesarean delivery is necessary. Neonatal support personnel are needed to attend to a neonate who may be severely compromised and to allow delivery room personnel to attend to the mother.

Treatment. Treatment is largely symptomatic. At the first signs of respiratory distress, oxygen is administered under positive pressure until endotracheal intubation can be accomplished. IV administration of blood components and heparin will be initiated. Close monitoring of cardiopulmonary status is essential; a central venous pressure line should be established to guard against the risk of fluid overload when blood components are being administered; this risk is especially great in the presence of right heart strain or failure. Respiratory and cardiac arrest is common, and cardiopulmonary resuscitation must be initiated immediately.

Implications for Nursing Care

Nursing responsibilities include prompt identification of early symptoms and initiation of emergency care, as discussed previously. Initial nursing actions include administration of oxygen under pressure, alerting staff and obtaining assistance, and monitoring maternal vital signs. This situation is often handled by delivery room staff assisted by the cardiopulmonary resuscitation team because of the complex nature of this emergency. The nurse assists in the emergency procedures described previously.

If the partner or other support persons are present, the nurse should make sure that they are escorted to a place where they can wait and that they are kept informed and supported while emergency care continues. If maternal or fetal death occurs, the nurse should immediately mobilize specialized support for family members, including the chaplain or another spiritual leader and other nursing staff whose attention can be directed solely to the family's needs during this catastrophic experience.

COMPLICATIONS INVOLVING UTERINE FUNCTION

Some of the most common and challenging intrapartal complications are associated with problems in uterine function. Abnormalities in uterine activity can result in dystocia (difficult labor) or preterm labor. Other uterine problems that may arise during labor include uterine rupture, inversion and prolapse, and uterine atony.

Complications Involving Uterine Function

Dystocia (difficult labor)
Preterm labor
Uterine rupture
Uterine inversion
Uterine atony

Preterm Labor and Birth

Etiology, incidence, and outpatient treatment of preterm labor are discussed in Chapter 19. In the event that preterm labor cannot be suppressed by use of bed rest and hydration at home, the woman may be hospitalized for more intensive treatment in an effort to suppress labor and delay delivery of the fetus. The primary mode of inpatient treatment for preterm labor is bed rest, careful monitoring of labor and fetal status, and use of tocolytics to suppress uterine activity.

When the patient is having contractions upon admission, bed rest and hydration with rapid infusion of intravenous fluids will expand blood volume and inhibit oxytocin release. On occasion, this therapy is all that is needed. When electronic monitoring shows that contractions continue to occur at a rate of more than 4 to 6 contractions per hour and/or cervical change is detected, tocolytic therapy is indicated.

Tocolytic Therapy. Various types of drugs have been used to arrest labor when bed rest and hydration prove insufficient. The most common group of tocolytics used are beta sympathomimetics, such as Terbutaline. Other drug categories include CNS depressants (magnesium sulfate and ethanol), calcium channel blockers (nifedipine), and prostaglandin inhibitors (Indocin). Each of these drugs may afford some degree of success, but each has side effects that must be monitored (Table 28–5).

Initiating Tocolytic Therapy. Before initiating therapy, the patient should be made comfortable and baseline maternal and fetal information recorded (see Nursing Alert: Basic Nursing Measures).

Beta Sympathomimetic Therapy. It is important that the patient be attended continuously during the initiation of beta sympathomimetics. Vital signs, FHR, uterine activity, and patient tolerance must be monitored and recorded every 10 to 15 minutes and just prior to the increase in medication dosage. Glucose levels may be ordered and monitored hourly with a dextrometer. The

Table 28–5   **Drugs Used in Treatment of Preterm Labor**

Drug	Dosage/Route/ Action	Maternal Side-Effects	Fetal Side-Effects	Nursing Implications
Ritodrine (Yutopar)	IV: 150 mg in 500 ml fluid yields concentration of 0.3 mg/ml Dosage: 0.05–0.1 mg/min, increasing every 10 min to maximum of 0.35 mg/min or until adequate response obtained Oral: 10 mg every 2 hr for 24 hr (often started 30 min before IV administration is discontinued), then decreased to 10–20 mg every 4–6 hr; not to exceed 120 mg/day Stimulates sympathetic beta 2 receptors; inhibits uterine contractility Metabolized by liver; 70%–90% excreted in urine in 10–12 hr	ECG changes and cardiac arrhythmia; dose-related tachycardia; decreased blood pressure; increased pulse pressure; flushing; sweating; nausea and vomiting; tremors; headache Pulmonary edema (more frequent when used concurrently with corticosteroids and in cases of multiple gestation) Positional hypotension (may be exacerbated by anesthesia) Transient increases in serum insulin, glucose, and free fatty acids; decrease in serum potassium Risk of overdose (signaled by exaggeration of cardiac and other side-effects) Maternal deaths reported (from pulmonary edema)	Drug crosses placenta; increased FHR; hypoglycemia (infrequently); cardiac arrhythmia (occasionally)	Closely observe blood pressure and maternal and fetal heart rates; maternal heart rate should not exceed 130 bpm. Check apical heart rate for arrhythmia. Observe closely for signs of pulmonary edema; monitor input and output; maintain fluid restrictions. Ritodrine therapy may unmask occult heart disease and must be used with caution in hypertensive, diabetic, and preeclamptic patients. Drug is contraindicated with active bleeding. Obtain maternal serum potassium, glucose, and ECG baselines before initiating IV therapy.
Betamethasone (Celestone) Dexamethasone Hydrocortisone Methylprednisolone	IM: 12 mg every 24 hr for two doses IM: 5 mg every 24 hr for two doses IV: 500 mg every 24 hr for two doses IM: 125 mg every 24 hr for two doses Increases lung maturity in fetus expected to be delivered preterm Thought to bind with glucocorticoid receptors in alveolar cells to increase production of surfactant Peak effect 48 hr after first dose; lasts 7 days	Increased white blood count; possibly decreased resistance to infection; increased risk of pulmonary edema if used concurrently with betamimetic therapy for preterm labor Possible production or exacerbation of maternal hypertension	Potential for fetal demise secondary to maternal HTN or placental insufficiency No documented long-term effects	All listed compounds *except* hydrocortisone are suspensions for IM use only; IV use is contraindicated. Monitor mother closely for signs of infection; ruptured membranes may be a relative contraindication, since medication may mask signs of developing infection.
Terbutaline (Brethine, Bricanyl): experimental — not currently approved by FDA for use as tocolytic	IV: 5 mg/500 ml fluid Initiate at rate of 1 mg/min to maximum of 8 mg/min; continue 8 to 12 hr; then subcutaneously 0.25 mg every 4 hr for 24 hr May be given orally for home management: 2.5 mg every 4 to 6 hr	Similar to those of ritodrine, but more severe	Similar to those of ritodrine	Similar to those of ritodrine

(continued)

Table 28–5   **Drugs Used in Treatment of Preterm Labor** (continued)

Drug	Dosage/Route/ Action	Maternal Side-Effects	Fetal Side-Effects	Nursing Implications
	Beta-adrenergic agent; supresses uterine contractility Partially metabolized by liver; excreted through gastrointestinal tract and kidneys			
$MgSO_4$	IV: 4 g loading dose in 100 to 250 ml of 5% dextrose in water (infused slowly at a rate 3–10 ml/min) Follow with maintenance dose of 1 to 4 g/hr to maintain uterine relaxation Standard solution is 20–40 g of $MgSO_4$ in 1000 ml of IV solution.	Central nervous system depression, skeletal and smooth muscle relaxation, resulting in: drowsiness, lethargy, ptosis, blurred vision, slurred speech, muscular weakness and generalized hypotonia, respiratory depression or paralysis, loss of deep tendon reflexes Vasodilation, resulting in: flushing, feeling of warmth, hypotension and possible cardiovascular collapse Other side-effects: nausea and increased thirst Pulmonary edema has been associated with $MgSO_4$ tocolysis. Exact etiology is unknown.	Possible decrease in FHR variability in preterm fetus	Monitor maternal vital signs closely during loading dose. Monitor maternal vital signs, DTRs, urinary output every 30 min to 1 hr until stable serum therapeutic level is achieved (4–7.5 mEq liter) Then monitor vital signs, as ordered, when client is stable. Notify physician of • Respirations <12/min • Urinary output <25–30 ml/hr • Absent DTRs • Signs of toxicity: increasing lethargy, hypotonia, hypotension, extreme thirst Limit intake to prevent pulmonary edema (usually 2000 to 3000 ml/24 hr). Have resuscitation equipment at bedside. Have antidote, 10% calcium gluconate, at bedside. Provide for continuous EFM and toco monitoring Prepare client for common side-effects of drug. Obtain serum Mg levels, as ordered.

patient should be advised of probable feelings of anxiety and observed for tremors, palpitations, sweating, and nervousness. Adverse cardiovascular reactions may limit the amount of medication that can be safely administered (see Nursing Alert: Beta Sympathomimetic Therapy). Hypotension may be corrected by:

• Displacing the uterus off the major vessels by repositioning the patient
• Elevating the patient's legs

• Increasing the intravenous fluid rate
• Decreasing or stopping the tocolytic infusion

A rapid respiratory rate and labored breathing may indicate developing pulmonary edema. The nurse should auscultate the lungs for rales and rhonchi hourly, or as indicated. Total fluid intake may be restricted to 2500 ml per day with 1500 ml limit for intravenous intake. A strict record of intake and output should be recorded for the

NURSING ALERT

Basic Nursing Measures Applicable to Labor Suppression Therapy

- Patient is on complete bed rest in the lateral position.
- External fetal monitor and pressure transducer are applied.
- Baseline vital signs, weight, and FHT are obtained.
- Clean-catch or catheterized urine for culture is obtained.
- Orders for cervical and vaginal cultures and lab studies, including CBC with differential, electrolytes, glucose, and blood type and hold, should be anticipated.
- An intravenous line using a large-bore indwelling catheter, microdrip, and infusion pump is established.

first 24 hours of therapy, and the patient weighed daily to prevent late detection of fluid overload.

Once a maintenance dose has been achieved and contractions cease, the tocolytic dose will be decreased to the lowest effective level. The physician may order an intramuscular or oral dose 30 minutes before discontinuing the intravenous tocolytic. If contractions do not resume and the patient tolerates the medication, she will be discharged on a maintenance oral dose until 36 or 37 weeks gestation. If contractions are not controlled with oral tocolytics, the patient may be discharged with a subcutaneous infusion pump for continuous therapeutic levels. Perinatal services which offer at-home infusion pumps also provide home care by perinatal nurses for continued monitoring of the patient and the safe use of tocolytic infusion.

Magnesium Sulfate.   Nursing care of the patient receiving magnesium sulfate is similar to that discussed

NURSING ALERT

Adverse Cardiopulmonary Reactions to Beta Sympathomimetic Therapy

Report the following findings to a physician immediately:

- Heart rate that exceeds 120 beats/min
- Systolic blood pressure level of <90 mm Hg
- Respiratory rate >30/min
- Shortness of breath, chest tightness, or pain

under beta sympathomimetics. Additionally, baselines for patellar reflexes and level of consciousness should be established by the physician, and the nurse should monitor the patient every 15 minutes for evidence of further depression of these signs (see Table 28–5).

Patency of the intravenous line must be carefully attended to because magnesium sulfate is extremely irritating to the tissue. If contractions cease with the use of magnesium sulfate, it is usually discontinued in 10 to 12 hours. With termination of magnesium sulfate, the patient will be maintained on oral beta sympathomimetic therapy, as described previously.

Ethanol.   Although this drug has primarily been replaced by beta sympathomimetics and magnesium sulfate, it is still applicable in some instances. The focus of nursing care is on continuous monitoring of mother and fetus, as described previously, and on providing a safe environment for the patient. The potential danger is maternal aspiration secondary to nausea and vomiting. Additionally, the patient may become confused and disoriented. Side rails should be up and padded, and the patient should be in view of the nurse at all times.

Before beginning therapy, the patient should be advised of the inebriating effects of ethanol. Observe the patient for the common side effects of nausea, vomiting, crying, restlessness, and urinary incontinence. As with magnesium sulfate, the patient's vital signs should be monitored for depression and reported to the physician immediately. Ethanol infusion is usually discontinued within 10 hours after contractions have ceased. If contractions recur within the 10-hour period, a loading dose is prepared and the patient begins another course of ethanol. As with all tocolytic therapy, if labor continues and delivery becomes imminent, preparations for delivery of a depressed infant are essential, since these drugs freely cross the placenta.

Experimental Drugs in Tocolytic Therapy: Calcium Channel Blockers.   Calcium channel blockers are being tested for effectiveness in tocolytic therapy. These medications inhibit utilization of calcium by smooth muscle, which inhibits contraction. Nifedipine is being used experimentally in some areas in combination with beta sympathomimetic agents. Side-effects include headache, flushing, pedal edema, and significant maternal hypotension.

Preparations for Preterm Delivery.   When preterm labor is advanced or is unresponsive to tocolysis, the health care team must prepare for delivery of a preterm infant. Several factors affect how preterm delivery is managed to optimize the chances for a viable neonate. An important factor is *fetal lung maturity* and the risk of *respiratory distress syndrome* (RDS).

If fetal lung immaturity is confirmed by a phosphati-

LEGAL/ETHICAL CONSIDERATIONS

Aggressive Management of Preterm Labor Between 23 and 26 Weeks of Gestation

Recent technologic advances make possible the survival of very low birth weight preterm infants. However, the possibility of long-term multisystem deficits (particularly neurological and cardiopulmonary) makes decision making regarding aggressive management of preterm labor between 23 and 26 weeks gestation difficult. Both legal and ethical dilemmas confront the birth attendant and nurse caring for women who present in irreversible labor in the late second trimester.

Central to the issue of management is the tremendous uncertainty regarding the final outcome for the very preterm infant; infants of the same gestational age and weight will experience very different postnatal outcomes. Moreover, women may present in advanced stages of labor and there may not be time to provide them with the information they require to make rational decisions regarding treatment options for the neonate. The nurse may be asked to implement care that she finds morally or philosophically objectionable.

It is crucial to include parents in the decision-making process and to encourage them to voice concerns, fears, and questions. It is often the primary nurse who is in the best position to help parents view issues from various perspectives. Recognizing the importance of parent preference is more likely to lead to a decision with which parents and care-givers will ultimately feel comfortable, regardless of the outcome.

Gates E: Obstetrical decision making in the delivery of the extremely premature infant. Neonatal Network 8:7–14, 1986

dylglycerol (PG) and lecithin/sphingomyelin (L/S) test, the physician may elect to administer corticosteroids (betamethasone) to the mother to enhance the process of fetal lung maturity and reduce the risk of RDS. Fetal lung maturation is known to occur more rapidly in response to maternal stress; corticosteroid administration mimics the physiologic stress response. To be responsive to this therapy, the fetus must be between 28 and 34 weeks of gestation and delivery must be delayed 24 to 48 hours. The fetal side effects and long-term consequences of fetal steroid treatment are not known; however, the risks of RDS are considered to outweigh these possible problems.

Another factor that must be considered in the manage-

ment of preterm labor is *membrane status*. Premature rupture of membranes occurs in 20% to 30% of cases of preterm labor. If membranes have been ruptured for 24 hours, a natural acceleration of lung maturity may occur, making the use of corticosteroids unnecessary. Further, since the anti-inflammatory action of corticosteroids suppresses signs of developing infection, it may mask early signs of chorioamnionitis and thus present more risk than benefit for patients with ruptured membranes.

Finally, *maternal and fetal status* must be considered. When preterm labor is a response to chorioamnionitis, suppression of labor is considered unwise for both mother and fetus. If the pregnancy is allowed to continue, the mother is at increasing risk for sepsis associated with the progressive intrauterine infection. The fetus is at risk while in the infected uterine environment and should be delivered in a tertiary care setting where intensive neonatal support is available. If maternal transport is necessary, labor may be suppressed long enough to ensure safe transport. Other maternal diseases, such as preeclampsia or severe renal or cardiovascular disease, may contraindicate labor suppression when both maternal and fetal status is threatened. In these circumstances maternal status will not improve until delivery, and the fetus may have a better chance of survival in an intensive care unit than in the unfavorable maternal environment.

The delivery itself is managed to minimize risk to the especially vulnerable premature infant. Use of analgesia is minimized to avoid further compromising respiratory efforts and the immature metabolism of the neonate. Rupture of the membranes is delayed until cervical dilatation of 6 cm or more has occurred, if possible, to afford additional protection for the soft skull of the preterm infant and to avoid additional risk of cord prolapse.

The fetal head is further protected by use of a generous episiotomy to avoid perineal pressure; outlet forceps may also be used to retract maternal soft tissue and guide the head over the perineum. Delivery must be attended by a neonatal support team skilled in providing immediate care to the preterm infant.

Implications for Nursing Care

Nursing responsibilities in providing care to the woman with preterm labor center on monitoring uterine activity and fetal status; monitoring maternal vital signs and intake and output while tocolytic therapy continues; and providing comfort measures and emotional support to the woman on bed rest and her partner.

The nurse assists in determining precise fetal age, based on information from the prenatal record (calculation of gestational age from LMP, measurement of fundal height, early sonogram reports, date of quickening, and first date of audible fetal heart tones). Sterile vaginal examination upon admission is necessary to determine cervical dilatation and effacement and membrane status. If membranes are shown to be ruptured, amniotic fluid may be aspirated to ascertain lung maturity. The nurse then minimizes vaginal examinations and helps the patient to maintain perineal hygiene and prevent ascending infection. A clean-catch urine specimen should be collected, since urinary tract infection is frequently associated with preterm labor. The nurse may also be ordered to initiate an IV line to hydrate the patient, since maternal dehydration is also associated with preterm labor.

The nurse then initiates close monitoring of uterine activity. External EFM is used to document the quality and frequency of uterine contractions. However, the nurse must remember that the tocodynamometer does not always accurately graph the onset and intensity of preterm labor contractions; thus, the nurse must ask the patient to indicate the onset of contractions so that information can be noted on the graphic strip, and she should also determine the intensity of the contraction by palpation to compare her own observation with the information about the strength of contractions provided on the monitor strip. If tocolytic therapy is initiated, the nurse must carefully monitor maternal vital signs, intake and output, and mental/emotional status throughout the course of therapy. The nurse must also educate the woman and her partner about potential side effects of the medication.

If labor cannot be suppressed, the nurse should inform the woman and her partner about preparations for delivery and care of the neonate. The nurse should assess the family's understanding of prematurity and provide anticipatory guidance about the preterm infant's appearance, needs, and care. The nurse should initiate parental contact with neonatal nursing staff as early as possible so that the process of parent–infant acquaintance after delivery can be facilitated (see Chapter 34 for nursing care of parents with high-risk neonates).

Uterine Problems

In addition to preterm labor and dystocia, which are complications reflected primarily in the pattern and timing of uterine contractions, the intrapartal patient may develop other uterine complications that involve trauma to the uterus or present the risk of excessive uterine bleeding immediately after delivery. Uterine trauma during the intrapartal period may occur as *uterine rupture* during labor or *inversion and prolapse of the uterus* soon after delivery. Absence of muscular contraction or *uterine atony* immediately after delivery predisposes the mother to excessive intrauterine bleeding and postpartum hemorrhage. Each of these problems may be life threatening if not detected and treated promptly.

Uterine Rupture

Rupture of the uterus during labor is potentially an obstetric catastrophe that threatens both mother and fetus (Fig. 28–12). Although uterine rupture is rare in the United States, occurring in approximately 1 in 1500 deliveries, it is more common in underdeveloped countries where home deliveries are the norm and obstetric care is limited. Even though improved obstetric management has improved maternal and fetal outcomes after uterine rupture, it is still responsible for 5% of all maternal deaths. When uterine rupture occurs, 50% of all instances result in fetal demise (Pritchard and Macdonald 1985).

Rupture of the uterus can be complete or incomplete. Complete rupture extends through the entire uterine wall, and the uterine contents are extruded into the abdominal cavity. Incomplete rupture extends through the endometrium and myometrium, but the peritoneum surrounding the uterus remains intact. Uterine rupture often occurs in the thinned-out lower uterine segment. Incomplete tears may occur along previous uterine scars. Another term used synonymously with incomplete rupture is *dehiscence,* the bursting open of a surgical scar.

Etiologic and Predisposing Factors. The most common predisposing factor for traumatic uterine rupture is a preexisting scar, which results in a weakening or defect in the myometrium that does not stretch as well as surrounding tissue. Rupture is considered more likely from a vertical (classic) cesarean incision; low transverse uterine incisions from previous cesarean deliveries are not as prone to rupture and thus do not preclude a subsequent normal labor (see Chapter 26 on vaginal birth after a cesarean delivery).

Rupture of the pregnant uterus may be classified as traumatic or spontaneous; either type can occur in the presence or absence of a uterine scar. *Traumatic uterine rupture* is usually associated with a previous uterine scar and the application of excessive force to the labor, sometimes from imprudent obstetric interference. Causes of traumatic uterine rupture include the following:

- Trauma from instruments (such as use of a uterine sound or curette or tools used to induce abortion)
- Obstetric intervention:
  Forceps delivery
  High vacuum extraction
  Excessive fundal pressure
  Tumultuous labor
  Violent bearing-down efforts
  Internal podalic version
  Forceps rotation
  Shoulder dystocia

(text continued on page 834)

NURSING CARE PLAN

The Woman in Preterm Labor

Nursing Diagnosis (Patient Problem) and Assessment Data	Nursing Interventions	Rationale
Complication: *preterm labor*		
• Pregnancy of 20 to 36 weeks of gestation	Place in Trendelenburg position or on bed rest on left side.	Trendelenburg position relieves pressure of presenting part on cervix. Bed rest will increase uterine perfusion, decrease uterine irritability, and calm patient, allowing for accurate assessment.
• Uterine contractions leading to cervical effacement and dilatation	Notify physician.	
• Significant cervical change (2 cm dilatation and 80% effacement) despite intact membranes		
• Reported feelings of pelvic pressure, backache, or cramping; diarrhea, or increased vaginal discharge	Maintain hydration by 300 ml IV fluid load	Dehydration causes oxytocin release by the pituitary, promoting contractions. Preterm labor contractions will stop with bed rest and hydration 50% of the time. A fluid load is required before initiation of tocolytic therapy if contractions do not stop.
	Test vaginal discharge for amniotic fluid with Nitrazine paper	Spontaneous rupture of membranes is positive indicator of preterm labor and will affect future management.
	Admit patient to high-risk unit:	
	• Obtain health history	One of the greatest risk factors for preterm labor is a prior history of preterm.
	• Obtain prenatal labor record for LMP, complications, allergies, and previous tests.	
	Assess patient's reason for suspecting preterm labor or rupture of membranes. If premature labor is suspected, use only sterile speculum exams.	
	If bleeding is present, do not allow vaginal exams unless prepared to perform an emergency cesarean delivery.	
	If PROM has occurred, perform sterile speculum exams.	Reduce the risk of introducing infection into uterus.
		Bleeding is a symptom of placenta previa; a vaginal exam could perforate the placenta and create an immediate emergency for the fetus and mother.
	Cervical examination is done on admission, then only when absolutely necessary.	Vaginal exam must be done to determine cervical changes.
		Frequent exams may induce infection.
	Facilitate lab tests:	To rule out infection. Urinary tract infections increase uterine irritability
	• CBC	

(continued)

NURSING CARE PLAN

The Woman in Preterm Labor (continued)

Nursing Diagnosis (Patient Problem) and Assessment Data	Nursing Interventions	Rationale
	• Urinalysis	and are a contributing factor in preterm labor.
	Prepare for possibility of: • Ultrasound • Amniocentesis	Ultrasound and amniocentesis may be ordered to verify gestational age and fetal lung maturity.
	• Tocolytic drug therapy • Steroid therapy	Tocolytic drugs inhibit uterine activity.
	Assess gestational age of fetus.	Accurate history taking from the patient, such as LMP, provides information necessary to determine fetal viability.

Expected Outcome:

Patient responds to appropriate treatment as evidenced by cessation of preterm labor signs.

Potential Complication:
fetal distress, as a result of preterm labor

	Initiate fetal monitoring.	To document frequency and duration of contractions and monitor fetal status.
		Some drugs used for treatment of preterm labor may affect the fetus. Fetus well-being is a criteria for continued management of preterm labor.
	Administer O$_2$ 8–12 liter/min by mask.	To optimize fetal oxygenation.

Expected Outcome:

Fetus responds to treatment as evidenced by normal monitoring results and pregnancy continues.

Nursing Diagnosis:
fear related to increased perinatal risk

	Discuss the plan of care with patient. Provide explanations as procedures are initiated. Provide emotional support to patient and family.	Decreases the patient's fears and increases patient's ability to participate in care.

(continued)

NURSING CARE PLAN

The Woman in Preterm Labor (continued)

Nursing Diagnosis (Patient Problem) and Assessment Data	Nursing Interventions	Rationale
	Assist patient and her family to ventilate feelings concerning preterm labor, anxiety, hospitalization, ambivalence about the pregnancy, or the lack of mobility.	A variety of emotions can be expected from patient and family.
	Assess parents for symptoms of grief or crisis. Provide grief counseling, crisis intervention, or referrals to appropriate counselors.	The stress of preterm labor can initiate a family crisis. Families without support may be prone to a crisis.
	If gestational age is less than 28 weeks, assist patient to verbalize desires concerning medical management to prevent premature delivery.	If extreme measures must be taken to prevent preterm labor, the patient should be informed of the benefits and risks of the medical management. Viability of the fetus can be a determining factor for the patient, particularly if life-style changes must be maintained for the duration of the pregnancy.
	Arrange for neonatal intensive care nurse or neonatologist to speak with both parents about what to expect from their preterm baby.	Anxiety may be lessened if the parents know what to expect from their baby.

Expected Outcome:

Patient verbalizes her fears and appreciation of staff support, further demonstrated by her cooperation with staff in care. The patient and her family experience a reduction in grief and anxiety as evidenced by verbalization of feeling less depressed/anxious, verbalization of understanding of medical procedures and expected neonatal outcome, and relaxed facial expressions.

Potential Complications Related to Tocolytic Therapy

Assess for contraindications: • Acute hemorrhage • Severe preeclampsia/eclampsia • Chorioamnionitis • Maternal cardiac disease • Pulmonary hypertension • Maternal hyperthyroidism • Uncontrolled diabetes • Fetal demise	If contraindications are present, prepare for management of high-risk premature labor and delivery: • Notify neonatology and anesthesia departments and pediatrician. • Manage labor and delivery according to standard of care. Explain to patient the reason for not prolonging pregnancy.	Contraindications to halting premature labor will increase the risk to mother and fetus, necessitating a team effort for optimal outcome.

(continued)

NURSING CARE PLAN

The Woman in Preterm Labor (continued)

Nursing Diagnosis (Patient Problem) and Assessment Data	Nursing Interventions	Rationale
	If no contraindications are present, administer tocolytic drugs as ordered by physician.	Maternal death can result from pulmonary edema.
	Calculate intake and output hourly.	Significant discrepancies between intake and output should be reported to physician.
	Monitor for signs and symptoms of pulmonary edema.	Shortness of breath or adventitious lung sounds should also be reported.
	Monitor maternal response to tocolysis.	A large number of patients report some side-effect to tocolysis. Toxicity may be indicated by an increasing maternal heart rate. Maternal heart should be below 140.
	If IV magnesium sulfate is administered, use IV pump for accurate measurement of drug fluid intake. Use hospital protocol for use of magnesium sulfate. Auscultate lung fields every hour. Check DTRs every hour. Calculate intake and output every hour. Draw blood labs as ordered to monitor for therapeutic level of the drug.	Overdosage may cause respiratory depression or cardiac arrest. The action of magnesium sulfate is not fully understood, but the therapeutic dose is 6–7 mEq/liter. Heart block or respiratory depression may result at higher serum levels.
	Start IV; run 300-ml fluid load	Fluid load decreases the hypotensive effect of tocolytic drugs, caused by peripheral vasodilation.
	Facilitate lab tests; glucose and electrolyte level, blood chemistry tests.	
	Obtain baseline ECG.	To monitor later ECG changes
	Regulate tocolytic drug via infusion pump.	
	Obtain protocol or doctor's order for specific procedure and guidelines:	The most commonly used drugs are betamimetics, such as ritodrine hydrochloride (Yutopar), isoxsuprine (Vasodilan), and terbutaline.
	• Check vital signs and intake/output every 15 min while increasing drug dose; hourly while patient is on maintenance dose.	Magnesium sulfate is also used to arrest labor. Institutional guidelines vary.

Nursing Diagnosis:
possible decreased maternal cardiac output

• Pulmonary edema	Monitor for adverse effects from	

(continued)

NURSING CARE PLAN

The Woman in Preterm Labor (continued)

Nursing Diagnosis (Patient Problem) and Assessment Data	Nursing Interventions	Rationale
• Ineffective breathing pattern secondary to magnesium sulfate toxicity	tocolytic drug therapy: • Maternal tachycardia: >130 bpm (betamimetics) • Severe hypotension • ECG changes indicative of myocardial ischemia • Pulmonary edema • Patient intolerance • Respiratory arrest ($MgSO_4$)	
	• Observe closely for side-effects: tremors, maternal and fetal tachycardia, headache, palpitations, anxiety, nausea/vomiting, hypotension, or widening pulse pressure	These side-effects are a normal response to beta adrenergic stimulation.
	Facilitate magnesium sulfate ($MgSO_4$) therapy if ordered: • Initiate drug dose as ordered; monitor reflexes and magnesium level every 8 hr × 4 or prn.	Magnesium toxicity is indicated by the absence of reflex response or by respirations below 10/min.
	If adverse effects occur: • Notify physician. • Discontinue drug • Provide physiologic support.	Untoward effects may result in morbidity. Selection of an alternative method may be necessary

Expected Outcome:

Patient experiences uneventful labor and birth and delivers a viable, stable, preterm neonate.

Nursing Diagnosis:
potential fluid volume excess

• Pulmonary edema related to steroid therapy.	Note that steroid therapy is contraindicated if delivery is anticipated in 24 to 48 hr.	Administration of steroids too close to delivery may mask signs of infection in the newborn.
	Administer drug as ordered *promptly* (Betamethasone 12 mg IM × two doses).	Steroids are most effective in increasing fetal lung maturation 48 hr after the first dose.

(continued)

NURSING CARE PLAN

The Woman in Preterm Labor (continued)

Nursing Diagnosis (Patient Problem) and Assessment Data	Nursing Interventions	Rationale
	Observe for side-effects: • Increased incidence of pulmonary edema when used with betamimetics. • Elevation of maternal WBC. • Increased incidence of infection. Monitor intake and output. Restrict 24 hr intake to 2400 cc when steroids combined with tocolytics.	Prompt treatment is imperative for optimal effect. Therapy is effective for 7 to 10 days after administration. To decrease risk of pulmonary edema.

Expected Outcome:

Patient experiences no complications related to medical management of preterm labor, as evidenced by equivalent intake and output, clear lung sounds, and adequate DTRs, and maintains pregnancy, or if therapy fails, after uneventful labor and birth, delivers a viable, stable preterm neonate.

Nursing Diagnosis:
diversional activity deficit related to hospitalization and bed rest

• Restlessness • Expressed boredom • Inability to maintain bed rest	Provide diversion if possible while the mother is hospitalized. If patient is discharged on PO tocolytics, review the signs and symptoms of preterm labor with her. Review when patient should contact health care provider. Inform of possible side-effects of tocolysis (rapid heart rate, anxiety). Review restrictions set by physician, such as strict bed rest or no sexual activity. Assist with problem solving related to activity restriction at home.	Depression and ambivalence may make compliance with preterm labor management difficult. Diversion may lessen these emotions. For successful intervention of preterm labor, the patient must seek medical attention before cervical dilation reaches 4–5 cm. Compliance of the prescribed medical management depends upon the patient's understanding of the regimen.

Expected Outcome:

Patient copes with decreased mobility as evidenced by statement of decreased boredom through increased quiet activities, verbalization of acceptance of bed rest regimen, or verbalization of understanding rationale for decreased mobility.

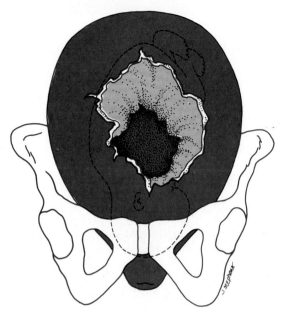

Figure 28–12. Uterine rupture. (Childbirth Graphics)

Induced uterine hypertonicity from oxytocin infusion
Manual removal of the placenta (rare)

Spontaneous uterine rupture before the onset of labor is rare. During labor it is most likely to occur under the following conditions:

- Previous uterine surgery, such as low-segment cesarean section, myomectomy, salpingectomy, curettage, or manual removal of the placenta
- Grand multiparity combined with the use of oxytocic agents to stimulate labor
- Cephalopelvic disproportion, malpresentation, or hydrocephalus

Uterine rupture that occurs in the absence of a scar is often an obstetric emergency. Maternal death from hemorrhage and shock may occur. On the other hand, uterine dehiscence or small ruptures may actually go undetected. Signs that reflect an abnormal thinning of the uterine wall may signal an impending uterine rupture. These signs include those listed in the display on the opposite page.

Symptoms of actual rupture may appear immediately or may not appear until the postpartum period, when anesthesia or sedation has worn off. This reflects the fact that signs and symptoms of uterine rupture may vary from very mild to severe and acute. Factors that determine when symptoms appear and their severity include the following:

- Site and extent of the rupture
- Degree of extrusion of the uterine contents
- Occurrence or absence of intraperitoneal spill of amniotic fluid and blood

Complete ruptures, those involving both the lower uterine segment and the body of the uterus, and those in which extrusion is marked or there is intraperitoneal spill are usually associated with rapid onset of severe symptoms. However, symptoms of uterine rupture are often difficult to differentiate from those of other pathologic events. Patients in labor may report an internal tearing sensation, which may or may not be painful, just before the actual rupture; this may be the most characteristic symptom of uterine rupture.

The most common symptom of uterine rupture is diffuse pain or pain localized to the umbilical and epigastric region, which may be referred to the shoulder (reflecting diaphragmatic irritation). Patients who have experienced uterine rupture prior to the onset of labor may experience continuous or intermittent pain that may easily be confused with labor.

When diagnosis of uterine rupture is not clear on the basis of these clinical signs, other diagnostic tests may be used. X-ray films of the abdomen may show the fetus lying abnormally high and outside the uterus. Free fluid or air may be seen in the abdominal cavity. Ultrasonography may show the absence of the amniotic cavity within the uterus. Culdocentesis (aspiration of fluid through the posterior vaginal fornix) may reveal the presence of blood in the abdominal cavity.

Maternal Implications.   Maternal risks associated with uterine rupture depend on the extent of the injury. Small tears may be asymptomatic; they may heal spontaneously and remain undetected until subsequent labor strains the scar, resulting in more serious damage. More severe ruptures present the risk of irreversible maternal hypovolemic shock or subsequent peritonitis.

Fetal Implications.   Maternal hypovolemia and fetal extrusion out of the uterus through the rupture with loss of placental circulation present major risks to the fetus. Anoxia is very common, and fetal or neonatal death occurs in 50% to 75% of all cases of complete rupture. Survival depends on prompt surgical delivery and immediate neonatal resuscitation.

Treatment.   Vaginal delivery is generally not attempted if signs of possible uterine rupture are present, since vaginal delivery will present greater risks to both mother and fetus. If symptoms of uterine rupture are not severe, an emergency cesarean delivery may be attempted with repair of the uterine tear, if possible. If symptoms of uterine rupture are severe, emergency laparotomy will be performed to attempt immediate delivery of the fetus, establish hemostasis, and allow for surgical repair of the uterus. The first concern is to monitor maternal status and to correct maternal hypovolemic shock, if present. The following procedures will be implemented in preparation for surgery:

NURSING ALERT

Signs and Symptoms in Uterine Rupture

Signs and Symptoms of Impending Uterine Rupture

- Restlessness, anxiety, severe lower abdominal pain
- Lack of progress in cervical dilatation or fetal descent
- Presence of a palpable ridge of uterus above the symphysis pubis or a retraction ring (indentation across the lower abdominal wall) between upper and lower uterine segments with acute tenderness above the symphysis
- Tetanic contractions

Signs and Symptoms of Incomplete Uterine Rupture

- Tenderness or pain in the abdomen associated with increasing uterine irritability prior to the onset of labor
- Small amounts of vaginal bleeding
- Persistence and intensification of abdominal pain and tenderness as labor progresses
- Restlessness and anxiety

- Rebound tenderness of the abdomen
- Abdominal distention beyond that expected in normal pregnancy
- Appearance of a retraction ring across the lower abdomen
- Thinning and ballooning of the lower uterine segment, similar in appearance to a full bladder
- Lack of progress in cervical dilatation

Signs and Symptoms of Complete Uterine Rupture

- Intense, sharp, tearing pain in the lower abdomen
- Palpation of fetal parts outside the uterine wall
- Abrupt cessation of uterine contractions
- Ascent of presenting part on vaginal examination relative to previous position
- Gross hematuria from bladder damage
- Rapid onset of signs of fetal distress or cessation of fetal heart tones
- Progressive signs of maternal hypovolemic shock

- Continuous monitoring of maternal blood pressure, pulse, and respirations and fetal heart rate, if present
- Institution of a central venous pressure catheter to permit assessment of blood loss and to monitor effects of fluid and blood replacement
- Insertion of an indwelling urinary catheter for precise evaluation of fluid balance
- Immediate blood studies to assess maternal acidosis
- Administration of oxygen and maintenance of an open airway

Surgical priorities will be to attempt to deliver the fetus before death ensues and to stop maternal hemorrhage. If uterine rupture is complete, the only hope for the fetus is prompt surgical delivery. The type of surgical procedure required will vary according to the extent of uterine damage. A repair of the uterine tear may be attempted, or hysterectomy may be required. Hysterectomy may be lifesaving for the mother if bleeding cannot otherwise be controlled.

Implications for Nursing Care

Nursing responsibilities begin with identification of maternal factors that may predispose a patient to uterine rupture and close monitoring of the labor pattern to iden-

tify uterine hypertonicity or signs of a weakening uterine muscle. The nurse must recognize signs of impending or overt uterine rupture and institute appropriate care by alerting the physician and calling for assistance, closely monitoring maternal and fetal status, taking steps to prevent or limit hypovolemic shock (see Shock earlier in this chapter), and preparing the patient for surgery. The nurse must respond in a calm, efficient manner and provide reassurance and support to the mother and her partner, explaining briefly what has happened and what can be anticipated. Once surgery has begun, the nurse should see that the partner and family members have staff support and are told when they will receive information about mother and neonate.

Uterine Inversion

Inversion of the uterus is a rare but dramatic complication occurring in between 1 in 2,000 and 1 in 12,000 deliveries. Uterine inversion occurs immediately following delivery of the placenta or in the immediate postpartum period and is evidenced by the uterus's turning either partially or completely inside out. Types of uterine inversion are characterized by the degree and the type of force causing the inversion; see the accompanying display on page 836.

Types of Uterine Inversion

- Complete inversion—collapse of the entire uterus through the cervix into the vagina
- Incomplete or partial inversion—inversion of the fundus, without extension beyond the external cervical os
- Forced inversion—inversion caused by excessive pulling of the cord or vigorous manual expression of the placenta or clots from an atonic uterus
- Spontaneous inversion—inversion due to increased abdominal pressure because of bearing down, coughing, or sudden abdominal muscle contraction

When uterine inversion is incomplete, it may only be detected when there is postpartum hemorrhage and the fundus cannot be palpated abdominally (Fig. 28–13) or when bimanual examination reveals a cup-shaped mass in the vagina. A completely inverted uterus will be seen as a bluish gray mass filling the vagina and extending from the vaginal orifice. In either case, early diagnosis is essential. Hemorrhage may result and, if untreated, lead to hypovolemic shock and death. In addition, early diagnosis allows prompt reinversion of the uterus and decreases the probability of long-term problems. When uterine replacement is delayed, the cervix becomes increasingly edematous and constricts around the body of the uterus, making reinversion difficult or impossible (Creasy and Resnik 1984).

Etiologic and Predisposing Factors.   Uterine inversion may be related to fundal implantation of the placenta. Thinning of the uterine wall at the placental site may allow invagination of the myometrium as the placenta separates, initiating the inversion process. Factors that predispose to uterine inversion include the following:

- Straining of the patient after delivery
- Precipitous delivery with patient in standing position
- Traction of the umbilical cord prior to placental separation

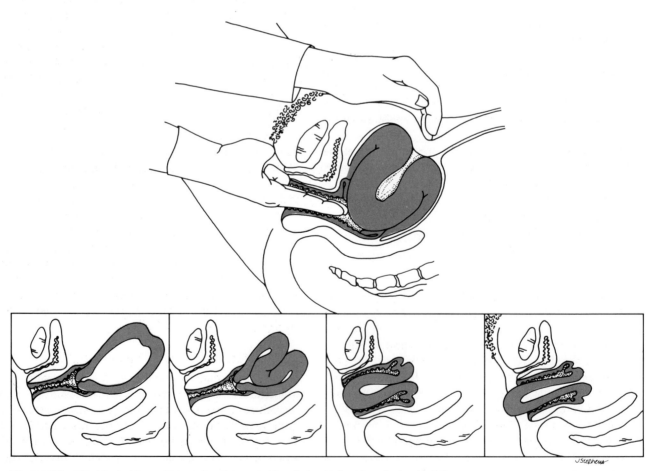

Figure 28–13. Uterine inversion can be diagnosed by abdominal and vaginal palpation. Lower diagrams show progressive degrees of inversion from slight to complete. (Childbirth Graphics)

- Vigorous kneading of the fundus to cause placental separation and expulsion
- Excessive manual pressure on the fundus — for example, during fundal massage
- Delivery of an infant with a coiled or short umbilical cord
- Manual separation and extraction of the placenta
- Rapid delivery with multiple gestation, or rapid release of excessive amniotic fluid

Maternal Implications.   When uterine inversion occurs, the unanesthetized patient will experience excruciating pain in conjunction with a sensation of extreme fullness extending into the vagina. Immediate manual replacement of the uterus at that time by the physician or nurse midwife will prevent its entrapment by the cervix. If reinversion is not promptly performed, blood loss may be rapid and extreme, resulting in hypovolemic shock.

Treatment.   Early diagnosis of uterine inversion should be followed by immediate measures to prevent hypovolemic shock (see Shock earlier in this chapter). The birth attendant will immediately attempt to replace the uterus manually in its normal position. When the uterus is successfully replaced, oxytocin is administered to stimulate uterine tone and avoid recurring inversion. If the inversion is complete, the attendant will keep a fist within the uterine cavity until the oxytocic drug causes the uterus to become well contracted. Antibiotic therapy may be initiated to prevent or minimize the risk of infection from exposure of the uterine lining and extensive manipulation.

If hypovolemic shock develops, late replacement of the uterus is delayed until the patient's condition is stabilized following blood and fluid replacement. General anesthesia may be needed to relax the uterus sufficiently to allow late replacement. In rare instances the uterus cannot be reinverted and emergency hysterectomy is necessary to prevent profound blood loss.

Implications for Nursing Care

The nurse is usually responsible for close patient monitoring during the third and fourth stages of labor; thus, the nurse must be alert for symptoms of uterine inversion. If the patient complains of pelvic pain and vaginal fullness or shows a dramatic increase in vaginal bleeding accompanied by increasing pulse and other signs of impending hemorrhage, the nurse must immediately institute steps to counteract hypovolemic shock and obtain help from other staff. The nurse assists the attendant in the attempt to replace the uterus, manually monitors maternal status, and administers fluid and oxytocin, as ordered. If manual replacement is not successful, the nurse must prepare the patient and the family for administration of general anesthesia and possible surgery.

Uterine Atony

Uterine atony is failure of the uterine muscle to contract after delivery. It is the most common cause of postpartum hemorrhage, accounting for 80% to 90% of episodes of excessive postpartum bleeding.

Etiologic and Predisposing Factors.   After delivery the uterus normally contracts, controlling bleeding by clamping severed blood vessels at the site of placental separation. Inadequate myometrial contraction permits patency of the vessels and the free flow of blood.

Predisposing factors in uterine atony include the following:

- General anesthesia
- Overdistention of the uterus as a result of hydramnios, a large fetus, or multiple gestation
- Previous hemorrhage from atony
- Prolonged or rapid labor
- High parity
- Vigorous oxytocin stimulation during labor

Maternal Implications.   Severe hemorrhage and shock may occur as a result of uterine atony. When maternal bleeding cannot be controlled by uterine massage or oxytocin stimulation, other sources of bleeding, such as genital tract lacerations or retained placental fragments, should be investigated. The mother will experience anxiety and require continuous close monitoring and support until her condition is stabilized.

Treatment.   Initial treatment in cases of uterine atony is to control uterine bleeding and stabilize the patient's vital signs. Immediate and frequent assessment of uterine tone is essential. When the uterus is soft, uterine massage is performed to cause it to contract (see Chapter 29 for a discussion of fundal massage). If the uterus contracts during massage but relaxes when it is discontinued, IV oxytocin infusion may be needed to stimulate and maintain uterine contractions. When bleeding continues, further vaginal and cervical examination is done to rule out trauma or laceration. Cervical curettage is necessary when retained placental fragments are responsible for excessive bleeding.

Implications for Nursing Care

The nurse plays a major role in the assessment and management of postpartum uterine bleeding. It is the nurse's responsibility to monitor and assess uterine contractions every 15 minutes for the first hour after delivery. Vital signs are checked every 15 minutes, or more often when bleeding is excessive. The patient's bladder should not be allowed to become distended, because it will push the uterus high into the abdomen, predisposing the patient to recurring uterine atony and increased bleeding.

When the nurse first notices that the uterus does not respond properly to uterine massage and that heavy bleeding is continuing, the attendant is promptly notified. IV oxytocin is ordered, and the nurse must continue to monitor the strength and frequency of uterine contractions to ensure that they are strong enough to prevent excessive bleeding without causing undue discomfort to the patient. The nurse must remain with the patient, monitoring vital signs frequently, until uterine bleeding becomes normal.

COMPLICATIONS INVOLVING THE REPRODUCTIVE TRACT

Intrapartal complications involving the reproductive tract can arise because of trauma to maternal tissue during delivery or because of preexisting structural abnormalities of the reproductive tract that affect uterine function or fetal descent through the birth canal.

Trauma to the Cervix, Vagina, and Perineum

During the intrapartal period the cervix, vagina, and perineum may experience trauma from laceration or from bruising and hematoma formation. Such trauma is often diagnosed in the immediate postpartum period and thus has no implications for the neonate; however, maternal implications are significant, and the nurse is responsible for prompt assessment and intervention when such trauma occurs. Lacerations may occur in the cervix,

---

Complications Involving the Reproductive Tract

Trauma to the Cervix, Vagina, and Perineum

- Laceration of the cervix
- Laceration of the upper vagina
- Laceration of the vulva and lower vagina
- Laceration of the perineum
- Hematoma

Structural Abnormalities of the Reproductive Tract

- Uterine abnormalities
- Cervical abnormalities
- Vaginal abnormalities

---

vagina, or perineum. In the last location, they are easily observed but lacerations of the vagina or cervix are often diagnosed after the nurse observes suggestive signs. Nursing responsibilities are similar regardless of the location of the laceration. Hematoma can occur in the vaginal wall, the vulva, or the perineum; thus, an important nursing responsibility is assessment and prompt identification.

Lacerations of the Cervix

During delivery small lacerations occur around the cervical os as it is stretched to its maximum dimensions. These are most commonly found at the 3- and 9-o'clock positions. Extensive or deep lacerations of the vascular lower uterine segment may cause severe hemorrhage and shock.

Regardless of size, cervical lacerations permanently alter the shape of the cervical os from its round nonparous configuration to the multiparous fish-mouthed shape. Predisposing factors for cervical laceration include the following:

- Operative delivery
- Precipitous delivery
- Rigid or scarred cervix
- Forceful delivery through an incompletely dilated cervix
- Breech extraction of a large baby

Maternal Implications. Cervical lacerations that remain undetected after delivery may continue to bleed. When bright red arterial bleeding persists in the presence of a well-contracted uterus, the cervix and vagina are reexamined for bleeding sites. The patient will be returned to the delivery room or surgery for repair of the bleeding cervix; delay in repair increases the risk of infection. In subsequent pregnancies the woman will be at higher risk for cervical lacerations.

Treatment. Careful repair of cervical lacerations larger than 1 cm is important for controlling hemorrhage and avoiding asymmetrical healing and scarring of the cervix.

Lacerations of the Upper Vagina

Lacerations of the upper vagina are more common with operative than with spontaneous delivery. Longitudinal tears are most common and may be bilateral. They tend to bleed profusely. Predisposing factors include the following:

- Congenital anomalies of the vagina
- Small or infantile vagina
- Lack of tissue elasticity (usually in the older primigravida)

- Scar tissue in the vagina
- Unhealthy vaginal tissue (*i.e.,* chronic infection)
- Forceps rotation and extraction
- Large infant

Treatment.   Repair of the upper vagina is performed after delivery of the placenta and the infusion of oxytocin. Careful suturing is necessary to ensure that all bleeding sites are staunched. When bleeding cannot be adequately controlled by suturing alone, the vagina is packed with a 5-yard gauze, which controls bleeding through pressure on the blood vessels. Packing also prevents hematoma formation. The packing is removed after 24 hours.

Lacerations of the Vulva and Lower Vagina

Superficial tears in the anterior vulva and lower vaginal wall are not serious. When the tissues are deeply torn, profuse bleeding occurs. Tissues that become lacerated in this area include the tissue surrounding the urethra, labia minora, side walls of the vagina, clitoral area, urethra, and bladder. See Chapter 24 for discussion of lacerations of the perineum.

Treatment.   Small, superficial lacerations of the vulva and lower vagina do not require repair, since the torn edges become approximated and heal spontaneously. Interrupted sutures to promote healing are used when large tears have to be repaired.

Deep lacerations always require repair to control bleeding and to approximate the torn tissue to ensure normal healing. When bleeding continues after suturing, a firm tamponade is applied against the bleeding site.

When tissues in the area of the urethra and clitoris are lacerated, hemorrhage can be excessive. Repair of the urethral area is difficult because of the danger of damage to the urethra. To avoid damage to the urethral canal during repair, a catheter is placed within it.

Implications for Nursing Care

Nursing responsibilities in the care of patients with lacerations of the genital tract include identifying the problem, facilitating prompt medical treatment, assisting with repair, and promoting comfort. The nurse should always be alert to the possibility of genital tract laceration, especially when delivery has been difficult and when vaginal bleeding occurs in the presence of a firm fundus. The nurse is also responsible for providing emotional support to the woman as diagnosis and treatment proceed.

Hematoma

Hematoma formation is caused by bleeding into loose connective tissue caused by trauma to underlying vessels. Hematomas enlarge progressively until bleeding stops. The cardinal symptom of hematoma formation is excruciating pain in the unanesthetized patient, described as a tearing sensation or as intense pressure. The pain may be localized in the site or may be referred to one leg. If the hematoma is high in the vagina, pain may be localized near the rectum.

Hematoma formation in the perineum may be anticipated if heavy bruising is present and the area is exquisitely sensitive to touch. However, vaginal hematomas may be detected only by gentle rectal or sterile vaginal examination, a procedure that must be done under analgesia to avoid causing the mother extreme pain.

Etiologic and Predisposing Factors.   Hematomas occurring in the vaginal walls, often near the ischial spines, may be associated with forceps delivery; they often occur in the perineum or vulva when hemostasis at the time of episiotomy is inadequate. Hematomas are also associated with difficult and prolonged second-stage labor in which the presenting part exerts pressure and causes local tissue necrosis in the vagina.

Maternal Implications.   Extreme pain is associated with hematoma formation. In addition, if the hematoma is large and bleeding continues, blood loss may be sufficient to produce signs of shock, and anemia may result subsequently. If large hematomas are not treated, infection may follow, and healing will produce calcification and scar tissue formation. Depending on the location, this scarring may permanently distort the anatomy.

Treatment.   If the hematoma is large (3 cm or more), the physician will open the hematoma, drain it, and ligate the bleeding vessel. The surrounding area may be packed to promote hemostasis.

Implications for Nursing Care

The nurse is responsible for monitoring the patient's condition and for further assessment if the patient complains of vaginal, perineal, or rectal pain in the immediate postpartum period. The nurse should examine the perineal area and should alert the birth attendant if hematoma formation is suspected. Maternal pulse and blood pressure should be assessed and observed for signs of excessive bleeding; such signs in the presence of a firm uterus and no excessive vaginal bleeding suggest the presence of a progressing hematoma. In severe cases, steps to prevent or limit hypovolemic shock may be necessary.

Structural Abnormalities of the Reproductive Tract

Structural abnormalities can occur in the uterus, cervix and vagina, affecting the process of labor and birth.

Etiologic and Predisposing Factors.   During fetal development, the female reproductive tract is formed by the fusion of the two müllerian ducts. Anomalies arise primarily from the alteration of the fusion process. Failure of the ducts to fuse normally results in two partially or completely separated tracts. Failure of one duct to mature results in a one-sided tract. Incomplete fusion of one or both ducts causes faulty canalization and formation of a transverse vaginal septum or, more rarely, absence of the vagina (Pritchard and MacDonald 1985). The cause of these disruptions in embryonic development is usually not known; however, some patterns of vaginal and cervical abnormalities have been identified in daughters born in the 1940s and 1950s to women who received diethylstilbestrol (DES) during pregnancy.

Uterine abnormalities are manifested in a variety of forms, but four simplified types are generally recognized (Fig. 28–14). The *septate uterus* appears normal from the exterior, but it contains a septum that extends partially or completely from the fundus to the cervix, dividing the uterine cavity into two separate compartments. The *bicornuate uterus* is roughly Y-shaped. The fundus is notched to various depths, and the patient may even appear to have a "double uterus"; however, there is only one cervix. A true *double uterus* results from a lack of midline

fusion, and two complete uteri, each with its own cervix, are formed. When both are fully formed, this anomaly may be referred to as *uterus didelphys*. Occasionally, one of the uteri will not fully form, remaining as a rudimentary organ without a cervix or uterine cavity. A single *hemiuterus* results when one müllerian duct fails to develop during embryonic growth, resulting in one uterine cavity and one oviduct.

Malformations of the uterus may cause difficulty when pregnancy occurs. Depending on its configuration, the uterus may not be able to stretch sufficiently to accommodate the growing fetus and permit it to assume a normal position. The hemiuterus in particular presents a variety of problems because of its small size. Abortion, preterm labor, uterine dysfunction, and pathologic lie are more common; uterine rupture may also be more common. Women with other uterine abnormalities may experience relatively few problems during labor and birth.

Cervical abnormalities may also affect the course of labor and birth. Three general types of cervical abnormalities have been identified. The *septate cervix* consists of a ring of muscular tissue partitioned by a septum that either extends downward from the uterus or upward from

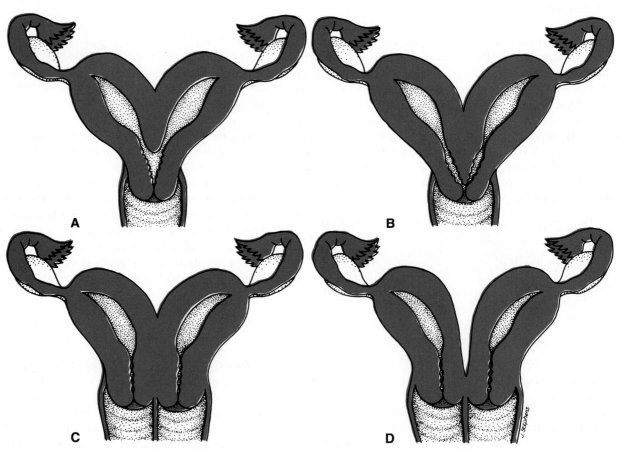

Figure 28–14. Abnormal uterine types. *(A)* Septate uterus. *(B)* Bicornuate uterus. *(C)* Double uterus. *(D)* Uterus didelphys. (Childbirth Graphics)

the vagina or is contained completely within the cervix itself. A *double cervix* has two separate cervices in one uterus. A *single hemicervix* or half-cervix results from incomplete and asymmetrical development in which only one müllerian duct matures.

Cervical abnormalities affect labor and birth to varying degrees, depending on the ability of the cervix to dilate and efface to permit delivery. In many cases cesarean delivery is necessary; the septate cervix may function adequately to permit vaginal delivery, but vaginal birth is accompanied by an increased risk of cervical rupture and hemorrhage.

Vaginal abnormalities also occur. The most common abnormality is the presence of *vaginal septa*. These usually do not present serious problems in terms of normal reproductive function. They are easily accessible and can be easily dilated or removed surgically, whereupon labor and birth may proceed normally.

Most vaginal and cervical abnormalities will be discovered antenatally. Previously undiscovered uterine abnormalities may be detected after onset of preterm labor or after the appearance of an abnormal pattern of uterine contraction in labor (Pritchard and MacDonald 1985).

Maternal and Fetal/Neonatal Implications. For women with minor reproductive tract abnormalities, chances for safe childbearing are good. When defects do not affect the maintenance of pregnancy and the normal development of the fetus, cesarean delivery may be selected to avoid the risk of dysfunction during labor. When uterine defects exist, perinatal loss is higher than among women without uterine abnormalities, in part reflecting a higher rate of spontaneous abortion. In addition, the incidence of low birth weight, due to problems in placental structure and function, and of preterm labor is three times greater than in the normal population (Pritchard and MacDonald 1985). The risk of uterine rupture during labor is also thought to be higher.

Treatment. Surgical treatment for structural abnormalities is generally done before conception, if possible. Intrapartal management focuses on close monitoring of labor pattern, uterine and cervical functioning, and fetal status. Cesarean delivery will be performed should structural abnormalities impede normal progress or threaten fetal status.

Implications for Nursing Care

Nursing responsibilities in the intrapartal care of women with reproductive tract abnormalities include assessment and close monitoring of labor progress and maternal and fetal status and providing support and anticipatory guidance about likely outcomes of labor. Patients with uterine abnormalities are more prone to preterm labor; the nurse must therefore carefully assess fetal gestational age by reviewing the patient record for LMP,

quickening date, and ultrasonography reports, when available, and by directly assessing the fundal height in centimeters. The nurse must also monitor the mother closely for signs of dystocia and impending uterine rupture. Nursing care for the patient with uterine complications, such as preterm labor, dystocia, and uterine rupture, is discussed earlier in this chapter. When vaginal delivery is being attempted, careful assessment of fetal descent and progress through the birth canal is especially important, as is close fetal monitoring.

The nurse should also recognize that women with reproductive tract abnormalities may feel guilt and anxiety about their effect on pregnancy outcome. By carefully assessing the woman's knowledge and feelings about her condition and providing information and encouragement about her progress in labor and possible obstetric interventions, the nurse can contribute to a more positive childbearing experience for the patient and her family.

LOSS AND GRIEF IN THE PERINATAL PERIOD: NURSING IMPLICATIONS

Although the outcomes of childbirth are usually positive, even among women who experience intrapartal complications, loss and the grief response to that loss are dynamics always present in the childbearing years, especially the immediate postpartum period. The phases of the grief response—that is, shock, protest and anger, disorganization, and reorganization—occur with any loss. The depth and extent of these emotional responses will vary according to the significance of the loss and the parents' coping resources.

The nurse in many conventional labor and delivery settings often does not have the opportunity for close, continuous contact with parents in the immediate postpartum period and so may not see the entire natural progression of grief and resolution take place. The nursing interventions suggested here can be initiated in the intrapartal period but should be extended into postpartum care.

Intrapartal Complications: Loss of the Anticipated Normal Birth

One of the most frequent losses parents may experience in the intrapartal period is the loss of the normal birth that they had anticipated and for which, perhaps, they had eagerly planned. The contemporary emphasis on preparation for childbirth and family participation in the birth event intensifies this natural anticipation and may deepen the parents' disappointment and feelings of loss when the birth does not go as expected. The nurse must remember that the important point is the parents' feelings and not how serious a particular failed expectation may appear to others.

For instance, if a woman strongly desires to avoid an episiotomy and has taken steps to achieve that goal only to require a generous episiotomy, she is likely to feel disappointment, and perhaps some anger, and will grieve for the change in her body image. Parents who prepare themselves extensively for a "natural" birth may experience feelings of loss if analgesia is required for labor and delivery. They may feel angry or guilty about their "failure" and will be preoccupied with these feelings until they can give up their wished-for birth and integrate the actual birth into their life experience.

The mother's sense of loss may center on body image if she has an abdominal or perineal incision, on her perception of her body as having "failed," on having missed the "perfect" birth she had been hoping for, and perhaps on having lost the support of her partner if his participation was cut short by intrapartal problems. Research suggests that the father's presence at birth, when planned for throughout the pregnancy, contributes to the mother's positive perception of childbirth, regardless of whether or not problems arose; when the father is unable to be present because of complications, mothers tend to view their birth experience more negatively. The father's sense of loss may focus more on having missed planned-for participation in the birth event or the opportunity for close contact with his wife and baby, or on a sense of having "failed" as a labor support person (May and Sollid 1984).

One particularly common intrapartal event, the need for cesarean delivery, is an excellent example. Even if maternal and neonatal outcomes are excellent, the mother may experience emotional shock related to the cesarean experience and, later, anger and guilt at her "failure" to give birth "naturally." She experiences the invasion of the body and permanent scarring of abdominal surgery, and her postpartum course is more painful and more stressful than normal. The father may experience shock at both the loss of the anticipated childbirth and the potential threat to his partner's life. Later, he may experience guilt at his "failure" as a labor coach, anger toward medical or nursing staff, worry about the well-being of his partner and newborn, and sorrow at missing the close family contact he may have been looking forward to. Research suggests that although not all parents respond to cesarean birth in this way, for many it represents a loss of the wished-for birth experience. For these parents, resolving the loss may take several weeks or months (Cranley, Hedahl, and Pegg 1983; May and Sollid 1984; Tilden and Lipson 1982).

No matter how trivial these issues may seem, parents will have to resolve these losses through a grief process. They will think about what they have lost, ask questions,

look for explanations, and relive the loss until their feelings are less intense and they can move on to the present. The nurse should recognize that the intensity of the parents' emotional reactions is proportional to the gap between their expectations and the actual birth. The nurse must guard against expressing such value judgments as "the important thing is that you and your baby are fine," or "things could have been much worse," as she cares for the family. Instead, the nurse should acknowledge their sense of loss, answer any questions they may have, allow them to express their feelings, and listen empathetically. Expressing their concerns and feelings will assist parents in resolving their loss and moving into the tasks of the postpartum period.

Implications for Nursing Care

Nursing care directed at the psychosocial needs of parents whose wished-for normal labor and birth were not possible should include the interventions listed in the accompanying display.

Consequences of Maternal Complications: Loss of Physical Health

Although they occur much less frequently than in years past, women still experience intrapartal complications, such as hemorrhage or infection, that jeopardize

---

Key Nursing Interventions in Loss of Anticipated Normal Birth

- Use caring touch and reassurance generously. Give frequent explanations about necessary procedures and mother's or newborn's status.

- Emphasize the unpredictability of some aspects of birth and remind parents that they coped as best they could in a difficult situation, giving specific examples, if possible.

- Allow parents to express their concerns or failed expectations and acknowledge their feelings with statements like: "It's disappointing to have problems during your childbirth."

- Spend ample time with parents. Do not give the impression that you are "too busy" to listen.

- Remember that physical pain and fatigue can play a large part in negative emotional states. Make sure that the mother receives adequate analgesia and comfort care before seeing the baby and remind her that she will begin to feel more like herself physically in a few days.

- Facilitate parent–infant interaction by promoting frequent and *enjoyable* contact with their baby as the parents express readiness for it.

their lives and lead to extended, more difficult postpartum recovery periods. A woman may experience temporary loss of physical health or permanent loss of function, such as occurs with an emergency hysterectomy.

Some mothers will express anger at their newborn for having caused the complication. This by itself is not evidence of disordered mother–newborn bonding, but an expression of the mother's anger and loss. Other mothers who have experienced intrapartal complications may be tentative about interacting with their newborn because they fear that they will fall asleep and drop the baby or because they feel too weak and unsteady to safely hold and care for the baby. The nurse should assess the mother's condition carefully if she seems unwilling to interact with her newborn. The unwillingness may be a sign that the mother needs more intensive nursing support and direct assistance during this time or that she needs rest more than she needs her baby. The nurse must observe several interactions before the presence or absence of a developing bond can be diagnosed with confidence. Thus, the labor nurse should report her observations of parent–infant interaction to postpartum staff carefully and without premature conclusions about the quality of the parent–infant bond.

The nurse should also recognize that the mother's extended recovery will disrupt individual and family adaptation in the postpartum period. Additional supportive services, such as postpartum home visits or referral to social services or a public health nurse, may be beneficial for some families and should be planned for early in the hospital stay.

Implications for Nursing Care

All of the nursing interventions listed earlier also apply to the woman who has experienced a significant change in her health status after childbirth and to her family. In addition, the areas of nursing care listed in the accompanying display are especially important.

Birth of a High-risk Newborn: Loss of the Anticipated Normal Newborn

A more obvious type of loss parents may experience is the birth of a sick infant or an infant with a defect and the consequent loss of the anticipated normal newborn. If the pregnancy was complicated, the birth of a sick infant or one with a defect represents the parents' worst fears and extends a long period of stress and uncertainty. When neonatal problems were unanticipated, the parents must deal with overwhelming shock and disruption on the heels of an exhausting and often stressful birth experience. Parental adjustments in the subsequent days and weeks consume huge amounts of time and energy, inflict great emotional pain, and require drastic reorganization

---

Key Nursing Interventions in Loss of Maternal Physical Health

- Organize care to support the mother physically and emotionally. The mother will need to focus her energy on her own recovery.
- Be sure that interaction with the infant is enjoyable and tailored to the mother's physical and emotional status.
- Be alert for the possibility that the father may interact with the newborn more often because of the mother's illness and may become more confident in his caretaking skills than the mother. This may increase the mother's insecurity. Provide for supportive mother–infant interaction without devaluing the father's participation.
- Help the parents relive their experience by offering information and answering questions.

---

of their plans, goals, and physical and social circumstances.

Implications for Nursing Care

The nurse has a major responsibility for providing support and information to the parents in the first few minutes after birth when neonatal problems are present. Parents usually detect the presence of problems immediately, either from the verbal and nonverbal interactions of staff in the first moments or, more clearly, from emergency measures that may be instituted. The labor nurse must first assist in initiating emergency care, as needed, but once she is relieved by pediatric or other delivery room staff, she should turn to the parents.

When neonatal problems occur, the infant is usually moved quickly from the delivery room to the admission nursery or neonatal intensive care unit. However, whenever the infant's condition permits, the parents should be given an opportunity for visual or physical contact, even for just a few moments, to allow them to have a sense that the infant is real. If there are visible defects, the nurse must make sure parents are prepared for the newborn's appearance. This can be done by describing the infant's appearance in simple terms first, calling attention to normal features, and making sure that the father or support person is seated and with the mother before the infant is brought to them. The nurse must also be aware of her own response to the newborn's appearance and take care not to exhibit distaste or pity by facial expression or verbal comments.

Once the infant is transferred and evaluated, the parents should be told as soon as possible about the nature of the problem and the infant's condition. Usually this is done by the physician, with the nurse present. The nurse should make provisions for the parents' privacy and comfort. Extreme care must be taken in discussing the infant's condition, since information given in the first hours may leave a lasting impression. For this reason, speculation about possible causes of the problem and future outcomes should be avoided, and such consequences as death or brain damage should be mentioned only when the probability of their occurrence is very high. Parents should not be rushed into making decisions at this time and should be given ample time to ask questions.

Once the parents have been informed, the maternity nurse should facilitate ongoing contact by the parents with neonatal medical and nursing staff. Until both parents can see the infant, an instant photograph of the infant in the nursery may be helpful in preparing the parents for what they will see, as well as being tangible evidence that the infant exists. The nurse must make herself available to the parents and avoid isolating them, even though interaction with them may be quite painful. The nurse's own sadness and tears are likely to be seen as kind, compassionate responses. The mother still requires close nursing observation in the postpartum period, and this routine care provides the nurse with many opportunities to listen and give emotional support and comfort measures.

Ongoing nursing care for parents with a high-risk newborn is discussed in Chapters 34 and 35. Listed in the accompanying display are nursing interventions in the immediate postbirth care of such families.

Fetal Death: Loss of the Anticipated Child

The most profound loss associated with childbearing is a perinatal death—the death of a fetus during labor or delivery. The nurse has a major responsibility in assisting parents in their grieving. Medical and nursing care of parents whose baby has died during labor or delivery is outlined in Table 28-6 and the accompanying Nursing Care Plan.

The challenge of providing care for these families is made even more difficult because the nurse and physician must first come to grips with their own feelings of guilt, anger, and sadness. One of the most painful responsibilities falls to the physician: informing the parents of their baby's death. Parents should be informed together and as soon as possible after the death is known. This should be done in an unrushed, quiet manner; delaying disclosure, sedating the mother, or initiating early transfer or discharge, while well intentioned, may interfere with the parents' normal mourning process.

The initial disclosure and subsequent interactions with parents whose baby has died will be uncomfortable for staff. Avoidance or isolation of the family, defensive reactions to normal parental anger, delegation to others of

---

Key Nursing Interventions in the Loss of an Anticipated Normal Newborn

- Avoid global reassurances ("Everything will turn out for the best") or comments that fail to acknowledge the parent's feelings ("I know just how you feel").
- Stress that the newborn is getting good care. Give factual information and help parents reduce their stress by providing them with sensitive care and reassuring them that you are available.
- Avoid giving conflicting information; this is a challenge when the parents may be asking questions of many staff members and remembering only part of what they are told. Verify the accuracy of your information before answering.
- Respect the parents' need for privacy and avoid pushing them into activities for which they are unready. Refusals to see the infant or speak with physicians or other care providers may reflect a need to take things at a slower pace.
- Do not personalize parental anger at staff and respond defensively; instead, allow them to ventilate their feelings and acknowledge their pain, disappointment, and feelings of helplessness.

---

face-to-face contact with the parents, and failure to acknowledge the death in each interaction with the family —all reflect the professionals' inability to deal with their own pain. When the professionals' ability to work with parents is compromised by their own response to the death, other staff should be brought in immediately to take over care of the family, and opportunities for the staff to discuss their feelings and come to some resolution should be provided.

Two nurse researchers who have studied bereaved parents and perinatal death, Patricia Estok and Ann Lehman, describe the principal needs of parents whose baby has died and the actions that parents found helpful. The display on the opposite page summarizes these findings.

Intrauterine Fetal Demise

Intrauterine fetal demise (IUFD) and its attendant medical and psychological stressors are extremely traumatic to the patient and her family. Not only does the long-awaited child die, but the patient must also undergo the process of labor and birth and postpartum involution. The fact that the fetus may remain in the uterus for some time after death has been confirmed places the mother at additional physical and emotional risk.

Categorization of fetal death is determined by the point in gestation when death occurs. When the fetus dies be-

---

The Care of Grieving Parents: Helpful Professional Behaviors

Acknowledging Shock and Grief

- Express your feelings about the baby's death with consoling words.
- Touch parents in a caring fashion; words are not always necessary.

Sharpening the Reality of the Baby's Death

- Provide as much factual information about the baby's death as is available.
- Describe the baby's appearance in factual and tender terms before bringing the baby to the parents.
- Encourage the parents to see and hold the baby. Stay with them as they examine the baby for the first time.
- Acknowledge the baby's death at first contact with the parents and daily thereafter; do not act as if the death has not occurred.
- Provide parents with physical tokens of the baby: wisp of hair, instant photograph, blanket, identification bracelet.

Assisting Parents in Grieving

- Encourage the parents to grieve openly.
- Spend extra time with the parents to review events surrounding the baby's death.

- Encourage the parents to make arrangement for a spiritual or religious ritual to mark the baby's death (baptism, funeral, memorial service).

Helping Parents to Prepare for Homegoing

- Suggest a "practice run" of the discharge process to help the parents work through their feelings about going home without a baby.
- Help parents prepare themselves for telling family and friends and responding to others who do not know of the baby's death.
- Involve other family members or support people in preparations for homegoing.
- Discuss possible difficult times: dismantling the nursery, renewing their sexual relationship, seeing other newborns.
- Provide referral to support services, such as parent support groups or counseling.
- Maintain postdischarge contact with parents through the first year.

Adapted from Estok P, Lehman A: Perinatal death: Grief support for families. Birth 10:17, 1983

---

fore 20 weeks of gestation and is not aborted spontaneously, the term "missed abortion" is used. After 20 weeks of gestation, the term "fetal death syndrome" may be used when labor does not begin within 48 hours of death.

Diagnosis of fetal death usually begins with the mother's observation that fetal movement has stopped. Diagnosis is confirmed when fetal heart tones are absent, uterine growth ceases, uterine size decreases, and fetal heart movement cannot be visualized by ultrasonography. When x-ray is used, fetal death is detected by the appearance of intravascular or intra-abdominal fetal gas (Roberts' sign). Collapse and angulation (deviation from the normal shape) of the fetal spine also indicates fetal demise.

In 75% of cases of IUFD, the woman will experience spontaneous onset of labor within 14 days of the estimated time of fetal death; this percentage increases to 89% by 21 days (Pritchard and MacDonald 1985). This extended period of waiting is particularly stressful to the woman and her family and may result in feelings of anxiety, depression, or guilt. However, it is difficult for the

family to grieve for their loss until after the actual delivery.

Etiologic and Predisposing Factors. It is frequently impossible to determine the cause of IUFD. However, it is often associated with severe and poorly controlled maternal diabetes mellitus, preeclampsia, erythroblastosis fetalis (Rh disease), premature separation of the placenta, and umbilical cord accidents.

Maternal Implications. When pregnancy is prolonged 5 or more weeks after fetal death without spontaneous onset of labor, the mother is at increased risk of hypofibrinogenemia or disseminated intravascular coagulation (DIC). Maternal fibrinogen levels begin to drop 3 weeks after fetal death, when fetal tissue degeneration begins and thromboplastin is released into the amniotic fluid and absorbed into the maternal circulation. However, thromboplastin levels rarely increase to the point of endangering the mother until 5 weeks after fetal death, when the risk of DIC is approximately 25%. Hemorrhage

Table 28-6   Medical Management of Missed Abortion/Intrauterine Fetal Demise

Medical Management	Rationale	Laboratory Studies	Nursing Implications
12 Weeks			
Confirmation of diagnosis	To diagnose fetal death as soon as possible	Ultrasound	Prepare patient for ultrasound.
Dilatation and curettage of uterine contents	To evacuate the uterus To decrease patient discomfort	Pregnancy test (converts from positive to negative)	Obtain repeat pregnancy test.
Prescription analgesic Blood studies	To control possible hemorrhage following uterine evacuation and curettage	Tests: • Hemoglobin (Hgb), hematocrit (Hct), white blood count • Fibrinogen • Platelets • Type and crossmatch	Order two units of blood, fresh frozen plasma, and cryoprecipitate before curettage. Routinely monitor postoperative vital signs. Monitor state of uterine contractions every 15 minutes and massage uterus to maintain firmness. Permit the patient's partner to remain to offer support. Prepare the patient for discharge when her condition stabilizes at 10 to 12 hr.
13–28 Weeks			
Confirmation of diagnosis	Medical intervention is not appropriate until after 3 weeks of fetal death: spontaneous labor begins in 89% of women during this period.	Ultrasound Weekly Hgb, Hct, and fibrinogen-level tests (if fibrinogen levels drop to 0.2 g%, delivery is indicated)	Prepare patient for ultrasound. Schedule weekly counseling visits. Obtain type and crossmatch for two units of whole blood. Order cryoprecipitate and fresh frozen plasma for emergency use.
After 3 weeks of fetal death, induction of labor with vaginal prostaglandin E_2 suppositories (20 mg)	Drop in fibrinogen causes risk of DIC		Assist patients who experience nausea and vomiting from prostaglandin use. Give medication before prostaglandin use to minimize side-effects.
Prescription of analgesic	To decrease patient discomfort from uterine contractions		Offer patient analgesic
Labor and delivery of products of conception (takes 10 to 12 hr) Prescription of Methergine	To enhance postoperative uterine contractions and reduce blood loss		Give IM Methergine 0.2 mg
Uterine curettage Cervical inspection for trauma from procedure	To ensure removal of all tissue	Hct and fibrinogen levels, collected 4 hr after uterine evacuation	
Discharge after 24 hours of stable vital signs	The patient will be eager for discharge. No further risk of DIC exists.		Prepare the patient for discharge. Schedule counseling session with a professional counselor for 2 weeks after discharge, or sooner if deemed necessary. Refer for genetic counseling regarding possible risk in future pregnancies. Refer to parent support group.
Greater than 28 weeks			
Confirmation of diagnosis	Medical intervention is not appropriate until after 3 weeks of fetal death.	Ultrasound	Offer support to grieving couple.
Scheduling of weekly visits	To monitor for early signs of DIC	Weekly Hgb, Hct, and fibrinogen level tests (if fibrinogen levels drop to 0.2 g/%, delivery is indicated)	Keep patient informed of need for close surveillance of her blood levels and signs of bleeding.

(continued)

Table 28–6   **Medical Management of Missed Abortion/Intrauterine Fetal Demise** (continued)

Medical Management	Rationale	Laboratory Studies	Nursing Implications
After 3 weeks, collection of blood coagulation studies every 6 hours	Patient is at greater risk for DIC.		Obtain type and crossmatch for two units of whole blood. Order cryoprecipitate and fresh frozen plasma for emergency use
Induction of labor	Low fibrinogen levels increase DIC risk.		Discuss need for induced labor with couple and answer questions.
Induction options: • Laminaria placed in cervix 12 hours before induction • Prostaglandin gel applied to cervix • Prostaglandin E$_2$ suppository inserted high in posterior vaginal fornix • Prostaglandin or oxytocin infusions	To speed cervical ripening or dilatation or to initiate labor		Assure couple that a nurse will be with them throughout procedure. Obtain type and crossmatch for two units of whole blood. Order cryoprecipitate and fresh frozen plasma for emergency use. Assist with insertion of laminaria or suppository, informing patient about what is happening and why. Establish an IV line with Ringer's lactate or similar solution. Collect equipment and assist with placement of pressure catheter. Place an external pressure monitor when amniotomy cannot be performed.
Amniotomy and insertion of transcervical pressure catheter between amnion and uterine wall Monitor vital signs every 2 to 4 hr.	To permit accurate monitoring of uterine pressure and reduce risk of uterine rupture	Coagulation studies collected every 4 hr	Ensure collection of blood specimen and expedite its transport to the laboratory.
Prescription of antiemetic and antidiarrheal medication	Nausea, vomiting, and diarrhea may occur with prostaglandin use.		Give patient medications before prostaglandin use to minimize side-effects.
Prescription of analgesic	To decrease patient discomfort from uterine contractions		Offer patient ordered analgesic. Encourage partner to support patient during labor and delivery.
Delivery of infant			Support couple and assist in their grieving process and its resolution. After delivery, infant should be cleaned, wrapped in a blanket, and given to parents to hold. They may prefer to be left alone at this time. Refer the couple to a parent support group if they desire. (See Nursing Care Plan: The Family Experiencing Fetal Demise)

resulting from DIC may be life threatening; see Disseminated Intravascular Coagulation earlier in this chapter.

Treatment.   Treatment of IUFD includes induction of labor if it does not begin spontaneously within 3 weeks of the estimated time of fetal death, monitoring of maternal coagulation studies to detect early signs of hypofibrinogenemia, and providing emotional support and initiating follow-up for the woman and her partner. Medical management of IUFD and nursing implications are described in Table 28–6.

(text continued on page 853)

NURSING CARE PLAN

The Family Experiencing Fetal Demise

Nursing Diagnosis (Patient Problem) and Assessment Data	Nursing Interventions	Rationale
Probable Complication: *intrauterine fetal demise*		
• Risk factors: Poorly controlled diabetes Rh isoimmunization Vaginal bleeding Previous stillbirth Known congenital anomalies Chorioamnionitis Umbilical cord prolapse	Explain to mother and family that you are unable to detect FHTs. Apply EFM, using an internal monitor (if membranes have ruptured), to search for FHTs.	Mother usually knows something is wrong. Hiding the facts only increases anxiety, anger, and mistrust. Open, tactful, careful honesty, while leaving some hope until death is verified, is the most helpful course. Attempt verification with EFM.
• Maternal report of decreased/absent fetal activity	Notify physician if no FHR is found.	To obtain orders.
• Absence of fetal heart tones by auscultation, EFM	Anticipate and prepare for ultrasound or amniotomy.	Real-time ultrasound will display fetal heart activity. Amniotomy will be used before application of internal EFM for verification of fetal death and to initiate labor.
• Fear related to fetal status		
	Remain with patient while verifying fetal status. Inform patient of known death once verified.	The patient and her family feel tremendous anxiety and helplessness. Nursing support and fostered trust and confidence are sometimes the only means available for honest communication. It is *never* advisable to withhold information while waiting for the physician, since this only sets up barrier between the patient and the nurse, who is the primary care-giver
	Provide emotional support; involve family, friends, pastor, or social worker as desired by patient.	It is important to relax regulations to alleviate the incredible grief that will overcome the patient. Initiation of the grieving process, beginning with shock, disbelief, and denial, can be augmented by including supportive others.

Expected Outcome:

The patient and her family express emotions, consider available options, and make choices about handling fetal death before, during, and after delivery.

Potential Complication:
coagulopathy

	Observe for signs of coagulopathy: • Hematuria	There is danger of disseminated intravascular coagulopathy (DIC) in

(continued)

NURSING CARE PLAN

The Family Experiencing Fetal Demise (continued)

Nursing Diagnosis (Patient Problem) and Assessment Data	Nursing Interventions	Rationale
	• Petechiae • Ecchymosis • Oozing at venipuncture sites Facilitate lab tests: • Complete blood count • DIC screen/coagulation studies • Typing and crossmatching of two units of blood	women who retain the fetus following IUFD. Often the time of fetal death is not known.
	Prepare patient for induction of labor • Amniotomy • Oxytocin infusion • Prostaglandin suppositories	Once fetal demise is diagnosed, most physicians will induce or augment labor to avoid DIC risk and reduce emotional trauma to mother who is carrying a dead fetus. The patient should be informed about procedures. Induction may be more aggressive than usual because there is no risk to the fetus. Usually no EFM is used or only a contraction to-cotransducer.
	Anticipate rapid labor and birth: *be prepared.*	A stillborn fetus is often delivered rapidly because the skull molds easily.

Expected Outcome:

Patient delivers stillborn fetus and maintains normal postpartum physiological status.

Nursing Diagnosis:
grieving related to fetal loss

• Denial • Disbelief • Anger • Numbness • Withdrawal	Explain and provide available options throughout the labor process, allowing adequate time for shared family decision making. Until absolutely necessary, avoid requesting a specific answer about the following: • Analgesic/anesthesia (narcotics, sedatives, epidural for labor, general anesthesia at birth).	The patient and her family will listen to options and usually discuss them in private. They may ask questions, request suggestions, and express uncertainty and feelings of loss of control. Time and understanding are essential. Some patients prefer total sedation for labor and birth; other prefer to use learned techniques, remaining awake and alert for birth. Use of a learned coping mechanism fosters a sense of control over labor, especially important when control over fetal outcome is impossible.

(continued)

NURSING CARE PLAN

The Family Experiencing Fetal Demise (continued)

Nursing Diagnosis (Patient Problem) and Assessment Data	Nursing Interventions	Rationale
	• Knowledge of sex of infant, time of birth.	The nurse should know and follow the patient's preference.
	• Desire to name baby (names may already be picked out).	Naming acknowledges the reality of the baby and pregnancy and allows parents to grieve over the loss of a named baby with an identity and personality.
	• Baptism at birth.	The nurse should follow the religious preference of the family.
	• Desire to see, hold, or touch baby at delivery or afterward (include the family in this offer).	Theory about prenatal attachment suggests that holding and touching the baby permits "detachment" and facilitates grieving.
	• Desire to have picture, baby cards, arm band, foot and hand prints, lock of hair.	Memorabilia acknowledge the reality of the birth and assist grieving. If patient declines, these items should be collected and held in the labor unit for 2 years for later retrieval if desired.
	• Willingness to permit autopsy.	The cause of most fetal deaths is unknown despite autopsy. Finding that the infant was normal may reassure parents (especially first-time parents) of the ability to produce normal offspring. Finding a genetic defect or congenital anomaly may allow parents to "justify" and accept the death.
	• Desire for funeral service or burial.	Funeral service is usually inexpensive for neonates. This may be a religious ritual and assist in grieving. Most institutions encourage burial by family if the fetus weighs over 500 g.
	• Encourage husband or support person to attend if desired.	Providing support for the mother will help the father to adjust to reality and cope.

Expected Outcome:

Parents/family support each other through communication, as evidenced by its various forms (talking, touching, etc.) and beginning normal steps of grieving.

(continued)

NURSING CARE PLAN

The Family Experiencing Fetal Demise (continued)

Nursing Diagnosis (Patient Problem) and Assessment Data	Nursing Interventions	Rationale

Nursing Diagnosis:
grieving related to delivery of neonate who is stillborn or dies shortly after birth

• Crying • Quiet viewing • Holding infant • Talking to infant • Anger • Speechlessness • Inability to respond to questions • Questioning about reason for IUFD • Denial • Withdrawal	Offer all options *again* as they arise (see above). Parents often change their mind once the birth is occurring.	Denial of reality and the grieving process cause aversion to making decisions that imply that the baby has died.
	Tell parents the baby is dead when born. Ask if they want to know the baby's sex, etc.	Patients will always continue to hope that there has been an error in diagnosis until the baby is actually born. They need verification of death.
	Encourage expression of emotions, crying, and communication between parents. Avoid comments that demean the significance of this baby, such as "You can have another," "Feel blessed you have one at home." Avoid saying, "It is God's will." Focus on support, quite touch, understanding and empathy. Acknowledge feelings of anger as normal response: *e.g.:* "It is very hard to lose a baby," or "You're right, it does seem unfair." Discuss explanations for siblings.	Communication encourages the grief process. Parents often view telling other children of baby's death as the most difficult task.
	Prepare baby for viewing: • Clean or bathe to remove delivery blood, meconium mucus. • Wrap in warm baby blankets; put on head cap. • Use cord clamp (not hemostat) on umbilical cord. • Inform parents how the baby will look before they see the newborn: bluish, mottled, areas of skin peeling, deformities.	Viewing may occur immediately in the delivery room or recovery room. Parents should be informed about the newborn's appearance to establish expectations and allow adjustment. A baby with congenital anomalies can be made more presentable by using clothing (*e.g.,* cap for anencephalic infant, T-shirt for one with omphalocele). Instruments should be removed.
	During the viewing: • Show parents the baby first; then ask if they would like to hold the baby; allow them to unwrap the blanket. • Point out individual characteristics, such as the amount and color of	Babies are nearly always beautiful and precious to their parents. Even a deformed child will have some attractive characteristics. Pointing out special attributes preserves family dignity and sense of self-worth; slowly parents will explore

(continued)

851

NURSING CARE PLAN

The Family Experiencing Fetal Demise (continued)

Nursing Diagnosis (Patient Problem) and Assessment Data	Nursing Interventions	Rationale
	hair, perfect fingers and toes, size, shape of mouth, etc. • Ask parents if they would like to be left alone. Instruct them to use call signal for your return. Be available to take the infant when requested and to answer questions. • Never limit the time or number of viewings available.	the infant, noting individual features, and often crying and talking to the infant. These behaviors are sometimes done in private, when parents say goodbye to their baby.

Expected Outcome:

Parents/family support each other through communication, as evidenced by its various forms (talking, touching, etc.) and beginning normal steps of grieving.

Nursing Diagnosis:
self-concept disturbance related to feelings of reality of loss, isolation

• Expressions of guilt, shame • Denial of magnitude of loss by self or family members	Provide the parents with memorabilia or file (footprints, arm band, baby cards, picture).	Acknowledge reality of the birth.
	Ask mother if she prefers a room on or off the maternity floor.	Most patients prefer to be away from other mothers with healthy infants. However, providing the choice promotes participation and feelings of control, and keeps the transferred patient from feeling that she is being shunned.
	Discuss normal physiologic changes that will occur postnatally even though baby is not alive: • Breast engorgement • Lochia (discuss perineal care) • Perineal pain • Urinary and bowel elimination	Patients forget that they will have to deal with these changes, which act as a constant reminder that they have given birth. Preparation for these events fosters adaptation.

Expected Outcome:

Parents demonstrate progressive adaptation to loss and acceptance of death, as evidenced by realistic statements of cause of baby's death and of recognition that they were not responsible for it.

(continued)

NURSING CARE PLAN

The Family Experiencing Fetal Demise (continued)

Nursing Diagnosis (Patient Problem) and Assessment Data	Nursing Interventions	Rationale

Nursing Diagnosis:
altered family process related to death of newborn

• Inadequate social support • Difficult communication among family members • Family history of disruption or multiple unresolved losses	Visit mother and family while still in the hospital. Discuss home help, returning to work, what to tell friends and coworkers, the baby's room, and future plans.	Patients feel isolated once moved away from the intense supportive care of labor and delivery staff to routine care. Continued support and visits assist the process of grieving and promote adjustments to reality.

Expected Outcome:

Family begins adaptation process to neonatal death as evidenced by open discussion with staff and each other concerning meaning of loss, methods of facing concerned friends, and plans for future children.

Nursing Diagnosis:
dysfunctional grieving

• Inability to acknowledge loss • Inability to mobilize and use available support	Provide parents and family members with brochures or phone numbers of area support groups for newborn death.	Brochures are usually provided free. Offering access to the number or name displays acceptance and caring.
	Following up with a phone call 1 week to 1 month after dismissal if possible.	Follow up allows continued assessment of and support for healthy grieving as well as an opportunity to answer questions.

Expected Outcome:

Parents begin adaptation process to neonatal death as evidenced by discussion with staff regarding what they learned about the grieving process and how it applies to them and by seeking information from or attending a support group.

Implications for Nursing Care. Caring for a couple who have experienced IUFD is one of the most emotionally demanding situations the maternity nurse must face. Nursing responsibilities include providing physical and emotional support for the couple through labor and birth, monitoring maternal physiologic status for signs of complications associated with the IUFD as well as those associated with induction or intrapartal analgesia or anesthesia, and establishing the groundwork for ongoing support of the family through their period of grief. Intrapartal nursing care for the family with IUFD is discussed in detail in the accompanying nursing care plan.

The nurse has the most continuous close contact with bereaved parents throughout the immediate postpartum period. In collaboration with medical personnel, social workers, and others involved with families experiencing perinatal loss, the nurse must assist in the grieving process, facilitate physical and emotional recovery, and initiate contact with other support services. (See the Nursing Care Plan, page 848.)

CHAPTER SUMMARY

Childbirth is ordinarily viewed as a happy, exciting event for women and their families, and family-centered maternity care allows for the full appreciation of that side of childbirth. However, birth is nothing if not unpredictable. Complications arise that can threaten maternal and fetal well-being and that require expert medical and nursing intervention to ensure positive outcomes.

The nurse plays a crucial role in the care of families at risk for or actually experiencing complications in the intrapartal period. The nurse assesses maternal and fetal status, detects early signs of developing complications, observes signs of impending danger, and often offers the first emergency interventions to preserve maternal and fetal well-being. A systematic approach to care, reflected in the nursing process, is required in order to ensure that nursing actions are based on accurate data and that care is provided in an orderly fashion, even in emergencies.

The constantly developing technology of perinatal care allows health care professionals greater precision and effectiveness in their treatment of complications associated with childbirth. The nurse is continually challenged to take the best from this technology and combine it with the best of humane nursing practice to improve the quality of maternal and neonatal outcomes and to preserve the dignity of the childbirth experience.

STUDY QUESTIONS

1. Why is a family-centered approach to intrapartal care especially important for high-risk women and their families? Describe some ways family-centered practices can be implemented when families experience intrapartal crises.

2. What are common causes for third-trimester bleeding? Describe each condition, the major maternal and fetal risks associated with it, and appropriate nursing care.

3. What are the major maternal and fetal risks associated with premature rupture of membranes? What can the nurse do to reduce these risks?

4. Why is umbilical cord prolapse an obstetric emergency? List essential nursing actions in the identification and treatment of cord prolapse.

5. What are the major nursing responsibilities during labor and birth in caring for the woman experiencing a post-term gestation?

6. Define the terms *preeclampsia* and *eclampsia*. Discuss the implications of these conditions in the intrapartal period and nursing responsibilities in providing care to patients with these conditions.

7. Describe the etiology and major maternal and fetal risks associated with shock and DIC. Outline emergency interventions for each condition and nursing responsibilities.

8. Define *preterm labor*. Discuss the major maternal and fetal implications and current modes of treatment. Outline nursing interventions appropriate to the care of the patient in preterm labor.

9. How is intrauterine fetal demise diagnosed? What implications does it have for the course of labor and delivery? What is the major physiologic complication associated with IUFD? Discuss its prevention and treatment.

10. Discuss nursing support for families experiencing intrauterine fetal demise. Identify some actions the nurse should avoid and explain why.

11. What types of grief and loss do families typically experience in relation to the intrapartal period?

12. How can the nurse provide support to families as they resolve these feelings? List the types of referrals available to the labor and delivery nurse for families returning home after experiencing loss and grief.

REFERENCES/BIBLIOGRAPHY

Arias F, Holcomb W: Abnormal fetal presentations and positions during labor. In Arias F (ed): High-risk Pregnancy and Delivery. St. Louis, CV Mosby, 1984

Benson R: Multiple pregnancy. In Benson R (ed): Current Obstetric and Gynecologic Diagnosis and Treatment, 6th ed. Los Altos, CA, Lange Medical Publications, 1987

Cranley M, Hedahl K, Pegg S: Women's preceptions of vaginal and cesarean deliveries. Nurs Res 32(1):10, 1983

Creasy R, Resnick R: Maternal–Fetal Medicine. Philadelphia, WB Saunders, 1984

Danforth D: Obstetrics and Gynecology, 5th ed. Philadelphia, JB Lippincott, 1986

Hibbard L: Complications of labor and delivery. In Benson R (ed): Current Obstetric and Gynecologic Diagnosis and Treatment, 5th ed. Los Altos, CA, Lange Medical Publications, 1987

Killan A: Amniotic fluid embolism. Clin Obstet Gynecol 28:32–35, 1985

Lacro RV, Jones KL, Benirschke K: The umbilical cord twist: Origin, direction, and relevance. Am J Obstet Gynecol 157:833–838, 1987

May K, Sollid D: Unanticipated cesarean birth: From the father's perspective. Birth 11:87, 1984

Oxorn H: Human Labor and Birth, 5th ed. New York, Appleton-Century-Crofts, 1985

Perrin E, Sanders C: How to examine the placenta and why. In Perrin E (ed): Pathology of the Placenta. New York, Churchill Livingstone, 1984

Pritchard J, MacDonald P: Williams' Obstetrics, 17th ed. New York, Appleton-Century Croft, 1985

Ratnoff R: Disseminated intravascular coagulation. In Ratnoff O, Forbes C (eds): Disorders of Hemostasis. Orlando, FL, Grune & Stratton, 1984

Tilden V, Lipson J: Cesarean childbirth: Variables affecting psychological impact. West J Nurs Res 3:127, 1982

Vintzileos AM, Campbell WA, Nochimson DJ, Weinbaum PJ: The use and misuse of the fetal biophysical profile. Am J Obstet Gynecol 156:527–33, 1987

SUGGESTED READINGS

Beckey RD, Price RA, Okerson M, Riley KW: Development of a perinatal grief checklist. J Obstet Gynecol Neonatal Nurs 14:194–199, 1985

Fisher LY: Nursing management of the pregnant psychotic patient during labor and delivery. J Obstet Gynecol Neonatal Nurs 17:25–28, 1988

Harvey CJ: Fetal scalp stimulation: Enhancing the interpretation of fetal monitor tracings. J Perinat Neonatal Nurs 1(1):13–21, 1987

NAACOG: Grief related to perinatal death. Washington, DC: OGN Nursing Practice Resource, 1985

Shannon DM: HELLP Syndrome: A severe consequence of pregnancy–induced hypertension. J Obstet Gynecol Neonatal Nurs 16:395–402, 1987

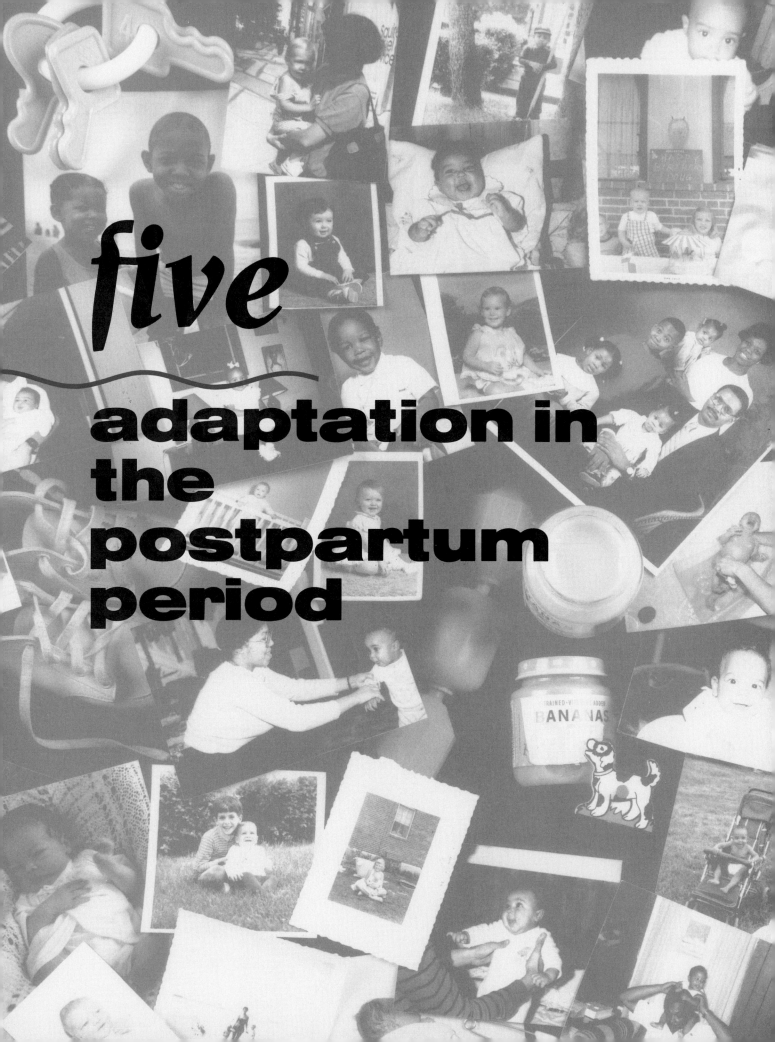

five

adaptation in the postpartum period

29

nursing care of the family in the postpartum period

KEY TERMS

Afterpains

Boggy uterus

Diastasis recti abdominis

Fundus

Involution

Lochia

Puerperium

Uterine atony

The postpartum period may seem anticlimactic in comparison with the 9 months of anticipation that accompany pregnancy and the intensity and wonder of the labor and birth experience. In reality, however, the postpartum period comprises an amazing variety of complex physiologic and psychological adaptations. The nurse's role is vital as she assists the new parents through these adjustments and supports them as they make a fresh start as a new family.

The nursing process serves as the framework for comprehensive postpartum care. Although most families deliver healthy newborns and progress through the postpartum period without significant difficulty, thorough and accurate assessments will give the nurse the information necessary to provide complete and appropriate care. Systematic assessments will also enable the nurse to identify potential or actual problems early, allowing prompt intervention should it be necessary.

The relatively short postpartum hospitalization of 1 to 3 days requires the nurse to plan effectively for necessary nursing interventions. Intervention includes provision of direct physical support to the mother, emotional support to the parents and family, and teaching for effective care of self and newborn. Patient and family teaching is especially important in the postpartum setting, since the postpartum nurse is often the last health professional with whom the patient has personal contact until her visit with her care provider 2 to 6 weeks after the birth. The postpartum nurse must identify major teaching needs and provide the information needed to allow parents to take good care of themselves and their new baby during the first weeks after childbirth.

THE POSTPARTUM PERIOD: THE BEGINNING OF A NEW FAMILY

Physiologic Adaptation

In the first hours and days after childbirth, the mother undergoes dramatic physiologic adaptation involving nearly every system of the body. Were changes of this magnitude to occur in a patient other than a postpartum woman, they would be cause for grave concern. For instance, the postpartum woman typically experiences a weight loss of 15 lb to 17 lb. Most of this loss (10–12 lb) is the result of the delivery of the infant, placenta, and amniotic fluid; in addition, 5 lb of excess fluid is lost through diuresis, and there is a blood loss of 500 ml or more. Fluid loss of this degree through diuresis or other mechanisms would likely pose a significant risk of hypovolemic shock to a nonmaternity patient.

Most postpartum women experience relatively little discomfort related to these physical changes and tend to

be more concerned about rest, perineal discomfort, and learning, with their partners and other family members, about their new babies. Nevertheless, these physiologic changes are of significance to the postpartum nurse and must be monitored. Deviations from the normal physiologic changes may signal postpartum complications, such as hemorrhage or infection.

The postpartum period is usually divided into three phases. The *immediate* postpartum period comprises the first 24 hours after birth; the *early* postpartum period, the first week; and the *late* postpartum period the second through sixth weeks. This division reflects the varying character of postpartum changes. The most dramatic and potentially hazardous changes occur in the immediate and early postpartum periods. The rate of change is much more gradual in the late postpartum period.

Vital Signs

Monitoring of temperature and blood pressure is of particular importance in the immediate and early postpartum periods. The woman's oral temperature within 24 hours of delivery may be as high as 100.4°F (38°C) as a result of muscular exertion, dehydration and hormonal changes. She should, however, be afebrile after the first 24 hours. Elevations over 100.4°F on any 2 of the first 10 postpartum days may suggest puerperal sepsis, urinary tract infection, endometritis, mastitis, or other infections. Breast engorgement on the second or third day was once thought to cause temperature elevations ("milk fever"); however, this is not a common cause of temperature elevations in newly delivered mothers, and if it occurs, it should not persist more than 24 hours.

Adaptations of the Cardiovascular System

Perhaps the most dramatic maternal changes in the postpartum period involve the cardiovascular system. Pregnancy-induced hypervolemia, which produces a 50% increase in circulating blood volume at term, allows the woman to tolerate a substantial blood loss at delivery without ill effect. Blood losses of 400 to 500 ml in a vaginal birth and 700 to 1000 ml in a cesarean birth are not uncommon. Bradycardia of 50 to 70 beats per minute may be considered normal, since the heart compensates for the decreased vascular resistance in the pelvis. Tachycardia is less common and may reflect a difficult, prolonged labor and birth, greater than normal blood loss, or significant postpartum hemorrhage.

Blood Pressure

Maternal blood pressure should remain stable after delivery. A decrease of 20 mm Hg or more systolic pressure when the mother moves from a supine to a sitting position probably reflects *orthostatic hypotension,* a temporary lag in cardiovascular compensation for the decreased vascular resistance in the pelvis. However, any decrease unassociated with position change may reflect continuing blood loss from hemorrhage and requires further assessment at once. An increase of 30 mm Hg systolic or 15 mm Hg diastolic pressure, especially when accompanied by headache or visual changes, may suggest preeclampsia. Therefore, the nurse should always evaluate the blood pressure of a postpartum patient complaining of headache before analgesia is administered. (See Chapter 30 for discussion of postpartum preeclampsia.)

Diaphoresis and Postpartum Chill

Mothers may experience a shaking chill immediately after delivery. This chill is thought to be caused by vasomotor instability and is not clinically significant if not followed by fever. Comfort measures, such as offering a warmed blanket or a warm beverage, are indicated. In the early postpartum period, mothers may also experience episodes of diaphoresis; these frequently occur at night, the mother awakening drenched in perspiration. Again, this diaphoresis, while uncomfortable, is not clinically significant unless it is accompanied by fever. Comfort measures, such as changing bed linens and clothing to prevent the mother from becoming chilled, and showers or sponge baths, if desired, are indicated.

Blood Components

The postpartum woman's hemoglobin, hematocrit, and erythrocyte count should remain near prelabor levels. A drop of four points in the hematocrit may reflect as much as 1 pint of blood loss in the intrapartal period. However, this drop may be masked by the hemoconcentration caused by the postdelivery diuresis. Leukocytosis with an increase in white cells of 15,000 to 30,000/mm³ is not uncommon; lymphocytes are usually reduced.

The body's blood-clotting mechanisms are activated in the immediate postpartum period and may persist for some time after delivery, putting the woman at increased risk for thromboembolism. The increased plasma fibrinogen and sedimentation rate observed during pregnancy usually continue for a week or more after delivery.

Adaptations of the Urinary Tract

During the birth process the bladder is subjected to trauma that can result in edema and a diminished sensitivity to fluid pressures. These changes can lead to overdistention and incomplete emptying of the bladder. It is not uncommon for the woman to experience urinary incompetence during the first 2 days after delivery.

Excess fluid accumulated in tissue during pregnancy is eliminated by diuresis, which usually begins within 24 hours after delivery. This diuresis can account for as much as 5 lb body weight lost in the early postpartum

period. Hematuria in the early postpartum period may reflect bladder trauma from delivery; later, urinary tract infection should be suspected. Acetonuria and mild proteinuria may also occur in the early postpartum period; acetonuria may reflect dehydration after prolonged labor, whereas proteinuria reflects catabolic processes involved in uterine involution. The renal plasma flow, glomerular filtration rate, and ureters gradually return to the prepregnant state in the first month after the birth.

Adaptations of the Endocrine System

The woman's endocrine system undergoes abrupt changes during the fourth stage of labor. Following delivery of the placenta, there is a sudden decrease in estrogen, progesterone, and prolactin levels. Prolactin levels will continue to decline to normal nonpregnant levels in the nonlactating woman over the first few weeks. Prolactin levels in the lactating woman will increase in response to stimulation from the infant's sucking.

Estrogen in the nonlactating woman gradually increases, reaching follicular phase levels by 3 weeks after delivery. Menstruation usually occurs by the 12th postpartum week in the nonlactating woman and by the 36th postpartum week in the lactating woman. The first menstrual cycle is often anovulatory. Although breast-feeding tends to delay the first ovulatory menstrual cycle, breast-feeding alone is not an effective method of contraception.

Breast Changes

Throughout pregnancy, the breasts are being prepared for lactation under the influence of estrogen and progesterone. Colostrum, a breast fluid that precedes milk production, may appear in the third trimester of pregnancy and continues into the first postpartum week. Colostrum is a thin, yellow fluid composed of protein, larger fat globules, and antibodies.

Breast milk production begins around the third postpartum day. Initial breast engorgement occurs with an increase in the vascular and lymphatic systems surrounding the breast. The breasts become larger, firmer, and tender or painful to touch. These changes will be experienced by most women, unless lactation-suppressant medication has been administered in the immediate postpartum period.

Milk production begins in the alveolar cells under the influence of prolactin. The let-down reflex, or the release of milk into the lactiferous duct by contraction of the myoepithelial cells, is dependent on endogenous oxytocin secretion, stimulated by suckling. If lactation is uninterrupted, the woman will experience milder episodes of engorgement related to overdistention of the breast lobes and increases in milk production until lactation is well established.

Adaptations of the Gastrointestinal System

Reestablishment of normal bowel function is delayed into the first postpartum week. This is due to decreased bowel motility, fluid loss, and perineal discomfort. The use of enemas in the first stage of labor and decreased abdominal muscle tone can also predispose the postpartum woman to constipation. Bowel function is usually reestablished by the end of the first postpartum week as the woman's appetite and fluid intake increase and perineal discomfort is reduced.

Adaptations of the Musculoskeletal System

The abdominal muscles are gradually stretched during pregnancy, causing diminished muscle tone, which is evident in the postpartum period. The abdomen is often soft, weak, and flabby. During pregnancy the rectus muscles may separate, a condition called *diastasis recti abdominis.* When this separation is present, the uterus and bladder can be easily palpated through the abdominal wall when the woman is supine.

Sensation in the lower extremities may be decreased during the first 24 hours after delivery if a regional anesthesic was used for the birth. The mother may also experience a decrease in muscular strength related to muscle strain and exertion from the birth process. Decreased activity and increased prothrombin levels predispose the postpartum woman to thrombophlebitis. If the woman suffered from edema of the extremities during pregnancy, it will diminish in the early postpartum period.

Muscles and fascia of the abdominal wall and pelvic floor that were stretched during pregnancy gradually regain their tone and approximate their prepregnant length over the last postpartum period. Vigorous exercise is not recommended until this natural healing has been allowed to take place.

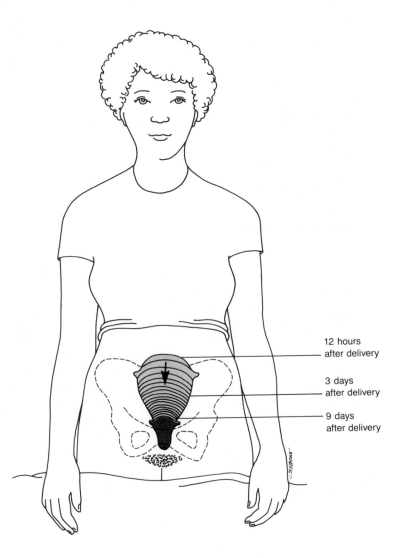

12 hours after delivery

3 days after delivery

9 days after delivery

Figure 29–1. The uterus involutes rapidly after delivery; by 2 weeks, the uterus is once again a pelvic organ, and by 6 weeks, it is only slightly larger than its nulliparous size. (Childbirth Graphics)

Table 29–1   **Stages in Uterine Involution**

Time Since Delivery	Position of Fundus	Uterine Weight	Lochia
1–2 hr	Midway between umbilicus and symphysis, on midline	1000 g	Rubra
12 hr	1 cm above or at umbilicus		Rubra
3 days	3 cm below umbilicus (continues descent at 1 cm/day)		Serosa
9 days	Not palpable above symphysis	500 g	Alba
5–6 weeks	Not palpable above symphysis; slightly larger than in nullipara		Not present

Adaptations of the Reproductive Organs

The involution of the uterus begins soon after delivery and proceeds rapidly (Fig. 29–1). After the placenta is expelled, the fundus of the uterus can be palpated midway between the symphysis and the umbilicus on the midline, or slightly higher. The contracted uterus in the immediate postpartum period is about the size of a large grapefruit. The uterine walls are closely approximated. The cervix is bruised, quite soft, and distensible in the first few hours; by 10 to 12 hours after delivery, the cervix has shortened and become firmer. Stages in uterine involution are summarized in Table 29–1.

Uterine Involution

By 12 hours after delivery, the fundus can be palpated at 1 cm (one finger breadth) above the umbilicus. Uterine contractions continue after delivery of the placenta. In primiparas, uterine tone is usually high, and the uterus remains firm. In multiparas, periodic uterine contraction and relaxation is more common causing "afterpains" that may be uncomfortable for 2 to 3 days and are likely to be intensified by breast-feeding.

Two days after delivery, the uterus begins to descend and shrink gradually. By the second or third day, the spongy layer of the decidua is sloughed off in the lochia. The outermost layer then becomes necrotic and also sloughs off. The innermost layer remains as the foundation for the new endometrium. By 2 weeks after delivery, the uterus has descended into the true pelvis and is not palpable above the symphysis. Superficial lacerations of the cervix are completely healed, and the external os has regained prepregnant tone. However, the shape of the os itself, now a lateral slit rather than a circular opening, is permanently changed. By 2 to 3 weeks, endometrial glands and stroma from interglandular connective tissue has proliferated, and the entire endometrium is restored, except for the placental site.

By 5 to 6 weeks the uterus has almost returned to its nonpregnant size. This change is due to a decrease in the size of individual cells, not to a reduction in the number of cells.

Lochia.   The uterus cleanses itself of debris after childbirth by a vaginal discharge called *lochia* (Table 29–2). *Lochia rubra,* the vaginal discharge of the first 3 days after delivery, is bloody and contains small clots. The presence of numerous large clots suggests unusual

Table 29–2   **Characteristics of Lochia**

Name	Approximate Time Since Delivery	Normal Discharge	Abnormal Discharge
Lochia rubra	Days 1 to 3	Bloody with clots Fleshy odor Increase in flow upon rising, with breast-feeding, with exertion	Numerous large clots Foul smell Saturated perineal pad
Lochia serosa	Days 4 to 9	Pink or brown with a serosanguineous consistency Fleshy odor	Foul smell Saturated perineal pad
Lochia alba	Day 10	Yellow to white Fleshy odor	Foul smell Saturated perineal pad Persistent lochia serosa Return to pink or red discharge Persistent discharge over 2 to 3 weeks

bleeding, and the patient should be further evaluated. Contraction of the uterus limits the amount of immediate postpartum bleeding through the compression of blood vessels by muscle fibers.

Continuous seepage of bright red blood when the fundus is firm suggests a bleeding cervical or vaginal laceration and the need for further evaluation. Lochia may appear to be heavier upon rising because of pooling in the vagina while the patient is recumbent. Flow may also be increased with breast-feeding or after exertion. After several days, the blood cell component of the lochia decreases, and the proportion of serous exudate increases. The flow becomes more pink or brown in color and has a serosanguineous consistency. This discharge is called *lochia serosa*. By the tenth day, the lochia *(lochia alba)* has become yellow to white and contains numerous leukocytes and cellular debris.

This progression of the discharge from bloody to pink to white or clear reflects the reestablishment of the uterine lining and the healing of the placental site. Persistent lochia serosa after 2 weeks, or a return to pink or red discharge after it has cleared, indicates subinvolution of the placental site (see the discussion in the following section) or late postpartum hemorrhage. Persistent discharge after 2 to 3 weeks may suggest endometritis, particularly when accompanied by pelvic tenderness or pain and fever. (These complications are dealt with in more detail in Chapter 30.)

Lochia has a fleshy odor similar to that of menstrual flow. A foul smell from the flow or from a used perineal pad suggests infection and the need for further assessment. Vaginal organisms are always present and can be found in the uterus as early as 2 days after delivery. In most cases, however, infection does not occur, perhaps because the organisms are not particularly virulent or because the uterine lining is already protected by a thin layer of granulating tissue.

Involution of the Placental Site.   The placental site heals by a different mechanism from the rest of the endometrium. The placental site is an area approximately 8 to 9 cm in diameter. Bleeding from this site is controlled by compression of vessels by the contracted uterine muscle fibers. The site contains thrombosed vessels, some of which will be replaced by new, smaller vessels. The site heals by exfoliation, which involves the undermining of the site by the growth of endometrial tissue from the margins and the proliferation of endometrial glands in the basal layer of the site. The undermined tissue becomes necrotic and sloughs off, usually around 6 weeks after delivery.

This process results in no fibrous scarring of the endometrium, which would limit the surface available for future implantation. Delay in healing or failure of the placental site to heal completely, called *subinvolution of the*

placental site, may result in persistent lochia and episodes of brisk, painless vaginal bleeding.

Vaginal Changes

Immediately after delivery, the walls of the vagina appear edematous and bruised, and small surface lacerations may be present. Vaginal rugae are absent. The hymen may have been torn in several places; the torn edges do not approximate. Small tags called *carunculae myrtiformes* will form along the torn edges. Congestion of the vaginal walls resolves within several days. Vaginal rugae begin to return by 3 weeks. The dimensions of the distended vagina gradually decrease; however, the vagina usually does not return to its previous nulliparous size. The vaginal mucosa remains atrophic until the hormonal cycle regulating menstruation is reestablished. The labia minora and labia majora appear slightly stretched and are less firm after the first vaginal birth.

Perineal Changes

The pressure of the descending fetal head stretches and thins the muscles of the pelvic floor. Common obstetric practice in the United States includes an incision in the perineum called an *episiotomy*. The rationale for this procedure is to prevent overstretching and weakening of the perineal muscles, which predisposes the woman to cystocele and rectocele, to prevent laceration of the perineum, and to expedite the delivery of the fetal head.

If an episiotomy has been performed, the edges of the incision should remain approximated and be free from ecchymoses, which can delay healing. The discomfort resulting from episiotomy varies according to the type of incision and repair, the length of the second stage and the degree of perineal pressure experienced, and the effectiveness of early management. Incisional discomfort or pain may persist as long as 5 to 6 weeks in some cases. Regardless of whether an episiotomy was performed, the perineum may become edematous and show some bruising in the early postpartum period. Muscle tone in the perineum will likely be reduced for several weeks and may be improved with specific exercises once the soft tissue has healed.

Psychological Adaptation

Along with the rapid and extensive physiologic changes experienced by the postpartum woman come a myriad of psychological adaptations. The simultaneous occurrence of these emotional changes with the biological ones makes the mother's adaptation quite complex. Although the father and other family members do not experience this physiologic reorganization, they must also adjust psychologically to the presence of the newborn. The mother's own psychological well-being depends in large part on how her partner and other family members respond to the birth of the new baby.

Therefore, the nurse must assist each patient's physical and psychological status and the psychological status of the father and other family members in order to provide appropriate and comprehensive nursing care. Knowledge of the basic psychological characteristics of maternal and paternal adaptation in the postpartum period provides the basis for nursing care.

Parental Adaptation

Parental adaptation in the postpartum period involves taking on new role responsibilities and behaviors, readjusting relationships with significant others, and beginning an acquaintance with the long-awaited newborn. This reorganization takes place on many levels and may be either enhanced or inhibited by the mother's physical state, the father's level of participation, and the nature and quality of their social supports.

Maternal Phases

Patterns have been observed in the progressive adaptation of women in the postpartum period. One of the first maternity nurses to engage in clinical research, Reva Rubin (1963a), observed the behavior of postpartum women as they took on the mothering role. She identified three phases in their behavior, summarized in the accompanying display. The nurse should recognize that many physical, psychological and cultural factors influence early maternal behavior and the timing of behavior change. Moreover, Rubin's work was done in the early 1960s; many aspects of maternity care have changed, as have women's expectations about the postpartum period. Contemporary nurse investigators find that most women progress through these phases much more rapidly than Rubin suggests. Thus, these phases are not strict guidelines for assessing maternal behavior; rather, they are useful as a way of observing progressions in maternal behavior.

Taking in: A Period of Dependent Behavior. The first maternal phase described by Rubin is called *taking in*. During this phase, the woman is primarily focused on herself and dependent on others. The inward focus of labor and birth persists, and the new mother's energy is centered on her own health and well-being, rather than on her infant. Her behavior may be passive and dependent, and she will readily accept assistance in meeting her physical and emotional needs. Decision making may be difficult, and assistance and support from care providers are greatly valued. Needs for rest and food are verbalized; the mother may have a large appetite. Emotionally, she is working to integrate the labor and birth process into her life experience. She may relive the events of labor and birth again and again, seeking details and comparing her

Rubin's Maternal Phases

Taking In: A Period of Dependent Behavior

- Focus on self
- Verbalization of need for sleep and food
- Reliving of birth experience
- Passive and dependent behavior

Taking Hold: Moving Between Dependence and Independence

- Widening of focus to include infant
- Independence in self-care activities
- Verbalized concern about body functions of self and infant
- Openness to teaching on care of self and infant
- Lack of confidence (mother is easily discouraged about caretaking skills)

Letting Go: Taking on New Role Responsibilities

- Increasing independence in care of self and infant
- Recognition of infant as separate from self
- Grief work for relinquished roles, expectations
- Adjustment of family relationships to accommodate infant

performance to her expectations, her previous birth experiences, or those of others. In Rubin's early description, the taking-in phase lasted for 1 or 2 days; contemporary clinicians may observe this behavior in the first hours after birth.

Taking Hold: Movement Between Dependent and Independent Behavior. Gradually, the woman's energy level increases. She feels more comfortable, and she is able to focus less on herself and more on her infant. The new mother is now more independent, initiating self-care activities and often voicing concerns about body functions. Control of bowel and bladder function as well as her ability to breast-feed, if she chooses to do so, are of concern. As she regains control of her body, she becomes more able to accept responsibility for the care of her newborn. Being successful as caretaker is vital to her; she responds enthusiastically to instruction and praise regarding her mothering skills.

For this reason, the phase Rubin labels *taking hold* may be ideal for teaching about infant and self-care. However, the nurse should be careful to avoid assuming the mothering role. The new mother may be anxious and easily discouraged. She may interpret the nurse's competence as a reflection of her own incompetence and see herself as a failure. If, instead, the mother is allowed to assume the care of her infant with appropriate guidance and frequent reassurance from the nursing staff, she will be more confident.

Letting Go: Moving to Independence in a New Role. The final phase, *letting go,* as described by Rubin, began near the end of the first week after delivery. Contemporary mothers may progress to this point sooner, but early postpartum discharge still makes it likely that the nurse will not see evidence of this maternal behavior. As the name implies, this is a time of relinquishment for the new mother. She must give up roles that are inconsistent with her new identity, such as that of the dependent new mother, the childless woman, or the mother of one child. She now must take on the responsibilities of the new role of mother of a newborn.

The new mother must also adjust to the physical separation of the baby and recognize that the baby is no longer a part of her body but a separate and unique individual. She must also give up her fantasized birth and infant and accept the real versions, as well as dealing with her partner's met and unmet expectations about the birth experience and their newborn. To accomplish this requires some grief work and a readjustment of her relationships with her partner and other family members. Feelings of being "let down" or mild depression in the early postpartum period may be a result of this grief work and reorganization of family ties.

Maternal Touch

Along with her observations on maternal phases, Rubin also observed and described the development of maternal touch (1963 b). Contrary to common belief, few mothers feel instantly close to their newborns. The relationship between a mother and her infant must develop over time, as does any relationship between two human beings who do not know each other. Initially, the mother touches her new infant tentatively, using her fingertips and touching only small portions of the baby's body (Fig. 29–2). Gradually, as she becomes more comfortable with herself as a mother and better acquainted with her infant, she will use her hand to stroke larger areas of the infant's body. Eventually, as her comfort and familiarity increase, the mother will enfold the infant in her arms and hold it close to her body.

Many psychological, physical, and cultural factors affect the progression of maternal touch. When Rubin made her first observations over 20 years ago, she noted that it often took a mother several days to fully develop maternal touch. At that time mothers and newborns were routinely separated for hours after birth. Newborns were kept fully clothed and wrapped and mothers often had access to them only at feeding time.

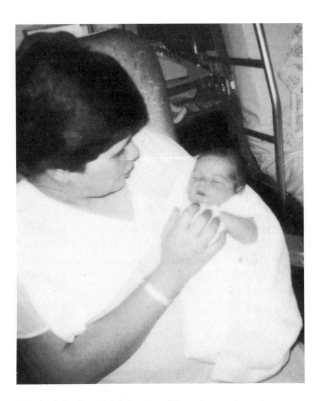

Figure 29–2. Acquaintance of mother and newborn through visual and tactile sense. (Photo: T. Mudrick)

A visit to a mother–infant recovery room in any hospital setting will show that this progression can be accomplished in a matter of hours, in part because of current practices that attempt to promote early contact between parents and their newborn. However, if complications arise for either mother or newborn that delay or interfere with the opportunity for parent–infant acquaintance, a slower progression in the development of maternal touch can be expected.

Postpartum Blues and Postpartum Depression

The nurse must be aware of the emotional swings commonly experienced by newly delivered women. The terms *postpartum blues* and *baby blues* are used to describe the transient feelings of depression experienced by up to 80% of women in the first 10 days after delivery (Hawkins and Gorvine 1985). Symptoms may include unexplained tearfulness, irritability, and disturbances in appetite and sleep patterns.

Many women are unprepared for these let-down feelings after having a baby because they have been socialized to expect that once the baby is born, the family will live "happily ever after." In reality, the adjustment to new parenthood is often difficult, and many factors may combine to bring on these feelings of depression. One stressor, commonly identified as a major contributor to mild depression, is the hormonal fluctuation that occurs after birth. Also contributing are the major psychological adjustments necessary during the transition to parenthood, perineal and breast discomfort, exhaustion, and the mother's disappointment about the appearance of her postpartum body.

The nurse must remember that postpartum or baby blues are self-limiting and that recovery is spontaneous. They most frequently occur during the first 6 weeks after delivery but may recur during the first year in response to the ongoing transition to the parental role and adjustments of family life to childcare. When depression continues for 2 weeks or more and leads to feelings of despondency and inability to cope with the demands of daily life, the condition is more serious and is accurately described as *postpartum depression*. Postpartum depression occurs in approximately 10% of new mothers (Hazle 1982). Postpartum depression responds best to active treatment. The nurse should be able to differentiate between the two conditions so that true depression can be identified and treated early. Postpartum blues and depression are further discussed in Chapter 30, which contains a Nursing Care Plan for dealing with them.

Paternal Responses

Little is known about the father's adaptation in the postpartum period because research has only recently begun on many aspects of expectant and new fatherhood. The father often experiences a fascination with the newborn, just as the mother does. However, many men are reluctant to hold or handle the newborn and will wait for encouragement from others.

Most men have a similar period of excitement after the birth and may express it in several ways. Some men experience a strong family bond at this time and want to stay close to their partner and the newborn; these men will often take advantage of hospital policies that allow them to stay overnight with the rest of their family. Others will communicate the news to other family members and friends or go out and "celebrate" in traditional ways.

The father's immediate postpartum response will depend in large part on his involvement in the birth process. Usually the father experiences fatigue and a need for sleep at about the same time that the mother does but may need to be encouraged to get rest. If problems arose during the birth or with the newborn, fathers often accompany the newborn to the nursery; in this situation, the father becomes the mother's most important source of information about the newborn. This role is one for which men are often not prepared; the father may experience worry and anxiety not only about the condition of his wife and baby but also about the need to stay on top of the situation.

Little is known about the process of paternal adaptation in the later postpartum period. Early research on new fathers suggested that those who were active participants in the birth process developed an earlier and stronger tie

to the newborn and that they perceived their relationship with their spouses as closer in the postpartum period. However, later research shows that although the birth experience is important for the father, his own personality, his readiness for fatherhood, and his previous relationship with his spouse determine his responses to his spouse and his infant. His presence at the birth or early contact with the infant do not appear to have as significant an effect as was once believed (May and Perrin 1985).

Nevertheless, *unrestricted access* to the spouse and newborn is important to fathers. Fathers who become demanding and angry with hospital staff are often those who have been kept from spouse and baby by hospital policy or have been made to feel as if they are in the way. Most hospitals now do not consider fathers as visitors on postpartum units; however, many facilities still restrict fathers' access to their partners during postsurgical recovery after cesarean birth or do not welcome them wholeheartedly into the newborn admission nursery. Fathers perceive when they are considered "necessary evils" and sometimes resent such treatment (May and Sollid 1984).

Recent research suggests that fathers also may experience postpartum "baby blues" and even depression (May and Perrin 1985). For fathers the cause is clearly not hormonal, as it may be in mothers. Sleep interruption, concerns about financial responsibilities, insecurity about parenting abilities, and difficulty adapting to the changes in the couple relationship are believed to be contributing factors.

Family Adaptation

The arrival of a newborn in a family requires that roles and relationships within the family unit be reorganized. Other children now have a younger sibling, parents become grandparents, and husband and wife now must share each other's attention with a demanding, dependent infant. In addition, family routines and living arrangements must be adapted to accommodate the newborn. Even the most well organized couple will find that patterns and schedules are totally disrupted during the postpartum period.

Most of this disorganization and reorganization is related to learning to care for and anticipate the needs of the new infant while continuing to meet the other demands of daily life. In family networks where there are many hands to help, this work may be easier and less of a strain on new parents. Where there is no extended network, the task of caring for a new infant and maintaining work, home, and family life is more difficult. The families who make an easier adjustment are those for whom extended support networks are available and those whose employment and household responsibilities are flexible.

As more women enter the work force and more men

FAMILY CONSIDERATIONS

Supporting Women Returning to Work After Childbirth

Increasing numbers of women are returning to work within weeks of the birth of their first infants. Nearly one half of new American mothers return to employment before their infants reach 1 year of age. Common concerns among employed mothers include conflicts between personal needs and family and career obligations, difficulties maintaining breast-feeding responsibilities, maternal fatigue and guilt, concerns about the adequacy of role performance and difficulties establishing and maintaining adequate external and marital support.

A needs assessment was conducted in the mid-Michigan area to determine the level of interest in a program designed to facilitate maternal adaptation after return to work. A program was then developed based on information available in the scientific and lay literature as well as on information gained from open-ended interviews with focus groups of women with infants or toddlers who anticipated returning or who had already returned to employment.

A six-session program was then developed, stressing self-assessment, strategies to reduce environmental stressors and to maintain individual and family well-being. Evaluation of the program suggests that a community-based program of nursing intervention can promote optimal adaptation for women by exploring issues that arise when combining employment and new motherhood and developing strategies to cope with multiple roles.

Collins C, Tiedje L: A program for women returning to work after childbirth. J Obstet Gynecol Neonatal Nurs 17(4):246–254, 1988

become actively involved in child care and household duties, some may assume that the division of labor in childbearing families is now less determined by gender. After the birth of a child, however, families tend to adopt more traditional divisions of labor, regardless of their members' previous attitudes toward male and female roles. In families with new infants, women continue to be the primary caretakers and to assume responsibility for household management and men continue to be wage earners with less involvement in child care.

In large part, this occurs because the woman requires a period of restoration after birth and because breast-feeding requires close, continuous contact with the newborn, at least for the first several months of life. A major task of families with new infants is to adjust to these shifts in roles and responsibilities while continuing to meet the needs of the individuals in the family. The adjustment each individual makes directly affects the well-being of the family as a unit, which in turn affects the well-being of the individual. For this reason the postpartum nurse must constantly keep in mind that although she may be providing direct care to the new mother and her newborn, her goal includes promoting optimal individual and family adaptation and her scope of responsibility includes the entire family.

Assessment

Assessment of the postpartum family encompasses a review of the prenatal and intrapartal records, physical assessment of the mother, and psychosocial assessment of the mother, father, and other important family members. The nurse must have a comprehensive knowledge of the changes that occur in the postpartum period in order to detect deviations from the norm and provide early treatment.

In reviewing the prenatal record, the nurse must take note of preexisting health problems as well as pregnancy-induced problems. Conditions such as anemia, pregnancy-induced hypertension, and diabetes can predispose the mother and, in some cases, her infant to complications in the postpartum period. The nurse must also review the intrapartal record for the following information:

- Length of labor and type of delivery
- Status of membranes and amniotic fluid
- Fetal response to labor
- Medications and analgesia/anesthesia used in labor
- Family members' (especially the father's) response to labor and birth

Once this information has been reviewed, the nurse conducts a systematic assessment of the mother's physical and psychological status as well as the father's psychological status and the family's response to the newborn.

Assessing Maternal Physiologic Status

The nurse must monitor the postpartum woman's physiologic status carefully in the immediate postpartum period. The emphasis should be on vital signs, maintenance of fluid balance, prevention of abnormal blood loss, and maintenance of urinary elimination.

Vital Signs

The mother's vital signs must be monitored frequently in the early postpartum period, primarily to assess cardiovascular adaptation and screen for infection. Generally, vital signs are taken every 4 hours for the first 24 hours, and every 8 hours thereafter. Fluctuations in blood pressure in the immediate postpartum period may be related to orthostatic hypotension or hemorrhage; changes after that time may be related to infection or late postpartum hemorrhage. An increase of 30 mm Hg systolic pressure or 15 mm Hg diastolic pressure over prelabor levels may suggest preeclampsia and requires further evaluation. Temperature elevations must be noted; two observations of temperature elevations above 100.4°F (38°C) suggest infection, and further assessment is required.

Uterine Tone, Position, and Height

The nurse assesses uterine tone, position, and height by abdominal palpation. In preparing the patient for this assessment, the nurse should explain the procedure and its purpose. The patient should be asked to empty her bladder prior to the examination to ensure a correct assessment of uterine tone and position. The head of the bed should be flat and the patient in a supine position.

To provide support to the lower uterine segment, the nurse places one hand just above the symphysis pubis and applies gentle downward pressure (Fig. 29–3). Support of the lower uterine segment helps to prevent prolapse of the uterus into the vagina, should excessive pressure be used in palpation of the fundus. With the other hand, the nurse gently palpates the abdomen to locate the fundus of the uterus. The involuting uterus will feel rounded and firm; a boggy or soft uterus increases the risk of hemorrhage. The position of the uterus should be noted; deviation from the normal midline position may suggest a distended bladder. Displacement of the uterus by a full bladder can predispose the mother to uterine atony and postpartum hemorrhage.

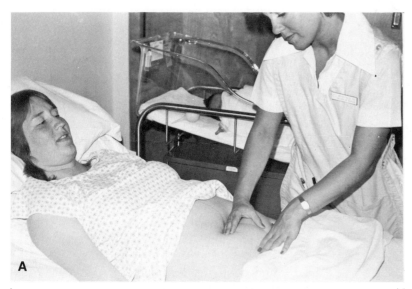

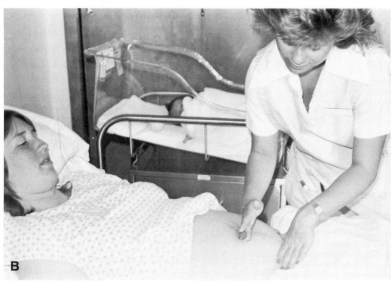

Figure 29–3. Assessing fundal position and height. *(A)* The nurse notes the position of the fundus. *(B)* The nurse assesses its height in centimeters from the umbilicus. (Courtesy of Samuel Merritt College of Nursing)

After noting the tone and position of the uterus, the nurse notes the height of the fundus in centimeters or (finger-breadths) from the umbilicus. If the nurse can place two fingers between the umbilicus and the fundus, she will chart uterine height as "2 FB below U," or "U/2." If the fundus is one finger-breadth above the umbilicus, that would be recorded as "1 FB above U," or "1/U." During this abdominal palpation, the nurse should note whether diastasis recti is present and, if it is, should measure the diastasis in finger-breadths.

Assessment of the mother with a cesarean incision will vary according to the type of incision, the degree of incisional pain she is experiencing, and the amount of surgical dressing covering the incision. The nurse may not be able to assess the position and height of the fundus, but uterine tone usually can be assessed by gently palpating the side of the uterus away from the surgical incision. The surgical dressing should be checked for drainage and bleeding; the surgical incision should be assessed for approximation of the wound edges, redness, drainage, and tenderness.

Generally, the mother's uterine tone, position, and height should be assessed every 4 hours for the first 24 hours after delivery. Assessment and recording of diastasis recti is necessary only once in the early postpartum period, since no change in that condition is likely to be noted in this period.

Type and Amount of Lochia

The nurse assesses lochial flow in conjunction with the fundal check. With the patient in a supine position, the nurse lowers the perineal pad and assesses lochial flow for amount, color, odor, and presence of clots. The nurse should question the patient to determine how frequently pads have been changed and the degree of saturation.

Lochial flow is described as heavy, moderate, or scant. A patient who saturates a pad every 2 hours is considered to be experiencing a heavy flow. If the amount of lochia is comparable to menstrual flow, it is considered moderate, whereas an amount less than that is considered to be scant.

Heavy lochial flow always requires further nursing assessment to determine the cause, if possible. The woman will experience what appears to be heavy flow of lochia upon rising after several hours in a recumbent position; this is the result of pooling of lochia in the vagina and lower uterine segment. Heavy flow may also be related to uterine atony and retained placental fragments. Brisk vaginal bleeding may occur as a result of cervical or vaginal lacerations and may be difficult to distinguish from lochia. Prolonged heavy lochia should be reported to the attending physician or nurse midwife.

Breast Changes

The breasts should be soft and not tender during the first 24 to 48 hours after delivery. They will gradually become firmer as they prepare for lactation. The nurse can assess for signs of engorgement by palpating the breast for firmness and questioning the patient about tenderness. Once engorgement has occurred, the nurse should assess the patient's comfort frequently. The nurse assesses the nipples of the breast-feeding woman regularly for signs of irritation that can lead to cracking and bleeding. If nipples are flat or inverted, the mother may need guidance in early breast-feeding. Breast assessment is recommended twice a day during the hospitalization period.

Condition of the Perineum and Rectum

Assessment of the perineum and rectum should be done every 4 hours for the first 24 hours and daily thereafter. The nurse should inspect the perineum by asking the patient to move into a side-lying position and draw the upper knee up toward the chest; the nurse can then gently separate the buttocks and examine both the perineum and the rectum. If the patient has had an episiotomy, the nurse assesses for redness, edema, ecchymosis, discharge, and approximation of the wound edges (REEDA). The patient who has not had an episiotomy should be assessed for perineal bruising and edema. The nurse should ask the patient about the degree of discomfort. A bruised, edematous, and painful perineum may be suggestive of a perineal hematoma, and further evaluation by the physician or nurse midwife is needed. The nurse can also assess the rectum for hemorrhoids, which are common in the postpartum period and usually resolve without further treatment.

Bladder Function

The nurse should assess urinary output in the postpartum patient to identify potential difficulty in voiding. The

NURSING ALERT

Review of HIV and Hepatitis Precautions

Latex gloves should be worn *for every patient* when

Inspecting the perineum

Changing or handling perineal pads

Changing soiled linen

Starting or discontinuing intravenous catheters

Anticipating contact with mucous membranes, blood, body fluids, or nonintact skin

first few voidings should be measured; frequent voiding of small amounts of urine suggests incomplete emptying of the bladder. This condition is verified if a straight catheterization immediately after a voiding produces 50 ml or more residual urine. Bladder distention without the sensation of needing to void is also common in the immediate postpartum period; the nurse should palpate the abdomen to determine whether the uterus is displaced from the midline by a full bladder. The woman should be encouraged to void every 3 to 4 hours to avoid overdistention and further decrease in bladder tone. All postpartum mothers should be instructed to report burning on urination, since this may be an early sign of urinary tract infection.

The mother with a cesarean birth will have an indwelling urinary catheter for the first 12 to 24 hours postpartum. Urine needs to be assessed for amount, color, and presence of blood, which suggests bladder trauma. After the catheter is removed, the first few voidings should be measured to assess bladder emptying.

Gastrointestinal Function

Assessment of gastrointestinal function in the postpartum patient includes listening for bowel sounds, observing for nausea and vomiting, and questioning the patient about flatulence or bowel movements. These assessments are generally recommended twice a day until normal function has been established. The normal postpartum diet should be well balanced and high in protein, with a fluid intake of around 3000 ml per day to promote tissue healing and prevent constipation.

Special attention should be given to the postcesarean patient, since return of normal gastrointestinal function is delayed. Bowel sounds should be present before the patient is advanced to solid food, to avoid exacerbation of a possible postoperative ileus (absence of peristalsis). Fluid intake and output of the postcesarean patient should also be carefully monitored.

Lower Extremities

The lower extremities should be assessed for sensation, strength, edema, and signs of thromboembolism in the immediate postpartum period. The presence of any of the following signs of thromboembolism requires the nurse to restrict the patient to bedrest and notify the physician immediately:

- Redness, warmth, and pain in the calf area
- Subjective feeling of heaviness in the affected extremity
- Positive *Homans' sign:* dorsiflexion of foot causes muscles to compress veins, producing pain if thrombosis is present.

Thromboembolism is discussed in more detail in Chapter 30.

Maternal Rest and Comfort

As part of her assessment, the nurse should inquire about the amount of rest and sleep the mother is getting and ask how she can assist in promoting rest during the hospitalization. Mothers may not anticipate having difficulty sleeping after the demands of labor and birth; however, excitement, the strange environment, and discomfort may seriously disrupt a sleep pattern that was probably already compromised by the period of labor. Mothers may hesitate to ask for assistance in this area and may not volunteer information because they think it is an unimportant problem.

Assessing Maternal Psychological Status

In the first 24 hours after delivery, the nurse assesses the mother's psychological status to monitor mood, her feelings about the birth experience, the responses of significant others to the infant, and the adequacy of the social support system available.

Immediately after a normal delivery, most women feel great excitement. Even a woman who has just completed a long and difficult labor will feel a rush of energy as she is flooded with joy at the birth of a healthy baby and relief that she has passed the ordeal of childbirth. Absence of this excitement in the newly delivered woman warrants further assessment.

Maternal Response to Birth

The nurse can employ this initial excitement phase to help the woman begin to integrate the birth into her life experience. Reviewing the labor and birth experience with the mother allows the nurse to determine whether the woman has predominantly negative or positive feelings about it. It is appropriate for the nurse to offer praise for a job well done and to convey understanding if the woman expresses disappointment or anger about some aspect of the process. A follow-up visit from the labor and delivery nurse involved in her care further enhances this integration process by allowing the mother to relive the birth with another participant and ask any questions she may have (Mercer 1981).

Maternal Perceptions of Family Responses

Another important aspect of the maternal psychological assessment is determining how the mother perceives the response of her significant others to the newborn. The mother's knowledge that the infant she has delivered is accepted by her mate, family, and friends serves to reinforce their acceptance of *her* as a woman and a mother.

NURSING RESEARCH

Postpartum Integration

Dyanne Affonso's research study (1977) of postpartum women revealed that women during the early postpartum period cannot recall all of the events that occurred during their labor and birth experience. Her subjects indicated a need to recall these vague events or "missing pieces," and they would spend considerable amounts of time reviewing the events of labor and birth by talking to others, asking questions, and dreaming about their experience. Affonso postulated that women need to reconstruct their labor and birth experience and fill in these "missing pieces" in order to continue in their transition to parenthood. She suggested that nursing staff can assist the woman in this reconstruction by providing information about the woman's labor and birth experience.

A recent study reexamined the concept of "missing pieces" in the process of postpartum psychological adaptation. Of 70 women interviewed between 24 and 72 hours postpartum, six described events during childbirth as being confusing and six identified "missing pieces," for a total of 17% of the sample. The latter six defined "missing pieces" as external events related to the use of technological equipment and directions from others. Those who said they were confused but experienced no feeling of missing pieces described global events, such as losing track of time. The incidence of confusion and missing pieces was only a fraction of the percentage Affonso reported in 1977 (90%), perhaps because mind-altering medication is used less frequently today or because women are better educated about modern management of labor and delivery. Nursing implications from this study include the importance of examining human behavior in context and recognizing the impact of patient education, societal change, and technological modes of intervention on psychological adaptation.

Affonso DD: "Missing pieces" — a study of postpartum feelings. Birth and the Family Journal 4:159, 1977

Stolte K: Postpartum 'missing pieces': Sequela of a passing obstetrical era? Birth 13(2):100, 1986

This acceptance seems to be particularly important to successful adaptation to the maternal role.

To assess this, the nurse can observe interactions between the mother, father, and other significant persons. The nurse may also ask, "How does your family feel about this baby?" If acceptance of the child by significant others is not clear, the nurse should provide extra support to this mother and observe for potential problems in the parent–infant relationship.

Finally, the nurse should assess whether the mother is receiving adequate emotional support. Depending on her individual circumstances, such support may come from the woman's mate or the father of the baby, her parents, or friends. Flowers, gifts, phone calls, and visitors are signals of support from others. The patient with no apparent support is at risk for problems in adaptation to motherhood and should receive extra support from the postpartum nurse as well as referral for follow-up upon discharge.

Ongoing Assessment of Maternal Psychological Status

During the remainder of the hospital stay, the nurse continues to assess the woman's adjustment to the maternal role. Her behavior with her newborn should be observed and any difficulties noted. The nurse should observe for any evidence of postpartum blues and for indications that maternal–infant acquaintance is not proceeding as expected. One useful sign to observe is evidence of healthy self-esteem in the new mother. Wearing makeup, arranging her hair, and donning an attractive gown for visiting hours are positive signs.

As always, the nurse must consider each patient as an individual. Many factors affect the psychological and emotional responses of a woman after birth. Some of these include the woman's age and parity, her cultural background, and the presence of complications in the intrapartal period. Nurses often assume that primiparas need more assistance and teaching postpartally than do multiparas (Mercer 1979) because the multipara has been through the experience before and knows what to expect. In reality, however, all new mothers need nursing support. The needs of the multipara are different in that she needs to find the energy to love and care for an additional child, may have lower physical and emotional reserves on which to draw, and must anticipate a greatly increased complexity in her family life.

Assessing Family Adaptation

The nurse may have contact only with the mother and father in the postpartum period and thus may not be able to assess the process of family adaptation directly. While working with the new mother, however, the nurse should keep in mind the family as the focus of care. The father of the baby is most often the mother's primary support person. The adaptation of each partner is largely dependent on that of the other.

Paternal Psychological Status

The nurse must recognize the psychological adaptation required of fathers in the postpartum period. Although men do not experience physiologic changes as their partners do, they experience similar needs to integrate the birth into their life experience, become acquainted with their newborn, and begin taking on the role of father of a newborn. In addition, most fathers are concerned about their partner's physical well-being and need information about her condition. Further, since most men have little or no experience in caring for newborns, fathers tend to need more information about infant care and are less confident about their ability to provide care to their newborn.

Reliving and Integrating the Birth Experience.
As men have become more actively involved in childbirth, new postpartum responses have been identified among new fathers. A father may need to relive the birth experience with his partner and with others, yet this need may not always be recognized. Some fathers find that they have little or no opportunity to discuss the birth with anyone other than their spouses. This may be troublesome for fathers who had planned to be active participants in the birth but were unable to fulfill that role because of complications during labor. Fathers frequently are excluded from cesarean deliveries. The nurse should be alert to the possibility that the father may feel disappointment, grief, or anger at "missing the birth," even as he feels relief that mother and baby received needed care. Fathers, especially those who had been involved in the labor process, may seek out someone with whom they can talk, often looking for reassurance that they could not have prevented the complications that required the cesarean birth (May and Sollid 1984).

Father–Infant Acquaintance.
Relatively little research has been done to date on the process of father–infant acquaintance. Observations of parent–newborn interaction suggest that patterns of touching and holding the infant in the first days of life are more alike than different among mothers and fathers. However, fathers tend to hold and touch newborns less when mothers are present, suggesting that men defer to their partners and see their role in care-giving as secondary to the mothers'.

Fathers vary in their comfort with involvement in infant caretaking. Some need encouragement, and others do not see infant caretaking as part of their role as husband and father; the latter view is more common among men from ethnic or cultural groups in which more traditional sex roles are valued. The nurse should assess each father's comfort in assuming caretaking responsibilities, recognizing that families will divide child-care duties differently. Regardless of how much actual caretaking the father will provide, however, the nurse should assess his knowledge about the newborn. This knowledge provides part of the basis for the father's interactions with his newborn. If it is inaccurate or limited, the father may be inhibited in establishing a positive relationship with his infant.

Disappointment and Paternal Adaptation.
The nurse should also assess the father's expectations about his partner's postpartum recovery and his infant on the one hand, and his actual circumstances on the other. Men are often ill-prepared for the demands of caring for a new infant and for the length of time their partners will require for postpartum recovery. If a man were looking forward to a quick return to his partner's prepregnant figure, high energy level, and sexual activity, he may be distinctly disappointed at the restorative time required. This disappointment may contribute to resentment, withdrawn behavior, and potential difficulties in establishing a relationship with the newborn and reestablishing the couple relationship after birth.

Other circumstances may predispose a father to feelings of disappointment in the postpartum period, such as complications in the birth process, maternal complications that delay recovery or threaten the mother's health, or the birth of an infant of the "wrong" sex or with a minor anomaly. Fathers often express a stronger desire than do mothers for a newborn of a particular sex and may respond with more shock to a minor physical anomaly, such as a visible birthmark. The nurse should be particularly alert to the father's responses to his newborn and his partner under these circumstances and should carefully assess the father's emotional status as part of her care.

Parental Caretaking

Along with the psychological assessments made in the postpartum period, the nurse should also assess the parents' ability to care for their newborn. In many cases, the nurse will have most contact with the mother, and the mother will be the primary caretaker for the newborn after discharge. However, family-centered care requires that the father be included as much as possible in providing and teaching about infant care.

The nurse will find that mothers will vary considerably in their knowledge and skill in infant care; some women are complete novices at feeding and caring for infants, whereas others are quite experienced and confident. Even an experienced mother, however, may encounter difficulties in caring for a new baby whose behavior is very different from that of her previous children. A multipara whose first two children were quiet and easily consoled may become very frustrated in caring for a third child who is active and less easily comforted.

Fathers are less variable, since it is quite rare for men to have had much contact or experience with infants. Even experienced fathers tend not to be confident in their caretaking with small infants, either because they had little involvement in caretaking when previous children were newborns, or because they feel more at ease with older infants. While breastfeeding is clearly the superior feeding method for most mothers and infants, it tends to exclude fathers from many caretaking activities; thus, the father may not have the opportunity to become expert in certain skills.

In order to assess parental caretaking, the nurse can observe parents as they provide newborn care and inquire about their previous experience in caring for babies. Often the parents' inexperience is obvious, and they will request assistance and reassurance. In other cases the nurse may need to give parents the opportunity to ask questions about aspects of care. She may say to more experienced parents, "Is there anything about caring for your baby that you aren't clear on? Is there anything about this baby that seems different from your other children?"

The nurse should be careful to assess parents' caretaking completely before offering assistance or showing them how to do something. The nurse's competence in infant care can be quite discouraging to new parents, who may be uncertain that they will ever be that skillful and then will stop trying to develop their own methods and skills.

Family Responses to the Newborn

The family's responses to the newborn are very important to both parents, especially to the mother. Responses of relatives, grandparents, and other children symbolize acceptance of them as parents and of their new family. The nurse should be especially alert to family responses that imply that there is something unusual about the childbirth or the infant. These responses may occur when the newborn has some benign physical variation, such as a molded head or a birthmark. Family responses may also be affected by differences in cultural or religious practices. For example, grandparents may be shocked to see an uncircumcised male infant. A sister may disagree with the new mother's decision to bottle-feed. In these situations, the nurse can expect the new parents to show some delay in their postpartum adjustment as they attempt to integrate family responses with their own thoughts and feelings about themselves and their newborn.

Family Support and Assistance After Discharge

The nurse should assess the level of family support and assistance available to the new parents on their return home. Usually such plans are made in advance of the birth and are of some importance to family members. New parents who anticipate no additional assistance in the first few weeks home with their baby may be at risk for a more difficult adjustment to parenting.

Diagnosis

Nursing diagnosis and planning for care in the postpartum setting are based on the accuracy and completeness of ongoing assessments. Many women and their families will encounter no problems in their postpartum adaptation and will require only supportive care and teaching for effective self-care and infant care. In some families, however, the nurse may identify both existing and potential problems in her physiologic and psychological assessments.

The following nursing diagnoses reflect possible problems in maternal status that may arise in the postpartum period. They may be addressed independently and may be useful in planning postpartum care to new families:

- Potential fluid volume deficit
- Altered patterns of urinary elimination
- Altered bowel elimination: constipation
- Altered comfort: pain
- Self-concept disturbance
- Potential for altered parenting
- Altered health maintenance: need for self-care/newborn information
- Self-care deficit

The nurse must also monitor for and provide supportive care directed at preventing complications. Such complications include the following:

- Postpartum hemorrhage
- Postpartum mood disturbance
- Postpartum infection

Such complications require collaboration with other members of the health care team and are discussed in the next chapter. Some of the interventions in this chapter, however, are directed at preventing complications.

Planning and Implementation

On the basis of identified patient needs, the postpartum nurse plans her care, taking into account the following factors:

- Condition of both mother and infant
- Anticipated length of hospitalization of both mother and infant
- Availability of the father for involvement in care and teaching

Based on the nurse's assessment of patient and family needs, a plan of care is developed and implemented. Nursing interventions in postpartum care center on monitoring, restoration, and patient education.

Monitoring and Supporting Maternal Physiologic Status

Monitoring and Care

The postpartum nurse must actively monitor and support the mother's physiologic status in the immediate and early postpartum periods.

Vital Signs

Fluctuations in blood pressure related to orthostatic hypotension can result in weakness and syncope. Patients experiencing orthostatic hypotension should be instructed to sit on the edge of the bed before standing and to rise slowly. The nurse should always accompany the postpartum mother on her first ambulation to provide assistance. If hypotension is accompanied by rapid pulse, further assessment of uterine tone and lochia is recommended to rule out early postpartum hemorrhage.

Temperature is monitored carefully to screen for the presence of infection. Elevations should be noted; if dehydration is the likely cause, the nurse should recommend an increase in oral fluid intake. If temperature elevation persists, antibiotic therapy is sometimes initiated prophylactically, even before a source of infection is identified. Usually, however, a culture to identify the source of infection is done first.

Monitoring and Promoting Optimal Uterine Tone

If the fundus feels soft or boggy, the nurse should gently massage it in a slow, circular fashion to avoid overstimulation of the uterine muscle. She should feel the fundal tone increase in a few moments. If the uterus does not respond to massage, the physician or nurse midwife should be notified, since an oxytocic agent may be required to facilitate restoration of uterine tone.

Monitoring Lochia

Heavy lochial flow is usually associated with uterine atony and can be controlled by fundal massage to restore uterine tone. If the uterus is firm and lochia remains heavy, the nurse should consult the physician or nurse midwife, who should inspect the cervix and vaginal walls for lacerations.

The mother should be taught what normal changes in lochia to expect and instructed to notify her care provider if symptomatic changes occur after discharge. Warning signs are listed in the display.

SELF-CARE TEACHING

Changes in Lochia to Report

The nurse should instruct every postpartum patient to report the following symptoms to her health care provider immediately:

- Foul-smelling lochia: suggests endometritis
- Heavy lochia: suggest uterine atony, retained placental fragments, or vaginal/cervical laceration
- Lochia rubra after the third postpartum day: suggests late postpartum hemorrhage
- Presence of clots: suggests retained placental fragments or hemorrhage

---

Monitoring Extremities for Thrombophlebitis

Early ambulation of mothers in the postpartum period has significantly reduced the incidence of thrombophlebitis. Once normal sensation and strength have returned to the extremities, the patient should be encouraged to begin walking and gentle stretching. Pain, warmth, or tenderness in the calf or a swollen, reddened area that feels thick are signs of thromboembolism and must be reported to the physician immediately. The extremity involved should be elevated on pillows and the patient confined to bed with movement of the leg minimized.

Expected Outcome: The postpartum woman returns to normal physiologic status as demonstrated by vital signs (including temperature) within normal range and lochia at expected stage by discharge and a firm uterus descending one finger-breadth per day.

Promoting Restoration of Bodily Function

A major nursing responsibility in the postpartum period is to help the mother restore normal body functions that have been disrupted by labor and birth.

Restoring Bladder Function

The nurse should encourage the patient to void every 3 to 4 hours to avoid overdistention of the bladder. Since the patient usually experiences some decrease in sensation, she may need to be reminded to void. If the patient experiences difficulty in voiding, privacy, warm water poured over the perineum, or the sound of running water may help initiate it. The postpartum patient must void within

12 hours to prevent overdistention and stasis of urine; if she cannot void spontaneously in that time, a straight catheterization is warranted.

Restoring Gastrointestinal Function

Nursing care should be directed at promotion of normal gastrointestinal functioning in the postpartum mother. In the immediate postpartum period, mothers, especially those recovering from cesarean birth, may experience nausea and vomiting. These patients are generally given no food by mouth or are given only clear liquids until nausea and vomiting subside. The postcesarean patient will generally be kept on intravenous fluids for the first 12 to 24 hours after the delivery. At that point she is often advanced to a clear liquid diet, as tolerated, until bowel sounds are reestablished and flatus is passed, when a regular diet can be started.

Decreased peristalsis, alterations in diet patterns, and concern about discomfort predispose the postpartum mother to constipation. A high-fiber diet and high fluid intake (3000 ml/day) will aid in decreasing constipation. Early ambulation, especially in the cesarean patient, is also important and will accelerate the return of normal peristalsis. Stool softeners are often administered to decrease potential perineal discomfort on defecation. Anticipated or actual pain associated with an episiotomy can delay the return of normal bowel function. The nurse can help reduce the patient's concern by listening to her fears and providing appropriate information and reassurance.

If bowel function is not reestablished by the third or fourth day, an enema may be considered. However, enemas are contraindicated for patients with third- or fourth-degree perineal lacerations because of the risk of trauma and of contamination of the perineal and rectal repair.

Expected Outcomes:

- The postpartum woman establishes normal bladder function as evidenced by complete emptying of the bladder, with the uterus in a midline position, by the end of the first 24 hours postpartum.
- The postpartum woman establishes gastrointestinal function as evidenced by normal bowel sounds, passing of flatus, and toleration of a regular diet by the end of the immediate postpartum period (first 24 hours) following a vaginal birth or by 48 hours following a cesarean birth.

Promoting Rest and Comfort

Another important nursing responsibility is the promotion of rest and comfort.

Promoting Rest

The nurse may need to be especially watchful for opportunities to promote rest for the postpartum mother. Following the birth, women usually experience an emotional "high" that can interfere with rest and sleep, as can visitors and phone calls, frequent nursing assessments, time spent with the newborn, and pain.

The nurse should encourage the mother to limit phone calls and visitors to certain periods so that she can rest uninterrupted. The nurse can organize her nursing care to permit unbroken periods for rest and sleep and can suggest use of relaxation techniques or offer comfort measures, such as a warm shower or a back rub, to promote rest. Analgesia and sedatives may also help the mother to achieve restful sleep.

The nurse should also explain the importance of rest once the mother is home with her newborn. She should be encouraged to sleep whenever the baby does for the first few weeks to help offset the loss of uninterrupted sleep at night. The mother should also be strongly encouraged to plan some relaxation for herself each day, such as reading or a relaxing tub bath.

Promoting Comfort

Discomfort and pain interfere with the mother's physiologic and psychological restoration and divert energy from other areas, such as learning about her newborn and reestablishing family relationships.

Discomfort and pain in the postpartum period are usually associated with perineal or rectal pain, breast engorgement and nipple tenderness, pain from uterine contractions ("afterpains"), muscle strain and fatigue from the birth process, and incisional or gas pain in the postcesarean mother. Nursing care for perineal or rectal pain and breast changes is described in the following sections.

Discomfort from Uterine Contractions.   If the patient experiences discomfort from afterpains, she should be reminded to keep her bladder empty, since bladder distention contributes to uterine relaxation, which, in turn, may intensify afterpains. Discomfort from afterpains may also be relieved by analgesics or by positioning the mother on her abdomen for a rest.

Discomfort from Muscle Strain and Fatigue.   The nurse can suggest gentle stretching, increasing fluid intake, and early ambulation to promote healing. Warm showers may be especially helpful, as are mild analgesics.

Pain in the Postcesarean Mother.   The nurse should be especially attentive to minimizing the pain and discomfort experienced by the postcesarean mother. The mother should be taught how to "splint" or support the incisional area with hands or pillows during coughing, deep breathing, or position changes for the first day. Infant care will be more difficult for this mother because of intravenous lines and incisional discomfort, and she should be encouraged to participate in infant care when she feels ready, usually after 24 hours.

The mother intending to breast-feed should receive analgesics that do not adversely affect the nursing infant; analgesics may be most effectively given an hour prior to feeding, so that she will be comfortable for that period. When the mother holds or feeds the infant, a pillow should be placed on her abdomen to avoid pressure on the incision. A side-lying position for breastfeeding may be most comfortable for the postcesarean mother.

Gas pain can be particularly annoying and distressing following any abdominal surgery, including cesarean birth. Gas pains are usually relieved by increased ambulation and deep abdominal breathing. Relaxation techniques, such as those learned in prepared childbirth classes, may assist the mother with the discomfort. If these measures are unsuccessful, use of a return-flow enema may be necessary to stimulate peristalsis and elimination of intestinal gas.

Providing Care of the Perineum and Rectum

Nursing interventions are directed at minimizing perineal discomfort and preventing trauma and infection to the area. Immediately after delivery, perineal ice packs should be applied for 12 hours to minimize edema and discomfort. The patient should be instructed to rinse the perineal area with warm water after voiding; most postpartum units have special appliances that mothers can use to direct warm, soapy water over the perineal area. The area should be patted dry gently from front to back to avoid contamination from the rectal area.

The mother should be instructed to change perineal pads frequently to maintain cleanliness; saturated pads can be a site for growth of microorganisms. Pads should be worn snugly to avoid friction and irritation. Sitz baths are often advised twice a day, starting 24 hours after delivery. Sitz baths promote healing by increasing circulation to the area and promote comfort by relaxing the tissues and decreasing edema.

To minimize the discomfort of sitting down, the mother should be instructed to tighten her buttocks before sitting to decrease the pressure and tension on the perineal area. Analgesics and topical anesthetics are often used to decrease perineal discomfort as well.

Providing Breast Care

The nurse's assessment of breast changes enables her to anticipate when a woman's breasts are becoming engorged and when comfort measures are likely to be needed. For the woman who intends to breast-feed, engorgement may be eased by hot showers to release the flow of milk or by suckling the infant. The mother should be encouraged to wear a nursing bra to provide support

NURSING RESEARCH

Sitz Baths and Perineal Pain

The effectiveness of cold sitz baths (rather than the customary warm baths) for relieving perineal episiotomy pain in the postpartum period was evaluated. Forty patients took both warm and cold sitz baths 6 hours apart with random assignment to the first type of bath taken. Patients rated the degree of perineal pain before and after each sitz bath and at half-hour and one-hour intervals after each bath. A 5-point pain scale was used, ranging from no pain to extreme pain. Analysis showed that cold sitz baths were significantly more effective in relieving perineal pain. The greatest amount of pain relief was experienced immediately after the cold sitz baths.

This study should be replicated, with special attention to the documentation of episiotomy incision and any effects the use of cold might have on hematoma formation or edema. Further, any aesthetic aversion on the part of nurses or patients to the use of cold sitz baths must also be examined, since it will likely affect its use.

Ramler D, Roberts J: A comparison of cold and warm sitz baths for relief of postpartum perineal pain. J Obstet Gynecol Neonatal Nurs 15(6):471, 1985

for her breasts (see Promoting Successful Lactation in Chapter 37).

Lactation Suppression. Women who do not wish to breast-feed will need assistance in suppressing lactation. Medications are sometimes freely used for this purpose. However, the nurse should recognize that medications designed to suppress lactation have side effects and some risks associated with their use (Table 29–3) and that mechanical methods of lactation suppression may work nearly as well without side-effects. Even with the use of lactation suppressants, the patient will still experience some degree of engorgement and may require comfort measures.

Mechanical methods of lactation suppression include the following:

- Wearing a tight-fitting bra or breast binder 24 hours a day until breasts become soft again
- Avoiding breast and nipple stimulation, such as suckling, heat, or massage

Fluid restriction is not helpful in suppressing lactation in the postpartum mother. Ice packs or analgesics may be used to ease breast tenderness. About 48 to 72 hours after engorgement, breast tenderness will ease. Complete involution may take up to 1 month.

Table 29-3   **Drugs Used in Postpartum Care**

Drug	Indication/Action	Dosage/Route	Potential Side-Effects	Nursing Implications
Rubella vaccine live	Indicated for women without signs of rubella or serologically negative (antibody titer 1:8 or less). Attenuated live virus causes antibody response to prevent fetal anomalies due to rubella exposure in future pregnancies.	0.5 ml SC	Temperature elevation, rash, transient arthralgia, polyneuritis, lymphade-nopathy; teratogenic during pregnancy	Advise patient of need to avoid pregnancy for 2 months after vaccination. Assess for allergy to neomycin.
HypRho-D, RhoGAM, Gamulin Rh	Indicated for Rh-negative postpartum women who may have had fetal–maternal transfusion of Rh-positive blood cells. Promotes lysis of fetal Rh-positive blood cells in maternal circulation before formation of maternal antibodies that would threaten future pregnancies	1 vial IM	Mild temperature elevation; soreness at injection site	Must be given within 72 hr of birth when following criteria are met: Mother is Rh_0 (D) or D^u negative and without antibodies. Baby is Rh_1 (D) or D^u positive with negative Coombs test. Verify lot numbers on cross-matched solution and preparation to be administered.
Deladumone OB	Lactation suppression; inhibits breast stimulation with synthetic estrogen. Not found to be consistently superior to mechanical methods of lactation suppression	2 ml IM at onset of second stage of labor	Flushing, acne, hirsutism; may contribute to thromboembolic disorders in puerperium	This long-acting estrogen is contraindicated for patients with signs of reproductive tract cancer or cardiac, renal, or hepatic disease. *Informed consent must be obtained.* Patient should wear tight-fitting bra and avoid breast stimulation.
Tace	Lactation suppression; inhibits breast stimulation with synthetic estrogen. Not found to be consistently superior to mechanical methods of lactation suppression	72 mg orally twice a day for 2 days	Nausea, vomiting, diarrhea, skin rash	See Nursing Implications listed for Deladumone OB.
Parlodel (bromocriptine)	Lactation suppression; prevents secretion of prolactin. Not found to be consistently superior to mechanical methods of lactation suppression	2.5 mg orally twice a day for 14 days	Hypotension, headache, dizziness, nausea and vomiting, fatigue	Administer at least 4 hr after birth and only if vital signs are stable. Take precautions for syncope on first ambulation. Monitor blood pressure, especially when other medications known to affect blood pressure are used. Patient should wear tight-fitting bra and avoid breast stimulation.

Expected Outcome: The postpartum woman states she is comfortable and demonstrates a satisfactory comfort level as evidenced by self-care and infant care by discharge.

Promoting Maternal Psychological Adaptation

On the basis of the nurse's assessment of each mother's individual situation, specific nursing support can be offered to facilitate psychological adaptation in the postpartum period. Women with special needs include adolescent and older mothers and mothers who experienced complications in the intrapartum period, especially those with cesarean births.

Mothers With Special Support Needs

Adolescent mothers typically have greater educational needs than older women, especially in terms of infant care and effective self-care after discharge. The nurse should discuss with the adolescent mother the arrangements she has made for help and support at home, and if social support seems inadequate, the nurse may initiate referral to community resources.

First-time mothers over 30 may also have special needs for nursing support. Frequently the older primipara is well educated and knowledgeable about pregnancy and birth but feels quite anxious about her knowledge of and skill in child care. Allowing her to express her feelings about the role change she is experiencing may be an important nursing intervention. In many cases, the older primipara has chosen to give up a career in order to become a mother, and some may find the adjustment difficult.

Mothers who experienced long, difficult labors, who were designated high-risk, or who developed complications during pregnancy or the intrapartal period need special nursing support in the postpartum period. Obviously, the physical recovery of a woman who has experienced complications or a cesarean birth will be delayed, compared to that of a woman with an uncomplicated vaginal birth. This delay will affect the woman's psychological adaptation in the early postpartum period. Often her own needs must be met before she can attend to the needs of her infant and family.

In addition, this woman may have negative feelings about the pregnancy or birth experience if she had planned a vaginal birth but had a cesarean delivery, or if her expectations for her partner's attendance at the birth, early breast-feeding, or an unmedicated birth were not met. The nurse must provide her with an opportunity to express these feelings and should assure her that her disappointment is quite normal.

Body Image Concerns

Many women are disappointed or distressed about their postpartum bodies. Although thrilled at the rapid weight loss after birth, they are still dismayed that they cannot wear prepregnancy clothes and must still wear maternity clothes for the first week or two after the birth. The nurse should stress that this is the rule, not the exception, and that few women leave the hospital in prepregnancy jeans or slacks after the birth of a child. The nurse should encourage the woman to have an attractive, loose-fitting dress or pants outfit brought for her to wear home.

The nurse should caution the breast-feeding woman against attempting to lose excess weight while lactation is being established. The nonlactating mother may adopt a low-calorie, high-protein diet in the postpartum period, as long as weight reduction and exercise are done in moderation (see Chapter 37).

A postnatal exercise program may improve the mother's self-esteem and assist her to regain the prepregnant figure (see Teaching for Effective Self Care, later in this chapter). The nurse should stress that vigorous exercise is to be avoided until after lochia has ceased. An increase in lochial flow or reappearance of lochia after it has ceased is an indication that activity may have been too demanding. However, gentle stretching and postnatal exercises, walking, and other physical activities may be introduced in the second or third week. The general rule should be avoidance of fatigue and muscle strain.

Expected Outcome: The postpartum woman states diet and exercise guidelines appropriate to restoring optimal health and prepregnant appearance by discharge.

Promoting Parenting
Promoting Parent–Infant Acquaintance

The nurse can facilitate and support the parent–infant acquaintance process by helping parents to become aware of the individuality of their newborn. Characteristics that indicate temperament can be identified and explained to the parent (see Chapter 31 on behavioral assessment of the newborn). As the nurse points out these characteristics, she can assist the parents in finding ways to respond to their child appropriately. For example, she can tell parents that the infant is able to see best at a distance of 8 to 10 inches and likes to gaze at the human face. The mother and father can then be encouraged to hold the infant close and to establish eye contact. The nurse's actions increase the parents' knowledge about their baby and promote the growing parent–infant relationship.

FAMILY CONSIDERATIONS

Parent – Infant Acquaintance

Events during the early hours and days following birth can affect the parent – infant acquaintance. Prolonged infant and parent separation, parental health status, and initial contact with the infant are factors that can have an influence on the parent – infant relationship. The nurse can foster parent – infant acquaintance by the following behaviors:

- Encouraging the couple to inspect their infant's body parts
- Comparing their infant's features to other family members
- Encouraging parental rest and relaxation
- Encouraging early breast-feeding
- Assisting the couple in a comfortable position for holding their infant
- Providing time alone with their infant
- Providing information on normal newborn characteristics, newborn growth and development, and newborn alertness and sleep patterns
- Praising the couple for their abilities to care for their infant

Promoting Parental Caretaking

The nurse provides information, encouragement, and support to parents as they learn how to care for their new baby. Usually she demonstrates basic care skills at the bedside for inexperienced parents. This teaching can then be reinforced in a group session on the postpartum unit.

It is important to give encouragement and praise. New parents are often very insecure about their ability and will have few opportunities to get direct feedback on their caretaking once they leave the hospital setting. All parents, whether experienced or not, benefit from praise and encouragement about their infant caretaking. (See Chapters 4 and 32 for a detailed discussion of parent teaching for newborn care.)

The nurse is the key person in assisting parents with both breast-feeding and formula feeding. Because of the increasing popularity of breast-feeding, nursing support of the breast-feeding mother is addressed in depth in Chapter 37. Formula feeding is discussed further in Chapters 32 and 37. The nurse should remember that mothers who choose formula feeding also need much nursing attention and support and should not assume that nursing time can be reduced because the patient does not require assistance with breast-feeding.

Expected Outcome:

- By discharge, parents demonstrate parenting techniques, as evidenced by holding infant close and *en face* while feeding or cuddling, making eye contact when infant is in quiet alert state, and calling infant by name.
- Parents indicate they have learned infant-care skills by demonstrating proper feeding of newborn and changing of diapers and clothing and by restating proper care techniques by time of discharge.

Promoting Family Adaptation

The nurse should teach other family members as much as possible about infant care. Siblings, grandparents, and others have great importance in the family unit; if they are well prepared for the arrival of the newborn in the home, the parents will be able to devote more of their energy to meeting their own needs and those of their infant (Fig. 29 – 4).

Supporting Paternal Adaptation

The father is usually the mother's primary support person throughout the childbearing cycle, yet the father's needs and appropriate nursing interventions have only recently received much attention. In part this reflects the nurse's relatively infrequent or irregular contact with the father. Effective intervention to support the father may require planning for his inclusion in postpartum teaching and baby care demonstrations as well as taking advantage of opportunities for talking with him about his own feelings, worries, and concerns. The nurse will be most effective in providing family-centered care if she remembers that mother, father, and newborn are all her patients and that family health can be promoted only if all members receive needed support in the adaptation period after childbirth.

Debriefing the Father About the Birth Experience. The nurse should remember that the father may need to talk about the birth experience as a way of clarifying events in his mind and integrating the birth into his life experience. This need may be especially strong if the father was an active participant in the labor and birth or if unexpected events, such as maternal or neonatal complications, arose. The nurse may be able to include both parents in an unhurried conversation about the birth as she monitors the mother's physiologic status closely in the hours just after birth.

The nurse can offer information to fill in gaps in memory or understanding. Both parents usually benefit from this, but the father may find it particularly helpful if he was absent for periods or hesitated to ask questions at the

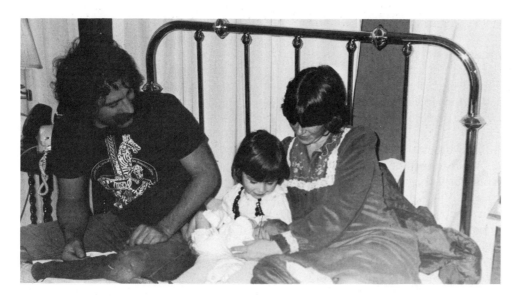

Figure 29 – 4. The postpartum period is a time for family closeness and readjustment. (Photo: Colleen Stainton)

time. The nurse should observe for behavior that suggests that the father has doubts about his effectiveness as his partner's labor support person. Often the mother will express her appreciation of his support, and the nurse can reinforce this reassurance, even if she has no direct knowledge of the labor. She can also reassure the father that his doubts are common, since fathers are often surprised by the unpredictability of birth and their feelings of "being out of control."

The nurse should be particularly alert to the needs of a father whose partner or newborn developed complications. Fathers sometimes mistakenly believe that they somehow should have prevented complications or could have prevented the need for medication or a cesarean birth if they had been more effective in their labor support. The nurse should explore this belief with the father and provide accurate information about the cause of the problem and ways of preventing it. She can reassure the father that it is unlikely that he could have done anything differently to influence the outcome and should point out any evidence she observes that his support was effective, such as the mother's appreciation, comments from labor and delivery staff, and so on.

In all cases, the nurse should acknowledge that both parents have completed a difficult task and congratulate them. New mothers are more likely to receive this acknowledgment from family and friends, but new fathers may not receive "credit" for having come through a challenging and exciting experience.

Anticipatory Guidance About the Postpartum Period.   Another important nursing intervention is providing accurate information about what the father should expect in the early postpartum period and through the fourth trimester of the childbearing year. The nurse should begin by asking the father if he has any questions

FAMILY CONSIDERATIONS

Supporting the Couple Relationship

The addition of a new member to the family unit can create a disruption in other relationships within the preexisting unit. The couple may sense a loss of togetherness due to the demands of caring for a newborn child. The couple's relationship can be enhanced by encouraging

- Open communication
- Time together without the newborn
- Discussion of roles and division of household tasks and newborn care
- Individual time for relaxation away from the newborn
- Awareness of each other's needs and desire for recognition

about going home with his new family. After answering his more pressing questions, the nurse can progress to other important areas.

One area that is often of importance to new fathers but that may not come up spontaneously is sexual activity after birth. The nurse should approach this area in a sensitive, matter-of-fact way as she outlines the woman's physiologic recovery in the first month after birth. The nurse should observe carefully to assess whether this information might be most appropriately discussed with husband and wife together or separately with the wife. In many cases, the nurse can explain the guidelines for resumption of safe and comfortable sexual activity with both spouses, reassuring them that this is a common area of concern and that she is willing to answer any questions they may have.

The nurse should also take this opportunity to stress that the couple relationship and each partner will require extra attention in the first months of parenthood. She should encourage the father to plan for activities as a couple in the first 2 weeks and point out that they were a couple before they were parents.

The nurse should also remind the father that both parents will need time for individual relaxation. She may need to stress that he will be his partner's primary support person for the next several weeks. Individual time away from work responsibilities is important for both spouses' self-esteem and emotional well-being. The nurse may want to reinforce the point that being at home with a new infant is in some ways more demanding than employment outside the home because the duties persist 24 hours a day. She can explain that the support the father provides for his partner in the early weeks will contribute to a faster physical restoration and will help protect the couple relationship from the inevitable strains posed by new parenthood.

Promoting Positive Father–Infant Interaction.

The nurse should encourage the father to hold and care for the newborn, while acknowledging the concerns and insecurity most new fathers feel. Many men will not ask to hold their newborns but are eager to do so and will respond favorably to sensitive encouragement. If a father seems nervous and unsure of himself, the nurse should take steps to promote confidence, such as having the father sit comfortably and handing the securely wrapped infant to him, showing him how to pick up and hold the infant and then staying close by as he does so, and reinforcing the fact that newborn care is a learned skill at which everyone is uncertain at first. The nurse should remember that men are usually even more unsure of their knowledge and skill than are their partners and so may need additional reassurance.

The nurse can also promote positive father–infant interaction by pointing out the newborn's unique capabilities and characteristics. Fathers are often "hooked" when they learn that newborns are not simply passive recipients of care but have special abilities and social responses. Some strategies for teaching include demonstrating the newborn's protective reflexes, ability to differentiate voices and follow visual and auditory stimuli, temperamental differences, and states of alertness.

The nurse can assist the father to think about and plan ways he can routinely participate in care, such as giving baths, bringing the baby to the mother for breast-feeding at night, or bottle-feeding the newborn for a particular feeding each day. Many new fathers want to be involved in taking care of their new infant but do not know how to start and lack role models. If the father participates little in early infant care, this pattern tends to persist; the father then has difficulty catching up with the mother's well-established competence and routines later.

The nurse may want to encourage the father to seek more information about infant care and fatherhood through classes, fathers' groups, or reading and educational television. Men sometimes assume that parenthood is instinctive or can be learned only through direct experience. The nurse can use the analogy of other learned skills, such as repair work or driving, in which a certain amount of information is acquired before actual practice begins. The nurse working in the postpartum setting should be aware of local resources for fathers and have access to educational pamphlets that provide practical information for fathers on infant care and infant development. This is especially important in settings where the nurse's contact with fathers is limited.

Supporting Sibling Adaptation

The arrival of a new baby brother or sister can stir mixed emotions in other siblings. The response of siblings will vary according to their age, the number of other siblings, and the extent of preparation for the baby. Even with the best prenatal preparation, older siblings will feel some loss of love and attention and will have periods of unhappiness at sharing parents with the new baby. The nurse should encourage parents to be sensitive to these

FAMILY CONSIDERATIONS

Easing Adaptation by Older Siblings

The addition of a new member to the family unit can create a disruption to other relationships within the preexisting unit. Older siblings often feel displaced and less loved following the birth of a new sibling. To ease adjustment by older siblings to the birth of a new baby, the mother can take the following measures:

- Encourage sibling visitation when hospital regulations allow it
- During hospitalization, call older children on the phone
- Plan for high-quality, uninterrupted time with the older children
- Let the father carry the baby on discharge from the hospital so that she can hug and hold other children
- Give a gift from the baby to the older children
- Request that visitors greet older children before focusing on the newborn
- Allow siblings to care for a doll while she cares for the infant

feelings and to the changes the older children are experiencing.

The parents may wish to take specific steps to ease the transition for older children. The accompanying display lists some ways this might be done.

The nurse should remind parents that young children do not have the judgment or skill to handle a newborn safely without supervision. The parents should not refer to the baby as "just like a doll," since this might be interpreted by the child as permission to play with it like a doll. Parents should be watchful when the older child is with the newborn; natural expressions of sibling jealousy may involve rough handling, burying the baby with toys or throwing them at it, attempting to take the newborn out of a crib or infant seat, and slapping or hitting.

Expected Outcomes:

- By discharge, new father states ways to support his partner during the postpartum recovery and ways he can participate in the care of his newborn child.

- By discharge, couple understands the impact of the newborn on older siblings, as evidenced by restating techniques to decrease sibling rivalry.

Promoting Health Maintenance by Discharge Teaching

Most women and their newborns will be discharged 2 or 3 days after delivery, whereas postcesarean mothers are usually discharged 5 days after the birth. Prior to discharge, the nurse should help the family to anticipate and plan for the changes that will occur during their first few weeks at home. The nurse should discuss with them the changes they are likely to experience in their relationship and in the family as a whole. She should stress the importance of maintaining their couple bond as well as developing their roles as parents.

The nurse should assess whether a home visit by a public health nurse or referral to a community agency for families with special needs would be helpful. She should also stress the importance of the well-baby check and postpartum check for the health of both mother and infant. She should verify that the parents have an infant car seat for use upon discharge from the hospital; if they do not have one and cannot afford to purchase their own, she should contact community car seat loan programs. She should stress strongly the importance of using an infant car seat for the *first ride home* and consistently thereafter.

The nurse should verify before discharge that the mother has received any needed immunizations (see Table 29–3) and that the infant has been screened for inborn metabolic errors (see Chapter 32). The nurse should also emphasize that the mother can call the nursing staff on the postpartum unit or at the newborn nursery at any hour if she has a question or concern.

Early Postpartum Discharge

With the advent of alternative birth centers and more flexible hospital policies in many areas, healthy mothers and their newborns may now be discharged within the first 24 hours after birth. Most settings have specific criteria for early discharge, such as the following:

- Uncomplicated pregnancy
- Uncomplicated labor and vaginal delivery
- Vital signs within normal limits
- Firm uterus with moderate lochia
- Voiding without difficulty
- Maternal hemoglobin and hematocrit within normal limits
- Absence of nausea and vomiting
- Healthy newborn
- Positive parent–infant interaction
- Availability of home visit in the first 5 days by a nurse or a representative of a community agency
- Adequate support system

Teaching for Effective Self-Care

The new parents' many learning needs must be met in order for them to care effectively for themselves, their newborn, and their family. Many postpartum units have teaching checklists to guide the nurse (see the Assessment Tool). Many of these points have already been discussed in detail in this chapter. In addition, each parent should be offered teaching in all aspects of infant care, as described in Chapter 32. Some self-care topics of particular interest and importance to new mothers are discussed here.

Postpartum Exercise

The nurse can teach the mother specific exercises that can be done in the early postpartum period to strengthen the abdominal muscles and promote relaxation and flexibility. These exercises can be started on the first day after delivery. Each should initially be done five times twice a day in a slow, smooth, and relaxing manner and should never make the patient feel sore or tired. The number of repetitions can be gradually increased until the mother feels stronger and, in 4 to 5 weeks, is ready to resume more active exercise. The postcesarean mother should consult her physician regarding an exercise regimen to meet her needs.

ASSESSMENT TOOL

Postpartum Teaching Checklist

Information packet given

Topic
1. Hygiene: (a) Pericare
            (b) Bathing/douching
2. Involution: (a) Rate
               (b) Massage
               (c) "Afterbirth" pain
               (d) Lochia
3. Exercise
4. Contraception — types discussed
   (a)
   (b)
   (c)
5. Nutrition — General/lactating
6. Emotions — "Baby blues"
7. Siblings — Preparation, rivalry
8. Discharge: (a) Assistance
              (b) Sleep, rest
              (c) Activity
              (d) Educational
                  (parent classes, etc.)

Date of instruction(s): _____

Evaluation of the level of understanding by the patient:

Instruction given by: _____

Courtesy of Merritt Peralta Medical Center, Oakland, CA

NURSING RESEARCH

Kegel Exercises

Nurses frequently instruct new mothers in the use of Kegel exercises (see Chapter 18) to strengthen pelvic floor muscles after childbirth. It is commonly believed that these exercises increase sexual response, decrease stress incontinence, and speed the recovery of the perineum after vaginal birth. A recent study by a team of investigators, which included two nurses, found that the circumvaginal muscles of women delivered vaginally are significantly weaker that those muscles in nulliparous women or women who had cesarean deliveries. This study of 98 women failed to find improved muscle strength in women who reported doing Kegel exercises. Although there is question as to the reason for this finding and more research is needed, the investigators suggest that nurses recommending Kegel exercises to their clients do so with the understanding that not all women may derive equal benefit from their use.

Samples J, Dougherty M, Abrams R, Batich C: The dynamic characteristics of the circumvaginal muscles. J Obstet Gynecol Neonatal Nurs 17:194, 1988

Abdominal Breathing. To perform abdominal breathing, the patient is in a supine position with legs slightly bent. She inhales slowly through her nose, letting her abdomen rise, then slowly exhales through her mouth, flattening her abdomen by contracting her abdominal muscles.

Head and Shoulder Raising. The patient begins head and shoulder raising in a supine position with legs bent and arms outstretched toward knees. She tucks in her chin, lifts her head and shoulders slowly, and holds to a count of five. She then slowly lowers her shoulders and head to the beginning position. The head and shoulders are lifted only as far as needed to clear the shoulder blades from the flat surface.

Arm Raises. For arm raises, the patient is in a supine position with legs bent and arms extended out from her sides at a 90 degree angle. With arms extended, the patient lifts them slowly to the center above the body and then slowly lowers them to the starting position.

Contraception and Sexuality

Each woman and her partner should receive teaching about contraception and sexuality during the postpartum period. Contraceptive teaching should include a review of information about the available methods so that the woman can make an informed decision before her postpartum checkup, usually scheduled at 4 to 6 weeks after delivery. Closely spaced pregnancies (one year or less apart) put a greater stress on the woman's body and place her at slightly higher obstetric risk. The mother may want to consider this if she is planning another pregnancy soon.

The nurse should ask what contraceptive methods were used in the past and remind the mother that breastfeeding is not a reliable form of contraception. If the woman used a diaphragm, she should be reminded that she needs to have it refitted or replaced. Contraceptive foam or cream used in combination with a condom is a good choice for birth control in the postpartum period.

While discussing contraception, the nurse can allow the woman to express any concerns she may have about sexuality. The nurse may use an opening such as "Most women have concerns about sex after they have had a baby. What are your concerns?" This communicates that the nurse is supportive and willing to listen. During such a discussion, the nurse can provide information as well as allow the patient to express her concerns. (See Chapter 6 for further information on sexuality.) The nurse can point out that it is common for women to have mixed feelings about sexual activity after the birth of a baby; perineal pain, fear of injury, and fatigue are some factors that may inhibit a woman's desire for sexual intercourse.

There is a common belief that intercourse must be delayed until after the 6-week postpartum checkup. However, intercourse may be initiated, as desired, once the episiotomy has healed and lochia has become light-colored and decreased in amount. A water-soluble lubricant or contraceptive cream may be used to compensate for decreased vaginal lubrication.

A lactating mother should be informed that she may experience sexual arousal from the suckling of her baby and that there is often a release of milk from the breasts with orgasm. This knowledge will allow the woman to accept these feelings and responses as normal.

The woman should also be encouraged to explore alternative methods of sexual expression with her partner until she feels ready to resume intercourse. The nurse should stress the importance of open communication with her partner; expression of fears and desires will greatly ease the reestablishment of the couple's sexual relationship.

Expected Outcomes:

- By discharge, mother shows understanding of postpartum physiologic adaptations by restating warning signs regarding lochia and thrombophlebitis to report to her health care provider, by verbalizing the importance of rest and comfort and maintaining perineal hygiene, by demonstrating postpartum exercises, and by demonstrating proper breast-feeding techniques if she is lactating.

- By discharge, the postpartum couple understands various methods of contraception, as evidenced by knowledgeable discussion and ability to state one method appropriate to their personal needs and cultural/religious beliefs.

Evaluation

Evaluating the effects of specific nursing interventions and the overall quality of postpartum nursing care re-

quires that the nurse identify specific objectives in her plan of care for each patient and then judge outcomes against those objectives. Many interventions in the postpartum period are focused on support and patient teaching. The long-term effects of patient teaching are more difficult to evaluate than are such easily observable outcomes as improved uterine tone or decreased perineal discomfort.

Evaluation of postpartum nursing care is complicated by the fact that postpartum stays have shortened. The postpartum nurse is challenged to deliver more thorough and comprehensive family-centered care in less time. However, maternity nurses continue to meet that challenge and contribute to the health and well-being of new parents and their newborn infants long after the excitement and change of the postpartum period.

CHAPTER SUMMARY

The postpartum period offers a unique opportunity for the nurse to observe individual and family adaptation to the arrival of a new mother. The nurse provides expert knowledge, assistance, and support to the new mother and father and other family members as they learn about the newborn and take on the responsibility of infant care.

The mother's physiologic restoration is of particular importance. Nursing assessment and intervention focus on the monitoring of normal physiologic changes, promotion of rest and comfort, and promotion of successful breast-feeding, if the mother so chooses.

Nursing assessment and intervention are also directed at identifying and meeting the educational needs of families in order to promote optimal individual and family adaptation and effective self-care. Patient teaching is of major importance in postpartum care. The nurse's sensitivity, knowledge, and ability to teach effectively can contribute to a relatively problem-free postpartum transition for most families.

STUDY QUESTIONS

1. Describe the components of the physiologic and psychological assessment of the postpartum patient. Identify physiologic and psychological signs that require further assessment of patient status.
2. List three interventions for care of the mother when mother–infant acquaintance is delayed.
3. Discuss the special postpartum needs of the family that experiences a cesarean birth.
4. Describe guidelines for effective patient teaching in the postpartum period.

(text continued on page 891)

NURSING CARE PLAN

The Family in the Early Postpartum Period

Nursing Diagnosis (Patient Problem) and Assessment Data	Nursing Interventions	Rationale
First 4 to 6 hours after delivery **Potential Complication:** *postpartum hemorrhage* • Decreasing BP • Increasing pulse • Excessive lochia • History of excessive bleeding • Long labor/difficult delivery • Large distended uterus (multiple gestation, polyhydramnios, large infant) • Placental abnormalities • Anemia	Monitor blood pressure, pulse, skin color, and uterine tone every 15 minutes for the first hour. Assess uterine position and lochial flow. Massage fundus as needed. Administer oxytocin as ordered. Explain need for continuous assessment. Instruct patient to do self-assessment of bleeding and uterine tone and fundal massage.	Postpartum hemorrhage is a major source of maternal perinatal morbidity. Bleeding from placental site is controlled by effective uterine contractions compressing torn vessels. Bleeding that soaks two pads or less without clots in the first hour is within normal limits; patient must understand difference between normal and abnormal bleeding for effective self-care.

Expected Outcome:

Mother maintains normal physiological status in immediate postpartum period as evidenced by stable vital signs and bleeding within normal limits in the first 6 hours postbirth.

Nursing Diagnosis: *altered comfort: acute pain* • Perineal edema, bruising episiotomy • Uterine contractions	Examine perineum and note changes in first 2–4 hr after delivery. Apply ice pack for first 8–12 hr. Encourage lying flat on abdomen. Administer analgesic as indicated. Explain reason for discomfort and usual duration (1–2 days).	Progressive discoloration and discomfort may signal hematoma formation. Ice pack promotes maternal comfort and decreases edema. Comfort measures and information about cause will ease discomfort and associated anxiety.

Expected Outcome:

Mother maintains control of discomfort with comfort measures as evidenced by normal bowel/bladder function and unhindered mobility in the immediate postpartum period.

(continued)

NURSING CARE PLAN

The Family in the Early Postpartum Period (continued)

Nursing Diagnosis (Patient Problem) and Assessment Data	Nursing Interventions	Rationale
Nursing Diagnosis: *potential altered patterns in urinary elimination*		
• Uterus displaced laterally • Inability to void • Excessive lochia	Assess for bladder distention during first 2–4 hr. Encourage early and frequent voiding. Measure first three voidings; explain rationale to patient.	Decreased bladder tone, sensation, and postdelivery diuresis may predispose to overflow. Voidings should be in amount of 100 ml or more (reflecting lowest normal urine output of 30 ml/h); frequent small voidings with other symptoms listed (see assessment data) suggest urinary retention and need for straight catheterization.

Expected Outcome:

Patient maintains normal voiding patterns, as evidenced by voiding normal amounts without assistance within 12 hr of delivery.

Nursing Diagnosis: *potential altered parenting*		
• Expressed displeasure at newborn appearance • Newborn opposite of desired gender • Unplanned pregnancy • Difficult labor/delivery	Promote early contact and interactions with mate, newborn, other family members as desired. Assist with feeding and infant care within 1–2 hr of delivery.	Early alert period in the neonate provides optimal opportunity for interaction and initiation of early breast-feeding.

Expected Outcome:

Parent and newborn begin attachment, as evidenced by parent's exploring newborn's body, touching, cuddling, and breast-feeding (if desired) in immediate postpartum period.

Ongoing care: (6 hr to 3 days after delivery)

Potential for Complication: *postpartum hemorrhage*		
• Early postpartum hemorrhage • Manual removal of placenta • Infection	Assess uterine tone and lochial flow every 8 hr. Begin pad count and closer monitoring if flow appears	To allow early identification of postpartum hemorrhage.

(continued)

NURSING CARE PLAN

The Family in the Early Postpartum Period (continued)

Nursing Diagnosis (Patient Problem) and Assessment Data	Nursing Interventions	Rationale
• Subinvolution of uterus	heavy—*i.e.*, more than one pad saturated from end to end in 1 hr, or sudden increase in flow after progressive decrease. Explain normal progression of lochia and warning signs to patient. Explain relationship of excessive activity to lochial flow.	To promote effective self-care.

Expected Outcome:

Mother maintains normal physiological status in postpartum period, as evidenced by stable vital signs and blood loss within normal limits in first 36 hours postbirth.

Nursing Diagnosis:
altered comfort: pain related to perineal trauma

• Maternal unwillingness to sit or ambulate • Concerns expressed about perineal healing, bowel function • Tenderness on palpation, at pad change	Encourage sitz baths—cool to cold baths for first day, with ice gradually added to cool water to tolerance; warm baths thereafter.	Sitz baths in cold water decrease circulation and edema in bruised pernieum and promote comfort. After the initial period of edema and inflammation, warm baths promote circulation to healing tissue.
	Advise patient to change perineal pad frequently and keep it securely fastened to avoid friction. Encourage patient to tighten buttocks before sitting and to sit on flat, padded surfaces. Examine perineum daily for signs of infection or delayed healing.	Use of foam "donut" or soft pillow may actually increase pressure on perirectal area and perineum. Perineal area is especially vulnerable to infection.

Expected Outcome:

Mother acknowledges pain relief as demonstrated by compliance with self-care techniques and no indication of infection prior to discharge.

Nursing Diagnosis:
potential for infection related to birth process

• Prolonged labor and/or difficult delivery • Manual removal of placenta	Monitor vital signs every 4–6 hr. Assess fluid intake; if less than 2000 ml/day, encourage additional fluids. Notify physician or midwife if	Temperature elevation may result from dehydration or be an early sign of infection.

(continued)

888

NURSING CARE PLAN

The Family in the Early Postpartum Period (continued)

Nursing Diagnosis (Patient Problem) and Assessment Data	Nursing Interventions	Rationale
• Elevation of temperature • Excessive uterine or perineal pain	temperature is elevated over 100.4°F (38°C) on any two observations. Assess lochia for odor; episiotomy for signs of infection.	Normal lochia has fleshy odor similar to menstrual blood; a change in odor may suggest endometritis.

Expected Outcome:

Mother remains free of infection, as demonstrated by mother's verbalization of comfort and nurse's assessment of stable vital signs, balanced fluid intake, output, and normal lochia discharge within first 36 hours postbirth.

Nursing Diagnosis:
bowel elimination: constipation related to decreased peristalsis and perineal pain

• Absent or decreased bowel sounds • Signs of dehydration • Use of regional or general anesthesia • Intrapartal enema received	Assess every 8 hr for flatus or bowel movement Encourage ambulation. Encourage increased fluids and roughage in diet.	Promotes peristalsis. Provides bulk to stimulate elimination.

Expected Outcome:

Mother returns to normal bowel function as evidenced by mother's verbalization of comfort and regularity of bowel movements and nurse's assessment of normal bowel sounds in 24 hr.

Nursing Diagnosis:
altered comfort: breast engorgement

• Breasts firm and tender to touch	Assess breasts for signs of lactation every 8 hr. If patient is breast-feeding • Encourage breast-feeding on demand. • Teach mother comfort measures: wearing support bra, warm showers, breast massage. • Administer analgesic as needed. If not breast-feeding • Apply ice packs and tight bra or binder. • Teach mother to avoid breast stimulation. • Administer analgesic as needed.	Warm showers and breast massage stimulate circulation and promote let-down of breast milk. Pharmaceutical lactation suppressants have side-effects, may pose small maternal risk due to estrogenic action, and have not been demonstrated to be superior to mechanical methods of lactation suppression.

(continued)

NURSING CARE PLAN

The Family in the Early Postpartum Period   (continued)

Nursing Diagnosis (Patient Problem) and Assessment Data	Nursing Interventions	Rationale

Expected Outcome:

Mother, who is breast-feeding on demand, verbalizes comfort and adapts breast care suggestions by discharge. Formula-feeding mother verbalizes comfort with nonmedicinal methods of lactation suppression, as demonstrated by decreasing tenderness of breasts by discharge.

Nursing Diagnosis:
potential altered health maintenance related to self-care

• Youthful, inexperienced parents • Inadequate or underutilized support system • Slow maternal physical adaptation	Institute discharge teaching plan, including both mother and support person. Include assessment of learning needs and review of important information on: • Expected changes in lochia and warning signs • Suggested exercise and activity level • Need for rest • Emotional aspects of postpartum period • Sexual relations and contraception • Breast and perineal care • Dietary recommendations	Knowledge and understanding of normal postpartum changes and recovery decreases stress and enhances parental adaptation.

Expected Outcome:

Mother and support person understand discharge teaching as evidenced by verbalization of their needs and discussion of health maintenance methods and return demonstration (where applicable) by discharge.

Nursing Diagnosis:
potential altered health maintenance related to newborn care

See above assessment data	Facilitate early parent–infant interaction. Plan adequate time to assess learning needs and readiness to learn. Allow parents to express feelings about birth and infant. Teach essentials of caretaking and point out infant characteristics as opportunity arises. Encourage	Maternal discomfort, emotional needs, unresolved feelings about the birth or infant, and the need to integrate the birth experience may delay learning readiness and parental involvement with the newborn. Teaching is more effective when tailored to the patient's expressed learning needs and when unhurried

(continued)

NURSING CARE PLAN

The Family in the Early Postpartum Period (continued)

Nursing Diagnosis (Patient Problem) and Assessment Data	Nursing Interventions	Rationale
	parents to take advantage of learning opportunities (bath demonstrations, infant care classes).	contacts allow rapport to develop and questions to be answered.
	Review routine baby care practices, well-baby care, and set date for return appointments for mother and baby.	Parent are usually eager for opportunities to review infant care, even if knowledge is not new to them.
	Encourage father to take active role as appropriate to family situation.	Fathers usually require some encouragement and additional teaching if inexperienced with newborns.
	Reinforce parental effort and give positive feedback.	
	Assess plans for discharge and availability of help for first days at home. Encourage phone contact with care providers for questions or concerns.	Contact with providers may assist family adaptation and provide situational support.

Expected Outcome:

Mother and support person understand discharge teaching as evidenced by their verbalization of confidence in providing care and their skill in doing return demonstrations of care by discharge.

---

5. Describe the normative changes in the family in the postpartum period.
6. Differentiate between postpartum blues and postpartum depression.

REFERENCES/BIBLIOGRAPHY

Affonso DD: "Missing pieces" — a study of postpartum feelings. Birth and the Family Journal 4:159, 1977

Hawkins JW, Gorvine B: Postpartum Nursing. New York, Springer Publishing, 1985

Hazle N: Postpartum blues. J Nurse Midwife 27:21, 1982

May K, Perrin S: The father in pregnancy and birth. In Hanson S, Bozett F (eds): Dimensions of Fatherhood. Beverly Hills, Sage Publishing, 1985

May K, Sollid D: Unanticipated cesarean birth: From the father's perspective. Birth 11:87, 1984

Mercer R: She's a multip . . . she knows the ropes. MCN 4:301, 1979

Mercer R: The nurse and the maternal tasks of early postpartum. MCN 6:341, 1981

Rubin R: Puerperal change. Nurs Outlook 9:753, 1963a

Rubin R: Maternal touch. Nurs Outlook 11:828, 1963b

SUGGESTED READINGS

Gorrie TM: Postpartal nursing diagnosis. J Obstet Gynecol Neonatal Nur 15:52, 1986

Huggins K: The Nursing Mother's Companion. Boston, The Harvard Common Press, 1986

Konrad CJ: Helping mothers integrate the birth experience. MCN 12:268, 1987

Rubin R: Maternal Identity and the Maternal Experience. New York, Springer Publishing, 1984

Tribotti S et al: Nursing diagnoses for the postpartum woman. J Obstet Gynecol Neonatal Nur 17:410, 1988

Wiley K, Grohar J: Human immunodeficiency virus and precautions for obstetric, gynecologic and neonatal nurses. JOGN Nurs 17:165, 1988

30 postpartum complications

LEARNING OBJECTIVES

After studying the material in this chapter, the student should be able to

- Identify the most common complications that occur during the puerperium

- Describe predisposing factors for infections of the reproductive and urinary tracts and modes of entry and diffusion of infections

- Discuss common causes of early and late postpartum hemorrhage

- Explain treatment modalities and common procedures used in the management of postpartum complications

- Discuss psychological and social problems encountered in postpartum women experiencing complications

- Identify the goals of nursing care, appropriate nursing interventions, and their rationale for women with postpartum problems

KEY TERMS

Bacteriuria

Curettage

Cystitis

Embolus

Endometritis

Iatrogenic

Induration

Mastitis

Necrosis

Parametritis

Peritonitis

Polymicrobial infection

Pregnancy-induced hypertension (PIH)

Puerperal sepsis

Pyelonephritis

Thrombophlebitis

Thrombosis

New parents are often stunned by the magnitude of the physical and psychological adaptations to be made following childbirth. In the case of a complicated postpartum period, these adjustments are intensified and family ties are tested.

Serious medical problems during the postpartum period impact on early family formation, breast-feeding, nutrition, and future maternal health. Concerns regarding the escalation of costs, combined with worry over the maternal condition, serve to heighten family anxiety and may kindle a family crisis. Families with unanticipated stressors, inadequate coping mechanisms, or inadequate support systems will require expert nursing care.

Postpartum complications may be the consequence of chronic or preexisting maternal disease, the result of pregnancy itself, or the direct result of obstetric treatment; that is, they may be iatrogenic. Postpartum complications add to the maternal mortality statistics. Maternal age, poverty, and ethnicity influence both the occurrence and outcome of complicated courses. Mortality rates from postpartum complications are lowest for adolescents. Women of black or other minority races have mortality ratios approximately 2.7 times greater than those of white women. About 46% of women dying during or after childbirth will have had a cesarean delivery (Rochat et al 1988; Buehler et al 1986).

Nursing care plays a critical role in the early recognition and treatment of postpartum complications. Family support, advocacy, teaching, and referral are goals to be incorporated into the care plan of severely ill postpartum women. The contribution of the family to the patient's recovery is frequently overlooked when highly technical nursing care is required. Exemplary nursing care incorporates concepts of "high-tech," "high-touch," and consideration for family needs and values.

This chapter discusses the most common and most lethal postpartum complications. The order of the topics reflects the prevalence of the complications: those topics toward the end of the chapter represent less frequent complications. Emphasis is placed on early recognition and action in the assessment–intervention process. This reflects the emergent nature of these events and serves as a reminder that, while the postpartum period is generally problem-free, the astute nurse remains aware of these threats to individual and family well-being.

POSTPARTUM HEMORRHAGE

Postpartum hemorrhage is defined conventionally as a blood loss of more than 500 ml following birth. Blood loss to this extent within the first 24 hours postdelivery is termed *early postpartum hemorrhage,* while hemorrhage occurring after the first 24 hours is called *late postpartum*

hemorrhage. Postpartum hemorrhage is a complication of pregnancy whose treatment requires judgment and skill, often rendered under emergency conditions. Most women enter labor with a normal blood volume and a normal hematocrit and are able to recover from a blood loss at delivery of less than 500 ml. The best method of detection of excessive blood loss is close observation by an experienced, knowledgeable nurse. Observation is the key in the initiation of prompt medical evaluation, treatment, and prevention of the more extreme consequences of hemorrhage.

Although hysterectomy may be required to control bleeding, women experiencing postpartum hemorrhage should survive. Death from postpartum hemorrhage is rare in current obstetric practice, but it remains more common under less favorable conditions aggravated by poverty. Women dying from obstetric causes, including hemorrhage, tend to be older, obese, black, and married. Estimates of mortality from hemorrhagic complications of pregnancy account for about one quarter to one third of maternal deaths (Rochat et al 1988). Postpartum hemorrhage lowers maternal resistance to infection and increases the likelihood of blood transfusion and prolonged convalescence.

Bleeding may not present as a sudden massive hemorrhage but as a steady trickle that persists until serious hypovolemia develops.

The normotensive woman may initially become somewhat hypertensive in response to hemorrhage whereas the chronic hypertensive woman may erroneously be judged as normotensive. Persistent tachycardia following delivery may be one of the best clues to major blood loss.

Etiology

Knowledge of the risk factors in postpartum hemorrhage helps the nurse and the health care team prevent its occurrence, minimize its magnitude, plan treatment, and focus observation skills.

Risk factors for early postpartum hemorrhage include uterine atony, trauma and lacerations, and hematoma. Risk factors for late postpartum hemorrhage include retained placental fragments, bleeding disorders, and infection. (The latter is discussed later in this chapter as a complication of itself.)

Early Postpartum Hemorrhage

Uterine Atony

Uterine atony accounts for 80% to 90% of cases of immediate postpartum hemorrhage. It occurs when the uterine corpus fails to contract, permitting continued blood loss from the placental site. The following conditions should alert the clinician to the possibility of immediate postpartum hemorrhage resulting from uterine atony:

- Overdistended uterus (hydramnios, multiple gestation, macrosomic infant)
- Oxytocin induction or augmentation of labor
- Precipitous labor and delivery
- Prolonged first and second stage of labor
- Grand multiparity (greater than five deliveries)
- History of uterine atony with previous delivery
- Uterine leiomyomas
- Sepsis

- Magnesium sulfate used in labor
- Bladder distention (Gilbert, Porter, and Brown 1987)

Anticipation of possible uterine atony with resultant hemorrhage allows preparatory measures to be taken. When risk factors are present, the nurse should prepare for delivery by making certain that intravenous access is available and that the patient's bladder is empty. In addition, the nurse should ensure that a clot of the patient's blood is held for possible type and crossmatching and that oxytocic drugs are ready for immediate use. Pitocin,

Table 30–1 **Oxytocic Drugs Used to Control Postpartum Atony and Hemorrhage**

Drug	Use	Dosage	Potential Side-Effects and Contraindications
Oxytocin injection			
(Pitocin, Syntocinon)	To induce rhythmic uterine contractions that reduce or prevent uterine atony and hemorrhage	SC, IM, IV: 10 U as necessary IV drip: 10 to 40 U in 500–1000 ml Ringer's lactate	Nausea, vomiting, uterine tetany, hypersensitivity, water intoxication, anaphylactic reaction

Nursing Implications

When oxytocic drugs are used, a physician or nurse-midwife should be immediately available to manage possible complications.
Fundal checks are done every 10 to 15 min to assess the quantity and quality of uterine contractions.
When an IV infusion is used, uterus should remain in a strong tetanic contraction. The patient will complain of uterine pain.
When the uterus remains atonic (not contracted), the rate or dose of the infusion may be insufficient to effectively control uterine bleeding.
Notify the physician or nurse-midwife immediately.

Ergonovine maleate			
(Ergotrate maleate)	To produce uterine contractions to reduce or prevent postpartum hemorrhage due to atony	IM: 0.2 mg every 2 to 4 hr up to a maximum of five doses Oral: 0.2 to 0.4 mg every 6 to 16 hr until atony passes (48 hr)	Nausea, vomiting, severe hypertensive episode, bradycardia, allergic reaction, shock Ergonovine is contraindicated in patients with hypersensitivity, infection, hypertension.

Nursing Implications

Closely monitor and record the character of uterine contractions.
IM injections may cause vigorous contractions for 3 hr or more. The patient may be very uncomfortable and may need analgesia for pain relief.
Monitor the patient's blood pressure, pulse, and uterine response for 1 to 2 hr or until she is stabilized. Report any sudden blood pressure increase, pulse changes, and frequent episodes of uterine relaxation.
Patients receiving this therapy become more sensitive to cold. Exposure of the patient is to be avoided.

Methylergonovine maleate			
(Methergine)	To induce tetanic uterine contractions that reduce or prevent uterine atony and hemorrhage (also used in management of subinvolution)	IM: 0.2 mg every 2 to 4 hr as necessary Oral: 0.2 mg three to four times daily for a maximum of 1 week	Same as ergonovine Check BP prior to administration as methergine causes abrupt increase in systolic BP

Nursing Implications

Monitor vital signs (particularly blood pressure) and uterine response during IV or IM use of this drug for 1 to 2 hr or until patient is stabilized.
If blood pressure suddenly increases or there are frequent periods of uterine atony, notify the physician.

Prostaglandins			
(Prostaglandin $F_2\alpha$)	To control severe hemorrhage secondary to atony when other therapies have failed	1 mg injected directly into myometrium, either transvaginally or transabdominally	Nausea, vomiting, pyrexia, bradycardia, bronchospasm. Contraindicated in patients with cardiovascular disease or asthma

Nursing Implications

Same as for Ergonovine

Berkowitz R, Coustan D, Mochizuki T: Handbook for Prescribing Medications During Pregnancy, 2nd ed. Boston, Little, Brown & Co, 1986

Methergine and prostaglandins are the most commonly used drugs to combat postpartum hemorrhage (Table 30–1).

Bleeding associated with a soft, "boggy" uterus on abdominal palpation is characteristic of uterine atony. If the uterus is atonic, massage is used to stimulate contraction so that the bleeding vessels at the placental site will be compressed and bleeding will stop (Fig. 30–1). It may be necessary to frequently check the consistency of the uterus since bleeding may recur once palpation has been discontinued. If the uterus fails to maintain contraction after massage, Pitocin may be given in dilute solution intravenously, intramuscularly, or by both routes. The nurse must continue to closely monitor the patient's vital signs, paying particular attention to the pulse rate and blood pressure to assess signs and symptoms of impending shock. Prompt and complete communication of abnormal findings to the patient's birth attendant is vital so that further treatment can be quickly instituted. An important aspect of nursing care is to keep the patient and her family members apprised of the situation; communication minimizes fear and apprehension and maximizes cooperation with emergency measures.

Trauma and Lacerations

Whenever bleeding persists in the presence of a firmly contracted uterus, lacerations of the cervix and vaginal vault must be considered. Hemorrhage associated with lacerations of the lower genital tract is frequently bright red and may be accompanied by signs and symptoms of shock. Early recognition with appropriate and prompt repair is the definitive treatment. Minor lacerations of the cervix and vagina occur to some degree in most deliveries. Many do not require repair, but all must be inspected.

Factors predisposing to hemorrhage from lacerations of the genital tract are as follows:

- Episiotomy cut too early
- Precipitous labor
- Instrumented delivery
- Abnormal presentation
- Macrosomia
- Hydramnios
- Multiple gestation
- Previous cesarean delivery
- Breech extraction
- Oxytocin use in labor
- Poor tissue integrity

Nursing care is directed at anticipation and recognition of predisposing factors, focused observation and report of the patient's condition, the gathering of materials needed for tissue repair prior to delivery, and communication with the patient to keep her informed and to enhance

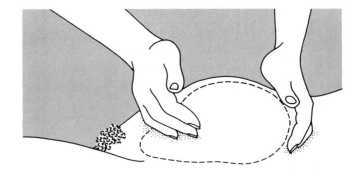

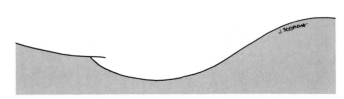

Figure 30–1. External fundal massage. Shown here are the enlarged uterus immediately after delivery and the maneuvers used to maintain its tone in order to prevent excessive bleeding and assist its involution. The right hand supports the lower portion of the uterus while the left hand gently palpates and massages the fundus. (Childbirth Graphics)

cooperation. As with most emergency situations, cooperation is the key to rapid and successful repair of profusely bleeding lacerations. When emergency procedures are instituted, rapport with and confidence in the nurse will help calm the patient. (See Chapter 24 for further discussion of cervical and vaginal repair.)

Hematoma

Hematomas are formed when blood escapes into connective tissue (Fig. 30–2). This usually occurs following injury to a blood vessel without laceration of the overlying tissue. Hematomas are more commonly associated with operative deliveries (forceps), inadequate repair of episiotomy, or pressure necrosis following spontaneous delivery. Occasionally hematoma formation is delayed and occurs as late hemorrhage, resulting from the sloughing of necrotic tissue.

Hematomas can occur anywhere along the birth canal. Most commonly they are perineal or vaginal. Less frequent are retroperitoneal and broad ligament hematoma formation. These latter sites are especially dangerous because massive hemorrhage into the tissues can go unrecognized for a prolonged period of time; in addition, these sites are more susceptible to infection, potentially leading to sepsis and death.

Hematomas form in loose connective tissue and follow

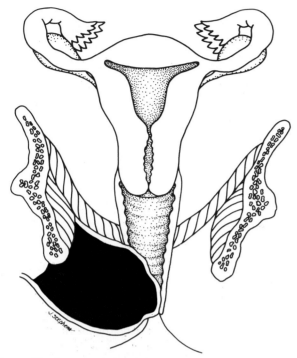

Figure 30–2. Paravaginal hematoma, showing the large amount of blood that can be contained within a hematoma and the pressure that it can exert on the tissues. The paravaginal hematoma extends over the vulva to the rectal area. (Childbirth Graphics)

the fascial folds. Excruciating tearing pain is the cardinal symptom. The pain may be described as intense pressure in the vagina, rectum, or perineum that radiates down the leg. Initial inspection may not confirm diagnosis, since external swelling and ecchymoses may not be immediately evident. It may be necessary to examine the woman under sterile conditions with sedation to identify high vaginal hematomas or to adequately assess vulvar hematomas. Treatment is accomplished by the physician, who opens the hematoma, evacuates the clots, and ligates bleeders. Large untreated hematomas are susceptible to infection. Broad-spectrum antibiotics are often added to the treatment plan. Small vulvar hematomas identified after leaving the delivery room may be managed with ice packs, pressure to the area, analgesics, observation and recording of hematoma size, and careful attention to signs of hypovolemia. Kegel exercises should be avoided until bleeding stops.

Late Postpartum Hemorrhage

Late postpartum hemorrhage is defined as blood loss of more than 500 ml occurring after the first 24 hours postdelivery. Diagnosis and treatment for such hemorrhage proceeds in the same way as in early hemorrhage.

This is the case whether bleeding occurs from retained placental fragments, infection, or subinvolution.

The signs and symptoms of hemorrhage include obvious vaginal bleeding, anemia, and perhaps shock. Management of acute bleeding is accomplished by means similar to those for early hemorrhage, that is, with massage, oxytocics, intravenous fluid volume replacement, and provision of external warmth until definitive treatment can be given. Bleeding that presents as a slow, reddish brown ooze or as occasional, irregular heavy bleeding accompanied by a soft, "boggy" uterus is treated by a course of oral Methergine. Methergine, unlike Pitocin, produces sustained contraction of the uterus. If the uterus is tender upon examination, a course of oral antibiotics may be prescribed. An uncontracted uterus that contains blood clots or placental fragments provides an excellent site for bacterial growth and infection. Often the body's own defenses are adequate to combat infection, but the presence of uterine tenderness should alert the health care provider that antibiotics are needed. The patient is reevaluated in 2 weeks; persistent bleeding after treatment indicates the need for dilation and curettage of the uterus (Herbert and Cefalo 1984).

Retained Placental Fragments

Placental separation and expulsion occurs within 30 minutes of delivery for all but about 6% of patients (Gilbert, Porter, and Brown 1987). Small retained placental fragments seldom cause immediate postpartum hemorrhage but are thought to explain a large proportion of late postpartum hemorrhages. Retention of all or part of the placenta interferes with normal uterine contraction, thus leaving bleeding sites open; bleeding continues until the rest of the placenta is separated and expelled. Routine examination of the placenta following delivery is necessary: if a portion of the placenta is missing, exploration of the uterus for the removal of the placental tissue should be made.

Bleeding Disorders

Any of the acquired or congenital blood dyscrasias can intensify hemorrhage from all causes. Afibrinogenemia may follow placental abruption, prolonged retention of a dead fetus, or amniotic fluid embolus (see Chapter 28). Preeclampsia also alters the clotting mechanism by reducing the platelet count. These conditions promote failure of the clotting mechanism, resulting in bleeding that cannot be controlled by the usual measures. For any woman with a history suggesting a disease process in which coagulopathy is a component, additional blood studies to assess platelet count and clotting ability should be done (Creasy and Resnik 1988).

Implications for Nursing Care

Postpartum hemorrhage should be readily identified except in rare instances where bleeding accumulates intravaginally and intraperitoneally. Differential diagnosis of the source of the bleeding is initially made on the presence or absence of uterine atony and the color of the blood. Every woman who has postpartum hemorrhage should survive, even though hysterectomy may be necessary to save her life under extreme circumstances (Clark et al 1985).

Skilled nursing care is recognized as pivotal in:

- Anticipation of factors predisposing to postpartum hemorrhage
- Observation for clinical signs of hemorrhage and changes in vital signs indicating impending shock
- Prompt initiation of treatment through timely report of findings
- Support and communication to the patient and family members present during an emergency situation, thus enhancing cooperation with resuscitative efforts
- Alert observation and care following the treatment of a woman with postpartum hemorrhage
- Providing follow-up instruction to patient and family regarding expectations for recovery

PUERPERAL INFECTION

Postpartum infection (puerperal sepsis) is a major cause of maternal morbidity and mortality. The pelvic cavity is the site of origin for the majority of postpartum infections. Other common sites of infection include the perineum and associated structures, the breasts, the urinary tract, and the venous system.

Puerperal infection is presumed to be present with a temperature of 100.4°F (38.0°C) or higher on any 2 of the first 10 days after delivery (exclusive of the first 24 hours).

Prior to the 1800s *childbed fever* was recognized but was infrequently reported. The beginning of the 19th century brought with it a shift from home childbirth to actively managed childbirth in hospitals and a concurrent, alarming increase in the incidence of puerperal infections.

In 1900 Louis Pasteur identified the primary microorganism, hemolytic streptococcus, and proposed that the female genitourinary tract was exceptionally vulnerable during the intrapartum period. Unfortunately, clinical practice did not change enough to significantly affect the high morbidity and mortality rates. It was not until the advent of sulfonamides and penicillin in the 1940s that the rate of complications from postpartum sepsis began to decrease.

Incidence

Current estimates of the incidence of puerperal infection range from 1% to 8%. There are a number of variables that may contribute to this variation. One is the increasingly common practice of early discharge. Other variables are the prophylactic administration of antibiotics and the rapid response to new broad-spectrum drugs. These changes in management obscure the temperature elevation that is the primary indicator of postpartum infection. Even though the risk during the postpartum period is limited, infection is still one of the primary causes of maternal death (Sweet and Gibbs 1987).

Etiology

Risk factors for puerperal infection can be identified throughout the childbearing cycle. The nurse can assist in early identification of an individual's susceptibility through careful history taking prior to or during the antenatal, intrapartum, and postpartum periods. Most common risk factors are shown in the accompanying display.

Cesarean delivery has increased the incidence of puer-

Risk Factors for Postpartum Infection

Antenatal Factors

- Poor nutritional status
- Low socioeconomic status and limited access to health care
- History of susceptibility to infection or preexisting medical conditions
- Vaginal Infections
- Obesity
- Anemia

Intrapartum Factors

- Long labor and premature rupture of the amniotic membranes
- Breaks in aseptic technique
- Genital tract trauma, lacerations, or hematomas
- Multiple vaginal examinations
- Internal fetal and uterine monitoring
- Urinary catheterization
- Operative deliveries
- Episiotomy
- Cesarean delivery

Postpartum Factors

- Manual removal of the placenta
- Hemorrhage

peral infections. With modifications in technique and the availability of antibiotics in the 1940s and 1950s, the safety of the cesarean procedure increased. Indications for the use of cesarean delivery changed to include not only the prevention of maternal mortality but also fetal mortality and maternal and fetal morbidity. Consequently, the incidence of the procedure in the US has increased from 5% of all deliveries prior to 1970 to current rates of 25% or greater. Rates of puerperal infection after cesarean delivery range from 5 to 30 times greater than vaginal delivery. The types of infection most commonly associated with cesarean deliveries, in order of occurrence, are endometritis, bacteremia, and wound infection.

Treatment

Diagnosis of infection is made from subjective report and objective observation of the patient. Signs and symptoms may include fever, malaise, body part pain, and purulent or foul-smelling discharges. Laboratory tests used for diagnosis include the complete blood count (CBC), venous blood cultures, urine cultures, and in some cases cultures of tissue taken from suspected infection sites, such as the endometrium or wounds.

The CBC yields much information. Hemoglobin, an indicator of the cells' oxygen-carrying ability, may be diminished by infection. An anemia not present antenatally or associated with blood loss may be suggestive of infection. More importantly, the CBC includes information about the status of the body's immune system and indicates whether there has been a recent challenge to the system. A normal white blood count (WBC) during pregnancy is 10,000 to 12,000/mm³. With an early infection the WBC count will rapidly or gradually increase to 20,000/mm³ or greater, and the differential count of cells will show an early response from the neutrophils or polymorphonuclear leukocytes.

Laboratory tests, including cultures and gram stains, allow identification of the many microbial agents found with postpartum infection. Gram's method of staining slides will identify gram-positive and gram-negative organisms and provide immediate direction for treatment, while the results of culturing the infectious agents will later determine the comprehensiveness of the chosen treatment. It is important to collect specimens for culture before antimicrobial treatment is begun in order to prevent confusion in the interpretation of clinical data (Dinsmoor and Gibbs 1988).

Moderate infections, represented by an increase in symptoms and verified by laboratory diagnosis, require that the patient remain hospitalized for antibiotic therapy. Depending on the history preceding the onset of symptoms, the patient receives intravenous antibiotic therapy that is continued for 24–48 hours after fever has subsided.

Because many of the infections that develop during the puerperium are polymicrobial, it is common practice to treat these infections with a combination antibiotic regimen (Dinsmoor and Gibbs 1988). The pathogens most commonly recovered are *Neisseria gonorrhoeae*, aerobic and anaerobic streptococci, anaerobic bacilli, Chlamydia trachomatis, and genital mycoplasmas. The drugs of choice for these pathogens are penicillin (or ampicillin), Cephalosporin, and aminoglycosides. (See Table 30–2 for the antibiotics commonly used to treat puerperal infection.)

Implications for Nursing Care

The first line of defense against infection is prevention. Whether or not a patient is identified at risk, there are basic nursing techniques that, when followed, will help to prevent or curtail infection.

The nurse must take special steps to:

- Monitor patient status to allow the earliest possible identification and treatment of infection
- Maintain a clean, well-ventilated environment
- Encourage a balanced diet, frequent fluids, and early ambulation (as appropriate to the individual situation)
- Teach and encourage the patient to follow aseptic techniques in her maintenance of personal hygiene, including new procedures that are necessary for perineal or wound care
- Remind the patient that caring for a newborn requires particular attention to hand washing and the disposal of soiled or contaminated objects

Once infection has been diagnosed, the nurse is responsible for monitoring aspects of antibiotic therapy. The nurse must determine if information about previous drug sensitivities or allergies has been gathered. If the patient reports symptoms of previous drug reactions, the nurse must clarify the exact nature of the reaction and ascertain if the physician or nurse-midwife was aware of this information prior to administering the drug. Once an antibiotic has been prescribed, the nurse must instruct the patient to report any symptoms suggestive of a drug reaction, that is, rash, swelling, itching, breathing difficulty, and must observe the patient for such symptoms after therapy is initiated.

Antibiotics work most effectively when serum concentrations are maintained at a constant level over a specified period of time. If the patient is recently postoperative or experiencing nausea and vomiting, gastrointestinal absorption may be limited, and intravenous administration may be necessary. If the patient is awakened for medications, the nurse should attempt to coordinate all other necessary care to limit sleep interruptions. Implications of antibiotic therapy for breast-feeding must be noted, and appropriate steps to support breast-feeding initiated.

Table 30-2   Antibiotic Drugs Commonly Used to Treat Puerperal Infection

Drug	Dosage	Potential Side-Effects	Nursing Implications
Ampicillin (Amcill) — penicillin group	Orally: 250 to 1000 mg q.i.d. IM or IV: 500 mg to 2 g every 6 hr	Allergic reaction as seen in penicillin hypersensitivity: rash, nausea, vomiting, dermatitis, anaphylactic reaction	Drug is not used in patients with penicillin allergy. 30% of hospital strains of *E. coli* are resistant to penicillin drugs. Drug appears in breast milk.
Carbenicillin (Geopen — synthetic penicillin	IM or IV: 1 to 2 g daily in divided doses	Allergic reaction as seen in penicillin hypersensitivity; vein irritation at point of injection	Unpleasant taste and dry mouth may occur; mouth care needed. Advise patient to report change in urine quantity, quality.
Cefoxitin (Mefoxin) — semisynthetic and related to penicillin	IM or IV: 3 to 8 g every 6 to 8 hr	Pain, tenderness, induration at IM injection site; thrombophlebitis at IV site; rash, fever, allergic reaction	Drug is not used in patients sensitive to penicillin or cephalosporins
Clindamycin (Cleocin)	Orally: 150 to 450 mg every 6 hr IM or IV: 300 to 600 mg every 6 to 8 hr, up to 2400 mg/day	Loose stools, diarrhea, nausea, vomiting, abdominal cramps, colitis, rash; abnormal liver function test following rapid IV injection	Drug is reserved for serious infections where less toxic antimicrobials are ineffective. It is the drug of choice in treating *Bacteroides fragilis*, a normal inhabitant of genital tract that causes infection when blood clots or necrotic tissue are present.
Chloramphenicol	Orally: 500 mg every 4 hr. IV: same as oral dose	Bone marrow depression, gastrointestinal disturbances, nausea, vomiting, bad taste in mouth. Neurotoxicity: headache, mental depression, confusion; optic effects: visual disturbances, contact conjunctivitis; hypersensitivity, fever, rash, topical itching	Shake medicine well. Drug is to be taken with water on an empty stomach 1 to 2 hr before or after a meal. Patient is hospitalized for close observation and lab tests. Observe closely for signs of toxicity. Patient should report sore throat, fatigue, petechiae, bleeding. Check temperature every 4 hr.
Metronidazol (Flagyl)	Orally: single 2-g dose IV for anaerobic infection: loading dose 15 mg/kg infused over 1-hr period; maintenance dose 7.5 mg/kg IV or orally every 6 hr	Anorexia, nausea, vomiting, diarrhea, epigastric distress, bad taste in mouth; possible carcinogenic, teratogenic, and mutagenic changes found in animal studies	Do not mix with another drug. Drug is contraindicated in patients with blood dyscrasias. Alcoholic beverages should not be consumed (drug is used in antiabuse therapy). Defer breast-feeding during treatment.
Streptomycin sulfate — aminoglycoside	15 to 25 mg/kg/day every 12 hr	Ototoxicity: labyrinth damage, auditory change; neurotoxicity: paresthesia, headache, inability to concentrate, muscular weakness; hypersensitivity	Drug is administered deep into large muscle mass to avoid irritation. Injections are painful. Avoid direct contact with drug — sensitization can occur. Advise patient to report unusual symptoms (esp. ear symptoms). Monitor intake and output.
Kanamycin sulfate — aminoglycoside	IM: 15 mg/kg in two to four equally divided doses IV: not to exceed 15 mg/kg body weight in two to three equal doses	Gastrointestinal effects: nausea, vomiting, diarrhea; nephrotoxicity: hematuria, proteinuria; ototoxicity: deafness, vertigo, tinnitus; neurotoxicity: paresthesia, optic or peripheral neuritis; hypersensitivity: pruritus, rash; changes in many blood studies	Drug is administered IM deep into upper-outer quadrant of buttock. Keep patient well hydrated (sufficient amount to produce 1500 ml urine/day). Postoperative patients should be monitored for respiratory and neuromuscular depression.
Gentamicin (Garamycin) — aminoglycoside	IM or IV: 3 to 5 mg/kg/day in three divided doses every 8 hr	Ototoxicity, nephrotoxicity; allergic reactions: rash, pruritus, fever, burning sensation of skin, local irritation of skin	Observe closely for signs of ototoxicity (headache, dizziness, nausea, ataxia, tinnitus). Monitor intake and output. Drug is not to be mixed with any other drug.
Tobramycin (Nebcin) — Aminoglycoside	IM or IV: 3 to 8 mg/kg/day, three equal doses every 8 hr	Ototoxicity, nephrotoxicity, rash, headache, nausea, vomiting, tremor, paresthesia	Observe for signs of toxicity. Keep patient hydrated. Monitor intake, output.

Complications Involving Uterine Infection

A large percentage of postpartum infections are not diagnosed as such during postpartum hospitalization but present as heavy postpartum bleeding or a low-grade fever. Uncontrolled postpartum infection may progress to life-threatening situations, such as parametritis, peritonitis, and septic shock (Shy and Eschenback 1979).

Superficial Endometritis and Endomyometritis

The terminology of puerperal infection associated with the uterus corresponds to the anatomical parts of the uterus involved. The most common infection in the postpartum period is an *endometritis* involving the superficial mucous or decidual layer. In its mildest form this infected layer of sloughing cellular material is simply passed away in the form of lochia, and normal involution continues.

If for some reason the patient's immunological resources are compromised and bacterial colonies continue to grow, infections will extend from the endometrium into the muscular layer, or myometrium, of the uterus and result in endomyometritis. Symptoms of a developing endomyometritis include the following:

- Onset usually occurs 24 hours after delivery
- Temperature range 100⁴ to 102F° (38 to 38°C)
- Tachycardia (averaging 100–120 beats per minute)
- Symptoms of malaise, fatigue, and anorexia
- Elevation of WBCs

- Reduction in size (involution) of the uterus does not occur
- Abdominal or uterine tenderness (Sweet and Gibbs 1987)

Implications for Nursing Care

Treatment is centered around supporting the body's natural response to pathogenic organisms, with the addition of antibiotic therapy when needed. Nursing responsibilities include those described in the previous sections on general nursing treatment of puerperal infection and nursing responsibilities with antibiotic therapy. Personal hygiene, pelvic rest, and promotion of recovery through diet, rest, and increased fluids should be emphasized. Patient education is of special importance with this type of infection so that an advancing infection may be recognized and an appropriate level of therapy initiated.

Prior to discharge the patient must be carefully instructed to recognize the symptoms of a progressive infection: changes in fever status, tenderness in body parts, changes in lochia, general malaise, and fatigue.

Parametritis

An undiagnosed or unsuccessfully treated infection of the endomyometrium will progress to involve the entire uterus and may spread to accessory pelvic structures, the main pathway constituted by the broad ligament (Fig. 30–3). The broad ligament is a double fold of peritoneum that encloses the uterus, fallopian tubes, ovaries, and round ligaments and attaches to the lateral walls of the

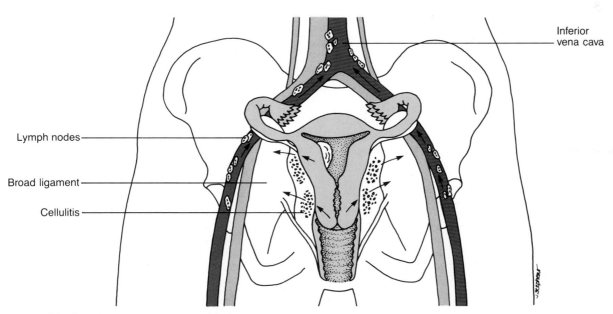

Figure 30–3. Puerperal infection extends to the structures around the uterus, resulting in pelvic cellulitis (parametritis). (Childbirth Graphics)

pelvic cavity. Contiguous with the broad ligament are the main arterial and venous circulation to the pelvis. An infection that spreads in this manner is known as *parametritis*. Untreated infections will organize into abscesses and continue to grow, threatening the peritoneum, abdominal cavity, and vascular systems. Symptoms of parametritis appear 24 hours or more after delivery and are more severe than those of endometritis; they include the following:

- Spiking temperatures to 104°F (40°C)
- Symptoms associated with elevated temperatures: chills, flushing, sweating
- Tachycardia, tachypnea
- Increasing uterine or abdominal tenderness, which may be accompanied by persistent or severe uterine cramping
- Change in consciousness, such as agitation, delirium, or disorientation
- Noticeable change in lochia: increase or decrease in amount, quality, and odor
- Pelvic exam reveals cervical or uterine tenderness and/or abscesses
- CBC demonstrates an elevation in WBCs (Sweet and Gibbs 1987)

Treatment

Treatment includes bed rest and an aggressive antibiotic regimen. If antibiotic treatment, including various combination therapies, is not successful, the physician may consider surgical intervention.

The endometrium is cleared using the procedure of curettage to remove retained infected tissue. Surgical resolution of an abscess is attempted with two methods. If there is a strong suspicion that the abscess is located in the *cul-de-sac* of Douglas (a recess or cavity created by an extension of the peritoneum between the uterus and vagina anteriorly and the rectum and uterus posteriorly), a colpotomy or incision is made to allow for drainage of purulent material (Fig. 30–4).

The second method involves the use of a laparotomy, or surgical opening of the abdomen, to identify the location and extent of the infection. Once this information has been ascertained, further surgery may be deemed necessary, including removal of the uterus and one or both of the ovaries and fallopian tubes (total abdominal hysterectomy with uni- or bilateral salpingo-oophorectomy).

Implications for Nursing Care

The patient's vital signs and intake and output are monitored. Pain relief is required as well as comfort measures to relieve fever symptoms. Patients are positioned for comfort and to diminish upward movement of the infection.

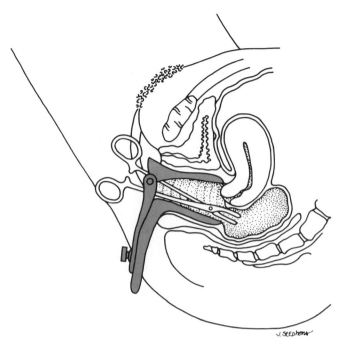

Figure 30–4. Posterior colpotomy. Draining a collection of localized pus in the cul-de-sac of Douglas. (Childbirth Graphics)

Patients with persistent obstetric infections require special attention, because they are compromised by the side-effects of illness at a time when it is frequently least expected. Family issues may arise and breast-feeding may be interrupted. Nurses need to set aside time to address these issues.

Threatened fertility is another concern associated with surgical interventions. The patient and her family must be well informed concerning the nature of the suggested surgery, the consequences, and the risks and benefits. This is the responsibility of the physician, but it frequently is the case that the patient uses the nurse to verify her understanding and to further explore the situation. Using active listening as a tool, the nurse can promote optimal adaptation by helping the patient work through her personal reactions to the situation and by acting as a resource person in referring the patient to others who can provide religious or psychological support or additional medical opinions concerning her condition.

Peritonitis

The peritoneum is a thin membranous tissue that extends from the pelvic cavity and is continuous with the abdominal cavity. Puerperal infections traveling from the pelvis usually do so through the lymphatic system (Fig. 30–5). The peritoneum produces a fibrous exudate in immediate response to the spread of infection. Generally, abscesses form between the fibrinous adhesions, which causes a localization of the infection. These adhesions

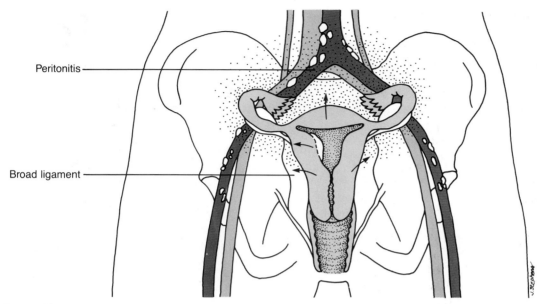

Figure 30–5. Puerperal infection extends to the peritoneum. Infection is extended by way of the lymph nodes and uterine wall. (Childbirth Graphics)

often disappear with adequate treatment of the infection. If unresolved, the adhesions may harden into fibrous bands that may later cause intestinal obstruction. A generalized peritonitis will diminish peristaltic activity and may ultimately lead to paralytic ileus and the loss of normal intestinal functioning. Peritonitis is a serious condition involving electrolyte imbalances, circulatory and/or renal compromise, and in some cases shock.

Symptoms of peritonitis vary according to the extent of the infection and the type of organisms involved. The most severe symptoms associated with nonlocalized infections that have affected other body systems include the following:

- Sudden rapid onset of symptoms
- Temperature spikes to 105°F (40.5°C)
- Shaking chills
- Abdominal pain and/or distention, tenseness, loss of bowel sounds
- Tachycardia, tachypnea, and shortness of breath
- Excessive thirst
- Fruity or foul-smelling breath
- Nausea, vomiting, diarrhea
- Oliguria
- Initial depressed leukocyte count followed by a leukocytosis
- Hyperglycemia followed by hypoglycemia
- Early symptoms of disseminated intravascular coagulation (DIC), evidenced by changes in the coagulation profile

Incidence

Overall, the reported mortality associated with septic shock ranges from 10% to 81%. Underlying the high mortality rate is the high incidence of coexisting debilitating diseases. In obstetrical populations this is less commonly so, and the maternal mortality rate associated with sepsis is estimated at 0% to 8% (Sweet and Gibbs 1987).

Treatment

Treatment is aggressive and comprehensive. Primary treatment is focused on maintenance of adequate circulation and intravascular volumes, maintenance of an adequate airway, diagnosis of infectious agent, and comprehensive antimicrobial therapy.

Implications for Nursing Care

Nursing responsibilities include careful monitoring of intake and output, central venous pressure and/or pulmonary artery pressure, electrolyte balance, and administration of pharmacologic agents. Output is monitored by frequent checking of urinary output and nasogastric emptying. Respiratory status is monitored by frequent checks of vital signs and assessment of lung sounds. Arterial blood gas readings are obtained to rule out the onset of adult respiratory distress syndrome (ARDS). General nursing care of the patient includes, in addition to frequent assessment of vital signs, checking for bowel sounds and abdominal distention. Attention is directed at measures of comfort, oral care, positioning, and providing medications for pain relief and anxiety.

Once specimens for culture have been obtained, antibiotic therapy is begun. The choice of drugs will vary with physicians but often include a penicillin, an aminoglycoside, and cephalosporin.

Usually peritonitis is very debilitating, and it will represent a crisis for the new mother and her family. Attention must be paid to keeping the woman's family informed about her condition. If healthy, the newborn may be ready for discharge before the mother. Issues of separation from the newborn may have emotional and psychological impact on the patient and should be approached carefully. It is of primary importance to determine how the patient feels about the separation and to give reassurance when appropriate.

Complications Involving Perineal or Vaginal Infection

Infection in the vagina usually involves the site of a laceration or episiotomy wound; it may spread to the fascia and internal structures. Untreated superficial fascial necrosis can lead to systemic involvement and a potentially fatal situation. Consequences of this complication include prolonged hospitalization and possible permanent anatomical damage as well as a mortality rate of 21% to 76% (Sweet and Gibbs 1987).

Superficial or Simple Infections

Infections of soft tissue are defined according to the depth of the infection. A simple or superficial infection involves only the skin, subcutaneous tissue, and superficial fascial edge. Symptoms include:

- Skin changes, including erythema and edema, that are frequently unilateral
- Pain at the wound site
- Exudate from the wound site

Implications for Nursing Care

Treatment includes the opening of the wound with exploration for possible hematomas and/or wall defects between the vagina and rectum, followed by debridement. Cultures are obtained at this time. Drainage alone may be sufficient but may be combined with antibiotic therapy. The wound is not sutured and will be allowed to heal by granulation.

Nursing responsibilities specific to the patient with a superficial infection involve close monitoring of the wound for symptoms of spread of the infection. The extent of edema (in centimeters) and the appearance of the tissue must be determined and charted at least once every 8 hours. Once the wound has been debrided, special care is given to promote drainage and provide a clean environment for healing. Perineal care includes sitz baths, exposure to air, and heat treatments. Analgesia is offered for

pain. If the wound is packed, the physician will write orders for removal of the packing. Special care should be taken to prevent contamination of the wound packing. Any contamination of the wound must be reported to the physician immediately.

Intermediate or Superficial Fascial Necrosis

In superficial fascial necrosis, infection extends to an intermediate level and usually involves both layers of the superficial perineal fascia. The infection may then spread along the fascia to the abdominal wall, thigh, or buttock. By this time the infection frequently involves necrosis, or a gradual degeneration or death of the tissue. When the infection involves the muscles below the deep fascia, the condition is called myonecrosis. A differentiating symptom is the existence of severe pain. Treatment for myonecrosis is similar to that for superficial fascial necrosis but may involve more disability if extensive dissection of muscle is involved. Symptoms of superficial fascial necrosis include:

- Acute onset with rapid course
- Skin changes, including edema and erythema with indistinct borders, skin color becoming blue or brown owing to an occluding of the vessels close to the surface of the skin, and the formation of bullae (blisters or skin vesicles filled with fluid)
- Tissue hypoesthesia (loss of sensation)
- Hemoconcentration
- Leukocytosis
- Localized pain

Systemic symptoms include those of septic shock, discussed in Chapter 28.

Implications for Nursing Care

Treatment includes rapid and aggressive antibiotic therapy. Group A and B streptococci are traditionally associated with this condition, but, as in other types of puerperal infection, multiple infectious agents may be present. For this reason, a polyantimicrobial regimen is followed. If the wound has not been debrided, this procedure is done; further surgical intervention may include dissection of much of the necrotic tissue.

Nursing responsibilities include those listed previously for superficial infections and those outlined for patients with systemic infection. In the case where extensive debridement or dissection is necessary, the nurse must take the time to help the patient deal with the impact of permanent changes to the anatomy in what is generally considered a sensitive or secret area of the body. Such changes may affect the way patient relates to her own sexuality and may have a lasting impact.

POSTPARTUM URINARY TRACT INFECTIONS

Bacteriuria is defined as the presence of 10^5 or more bacterial colonies per milliliter of urine on two consecutive, clean, midstream, voided specimens. Because of the structure and physiologic processes of the female urogenital tract, bacteriuria is a fact of life for many women. Normal changes of pregnancy that contribute to an increased risk for urinary tract infection (UTI) include the following:

- Uterine compression of the ureters at the pelvic inlet
- Dilatation and diminished tone of the ureters as a result of hormonal effects

When these risk factors are combined, urinary stasis promotes bacterial growth. Normal occurrences during the birthing process lead to a decreased bladder tone; therefore, UTI is one of the most common causes of postpartum infections.

Recent research indicates that women with a previous history of bacteriuria who are symptomatic with lower bacterial counts (10^2 or greater) may have urinary tract infections. The most common offending bacterium is *Escherichia coli,* followed by *Klebsiella* organisms, *Proteus* organisms, coagulase-negative staphylococci, and pseudomonads (Sweet and Gibbs 1987).

Etiology

The urogenital tract is made more vulnerable to infection during childbirth by trauma, urinary stasis, and catheterization. Unlike many other infections, UTIs can be present asymptomatically (asymptomatic bacteriuria) or may present with primary symptoms representing an infection that has ascended the urinary system.

In many cases postpartum women are screened for UTIs only in the light of recognizable symptoms. The consequences of not recognizing early infection include the progression of the infection along the urinary tract, escalating the severity of symptoms and ultimately resulting in an infection directly involving the kidneys (pyelonephritis), which may threaten permanent kidney damage and/or systemic infection.

Cystitis

Cystitis is an inflammation of the urinary bladder; often it is the result of a bacterial infection. Symptoms indicating cystitis include:

- Urinary urgency
- Urinary frequency
- Dysuria
- Suprapubic pain
- Hematuria (not always present)

If symptoms are vague, a routine urinalysis is done to observe first-line indicators of infection, including an increase in WBCs, protein and/or blood in the urine.

When infection is suspected, laboratory identification of the microorganism is obtained by urine culture, and antibiotic sensitivity tests are performed so that appropriate drug therapy can be initiated as quickly as possible. Primary treatment includes the use of appropriate antibiotic therapy. If the antibiotic used is appropriate for the organism, symptomatic relief should be obtained within 24 hours (Stamm 1988).

Implications for Nursing Care

Teaching is a primary key to prevention of any urinary tract infection and should include the following topics:

- Routine measures for urogenital cleanliness
- The use of cotton underclothing
- Maintenance of adequate fluids
- Frequent voiding
- Voiding before and after intercourse
- Early treatment of vaginitis

Nursing responsibilities of the hospitalized postpartum woman with cystitis includes observing for symptoms of an ascending infection, encouraging fluids, observing fluid intake and output, and teaching concerning proper use of antibiotics. Once symptoms are relieved, the patient will probably be sent home. The importance of continuing antibiotic therapy and completing the follow-up assessment with a urine culture to test for antibiotic cure should be stressed.

Pyelonephritis

Pyelonephritis is an inflammation of bacterial origin of one or both of the kidneys. The incidence in pregnancy, including puerperium, is 1% to 2.5%, with a recurrence rate of 10% to 18%. Symptoms of pyelonephritis are:

- Spiking temperature and shaking chills
- Flank pain; positive costovertebral angle tenderness (CVAT)
- Nausea and vomiting
- History of asymptomatic bacteriuria or cystitis
- Urgency, frequency, dysuria
- Back pain

Laboratory tests can confirm:

- Bacteriuria
- Increased serum WBCs
- WBCs, RBCs, and protein in the urine

Treatment of pyelonephritis necessitates continued hospitalization and aggressive treatment with antibiotics.

Cultures are obtained and broad-spectrum antibiotics are begun without waiting for culture and sensitivity lab reports; rapid treatment is necessary to prevent permanent kidney damage. Relief of symptoms is usually obtained in 24 to 48 hours. Drugs are then adjusted according to sensitivity reports.

Implications for Nursing Care

Nursing responsibilities include close observation of the patient and maintenance of fluid intake and output. The patient will have an IV and may also require a Foley catheter. Vital signs are monitored carefully for evidence of a developing bacteremia. Relief measures are provided for the discomforts of fever and kidney pain.

THROMBOPHLEBITIS AND THROMBOSIS

Thrombophlebitis is an inflammation of a blood vessel with a possible concurrent development of a thrombus. Thrombus formation results when blood components (cells, platelets, and fibrin) combine to form an aggregated body. Once formed, these thrombi may become detached (emboli), flowing freely through the vascular system until they are either lysed or become lodged in another area (Fig. 30–6).

Circumstances that lead to thrombi formation include injury to the vessel wall, diminished vascular flow, and changes in clotting factors. The pregnancy state predisposes a woman to these circumstances through two main mechanisms. First, normal hormonal changes produce a vascular system response of a loss of tone or contractibility in the veins and a state of hypercoaguability. Second, the enlarging uterus imposes a restriction of blood return from the lower extremities, creating a higher incidence of stasis.

Incidence

The incidence of postpartum thrombophlebitis is reported to be between 0.1% and 1%. When a thrombosis is not treated, up to 24% of these women will proceed to develop a pulmonary embolism, with an approximate fatality rate of 15%. Studies report that treatment with anticoagulants decreases the incidence of embolisms to 4.5%, with a mortality rate of less than 1%. These statistics stress the importance of early diagnosis and treatment. Risk factors associated with this disease include:

- Prior history of thrombophlebitis
- Obesity

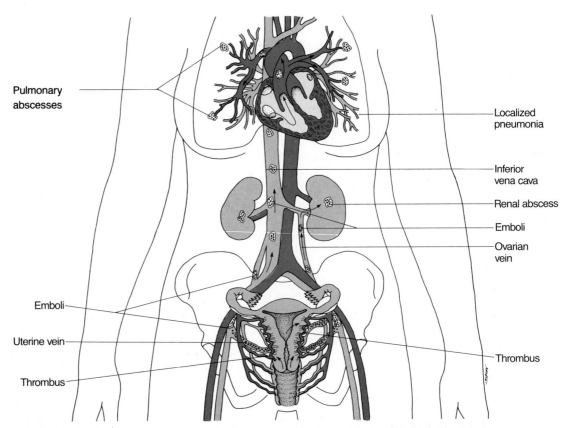

Figure 30–6. Extension of puerperal infection in pelvic thrombophlebitis. (Childbirth Graphics)

- Cesarean delivery (the risk is 9 times greater than in vaginal delivery)
- Forceps delivery
- Older maternal age
- Increased parity
- Recent infection
- Lactation suppression with estrogens
- Varicosities
- Anemia and blood dyscrasias

Conditions that involve embolisms present the greatest risk to the woman. These conditions include pulmonary embolism, which may cause respiratory distress and cardiac arrest and embolisms to the brain, which may cause cerebral vascular occlusions resulting in death or serious disabilities. (See section later in this chapter.) Ovarian embolisms may lead to conditions including cor pulmonale and septic shock.

Superficial Thrombophlebitis

The most common site of superficial thrombophlebitis is within the saphenous venous system. Symptoms include:

- Mild calf pain
- Tenderness
- Induration along the vein

In its simplest form symptoms are mild, and the involved veins are visible or palpable. Symptoms of erythema and swelling (edema) are not frequent.

Treatment consists of an increase in fluids, the use of support stockings and anti-inflammatory and analgesic medications, and close observation of the symptoms. Bed rest is recommended until symptoms subside, which usually occurs within 48 hours.

Implications for Nursing Care

Nursing responsibilities include continuing evaluation of vital signs and checking of the extremities for signs of inflammation, swelling, and a positive Homans' sign (pain in the calf on passive dorsiflexion of the foot that may represent a deep vein thrombosis). Warm moist packs are applied to the site to encourage blood flow. Caution should be taken to make sure that the patient is not given estrogens for lactation suppression, since estrogen may encourage the formation of clots.

Patients must be taught those everyday habits important to all women that will help prevent venous stasis. These measures include:

- Maintenance of adequate fluid intake
- Avoiding constriction or pressure to the popliteal area of the legs

- Avoiding crossing the legs at the knee while sitting
- Elevating the feet while sitting when possible
- Ambulating periodically throughout the day

Deep Vein Thrombosis

Deep vein thrombosis (DVT) is associated with the deep venous system located in the legs and pelvis. The larger veins there present more immediate access to the central venous system, thus increasing the risk of potentially fatal complications. The symptoms of DVT include:

- Muscle pain
- Tenderness to touch
- Positive Homans' sign
- Swelling in the affected limb

The clinical diagnosis of thrombophlebitis is sometimes difficult, since some of the symptoms listed may be a result of normal changes experienced with pregnancy and birth. The definitive tool for diagnosis of DVT is venography (the use of radiographic dyes to ascertain venous flow). Other methods used for diagnosis are isotope scanning, impedance plethysmography and Doppler ultrasound (Brown et al 1986).

Treatment of DVT consists of a regimen similar to that for superficial thrombosis (elevation of the affected extremity, warm moist packs, support hose, and analgesics) but also includes the addition of anticoagulant therapy. When symptoms have been relieved, the woman is encouraged to ambulate to facilitate venous flow.

Implications for Nursing Care

Nursing measures similarly follow those used for superficial thrombosis: encouraging bed rest, adequate fluid intake, and support hose and monitoring for symptoms of infection or embolism. Special attention is paid to positioning the patient so that flexion at the femoral junction is prevented. This is achieved by placing the bed in Trendelenburg's position. Measures taken to prevent complications of bed rest include use of a footboard, passive/active exercise, frequent shifts in position, and adequate fluid intake and output. Anticoagulant therapy is the cornerstone of treatment and will be discussed in the section on pulmonary embolism.

Pulmonary Embolism

Pulmonary embolism is the condition in which a clot traveling through the venous system becomes lodged within the pulmonary circulatory system, causing an infarction or occlusion. If the infarction is peripheral, the symptoms observed are pleuritic. A large central embolism causes symptoms that are similar but may lead to cardiac infarction and/or right-sided heart failure. A pulmonary embolism is heralded by the symptom of dyspnea and is followed by:

- Tachypnea
- Pleuritic pain
- Apprehension
- Cough
- Tachycardia
- Hemoptysis
- Temperature ($>37°C$)

When a pulmonary embolism is accompanied by a systemic infection, additional symptoms include:

- Spiking temperatures
- Severe abdominal pain
- Hypotension
- Tachycardia
- Severe chills
- Paleness and cyanosis

Diagnosis of a pulmonary embolis is verified by electrocardiogram, arterial blood gas studies, coagulation studies, CBC, blood cultures, lung scanning, and pulmonary arteriography.

The two primary goals of treatment are anticoagulation and treatment of infection. Anticoagulation therapy is most often provided by heparin and coumarin derivatives. Heparin is the most frequent drug of choice for initial treatment and is followed by the use of coumarin for long-term treatment in a nonlactating mother.

Implications for Nursing Care

Nursing responsibilities include gathering baseline laboratory information before the initiation of therapy. This includes CBC, platelet count, prothrombin time, and partial prothrombin time. An initial loading dose of heparin is given and is followed by a maintenance dose administered by a continuous infusion pump (Table 30–3). Maintenance of the dosage is determined by serial laboratory observation of clotting factors. Patients must be monitored for symptoms of bleeding and allergic reactions. The antidote *protamine sulfate* should be readily available in a dosage of 1 mg per 100 units of heparin. It is important to note that heparin is incompatible with a number of antibiotics.

Intravenous therapy is continued until symptoms have disappeared, usually in 1 to 2 weeks. At this time the woman is shifted to subcutaneous heparin therapy or oral coumarin. Therapy for DVT is continued for up to 6 months. When pulmonary embolism occurs, therapy may last up to 12 months.

INFLAMMATION OR INFECTION OF THE BREAST

Infectious complications involving the breast range from benign inflammations to breast abscesses. During the period of lactation, the breast changes from an essentially nonfunctioning to a complex functioning organ of the body. Because the developing multiductal system necessitates high volume circulation, the breast becomes a rich environment for the growth of bacteria.

Injury to the breast is the primary predisposing factor for infection in the breast. Injury in the lactating breast may be the result of overdistention, stasis, or cracking of the nipples. Injury results in a loss of circulation and a portal to the internal structures. Once pockets form and

NURSING ALERT

Patient Teaching and Anticoagulant Therapy

The nurse must stress the following points in discharge teaching for a patient on anticoagulant therapy. The patient should:

- Take the medication at the same time each day.

- Keep follow-up appointments to allow care providers to monitor clotting time and adjust medication.

- Stop taking other medications unless physician approves.

- Be aware of signs of overdose, such as bloody stools, hematomas, widespread bruising, bleeding gums, bleeding into joints. If symptoms occur, discontinue the drug and call the physician.

- Avoid trauma or injury that might cause bleeding, such as brushing teeth, contact sports, shaving the legs (use an electric razor).

- Avoid marked changes in eating habits or life-style.

- Avoid aspirin and ibuprofin. They inhibit platelet adhesiveness and increase the anticoagulant effect of heparin.

- Understand that stools may change color to pink, red, or black as a result of coagulant use.

- Wear a Medic-Alert bracelet or necklace indicating the anticoagulant drug being used.

Table 30–3   Anticoagulants Commonly Used in Puerperal Thromboembolic Disease

Heparin Sodium	Coumadin Derivatives	
	Warfarin Sodium (Coumadin, Panwarfin)	*Dicumarol*
Dose		
IV, SC: 5,000 to 30,000 U May be ordered as a drip over 24 hours Prophylactic dose: 5000 U SC every 12 hours	IM, IV: 50 mg per vial with diluent Orally: 2.5, 5, 7.5, 10, 25 mg tablets	Initial, oral: 100 mg; second day: 200 mg; subsequent days: as indicated by prothrombin time Maintenance dose: 25 to 100 mg/day orally
Mechanism of Action		
Inhibits conversion of prothrombin to thrombin Decreases agglutination of platelets Prolongs clotting time Has no effect on existing clots but prevents extension of old clots and formation of new ones	Inhibits prothrombin synthesis in liver by interfering with the action of vitamin K Acts more quickly than dicumarol, but effects last for a shorter time	Suppresses activity of liver in formation of prothrombin Prolongs clotting Takes 12 to 14 hr to take effect Action persists 24 to 72 hr after drug is discontinued Slower-acting but more prolonged in effect than heparin Used for maintenance
Therapeutic Uses for Postpartum Patients		
Lowering prothrombin time until slower-acting oral anticoagulants can take effect Prophylaxis and treatment of venous thrombosis and its extension Prophylaxis and treatment of pulmonary emboli	Prophylaxis and treatment of pulmonary thrombosis Prophylaxis and treatment of extension of venous thrombosis	Treatment of thrombophlebitis and pulmonary embolism (especially valuable in treatment of thrombosis and embolism)
Contraindications		
Not to be used in patients sensitive to heparin Not to be used in patients with any uncontrolled bleeding Not to be used in patients who cannot be supervised Incompatible with many antibiotics: check before use No IM injections because of risk of hematoma formation	Not to be used in patients with history of coumadin sensitivity Not to be used in patients with any bleeding conditions Not to be used in patients who cannot be supervised Must be used with caution in patients at risk for occupational injury	Same as warfarin sodium
Nursing Implications		
Monitor patients constantly for bleeding. Coagulation time determinations should be checked frequently (normal prothrombin time is 11–13 sec; levels above this are set for individual patients by physician). Rotate administration sites and check for hemorrhage. Avoid massaging IV site. Observe women for hemorrhage during postpartum period. Breast-feeding may continue; heparin does not appear in breast milk.	Monitor patients constantly for bleeding. Significant decreases in coagulant activity occur in patients taking estrogens, barbiturates, and oral contraceptives. Abdominal or lumbar pain may be due to hemorrhage and thus should be promptly reported. Hemorrhage may be treated with vitamin K or whole blood. Clotting status is monitored by prothrombin time.	Vitamin K should be available as an antidote. Frequent dose adjustments are necessary in first 2 weeks of therapy (drug absorption is variable). Patients on maintenance doses may be checked semiweekly, weekly, or at 2- to 4-week intervals, depending on response to drug.

fill with infectious exudates, circulation within the breast is interrupted, leading to the symptoms of fullness and pain. Because of the high circulatory profile of the breasts, infections must be treated promptly or the infection may spread systemically.

Etiology

The incidence of mastitis has not been reported definitively, but the probable origins of infection may be divided into two categories. *Epidemic* mastitis is derived from a nosocomial or care center source. This infection is commonly associated with the bacterium *Staphylococcus aureus* and localizes in the lactiferous glands and ducts. It occurs among women who have been hospitalized where babies are cared for in a central nursery. The second source is one of *endemic* infection, which occurs randomly and localizes in the periglandular connective tissue. This infection is frequently associated with a break in the integrity of the nipple surface (Lawrence 1984).

Superficial Mastitis

A superficial mastitis is characterized by a localized redness and tenderness to palpation. It is not uncommon that the woman also suffers from symptoms of engorgement, including fullness to the point of dermal tautness and breast/nipple tenderness.

Women must be encouraged to practice personal hygiene measures that will help to protect against mastitis. These measures include:

- Adequate around-the-clock nonconstrictive support of the breasts
- Gentleness during care
- Breast cleanliness and avoidance of irritating cleansing agents
- Avoidance of decrusting the nipple
- Frequent changing of pads
- Intermittent exposure of nipples to the air
- Avoidance of known sources of infection
- Frequent hand washing

The symptoms that herald an infection have a usual onset at 7 to 14 days postpartum and include a low-grade fever and mild pain in a localized segment of the breast that are commonly initiated by breast-feeding.

This type of symptomatology can be treated conservatively. The mother is encouraged to increase her fluid intake to eight to ten 8-ounce glasses per day, mostly of water. Breast-feeding is encouraged at frequent intervals in order to promote milk flow through the breast. Heat packs or hot showers are used to promote circulation to the area, and mild analgesics are used for the relief of pain. The mother is instructed to take her temperature every 4 hours and is reassessed in 24 hours or less, depending on changes in symptoms.

Infectious Mastitis

Symptoms that signify an established mastitis include:

- Rapid rise in temperature up to 104°F (40°C)
- Tachycardia
- Chills
- Reddened, exquisitely tender breast tissue
- Palpable, hard masses in the breast

Diagnosis and treatment are based on the symptomatology. Under circumstances of persistent infection, white cell counts and cultures and sensitivity tests of breast milk are used for a definitive diagnosis of the offending organism.

Treatments of established mastitis include those listed for a superficial mastitis, with the addition of antibiotics. The drug of choice is a penicillinase-resistant penicillin. Antibiotic treatment continues for 10 days. Relief of symptoms often occurs 24 to 48 hours after initiation of treatment. Women must be encouraged to follow through on the complete regimen of therapy.

Breast Abscess

Breast abscess presents a serious threat to the lactating woman. Systemic spread and possible tissue damage may result.

Symptoms include all those previously listed for mastitis as well as the following:

- Discharge of exudates
- Persistent, chilling fevers
- Masses or reddened areas that may develop a bluish hue possibly representing the accumulation of exudates

Treatment of a breast abscess includes the use of antibiotics and incision and drainage of the abscess.

Opinions vary concerning whether the woman with a breast abscess should continue to breast-feed. If the mother is advised to discontinue breast-feeding, support must be given for suppression of lactation. It should be remembered that breast-feeding is frequently an emotionally laden issue, and support may be needed. If breast-feeding is to be resumed following the infection, a woman will need support in the pumping of her breasts (Lawrence 1984).

POSTPARTUM PREECLAMPSIA

Pregnancy-induced hypertension (PIH), including preeclampsia and eclampsia, refers to a clinical spectrum of disease ranging from mild to severe. Preeclampsia rarely occurs before the 20th week of gestation and usually resolves within 48 hours of delivery of the infant. (See Chapter 19 for a discussion of PIH in the antenatal period and Chapter 28 for a discussion of intrapartal care.) Twenty percent of maternal mortality is attributed to hypertensive disease and another 5% to cerebral vascular accident. Preeclampsia/eclampsia contributes to these statistics (Rochat, Koonin et al 1988).

Since delivery does not immediately reverse the pathophysiology of preeclampsia, it is necessary to continue therapy into the postpartum period. Usually this therapy consists of intravenous magnesium sulfate for 24 hours postpartum and is accompanied by monitoring of urinary output, deep tendon reflexes, and blood pressure. The goal of therapy in the postpartum period is to prevent eclamptic seizures and subsequent neurological damage to the mother.

Incidence

It is estimated that as many as one third of patients who experience convulsions as a consequence of PIH will do so in the postpartum period. Of those who convulse in the postpartum period, most will convulse within the first 24 hours; the risk of convulsions is virtually eliminated after 48 hours postpartum.

The patient with preeclampsia during the intrapartum period is at greater risk for postpartum hemorrhage secondary to her disease and to drug therapy (magnesium sulfate may impair uterine contractility following delivery). In addition, these patients have contracted blood volumes, altered liver enzymes, and lowered platelet counts, which contribute to coagulopathy and poor tolerance of blood loss (Sibai and Moretti 1988). Intensive nursing care with absolute attention to detail in the monitoring of physical parameters and in the administration of medications and treatments is required.

Implications for Nursing Care

Magnesium sulfate is generally continued as the drug of choice for the prevention of postpartum seizures. Initiating other forms of drug therapy is undesirable because of the numbers of hours needed to reach therapeutic serum levels and because respiratory or cardiac arrest may occur from overly rapid intravenous infusion of anticonvulsant medications.

Medications are generally started during the intrapartum period and are maintained into the postpartum period. Rarely, the first diagnosis of preeclampsia is made after the delivery. In this case initiation of treatment remains the same, but maintenance of serum magnesium concentration at therapeutic levels with usual dosages is difficult. Serum magnesium levels decrease with increased urinary output, and the usual postpartum diuresis makes it unlikely that therapeutic levels can be maintained. Despite these problems convulsions rarely occur while patients are under treatment. (See Chapter 28 for drug schedules in patient treatment of PIH.)

In addition to the magnesium sulfate infusion, intravenous electrolyte solution is administered slowly. Urinary output is measured with an indwelling Foley catheter in place. The goal is to maintain urinary output at approximately 30 ml/hour. The urine is checked for protein and specific gravity at hourly intervals. Output may be maintained with the use of diuretics.

Blood pressure determinations are made every 15 minutes during the acute phase of treatment and observation. If the blood pressure continues to rise or the diastolic pressure is greater than 110 mm Hg, drug therapy is indicated. Since prompt control is indicated, antihypertensive drugs may be given by continuous infusion (ACOG 1986).

Sustained postpartum treatment usually prevents seizures. When an eclamptic seizure does occur, it is a frightening, life-threatening emergency. When the seizure is recognized, there are certain steps to be followed to ensure safety to the patient:

- Call for assistance
- Prevent maternal injury.
  Place the woman on her side, if possible, to prevent aspiration of vomitus.
- Maintain adequate oxygenation.
  After the convulsion has ceased, check for return of respirations; administer oxygen by mask.
- Administer medications, as ordered, to control seizure and correct acidemia.
  Closely monitor vital signs and level of consciousness.
  Obtain laboratory studies as ordered.

(See Chapter 28 for further discussion of eclampsia and emergency care.)

Treatment and monitoring of these patients requires expert nursing care. Communication with the patient's family regarding her status is important, since the acute nature of this complication is cause for great concern. Astute observation and the reporting of clinical signs that indicate progression of disease are crucial in the prevention of complications.

POSTPARTUM PSYCHOSIS AND MOOD DISORDER

Postpartum psychosis or *puerperal psychosis* is a relatively rare psychiatric disorder that usually occurs in the first 3 months following childbirth. Most commonly the signs of psychosis appear within the first 2 weeks postpartum with symptoms similar to general psychotic reactions. Confusion, fatigue, agitation, feelings of hopelessness and shame, and alterations of mood are prominent. Most importantly, delusions, auditory hallucinations, and hyperactivity with rapid speech or mania may be present. These latter symptoms are hallmarks that differentiate psychotic reactions from postpartum "blues" or a chronic major affective disorder (Inwood 1985). Mood disturbances following childbirth may be conceptualized as a continuum, with postpartum "blues" being self-limiting and more frequent and less severe than chronic affective disorders or postpartum psychosis.

The patient with puerperal psychosis may often exhibit suicidal or homicidal ideation. Since such a patient requires treatment by hospitalization and intervention by child-protective services, astute observation by the nurse in the early postpartum period may provide opportunity for prompt diagnosis and institution of therapy. Prognosis for recovery from postpartum psychosis is good, but the condition may recur following subsequent deliveries.

Incidence

The incidence of puerperal psychosis is approximately 1 per 1000 deliveries. Onset is acute and often occurs abruptly following a symptom-free period. Eighty percent of all cases occur between 3 to 14 days postpartum. Incidence rates for postpartum psychosis have remained unchanged since the 1850s even though diagnostic criteria and recording techniques have varied. This seems to indicate relatively stable rates for the complication over the past 130 years. Risk factors to consider are

- Previous history of puerperal psychosis
- History of manic-depressive disorder
- Delirium, hallucinations
- Rapid mood change, agitation or confusion
- Potential for both suicide and infanticide

Management includes hospitalization, neuroleptic drugs, social support, and psychotherapy (Spitzer 1980).

Moderate depression, or postpartum major affective disorder, is more variable in time of onset but usually presents within 2 weeks to 3 months postpartum. The incidence may range from 30 to 200 per 1000 deliveries. Symptoms include

- Depression
- Ambivalence about the pregnancy
- Feelings of inadequacy
- Marital discord
- Guilt and irritability

Suicide is potentially possible, but to a lesser degree than in the patient with postpartum psychosis. Medication, psychotherapy, and social support are necessary to promote recovery. The prognosis for these patients depends upon the severity of the depression, the patient's prior history, and the patient's support system.

The third and most common form of postpartum mood disorder, the baby "blues," occurs in approximately 50% to 80% of gravidas. Spontaneous remission of symptoms follows supportive actions from family and health care providers. (This common problem of the postpartum is discussed in more detail in Chapters 29 and 36.)

The skill of the practitioner is crucial in differentiating normal transitory "blues" from more serious mood disorders, initiating appropriate follow-up, and preventing serious complications.

Principles of treatment of psychiatric disease in the postpartum period (Inwood 1985) include the following:

- Liberal use of hospitalization
- Explanation to the patient of all procedures to be performed
- Mobilization of social support systems for child care
- Anxiety reduction by exploration of fantasies and by reassurance

---

Factors Postulated to Explain Postpartum Psychosis

Hormonal Factors

- Progesterone level declines from 140 ng/ml during pregnancy to 2 ng/ml by postpartum day 10
- Estrogen level drops from 2100 ng/ml during pregnancy to 10 ng/ml by postpartum day 9
- Corticosteroids are elevated in pregnancy and fall during the early postpartum period
- Elevation of prolactin level early in postpartum period

Biological Factors

- Previous history of menstrual cycle distress
- Sleep disorder
- Consanguineous relative with psychiatric disorder
- Labor complications
- Maternal role conflicts

Psychoanalytic Factors

- Unresolved Oedipal conflicts
- Narcissistic personality
- Frustration of oral and dependency needs
- Disturbance of ego control

Psychological Factors

- Poor relationship with own mother
- Inadequate housing
- Reduced social support networks
- Poor marital relationship
- Sexual identity conflict

Affonso DD, Domino G: Postpartum depression: A review. Birth 11(4):231–235, 1984

Etiology

Theories shown in the accompanying display (page 912) have been proposed to account for the occurrence of postpartum psychosis (Affonso and Domino 1984).

Postpartum psychiatric illness is presently categorized under the diagnostic category with which the presenting symptoms are consistent. Controversy exists as to whether it is appropriate to have a separate category in the *Diagnostic and Statistical Manual of Mental Disorders (DSM-III)* for women with postpartum illness.

Implications for Nursing Care

Postpartum women may suffer from grades of mood dysphoria following childbirth. This implies that astute observation and differentiation of symptoms are key to the success of treatment and subsequent outcome. Early nursing care observations are valuable in the assessment of the new mother's general mood. It has been suggested that inquiries regarding the new mother's state of mind be made by asking questions regarding the infant's behavior if direct inquires are ineffective. Often women who are feeling acutely distressed will answer by stating that the infant is very fussy, not easily consolable, or irritable. These statements may be viewed as clues needing further exploration. The new mother may be remarkably sensitive to the words and actions of all those involved in her treatment. Communication of abnormal or worrisome findings should be made to the health care provider. Once discharge from the hospital has occurred, symptoms may go unrecognized or unreported unless they become extreme enough for the family to communicate them to the provider. Most women are not reevaluated by their health care provider until the 6-week postpartum visit. For these reasons, nursing care must include:

- Recognition of predisposing factors
- Observation of clues in behavior that may indicate need for intervention
- Prompt report of symptoms to patient's health care provider

Postpartum or puerperal psychosis is a rare but dramatic event that responds well to early appropriate intervention. Hospitalization of the mother is often necessary because of the risk of suicide and infanticide. Medications used in psychiatric treatment have some associated risks for the breast-feeding woman. Cooperation of the health care team and the patient's family are crucial to the treatment of the woman.

Patients with postpartum psychosis are different from other psychiatric patients. The new mother is faced with the responsibility of caring for her infant, and she is not able to fulfill that function. She is experiencing extremely uncomfortable symptoms of insomnia, exhaustion, con-fusion, frightening hallucinations, and depression. In her mind there is no explanation for the sudden onset of illness. These women tend to view themselves as inadequate mothers, abnormal women who cannot perform a normal female function. This cluster of symptoms demands the skill and effort of a coordinated, knowledgeable health care team.

A family conference held by the psychiatrist begins the process of therapeutic management. The development of symptoms and the severity and direction of illness are assessed. The hazards, nature, and prognosis of the illness are discussed with the family. The family is informed of the responsibilities it will be called upon to assume. Decisions regarding hospitalization of the mother are made at this time. All efforts should be made to communicate with the family in a way that encourages maximal awareness and cooperation. An in-depth interview of the mother is done by the psychiatrist to ascertain the severity of illness, particularly the patient's attitude toward the baby. Responsibility of the nursing staff includes formulation of a comprehensive nursing care plan that stresses the following:

- Continuity of care
- Specifically outlined therapeutic goals
- Open communication with the patient's physician, midwife, psychiatrist
- Coordination of social services
- Family participation and involvement in the care plan

Medications may be administered to rapidly relieve symptoms, make the patient more comfortable, and to promote sleep at night. If the patient is highly agitated or violent, more specific drugs may be used. Neuroleptic medications (Thorazine, Prolixin, Mellaril, Haldol) are employed for initial management of hallucinations. Breast-feeding while taking these medications is appropriate if prolonged, frequent contact with the infant is deemed therapeutic or safe. When a bipolar or manic component to the illness is present, lithium is the drug of choice. Patients taking lithium may be discouraged from breast-feeding. Lithium is excreted into breast milk at about 40% of maternal serum concentration. Although no toxic effects have been reported, long-term studies have not been done. Tricyclic antidepressants have not been well studied in breast-feeding women. Minute quantities are found in the milk of mothers taking these drugs, but the amount seems insufficient to affect the infant. Close monitoring and caution are warranted when these drugs are used during lactation. Appropriate nursing care includes suppression of lactation if indicated, maintenance of the medication schedule, and observation of mother and baby for signs of toxicity.

When the acute episode of the illness has been treated,

follow-up visits at progressively lengthened intervals are scheduled. The final visit is generally at about 6 months postpartum. As the patient recovers, she and her family should be informed of the hazard of recurrence of postpartum psychosis with subsequent pregnancy, the risk of recurrence after one episode of postpartum psychosis being approximately 1 in 3 or 4 (Spitzer 1980).

CHAPTER SUMMARY

Nursing care takes on additional importance in the immediate postpartum period. Postpartum complications are disruptive to the patient's mental and physical well-being as well as to the integration of the new infant into the family. When the nurse can identify early signs of possible illness in the postpartum woman and intervene to affect early resolution of the problem, she will help the family unit both economically and emotionally.

STUDY QUESTIONS

1. What are some factors that predispose women to puerperal infection?
2. What are some of the most common organisms responsible for puerperal infection?
3. As a nurse, how can you help detect infection before it becomes acute?
4. Discuss factors that may predispose postpartum women to hemorrhage.
5. Why are postpartum women so prone to thrombophlebitis? What complications can develop?
6. The breast-feeding mother with postpartum complications presents special challenges to nursing care. What are these challenges and how can the nurse intervene to ensure that lactation and breast-feeding are uninterrupted?
7. Mrs. M. developed symptoms of a urinary tract infection soon after delivery. Her symptoms resolved with treatment and she is being discharged. What counseling would you give Mrs. M.?
8. Two days after delivery you find a new mother in the bathroom sobbing with a towel over her face to muffle the sound. What would you do?

REFERENCES/BIBLIOGRAPHY

A.C.O.G: Management of preeclampsia. ACOG Technical Bulletin, No. 91. Washington, DC, The American College of Obstetricians and Gynecologists, 1986

Affonso DD, Domino G: Postpartum depression: A review. Birth 11(4):231–235, 1984

Brown CE et al: Puerperal pelvic thrombophlebitis: Impact on diagnosis and treatment using x-ray computed tomography and magnetic resonance imaging. Obstet Gynecol 68(6):789–794, 1986

Buehler JW, Kaunitz AM, Hogue JR, Hughes JM, et al: Maternal mortality in women aged 35 years or older: United States. JAMA 255(1):53–57, 1986

Clark SL, Yeh S, Phelan JP, Bruce S et al: Emergency hysterectomy for obstetric hemorrhage. Obstet Gynecol Surv 40(2):82–83, 1985

Creasy RK, Resnik R (eds): Maternal–Fetal Medicine, 2nd ed. Philadelphia, WB Saunders, 1988

Dinsmoor MJ, Gibbs R: The role of the newer antimicrobial agents in obstetrics and gynecology. Clin Obstet Gynecol 31(2):423–434, 1988

Gilbert L, Porter W, Brown VA: Postpartum hemorrhage—A continuing problem. Obstet Gynecol Surv 42(2):509–510, 1987

Herbert WNP, Cefalo RC: Management of postpartum hemorrhage. Clin Obstet Gynecol 27(1):139–147, 1984

Inwood DG: Recent advances in postpartum psychiatric disorders. In Inwood DG (ed): Clinical Insights. Washington, DC, American Psychiatric Press, 1985

Lawrence R: Breastfeeding: A Guide for the Medical Profession, 2nd ed. St. Louis, CV Mosby, 1984

Rochat RW, Koonin LM, Atrash HK, Jewett JF, The Maternal Mortality Collaborative: Maternal mortality in the United States: Report from the Maternal Mortality Collaborative. Obstet Gynecol 72(1):91–97, 1988

Shy K, Eschenback D: Fatal perineal cellulitis from an episiotomy site. Obstet Gynecol 54(3):292, 1979

Sibai BM, Moretti MM: PIH: Still common and still dangerous. Contemp OB/GYN February: 57–70, 1988

Spitzer RL: Diagnostic and Statistical Manual of Mental Disorders, 3rd ed. Washington DC, American Psychiatric Association, 1980

Stamm WE: Dysuria: Establishing a diagnostic protocol. Contemp OB GYN 32(4):81–93, 1988

Sweet R, Gibbs R: Infectious Diseases of the Female Genital Tract. Baltimore, Williams & Wilkins, 1987

SUGGESTED READINGS

Balkam J: Guidelines for drug therapy during lactation. J Obstet Gynecol Neonatal Nurs 15(1):65–70, 1986

Hans A: Postpartum assessment: The psychological component. J Obstet Gynecol Neonatal Nurs 15(1):49–52, 1986

Inturrissi M, Camenga C, Rosen M: Epidural morphine for relief of postpartum post-surgical pain. J Obstet Gynecol Neonatal Nurs 17(4):238–246, 1988

Shannon D: HELLP syndrome: A severe consequence of pregnancy-induced hypertension. J Obstet Gynecol Neonatal Nurs 16(6):395–404, 1987

31

assessment of the neonate

LEARNING OBJECTIVES

After studying the material in this chapter, the student should be able to

- Describe the major physiologic adaptations required of the neonate in the first 24 hours of life

- Describe the major behavioral adaptations required of the neonate in the first 24 hours of life

- Outline essential steps in the process of newborn assessment

- Describe normal physical and behavioral findings in the newborn

- Explain the purpose of a gestational age assessment and describe the components of this assessment

KEY TERMS

Alveolar surface tension

Ductus arteriosus

Foramen ovale

Functional residual capacity

Lung compliance

Meconium

Neck webbing

Neonate

Reflex

Viscosity of lung fluid

Before the neonatal period is safely concluded at the 28th day of life, major physiologic and behavioral adaptations must be made. The extrauterine adjustments made during the first 24 hours are particularly critical to the newborn's chances for survival.

This chapter discusses the major physiologic and behavioral adaptations the neonate must undergo after birth. Normal newborn characteristics and common variations in physical appearance and behavior are also described. Essential aspects of the nursing assessment of the newborn are delineated to assist the beginning practitioner.

NEONATAL ADAPTATION TO EXTRAUTERINE LIFE

The nurse is in a unique position to aid the newborn in the stressful transition from a warm, dark, fluid-filled environment to an outside world filled with light, sound, and novel tactile stimuli.

Depending upon the type of birthing facility the parents choose, a certified nurse midwife or delivery room nurse may actually present the parents with their new family member. The nurse performs an initial assessment to evaluate the neonate, its immediate postbirth adaptations, and the need for further support. Later, a pediatric or neonatal nurse practitioner or nursery nurse will conduct a comprehensive assessment to determine the infant's status and to identify internal and external stressors that might jeopardize successful adaptation.

Physiologic Adaptations
Preparation for Birth

The major adaptation to extrauterine life required of the neonate is the ability to breathe. This ability depends upon a variety of factors related to fetal growth and development. In preparation for the tremendous demands placed upon its respiratory system at the moment of birth, the fetus normally begins breathing movements *in utero*. To facilitate full expansion of alveoli with air when the first breath is taken, fetal alveoli are filled with fetal lung fluid, which stretches the tissues and improves lung compliance. Fetal lungs must also have reached maturity. At birth, Type II alveolar cells must be present for the production of surfactant, a complex of phospholipids that reduces surface tension in the alveoli and prevents their collapse on expiration. The pulmonary vascular bed must be developed and in proximity to lung tissue for gas exchange to occur. Lastly, the newborn must possess an intact central nervous system to initiate and coordinate respiratory efforts.

Initiation of Respiration

Many stimuli during labor and delivery contribute to the initiation of respiration in the newborn. Four major categories of stimuli have been identified. Figure 31–1 illustrates how these stimuli interact to influence the onset of respiration.

Chemical Stimuli.   The fetus experiences a transient asphyxia as a result of interruptions in placental blood flow during uterine contractions and with compression and severing of the umbilical cord at birth. Chemoreceptors in the carotid artery and aorta are stimulated by the lowered arterial oxygen tension (P_aO_2), the elevated arterial carbon dioxide tension (P_aCO_2), and the decrease in arterial pH. Impulses triggered by these chemoreceptors stimulate the respiratory center in the medulla.

Sensory Stimuli.   The newborn is bombarded with a variety of new stimuli during labor and delivery. Even when the tactile, visual, auditory, and olfactory stimuli are reduced, as in gentle birthing environments, their combined effects still contribute to the initiation of respiration.

Thermal Stimuli.   Cold appears to be a powerful stimulus to the initiation of breathing in the newborn. When the infant's wet body is delivered, evaporation causes an immediate drop in the skin temperature. Thermal receptors, particularly on the face and chest, relay impulses to the medulla, triggering the first breath. Profound cooling can cause a drop in the core temperature and lead to respiratory depression.

Mechanical Stimuli.   During the passage through the birth canal, approximately 30% of the fetal lung fluid filling the airways and alveoli is squeezed out. It is estimated that up to 30 ml of tracheal fluid is expelled through the oropharynx before birth. As the chest is delivered, recoil of the chest wall occurs, drawing air into the partially cleared passages. Infants born by cesarean delivery do not experience this compression of the thorax and may suffer from transient respiratory distress due to retained fetal lung fluid.

Factors Opposing the First Breath

Several factors oppose the newborn's efforts to take the first breath, including *alveolar surface tension, lung fluid viscosity,* and *lung compliance.* The diaphragm must descend forcefully to create a negative intrathoracic pressure powerful enough to overcome these forces (40–80 cm H_2O pressure). Air then rushes in, expanding the alveoli, reducing surface tension, and forcing the remain-

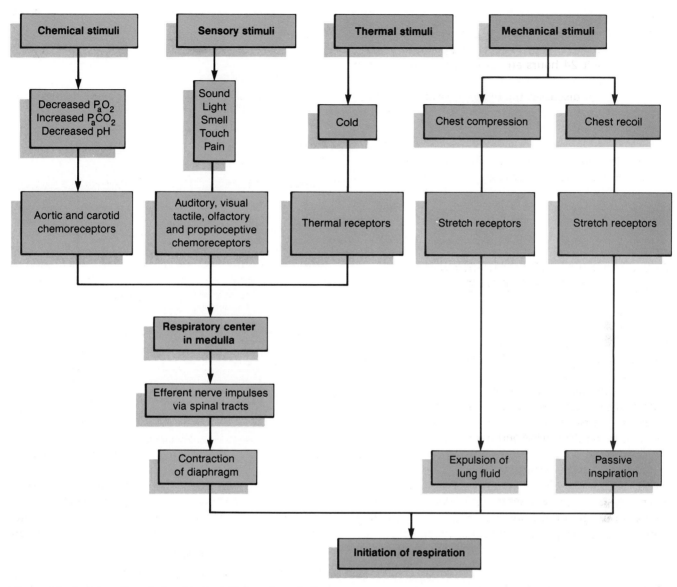

Figure 31–1. Interaction of stimuli in the initiation of respiration.

ing lung fluid out through the pulmonary capillaries and lymphatic system. A functional residual capacity is established so that alveolar sacs remain partially expanded on expiration. Thus, subsequent breaths require less effort and lower pressure (6–8 cm H_2O). Figure 31–2 illustrates the effects of the first breath on pulmonary circulation and gas exchange in the lungs.

The pulmonary vascular bed, which was constricted during fetal life, must now dilate to allow adequate perfusion of lung tissue and effective gas exchange. With the first breath, the rise in alveolar oxygen tension (PaO_2), decrease in arterial pH, and an increase in the level of blood bradykinin, a vasoactive peptide protein, results in dilatation of the pulmonary arteries, decreasing pulmonary vascular resistance. This increased pulmonary perfusion facilitates oxygen and carbon dioxide exchange.

Persistent hypoxemia and acidosis lead to constriction of the pulmonary arteries; this decreases pulmonary perfusion and can reverse those critical pulmonary adaptations in the newborn, resulting in respiratory distress. Figure 31–3 illustrates the changes in pulmonary vascular resistance following initiation of respiration and the resulting cardiovascular adaptations. Table 31–1 illustrates changes in blood gas and pH values during the first hour of life.

Pulmonary artery pressure normally decreases to approximately 50% of systemic arterial pressure within 24 hours of birth. Persistent elevation in pulmonary artery pressure may occur in infants born with an abnormal thickening of the medial muscle layer of pulmonary arterioles. Chronic intrauterine hypoxemia has been implicated in hypertrophy of pulmonary artery musculature.

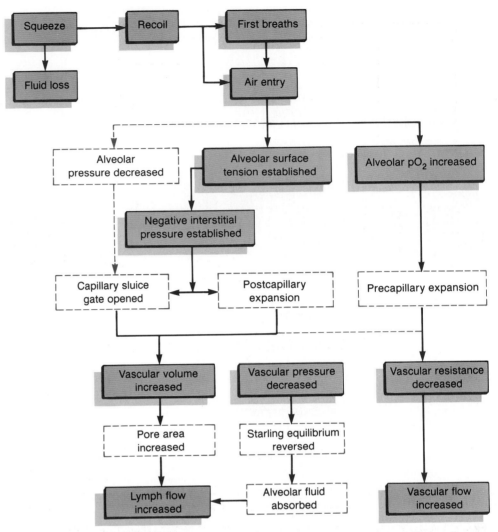

Figure 31–2. Effect of first breath on pulmonary circulation and gas exchange. Broken lines indicate hypothesized mechanisms involved in the transition to extrauterine pulmonary function. (Smith C, Nelson N: The Physiology of the Newborn Infant, 4th ed. Springfield, IL, Charles C Thomas, 1976)

Cardiovascular Adaptations

With clamping of the umbilical cord and initiation of the first breath, dramatic changes occur in the cardiovascular system of the neonate.

Closure of the Foramen Ovale. As the pulmonary arteries dilate in response to oxygenation of lung tissue, pulmonary vascular resistance decreases and pressure drops in the right side of the heart. Simultaneously, pressure rises in the left side of the heart. This leads to functional closure of the foramen ovale within several hours of birth. Permanent closure of this bypass is not accomplished for several months. Right-to-left shunting of blood may occur until that time, and this accounts for the nonpathologic murmurs heard in some neonates.

Closure of the Ductus Arteriosus. The *ductus arteriosus* is sensitive to changes in arterial oxygen tension. As blood oxygen tension (P_aO_2) levels rise with the first breath, the ductus arteriosus constricts. Functional closure usually occurs within 15 hours of birth, and permanent closure is accomplished by 3 weeks. Hypoxemia leads to continued patency of the ductus and shunting of blood through this fetal circulatory bypass.

The clamping of the umbilical cord results in closure of the *ductus venosus*. Fibrosis of this fetal circulatory bypass occurs within a week.

Systemic blood pressure rises with the clamping of the umbilical cord because elimination of the large placental vascular bed results in increased systemic resistance. Concomitantly, the severing of the placental circulation

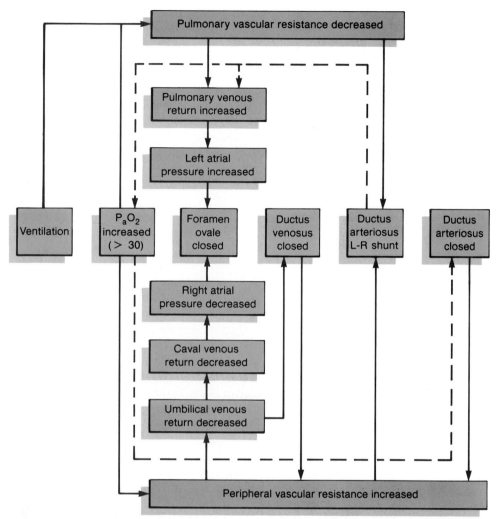

Figure 31–3. Alterations in pulmonary vascular resistance and neonatal circulation following initiation of respiration. Broken lines indicate hypothesized mechanisms involved in alterations in pulmonary vascular resistance. (Smith C, Nelson N: The Physiology of the Newborn Infant, 4th ed. Springfield, IL, Charles C Thomas, 1976)

Table 31–1   **Oxygen Tension, Carbon Dioxide Tension, pH and Base Excess Values in Cord Blood and Arterial Blood During the First 24 Hours of Life**

	Birth		5–10 Minutes	30 Minutes	60 Minutes	24 Hours
	Umbilical Vein	*Umbilical Artery*				
PaO_2 (mm Hg)	27.5	16	50	54	63	73
$PaCO_2$ (mm Hg)	39	49	46	38	36	33
*p*H	7.32	7.24	7.20	7.29	7.33	7.36
Base excess	−5.5	−7.2	−9.8	−7.8	−6.5	−5.2

and the consequent decreased blood return via the inferior vena cava contribute to a lowered venous blood pressure.

Hepatic Adaptations

Normal development of liver tissue and the biliary ducts is essential for hepatic function at birth. Although the neonatal liver is immature, it is capable of performing vital functions, including bilirubin conjugation, production of coagulation factors, iron storage, and carbohydrate metabolism.

Bilirubin Conjugation

Indirect (fat-soluble) bilirubin is a breakdown product of red blood cell lysis. It is converted by a liver enzyme, *glucuronyl transferase,* into a water-soluble form *(direct bilirubin)* that can be excreted in urine and stool. In the newborn, because the liver is immature, the ability to conjugate (convert) indirect bilirubin is limited. This, coupled with the high red blood cell count in the newborn and the increased hemolysis resulting from the shorter lifespan of fetal red blood cells, accounts for the frequent appearance of jaundice between 48 and 72 hours after birth.

Indirect bilirubin, because it is fat-soluble, has an affinity for certain types of body tissue. Accumulation of indirect bilirubin in subcutaneous tissue gives the familiar jaundiced appearance. A more serious consequence of high levels of indirect bilirubin can be accumulation in brain tissue, a condition called *kernicterus.* This condition can cause permanent brain damage and retardation; for this reason, the newborn's bilirubin levels are monitored closely. If necessary, steps are taken to facilitate the conversion of indirect bilirubin to direct bilirubin, which can

then be excreted by the kidneys. (See Chapter 32 for preventive nursing interventions and Chapter 34 for treatment modalities for hyperbilirubinemia.)

Physiologic jaundice is observed in approximately 50% of full-term newborns. Serum levels of bilirubin may range from 4 mg/dl to 12 mg/dl at 3 days; the average peak serum level is 6 mg/dl followed by a rapid decline to 3 mg/dl by the fifth day of life (Fig. 31–4). Physiologic jaundice is differentiated from pathologic jaundice by the time at which the jaundice appears. *Pathologic* or *nonphysiologic jaundice* occurs within the first 24 hours of life and can be caused by a variety of problems, including blood incompatibilities, inherited metabolic disorders, and severe birth asphyxia. *Physiologic jaundice* occurs after the first 24 hours of life and usually resolves with hydration and frequent feedings, which promote elimination of direct bilirubin.

Breast milk jaundice occurs around the third or fourth day of life when the mother begins producing greater amounts of breast milk. Although the etiology is unknown, several factors have been implicated in the development of breast milk jaundice. Pregnanediol, an enzyme that interferes with the release of conjugated bilirubin from neonatal liver cells, has been suggested as a possible contributing factor. More recent research has also implicated the presence of elevated lipase levels in the breast milk of mothers of infants exhibiting breast milk jaundice. Increased lipase activity may result in high levels of free fatty acids, which may inhibit bilirubin conjugation in the newborn. Dangerous elevations in serum bilirubin rarely occur, but when levels do exceed 16 mg/dl, breastfeeding is usually stopped for several days. The mother is instructed in the manual expression or hand pumping of breast milk so that her milk supply does not diminish. Nursing can usually be resumed when the bilirubin level

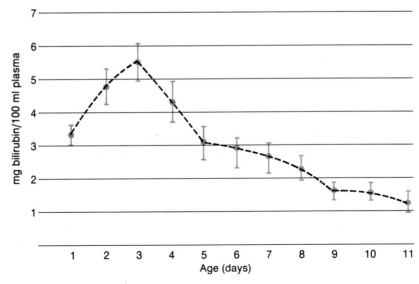

Figure 31–4. Average serum unconjugated bilirubin levels in full-term neonates. (McMillan J, Stockman J, Oski F: The Whole Pediatrician Catalog. Philadelphia, WB Saunders, 1982)

falls to within normal limits. An alternative therapy to the total cessation of breast-feeding that promotes maternal efforts to nurse her infant is to alternate breast milk with formula until bilirubin levels decrease.

Production of Blood Coagulation Factors

Coagulation factors are essential elements in the process of hemostasis. Maternal coagulation factors do not cross the placenta. Furthermore the infant's liver is immature at birth. Therefore, newborn infants suffer a temporary deficit in coagulation factors that are synthesized in the liver, and they have prolonged blood coagulation time. Four of the factors (II, VII, IX, and X) are activated under the influence of vitamin K produced by bacteria in the gut (Fig. 31–5). However, since the gastrointestinal tract is sterile until birth and normal intestinal flora is not established until the neonate begins to ingest milk, vitamin K levels remain low for several days. The newborn is therefore at special risk between the second and fifth days of life for a bleeding disorder referred to as *hemolytic disease of the newborn*. For this reason, vitamin K is usually given prophylactically to protect the newborn.

Iron Storage

The neonate is born with iron stores accumulated during fetal life. If the mother's iron intake was adequate, the infant will have sufficient iron to produce red blood cells until about 5 months of age. As fetal red blood cells are lysed after birth, iron is recycled and stored in the liver until needed for new red blood cell production.

Carbohydrate Metabolism

Gluconeogenesis occurs in neonatal hepatic cells immediately after birth, although less efficiently than in adults. The newborn stores glucose in the liver as glycogen. Glucose is the major energy source in the first hours after birth before feedings begin. The brain is an obligate glucose utilizer as are peripheral nerves, red and white blood cells, and the medulla of the kidney. As blood glucose levels drop, glycogenolysis occurs and glucose is released into the newborn's bloodstream in order to maintain a blood glucose level of approximately 60 mg/dl. Glycogen stores can be rapidly depleted in the presence of stressors such as birth asphyxia or hypothermia (Fig. 31–6). Ninety percent of hepatic glycogen stores may be consumed by the third to fourth hour of life.

Insulin, glucagon, and growth hormone, the three major hormones involved in glucose homeostasis, are present at birth. Normal serum insulin levels in fasting newborns range from 6 to 24 microunits/ml. Neonatal insulin secretion is sluggish during the first two weeks of life owing to immaturity of the endocrine system; thus, effective glucose utilization is limited.

Gastrointestinal Adaptations

To undergo the normal rapid growth and development, the newborn must ingest, digest, and absorb sufficient nutrients. The gastrointestinal tract, although both structurally and functionally immature, is capable of digesting and absorbing breast milk and modified cow's milk and

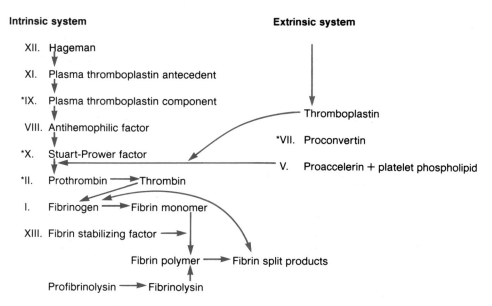

* Clotting factors activated under the influence of Vitamin K in neonatal intestine.

Figure 31–5. The normal system of clot promotion, stabilization, and lysis in the neonate. Asterisks indicate clotting factors activated under the influence of vitamin K in neonatal intestine. (Gross S: Hematologic problems. In Klaus M, Fanaroff A [eds.]: Care of the High-Risk Neonate. Philadelphia, WB Saunders, 1979)

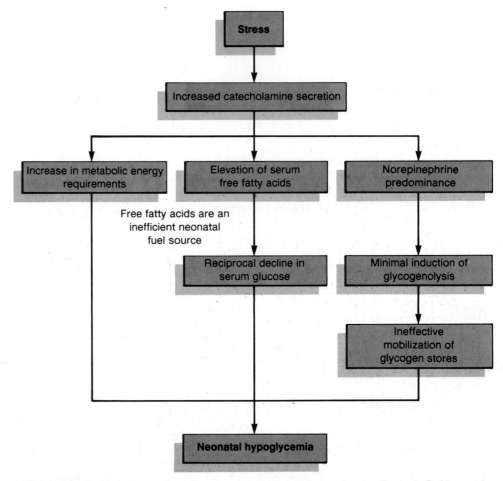

Figure 31–6. The effects of stress on neonatal serum glucose levels. (Fantazia D: Neonatal hypoglycemia. JOGN 13:298, 1984)

eliminating waste products. The mouth is shaped to facilitate breast-feeding. Ridges and corrugations on the hard palate, strong sucking muscles in the mouth and jaw, and fat-pads in the cheeks assist the newborn to grasp the nipple and compress the areola of the breast during nursing. Tastebuds located primarily on the tip of the tongue can distinguish between sweet and sour. Salivary glands are immature and saliva production is scant.

Gastric capacity is limited in the first day of life to approximately 40 to 60 ml. Because the stomach is distensible, capacity increases when feedings are introduced. It reaches 90 ml in many infants by 3 to 4 days of age. *Pepsinogen* is present and begins the digestion of milk when it enters the stomach. Stomach emptying time is approximately 2 to 4 hours. The *cardiac sphincter* is immature, and slight regurgitation of milk after feedings is common in the newborn.

The newborn's intestinal tract is proportionately longer than that of an adult and has a large absorption surface. Enzymes essential for protein digestion are present in the newborn. Fats are digested and absorbed

less effectively because there are inadequate amounts of *pancreatic lipase*. The fats in breast milk are more easily digested than those in cow's milk because of their composition and because breast milk contains lipase.

The content of the fetal bowel is called *meconium*. Most newborns (94%) pass the first meconium stool within 24 hours of birth. Meconium is an odorless, thick, dark-green substance composed of bile, fetal epithelial cells and hair, and amniotic fluid. Once feedings are introduced, the consistency, color, and odor of the stools change. *Transitional stools,* which are observed after 2 to 3 days of milk ingestion, are greenish brown in color and less viscous than meconium. By the fourth day of life, breast-fed infants pass a sweet-smelling, golden-yellow, loose stool, while formula-fed infants produce stools that are pungent, pale yellow, and pasty. Bowel movement patterns vary among infants, with breast-fed babies often passing stools more frequently. Once the infant establishes a regular feeding schedule, bowel movements may range from one stool every 2 to 3 days to as many as ten stools a day.

Renal Adaptations

Although urine is produced and excreted into the amniotic fluid by the fetus from the fourth month of gestation, the kidney is still immature at birth. Nephrons continue to develop in the first years of life and *glomerular filtration* rate is low in the neonate. The tubules are short and narrow, which limits the effectiveness of tubular reabsorption and urine concentration mechanisms. Amino acids and bicarbonate may be lost in the urine. The newborn is extremely susceptible to dehydration, acidosis, and electrolyte imbalance if normal fluid intake is restricted or vomiting or diarrhea occur.

Most newborns (92%) void within 24 hours after birth. The first voiding may be dark amber and cloudy owing to the mucus and urate content. *Uric acid crystals* excreted in the urine leave peach-colored crystals or "brick-dust" stains in the diaper, a sign with no clinical significance. The urine will become clear, straw-colored, and less concentrated with increased fluid intake. Urine output may be scanty during the first few days of life as the newborn adjusts to feedings. The volume of urine output in the full-term neonate ranges from 15 to 60 ml/24 hours, depending upon fluid intake and the solute load of feedings. Frequency increases from two to six voidings the first day to up to 20 voidings per day once the infant's intake improves.

A *weight loss* of between 5% and 15% of birth weight may occur in the newborn during the first 4 to 5 days. This weight loss results from continued voidings and stool passage, limited intake, insensible water loss, and a high metabolic rate. Weight loss should stabilize by about the fifth day and a weight gain of approximately 1 oz (30 g) per day will occur with adequate fluid and caloric intake.

Neurologic Adaptations

Although the sophisticated physiologic functioning and behavioral capabilities of the neonate are evidence of an intact neurologic system, the system is immature at birth. The brain is only 25% of its adult size and myelinization of nerve fibers is incomplete. The newborn exhibits many primitive reflexes (see Table 31–6) that later disappear as the nervous system develops. Transient tremors, frequent startles, and incoordinate motor activity can also be observed. Although the nervous system is immature, it is sufficiently integrated to support neonatal adaptations at birth. The autonomic nervous system and brain stem coordinate vital respiratory and cardiac functions, and sensory capabilities are well developed. Protective, feeding, and social reflexes are present and provide the neonate with a repertoire of behaviors that greatly improve chances of survival. Growth occurs in a cephalocaudal, proximal-distal fashion. Gross motor skills are mastered before those requiring fine motor coordination.

NURSING RESEARCH

Neonatal Pain Perception and Adaptation

Until relatively recently many health care professionals did not believe that neonates could feel pain (or perceive pain to the same degree as adults). This was based upon the false assumption that pain impulses could not be carried by unmyelinated nerve fibers. It is now recognized that pain impulses may be transmitted by unmyelinated c-polymodal fibers, although at a slower rate.

Nurse researchers have begun to explore the pain behaviors and responses of infants. Alterations in respiratory rate, systolic blood pressure, and blood oxygenation have been observed in infants exposed to activities that are considered painful, such as circumcision and heel sticks.

It is suggested that physiologic changes in response to painful procedures may adversely affect adaptive processes in the neonate and place the already compromised infant at greater risk. Further research is required; however, current findings have begun to alter practice, and clinicians are attempting to ameliorate and limit painful experiences for the neonate through both pharmacologic and nonpharmacologic interventions.

Brown L: Physiologic responses to cutaneous pain in neonates. Neonatal Network 6(3):18–22, 1987

Endocrine and Metabolic Adaptations

The endocrine system coordinates the newborn's adjustments to extrauterine life. Hormones synthesized and released by endocrine glands support major metabolic functions and mediate responses to internal and external stressors. Endocrine activity is linked with the nervous system in a complex arrangement of feedback loops. Three major neuroendocrine pathways supporting neonatal adaptations are the hypothalamic–anterior pituitary axis, the hypothalamic–posterior pituitary axis, and the parasympathetic–adrenal medulla path. Major neurohormonal systems are intact at birth, and hormones essential for neonatal adaptations, including growth hormone, thyroid-stimulating hormone (TSH), adrenocorticotropic hormone (ACTH), cortisol, and catecholamines, are secreted.

Thermoregulation

Thermoregulation, the ability of the neonate to produce heat and maintain a normal body temperature, is a vital metabolic function mediated by the neuroendocrine system. Neonates are especially susceptible to heat loss

Table 31–2 **Environmental Factors Contributing to Neonatal Heat Loss**

Major Mechanisms	Environmental Factors
Evaporation Loss of heat when water on the infant's skin is converted to a vapor	Wet blankets or diapers in contact with skin Water or urine on skin
Convection Transfer of heat when a flow of cool air passes over the infant's skin	Drafts from open windows Drafts from open portholes on isolette Drafts from air-conditioning ducts Flow of unheated oxygen over face
Conduction Transfer of heat when the infant comes in direct contact with cooler surfaces and objects	Cold mattresses, cold sidewalls in crib or isolette Cold blankets, shirts, diapers Cold hands of care-giver Cold weight scale Cold stethoscope
Radiation Transfer of heat from the infant to cooler surfaces and objects not in direct contact with the infant	Cold sidewalls of crib or isolette Cold outside building walls and windows Cold equipment in infant's environment

because of a combination of unique anatomical features and environmental factors surrounding birth.

Factors Contributing to Heat Loss. Neonates are prone to heat loss because they have a large surface area in relation to their weight. In addition, because they have less adipose tissue for insulation, thinner skin, and blood vessels in closer proximity to the skin surface, newborns experience a greater transfer of heat to the external environment. The newborn's skin is wet at birth, and the ambient temperature at birth is much cooler than that of the intrauterine environment. The low humidity and fast air currents found in many delivery rooms as a result of air conditioning systems also increase heat loss. Table 31–2 describes the four major mechanisms of heat loss and heat transfer to which the newborn is susceptible and environmental factors contributing to hypothermia.

Neonatal Responses to Hypothermia. The infant responds to cold stress in a variety of ways (Fig. 31–7). Heat loss is decreased by vasoconstriction of vessels. Heat production occurs through an increase in metabolic rate and muscular activity. Shivering, a major mechanism of heat production in adults, is rarely seen in newborns. *Nonshivering thermogenesis* is the primary method of heat production in neonates.

When skin temperature begins to drop, thermal receptors transmit impulses to the central nervous system. The sympathetic nervous system is stimulated and norepinephrine is released by the adrenal gland and at nerve endings located in a special type of adipose tissue known as brown fat. *Brown fat* is very dense, highly vascular adipose tissue that is metabolized to produce heat. Found only in infants, brown fat is located in the intrascapular area, the neck, thorax, and axilla, and around the kidneys and adrenal glands.

Although nonshivering thermogenesis and an increased metabolic rate are effective means of heat production in the newborn, they result in increased demands for oxygen and glucose. Healthy full-term infants will have no difficulty in meeting these demands initially by increasing the respiratory rate and releasing liver stores of glucose. With prolonged cold stress or in compromised neonates, brown fat sources and glucose stores may be depleted, which can result in decreased surfactant production and increased pulmonary vascular resistance. These infants must then rely on external sources of heat to maintain their body temperatures.

Neonatal Responses to Hyperthermia. The newborn infant will respond to an elevation in temperature by dilating blood vessels to dissipate heat. Although sweat glands are less active than in an adult, a full-term infant will also sweat and lose heat through evaporation. Metabolic rate, oxygen consumption, and insensible water loss also increase significantly with hyperthermia in the newborn (Te Pas 1988). Figure 31–8 illustrates the rise in oxygen consumption with hyperthermia.

Immunologic Adaptations

Although there is some controversy over the extent to which the immune system of the neonate is impaired, it is generally accepted that the infant's response to infection is limited at birth. Phagocytosis and localization of infection appears limited and low levels of a particular anti-

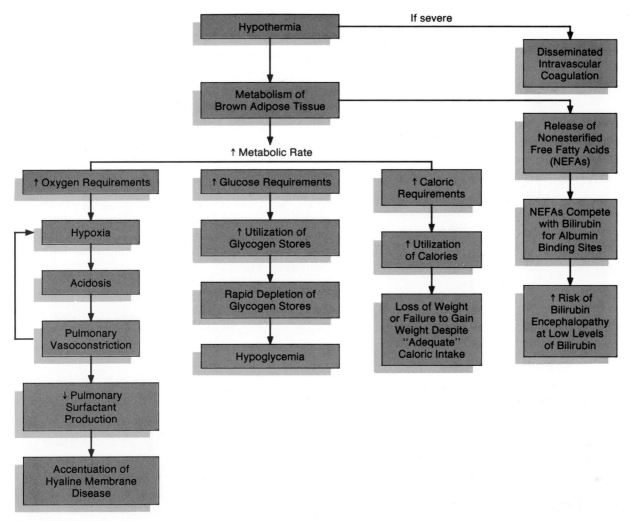

Figure 31–7. Deleterious effects of hypothermia in the neonate. (Streeter N: High-risk Neonatal Care, p 101. Rockville, Maryland, Aspen Publishers Inc., 1986)

body, immunoglobulin M (IgM), may be responsible for the infant's susceptibility to gram-positive infections.

The fetus is capable of synthesizing small amounts of certain immunoglobulins by the 20th week of gestation (IgM, IgG, and IgE), and passive immunity is acquired against many bacterial and viral diseases to which the mother has developed antibodies, including diphtheria, poliomyelitis, tetanus, measles, and mumps. This is accomplished by the passage of IgG across the placenta in the third trimester.

IgM is the largest immunoglobulin. It does not cross the placenta, and elevated levels in the newborn may indicate a fetal response to such intrauterine infections as toxoplasmosis, syphilis, rubella, cytomegalovirus infection, or herpes. These infections are often referred to as the TORCH infections. The infant born with one of the TORCH infections may show signs of chronic intrauterine infection (small brain size, retardation, and hepatomegaly) and may continue to shed live virus for months.

IgA is not normally produced *in utero* but is secreted in colostrum. It has been suggested that IgA confers passive immunity to certain gastrointestinal and respiratory infections in the breast-fed infant.

Hematopoietic Adaptations

At birth the bone marrow constitutes the major hematopoietic organ. Changes in red blood cell count, white blood cell count, and hemoglobin concentration occur slowly during the first 6 months of life.

Red Blood Cell Production. In order to compensate for the relatively low blood oxygen concentration *in utero*, the fetus has a much higher erythrocyte and hemoglobin count than an adult. The newborn's erythrocyte count ranges from 5.0 to 7.5 million/mm³. The hematocrit count is also high, with a range of 45% to 65%. Immediately after birth, as the lungs assume responsibility for tissue oxygenation, blood oxygen saturation rises and

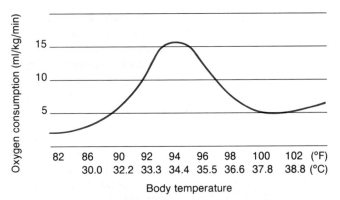

Figure 31-8. Alterations in neonatal oxygen consumption related to body temperature. (Graven S: Heat and body temperature. In Dahl N, Frazier S, Duxbury M [eds]: Neonatal Thermoregulation. White Plains, NY, The National Foundation/ March of Dimes, 1976)

erythropoietic activity is suppressed. *Erythropoietin,* the renal hormone that mediates red blood cell production, is barely detectable for 8 to 12 weeks. By the first week of life, red blood cell production is less than one tenth the level *in utero.* Furthermore, the life span of fetal erythrocytes (80-100 days) is shorter than that of an adult (approximately 120 days), and the red blood cell count begins to decline shortly after birth. This decline continues to a low of 3 to 4 million/mm³ by the 8th to 10th week after birth, when erythropoietic activity increases.

Hemoglobin Concentration. Several types of hemoglobin are detectable in the newborn. Fetal hemoglobin (Hgb F), which has a greater oxygen-carrying capacity than adult hemoglobin (Hgb A), is the predominant form (70% to 80%). After birth, the concentration of Hgb A slowly increases as the production of Hgb F ceases. The newborn's hemoglobin level ranges between 15 g/dl to 20 g/dl. As the red blood cell count drops, the hemoglobin level also decreases, reaching 10g/dl to 11 g/dl at its nadir.

White Blood Cell Concentrations. In the neonate, white blood cells, or leukocytes, function as the body's internal defense against infection. Polymorphonuclear cells (neutrophils) are the predominant form of leukocyte (40% to 80%) found in the newborn. The lymphocyte count (approximately 30%) slowly rises from birth and surpasses the neutrophil count by 1 month of age. The total white blood count is high (9,000-30,000/mm³). Leukocytosis is a normal response to the stress of birth. The white blood count does not always rise in response to infection. An increase in the number of immature leukocytes and *neutropenia* (a decrease in the number of neutrophils) is not uncommon in neonatal sepsis.

Platelet Count. Platelet function is adequate in the newborn (range 150,000 to 400,000/mm³). Thrombocytopenia may be found in the presence of neonatal sepsis.

Reproductive-Sexual Adaptations

Physical signs of sexual-reproductive adaptation in the neonate may appear several days after birth. The uterus in the female neonate, which has been stimulated by maternal estrogens during pregnancy, involutes and may produce a blood-tinged mucoid vaginal discharge *(pseudomenstruation)* several days after birth. Both male and female newborns may exhibit temporary breast engorgement, a result of estrogen stimulation. Fluid, sometimes called "witch's milk," may be discharged. The testes have descended into the scrotal sac in 90% of full-term male infants.

In most Western cultures it is accepted as fact that a capacity for sexual pleasure either does not exist in infancy or remains dormant until puberty. However, research suggests that infants are born with the potential

NURSING RESEARCH

Postnatal Adaptations and Crying in Neonates

Crying in neonates during the transitional period has been regarded as a normal behavior, and many clinicians have even considered crying beneficial during the first hours of life. Physiologic research, however, suggests that crying may actually be harmful. Recent studies have demonstrated reestablishment of fetal circulation with shunting of unoxygenated blood through the foramen ovale secondary to increased intrathoracic pressure during crying.

Nurse scientists are now studying crying behaviors and strategies to prevent or reduce the duration of crying episodes in the neonate. Crying has been found to be reduced when infants received nurturing support between 0.5 and 4 hours postbirth. They also achieved physiologic stability more rapidly. The newborn exhibits pre-cry cues that may alert care-givers to crying (grimace, red face, body tension, and clenched fists). Further research is indicated but it appears appropriate at this time to recommend that clinicians observe infants for crying cues and attempt to reduce the intensity and duration of crying episodes.

Gill NE, White MA, Anderson CG: Transitional newborn infants in a hospital nursery: From first oral cue to first sustained cry. Nurs Res 33(4):213-217, 1984

for sexual pleasure and expression. Penile erection, vaginal lubrication, and pelvic rocking have been observed in young infants, and it has been suggested that infants may experience orgasm (Crooks and Baur 1980). Self-pleasuring activity appears in conjunction with the development of other motor skills in the older infant and remains a more or less observable behavior throughout childhood, depending on parental response to the activity.

Behavioral Adaptations

Periods of Reactivity

In the period immediately after birth the neonate progresses through a series of predictable behavior patterns known as *periods of reactivity*. These distinct stages are characterized by waking and sleep states and by rapid changes in physiologic functioning (Fig. 31–9). The infant may need specialized nursing care during each period, since adaptations, especially respiratory and temperature adjustments, are not always accomplished smoothly.

First Period of Reactivity. This period, which lasts 15 to 30 minutes, is characterized by a state of alert awareness alternating with episodes of vigorous activity,

crying, and rapid irregular respirations and heart rate. Because the neonate's eyes are open at times and a strong sucking reflex is frequently present, this is an excellent time for the nurse to assist the parent–infant acquaintance process and for initiating breast-feeding. Although bowel sounds are normally still absent, breast-feeding at this time is often successful and satisfying to both mother and infant.

Period of Inactivity. After approximately half an hour, the neonate becomes progressively quieter and eventually enters a sleep phase. This period of inactivity lasts 2 to 4 hours, and difficulty may be encountered in waking the infant or initiating breast-feeding during this period. Respiratory and cardiac rates slow to resting or baseline rates. The temperature may drop to its lowest point and bowel sounds become audible.

Second Period of Reactivity. Gradually the infant awakens and enters the second period of reactivity, which lasts from 4 to 6 hours. Although the neonate attempts to reach physiologic stability during this period, this phase may evidence the most variability in behavioral responses. Respiratory and cardiac rates may change rapidly; periods of tachypnea, gagging, regurgitation of

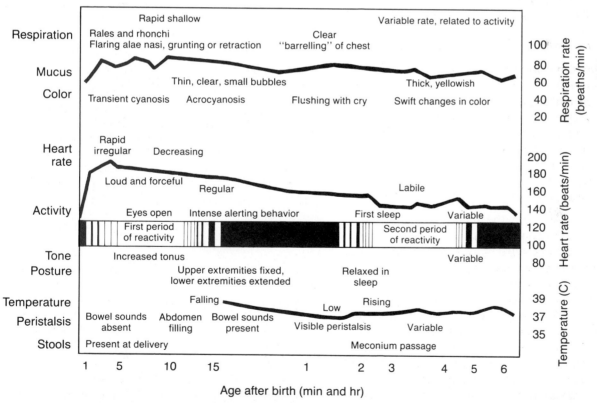

Figure 31–9. Periods of reactivity. (Adapted from Arnold HW, Putnam NJ, Barnard BL et al: Transition to extrauterine life. Am J Nurs 65(10):78, 1965)

mucus, and transient cyanosis may alternate with episodes of quiet sleep. The infant may even experience apnea. Bowel sounds increase, meconium may be passed, and the newborn again demonstrates interest in feeding.

By about 6 to 8 hours after birth, most healthy full-term infants have achieved a state of equilibrium. The transition from intrauterine to extrauterine environment is successfully accomplished, and the newborn settles into a less dramatic routine of sleep followed by wakefulness interspersed with periods of crying. The development of circadian and diurnal rhythms begins but is strongly influenced by the newborn's environment (Anders and Keener 1985). The need for careful, frequent monitoring usually ends at about 8 hours after birth. The infant is normally then ready to move into the mother's room or a central nursery.

ASSESSMENT OF THE NEONATE

The nurse is often the first health care professional to perform a thorough assessment of the newborn. Although an immediate evaluation is made by the birth attendant (certified nurse midwife or physician), the nurse is usually responsible for monitoring the infant during the 6- to 8-hour transition period and for completing the initial assessment, including the estimation of gestational age. The nurse evaluates the continuing adaptations to extrauterine life while the neonate remains in the hospital or birthing center. Nursing responsibility for the newborn assessment is being extended to the community as the number of home births and early hospital discharges continues to rise.

Neonatal Health History

The newborn assessment should be completed in an organized manner. Before beginning the actual physical examination of the neonate, the nurse should collect pertinent historical data about the mother's pregnancy, labor, and delivery. The delivery room nurse should provide a verbal report of the birth, the 1-minute and 5-minute Apgar scores (see Table 24–1), and any significant findings (birth injuries or anomalies) and should describe any resuscitative measures performed. Arm and leg identification bands are rechecked to verify the newborn's identity before the assessment is conducted or care is initiated.

It is essential that the nurse have as comprehensive a knowledge of the pregnancy, labor, and delivery history as possible in order to understand the significance of findings and to modify the initial care. The infant's size, head circumference, skin color and turgor, and posture are all affected by medical and obstetric complications of pregnancy. Behavioral responses and Apgar scores will be influenced by drugs administered to the mother during labor and by any degree of birth asphyxia. The postnatal risks of infection and respiratory complications are influenced by the extent of interval between rupture of membranes and birth and the presence of meconium in the amniotic fluid. Table 31–3 lists significant data to be included in the initial health history of the neonate.

Neonatal Physical Assessment

Once the nurse has an adequate data base from which to start, the assessment is begun with a general inspection of the infant for posture, color, and respiratory effort. Vital signs are measured. The physical examination is performed in a cephalocaudal manner or by systems and includes the four major components of assessment: inspection, auscultation, palpation, and percussion.

The nurse usually uses a newborn assessment tool provided by the health care facility to complete her admission examination and document her findings. A sample of such a form is shown in the display on page 931. Subsequent assessments are conducted in the same organized fashion. Documentation of the infant's condition varies among health care facilities and can include flow sheets, checklists, graphs, and problem-oriented nurse's notes.

The nurse should conduct the assessment in a warm, well-lighted environment that is free of drafts. The admission examination is often completed under an overhead radiant warmer to minimize cold stress during the transition period. It may be possible to perform the admission assessment at the mother's bedside if the hospital provides alternative birthing rooms or has a mother–infant recovery room. If the infant is transferred to a central admission nursery, encouraging the father to accompany the newborn and observe the assessment is an excellent way to initiate the father–infant acquaintance process. An effort should be made to conduct subsequent daily evaluations at the mother's bedside, since they provide an excellent opportunity for parent teaching and support.

General Appearance

The nurse begins her assessment by evaluating posture, color, respiratory effort, and appearance of the skin. This inspection gives information about the neurologic, cardiac, respiratory, and nutritional status of the neonate. The general appearance of the newborn can change dramatically in response to stress. A pink, healthy infant with well-flexed extremities can suddenly become cyanotic and flaccid if he or she is unable to clear the airway of

Table 31–3   **Essential Elements of the Neonatal Health History**

Major Categories of Data Obtained	Specific Elements of Health History

Maternal Prenatal Care	Extent of prenatal care:
	  Number of visits
	  Degree of compliance with care plan
	Type of facility (clinic, health department, private practice)
	Type of prenatal education

Maternal Prenatal History	Last menstrual period (LMP) Estimated due date (EDC) Weight gain in pregnancy Obstetric complications Medical complications Types of treatment received Types of medication received History of hospitalization
Maternal Blood Type and Rh Factor	History of isoimmunization (Rh or ABO incompatibilities) Antibody titers
Maternal Screening Test Results	Rubella titer Hepatitis antigen screening Chlamydia screening VDRL Gonorrhea cultures Herpes cultures HIV screening

Labor History	Onset of labor
	Length of labor
	Length of gestation at time of labor
	Obstetric complications
	Medication administration
	  Types and amount
	  Time of last medication
	Anesthesia received in labor

Rupture of Membranes	Length of time between rupture of membranes and onset of labor Amount of fluid Presence of meconium
Fetal Monitoring Record	Indication for monitoring Internal or external monitoring Abnormal FHR patterns Evidence of fetal distress Fetal scalp sampling Blood gas analysis results

Delivery History	Length of second stage
	Type of delivery
	  Vaginal
	  Cesarean
	Place of delivery
	  Delivery room
	  Alternate birthing room
	  Labor room
	  Home birth
	    Planned
	    Unplanned
	  Other locations
	Anesthesia administered
	Medication administered
	Use of forceps/vacuum extractor
	Fetal heart rate pattern in second stage

(continued)

Table 31–3   **Essential Elements of the Neonatal Health History**   (continued)

Major Categories of Data Obtained	Specific Elements of Health History
	Fetal position at birth
	Shoulder dystocia
	Compound presentation
	Breaks in sterile technique
Postnatal History	Delay in cord clamping
	Respiratory effort at birth
	Assisted
	Unassisted
	Need for resuscitation
	Type and extent of 1- and 5-minute
	Apgar scores
	Medications administered to neonate
	Cord blood gas analysis
	Parent–infant interaction
	Quality
	Extent
	Evidence of birth injury
	Evidence of narcosis
	Passage of urine or stool
	Other significant physiologic or behavioral responses
	Other significant procedures performed
	Gastric aspiration
	Laryngoscopy and tracheal suctioning
	Others
Significant Social History	Family structure
	Anticipated versus actual birth experience
	Presence of significant others at birth
	Evidence of social support system
	Significant cultural variables
	Ethnic background
	Primary language
	Religious practices related to infant care
	Plans for infant feeding
	Plans for rooming-in
	Anticipated length of hospital stay
	Early discharge
	Traditional length for recovery
	Significant social problems
	Lack of social support system
	Language barrier
	History of substance abuse
	Lack of adequate housing
	Financial distress
	Others

mucus or aspirates regurgitated milk. Such changes are indications that immediate help is required. Because the newborn's vocal expressions of discomfort or distress are limited to crying, the nurse must become skilled in making rapid appraisals of the neonate's general appearance.

Posture

The posture of the infant is influenced by the position maintained *in utero,* neurologic status, and gestational age. The healthy full-term newborn assumes a flexed posture. Muscle resistance is evident when attempts are

made to extend the extremities and there is rapid recoil to the flexed position. Infants who have been in a breech position *in utero* may exhibit temporary extension of the lower extremities. However, the normal state of flexion will be assumed in several days. Infants who have sustained neurologic injury at birth as a result of trauma or asphyxia will demonstrate varying degrees of muscle flaccidity and extension of extremities. These neonates are often described as "floppy" babies. Decreased muscle tone will also be evident in premature infants. The degree

(text continued on page 933)

ASSESSMENT TOOL

Newborn Admission History

Name		
Sex Male Female Amb.	**Birthdate**	**Admission Date**
Admitting Diagnosis		
Inborn	**UC Setup**	**Outborn**

II. INFANT HISTORY

Apgars   1″ _____   5″ _____

G.A. _____   Birthweight _____

Delivery Complications

☐ None   ☐ FHR Abnormality

☐ Meconium   ☐ Nuchal Cord/Prolapse

☐ Other _____

III. MATERNAL HISTORY

Age	Gravida	Para	AB

Delivery ☐ Vaginal   ☐ Cesarean section-reason:

Pregnancy Complications:

☐ None   ☐ Preeclampsia/Toxemia

☐ No Prenatal Care   ☐ Suspected sepsis

☐ PROM > 24°   ☐ Pre/Post-term labor

☐ Abruptio/Placenta previa

☐ Other: _____

IV. PHYSICAL ASSESSMENT

Instructions: Check the appropriate descriptive term for all the following items. Asterisked items need not be completed for infants in Admit Nursery. Please describe all abnormal findings objectively; use comment column if necessary.

1. Reflexes (Check if present and normal)

   Moro _____   Grasp _____   Suck _____

2. Tone/Activity

   a. Active _____ Quiet _____ Lethargic _____

   Flaccid _____ Paralyzed _____ Tremors _____

   Seizure Activity _____

   b. Cry Vigorous _____ Weak _____

   High Pitched _____ Difficult to elicit _____

3. Head/Neck

   a. Anterior Fontanelle   soft _____ firm _____

   flat _____   bulging _____ depressed _____

   b. Sagittal Suture: approx. _____ sep. _____ overriding _____

   c. Facial Features: symmetrical _____ asymmetrical _____

   d. Scalp molding _____

   caput succedaneum _____ cephalohematoma _____

4. Eyes

   clear _____   drainage _____

5. ENT

   a. Ears   normal _____ abnormal _____

   b. Nares patent bilaterally ___ obstructed ___ flaring _____

   c. Palate   normal _____ abnormal _____

6. Abdomen

   a. soft _____ firm _____ flat _____ distended _____

   *girth _____ cm.

   *b. liver   down ≤ 2 cm. Ⓡ CM _____

   down > 2 cm. Ⓡ CM _____

IV. PHYSICAL ASSESSMENT

7. Thorax   a. symmetrical _____ asymmetrical _____

   b. retractions   0-1 _____   1+ _____

   1-2+ _____   2+ _____

   c. clavicles   normal _____   abnormal _____

8. Lungs

   a. Breath sounds equal bilat. _____ Br. Sounds unequal _____

   b. Breath sounds audible in all lung fields _____

   inaudible _____   diminished _____

   c. Breath sounds clear _____ rhonchi _____

   rales _____ wheezing _____ secretions _____ grunting _____

   d. Respirations: spont. _____ rate _____ FIO$_2$ _____ hood _____

   Assisted ventilation CPAP _____   MV _____

   F1O$_2$ _____   PIP/PEEP _____ Rate _____

9. Heart a. Sounds NSR _____   Ectopics _____

   Murmur _____ PMI _____

   b. Rate _____

   c. Capillary Filling Time: Trunk _____ Extremities _____

10. Extremities a. moves all extremities _____

   limited range of motion _____ unable to assess _____

   b. Peripheral pulses

		STRONG	WEAK	ABSENT
Ⓡ	brachial			
Ⓛ	brachial			
Ⓡ	femoral			
Ⓛ	femoral			
Ⓡ				
Ⓛ				

   Upper & lower extremities   equal _____ unequal _____

   c. hips   normal _____ abnormal _____

   unable to assess _____

11. Umbilicus   normal _____   abnormal _____

   inflamed _____   drainage _____

   number of cord vessels _____

12. Genitals

   normal female _____ normal male _____ ambiguous _____

13. Anus   patent _____   imperforate _____

14. Spine   normal _____   abnormal _____

15. Skin

   a. color   pink _____ plethoric _____   pallor _____

   jaundice _____ cyanosis trunk _____   nailbeds _____

   circumoral _____   periorbital _____

   b. rash _____

   c. birthmarks _____

16. Temperature

   a. environment

   radiant warmer _____   temperature set _____

   incubator _____   ambient temperature _____

   open crib _____

   b. skin temperature _____

(continued)

ASSESSMENT TOOL (continued)

Comments:

V. SOCIAL HISTORY

Parents   Ages

Address

Phone: where parents can be reached

Employment

Parent/Infant Bonding

Mother		Father
	touched	
	held	
	spoke to	
	visited	
	named	
	eye contact	

Other significant social information

Parents response to prior experiences of illness &/or hospitalizations

Other children

Support systems (or significant others) for parents:

Introduction to Unit

    Instruction Booklet

    Tour of Unit

    Parent Support Group Info

    Photo of Infant Given

Date_____ Signature_____

to which muscle tone is decreased correlates with the degree of immaturity and is a result of incomplete neuro-muscular development.

Color

Because of the large number of red cells present at birth, caucasian and oriental newborns will have a pale pink skin tone. When the infant cries or passes stool, the color changes to bright pink or beefy red. Black infants have a warm brown skin color at birth and also become obviously ruddy with crying. Variations in skin color are observed in the newborn and are due to physiologic insta-bility and immaturity of organ systems. *Acrocyanosis,* localized cyanosis of the hands and feet, is common in the newborn. It is a result of the sluggish peripheral circula-tion in the neonate and is exacerbated when the infant is cold. *Circumoral cyanosis,* localized transient cyanosis around the mouth, is sometimes observed in the infant during the transition period. Circumoral cyanosis that persists or occurs with feeding and crying is abnormal and may indicate cardiac anomalies. *Mottling,* a transient pat-tern of pink and white lacelike blotches on the skin (seen especially when the infant is cold), is a result of vasomotor instability. In *Harlequin's sign,* a distinctive color pattern caused by vasomotor instability, one side of the body is pink while the other side is pale. (It is named for the clown character "Harlequin," who wore a multicolored cos-tume.) *Jaundice (icterus neonatorum)* is a yellow cast to the skin and sclera. Physiologic jaundice occurs after the first 24 hours of life, first appearing on the head and progressing caudally. It is often more observable in the sclera and in skin surfaces or mucous membranes that have been blanched. *Plethora,* a deep-red coloration of the skin, often exaggerated with crying, is caused by the in-creased number of red blood cells in the neonate (polycy-themia).

Respiratory Effort

At rest, the normal newborn's respiratory pattern is quiet, shallow, and irregular. The mouth remains closed and air moves in and out of the nose without *flaring* of the nares. Respiratory movements are abdominal, and chest expansion, while shallow, is synchronous with the rise and fall of the abdomen. There is no retraction of the chest wall with inspiration and expiratory *grunting* is not audi-ble. A complete discussion of normal respiration is pre-sented later in this chapter.

Appearance of the Skin

The skin provides a visible record of the newborn's intrauterine history, birth experience, and gestational age. The full-term infant with an uneventful gestation has pink, smooth, intact skin with good turgor at birth. Some loss of turgor and superficial peeling of skin occurs after several days as a result of limited fluid intake, fluid shifts,

and continued elimination of wastes. Greenish-yellow staining of the skin and nails indicates passage of meco-nium *in utero* related to hypoxia and fetal distress. Loose, wrinkled skin with poor turgor occurs with chronic intra-uterine malnutrition.

Ecchymoses and *petechiae* are visible when labor has been precipitous or delivery difficult. *Forcep marks* (facial bruising) may be evident when forceps are used during delivery. Small scalp lacerations are common when an internal fetal monitor has been applied during labor or capillary blood samples have been obtained from the scalp. There may be a bright red, circular, raised mark over the presenting part if a vacuum extractor was applied to the head to facilitate delivery of the fetus.

A full-term neonate's skin is relatively opaque. Few veins are visible and many creases cover the soles of the feet. Thick parchment-like skin that is peeling at birth is indicative of postmaturity. Premature infants have a transparent skin with many visible veins, and the skin on the soles of the feet is shiny with few creases.

The nurse can observe a variety of unique skin charac-teristics and birth marks in the neonate.

Vernix Caseosa. *Vernix caseosa* is the white, cream cheese-like substance that serves as a protective skin covering *in utero.* It may form a thick covering between 36 and 38 weeks of gestation but by 40 weeks, vernix is usually found only in skin folds of the axilla and groin. Vernix is gradually absorbed by the skin and may be gently removed during bathing.

Milia. *Milia* are small white papules on the nose, chin, and cheeks that are formed by plugged *sebaceous glands.* They are commonly mistaken for blemishes by parents. They should not be squeezed and will disappear spontaneously within the first few weeks of life.

Lanugo. *Lanugo* is the fine, downy hair that covers the fetus *in utero.* It begins to thin before birth and by 40 weeks of gestation is normally found only on the shoul-ders, back, and upper arms. It is gradually removed by the friction of clothing and bed linen.

Erythema Toxicum. *Erythema toxicum* is a benign maculopapular rash with an erythematous base and a pale yellow papule. It may appear on any part of the skin surface except the palms of the hands and the soles of the feet. This rash occurs in 30% to 70% of newborns and peak incidence is the second and third day of life. It usually resolves in 48 to 72 hours. Its cause is unknown and no treatment is indicated.

Birthmarks. Birthmarks fall into two categories: vascular and pigmented nevi. *Pigmented nevi* are lesions containing cells colored by melanin. They range from yel-low to black in color. *Vascular nevi* are lesions containing enlarged blood vessels. They are usually reddish or purplish in color.

Nevus flammeus (port-wine stain), a vascular nevus, is a capillary angioma located below the dermis. It is a flat, sharply demarcated purple red birthmark commonly found on the face. This birthmark does not enlarge after birth, nor will it fade. Recent advances in laser technology make removal of the birthmark possible. Although normally an isolated finding, nevus flammeus may be associated with a life-threatening genetic disorder known as Sturge-Weber syndrome.

Nevus vasculosus (strawberry mark), a vascular nevus, is a capillary angioma located in the dermal and subdermal layers of the skin. It is a raised, sharply demarcated, rough-surfaced birthmark. Strawberry marks continue to grow after birth and then recede after the first year of life. They may completely disappear by 10 years of age.

Telangiectatic nevi (stork bites) are also vascular nevi. They are pale pink, flat lesions of dilated capillaries frequently found on the nose, eyelids, and nape of the neck. Stork bites blanch with pressure, slowly fade during infancy, and eventually disappear by 2 years of age.

Mongolian spots are bluish gray pigmented nevi found primarily on the skin of the sacrum and buttocks of oriental and black babies. They are frequently mistaken for bruises by concerned parents. Mongolian spots slowly fade and disappear in childhood.

Moles are pigmented nevi. They have no clinical significance in the neonate.

Vital Signs and Measurements

After the general inspection, the nurse proceeds to take vital signs and obtains important measurements.

Respiratory Rate. Normal rate ranges from 30 to 60 breaths per minute. Respirations are counted for 1 full minute by observing the abdomen. Auscultation of breath sounds is discussed later in the chapter.

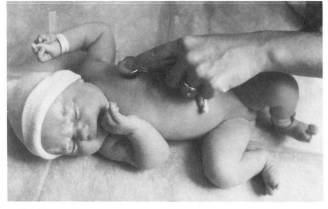

Figure 31–10. Auscultation.

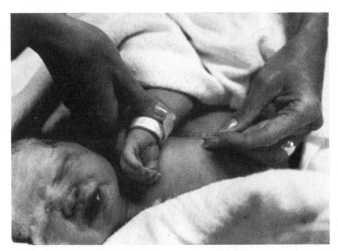

Figure 31–11. Axillary temperature measurement.

Heart Rate. Normal rate ranges from 120 to 160 bpm. The rate may drop to 100 bpm during sleep and rise to 180 bpm with crying. The heart rate should be auscultated for 1 full minute over the cardiac apex, which is normally located at the third or fourth intercostal space (Fig. 31–10). (Auscultation of heart sounds is discussed later in this chapter.)

Temperature. Accurate monitoring of the neonatal temperature is essential to determine the adequacy of postbirth adaptations. Axillary measurement is used if possible; there is a risk of traumatizing or perforating rectal mucosa when rectal temperature is taken. The thermometer is held in the axillary fold for 10 minutes (Fig. 31–11). If rectal measurement is needed, the thermometer should be inserted no further than 0.25 to 0.5 inch into the rectum and the infant's legs should be held to prevent dislodgment or breakage. Normal temperature ranges from 97.5°F to 99°F (36.4°C to 37.2°C).

Weight. Average full-term weight is 3400 g (7 lb 8 oz); 95% of newborns weigh between 2500 g and 4250 g. The infant should be weighed at the same time each day, preferably before feeding. The infant should be undressed completely, including diaper, and placed on the scale in the supine position. A protecting hand should be placed just above the infant while reading weight (Fig. 31–12).

Length. Average full-term length is 49.5 cm (19.5 inches). The length from bregma (anterior fontanelle) to heel should be measured. The infant should be placed on a flat surface and care taken to extend the legs fully before measuring length (Fig. 31–13).

Head Circumference. Average head circumference is 35.5 cm. Normally it is approximately 2 cm larger than the chest. The tape measure should be placed above the

NURSING RESEARCH

Assessment of Neonatal Temperature

In the monitoring of neonatal temperature, nurse researchers have evaluated optimal thermometer placement time, defined as the duration of time required for the temperature to be accurately recorded in 90% of infants. Although findings have been somewhat contradictory, it appears that significant differences do exist in the duration of time required for stable temperature readings for evaluating neonatal temperature among four possible sites: rectal, axilla, femoral fold, and skin-to-mattress.

Kunnel and her co-researchers found the following optimal placement times for using a mercury thermometer in neonates: rectal, 5 minutes; axilla, 11 minutes; femoral fold, 11 minutes; skin-to-mattress, 13 minutes. Other researchers have reported 90% stabilization in axillary temperature in 5 minutes and in rectal temperature in 2 minutes. Until further research resolves these contradictions in findings, it may be more appropriate to place the thermometer for the longer period of time reported by Kunnel and associates. In order to use nursing time effectively, the nurse may conduct other bedside activities while obtaining accurate temperature readings.

Kunnel MT, O'Brien C, Munro BH, Medoff–Cooper B: Comparisons of rectal, femoral, axillary, and skin-to-mattress temperatures in stable neonates. Nurs Res 37(3):162–164, 1988

NURSING ALERT

Rectal Temperature Assessment

It has been a standard practice to take neonatal rectal temperatures upon admission to the nursery. A serious contraindication to this practice is the potential for rectal perforation secondary to idiosyncracies of neonatal anatomy. The newborn's colon changes acutely from an anterior to posterior angle at a depth of 3 centimeters (approximately 1 inch). Although perforation is rare, the mortality rate may reach 70% when it occurs.

When a rectal temperature must be taken, the nurse must take care to stabilize the infant's lower extremities with one hand while inserting the lubricated thermometer bulb to a depth no greater than 0.25 to 0.5 inch or 1 centimeter. The infant must *never* be left unattended while the thermometer remains in the rectum. Accurate temperature measurement can be obtained by the axillary, femoral, and skin-to-mattress mode, and these are preferable to the high-risk practice of obtaining a rectal temperature.

the nipples. Average chest circumference is 33 cm. It is approximately 2 to 3 cm smaller than the head.

Blood Pressure.   Average blood pressure at birth is 80/46. However, blood pressure may not be routinely measured. The ultrasound (Doppler) method is the most accurate and most commonly used method of blood pressure measurement in neonates. It uses a Doppler device on an inflatable cuff attached to the infant's arm or leg to obtain an electronic reading of systolic, diastolic, and mean arterial pressure. Several cuff sizes are available and the neonate's extremity should be measured so that

eyebrow, over the top of the ears and around the fullest part of the occiput (Fig. 31–14).

Chest Circumference.   The tape measure should be placed across the lower border of the scapulae and over

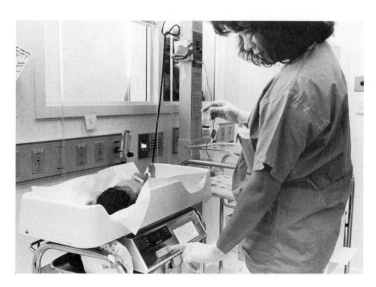

Figure 31–12. Weight measurement.

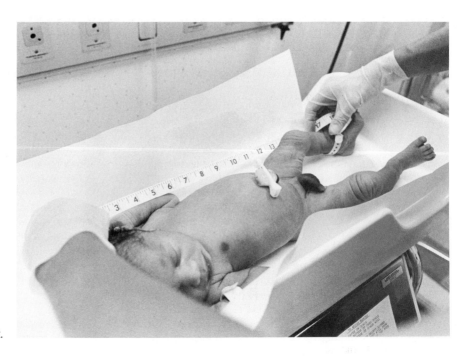

Figure 31–13. Length measurement.

the appropriate cuff is utilized for accurate blood pressure measurement. Infant movement can also affect the accuracy of the blood pressure measurement, so the Doppler device should be used when the infant is quiet.

Detailed Physical Assessment

A detailed physical assessment gives the nurse important information about the neonate's progress in adapting to extrauterine life and about the infant's particular capabilities and level of maturity.

Table 31–4 summarizes normal and unusual physical findings in the neonatal assessment. Normal variations are rarely charted in the neonatal record but should be explained to parents if they have questions or concerns. The nurse should note any unusual findings and ascertain if they have been recorded by other examiners in the neonate's chart. If *not,* the nurse should chart her findings according to that setting's protocol and bring them to the physician's attention.

(text continued on page 944)

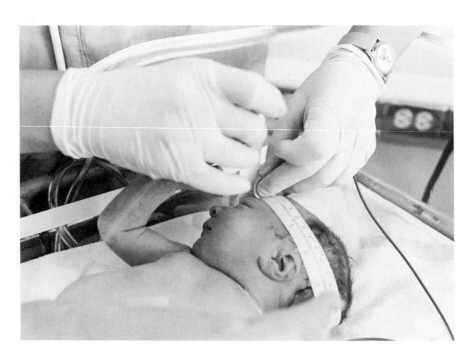

Figure 31–14. Measurement of head circumference.

Table 31-4   **Physical Findings in the Assessment of the Neonate***

Normal Findings and Common Variations	Unusual Findings and Significant Deviations	Possible Causes and Potential Problems
Integument		
General Appearance and Texture		
Skin smooth and pliant, with good turgor and visible layer of adipose tissue below	Skin thick and leathery, cracked with generalized peeling Long nails	Postmaturity
Superficial peeling after first 24 hours Veins rarely visible Milia over nose, chin, and forehead Vernix only in skin creases or absent	Skin thin and transparent with minimal adipose tissue, and many visible veins Thick layer of vernix or lanugo Nails thin and incompletely developed	Prematurity
Lanugo patchy or absent Nails soft and pliant but well formed	Skin wrinkled with poor turgor and minimal adipose tissue Umbilical cord thin Skin, umbilical cord, and nails stained with meconium	Intrauterine growth retardation Chronic maternal malnutrition
	Generalized edema	Severe erythroblastosis fetalis
Color		
Skin pink, with incomplete pigmentation in dark-skinned races at birth Acrocyanosis	Pallor	Anemia Asphyxia Shock Sepsis Hypothermia Congenital heart disease
Mottling Harlequin's sign	Cyanosis	Asphyxia Anoxia Congenital heart anomaly
Jaundice (after first 24 hours)		Hypoglycemia
	Plethora	Polycythemia
	Jaundice (within first 24 hours)	Blood incompatibilities Sepsis Biliary obstruction Drug reactions
Integrity		
Skin intact, with petechiae over presenting part	Lacerations or punctures	Accidental incision of skin with surgical scalpel during cesarean delivery Application of fetal scalp electrode during labor Fetal scalp sampling
	Generalized petechiae	Clotting disorders Sepsis
Ecchymosis secondary to application of forceps	Ecchymosis secondary to birth trauma or manipulation during delivery of infant	Cephalopelvic disproportion Shoulder dystocia Breech presentation at birth Precipitous delivery
Rashes		
Erythema toxicum Diaper rash	Skin pustules	Staphylococcal or beta-hemolytic streptococcal skin infection
	Vesicles	Congenital syphilis Herpesvirus infection

* This table summarizes normal and unusual physical findings in the neonatal assessment. Normal variations are rarely charted in the neonatal record but should be explained to parents if they have questions or concerns. The nurse should note any unusual findings and ascertain if they have been recorded by other examiners in the neonate's chart. If not, the nurse should chart her finding according to that setting's protocol and bring the finding to the physician's attention.

(continued)

Table 31–4   **Physical Findings in the Assessment of the Neonate**   (continued)

Normal Findings and Common Variations	Unusual Findings and Significant Deviations	Possible Causes and Potential Problems
	Perianal eruptions	Yeast infection (*Candida albicans*)
	Spreading diaper rash-like skin eruption	Congenital rubella
	Generalized scaling	Genetic disorders
Vascular and Pigmented Nevi Nevus vasculosus	Nevus vasculosus	Genetic disorders (Sturge-Weber syndrome)
	Nevus flammeus	
	Cavernous hemangiomas	Genetic disorders
Mongolian spots	Café-au-lait spots	Neurofibromatosis
	Hypopigmentation	Genetic disorders
Head **Size**		
	Microcephaly	Intrauterine growth retardation Genetic disorders Fetal alcohol syndrome
	Macrocephaly	Hydrocephalus
Shape Head rounded, with mild to moderate molding Plagiocephaly	Severe molding	Cephalopelvic disproportion
Caput succedaneum	Brachycephaly with flat occiput	Down syndrome
	Cephalhematoma	Head trauma secondary to labor dystocia, cephalopelvic disproportion, or forceps application
	Craniotabes	Postmaturity
Fontanelles Anterior fontanelle diamond-shaped, 3–4 cm by 2–3 cm wide (closes by 12–18 months)	Bulging, tense fontanelle	Hydrocephalus Meningitis
Posterior fontanelle triangular-shaped; may be closed at birth due to molding (closes by 8 to 12 weeks)	Abnormally large, flat open fontanelle	Hypothyroidism Intrauterine growth retardation Prematurity
	Depressed fontanelle	Dehydration
Sutures Sutures slightly separated or overlapping at birth due to molding	Widely separated sutures	Hypothyroidism Hydrocephalus Prematurity Intrauterine growth retardation
	Premature closure of sutures (craniosynostosis)	Genetic disorders
Hair Hair silky; may be curly or kinky based on familial and racial traits	Fine and wooly, sparse	Prematurity
	Coarse, brittle	Endocrine disorders Genetic disorders Intrauterine growth disorders
	Lowset hairline, low forehead	Genetic disorders
Eyes **Appearance and Position** Eyes symmetrically spaced, less than 3 cm apart, clear,	Agenesis (failure to develop)	Genetic disorders Teratogenic injury

(continued)

Table 31–4   **Physical Findings in the Assessment of the Neonate**   (continued)

Normal Findings and Common Variations	Unusual Findings and Significant Deviations	Possible Causes and Potential Problems
with transient discharge secondary to chemical conjunctivitis	Hypertelorism (abnormal width in eye spacing)	Genetic disorders
Pseudostrabismus	Persistent purulent discharge	Ophthalmia neonatorum Chlamydia conjunctivitis
Cornea and Lens		
Eyes clear, without clouding	Large or uneven cornea Corneal ulcerations Clouding or opacity of lens	Congenital glaucoma Herpesvirus infection Cataracts (rubella infection)
Sclera and Conjunctiva		
Sclera white or with faint blue tinge	True blue sclera	Osteogenesis imperfecta
Icteric after first 24 hrs	Icteric within first 24 hours	Pathologic jaundice
Chemical conjunctivitis	Persistent purulent eye discharge	Ophthalmia neonatorum Chlamydia conjunctivitis
Subconjunctival hemorrhage		
Iris		
Slate gray or brown in color	Pink iris Colobomas (lesions or clefts in structures) Brushfield's spots	Albinism May be benign or may be associated with genetic disorders Down syndrome
Pupils		
Pupils equal and reactive to light	Anisocoria (unequal pupil size) Nonreactive, fixed	Neurologic injury
Retina		
Presence of red reflex	Absence of red reflex	Congenital cataracts
Eyelids and Lacrimal Glands		
Eyelids close completely Transient edema	Eyelids fused closed	Genetic disorders Severe prematurity
Transient erythema and petechiae	Ptosis	11th cranial nerve injury
Epicanthal folds in Oriental infants and in 15–20% of non-Oriental infants	Shortened palpebral fissures	Fetal alcohol syndrome
	Epicanthal folds in non-Oriental infants	Down syndrome in conjunction with other physical findings
	Absence of eyelashes	Genetic disorders
Eyelashes		
Absence of tears, scant tearing	Excessive tearing	Plugged lacrimal duct
Neuromuscular Function		
Transient tracking and fixation ability	Persistent strabismus	Neuromuscular disorder
Transient strabismus	Vertical nystagmus	Seizure disorder
Doll's eye movement	Setting sun sign	CNS injury/disorders
Blink reflex	Blink reflex absent	CNS injury Neuromuscular disorder
Ears		
Ears normally placed with pinna at or above level of line drawn from canthus of eye	Lowset ears	Genetic abnormalities
Ears well formed and firm with good recoil if folded against head	Soft, unformed ear with little cartilage	Prematurity
Auricular skin tags	Preauricular sinus	Failure of embryonic closure of branchial cleft; may lead to infection

(continued)

Table 31–4   **Physical Findings in the Assessment of the Neonate**   (continued)

Normal Findings and Common Variations	Unusual Findings and Significant Deviations	Possible Causes and Potential Problems
Nose		
Nose in midline with wide flat bridge	Short, upturned with hypoplastic philtrum	Fetal alcohol syndrome
Infant is obligate nose breather	Nasal flaring, grunting	Nasal obstruction, choanal atresia
Scant nasal discharge	Copious nasal discharge	CNS anomalies
		Tracheoesophageal fistula
		Infection
Occasional sneezing	Frequent sneezing	Drug withdrawal
	Snuffles	Congenital syphilis
Mouth and Chin		
Mouth moist and pink with scant saliva production	Fusion of lips, atresia, or agenesis of oral structures	Genetic disorders
Symmetrical movement with crying and sucking	Asymmetry of mouth with sucking or crying	Teratogenic injury
Inclusion cysts, Epstein's pearls		Facial nerve injury
Lips intact; labial tubercles present	Cleft lip	Genetic disorders
		Teratogenic injury
Tongue mobile with short frenum	Macroglossia (hypertrophied tongue)	Genetic disorders
		Prematurity
Sucking fat pads in cheeks	White plaques on tongue, gums, buccal cavity	*Candida albicans* infection
	Hypertonic suck	Drug withdrawal
	Weak, uncoordinated suck	Prematurity, Neuromuscular disorders
		Asphyxia
Palates intact	Cleft palate	Genetic disorder
	Uvula not in midline	Teratogenic injury
Presence of rooting, sucking, swallowing, gagging reflexes	Absence of reflexes	Prematurity
		Asphyxia
		CNS injury/disorders
Vigorous cry	High-pitched cry	CNS disorders
	Crowing cry	Laryngeal disorder
	Natal teeth	Potential for aspiration if dislodged
Neck and Shoulder		
Neck short, in midline, with head maintained in midline	Abnormally short	Genetic disorders (Turner's syndrome)
	Deviation from midline	Congenital torticollis
	Lateral flexion	
Range of motion normal	Limited range of motion	Meningitis
	Nuchal rigidity	
Ability to raise head momentarily	Inability to control head	Prematurity
	Severe head lag	Asphyxia
		CNS injury
		Neuromuscular disorders
Trachea in midline	Trachea deviated	Neck mass
Thyroid not palpable	Enlarged thyroid	Hyperthyroidism
		Hypothyroidism
	Lump or crepitus over clavicle	Fracture of clavicle
Chest		
Lung		
Normal respiratory rate	Tachypnea	Sepsis
		Respiratory distress
		Hypothermia
		Hypoglycemia
Symmetrical respiratory	Seesaw breathing	Diaphragmatic hernia

(continued)

Table 31–4   **Physical Findings in the Assessment of the Neonate**   (continued)

Normal Findings and Common Variations	Unusual Findings and Significant Deviations	Possible Causes and Potential Problems
excursion	Retractions	Respiratory distress
	Grunting	Prematurity
Breath sounds clear and	Rales	Atelectasis
equal bilaterally	Rhonchi	Meconium aspiration
Transient rales at birth		
	Decreased breath sounds	Atelectasis
		Pneumothorax
	Hyperresonance	Air trapping
Shape		
Chest rounded, symmetrical	Asymmetrical chest	Pneumothorax
Transient breast engorge-	Unilateral chest bulging	Air trapping
ment and nipple discharge		
(nonpurulent)		
	Supernumerary nipples	Benign finding, but potential cosmetic concern in later life
Heart		
Heart rate normal	Tachycardia	Prematurity
		Anemia
		Shock
		Sepsis
		Congenital heart anomalies
Sinus rhythm with transient	Persistent arrhythmias	Congenital heart anomaly
arrhythmias		
Transient murmurs	Persistent murmur	Persistent fetal circulation
		Congenital heart anomaly
		Fluid overload
Quiet precordium	Active precordium	Persistent fetal circulation
		Congenital heart anomaly
		Fluid overload
		Congestive heart failure
Back, Hips, and Buttocks		
Back straight, spine intact,	Pilonidal dimple	Possible CNS anomaly
posture slightly flexed	Pilonidal sinus	Possible CNS anomaly
		Possible infection
	Hairy nevus at base of spine	Possible CNS anomaly
	Meningomyelocele	CNS anomaly
	Hip clicks	Congenital hip dysplasia
Symmetrical buttock folds	Asymmetrical buttock folds	Congenital hip dysplasia
Mongolian spots on buttocks		
Transient ecchymosis of		
buttocks after		
breech delivery		
Anus patent	Absence of stools after 24 hours	Imperforate anus, GI obstruction
	Anal fissures	Potential infection
Abdomen		
Abdomen full, rounded, and	Scaphoid abdomen	Diaphragmatic hernia
soft	Flat abdomen with horizontal wrinkles	Intrauterine growth retardation Chronic malnutrition
Bowel sounds	Hyperactive bowel sounds	Drug withdrawal
		Bowel obstructions
	Visible peristaltic waves	Pyloric stenosis
	Hypoactive bowel sounds	Sepsis
	Abdominal distention at birth	Abdominal masses
		GI obstruction
		Malrotation of bowel
		Hydronephrosis

(continued)

Table 31–4   **Physical Findings in the Assessment of the Neonate**   (continued)

Normal Findings and Common Variations	Unusual Findings and Significant Deviations	Possible Causes and Potential Problems
	Development of abdominal distention after birth; no passage of stools	GI obstruction Meconium plug Meconium ileus Hirschsprung's disease Imperforate anus
	Presence of fecal smears in diaper without passage of stool through anus	Rectovaginal fistula
Liver palpable 1–2 cm below right costal margin Linea nigra	Hepatosplenomegaly	Intrauterine infection
Umbilical cord		
Umbilical cord white with Wharton's jelly	Thin, meconium-stained cord	Fetal distress Intrauterine growth retardation
	Urine drainage around umbilical cord	Patent urachus
	Oozing of blood at base of cord	Premature detachment of cord stump Trauma to base of cord
	Purulent discharge at base of cord, foul odor, red streaking from base of cord across abdomen	Omphalitis
Two arteries, one vein	One artery, one vein	Congenital heart anomaly
	Intestine palpated in abdominal area at base of umbilical cord	Umbilical hernia
	Protrusion of abdominal contents on surface of abdomen at umbilicus	GI anomaly (omphalocele)
	Protrusion of abdominal contents on surface of abdomen, but not involving umbilicus	GI anomaly (gastroschisis)
	Bladder distention	Meatal stenosis
Presence of helix or twist; majority twist to left	Absence of helix or twist	Multiple gestation Single umbilical artery
Genitals		
Female		
Labia majora large (may be slightly edematous), covering clitoris and labia minora Transient mucoid vaginal discharge Pseudomenstruation Hymen tag visible	Ambiguous genitalia	Genetic disorder
First void within 24 to 48 hours	Absence of full stream	Meatal stenosis
	Absence of urination	Meatal stenosis Renal disorder
Uric acid crystals present		
Male		
Penis with foreskin intact (if no circumcision)	Ambiguous genitalia	Genetic disorder
Foreskin covers glans	Inability to retract foreskin to any degree	True phimosis
Meatus in center of glans at tip of penis	Meatus located on dorsal surface of penis	GU anomaly (epispadias) GU anomaly (hypospadias)

(continued)

Table 31–4   **Physical Findings in the Assessment of the Neonate** (continued)

Normal Findings and Common Variations	Unusual Findings and Significant Deviations	Possible Causes and Potential Problems
Full urine stream Glans clean, erythematous, with nonpurulent serous membrane postcircumcision Uric acid crystals present in urine	Meatus located on ventral surface of penis Spurts or dribbling of urine Purulent discharge and foul odor	Meatal stenosis Infection
Scrotum large, pendulous, many rugae Testes descended Transient edema of scrotal sac after birth	Small, shiny scrotum with few or absent rugae Testes undescended	Prematurity Cryptorchidism Prematurity Genetic disorder
	Fluid in testes Presence of intestine in inguinal canal	Hydrocele Inguinal hernia

Extremities

Arms

Posture of flexion at rest	Extension of arm from shoulder or elbow	Brachial plexus injury
Symmetrical movement	Asymmetrical movement of arms or guarding of extremity	CNS injury Fracture of long bone Brachial plexus injury
	Repetitive rowing motions	Seizure disorder
Strong muscle tonus and good recoil with extension of arm	Weak or absent tonus	Prematurity CNS injury Neuromuscular disorder Genetic disorder
Palpable brachial and radial pulses	Bounding pulses Absence of radial pulse	Fluid overload Congenital absence Spasm or obstruction

Hands and Fingers

Fingers flexed at rest Strong grasp reflex	Hand relaxed Absence of grasp reflex	CNS injury Neuromuscular disorder Brachial nerve injury
Symmetrical hand movement	Asymmetrical hand movement	Fracture, soft tissue injury, CNS injury
Multiple palmar creases	Simian crease	Down syndrome (in conjunction with other findings)
Five fingers, flexed but straight and separate	Polydactyly Syndactyly	Familial trait Familial trait Genetic disorder
Nails firm, pliant, well formed	Incurving of little finger Thin, incompletely formed nails	Down syndrome Prematurity
Moro reflex symmetrical	Meconium-stained nails Asymmetrical Moro	Fetal distress CNS injury Brachial nerve injury Fracture of long bone or clavicle

Legs

Legs well flexed at rest	Amelia or phocomelia	Genetic disorder Teratogenic injury
Slightly bowed appearance	Shortened long bones	Genetic disorder (dwarfism or achondroplasia)

(continued)

Table 31–4   **Physical Findings in the Assessment of the Neonate**   (continued)

Normal Findings and Common Variations	Unusual Findings and Significant Deviations	Possible Causes and Potential Problems
Muscle tonus strong with good recoil when legs are extended	Weak or absent muscle tone	Prematurity Neuromuscular disorder CNS injury
	Asymmetrical movement or guarding of extremity	Fracture of long bone Soft-tissue injury CNS injury
Femoral pulses palpable	Differential between pulses in upper and lower extremities	Coarctation of aorta
	Blanching of one extremity	Thrombosis, arterial spasm
Feet and Toes		
Feet have fat pad on sole	Rocker-bottom soles	Genetic disorder
Sole crease over at least anterior two thirds of foot	Absence of creases or few sole creases	Prematurity
Ankle mobile, with full range of motion	Abnormal positioning or rigid fixation of ankle or heel	Congenital clubfoot (talipes deformity)
	Deformity of arch of foot	Congenital clubfoot (talipes deformity)
Pedal pulses palpable	Differential in pulses between upper and lower extremities	Coarctation of aorta
Five toes	Polydactyly	Familial trait
	Syndactyly	Familial trait Genetic disorder
Toenails well formed	Thin, poorly developed nails	Prematurity
Presence of plantar grasp	Absence of grasp	CNS injury
Positive Babinski's reflex	Negative Babinski's reflex	Neuromuscular disorder

Head and Face

The nurse examines the size and shape of the head first. The newborn head is large (approximately 25% of the total body size), with a prominent cranium and forehead. The face appears small in comparison and has a receding chin. The shape of the head may be asymmetrical or elongated because of *molding,* an overlapping of the cranial bones that occurs as the fetus moves through the birth canal. Molding is temporary and the head will assume a rounded appearance several days after birth.

The general appearance of the face is evaluated. The nurse inspects for signs of facial paralysis (best assessed when the infant is crying). The distance between the eyes is noted. *Ocular hypertelorism* is the excessive spacing of the eyes and is defined as a distance of greater than 3 cm between the inner canthi of the eyes in full-term infants. The size and shape of the nose are assessed. The bridge of the nose normally is low, and the nose may appear flat as a result of labor and delivery. The presence of birth marks, bruising, petechiae, lacerations, or edema is noted. *Plagiocephaly,* or facial asymmetry, may also be noted. It occurs with persistent positioning of the fetal head against the maternal pelvis and results in premature closure of a cranial suture. The face and head usually resume a symmetrical appearance when pressure is relieved after birth and concomitant molding resolves.

Palpation.   Palpation of the cranium follows inspection. The cranium is composed of seven bones (two parietal, two temporal, two frontal, and one occipital), which are not fused together at birth. Palpation of the suture lines, the separating lines between the bones, may reveal overlapping due to molding. The cranial bones are pliable. Palpation may reveal the presence of *craniotabes,* a rare abnormal localized softening of the bones.

Fontanelles.   The *fontanelles* are the membranous openings at the juncture of three cranial bones. The largest is the *anterior fontanelle,* or *bregma,* which is located at the junction of the frontal bone and the parietal bones. It is diamond-shaped and measures approximately 3 cm to 4 cm long by 2 cm to 3 cm wide. It remains open for 12 to 18 months. The *posterior fontanelle* is smaller, triangular in shape, and located at the junction of the occipital bone and parietal bones. The posterior fontanelle may actually be closed at birth due to molding but can be palpated again after several days. It closes within 8 to 12 weeks.

The nurse palpates the anterior fontanelle to assess changes in intracranial pressure and the degree of hydration. A sunken fontanelle may indicate dehydration, whereas a tense or bulging fontanelle suggests increased intracranial pressure. The infant should be in a sitting position and quiet when the fontanelles are palpated because they may bulge slightly with crying. It is normal to feel pulsations through the membrane, especially when the infant is lying down.

A hand is passed over the scalp to assess the location, degree, and extent of any noted swellings. A localized soft-tissue edema of the scalp, *caput succedaneum,* may be present. Caput, which results from sustained pressure of the presenting part against the cervix during labor, feels spongy and may cross suture lines. It resolves within 24 to 48 hours of birth. *Cephalhematoma* is a collection of blood between the periosteal membrane and the cranial bone. It will produce a soft, fluctuant, localized swelling on the head that does not cross suture lines. It may take up to several months for all the blood in a cephalhematoma to be reabsorbed. If the cephalhematoma is large, a considerable number of red blood cells will be hemolyzed, contributing to the development of jaundice in the neonate. Table 31–5 outlines differences between caput succedaneum and cephalhematoma.

The scalp is inspected carefully for bruising, redness, or lacerations. If an internal fetal scalp electrode was attached to monitor the fetal heart rate or if fetal scalp sampling was performed, small lacerations will be present on the infant's head. The texture and amount of hair is noted. Whether the hair is curly or straight, it should have a silky texture without coarseness or brittleness.

Eyes

It may be difficult to inspect the eyes of the newborn immediately after birth because of edema of the eyelids. The sclera has a bluish tinge due to the relative thinness of the membrane. The iris is normally slate gray or blue. (The permanent color cannot be ascertained until the infant is approximately 3 months of age.) Small *subconjunctival hemorrhages* may appear in the sclera as a result of changes in ocular pressure during birth.

The eyes should be clear and without discharge. Tearing is uncommon because the lacrimal glands are imma-

ture. Some newborns experience a *chemical conjunctivitis* after the instillation of silver nitrate drops. Sometimes these drops are given as prophylaxis against gonococcal infection of the eye. In these newborns greenish yellow discharge is observed for 24 to 48 hours after administration of the drops. Many nurseries now apply erythromycin ointment to the eyes instead of silver nitrate to reduce the incidence of conjunctivitis. Additionally, erythromycin ophthalmic ointment is effective in the prevention of chlamydial infection, which is now the most common sexually transmitted disease in the United States. There is usually less drainage or discharge after use of ointment; if discharge occurs, it may be suggestive of infection.

An ophthalmoscope is used to examine the pupil, lens, cornea, and retina. Bringing the infant to a sitting position often causes the eyes to open and assists the nurse with assessment. The *pupillary* and *blink* reflexes are present at birth and should be symmetrical. The pupil and cornea are round. When light is directed at the pupil, it should appear clear of opacities or cloudiness (*cataracts*). A red-orange flash of light will be observed (*red reflex*) as the light reflects off the retina.

Sensory perception and neuromuscular coordination are limited, but recent research has revealed greater visual capabilities in newborns than was once recognized. They have *binocular vision* and can *fixate* for up to 10 seconds on near objects. *Acuity,* or clarity, of vision is best within a distance range of 9 to 12 inches. Neonates seem most interested in the human face but also show interest in geometric shapes (circles, squares, and dots) at least 2 to 3 inches tall, in patterns of medium complexity, and with sharp black and white contrast. They fixate longest on colors of medium intensity (medium pinks, yellows, and greens). *Accommodation,* the ability of the eyes to adjust for distance, is absent for the first month, but *conjugation,* the ability of the eyes to move together, is present.

Muscular control of ocular movement is imprecise, and transient *strabismus* and *nystagmus* are common. *Transi-*

Table 31–5 Comparison of Caput Succedaneum and Cephalhematoma

Caput Succedaneum	Cephalhematoma
Appears at birth; no increase in size	Appears several hours after birth; increases in size for 2–3 days
Disappears several days after birth; outline is vague, poorly defined	Disappears approximately 6 weeks after birth; outline is well defined
Sometimes crosses suture lines	Never crosses suture lines
Caused by diffuse, edematous swelling involving the soft tissues of the scalp	Caused by subperiosteal hemorrhage
Complications; rarely, anemia	Complications: jaundice, underlying skull fracture, intracranial bleeding, shock

Adapted from Waechter EH, Phillips J, Holaday B: Nursing Care of Children, 10th ed. Philadelphia, JB Lippincott, 1985

tory strabismus is due to immature neuromuscular control. *Pseudostrabismus* or "cross-eyed" appearance is an illusion created by the large epicanthal fold many infants have covering the inner canthus of the eye. This skinfold narrows the visible width of the sclera medial to the iris, creating the impression of strabismus. *Doll's eye phenomenon* may also be observed when the head is turned quickly and eye movement lags behind.

Nose and Mouth

The nasal passages in the neonate are narrow and have a delicate mucosal lining. Because the infant is an obligate nose breather, any obstruction (such as mucus or edema) can lead to respiratory distress. The nurse checks for *choanal atresia,* a rare congenital blockage of the nasal passage. Patency of the nasal passage is evaluated by closing the infant's mouth and compressing one naris at a time. A wisp of cotton can be placed at the open naris to check for movement of air. Routine passage of catheters to assess patency is not recommended because of risk of trauma to the mucosa. Sneezing occurs occasionally and is the infant's method for clearing the nose of mucus or milk.

Although the newborn should have moist, pink mucous membranes, salivary glands are immature and saliva production is scant. Heavy drooling or constant bubbling of oral mucus is abnormal and may indicate a *tracheoesophageal fistula.* The lips are sensitive to touch, and stimulating them causes the infant to suck. *Labial tubercles,* or sucking calluses, may actually be present at birth as a result of strong sucking activity *in utero.*

Next, the gums, hard and soft palate, and tongue are assessed. Firm, rounded *inclusion cysts* may be found on the gums and are benign. Occasionally, *precocious teeth* are also discovered at birth; if they are loose they may be removed to prevent accidental aspiration. If they are true primary teeth and not loose, they sometimes will be left in place. The tongue is short but mobile, and the *frenulum* attached from the base of the tongue to the base of the mouth is also short, giving the newborn the appearance of being "tongue-tied". The frenulum should not be clipped and will lengthen with growth and development of the infant. The tongue and cheeks should be examined for evidence of *thrush,* a yeast infection caused by *Candida albicans,* which can be acquired by the infant during passage through an infected vagina. The infection is characterized by white, adherent, curdlike patches on the tongue and cheeks.

Using a good light source and a tongue blade, the nurse should carefully examine the hard and soft palate. *Cleft palate* may extend the entire length of the hard palate or may involve only the soft palate or uvula. Small, firm, white inclusion cysts *(Epstein pearls)* may also be found on the palate and are benign.

Ears and Neck

The full-term newborn's ears *(pinna)* are soft and pliable but recoil readily when bent toward the head. The nurse must evaluate the ears for placement, size, shape, and firmness of ear cartilage. The top of the ear should be at or above the level of an imaginary line drawn from the inner and outer canthus of the eye to the ear. Low-set ears may be indicative of certain chromosomal abnormalities or organ anomalies (particularly renal anomalies, since the ears and kidneys develop concurrently *in utero*). *Preauricular skin tags* or *dermal sinuses* may be found immediately in front of the ear. They are often isolated findings and can be removed or repaired. Visualization of the tympanic membrane with an otoscope is not usually attempted immediately after birth because the ear canal is obliterated with vernix and blood.

Hearing is well developed once the eustachian tube is aerated and the outer ear is free of blood, vernix, and mucus. The infant will show a startle reflex to a sudden loud noise and in the alert awake state will attend to auditory stimuli, such as the ringing of a bell. Studies of newborn auditory capacity suggest that infants prefer high-pitched voices (high frequency range) to low-pitched voices.

Many nurseries are now screening infants to identify those at risk for hearing loss. The following risk factors are associated with hearing loss:

- Defects in the ears, nose, or throat
- History of hearing loss before age 50 in a family member
- Suspected maternal rubella infection during pregnancy
- Birth weights of less than 1500 g

The neck is short and has several thick folds of skin. The muscles that control and support head movement are not fully developed and the head lags when the infant is pulled from a supine to a sitting position. When placed on the abdomen, the full-term infant can raise its head momentarily and turn it from side to side. The nurse must evaluate the neck for evidence of webbing, which is associated with chromosomal abnormalities, and for range of motion. Nuchal rigidity may suggest damage to the sternocleidomastoid muscle *(congenital torticollis)* or central nervous system disorder, including meningitis.

Since the clavicle is the bone most frequently fractured during delivery, the nurse must carefully palpate both clavicles for evidence of a lump or *crepitus* (a snapping or crackling feeling). The nurse should also elicit the Moro (startle) reflex at this point. If a clavicle is fractured, the Moro reflex is absent or diminished on the affected side. The assessment of reflexes is discussed in detail later in this chapter.

Chest

The nurse now places the infant in a supine position on a flat surface and inspects the chest. The infant's chest is round, slightly smaller than the head, and symmetrical. The sternum is in the midline and the xiphoid cartilage is visible under the skin as a nodule. The nipples and areola are pigmented in the full-term infant. Buds of breast tissue approximately 10 mm in size can be palpated below the nipple. *Breast engorgement* may be evident 2 to 3 days after birth due to the effects of withdrawal of maternal estrogen, and a cloudy fluid discharge (witch's milk) may be secreted from the nipple. Accessory nipples *(supernumerary nipples)* may be noted below and medial to the nipples. Accessory nipples are fairly common and are benign.

Shallow symmetrical chest expansion is noted with respirations (30/min to 60/min). This should be synchronous with abdominal movement. The sternum and intercostal muscles should not retract (collapse in toward the spine) with inspiration.

The intensity of heart action is estimated by placing a hand on the precordium and feeling the heart impulse through the chest wall. Slight chest movement over the *point of maximum impulse* may be observed and is normal.

Breath Sounds.   Auscultation of the breath sounds requires practice and often has limited usefulness in neonates because sound emanating from one lung may be transmitted to the other. Furthermore, bowel sounds and upper airway noises (created by the movement of air over the soft tissues of the upper airway and mouth) are heard over the chest wall and make auscultation difficult.

The nurse should auscultate the breath sounds over the anterior and posterior chest. *Rales,* identified as crackling noises predominantly on inspiration, may be heard in the transition period immediately after birth and indicate retained fetal lung fluid and areas of atelectasis. Rales should be absent within several hours of birth as lung fluid is absorbed through the lymphatics. Clearing of fluid can be facilitated by chest percussion and suctioning. However, chest physiotherapy must be performed carefully and cautiously because of the association of this procedure with systemic blood pressure changes and intraventricular hemorrhage in preterm infants. *Rhonchi,* identified as coarse rattling noises, are less frequently heard. Rhonchi indicate fluid, mucus, or meconium in the larger bronchi and may be associated with more life-threatening conditions, such as meconium aspiration syndrome. (Meconium aspiration syndrome is discussed in Chapter 34.)

Heart Sounds.   Heart sounds should be auscultated when the infant is quiet. Beginning at the point of maximum impulse (normally the apex), the stethoscope should be moved slowly over the entire precordium, below the left axilla, and posteriorly over the left scapula. If a murmur is auscultated, the nurse determines whether it occurs after the first heart sound (caused by closure of the mitral and tricuspid valves) or the second heart sound (caused by the closure of the pulmonic and aortic valves). In neonates, 90% of all murmurs are transient and are related to incomplete closure of the foramen ovale or ductus arteriosus. The nurse also listens for the presence of the splitting of heart sounds, thrills, and gallops. Any irregularity in heart rhythm is noted, as well as any shift in the point of maximum impulse, which might indicate pneumothorax or diaphragmatic hernia. However, many full-term health infants experience some dysrhythmia during the first 6 to 12 hours of life, including sinus tachycardia and premature ectopic beats of supraventricular and ventricular origin. They are generally asymptomatic and require no treatment but should be monitored carefully.

Abdomen

The inspection of the abdomen is begun with the infant in a supine position and quiet. The shape is rounded and protuberant because of the weakness of the abdominal musculature. The skin should be smooth with few visible veins. It should not appear stretched or shiny. A shrunken or *scaphoid abdomen* may indicate diaphragmatic hernia (displacement of intestinal contents into the thoracic cavity through a defect in the diaphragm). A flat abdomen covered by loose, wrinkled skin is suggestive of chronic intrauterine malnutrition.

The umbilical cord normally appears white and gelatinous in the first few hours of life. It is clamped about an inch from the surface of the skin, and the three vessels (one vein and two arteries) may be visible at the cut edge. The umbilical cord begins to dry after a few hours, shrinks in size, and turns brownish black. It begins to separate from the skin, and usually falls off between the sixth and tenth day of life. Oozing of blood or purulent discharge from the cord is abnormal and may indicate loosening of the cord clamp, trauma to the cord, or omphalitis. In a small percentage of infants (especially black infants) an umbilical hernia may be noted. This is due to incomplete closure of the abdominal muscles and requires no special care at birth. Most hernias close without surgical intervention within the first 2 years of life.

Unless immediately indicated, auscultation and palpation of the abdomen can be deferred until the period of inactivity, approximately 30 minutes after birth, when the infant is relaxed and less responsive to external stimuli and bowel sounds are audible. Auscultation should be done first, since palpation may cause a transient decrease in the intensity of bowel sounds.

The abdomen feels soft, without distention or tenderness. The edge of the liver may be palpated 1 to 2 cm below the right costal margin. The spleen may be palpated 1 to 2 cm below the left costal margin. The kidneys, most easily identified before the intestines fill with air and digested milk, feel like firm oval masses about the size of walnuts. They are located by deep palpation 1 to 2 cm above and slightly lateral to the umbilicus. The bladder is also an abdominal organ in the newborn because of the smallness of the pelvis, and it may be palpated when filled with urine.

Genitalia

Female Genitalia.   The external genitalia of the female infant reflect gestational age as well as nutritional status at birth. In the full-term newborn the labia majora are large, may be swollen as a result of the influence of maternal hormones, and completely cover the labia minora. By contrast, the preterm female has little adipose tissue in the labia majora. The labia minora are visible but are small and incompletely developed. The clitoris is prominent and the urinary meatus is located just below it. The vaginal opening should be identified. Many females have a mucoid vaginal discharge, which may be blood-tinged *(pseudomenstruation)* as a result of maternal hormonal influence. A hymenal tag may protrude from the vaginal opening. Vernix and smegma may be found in the creases of the labia and are gently washed away with bathing.

Male Genitalia.   The male genitalia also reflect the degree of maturity at birth. The penis is relatively small and the foreskin covers the glans. The prepuce (foreskin) may not retract easily from the glans, but true *phimosis,* the inability to retract the foreskin at all, is rare. The foreskin may be removed surgically by circumcision, and in those infants the glans will be exposed, slightly edematous, and erythematous for the first few days after the procedure. A yellow exudate may be formed over the glans following circumcision, but bleeding or the presence of purulent discharge is abnormal.

The nurse locates the meatal opening, which is normally on the tip of the glans. *Hypospadias* is a congenital anomaly in which the urethral meatus is located on the ventral surface of the penis. *Epispadias* occurs when the meatal opening is on the dorsal surface. Both may be repaired surgically. In both male and female infants, the urine stream should be observed to eliminate the possibility of meatal stenosis. The bladder empties when approximately 15 ml of urine is collected. In the male the stream is forceful and can project 6 to 8 inches upward in an arc. In the female a full stream should also be noted, although it does not project more than ¼ to ½ inch beyond the labia majora.

In the full-term male infant, the scrotum is large and pendulous and the skin is rugous. The nurse palpates the scrotum gently. The testes are normally descended (in 90% of males) and palpable in the scrotal sac. *Cryptorchidism,* failure of the testes to descend into the scrotal sac of the full-term neonate, is rare but requires medical attention to identify the cause and, if possible, correct the condition. Edema and *hydrocele,* a collection of fluid in the testis, are common and usually benign findings that resolve spontaneously. By contrast, the scrotal sac of the preterm infant is small, smooth, and shiny and the skin is smooth. The testes, which do not descend until the 36th week, may not be palpable.

Back and Buttocks

The newborn is placed in a prone position so that the back and buttocks can be examined. The back appears rounded because of the normal flexed posture, but the spine is straight and does not develop the lumbar and sacral curves until the infant begins to sit upright and walk. The finger is passed slowly along the spine to ascertain its shape, and it is both inspected and palpated for masses and openings. The sacrum and base of the spine are examined for tufts of hair or small indentations, which may indicate *spina bifida occulta* (incomplete closure of the vertebral column). If a *pilonidal dimple* is present (a fold of skin located in the midline of the sacrococcygeal area) it should be inspected for evidence of a sinus tract.

The buttocks should be separated and the anal opening inspected for patency (no membrane evident over the opening). Anal fissures may be present. They are often identified by the presence of slight, bright-red bleeding from the rectum. Small fissures often heal quickly if the anal area is carefully cleansed after each bowel movement and periodically exposed to air. The anal area should also be examined for fistulas, which appear as small openings or dimples in the skin.

Hips

While the infant remains in a prone position the hips are examined. The symmetry of buttock skinfolds are assessed. They should be symmetrical. Uneven folds may indicate *congenital hip dysplasia,* which is a congenital deformity of the pelvis that is often accompanied by hip dislocation. The infant is then placed in a supine position and *Ortolani's maneuver* is performed. In this maneuver the infant's knees are flexed. The thighs are held with the examiner's thumbs on the inner aspect of the thighs and the fingers along the outer thighs from the knees to the greater trochanters. The thighs are adducted, internally rotated, and then abducted at least 175 degrees so that they lie almost flat against the mattress. If a jerk is felt or a clunking sound heard, it is a result of the head of the femur moving into the acetabulum and is a significant indication of hip dysplasia. A "click" unassociated with a sense of movement may be felt in approximately 25% of infants and is a result of minor joint incongruities. Finally, the hips and knees are flexed and the infant's feet are placed flat on the mattress. If hip dislocation is present, the knee on the affected side will be higher *(Allis's sign)*.

Upper Extremities

The arms are normally well flexed and should move symmetrically in the full-term newborn. When the arms and hands are fully extended the fingertips should reach to approximately the midthigh. The hands are plump and the fingers are tightly flexed. The fingernails are soft and extend beyond the tips of the fingers and should not be stained. Three palmar creases normally extend across the palm at a slight angle.

The symmetry and strength of muscle resistance to extension of the arms are assessed, as is the range of motion of the joints. The arm is palpated for lumps, evidence of trauma, or limitation in movement because the humerus is the second most frequently fractured bone during delivery. The brachial and radial pulses are palpated and their strength is assessed.

Partial or complete flaccidity of the arm may indicate trauma to the brachial plexus, which also occurs during delivery. *Erb-Duchenne paralysis,* a result of injury to the fifth and sixth cranial nerves, is characterized by partial paralysis of the arm. In this condition, the elbow is extended and the forearm pronated. The Moro reflex cannot be elicited on the affected side. Complete paralysis of the arm results from injury to the entire plexus and is rare. Return of function in either type of paralysis depends upon the severity of injury.

The grasp reflex is elicited by placing a finger in each palm and then slowly raising the infant toward a sitting position. The normal newborn can hold onto the examiner's finger long enough to achieve a momentary upright position. The palms should be inspected for evidence of a single *simian crease,* which runs straight across the hand, and an incurving of the small finger. These signs are frequently present in infants with *Down syndrome. Polydactyly,* extra digits, may occur as a benign inherited phenomenon or may be associated with genetic disorders. *Syndactyly* (webbing) is the presence of a membrane between fingers and is rare.

Lower Extremities

The legs are short, appear bowed, and are usually well flexed. In a prone position the knees are flexed and the thighs are tucked up against the abdomen. The feet also appear plump and in the full-term infant the sole is creased from toes to heel. An inward turning of the foot *(varus deviation)* may be evident and is frequently the result of a position maintained *in utero.* If the foot can be brought to the midline without force, no orthopedic correction is necessary. *Talipes deformity* (clubfoot) requires surgical correction.

After the lower extremities are inspected, muscle tone and symmetry of movement are assessed. Strength of resistance to extension of the legs and range of motion of the joints are evaluated. The toes are examined for polydactyly and syndactyly. Unusual spacing of the big toe from the others may indicate a chromosomal abnormality. Finally, pulses (femoral and pedal) are palpated and their strength is assessed.

Assessment of Neuromuscular Integrity

Although a general evaluation of neurologic status is conducted at the outset when posture, head size, and the fontanelles are being assessed, a systematic assessment of neuromuscular integrity should be performed before the examination of the newborn is completed. A readily apparent sign of neuromuscular status in the newborn is the sound of the cry. The full-term newborn has a loud, lusty cry. A shrill, high-pitched cry is indicative of central nervous system injury or abnormality.

Neonatal Reflexes

Although several reflexes may already have been elicited during the assessment, a complete evaluation of reflexes should be done at this time. Blink, cough, sneeze, and gag reflexes are present at birth and remain unchanged into adulthood. However, some reflexes reflect the neurologic immaturity of the neonate and disappear in the first year of life. Table 31–6 lists these neonatal reflexes and how to elicit them.

Assessment of Gestational Age

A major determinant of a newborn's ability to survive is the degree of maturity at birth. Historically, the estimation of gestational age was based on the mother's estimated due date calculated from her last menstrual period. The infant's birth weight has also been used to classify the newborn as premature, mature, or postmature. These methods were found to be unreliable. Many women are unable to provide precise dates for their last menstrual period, and the infant's birth weight can be significantly above or below the norm for a particular gestational age as a result of maternal nutritional status, disease processes, exposure to environmental hazards, and inherited disorders in the fetus. As a result, the need for an objective tool for assessing gestational age became apparent. One tool developed to address this need is the *Dubowitz scale,* which allows a detailed, systematic assessment of physical signs and neurologic traits that can be used to accurately estimate gestational age in infants between 28 and 42 weeks of gestation.

An assessment using the complete Dubowitz scale, however, takes a skilled examiner 15 to 20 minutes to

Table 31-6 **Assessment of Neonatal Reflexes**

Reflex	Category	How Elicited	Normal Response	Abnormal Response	Duration of Reflex
Rooting and sucking (Fig. 31-15)	Feeding	Touch cheek, lip or corner of mouth with finger or nipple.	Infant turns head in direction of stimulus, opens mouth, and begins to suck.	Weak or absent response seen with prematurity, neurologic deficit or injury, or CNS depression secondary to maternal drug ingestion (*e.g.,* narcotics)	Diminished by fifth to sixth month; disappears by 1 year
Swallowing	Feeding	Place fluid on back of tongue.	Infant swallows in coordination with sucking.	Gagging, coughing, or regurgitation of fluid; possibly associated with cyanosis secondary to prematurity, neurologic deficit, or injury Often seen after laryngoscopy	Does not disappear
Extrusion	Feeding	Touch tip of tongue with finger or nipple.	Infant pushes tongue outward.	Continuous extrusion of tongue or repetitive tongue thrusting seen with CNS anomalies and seizures	Disappears by about fourth month
Moro (Fig. 31-16)	Postural	Change infant's position suddenly or place on back on flat surface.	Bilateral symmetrical extension and abduction of all extremities, with thumb and forefinger forming characteristic "C," followed by adduction of extremities and return to relaxed flexion	Asymmetrical response seen with peripheral nerve injury (brachial plexus) or fracture of clavicle or long bone of arm or leg No response with severe CNS injury	Diminished by fourth month; disappears by sixth month
Stepping	Postural	Hold infant in upright position and touch one foot to flat surface.	Infant will step with one foot and then the other in walking motion.	Asymmetrical response seen with CNS or peripheral nerve injury or fracture of long bone of leg	Disappears within 1-2 months
Prone Crawl	Postural	Place infant on abdomen on flat surface.	Infant will attempt to crawl forward with both arms and legs.	Asymmetrical response seen with CNS or peripheral nerve injury or fracture of long bone	Disappears within 1-2 months
Tonic Neck or "Fencing" (Fig. 31-17)	Postural	Turn infant's head to one side when infant is resting.	Extremities on side to which head is turned will extend and opposite extremities will flex. Response may be absent or incomplete immediately after birth.	Persistent response after fourth month May indicate neurologic injury Persistent absence in CNS injury, neuromuscular disorders	Diminishes by fourth month.

(continued)

Table 31–6   **Assessment of Neonatal Reflexes**   (continued)

Reflex	Category	How Elicited	Normal Response	Abnormal Response	Duration of Reflex
Startle	Protective	Expose infant to sudden movement or loud noise.	Infant abducts and flexes all extremities and may begin to cry.	Absence of response may indicate neurologic deficit or injury. Complete, consistent absence of response to loud noises may indicate deafness. Response may be absent or diminished during deep sleep.	Diminishes by fourth month
Crossed Extension	Protective	Place infant in supine position and extend one leg while stimulating bottom of foot.	Infant's opposite leg will flex and then extend rapidly as if trying to deflect stimulus to other foot.	Weak or absent response seen with peripheral nerve injury or fracture of long bone	Disappears by 4–6 months
Glabellar "Blink"	Protective	Tap bridge of infant's nose when eyes are open.	Infant will blink with first four or five taps.	Persistent blinking and failure to habituate Suggestive of neurologic deficit	
Palmar Grasp (Fig. 31–18)	Social	Place finger in palm of infant's hand.	Infant's finger will curl around object and hold momentarily.	Diminished response with prematurity Asymmetry with peripheral nerve damage (brachial plexus) or fracture of humerus No response with severe neurologic deficit	Diminishes by fourth month
Plantar Grasp (Fig. 31–19)	Social	Place finger against base of toes.	Infant's toes will curl downward.	Diminished response with prematurity No response with severe neurologic deficit	Diminishes by fourth month
Babinski (Fig. 31–20)	Not categorized	Stroke one side of foot upward from heel and across ball of foot.	Infant's toes will hyperextend and fan apart from dorsiflexion of big toe.	No response with CNS deficit	Disappears by 1 year

complete. When a prompt assessment of gestational age is needed on a neonate requiring immediate care, a modified version of the scale, the Ballard scale, is used.

The Ballard Scale

The Ballard scale is a simplified version of the Dubowitz that allows a quick assessment of gestational age and is suitable for use with a neonate requiring immediate treatment. The neonate is given a score ranging from 0 to 4 on each of 13 traits. The score is totaled, and a maturity rating in weeks of gestation is determined using the scor-

ing guide, as shown in the accompanying Assessment Tool, page 954.

Physical Characteristics

Skin.   The skin is inspected for thickness, integrity, color, and the presence of visible veins. The skin of the preterm infant is thin, red or pink, and smooth, with veins quite visible. The full-term newborn has a thicker skin that is opaque and has few visible veins. Superficial peeling may be evident. After 42 weeks of gestation, the skin becomes thick and leathery with deep cracking and significant peeling (Fig. 31–21). Veins are not visible.

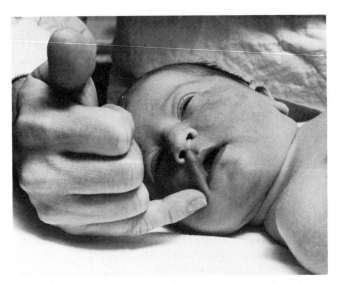

Figure 31–15. Rooting reflex (Sullivan R, Foster J, Schreiner RL: Determining a newborn's gestational age. Am J Matern Child Nurs, pp 38–45. Jan/Feb 1979)

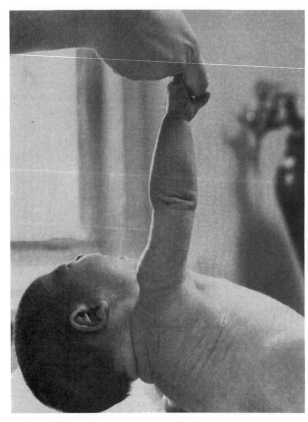

Figure 31–18. Palmar grasp reflex. (Courtesy of Mead Johnson)

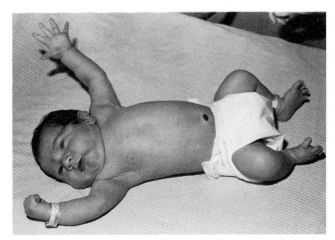

Figure 31–16. Moro reflex.

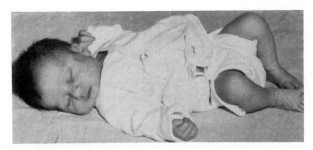

Figure 31–17. Tonic neck reflex.

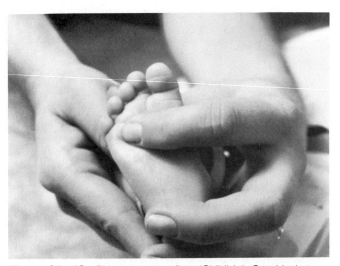

Figure 31–19. Plantar grasp reflex. (Childbirth Graphics)

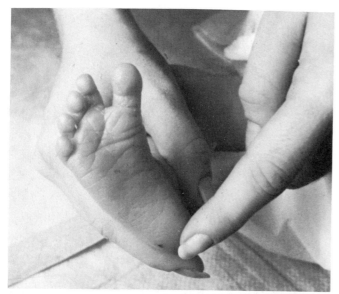

Figure 31–20. Babinski reflex. (Childbirth Graphics)

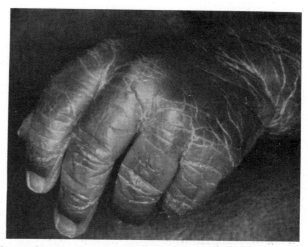

Figure 31–21. Post-term infant's hand. Note dry, peeling, cracked skin. (Sullivan R, Foster J, Schreiner RL: Determining a newborn's gestational age. Am J Matern Child Nurs, pp 38–45. Jan/Feb 1979)

Lanugo. The presence and amount of lanugo is assessed (see Fig. 31–24). The very premature infant (under 28 weeks) has a fine, barely visible covering of lanugo. Lanugo becomes thickest between 28 and 30 weeks of gestation and slowly disappears so that the full-term infant has only small amounts along the shoulders and scapular area.

Plantar Creases. The creases on the sole of the foot are examined. Sole creasing develops first at the anterior portion of the foot and proceeds to the heel. The full-term infant has plantar creases over the entire sole (Fig. 31–22). The sole creases must be assessed in the first 12

hours of life because superficial cracking and peeling occurs as the skin begins to dry after birth.

Breast Tissue. The amount of breast tissue (not adipose tissue) is evaluated. The presence of a nipple and development of the areola are checked. The breast tissue *under the nipple* is placed between the forefinger and the middle finger to assess the size of the breast bud. The premature infant has no perceptible breast bud. A small bud (1 to 2 mm) is felt at approximately 36 weeks of gestation and this increases to approximately 5 mm in size by 40 weeks of gestation. It continues to increase in size with increasing gestational age. The nipple and areola are not visible in the very premature infant. The areola becomes

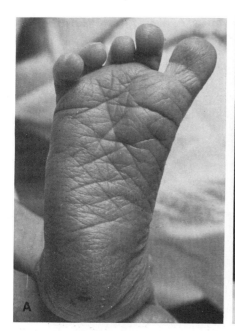

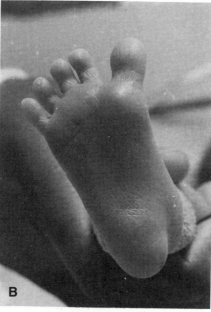

Figure 31–22. A comparison of the sole creases on the foot of a term infant *(A)* with those of a preterm infant *(B)*. At 40 weeks of gestation, the entire foot, including the heel, is crisscrossed with creases. (Sullivan R, Foster J, Schreiner RL: Determining a newborn's gestational age. Am J Matern Child Nurs, pp 38–45. Jan/Feb 1979)

ASSESSMENT TOOL

Estimation of Gestational Age

Scoring system: Ballard JL *et al*: A Simplified Assessment of Gestational Age. Pediatr Res 11:374, 1977. Figures adapted from "Classification of the Low-Birth-Weight Infant" by AY Sweet in Care of the High-Risk Infant by MH Klaus and AA Fanaroff, WB Saunders Co, Philadelphia, 1977, p. 47.

NEUROMUSCULAR MATURITY

	0	1	2	3	4	5
Posture						
Square Window (Wrist)	90°	60°	45°	30°	0°	
Arm Recoil	180°		100°-180°	90°-100°	< 90°	
Popliteal Angle	180°	160°	130°	110°	90°	< 90°
Scarf Sign						
Heel to Ear						

PHYSICAL MATURITY

	0	1	2	3	4	5
SKIN	gelatinous red, transparent	smooth pink, visible veins	superficial peeling &/or rash, few veins	cracking pale area, rare veins	parchment, deep cracking, no vessels	leathery, cracked, wrinkled
LANUGO	none	abundant	thinning	bald areas	mostly bald	
PLANTAR CREASES	no crease	faint red marks	anterior transverse crease only	creases ant. 2/3	creases cover entire sole	
BREAST	barely percept.	flat areola, no bud	stippled areola, 1–2 mm bud	raised areola, 3–4 mm bud	full areola, 5–10 mm bud	
EAR	pinna flat, stays folded	sl. curved pinna, soft with slow recoil	well-curv. pinna, soft but ready recoil	formed & firm with instant recoil	thick cartilage, ear stiff	
GENITALS Male	scrotum empty, no rugae		testes descending, few rugae	testes down, good rugae	testes pendulous, deep rugae	
GENITALS Female	prominent clitoris & labia minora		majora & minora equally prominent	majora large, minora small	clitoris & minora completely covered	

Gestation by Dates _____ wks

Birth Date _____ Hour _____ am / pm

APGAR _____ 1 min _____ 5 min

MATURITY RATING

Score	Wks
5	26
10	28
15	30
20	32
25	34
30	36
35	38
40	40
45	42
50	44

SCORING SECTION

	1st Exam=X	2nd Exam=O
Estimating Gest Age by Maturity Rating	_____ Weeks	_____ Weeks
Time of Exam	Date _____ am / Hour _____ pm	Date _____ am / Hour _____ pm
Age at Exam	_____ Hours	_____ Hours
Signature of Examiner	_____ M.D.	_____ M.D.

Scoring system: Ballard JL et al: A Simplified Assessment of Gestational Age. Pediatr Res 11:374, 1977. Figures adapted from "Classification of the Low-Birth-Weight Infant" by AY Sweet in Care of the High-Risk Infant by MH Klaus and AA Fanaroff. Philadelphia, WB Saunders, 1977.

raised at approximately 34 weeks of gestation and increases in size as the nipple bud increases (Fig. 31–23).

Ears. The degree of cartilage distribution and the resulting ear form are assessed. The external ear is relatively shapeless and flat before 34 weeks of gestation (Fig. 31–24). If the ear is bent forward against the side of the head, it will remain in that position. By 34 to 36 weeks there is some cartilage formation and slight incurving of the upper pinna. By 40 weeks there is incurving over two-thirds of the pinna, and if the ear is bent forward, it quickly recoils to its original position. The firmness of the ear increases after 40 weeks, and the ear stands erect and away from the head.

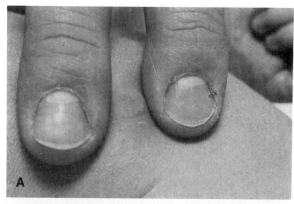

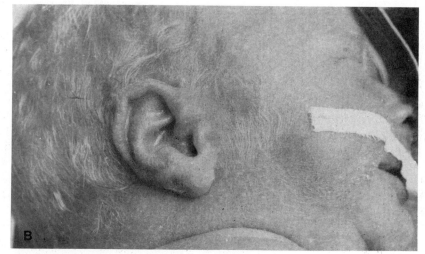

Figure 31-23. Note the relatively distinct areola and underlying breast bud of the term infant *(A)* when compared to the preterm infant *(B)*. (Sullivan R, Foster J, Schreiner RL: Determining a newborn's gestational age. Am J Matern Child Nurs, pp 38–45. Jan/Feb 1979)

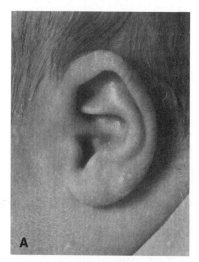

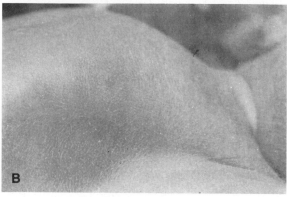

Figure 31-24. Cartilage is well developed in the term infant *(A)* and the ear is erect, away from the head, whereas the ears of the preterm infant *(B)* lie flat against the head. Also note the matted hair and the presence of lanugo on the face of the preterm infant. (Sullivan R, Foster J, Schreiner RL: Determining a newborn's gestational age. Am J Matern Child Nurs, pp 38–45. Jan/Feb 1979)

Male Genitalia. The male genitalia are assessed to determine the size of the scrotum and degree of rugation and whether the testes have descended (Fig. 31–25). In the premature infant the scrotum is small and has very few rugae, and the testes remain high in the inguinal canal. Rugation increases with gestational age. By 40

weeks of gestation, the scrotum is large, pendulous, and heavily rugous, and the testes have descended into the lower scrotum.

Female Genitalia. The female genitalia are examined to determine the amount of subcutaneous fat depo-

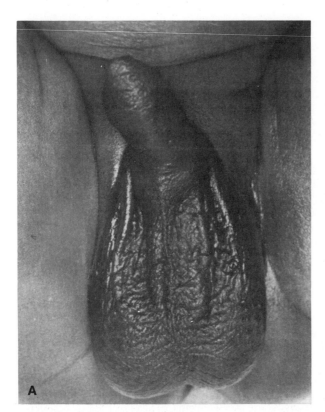
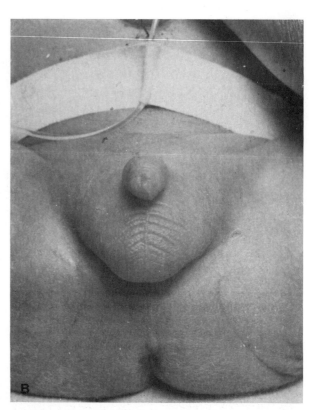

Figure 31–25. In the term infant *(A)* the testes are well descended into the scrotal sac and the scrotum is covered with numerous rugae. In the preterm infant *(B)* the testes remain high in the inguinal canal and the rugae are largely undeveloped. (Sullivan R, Foster J, Schreiner RL: Determining a newborn's gestational age. Am J Matern Child Nurs, pp 38–45. Jan/Feb 1979)

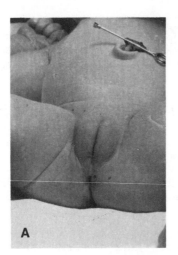
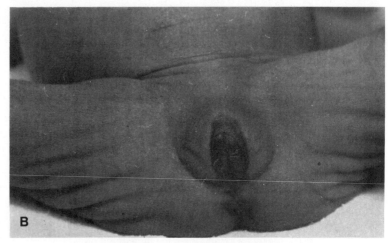

Figure 31–26. The labia majora of the term infant *(A)* completely cover the labia minora and clitoris while they are small and widely separated in the preterm infant *(B)*. Also note the loose skin folds on the posterior thighs of the preterm infant. (Sullivan R, Foster J, Schreiner RL: Determining a newborn's gestational age. Am J Matern Child Nurs, pp 38–45. Jan/Feb 1979)

sition in the labia majora and the prominence of the labia minora and clitoris (Fig. 31–26). Because the amount of adipose tissue also depends on the provision of adequate nutrients *in utero,* the size of the labia majora will be affected by factors other than gestational age. Before 36 weeks of gestation, the labia majora are small and widely separated and the labia minora and clitoris are prominent. After 36 weeks the labia majora begin to cover the internal structures, and by 40 weeks the labia minora and clitoris are completely covered.

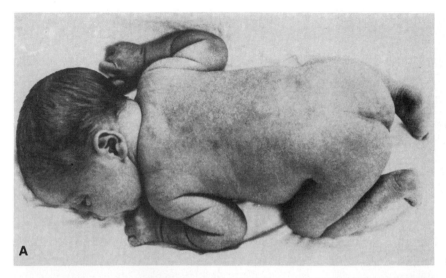

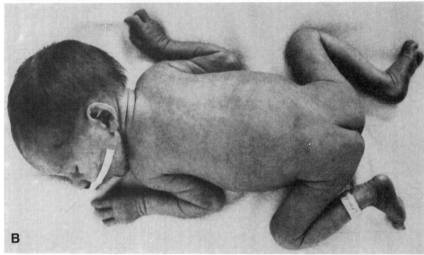

Figure 31–27. Resting posture. Note the flexion of the extremities in the term infant *(A)* compared to the partial flexion in the preterm infant *(B)*, resulting in a froglike resting posture.

Neuromuscular Characteristics

After the assessment and scoring of physical characteristics has been completed, the neurologic evaluation is conducted. The degree and strength of muscle tonus and flexion is assessed. The Ballard scale lists six neuromuscular traits.

Posture. The resting posture of the infant is assessed (Fig. 31–27). In the very premature infant (under 30 weeks of gestation), the extremities are in full extension. By approximately 34 to 36 weeks, partial flexion of both upper and lower extremities is evident. The full-term infant assumes a posture of complete flexion of all extremities.

Wrist Flexion ("Square Window"). The extent of wrist flexion is evaluated (Fig. 31–28). The nurse flexes the infant's wrist down toward the ventral forearm. The angle between the hypothenar eminence and the forearm is measured. A 90-degree angle is observed in infants below 32 weeks of gestation. A 30-degree angle is noted in infants between 38 and 40 weeks. The palm and forearm can be approximated (0 degrees) in the infant after 40 weeks of gestation.

Arm Recoil. The degree of elbow flexion is assessed. The infant is placed in a supine position. The nurse completely flexes both elbows, holds the position for 5 seconds, fully extends the arms, and then releases them. In the full-term infant, rapid recoil to flexion is the normal response to this maneuver. The angle formed at the elbow upon recoil is less than 90 degrees. The premature infant demonstrates slow recoil and a greater angle with flexion (greater than 90 degrees).

Popliteal Angle. The degree of knee flexion is evaluated. The infant is placed in a supine position. The nurse flexes the thigh on the abdomen. While holding the thigh against the abdomen with one hand, the nurse places the index finger of the other hand behind the infant's ankle and extends the lower leg until resistance is met. In the

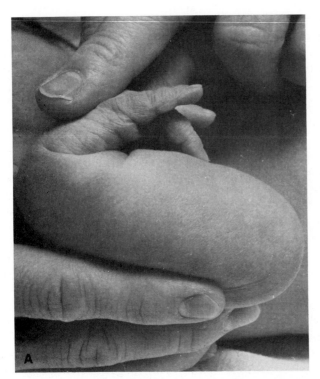
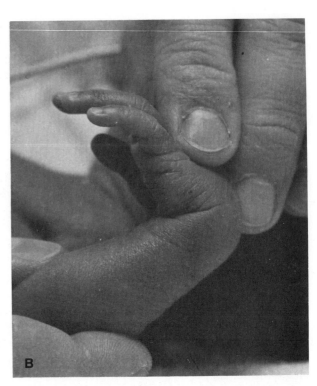

Figure 31–28. Wrist flexion. In the term infant *(A)* the wrist can be flexed onto the arm, but the wrist can only be flexed to an angle of about 90° in the preterm infant *(B)*. (Sullivan R, Foster J, Schreiner RL: Determining a newborn's gestational age. Am J Matern Child Nurs, pp 38–45. Jan/Feb 1979)

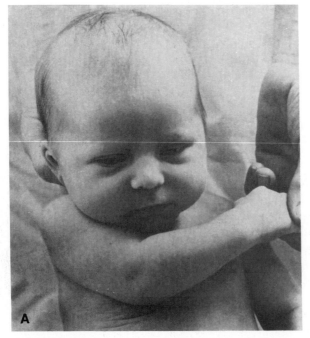
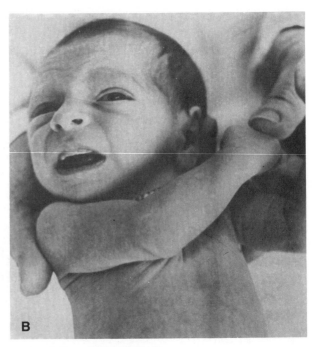

Figure 31–29. Scarf sign. In the term infant *(A)* the elbow will not reach the midline, but in the preterm infant *(B)* the elbow will reach across the midline. (Courtesy of Mead Johnson)

full-term newborn, resistance to extension of the knee is strong and the angle formed behind the knee is less than 80 degrees. In the premature newborn the angle is increased (greater than 90 degrees) and there is less resistance to extension.

Scarf Sign.   The extent of shoulder flexion is assessed (Fig. 31–29). The infant is placed in a supine position. The arm is drawn across the chest as far as possible until resistance is met. It is permissible to lift the elbow across the body as the arm is extended. The location of the elbow is noted. In the premature infant (before 36 weeks of gestation) the elbow can be drawn past the midline. Between 36 and 40 weeks of gestation the elbow reaches the midline and after 40 weeks the elbow cannot be drawn to the midline.

Heel-to-Ear Extension.   The degree of knee extension and the ability to draw the foot to the head are assessed (Fig. 31–30). The infant is placed in a supine position. While stabilizing the hips on the mattress, the nurse draws the foot toward the ear on the same side. The distance between the foot and head is noted as well as the degree of extension at the knee. There will be marked resistance in the full-term neonate. The popliteal angle will be 90 degrees or less. The foot cannot be drawn much farther toward the head than the umbilicus. The premature infant will demonstrate less resistance and the foot can be drawn closer to the head. This maneuver may be less accurate in neonates delivered in frank breech presentation.

Obtaining and Interpreting the Ballard Score

Once the nurse obtains a score for the neuromuscular assessment, it is added to the score calculated for the physical assessment portion of the rating scale. The sum

of the two scores is matched against a column listing gestational age. Once the gestational age is determined, the infant can be identified as premature (preterm), mature (full-term), or postmature (postterm) and a determination can be made of whether size (birth weight, head circumference, and length) is appropriate for estimated gestational age (Fig. 31–31). This determination is important because infants who are either *small for gestational age* (SGA) or *large for gestational age* (LGA) have special needs and problems. Definitions of important terms in estimating gestational age are shown in the accompanying display. Because of the major adaptations required of the neurologic system during the first days of life, the gestational age rating should be performed twice in order to fully evaluate the neuromuscular component. The first evaluation should be performed within the first 6 hours of life, before the skin begins to dry and crack. The second assessment is conducted between 24 and 48 hours after delivery. If the infant is sick, has sustained neurologic injury, or is heavily sedated as a result of medication given to the mother during labor and delivery, the neurologic assessment is postponed. A skilled examiner may still be able to estimate gestational age by evaluating only the physical characteristics; this type of assessment is essential if the infant is sick and requires immediate treatment.

Assessment of Behavioral Capabilities

In the not so distant past the newborn was considered to be merely a passive recipient of care, with limited sensory perception and behavioral capabilities. Researchers interested in the newborn have shattered this assumption. Each infant is now known to possess unique behav-

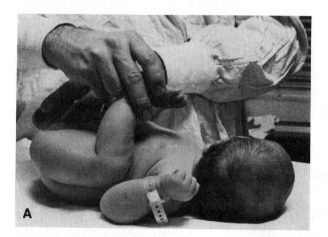 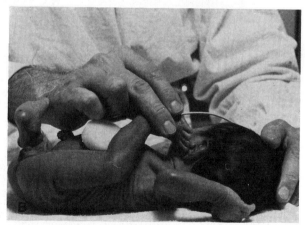

Figure 31–30. Heel to ear test. In the term infant *(A)* there is a marked resistance in the leg as the foot is gently drawn toward the ear, whereas in the preterm infant *(B)* very little resistance is noted. (Sullivan R, Foster J, Schreiner RL: Determining a newborn's gestational age. Am J Matern Child Nurs, pp 38–45. Jan/Feb 1979)

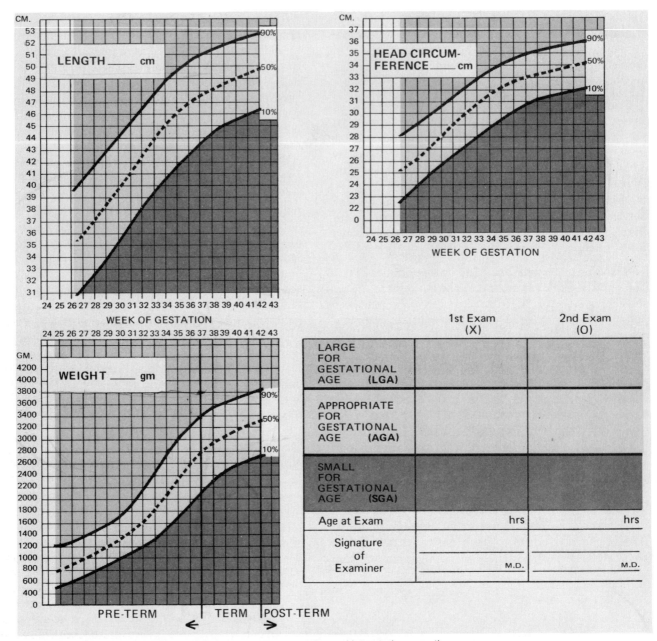

Figure 31–31. Classification of newborns based on maturity and intrauterine growth. (Lubchenco LC, Hansman C, Boyd E: Pediatrics 37:403, 1966; Battaglia FC, Lubchenco LC: J Pediatrics 71:159, copyright American Academy of Pediatrics, 1967)

ioral competencies that exert a powerful effect on parent–infant interactions and increase the neonate's chance of survival by engaging the caretaker's attention.

Temperamental differences are reflected in differing reactions to external events. Two major temperament types in infants have been described. The "easy" infant is characterized by regular body functions, a positive mood, and quick adaptability in new situations, whereas the "difficult" infant shows irregular body rhythms and intense, generally negative responses to new situations.

Brazelton Neonatal Behavioral Assessment Scale

T. Berry Brazelton, a pediatrician, created an assessment tool to assist in the evaluation of newborn behavioral competencies (Als et al 1982). The Neonatal Behavioral Assessment Scale is composed of 27 behavioral items and 20 measures of reflexes that are elicited during the evaluation to determine the newborn's capabilities. For each item, if the first response is less than optimal, the

Definitions of Terms in Gestational Age Assessment

Premature infant: an infant born before 37 weeks of gestation

Mature (full-term) infant: an infant born between 38 and 42 weeks of gestation

Postmature infant: an infant born after 42 weeks of gestation

Small-for-gestational-age (SGA) infant: a newborn whose weight is below the 10th percentile for estimated week of gestation or two standard deviations below the mean

Appropriate-for-gestational-age (AGA) infant: a newborn whose weight falls between the 10th and 90th percentile for estimated gestational age or within two standard deviations from the mean

Large-for-gestational-age (LGA) infant: a newborn whose weight is above the 90th percentile for estimated gestational age or two standard deviations above the mean

NURSING RESEARCH

Neonatal Assessment

Although traditional pediatric evaluation tools identify gross problems, they may fail to detect behavioral dysfunction or very early signs of physiologic destabilization. Skilled nurse clinicians may be able to identify subtle signs of dysfunction in neonates before obvious illness or neurologic abnormality is evident. These infants are often labeled as "unusual," "funny-looking," "funny-acting," or "different". Recent nursing research indicates that while nurses often have difficulty articulating their suspicions of dysfunction, they do possess the ability to accurately identify problems. Nurses focus on interactive competencies (responsiveness, irritability, and posturing), and repeated contact with infants provides them with opportunities to note very subtle changes in functioning.

An assessment instrument that may more accurately assist nurses in objectively documenting behavioral abnormalities is the Brazelton Neonatal Behavioral Assessment Scale (BNBAS). It is suggested that nurses learn to discern behavioral traits assessed by the BNBAS and persist in alerting physicians when they suspect problems, even if they are not able to clearly articulate their impressions.

Maloni JA, Stegman CE, Taylor PM, Brownell CA: Validation of infant behavior identified by neonatal nurses. Nurs Res 35(3):133–138, 1986

test is repeated. The infant is scored on the best performance rather than on an average response to each test. Because the infant passes through periods of behavioral disorganization during the first few days after birth, it is recommended that the assessment be done on the third day after delivery. This creates a problem in many settings because of increasing numbers of normal neonates being discharged before 72 hours of age. The assessment, which takes approximately 30 minutes, should be conducted in a quiet, dimly lit area. The examiner must complete training in the use of the Brazelton tool before performing the assessments. Brazelton and associates have also developed an instrument for the assessment of the preterm infant's behavior, the APIB (Als et al 1982).

The behaviors on the Brazelton assessment scale are divided into the following six categories.

Habituation.   *Habituation* is the ability of the newborn to diminish a response to specific repeated stimuli. In response to sound, light, or a pinprick to the heel, a normal newborn will startle. As the stimulus is repeated, the newborn will shut it out and stop responding. Immature neonates and those with central nervous system anomalies or injury may respond in an erratic or unpredictable manner to stimuli. They may never fully habituate, thus making it very difficult for parents to anticipate or predict their response to specific care-giving activities.

Orientation.   *Orientation* refers to the newborn's ability to attend to visual and auditory stimuli. When alert, normal newborns will attend to voices and fixate

and follow visual stimuli. By the third day of life, they can turn their head toward the light or sound. Recent research indicates that preterm infants have a limited ability to orient and attend to visual stimuli and a limited attention span. Attempts to attract the preterm neonate's attention for even short periods may lead to episodes of bradycardia and/or apnea. Parents and care-givers must minimize environmental stimuli and plan periods of interaction and stimulation that recognize the individual neonate's limitations.

Motor Maturity.   *Motor maturity* is reflected in the newborn's ability to control and coordinate motor activities. Normal full-term newborns demonstrate smooth, free movements within restricted arcs. Occasional tremors and startles can also be noted. Preterm infants and those with central nervous system anomalies or injury may move their extremities in very wide, uneven arcs. Movements are frequently jerky.

Self-Quieting Ability.   *Self-quieting ability* is the ability of newborns to utilize their own resources to quiet and comfort themselves. The normal newborn demonstrates a variety of self-consoling behaviors, such as hand-to-mouth movements, sucking on fist or tongue, and attending to external stimuli. Infants with neurologic injury or anomalies may be unable to engage effectively in self-quieting activities and require more frequent comforting from care-givers when aroused.

Social Behaviors. *Social behavior* in neonates refers to the extent to which infants need and respond to cuddling and how often they smile. Newborns vary in their need for and response to being held. Some infants are "cuddlers" who seek and enjoy being held. Others are less tolerant of restraint and stiffen when attempts are made to cuddle them. Neonates with central nervous system injury or anomalies may be very resistant to any form of cuddling or comforting behavior initially. These infants require consistent care-givers who can assist them in gradually developing tolerance to close physical contact.

Sleep/Awake States. Two sleep states and four awake states have been identified in neonates. Recognizing these states and their patterns, how long newborns remain in a state, and how frequently they move from one state to another is critical in understanding their individual behavioral capacities. It is also important in helping new parents become acquainted with the unique characteristics of their infant. Identification of the neonate's state of consciousness (sleep or awake) is an essential component of Brazelton's Neonatal Behavioral Assessment Scale.

When the infant is in *deep sleep*, eyes are closed, there is no eye movement, breathing is regular, and there is no spontaneous activity except for occasional startles. Startles are not easily elicited by external stimuli and are quickly suppressed. Even very loud noises may not disturb the infant, and attempts at arousal (*e.g.,* for nursing) may be met with frustration. State changes are less likely during deep sleep than in any other state.

In *light sleep*, the infant's eyes are closed, there is rapid eye movement, and respirations are irregular. Random movements, occasional sucking, and startles can be noted. Startles can be elicited with less difficulty and often result in state changes.

When the infant is in the *drowsy state*, eyes can be open or closed, and eyelids may flutter. Intermittent motor activity and occasional startles can be noted. The infant is reactive to sensory stimuli but response is delayed. State changes can frequently be noted after stimulation. Movements are usually smooth.

When in the *quiet alert state*, the infant has a bright look and focuses attention on the source of stimulation. This is an ideal state for parent–infant interactions because the infant is able to attend to vocal and visual stimuli for relatively long periods. Other stimuli may eventu-

ally interrupt concentration, but response is delayed. Motor activity is minimal.

In the *eyes open state*, the infant demonstrates considerable motor activity with thrusting movements of the extremities and occasional startles. The infant reacts to external stimulation with increased startles and motor activity. Discrete reactions are difficult to distinguish because of the generally high activity level.

In the *crying state* the infant cries loudly and does not respond to outside stimuli readily. It may take some time to calm the infant so that it will attend to other activities, such as feeding.

The nurse uses knowledge about neonatal behavioral capabilities in planning and providing care for the newborn. Interventions can focus on acquainting parents with the unique behavioral competencies and state patterns of their infant. They can be taught when and how best to interact with the neonate. The nurse supports early parenting efforts in this manner, thus facilitating parent–infant attachment.

CHAPTER SUMMARY

Extrauterine adjustments made during the first 24 hours are critical to the newborn's chances for survival. The nurse is in a unique position to aid the newborn in these adjustments. The nurse must develop a sound knowledge base for assessing the normal newborn and identifying problems.

Definite physiologic and behavioral adaptations are made by the normal neonate. Various stimuli work together to initiate respiration, which begins a chain of cardiovascular events and other physiologic adaptations. Each system begins functioning. Periods of reaction can be noted, and general characteristics for the normal neonate can be observed.

Comprehensive nursing assessment of the neonate's physical status and behavioral capabilities forms the foundation for subsequent nursing care of the normal neonate. Because the neonate is unable to express needs except through crying, the nurse must be skilled in assessment in order to collect the data needed for planning and implementing care.

STUDY QUESTIONS

1. What factors are responsible for initiation of respiration in the newborn?
2. What are the four major mechanisms of heat loss/heat transfer in the neonate?

3. What is the significance of cold stress in the neonate, and how can the nurse prevent it?
4. What is physiologic jaundice, and how is it distinguished from pathologic jaundice in the newborn?
5. How are the neonate's behavioral responses affected by the periods of reactivity/inactivity?
6. What is the significance of the gestational age assessment for the neonate?
7. What is the Brazelton Neonatal Behavioral Assessment Scale, and what is its significance?
8. How do the sleep/awake states influence parent–infant interactions?

REFERENCES/BIBLIOGRAPHY

Als H, Lester B, Tronick E, Brazelton B: Manual for the assessment of preterm infant's behavior. In Fitzgerald HE, Lester BM, Yogman MW (eds): Theory and Research in Behavioral Pediatrics. New York, Plenum, 1982

Anders TF, Keener M: Developmental course of nighttime sleep–wake patterns in full-term and premature infants during the first year of life. I. Sleep 8(3):173–192, 1985

Ballard JL, Novak LK, Driver M: A simplified score for assessment of fetal maturation of newly born infants. J Pediatr 95:769, 1979

Cole FS, Cloherty JP: Infection — prevention and treatment. In Cloherty JP, Stark AR (eds): Manual of Neonatal Care. Boston, Little, Brown and Co, 1985

Crooks R, Baur K: *Our Sexuality.* London, Benjamin/Cummings Publishing, 1980

Te Pas KE: Thermoregulation in newborns. Module 1. White Plains, NY, The National Foundation/March of Dimes, 1988

SUGGESTED READINGS

Banta SA: Transition to extrauterine life. Neonatal Network 3(6):35–39, 1985

NAACOG: Physical assessment of the neonate. Washington, DC, OGN Nursing Practice Resource, 1986

32 nursing care of the low-risk neonate

LEARNING OBJECTIVES

After studying the material in this chapter, the student should be able to

- Discuss how hospital environments influence neonatal adaptation

- Describe specific nursing interventions that facilitate stabilization of physiologic functions in the transitional stage

- Discuss nursing interventions that support the establishment of normal feeding patterns in neonates

- Describe specific nursing interventions that promote the parent–infant interaction

- List common nursing interventions employed to prevent potential neonatal complications

- List essential components of the nursing care plan for daily care of the neonate

- List topics normally included in the parent-teaching discharge plan

- Describe newborn screening tests and discuss their importance in preparation for discharge

- Discuss the risks and benefits of circumcision

KEY TERMS

Aspiration

Attachment

Circumcision

Cradle cap

Demand feeding

Diurnal rhythm

Football hold

Heel stick

Hyperbilirubinemia

Hypoglycemia

Hypothermia

Ophthalmia neonatorum

Prophylaxis

Regurgitation

Taking-hold phase

Taking-in phase

Transitional care

Nursing care for the low-risk neonate may take place in a variety of settings, and duration of care may range from just a few hours to several days. The number of settings in which care is delivered and the variation in length of hospital stay require careful planning for nursing care.

The nurse can make the newborn's adjustment to extrauterine life less traumatic by manipulating the environment, providing individualized nursing care, and facilitating the development of ties between newborn and parents. These interventions are best accomplished by adherence to principles of family-centered maternity care and use of the nursing process in organizing the pattern of care.

Assessment of the newborn has been discussed in Chapter 31. This chapter discusses possible nursing diagnoses, specific nursing interventions employed in care, and expected outcomes during transition and for ongoing care. Because of the increase of nontraditional settings, this chapter deals with nursing care designed to support physiologic and behavioral adaptation and to facilitate the parent–infant attachment process in a variety of settings. Suggestions for teaching in preparation for discharge are delineated.

ENVIRONMENTAL CONSIDERATIONS IN NEWBORN NURSING CARE

Of particular importance in planning and implementing effective nursing care is an understanding of how the hospital environment influences neonatal adaptation and the provision of neonatal nursing care (Table 32–1).

Birthing Room and Labor–Delivery–Recovery Room

The birthing room may offer the low-risk family the optimal environment for birth and the immediate postdelivery period within the hospital setting. This private, homelike room introduces the infant to a quiet, dimly lit extrauterine environment. Parents and infant can get acquainted at leisure in comfortable surroundings. Siblings may be allowed to participate in the experience. The nurse should recognize the nature of this intimate family event, providing parents with guidance and support, as needed, but also offering opportunities for privacy.

Because the birthing room simulates the home environment, equipment used for resuscitation and monitoring of the infant is placed out of sight or outside the room but must be immediately available. Birthing room light sources used for inspection of the infant may be inadequate. Because the newborn is usually placed against the

mother's skin and covered with blankets directly after birth in a birthing room, it is difficult for the nurse to assess subtle changes in skin color and respiratory effort. The nurse must be skillful in balancing her need to monitor vital signs closely against the family's need for a personal experience free of interruption and unnecessary technologic intervention.

Maternal–Neonatal Recovery Room

The maternal–neonatal recovery room provides the family with an opportunity to remain together during the first 4 to 6 hours after birth. Parents can become acquainted with their infant while the neonate is awake and particularly alert to external stimuli. Because the infant is frequently placed under a radiant warmer and attached to an electronic temperature probe in this setting, the nurse can easily monitor skin temperature and color. Adequate light sources for inspection and resuscitation equipment are also available. The nurse remains in the recovery room and can observe the infant frequently.

Because the recovery room is a more institutional, less intimate environment than a birthing room, more care must be taken to foster a meaningful family experience. Curtains may be drawn around the family to provide privacy. Noise levels should be minimized. Care should be taken to limit interruptions of the family–infant acquaintance process. The nurse may also use the opportunity provided by the neonatal assessment to acquaint the parents with the unique characteristics of their baby.

Admission Nursery

An admission nursery is frequently used when the mother or infant is ill and requires special care immediately after birth. A normal newborn may also be placed in the nursery after delivery by cesarean birth while the mother remains in the postsurgical recovery room. The admission nursery has special resuscitation and monitoring equipment that may be required during the transition period. The newborn is usually placed under a radiant warmer and a temperature probe is attached to the skin. The nurse monitors the neonate and is responsible for the infant's care and emotional support.

The nurse must be creative in planning family-centered care for the newborn placed in an admission nursery. If possible, the father can accompany the infant to the nursery. The admission procedures can be explained and teaching can be done during the admission assessment to facilitate father–infant acquaintance. The father can be encouraged to hold the newborn while the infant is awake, alert, and receptive to external stimuli. A continual effort must be made to provide the mother with information about her infant. It is important that both parents feel that the nurse caring for their baby is sensitive to the infant's needs for comfort and love.

Table 32–1   Environmental Factors That Influence the Quality of Family-Centered Neonatal Nursing Care

Type of Environment	Advantages	Disadvantages
Birthing center (separate from hospital)	Homelike environment Elimination of "high-tech" atmosphere Low-stress environment for staff and client Good opportunity for personalized nursing care Mother and infant may remain together during sensitive alert period right after birth Low exposure to pathogens found in hospital environment Cost effectiveness for low-risk clients Good opportunity for mother to breast-feed when infant demonstrates readiness	Absence of advanced life-support equipment Little opportunity for frequent monitoring of neonate Potential separation of parents from infant if neonatal transport is necessary Not universally available for clients with limited income
Alternative birthing room (Labor–Delivery–Recovery Room)	Homelike environment Elimination of "high-tech" atmosphere Low-stress environment for staff and client Advanced life-support equipment available in most facilities Good opportunity for family privacy Good opportunity for early discharge Mother and infant may remain together during sensitive alert period right after birth Good opportunity for mother to breast-feed when infant demonstrates readiness	Life-support equipment frequently not in room if needed Less than optimum conditions for immediate resuscitation of neonate (oxygen, adequate light) Potential for disruptions in bonding due to interruptions by hospital staff Exposure to hospital pathogens Little opportunity for close monitoring of infant (poor lighting, request for privacy, bundling of infant)
Mother–infant recovery room	Resuscitation and life-support equipment in room Good opportunity for frequent monitoring of neonate Mother and infant remain together during sensitive alert period right after birth Good opportunity for mother to breast-feed when infant demonstrates readiness	New family remains in "high-tech" environment Few opportunities for family privacy Sensory stimuli may decrease or otherwise alter neonatal behavioral responses Exposure to hospital pathogens Little opportunity for personalized nursing care
Admission nursery; central nursery	Resuscitation and life-support equipment available in room Continual monitoring of neonate possible Efficient use of nursing staff Nursing staff can care for neonate if mother ill or fatigued	Parents and infant are separated during sensitive alert awake period right after birth Sensory stimuli may decrease or otherwise alter neonatal behavioral responses Little opportunity for personalized nursing care Exposure to hospital pathogens Little opportunity for mother to breast-feed when infant demonstrates readiness Risk of iatrogenic illness due to invasive monitoring

NURSING RESEARCH

Infant Rooming-In and Maternal Sleep

The limited practice of rooming-in in some hospitals appears related to the belief that placing the infant in the nursery at night provides the new mother with an opportunity for better rest and undisturbed sleep. A study by Keefe (1988) challenges this assumption. The impact of rooming-in on maternal sleep was examined. Ten women returned their infants to the nursery at night, but infants were brought out for feeding if requested. Eleven women kept their infants during the night. A self-report form completed by the subjects found no significant differences in the number of hours slept or the quality of sleep between the two groups. Further research is indicated to support these findings, particularly with groups of women who do not request that infants be brought to them at night for feeding.

Keefe MR: The impact of infant rooming-in on maternal sleep at night. J Obstet Gynecol Neonatal Nurs 17(2):122–126, 1988

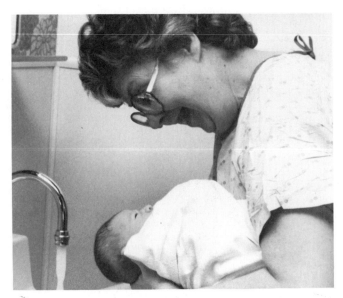

Figure 32–1. The nurse provides individualized care, comfort, and stimulation for the newborn. (Photo: BABES, Inc.)

Rooming-In

The majority of hospitals in the United States today provide mothers with the opportunity to keep their infants with them in the postpartum unit. This arrangement, known as *rooming-in,* allows mother and infant to become acquainted through continuous contact 24 hours a day. The nurse caring for the infant plans to perform as much of her care as possible at the mother's bedside. She uses this time to teach parents and to facilitate the acquaintance process. The nurse can also help build the mother's self-confidence in her new role by guiding her initial efforts in infant care and providing her with frequent positive feedback. The father should be welcome in this environment; he should be included in teaching sessions and encouraged in his efforts to learn parenting skills.

Central Nursery

Hospitals frequently provide parents with a central nursery where the infant can be cared for if the mother is ill during the postpartum period. A mother who is rooming-in may also use the central nursery during visiting hours or when she feels she would like a night of uninterrupted sleep before returning home with her new baby. The nurse is responsible for the care and emotional support of the newborn while he or she remains in the nursery (Fig. 32–1). Care should be organized to allow the infant periods of quiet sleep between feedings and assessments. If the mother is ill, the nurse should make every effort to incorporate visits with her infant into the plan of care. The nurse must keep the mother informed of her infant's condition; she should also encourage the father to visit the infant in the nursery and support him in his efforts to care for the baby.

CARE OF THE NEWBORN DURING TRANSITION TO EXTRAUTERINE LIFE

The nurse is in a unique position to help the neonate make major physiologic and behavioral adaptations following birth (Fig. 32–2).

In most postpartum health care settings the nurse is the health team member who provides direct care to the infant immediately after birth. Although the majority of infants successfully accomplish the transition to extrauterine life, the first hours after birth are a critical period of adjustment.

Assessment

The nurse must know the mother's prenatal history and the course of her labor and delivery in order to support the neonate's extrauterine adaptation effectively. Maternal

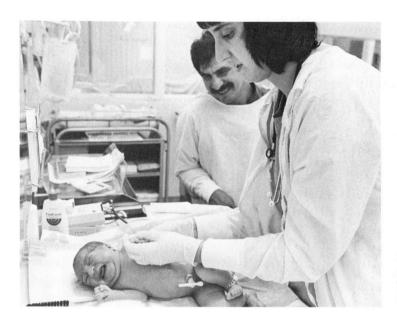

Figure 32–2. The nurse assists the newborn with its initial physiologic and behavioral adaptations to extrauterine life. (Courtesy of John B. Franklin Maternity Hospital, formerly Booth Maternity Center, Philadelphia)

NURSING ALERT

Universal Precautions for Neonatal Nurses

Since the prenatal history, physical exam, and laboratory tests cannot reliably identify all women infected with the human immunodeficiency virus (HIV) or other blood-borne pathogens, such as hepatitis, the US Department of Health and Human Services has recommended universal body substance precautions be established in *ALL* settings for *ALL* patients.

1. All health care workers should use appropriate barrier precautions to prevent skin and mucous membrane exposure to blood and body fluids. (All nurses should carry a clean pair of gloves in their pocket to quickly apply in emergency situations when gloves are *not* readily available.)
   (a) Gloves and protective skin coverings (gowns, plastic aprons) should be used when handling newborns before and during the first bath.
   (b) Gloves should be worn during venipuncture, heel stick and IV insertion procedures.
   (c) Gloves should be worn when applying pressure to accomplish hemostasis after venipuncture, heel stick, or IV removal procedures.
   (d) Gloves should be worn when changing diapers and when collecting and testing urine or stool samples.
   (e) Gloves should be worn when suctioning infants.
   (f) Eye goggles or face masks should be worn during procedures that are likely to generate splashing, such as the neonate's first bath and circumcision.

2. Hands, skin surfaces, eyes, and mucous membranes

should be washed immediately if contaminated with body fluids.

3. Precautions should be taken to prevent injuries caused by needles or other sharp instruments.
   (a) Needles should not be recapped or purposely bent or broken after use but placed directly into a puncture-resistant container (*e.g.*, after vitamin K administration).
   (b) Heel stick lancets should be disposed of immediately after use in a puncture-resistant container.
   (c) Reusable sharp instruments, such as circumcision instruments, should be placed in puncture-resistant containers for transport to the reprocessing area.

4. Resuscitation bags and infant masks should be available for use in all infant care areas to minimize the need for mouth-to-mouth resuscitation.

5. Manual suction devices, such as the De Lee Mucus Trap, should no longer be used to aspirate mucus, blood, or meconium from the neonate's airway. Meconium aspirators and mechanical suction equipment should be available in all infant care areas. Adaptors are available to connect mucus-trap catheters to wall suction if aspiration is needed for testing.

6. Health care workers who have exudative lesions or weeping dermatitis should refrain from all direct patient contact and patient equipment contact until the condition resolves.

illness, poor nutrition, and even psychosocial problems during pregnancy may have a direct effect on the infant's condition at birth. Obstetric complications and drugs administered during labor and delivery will also affect the newborn's responses immediately after birth. The nurse should know the infant's 1- and 5-minute Apgar scores and the type of delivery room care the mother received (see Chap. 24). It is particularly important for the nurse to note if there was any evidence of asphyxia at birth.

The infant is weighed and measured, and the first set of vital signs is taken soon after birth. Temperature, apical heart rate, and respiratory rate are recorded and reassessed at least every 30 minutes for the first hour and then once an hour for the next 4 to 6 hours. A blood pressure may be included in the initial assessment.

Once the nurse has completed assessment of the neonate (as discussed in Chapter 31) and has identified any problems, a nursing care plan is initiated. Many institutions have developed standardized care plans that can be adapted to the individual needs of each infant.

Diagnosis

Based on her review of labor and delivery records as well as other elements of the nurse's assessment upon admission (see previous chapter), the nurse formulates applicable diagnoses. The following are nursing diagnoses that reflect possible problems that may arise in transitional care of the newborn and may be addressed independently. Priorities in care may be established based on these diagnoses.

- Ineffective thermoregulation
- Ineffective airway clearance
- Altered cardiac output: decreased
- Altered nutrition: less than body requirements
- Altered parenting

Complications requiring collaboration with other members of the health care team may arise during transitional care. Such complications include infection, hypoglycemia, hemorrhage, and hyperbilirubinemia. Thus, in addition to routine care, the nurse is responsible for monitoring for potential complications. Monitoring for these complications is discussed at the end of this section on transitional care.

Planning and Implementation

When planning nursing care to meet identified patient needs, the nurse must take into account the length of time the mother and newborn are likely to be hospitalized, the mother's physical condition, the emotional state and learning needs of parents and other family members, and the physiologic adaptations required of the newborn. Nursing care planning may be based on standards of care or standardized care plans for the nursery. Nursing interventions in the transitional period focus on prevention and early identification of physiologic complications, assessment of extrauterine adaptation, establishment of a feeding pattern, and support of the parent–infant attachment. Preparation for discharge is begun early when the teaching plan is initiated shortly after birth. Procedures during this period are routine and must be anticipated and planned for in the care plan.

Promoting Physiologic Adaptation

Promoting Adaptation to Environmental Temperature

Thermoregulation is discussed in detail in Chapter 31. The nurse must carefully dry the infant to prevent heat loss by evaporation. Particular attention should be paid to drying the head, which is 25% of the total body length. If the neonate is to remain with the mother in a birthing room, he or she should be double-wrapped in warm, dry blankets, and a stockinette cap should be placed on his or her head. The room should be free of drafts.

The infant's temperature is taken at the beginning of the admission assessment and then at least every hour for the next 4 to 6 hours. If the infant is hypothermic (has a temperature below 97.5°F [36.4°C]), it may be necessary to temporarily place him or her under a radiant warmer or in an isolette. Direct skin-to-skin contact with the mother is also an excellent method for preventing hypothermia and heat loss. Use of a radiant warmer requires attachment of an electronic skin probe to the infant's skin surface to monitor the temperature (Fig. 32–3). Axillary temperature should also be taken every 30 minutes for the first 2 hours of use of the radiant warmer to preclude the development of hyperthermia.

If vital signs remain stable, the infant is usually bathed to remove vernix, dried blood, and mucus from the skin and hair and then moved to an open crib and placed in his or her mother's room or a central nursery. A 3% hexachlorophene solution may be used once to decrease the risk of staphylococcal skin infection; however, this is not done routinely since it is absorbed through the skin and is neurotoxic. Care should be taken to prevent hypothermia during the bath. The infant should be bathed quickly. Afterward, if his or her temperature has not dropped below 97.5°F (36.4°C), the infant is double-wrapped in warm blankets with a stockinette cap on his or her head and placed in an open crib. If his or her temperature is low, the infant is placed back under the radiant warmer until it has stabilized.

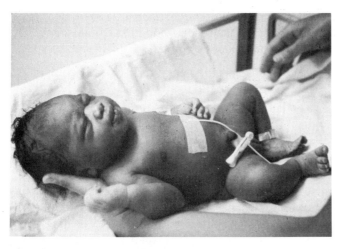

Figure 32-3. The neonate is placed in a radiant warmer and a heat sensor is taped to the abdomen to monitor skin temperature. (Photo: Childbirth Graphics)

Expected Outcome: Newborn maintains a stable temperature as evidenced by axillary temperature of 36.4 to 37.2°C within 1 to 2 hours of birth.

Promoting Respiratory Adaptation

The neonate may need assistance with respiratory adaptations immediately after birth, since regurgitation of mucus may lead to obstruction of the airway. A bulb syringe should be available for clearing the nose and mouth (Fig. 32-4). An 8 or 10 French catheter attached to wall suction (low-pressure setting) should be available since stomach contents are sometimes aspirated to prevent regurgitation of gastric fluids.

Immediately after delivery the newborn may be placed in Trendelenburg's position (supine, with the head tilted down) to facilitate drainage of fluids.

NURSING ALERT

Prevention of Aspiration

If the infant begins to gag or choke or becomes suddenly cyanotic:

1. Turn the infant on his or her side or abdomen with the head slightly lower than the feet (10–15 degree angle).
2. Pat the infant firmly on the back to encourage drainage of fluids from the mouth and nose.
3. Insert a bulb syringe* or suction catheter attached to wall suction (on low pressure) into the mouth first and remove all secretions.
4. Suction both nares.
5. If the infant is apneic or remains cyanotic after secretions are removed from the mouth and nose, apply 100% oxygen by resuscitation bag and mask apparatus until color improves and breathing is resumed.

* Be sure to compress the bulb first before placing the tip of bulb syringe into the infant's mouth or nares. Several compressions/insertions with a bulb syringe may be needed to clear the mouth completely.

The use of Trendelenburg's position is controversial, and a side-lying position without a tilt may be just as effective. The head down position causes increased intracranial pressure and may increase the risk of intraventricular hemorrhage, especially if there was cephalopelvic disproportion, prolonged labor, or forceps or vacuum extraction. If this position is used, there should not be more

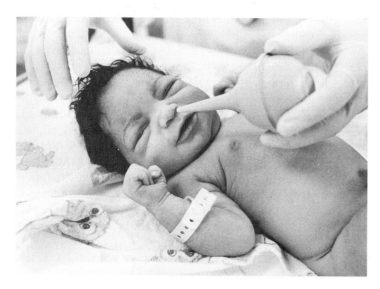

Figure 32-4. A bulb syringe is used to suction mucus from the neonate's nose and mouth. The bulb is compressed before insertion into the nares or mouth and then released to create suction. (Photo: Childbirth Graphics)

NURSING RESEARCH

The Use of Cover Gowns: A Nursery Ritual

An almost universal ritual found in American newborn nurseries is the practice of requiring all persons entering the well-baby nursery to don cover gowns (including the neonate's parents). Recently, the efficacy of this practice is being reevaluated. The majority of studies have concluded that the risk of transmission of infectious agents to the infant by the clothing of nurses or the newborn's parents is negligible (less than 2 per 10,000 infants). It was also discovered that while the gowning policy is scrupulously adhered to, nursery staff often fail to wash their hands before and after contact with the infant. Handwashing is the single most important preventative measure in controlling infection.

In this age of cost control and consumer awareness of rising health care costs, it is essential that nurses evaluate the fiscal consequences of all nursery practices. Further research to confirm preliminary findings regarding gowning policies is required, but it appears appropriate at this time to revise current thinking regarding who should gown and when. Several medical centers across the country have eliminated the requirement of cover gowns for personnel who enter the well-baby nursery but do not come in direct contact with the neonate. This has resulted in the savings of thousands of dollars per month in gown supplies and laundry costs.

Larson E: Rituals in infection control: What works in the newborn nursery? J Obstet Gynecol Neonatal Nurs 16:411–415, 1987

than a 15-degree incline. Once stabilized, the newborn should be positioned on his or her side. The infant should never be left unattended in a supine position, since in this position there is the danger of aspiration of mucus or fluid regurgitated from the stomach.

Respiratory function is directly affected by body temperature. Infants who are chilled are most likely to suffer respiratory complications for several reasons. First, hypothermia leads to increased oxygen consumption and tachypnea. Second, cold drafts over the neonate's face and chest can cause apnea. Finally, cold stress leads to a decrease in surfactant production.

Neonates may regurgitate mucus or milk at any time but are particularly likely to do so during the second period of reactivity, when the gastrointestinal and central nervous systems are in a state of hyperactivity. (Periods of reactivity are discussed in Chapter 31.) As a result of their physiologic and anatomic immaturity, infants are at risk

of aspiration when they suddenly regurgitate large amounts of fluid. The following nursing actions should minimize the risk of aspiration:

- Have available emergency resuscitation equipment, including wall suction and oxygen.
- At the time of admission place a bulb syringe in the infant's crib, where it is easily visible and readily available.
- Evaluate the sucking and swallowing reflexes of the infant before the first feeding.
- Test the patency of the esophagus and rule out esophageal and tracheal anomalies by giving the infant a small amount of sterile water before the first feeding.
- Avoid overfeeding the formula-fed infant.
- Carefully bubble the infant after each feeding.
- Always position the infant on his or her side or abdomen when placing him or her in the crib.
- Teach the mother about proper feeding, burping, and positioning of the infant.
- Demonstrate proper use of the bulb syringe to the mother (instructions for use are given later in the chapter, page 989).

Expected Outcome: Newborn breathes without assistance as evidenced by normal respiration between 40 and 60 breaths/min within 2 hours of birth.

Promoting Circulatory and Cardiac Adaptation

The nurse can best support circulatory and cardiac adaptation by maintaining the infant's temperature within normal limits and clearing all mucus from the airways so that the respiratory system is not compromised. She should examine the umbilical cord to make sure that the cord clamp is secure and that there is no bleeding from its base.

The brachial, radial, femoral, popliteal, and dorsalis pedis pulses are palpated in the neonate. The pulses are assessed for equality, amplitude, and rhythmicity. Simultaneous palpation of right and left pulses and lower and upper pulses assists the nurse in evaluating structural integrity of the cardiovascular system. Obstruction between the right and left subclavian arteries will result in stronger pulses in the right arm. Diminished strength in lower extremity pulses is associated with coarctation of the aorta, hip dysplasia, and thrombus formation secondary to placement of an umbilical artery catheter. Bounding pulses may indicate patent ductus arteriosus.

The quality of pulses is normally documented using a numerical scale. Although several different scales have been devised to assist clinicians in the assessment of pulses, the scale recommended by the American Association of Critical-Care Nurses is described here because it recognizes the full range of pulse amplitude that may be palpated in the neonate: 0 = absent pulse, 1+ = palpable pulse, 2+ = normal pulse, 3+ = full pulse, and 4+ = bounding pulse.

The skin on the infant's trunk and extremities is blanched periodically for assessment of central and peripheral capillary fill time (CFT), an indirect evaluation of tissue perfusion. Central CFT is normally 3 seconds or less. Peripheral CFT may be longer owing to the normally sluggish peripheral perfusion of the newborn. *Polycythemia* is a condition that exacerbates the normally sluggish peripheral perfusion of the newborn and may lead to thrombosis in brain tissue or other organs. An exchange transfusion is usually performed to prevent circulatory compromise to vital organs when the hematocrit is greater than 70%. (See Chap. 34 for further information on polycythemia.)

Expected Outcome: Newborn demonstrates normal cardiac output as evidenced by a regular heart rate of 120–160 beats per minute within 2 hours of birth.

Promoting Newborn Nutrition

Many infants breast-feed immediately after birth or some time during the transition period. If the neonate has not nursed or is to be bottle fed, the nurse initiates the feeding process. The infant is usually given a small amount of sterile water initially for assessment of the integrity of the suck, swallow, and gag reflexes. If the infant has difficulty with this feeding and aspiration occurs, the use of sterile water minimizes potential lung damage. Glucose water is not an acceptable test fluid for the first feeding, because it is as traumatic to lung tissue as is formula. A small amount of water is sufficient; if the baby has no problem, formula can be substituted immediately, thereby preventing a delay in feeding.

The patency of the esophagus is also assessed during the initial sterile water feeding. A very small number of infants are born with an abnormal connection between the esophagus and trachea (tracheoesophageal fistula, or TEF). The esophagus itself may end in a blind pouch. Infants with this condition are often identified by excessive drooling or episodes of cyanosis even before the introduction of formula or breast milk. If any infant presents with these signs or gags and becomes cyanotic during the first feeding, a thorough examination of the upper gastrointestinal tract must be performed to rule out TEF. An infant who is breast-fed before the sterile water feeding should be observed closely for evidence of choking or cyanosis.

Breast-feeding, formula feeding, and nursing care related to maternal and infant nutrition are discussed in Chapter 37. However, the following sections on demand feeding and safety considerations apply to both breast-fed and bottle-fed infants in the hospitalization period.

Demand Feeding. A frequent question is "How will I know when my baby has had enough milk?" The concept of demand feeding should be discussed with both breast-feeding and formula-feeding mothers. The normal newborn stops sucking and frequently falls asleep when full and satisfied. The infant can be expected to wake as often as every 2 hours, especially in the first few days after birth while the lactation process is being established. Breast-feeding is most successful and mothers experience fewest engorgement and nipple problems when they nurse their infants frequently (every 2 to 3 hours).

The formula-fed baby normally remains satisfied for longer (4 hours or more) than the breast-fed infant owing to slower digestion of formula than breast milk. When feeding her infant, the mother should watch for signs of satiety. The infant will slowly cease sucking and may actually let his or her mouth drop open slightly or push the nipple forward with his or her tongue. If the infant is full, small amounts of formula may drool from the corner of the mouth as he or she relaxes and stops sucking. As the infant begins to drift off to sleep, efforts to stimulate further feeding by jiggling or pumping the nipple should be avoided. By the third day of life most full-term neonates are taking 2 to 4 oz of milk per feeding (Fig. 32–5).

Safety Considerations During Feeding. Basic rules of safety should be discussed with the mother during and after feeding and reinforced with subsequent teaching. The mother should be instructed in the use of the bulb syringe to clear the nose and mouth if milk is regurgitated. Proper positioning of the infant on his or her side or stomach after feeding to avoid aspiration of regurgitated milk should also be demonstrated.

The nurse should discuss with the mother the dangers of "bottle propping," laying an infant on his or her back with the bottle propped in his or her mouth. Bottle propping deprives the infant of close physical contact essential for normal growth and development and increases the risk of aspiration. It is particularly important that the nurse stress the danger of aspiration and caution the mother never to leave her infant unattended during a feeding.

Formula Feeding. The nurse should also assist the mother who is formula feeding with the first feeding. Principles of positioning for comfort are similar to those applied to breast-feeding mothers. The mother is usually helped to a sitting position and the infant placed in her

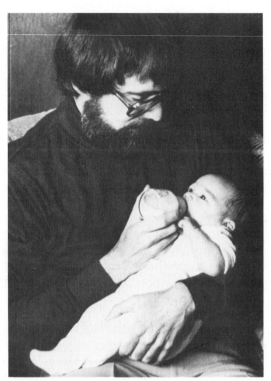

Figure 32-5. If the newborn is to be bottle fed, the nurse can encourage the father's involvement by assisting him in feeding. (Photo: BABES, Inc.)

arms with his or her back at approximately a 45-degree angle. She is then guided in eliciting the rooting reflex and placing the nipple well into the baby's mouth. The bottle is then positioned so that the neck and nipple are always filled with formula. This prevents the infant from swallowing excessive amounts of air.

The amount of formula to be given at the first feeding should be discussed with the mother; immediately after birth the newborn may take only 20 to 30 ml (1 oz) of formula owing to a limited stomach capacity. Burping techniques should be demonstrated. The infant can be placed in a sitting position with head and neck supported while the back is gently patted and massaged; alternatively, the newborn may be placed against the mother's shoulder or across her lap in a prone position.

All questions should be answered and positive reinforcement and praise given frequently during the feeding. The amount of information given to the mother at this time should be confined to basic instructions so that she is not overwhelmed and can enjoy this special time with her new baby. Instruction regarding methods for sterilization of bottles and nipples should be planned for subsequent feedings as part of the nurse's discharge teaching (see later in this chapter).

Expected Outcomes: Mother demonstrates ability to feed newborn by discharge. Newborn begins to take nourishment within 4 to 8 hours.

Promoting Behavioral Adaptation

Promoting Parent–Infant Interaction

Because the infant is awake and particularly alert to visual and auditory stimuli during the first period of reactivity (up to 1 hour after birth), this is an ideal time for the nurse to foster parent–infant interaction (Fig. 32–6). Eye prophylaxis can be delayed up to 1 hour to enhance the quality of early contact with parents. The new family should be offered privacy but with the understanding that a nurse is close by if she is needed.

Klaus and Kennell (1982), from their studies of early parent–infant interaction and an extensive review of related research, conclude that the first few hours after birth may be a particularly sensitive period for the formation of bonds between parents and infant. Certain types of nursing intervention may facilitate the formation of these ties. Skin-to-skin contact between mother and infant may enhance the quality of early interaction and can be combined with breast-feeding if the mother plans to nurse the newborn.

Health professionals should reassure concerned parents who have not had an opportunity for early contact that infants are quite adaptable and that the parent–infant relationship evolves over time as a result of repeated, mutually satisfying encounters.

Parent–infant interactions should be observed and significant findings recorded in the newborn's chart. Once the neonate's condition is stabilized, the nurse should provide the parents and their newborn with further opportunities to become acquainted; for example, rooming-in or extended periods of contact during the day

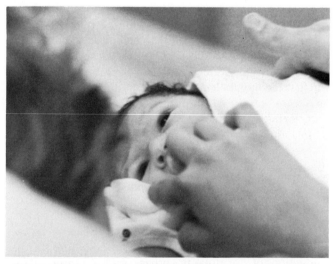

Figure 32-6. An alert newborn sucks on his mother's finger and gazes at her face only minutes after delivery. The nurse should facilitate this type of close contact in the first hour of life as the parents wish and as the newborn's condition allows. (Photo: BABES, Inc.)

can be encouraged. The nurse should facilitate the acquaintance process through teaching and support. Using principles of adult learning, the nurse begins with simple tasks that can be easily accomplished by new parents and moves on to more complex activities as the parents gain confidence in their ability to care for their infant. The subjects of cord care and diaper changing thus precede taking and reading the infant's temperature or bathing the infant. The nurse who is expert in handling and caring for newborns must be especially patient with first-time parents and avoid taking over when parents are slow and uncertain.

Another important nursing activity that facilitates the parent–infant acquaintance process is teaching about normal newborn characteristics and each infant's unique capabilities. Several studies suggest that teaching a mother about her infant's unique behaviors makes a positive difference in her sensitivity to the newborn's cues and her response to her infant's distress signals (Furr and Kirgis 1982; Riesch and Munns, 1984).

The nurse should use every opportunity to point out infant behaviors to the parents and describe their meaning and purpose. As much infant care as possible should be done at the mother's bedside to increase opportunities for teaching and reinforcement of parenting skills. An excellent strategy for facilitating the acquaintance process is to have the parents present when the neonate is examined by the nurse practitioner or pediatrician. Parents can also be invited to observe the Brazelton Neonatal Behavioral Assessment of their infant if it is done in the nursery.

Expected Outcome: Newborn and parents demonstrate interaction evidenced by touching, eye contact, and responding to each other.

Monitoring for Complications

Optimum physiologic adaptation to extrauterine life is the primary goal of the transitional period. The nurse has the responsibility of monitoring the newborn for potential complications. The nurse caring for the normal neonate is responsible for monitoring and preventing, as far as possible, the following complications.

Infection

The nurse caring for the neonate is responsible for minimizing the newborn's exposure to pathogenic organisms.

It is essential that each person coming in contact with the newborn observe principles of asepsis. *Handwashing is the single most important preventive measure.* Health

personnel providing direct care should remove all rings, bracelets, and wristwatches before handling the infant, because such pieces of jewelry are common fomites. Other procedures to be followed in the prevention of infection include the following:

- Providing separate supplies for each infant (*e.g.,* cotton balls, diapers, blankets)
- Limiting the number of infants placed in the nursery to allow adequate space between cribs (they should be at least 18 inches apart, and aisles should be at least 3 feet wide)
- Limiting the number of personnel who may enter the nursery
- Providing cover gowns for non-nursing personnel who enter the nursery
- Following established guidelines regarding the restriction of personnel with infections (respiratory tract infections, diarrhea, open wounds, infectious skin rashes, herpesvirus, and other communicable diseases)
- Encouraging frequent and prolonged contact between mother and infant (*e.g.,* rooming-in, skin-to-skin contact, and breast-feeding)

Eye Prophylaxis.   Eye prophylaxis is an essential aspect of care. Before institution of the practice of instilling silver nitrate drops in newborns' eyes, thousands of infants suffered permanent blindness as a result of *ophthalmia neonatorum,* a severe ocular infection due to gonorrhea. Today most states require the administration of a prophylactic agent in the eyes of all neonates to pre-

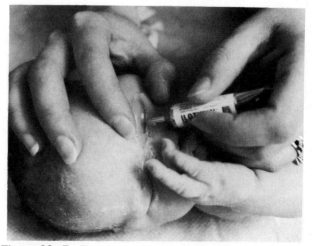

Figure 32–7. The nurse administers either silver nitrate solution or erythromycin ophthalmic ointment to prevent ocular infection. Administration may be delayed several hours after birth to allow the infant to see clearly during its first period of reactivity immediately after birth. (Photo: Childbirth Graphics)

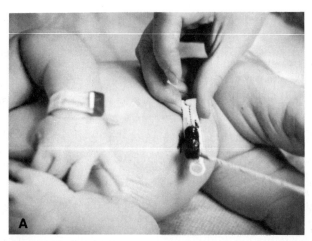
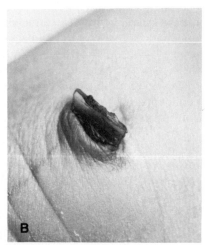

Figure 32–8. The umbilical cord stump may be painted with antibacterial solution after birth *(A)*. Special care must be taken to avoid risk of infection until the clamp has been removed and the cord stump has dried *(B)*. (Photo: Childbirth Graphics)

vent infection and blindness. Acceptable agents that prevent gonococcal ophthalmia neonatorum include: silver nitrate solution (1%), erythromycin (0.5%) ophthalmic ointment or drops, and tetracycline (1%) ophthalmic ointment or drops (Fig. 32–7).

Silver nitrate solution is a caustic chemical that can cause irritation of ocular mucous membranes and, in a small percentage of cases, a severe conjunctivitis with purulent eye drainage. As a result, many health care facilities have begun using a less irritating drug, erythromycin, for eye prophylaxis. Because use of either agent temporarily interferes with the infant's ability to see clearly, it is recommended that instillation of the drug be delayed for one hour after birth to allow the neonate unimpaired eye contact with the parents.

Cord Care.   Another aspect of preventive nursing care is special care of the umbilical cord (Fig. 32–8). Many nurseries apply an antibiotic ointment (*e.g.,* bacitracin) or an antibacterial solution (Triple Dye) to the umbilical cord after birth and each day thereafter to reduce the chance of omphalitis, an inflammation of the umbilical cord. This practice is frequently abandoned in birthing units, since infection is much less likely to develop in a rooming-in setting than in a central nursery with a large number of infants.

In the majority of health care facilities, the umbilical cord is swabbed with alcohol at each diaper change to remove urine and stool and to facilitate the desiccation process. The diaper should be folded below the cord. Although no method of cord care has been proven to effectively prevent omphalitis, there is general agreement that the umbilical area should be kept clean and exposed to air to promote healing and drying (Mugford et al 1986).

Hypoglycemia

Because the newborn's brain is almost entirely dependent on glucose for its metabolic functioning, early detection of hypoglycemia is essential for prevention of neurologic impairment and injury. *Hypoglycemia* is defined as a blood glucose level under 30 mg/dl whole blood during the first 72 hours of life in the full-term neonate.

Many nurseries obtain a heel stick capillary blood sample for hematocrit determination (see the display, opposite page, and Fig. 32–9). Prior to the procedure, the infant's heel is warmed to increase capillary blood flow. A warm, moist compress or a chemical heat pack specifically designed for neonatal heel stick procedures is ap-

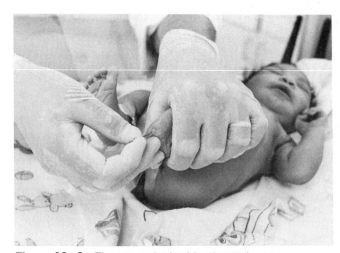

Figure 32–9. The nurse obtains blood samples to assess blood glucose levels and for other screening tests, using a heelstick procedure. (Photo: Childbirth Graphics)

NURSING ALERT

Appropriate Site for Heel Stick

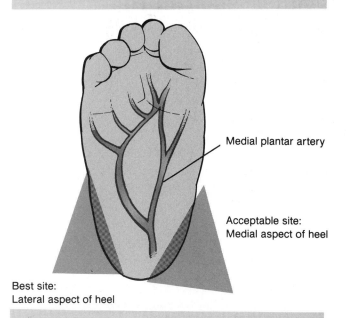

Medial plantar artery

Acceptable site:
Medial aspect of heel

Best site:
Lateral aspect of heel

Heel Stick Procedure

1. Warm infant's heel for about 10 minutes, using a warm, moist wrap or a specially designed chemical heat pad.
2. Stabilize the infant's foot by placing your thumb behind the heel and dorsiflexing the foot against the shin.
3. Circle the heel stick site firmly with hand but *do not squeeze.*
4. Cleanse selected heel stick site with alcohol and blot dry with sterile gauze.
5. Using microlancet (pediatric size), puncture skin with one quick downward movement toward heel.
6. Allow small drop of blood to form and then wipe away with sterile gauze to remove skin cells from puncture site.
7. Allow second large drop to form (avoid squeezing) and fall onto the glucose-sensitive strip.
8. Follow manufacturer's direction for timing of test and interpretation of results.

Art from Childbirth Graphics

plied for approximately 10 minutes. The puncture site is cleansed with alcohol and dried thoroughly with a gauze pad so that the blood will form a discreet drop. The first drop of blood obtained is wiped away to reduce the chance

of sample dilution with tissue fluid. Squeezing the puncture site is also avoided for the same reason.

After the sample is obtained, the bottom of the hematocrit tube is sealed to prevent leakage. It is then placed in a centrifuge. The specimen is spun for approximately 4 to 5 minutes, and then read using a graph or measuring device that estimates the percentage of red blood cells. A hematocrit above 65% to 70% may be indicative of polycythemia. A venous blood sample is obtained in this instance to confirm the diagnosis of true polycythemia, defined as a central hematocrit value greater than 65%.

Early feeding and prevention of cold stress reduce the risk of hypoglycemia. Immediate intervention is necessary when hypoglycemia is diagnosed to prevent depression of vital functions controlled by the central nervous system. Seizures and apnea are potential complications of untreated hypoglycemia. Treatment consists of a slowly administered intravenous bolus of 10% to 25% glucose followed by administration of a continuous intravenous infusion of 10% glucose until blood glucose levels are stabilized. Further discussion of hypoglycemia can be found in Chapter 34.

Hemorrhage

Because intrauterine circulating stores of vitamin K are depleted and enteric production is still low at birth, the newborn experiences a transient deficiency in the vitamin. This places the newborn at risk for hemorrhage from 2 to 5 days after birth, with bleeding problems most common on the second or third day of life. To prevent bleeding, a 0.5 mg to 1 mg dose of vitamin K (phytonadione) is administered intramuscularly after birth. The vastus lateralis or rectus muscle of the anterior thigh is the preferred site of injection (Fig. 32–10).

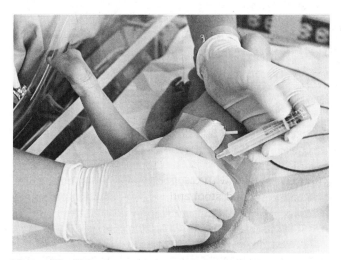

Figure 32–10A. Intramuscular injection of vitamin K prevents excessive bleeding in the neonatal period when endogenous production of the vitamin is still low. (Photo: Childbirth Graphics)

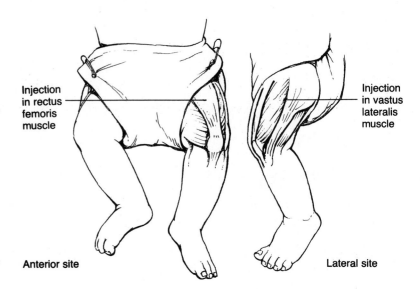

Figure 32–10B. Sites for intramuscular injections in infants.

Injection in rectus femoris muscle

Injection in vastus lateralis muscle

Anterior site

Lateral site

Hyperbilirubinemia

Nursing care is also directed at reducing the incidence and severity of neonatal physiologic jaundice. Bilirubin conjugation and jaundice are discussed in Chapter 31.

Because artificial lighting and colored walls in the nursery hinder accurate evaluation of skin color, detection is best accomplished by careful inspection of the infant in natural light. Jaundice first appears on the head and over the face and then spreads toward the lower extremities. In fair-skinned infants the face and sclera should be inspected first. The skin over the bridge of the nose should be blanched to reveal underlying jaundice. In newborns with dark skin pigmentation, the gums and buccal mucosa should be examined. The nurse should then proceed toward the toes, blanching the skin over bony prominences to determine the extent of icterus.

Specific nursing actions that aid in the prevention of jaundice and decrease serum bilirubin levels are the following:

- Prevention of cold stress
- Initiation of early and frequent feedings
- Promotion of adequate hydration

Controversy still exists about whether breast-fed infants characterized as "slow" or "poor" feeders should receive formula or sterile water supplementation when jaundice develops. The nurse should make every effort to support the breast-feeding mother who desires to meet her infant's fluid and nutritional needs through breast milk alone. If bilirubin levels continue to rise and fluid or formula supplementation or phototherapy is deemed necessary, the mother should be encouraged to continue frequent nursing of the infant to speed reduction of bilirubin levels. See the accompanying Nursing Care Plan for low-risk infant with hyperbilirubinemia. Further treat-

ment and care of the high-risk newborn with jaundice is discussed in Chapter 34.

Expected Outcome: Newborn remains free of signs of hyperbilirubinemia, or signs resolve without further complications within 12 to 24 hours.

Evaluation of Transitional Care

The nurse is responsible for the ongoing evaluation of the appropriateness and effectiveness of transitional care during the neonate's adaptation to extrauterine life. Many units have standards of care to which the nurse is accountable in determining a neonate's readiness for transfer to the mother's room or central nursery. Such evaluation criteria include the following: absence of signs of respiratory distress; evidence of adequate thermoregulation; absence of signs of infection, hypoglycemia, or hyperbilirubinemia (including completion of laboratory work, as ordered); administration of prophylactic antibiotics and vitamin K, as ordered; and provision of support for early parent–neonate interaction. When these criteria are met, the nurse implements the plan for daily care of the newborn awaiting discharge.

ONGOING NEWBORN CARE

Many normal neonates spend the majority of their waking hours with parents in a modified rooming-in situation. Their internal regulatory mechanisms are able to main-

(text continued on page 983)

NURSING CARE PLAN

The Full-Term Newborn With Hyperbilirubinemia Receiving Phototherapy Treatment

Nursing Diagnosis (Patient Problem) and Assessment Data	Nursing Interventions	Rationale
Potential Complication: *hyperbilirubinemia* *Risk factors:* • Rh negative sensitized mother • ABO incompatibility of mother • Cephalhematoma/bruising of infant • Asphyxia • Infection premature rupture of membranes • Diabetes mellitus • Small for gestational age • Prematurity • Gastrointestinal obstruction in infant • Polycythemia • G_6PD deficiency	Observe infants with any of these risk factors for jaundice in the first 24 hr of life. When the mother is Rh negative or 0^+, check the infant's cord blood results for type and direct Coombs' test. If direct Coombs' is positive, notify the physician.	To promptly identify those infants at risk for hyperbilirubinemia. For the physiologic mechanisms of action for each indication, see Chapter 34.

Expected Outcome:

Newborn responds to feedings, hydration, and maintenance of temperature as evidenced by normal vital signs and normal color within 3 to 7 days of birth.

Probable Complication: *hyperbilirubinemia* • Jaundice of any amount in first 24 hr or development of pronounced jaundice after 24 hr	Notify the physician. Observe infant's color every 4 to 8 hr. Observe infant for lethargy. Prepare for laboratory determination of total/direct bilirubin. Begin phototherapy as ordered based on bilirubin. For full term infants, guidelines for initiation of phototherapy are:	Early identification of jaundice with monitoring and appropriate intervention is necessary to prevent high levels of indirect bilirubin from damaging the infant's central nervous system. Indirect bilirubin is photodegraded to water soluble direct bilirubin by the phototherapy light. In this form it can be readily excreted in the stool

(continued)

NURSING CARE PLAN (continued)

The Full-Term Newborn With Hyperbilirubinemia Receiving Phototherapy Treatment

Nursing Diagnosis (Patient Problem) and Assessment Data	Nursing Interventions	Rationale
	Total bilirubin >5 mg/dl >4 hr; 10–14 mg/dl at 24–48 hr; or total bilirubin increased >5 mg/dl per day (if direct bilirubin <50% of the total bilirubin)	and urine and helps prevent development of kernicterus (bilirubin encephalopathy)

Expected Outcome:

The neonate with hyperbilirubinemia responds to treatment and remains free of complications.

Potential Complication:
hypothermia/hyperthermia related to phototherapy

Risk factors: • Nudity • Frequent wet diapers leading to heat loss • External heat source and potential for malfunction	Undress the infant and place in warmed isolette. Check vital signs every 4 hr. Place the isolette with the nude infant in it under the phototherapy light source at a distance of 18 in.	To maintain neutral thermal environment. To monitor for temperature instability and hyperthermia. Nudity and frequent turning are necessary to provide maximum cutaneous exposure to the light for photodecomposition.
	A phototherapy light is either a Cavitron high-intensity tungsten lamp at 6–10 μw/cm^2 or a bank of fluorescent lights with a wavelength of 420 to 550 mm. Turn the infant every 2 hours.	

Expected Outcome:

Newborn maintains stable temperature as evidenced by axillary temperature of 36.4°C to 37.2°C throughout treatment.

Nursing Diagnosis:
potential for fluid volume deficit related to abnormal loss

Risk factors: • Increased insensible loss from heat source	Offer infant 5% dextrose in water or sterile water; 2 oz between feedings. Note number and characteristics of voidings and stools.	Provides increased hydration to facilitate excretion of direct bilirubin To ensure adequate elimination

Expected Outcome:

Newborn maintains adequate hydration throughout treatment.

(continued)

NURSING CARE PLAN (continued)

The Full-Term Newborn With Hyperbilirubinemia Receiving Phototherapy Treatment

Nursing Diagnosis (Patient Problem) and Assessment Data	Nursing Interventions	Rationale

Nursing Diagnosis:
potential for impaired tissue integrity related to diarrhea and frequent voiding

Risk factors: • Loose stools • Frequent wet diapers from increased fluids	Keep diaper area clean and dry. Avoid oil-based ointments that can cause burns when used with photo-therapy. Monitor serum sodium, potassium, and chloride.	Prevents perianal skin breakdown Increased electrolyte loss with diarrhea

Expected Outcome:

Newborn demonstrates normal tissue integrity as evidenced by normal tissue turgor and no skin breakdown throughout treatment.

Nursing Diagnosis:
potential for impaired (eye) tissue integrity related to phototherapy

	Cover the infant's eyes with protective patches.	To prevent retinal damage from light

Nursing Diagnosis:
sensory-perceptual alterations, visual, related to placement of eye patches

	Remove eye patches and examine the infant's eyes at least every 8 hr. This is done in conjunction with feedings.	To check for signs of conjunctivitis and provide visual sensory stimula-tion

Expected Outcome:

Newborn demonstrates no adverse effects related to phototherapy treatment

Potential Complication:
kernicterus (bilirubin encephalopathy)

Risk factors: • Documented increasing levels of serum bilirubin despite treatment • Delayed or nonexistent care in immediate postbirth period	Monitor for rising levels of serum bilirubin: Total bilirubin ≥ 10 mg/dl at 24 hr or 18 to 20 mg/dl after 24 hr. Direct bilirubin <50% of total bilirubin.	High levels of unconjugated bilirubin cross blood–brain barrier and bind with neurons, resulting in • Lethargy • Convulsions • Opisthotonos • Hypoxia • High-pitched cry

(continued)

The Full-Term Newborn With Hyperbilirubinemia Receiving Phototherapy Treatment

Nursing Diagnosis (Patient Problem) and Assessment Data	Nursing Interventions	Rationale
	Notify the physician. Transfer the infant to the intensive care nursery and prepare for an exchange transfusion (see Chapter 34).	Phototherapy alone is not enough to reduce dangerous levels of indirect bilirubin.

Expected Outcome:

Newborn demonstrates a total bilirubin of 1 gm/dl when treatment is discontinued and no signs of bilirubin encephalopathy.

Nursing Diagnosis:
potential for altered parenting related to anxiety and impaired attachment

Risk factors: • Parents uninformed about hyperbilirubinemia and alarmed by their baby's jaundice • Parents fearful and unwilling to participate in infant care.	Inform the parents about physiologic jaundice and other predisposing conditions their infant may have. Provide written materials that have been developed for parents. Describe the phototherapy to the parents and explain their infant's care. Show them the location of their infant's isolette.	Reduce parental anxiety.
	Encourage the mother and father to visit the nursery as often as desired and to sit by their infant receiving phototherapy.	Allow time for parental–infant bonding and for visual stimulation and socialization of the infant
	Remove the infant from the isolette every 4 hr for 30 min at a time to allow the parents to feed the baby. The infant may be taken to the mother's room, or she can be given a private place for infant feeding. Allow the mother to offer water between feedings while the infant is in the isolette	

Expected Outcome:

Parents verbalize their concerns for baby and demonstrate they understand the condition by repeating correct information and by participating in care.

tain physiologic adaptations made in the first hours of life with little if any support from care-givers. Infants begin to eat, sleep, and eliminate wastes with amazing regularity, and a watchful observer can see an impressive range of newborn reflexes demonstrated throughout the day, including rooting, sucking, sneezing, blinking, and the fencing and Moro reflexes.

Assessment

The nurse continues to evaluate the neonate at periodic intervals throughout the day, monitoring vital signs, fluid and caloric intake, elimination patterns, and weight gain or loss. Most institutions use a combination flow sheet–graphic record to note neonatal parameters of healthy adaptation. In addition, the infant is observed for evidence of the development of regular behavioral patterns (feeding, sleeping, and elimination) and for indications of his or her temperament.

Diagnosis

Ongoing nursing care of the normal neonate focuses on supporting ongoing physiological and behavioral adaptations as well as monitoring and supporting the neonate during procedures that may be done before discharge. The following nursing diagnoses reflect priorities useful in directing care:

- Fluid volume deficit
- Altered nutrition: less than body requirements
- Altered bowel elimination: constipation/diarrhea
- Altered parenting
- Altered health maintenance

Although the newborn may be normal in all aspects, monitoring for and preventing potential complications remains a priority in care. Potential complications for which the nurse monitors are poor adaptation of body systems, phenylketonuria (PKU), other inborn errors in metabolism, and congenital hypothyroidism.

Planning and Implementation

The nurse implements a plan of ongoing care for the normal newborn, recognizing that the discharge may occur as soon as 6 hours after birth. Further, since the neonate will ideally spend much of that time with the parents, the nurse must plan care to include ongoing assessment of the neonate's status, involvement of parents in care, and discharge teaching. Plans must also be initiated at this time if home follow-up is desirable, and a written discharge plan is completed as necessary.

Promoting Physiologic Adaptation
Promoting Hydration and Nutrition

The infant is weighed at the same time each day, usually in the morning before an early feeding so that an accurate estimate of weight gain or loss can be made. All clothing and the diaper are removed before the infant is weighed, and light-weight barrier paper (scale paper) is placed between the infant and the scale to prevent cross-contamination. The nurse must be careful to keep one hand just above the infant during the weighing process to prevent an accidental fall.

The infant can be expected to lose between 5% and 15% of his or her body weight in water during the first 4 to 5 days of life. A 1-oz or 30-g weight gain occurs each day thereafter if the infant ingests a sufficient amount of fluids and calories. Daily caloric requirements for the neonate are approximately 115 to 120 kcal per kg of body weight. Daily water requirements are approximately 105 ml per kg of body weight. Parents should be reassured that the initial weight loss is normal; a mother who is breast-feeding for the first time may be concerned that she does not have sufficient breast milk.

Careful monitoring of the infant's fluid and caloric intake will assure both nurse and parents that the infant is healthy and receiving adequate nutrients. A formula-fed infant can be expected to take between 2 and 4 oz (60–120 ml) of formula every 3 to 4 hours in a 24-hour period for a total of approximately 24 oz per day.

The breast-fed infant will nurse vigorously for 15 to 20 minutes and then will fall asleep for 2 to 3 hours. If the physician or nurse practitioner is concerned about whether the fluid intake of a breast-fed infant is adequate, the newborn can be weighed before and after each feeding, in which case the diapers should also be weighed.

Expected Outcome: Newborn regains birth weight by 7 to 14 days of life.

Promoting Normal Elimination Patterns

Infants demonstrate a wide variation in elimination patterns during the first few days after birth. Urine output slowly increases with increasing fluid intake so that by the end of the first week of life a neonate may void as frequently as 20 or 30 times a day. Parents are often amazed by the number of wet diapers they discover. However, six to eight wet diapers per 24-hour period indicates adequate hydration.

Stool patterns also vary, depending on the type and frequency of feeding and amount taken. The thick, greenish black, viscous meconium stool slowly gives way to the yellowish green transitional stool within 2 to 3 days of birth. Some infants pass very large stools with much force and vocalization after each feeding, soiling themselves from their heels to the napes of their necks. Others pass few stools initially and show a slower, more gradual change to formula or breast-fed stools after 3 or 4 days. New parents may be intitially alarmed by their infant's redness and the straining that accompanies passage of stool and need reassurance that this is normal.

The nurse should observe stools for evidence of normal patterns as well as for signs of abnormality. The absence of stools, or the presence of only small stool streaks on the diaper, may indicate intestinal blockage. The passage of blood or mucus in the stool is also abnormal. Diarrhea, which can result from bacterial infection or formula intolerance, is an extremely dangerous sign in the neonate, since it can lead to rapid depletion of fluid and electrolytes. Whenever diarrhea occurs, all diapers should be weighed to determine the extent of fluid loss. The infant should be placed under isolation precautions as well.

Expected Outcome: Newborn demonstrates urinary and bowel elimination patterns within normal limits for mode of feeding.

Promoting Behavioral Adaptation

Providing Individualized Care for Parenting

Daily physical care, including bathing, diapering, and feeding, can be provided by parents and nursing staff. Encouraging parents to assume an increasingly large share of the care is the nurse's ultimate goal; by the time of discharge the parents should feel comfortable with their new baby, be aware of his or her capabilities and limitations, and be able to meet his or her basic physical and emotional needs.

The mother who has several children may wish to spend time resting and simply enjoying her new infant. She will not be anxious to be shown skills with which she is already familiar. Nursing staff should recognize and respect her desire for assistance with the routine day-to-day care of the neonate and help her enjoy a short reprieve from her busy routine at home.

Expected Outcome: Parents demonstrate growing comfort and ease in handling newborn by time of discharge.

Promoting Health Maintenance Through Discharge Teaching

A major goal of nursing care of the neonate is the creation and implementation of an individualized discharge teaching plan that will prepare the parents to meet the physical and emotional needs of their infant when they return home. For nurses working in the traditional hospital setting, discharge planning is initiated when the infant is admitted to the newborn unit and is completed by the traditional discharge date 2 to 3 days after delivery. For nurses working in birthing units where early discharge (6 to 24 hours after birth) is possible, discharge teaching is initiated in the unit but completed in the community during follow-up care of the family.

Most postpartum settings have organized parent teaching procedures, including classes, demonstrations, and discharge teaching guides. Topics of common concern to most parents, such as the subjects listed in the

LEGAL/ETHICAL CONSIDERATIONS

The Ethics of Parent Education

The neonatal nurse will inevitably encounter parents who are unreceptive to information about infant care and safety. This may present the clinician with an ethical dilemma. Leff (1986) suggests that at issue is patient autonomy versus the professional nurse's responsibility to promote health and safety. When an individual is unwilling to take advantage of any opportunity to learn about parenting, the nurse must attempt to determine the reason for and consequences of this decision.

Once a comprehensive assessment is completed, the individual's right to autonomy may be overridden if the nurse concludes that the infant is at risk for injury or abuse. This decision must be supported by objective documentation that can withstand the scrutiny of representatives of the legal system. The nurse must discuss her concerns with the primary health care provider, and a referral for evaluation and follow-up (social service, psychiatric service, or public health nurse) should be made as soon as possible.

In many instances initial resistance to health education may be overcome when the nurse establishes a trusting relationship with the parents. Recognition of individual differences in cultural values and socioeconomic and educational status will facilitate this process.

Leff EW: Ethics and patient teaching. MCN 11: 375–378, 1986

Infant-Care Teaching:

Common Concerns of Parents

The nurse is responsible for instructing parents on the following points:

- Bathing
- Cord care
- Care of the uncircumcised male
- Circumcision care
- Diapering and clothing the infant
- Crying
- Formula preparation
- Sterilization methods
- Feeding
- Burping
- Elimination patterns
- Prevention and care of diaper rash
- Swaddling or wrapping
- Handling and carrying
- Taking a temperature
- Safety considerations
- Signs and symptoms of illness

accompanying display (above), are often addressed. Some subjects have also been discussed in prenatal classes, and the nurse should build on those, where applicable.

Although the nurse can provide parents with basic knowledge in the areas of infant care and behavior, it is impossible for her to cover all areas of care. Parents can obtain additional information from child care reference books, community health nurses, and parent education groups. The nurse should be familiar with the variety of materials available in her institution for parent teaching; she should also have a general knowledge of the popular literature on infant care available to the parents and of community resources for parent education and support.

Bathing

The bath should be a pleasant, relaxing time for parent and baby. Some infants require time to get used to the bathing routine, but as both parent and child become comfortable with the activity, it becomes a time for loving interaction and play.

All necessary equipment is collected beforehand to avoid having to carry a wet baby around while gathering forgotten supplies. The infant should never be left unattended during the bath–on the countertop or in the water. The room should be draft-free and warm (75°–80°F [24°–27°C]) and the water comfortable when tested with the elbow (98°–100°F [37°–38°C]).

First the infant's eyes should be washed with clear water; care should be taken to wipe from the inner to the outer canthus, and a new area of the washcloth or a new cotton ball should be used with each wipe to prevent cross-infection of the eye. The nares and the outer ear should be cleaned with the tip of the washcloth or a cotton-tipped swab. Nares and ear canals should not be probed with swabs, which can damage fragile tissues.

While the infant is still clothed the head can be shampooed (hand soap or mild baby shampoo may be used). The scalp should be washed daily and then brushed with a soft-bristled brush to prevent the development of "cradle-cap," a grayish white, crusty scalp disorder (seborrheic dermatitis). The "football hold" is recommended for washing the head, since it provides the parent with a free hand to massage and rinse the scalp.

Once the infant's head is dried, he or she can be undressed and placed in the water. Soap should be used sparingly and may be applied before the infant is placed in the water to be rinsed. New parents may find the infant quite slippery. Wrapping the baby in a towel and then placing him or her in the water is an easy way to prevent slipping. The towel then serves as an additional cushion in the bottom of the sink or tub.

The bath should proceed from the cleanest to the most soiled areas, the genitals and perianal area being washed last. Special care should be taken to clean skin folds. Female genitals should be washed from front to back. In an uncircumcised male infant, it is not necessary to retract the foreskin for the first 3 to 6 months.

Baby lotion may be lightly applied to the skin after the bath. Baby oils are not recommended, since they may clog pores and irritate the skin. Baby powder should never be used with lotions, since it will cake on the skin. If powder is used, it should be applied sparingly and not near the face, where it can be inhaled or enter the infant's eyes.

The newborn may not require a complete bath every day, especially during the winter months when skin is likely to become dry with too frequent bathing. Even if a complete bath is not given, the face, neck, genitalia, and perianal area should still be washed daily. The baby may be bathed at any time during the day; many mothers like to give the bath when the father is at home. A variety of infant tubs are available commercially; but a clean kitchen sink padded with a towel is quite adequate. A clean washcloth and towel are needed, and a mild, nondeodorant hand soap can be used (*e.g.,* Ivory, Castile, or Neutrogena).

Cord Care

The umbilical cord stump will usually dry and fall off 7 to 10 days after birth. Parents are encouraged to keep the diaper folded down away from the area of the cord and to use a small amount of rubbing alcohol at the base several times a day to keep the cord clean and dry. Parents can

FAMILY CONSIDERATIONS

Care of the Umbilical Cord

Cultural beliefs regarding appropriate postnatal care of the umbilical cord vary widely. In some cultures a "belly band," a tight swaddling cloth often colorfully embroidered, encircles the abdomen over the cord area. This practice is believed to prevent umbilical hernias or infection. Other groups place a coin or flat stone over the umbilical stump and secure it with a swaddling band. Some families desire to keep the desiccated cord when it separates from the abdomen as a memento or to prevent evil spirits from obtaining any part of the infant's body.

It is important for the nurse to recognize and respect these cultural beliefs. While information should be given regarding routine cord care, there is usually no contraindication to family practices that deviate from American medical practice. The nurse should encourage families to use clean fabrics and coins that will come in contact with the umbilical stump and to visually inspect the area daily for signs of healing or infection.

sponge-bathe the baby until pink granulation tissue covers the site of detachment.

Care of the Uncircumcised Male

If the newborn will not be circumcised, the nurse should include instructions on how to care for the male infant. Daily bathing should include washing of the external genitalia without efforts to retract the foreskin or expose the glans. Natural loosening of the foreskin from the glans begins at birth owing to several factors, including spontaneous erections; nevertheless, the foreskin is retractable in only 50% of all male 1-year-olds.

Parents should be advised against vigorously or forcefully retracting the infant's foreskin, since it may be difficult to return it to its normal position owing to swelling of the glans. If the foreskin remains too tight as the infant grows, a surgical incision in the foreskin may be necessary to loosen the retracted tissue.

Diapering and Clothing

The infant voids and defecates with amazing frequency. Diapers should be checked often and changed when wet or soiled. It is not necessary to cleanse with soap and water after each voiding; clear warm water is adequate. Soap and water washings can be reserved for when the infant defecates. Premoistened wipes, which are convenient to use and save time for busy parents, are commercially available for perianal cleansing. But they may be an unnecessary expense for families with limited resources.

The infant's skin is tender, and diaper rash, which results from ammonia irritation, develops quite rapidly if the area is not cleansed. A and D ointment or zinc oxide may be applied after washing and careful drying if the infant's skin is especially sensitive. Exposure to air is recommended. If cloth diapers are used, they should be laundered with a nondetergent soap and rinsed twice to eliminate all traces of ammonia. Many parents choose to use disposable diapers. Occasionally an infant develops a rash where the skin comes in contact with the plastic on these diapers. If this occurs, the parents should switch to cloth diapers.

Parents often ask about their infant's need for clothing. As a general rule neonates are comfortable with several layers of light, loose clothing (diaper, T-shirt, and medium-weight neck-to-toe coverall) in an environment with an ambient temperature of 68° to 75°F (20°–24°C). If a parent feels cold and requires a sweater, the infant should also be dressed in an additional layer of clothing. Hats or caps should be worn outdoors in cool or cold weather. In hot weather babies feel most comfortable in a lightweight T-shirt and diaper. A sun hat should be worn in the sun, and care should be taken to protect the skin from sunburn.

Crying

If the mother has been rooming-in with her infant, she will be aware that he or she frequently cries when hungry or wet. Crying is the newborn infant's only means of communication. Most babies cry an average of about 2 hours each day, but some infants cry more often in response to discomfort, boredom, or exposure to new experiences. When the infant cries, the parents should try to discover the source of distress. It is perfectly acceptable to pick the infant up and comfort him or her; there is no basis in truth to the belief that babies will be spoiled if they are picked up when they cry (Pritchard 1986). Newborns need a tremendous amount of loving attention, and crying is their request for it. However, an exhausted mother who has spent hours trying to soothe a healthy but irritable baby should not feel guilty about laying the infant down in a crib, closing the door, and spending some time in the next room recouping her energy. Parents should be advised to find someone who can occasionally relieve them of caretaking to decrease their stress levels in this situation.

Formula Preparation

If the newborn is bottle-fed, specially prepared cow's or soy milk, known as *formula*, is used. Unmodified cow's milk is not recommended for the first year of life because of its high sodium and saturated fat content and the risk of causing gastrointestinal bleeding in infants. Commercial formula can be purchased in ready-to-use single feeding bottle or large cans that provide enough formula for a 24-hour period; concentrated liquid and powders, which are less expensive than the ready-to-use formula, can also be purchased. The nurse should make sure that new parents, expecially those whose first language is not English, understand that concentrated formula and powder must be properly diluted with water to prevent severe fluid and electrolyte imbalance in the infant.

With improved sanitary conditions and water purification procedures in this country, routine sterilization of formula and equipment is often not necessary. Washing of bottles and nipples with hot, soapy water before use is normally sufficient. Dishwashers are excellent for bottle washing. Large cans of formula should be refrigerated once opened and any unused portion discarded after 24 hours. (See Chapter 37 for further discussion of infant nutrition.)

Sterilization Methods

The nurse should be aware of the special needs of parents living in areas that do not have purified water; they will require additional instruction in the sterilization of formula and bottles.

Aseptic Technique. In this method, formula and equipment are sterilized, and then bottles are filled and sealed. The bottles, nipples, and equipment needed to open and measure the formula are sterilized first by boiling in a pan of water for 5 minutes. The water needed to dilute concentrated formula is boiled in a second pan for the same amount of time. The formula is then mixed and poured into the bottles using aseptic technique. This method is less frequently used than the terminal heat method because it requires a good understanding of aseptic technique and has a greater risk of contamination.

Terminal Heat Method. In this method, formula is placed in clean bottles first and then sterilized. Approximately 4 oz of formula is placed in each bottle (diluted if concentrate or powder is used). The caps and nipples are applied loosely to prevent explosion, and then all bottles are placed in a bottle sterilizer or a large kettle in about 3 inches of water. They are boiled gently, to prevent cracking, for 25 minutes. When the water in the sterilizer has cooled, the bottles are removed and refrigerated until used.

Feeding

The mother who plans to bottle-feed will also require instruction and support; the father should be included in teaching and given opportunities to feed his new infant.

Burping

All infants swallow air as they feed (bottle-fed infants swallow more than breast-fed infants), and burping allows the swallowed air to escape from the stomach.

FAMILY CONSIDERATIONS

The Father and Infant-Care Teaching

Nurse researchers have increasingly focused on the extent of father involvement in infant care and the impact of specific nursing interventions on father–infant interaction. While men's attitudes toward fathering have changed, the extent of participation in newborn care among fathers varies by age, ethnic background, and socioeconomic status. It has also been found that father involvement is determined in part by the mother's attitudes about parenting roles.

An exploratory study (Taubenheim 1981) demonstrated that fathers who engaged in such caretaking activities as infant feeding during the first days of life scored highest on bonding behaviors. Fathers who reported greater involvement in baby care also reported more signs of depression, irritability, sleep disturbance, and fatigability in an investigation by Hangsleben (1983).

While nurses are encouraged to include fathers in the discharge teaching plan and to support their participation in infant care, this may not be an appropriate intervention with all men. Much more research must be conducted before specific models for practices that promote father involvement in newborn care can be developed and endorsed. Until models evolve, clinicians should carefully assess the individual father's interest in and desire to care for his infant before they initiate the discharge teaching plan.

Hangsleben KL: Transition to fatherhood. J Obstet Gynecol Neonatal Nurs 12:265-270, 1983

Taubenheim AM: Paternal–infant bonding in the first-time father. J Obstet Gynecol Neonatal Nurs 10:261-264, 1981

When the infant is bottle-feeding, the nipple should be kept full of fluid so the baby does not take in air with each swallow. Feeding the baby in a nearly upright position allows air naturally to rise to the top of the stomach, where it can readily be brought up without much milk being brought up with it.

Newborns may not always burp after a feeding; if after 3 minutes of gentle patting and rubbing, a baby has not burped, he or she may not need to. Burping the baby is best done with the baby held upright against the adult's shoulder. Holding the baby on his or her stomach on the lap for burping is likely to bring up milk when air escapes. Holding the baby in a sitting position may also not work well because air may not be able to escape from the stomach.

Elimination Patterns

The nurse should discuss expected changes in stool consistency and frequency of elimination in the neonate. This is especially important with new parents who are unfamiliar with normal newborn stool characteristics and patterns of elimination. If the mother is encouraged to change the infant's diapers during her hospital stay, she will gain confidence in her ability to recognize normal variations in her baby's stools and habits.

Prevention and Care of Diaper Rash

Diaper rash is a localized cutaneous reaction due primarily to the ammonia found in urine as well as to detergents used in the laundering of cloth diapers. As mentioned earlier, the best preventive measures include frequent diaper changes and thorough rinsing of the skin and skin folds with warm water with each diaper change. If cloth diapers are used, a nondetergent soap specifically created for laundering diapers should be used, and the diapers should be rinsed twice to remove any soap residue.

Even with the best care, some infants are prone to diaper rash. If a rash occurs, the infant should be placed in cloth, not plastic disposable, diapers. The buttocks should be exposed to air and sunlight several times a day for 20 minutes or so, and an ointment specifically formulated for diaper rash protection (such as A and D ointment) should be used on the tender area to decrease exposure of the skin to urine. At no time should a skin powder and ointment be used together; this combination cakes on the skin surface and exacerbates the irritation of delicate skin tissues.

Swaddling or Wrapping

Wrapping the baby securely can help meet the baby's need for contact comfort and provide a relaxing arrangement for sleep. Wrapping the baby also prevents his or her own jerky movements from disturbing sleep and keeps the baby warm. The baby can be wrapped in a soft baby blanket, with the edges of the blanket tucked smoothly under the baby to secure the blanket in place. A wrapped infant may also be easier for new parents to lift and carry, because the blanket helps support the extremities and limits the baby's movements.

Handling and Carrying

Newborns have an inborn fear of being dropped; this is apparent in their distress when their heads or extremities are left unsupported or their position is suddenly changed. To avoid startling the newborn when picking him or her up, talk to the newborn and put your hands under his or her body for a second or two before lifting. The newborn may also feel more secure if securely wrapped in a blanket while being carried.

Parents should be advised to carry the newborn in a "football" hold (baby's head supported by adult's hand, baby's body supported on adult's lower arm and securely held against adult's body) or securely braced against the shoulder with the hand supporting the baby's head when going up and down stairs; this leaves one hand free to manage doors, use handrails, and so on

Taking a Temperature

If the nurse takes the infant's vital signs at the mother's bedside as part of the daily assessment, she can then teach both axillary and rectal temperature-taking techniques described earlier in this chapter. The mother should be able to state the normal temperature range and demonstrate correct temperature-taking and reading techniques before she leaves the hospital. Some parents have never used a thermometer. If they are unable to consistently read a temperature accurately, the nurse might suggest that they purchase plastic temperature strips. Such strips are placed on the skin surface and provide an approximate temperature reading; these are an acceptable alternative if parents cannot read a mercury thermometer accurately.

Safety Considerations

An important safety factor is use of the bulb syringe when regurgitated milk or mucus occurs in the infant's airway. Parents should be taught this safety feature (see the accompanying Infant-Care Teaching display).

Because accidents are the leading cause of death in children from 1 month of age through adolescence, the nurse should cover the topic of accident prevention in depth and reinforce information at every opportunity.

The importance of using an infant car seat should be stressed. Automobile accidents are the leading cause of infant death, and some neonates are injured or even killed during their first car ride on the way home from the hospital. An increasing number of states have enacted mandatory auto passenger restraint laws requiring that all infants and children be placed in specially designed car seats (not infant carriers). The nurse should encourage parents to obtain and use an infant car seat. Many local public health departments offer car seat rental or loan programs for parents with limited economic resources (Davis 1985).

Parents should be told that poisoning is second only to auto accidents as the leading cause of death in older infants and children. Parents should begin to "childproof" their home before their infant is old enough to crawl and begin to explore the environment. Cleaning solutions, medications, cosmetics, and other toxic substances should be placed in locked cabinets. Specially designed easy-to-install locks are available as part of a "childproofing" kit that can be purchased in hardware and infant specialty stores. All electrical outlets should have covers,

Infant-Care Teaching
How to Use the Bulb Syringe

In order to quickly and safely clear the infant's airway when regurgitation of milk or mucus occurs, the following steps in suctioning the mouth and nares with the bulb syringe are used:

Action	Rationale
1. Place the infant in a football hold.	To free one hand to use the bulb syringe
2. Place the head downward.	To facilitate drainage of fluids
3. Compress the bulb syringe quickly before placing into mouth and nares.	To prevent blowing the fluids deeper into oropharynx or trachea
4. Insert tip of bulb syringe FIRST into mouth in area between cheek and gums.	Placing tip of syringe into nares first may stimulate gasp, drawing fluids deeper into oropharynx or trachea.
5. Slowly release compression of bulb.	To create vacuum and to aspirate fluids from mouth
6. Remove tip of syringe from mouth, compress bulb, and reinsert in mouth to remove remaining liquids.	To expel aspirated fluids from bulb; To remove remaining fluids
7. Repeat steps 4, 5, and 6 until mouth is clear.	
8. Compress bulb and gently place tip of syringe into nares.	To remove any fluids regurgitated into nares
9. Repeat procedure until nares are clear.	

and cords should be out of sight and out of reach as much as possible. Many houseplants are also poisonous. Local poison control centers have information on plants and can help parents identify those that are harmful. Parents should have with them the phone number of the local poison control center when they leave the hospital and should place it near their phone along with other emergency numbers.

Other areas of safety the nurse should discuss with parents are prevention of falls, aspiration, and electric shock. The nurse should stress that an infant must never be left unattended on any unguarded surface; newborns can roll over and fall with amazing speed. Choking and aspiration are other major causes of death in infancy. To prevent this, bottle propping should be avoided, and the infant should be placed on his or her side or abdomen after being fed. Because the neonate is capable of random hand-to-mouth movements, all objects small enough to fit into his or her mouth should be kept out of reach. As toys are purchased, care should be taken to identify the age range for which they are intended, and those with sharp edges or small pieces that can be broken off and aspirated should be avoided.

The infant's sleep environment should be discussed with the parents. Pillows should not be used for infants because they can cause suffocation. If parents intend to purchase an old crib, they should be told that such cribs do not always meet contemporary safety standards, which require use of a nonlead paint and provide guide-

lines for the distance between slats. Other types of old infant furniture may also be hazardous to the infant and should be used with caution.

Controversy exists about the safety of having an infant sleep in the parents' bed. In many cultures infants automatically sleep with their mothers until they are no longer nursed or are old enough to sleep with siblings. However, some health professionals fear that infants may be accidentally suffocated by the weight of their sleeping parents. While respecting the mother's cultural values, the nurse should nevertheless suggest that the mother provide her infant with a simple sleeping crib with sides. Such a crib can be placed next to the mother's bed so that she can nurse the baby easily.

Signs and Symptoms of Illness

First-time parents may be especially concerned about being able to recognize signs and symptoms of illness in their baby. The nurse can provide them with a simple but descriptive list of significant signs:

- Lethargy—difficulty in waking the baby
- Fever—temperature above 100°F (37.2°C)
- Vomiting—spitting up of a large part or all of a feeding two or more times
- Diarrhea—three or more green, liquid stools in succession
- Loss of appetite—refusal of two feedings in a row

If parents observe any of these signs or symptoms, they should call their nurse practitioner or physician. If they are unable to contact their health care provider and the baby's condition is getting worse, they should take the baby to a clinic or emergency room.

Expected Outcomes: Parents state correctly signs of illness and sources of injury in newborns by time of discharge. Parents perform return-demon-strations of techniques that were covered in discharge teaching.

Monitoring for Complications

The newborn should continue to make physiological adaptations to extrauterine life. It is especially important for the nurse to continually evaluate the newborn's body systems for danger signals. The nurse is in a position to

Table 32-2   **Danger Signs in the Neonate**

Affected System	Presenting Signs	Potential Neonatal Disorder
Central nervous system	Jitteriness	Hypoglycemia, hypocalcemia, hypomagnesemia, drug withdrawal (maternal use)
	Diaphoresis	Chromosomal anomalies
	Abnormal cry	Asphyxia
	Excessive irritability	Intracranial hemorrhage
	Twitching	Brain edema
	Convulsions	Neuromuscular anomalies
	Hypotonia	Sepsis
		Chronic intrauterine infection
		Chromosomal anomalies
	Small head size	Fetal alcohol syndrome
	Bulging fontanelle, large head size	Hydrocephalus
Cardiovascular and respiratory systems	Apnea	Congenital heart anomaly
	Rapid, slow, or irregular pulse	Persistent fetal circulation
	Cyanosis	Hypoplastic lung
	Rapid respiration, chest retraction	Respiratory distress syndrome (type I or type II)
	Grunting	Meconium aspiration syndrome
	Flaring	Tracheal malacia
	Stridor	Aspiration
	Pallor	Pneumothorax
	Plethora	Polycythemia
	Single umbilical artery	Congenital heart anomaly
Gastrointestinal system	Vomiting	Gastrointestinal obstruction
	Abdominal distention	Gastrointestinal obstruction
	No meconium stool (beyond 48 hours after birth)	Imperforate anus, gastrointestinal obstruction
	Diarrhea	Sepsis
	Jaundice (within first 24 hours of life)	Hemolytic disease of newborn, biliary atresia
	Excessive salivation	Tracheoesophageal fistula
Genitourinary system	Delayed/inadequate voiding (beyond 48 hours after birth)	Genitourinary anomalies, renal failure secondary to hypoxia
Musculoskeletal system	Hypotonia	Congenital neuromuscular anomaly
	Uneven thigh or buttock folds	Congenital hip dysplasia
	Facial asymmetry with crying	Facial nerve injury
	Limited movement of arm	Brachial palsy
Integumentary system	Purulent discharge from cord	Omphalitis
	Skin pustules	Staphylococcal skin infection
	Rash	Congenital rubella, congenital syphillis
Hematologic system	Bleeding or oozing from cord, petechiae	Hemorrhage
Immunologic system	Hypothermia	Sepsis
	Fever	Intracranial hemorrhage

detect specific signs of complications in the earliest stages. Table 32–2 discusses presenting signs of body system complications and potential disorders.

Newborn Screening Tests

The majority of states require that all infants be screened for the presence of phenylketonuria (PKU) before being discharged from the hospital. PKU is an inborn error of metabolism in which the infant is unable to metabolize *phenylalanine,* an amino acid common in many foods. If an infant with PKU is fed normally, a biochemical buildup leads to progressive mental retardation. If the disorder is diagnosed by a simple blood test done shortly after birth, brain damage and retardation can be prevented by limiting the amount of phenylalanine in the diet.

It is important that the infant have had 2 to 3 days of milk or formula ingestion before the blood sample for the serum phenylalanine screening test is obtained. If initial feeding of the neonate has been delayed or early discharge is planned for the infant, arrangements must be made for the PKU test to be performed in a clinic or in the pediatrician's office after 3 full days of milk feedings. Performance of the screening test before adequate amounts of milk have been ingested may lead to a false-negative test result.

When the PKU screening is done, the newborn can also be tested for other inborn errors of metabolism, including galactosemia, maple syrup urine disease, and homocystinuria. Because congenital hypothyroidism occurs with greater frequency than PKU and can also lead to permanent neurologic impairment, many states now require that infants also be screened for this disorder. (See Chapter 9 for further information on these disorders.)

Expected Outcome: Newborn continues to make physiologic and behavioral adaptations, and is screened for congenital conditions as appropriate within the first week of life.

CIRCUMCISION

Circumcision is the surgical removal of the foreskin of the penis (Fig. 32–11). The procedure has its origins in religious tradition or the cultural practice of rite of passage to manhood. But the practice of routine circumcision in United States hospitals is based on commonly held misperceptions about penile hygiene and the relationship between the uncircumcised penis and a variety of diseases. Many parents choose circumcision when the father has been circumcised so that the male child's penis will "look like daddy's." In 1975 the American Academy of

LEGAL/ETHICAL CONSIDERATIONS

Role of the Nurse in the Parental Decision Regarding Circumcision

Nurses have a moral obligation to promote the physical and psychological well-being of the neonate. A growing ethical dilemma for many clinicians centers around the issue of circumcision. In 1975 the American Academy of Pediatrics stated that there was no absolute medical indication for circumcision. Researchers have discovered altered sleep patterns and circadian rhythms in circumcised infants. Recognition of the infant's ability to perceive pain and evidence in some newborns of posttraumatic behaviors further support arguments against circumcision. Finally, each year a small percentage of newborns suffer major complications from this procedure, including infection, hemorrhage, permanent disfigurement of the penis, and in rare instances even death.

Another moral principle observed by nurses is that infants have rights but cannot speak for themselves. What would they choose? When the parent's choice is motivated by religious convictions, nurses may feel less conflicted, but in other circumstances to what extent should the nurse involve herself in the decision-making process?

The primary responsibility of the practitioner is to fully inform parents, answer all questions, and provide them with all available resources in making their decision. Finally, the nurse must respect the parent's ultimate decision.

If a nurse strongly opposes circumcision, he or she can work through professional organizations to educate parents and physicians and can attempt to influence legislators and insurance companies to reduce or eliminate financial reimbursement for circumcisions.

Pediatrics reviewed all research literature on this issue and published a new position statement; they found no valid medical indication for circumcision of the newborn. Furthermore, recent research has demonstrated adverse physiologic responses in neonates who were circumcised, including agitation and changes in sleep patterns and serum cortisol levels (NAACOG 1985).

Although fewer parents request elective circumcision today than in the past, over 50% of all male newborns in the United States are still circumcised. The nurse assists the physician during the procedure and supports and cares for the infant afterward. A consent form must be signed by parents that explains the technique to be used and carefully enumerates potential risks. Infection, hemorrhage, and even death are associated with neonatal cir-

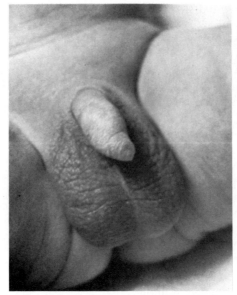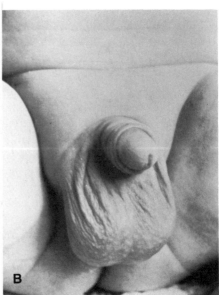

Figure 32–11. *(A)* Uncircumcised male infant. *(B)* Circumcised infant. Although circumcision is no longer recommended and is considered unnecessary surgery, parents may still choose to have their male infants circumcised for religious reasons or because of their unfamiliarity with the appearance or care of an uncircumcised male child. (Photo: Childbirth Graphics)

cumcision. The infant is not fed for 2 to 4 hours before the surgery to reduce the risk of vomiting and aspiration during the procedure.

Circumcision Methods

The newborn is positioned on a specially designed molded plastic board (circ board), and his limbs are restrained (Fig. 32–12). Care is taken to prevent cold stress. Anesthesia is usually not used, since the risks associated with it are considered greater than those associated with the pain and trauma of the procedure. Two methods are commonly used for circumcision; they are briefly described here.

Gomco (Yéllen) Clamp. The adherent prepuce is separated from the glans with a surgical probe. The prepuce is then stretched and drawn over a metal cone, and a clamp is applied with sufficient pressure to ligate blood vessels and prevent bleeding. After 3 to 5 minutes the prepuce above the clamp is removed with a surgical scalpel (Fig. 32–13).

Plastibell. The prepuce is separated from the glans and the Plastibell positioned over the glans. Next a suture is tied around the prepuce at the rim of the Plastibell, and the prepuce above the area of ligation is then removed with a scalpel. The plastic rim of the bell remains in place 2 to 3 days and falls off with healing of the tissues (Fig. 32–14).

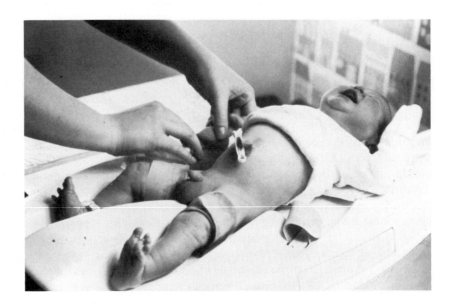

Figure 32–12. The infant is restrained in a specially designed circumcision board during the procedure. (Photo: Childbirth Graphics)

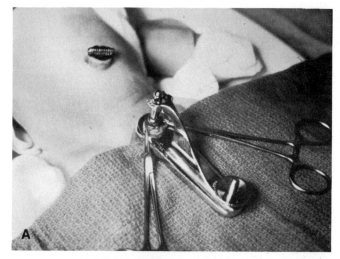

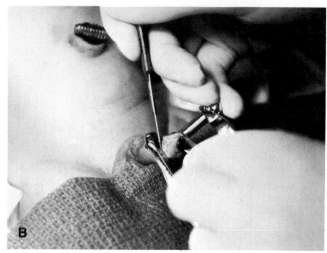

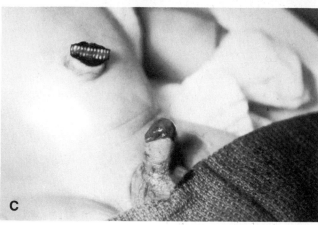

Figure 32–13. The prepuce, or foreskin, is stretched and drawn through a metal clamp *(A)*, which is applied with pressure to ligate vessels and prevent bleeding. The foreskin is then cut away with a scalpel *(B and C)*. (Photo: Childbirth Graphics)

Assisting at the Procedure

Possible nursing diagnoses resulting from the circumcision procedure are the following:

• Potential for infection
• Altered comfort: pain
• Altered urinary elimination pattern

A potential complication includes hemorrhage.

During the procedure the nurse assists the physician by preparing equipment and placing necessary supplies on the circumcision tray. The infant may be soothed by use of a pacifier or strokes on his cheek. After the circumcision parents should be encouraged to support the infant by holding and rocking him and by offering him the mother's breast or formula. Postoperative checks for bleeding are done by the nurse every 15 minutes for the first hour and then every 30 minutes for the next 3 to 4 hours. The first voiding is also noted. A petroleum jelly gauze may be applied to the glans when the foreskin is removed. It is replaced by clean gauze and a liberal amount of petroleum jelly with each diaper change.

Teaching Circumcision Care

Because infants are sent home shortly after circumcision, the nurse must prepare parents to observe for bleeding and signs of infection in their circumcised sons. They should be aware that a yellow exudate often forms over the surgical site but that a foul-smelling purulent exudate is abnormal and should be reported to the nurse practitioner or pediatrician at once. Before the petroleum jelly gauze is removed, it can be soaked with warm water to prevent trauma to tissues that have adhered to it. Each time a diaper is changed, the penis should be washed with clear, warm water gently squeezed from a cotton ball. Alcohol should never be used on the site; this would be extremely painful to the infant. A large dab of petroleum jelly may be placed in the diaper over the area that comes in contact with the penis. If the Plastibell method is used, no special gauze dressing or ointments are applied to the site; however, warm water may be used for cleansing, as described above. This special care should continue until the site is completely covered with clean, pink granulation tissue.

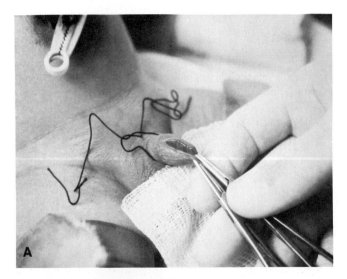

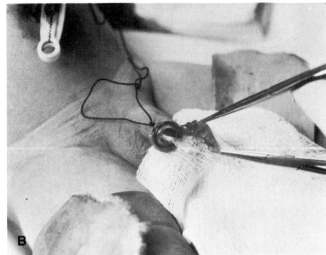

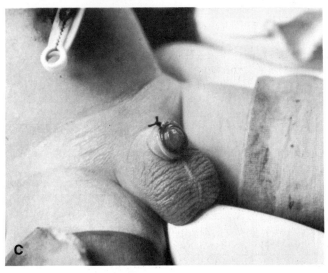

Figure 32–14. Circumcision by Plastibell. *(A)* The foreskin is slit and the Plastibell is positioned over the glans penis. *(B)* A suture is tied around the foreskin at the rim or base of the Plastibell, and the skin above the rim is cut away. *(C)* The plastic rim of the bell remains in place for 2 or 3 days and falls off as the tissues heal. (Photo: Childbirth Graphics)

Evaluation of Ongoing Newborn Care

The nurse is responsible for evaluating the neonate's physiological and behavioral adaptation as well as progress in the parent–neonate acquaintance process in preparation for discharge. In general, evaluation criteria include the following: successful initiation of feeding; establishment of normal elimination patterns; completion of required newborn screening tests or provisions to complete these tests after discharge; absence or resolution of complications from procedures; ability of parents to describe signs and symptoms of infant illness, normal developmental changes in the newborn, and normal psychological changes associated with parenthood; and the

ability of parents to perform appropriate infant care practices.

CHAPTER SUMMARY

Nursing care of the normal neonate is based on knowledge of the major physiologic and behavioral adaptations of the newborn to extrauterine life and on the needs of parents to learn about and care for their infant in preparation for their life together. Nursing interventions focus on supporting the neonate's physiologic adaptation, preventing potential neonatal complications, and facilitating parent–infant interaction. The nursing process is used to ensure systematic assessment, appropriate nursing diagnoses, careful planning, relevant intervention, and accurate evaluation of the newborn and family.

STUDY QUESTIONS

1. How do different neonatal environments influence the type of nursing care provided the newly formed family?
2. What are major nursing considerations in the prevention of aspiration in the newborn?
3. What are major nursing considerations in the promotion of breast-feeding and bottle-feeding?
4. What is the major nursing action performed to prevent infection in the newborn?
5. What is hypoglycemia and how can it be detected in the neonate?
6. What is hemorrhagic disease of the newborn and how is it prevented?
7. How does early feeding reduce the likelihood of hyperbilirubinemia in the newborn?
8. What are the normal fluid and caloric requirement of the newborn, and how does the nurse determine the individual neonate's requirements?
9. What are major topics to be included in the discharge teaching plan for parent education?
10. What are major nursing responsibilities in the care of the circumcised neonate?

REFERENCES/BIBLIOGRAPHY

Davis DJ: (1985). Infant car safety: The role of perinatal caregiver. Birth 12(3):21–27, 1985

Furr PA, Kirgis CA: A nurse–midwifery approach to early mother–infant acquaintance. J Nurse-Midwif 27(5):10, 1982

Klaus MH, Kennell JJ: Parent–infant bonding, 2nd ed. St. Louis, CV Mosby, 1982

Mugford M, Somchiwong M, Waterhouse I: Midwifery treatment of umbilical cords: A randomised trial to assess the effect of treatment methods on the work of midwives. Midwifery 2(4):177–186, 1986

NAACOG: OGN Nursing Practice Resource: Nurses' Role in Neonatal Circumcision. Washington, DC, NAACOG, 1985

Pritchard P: An infant crying clinic. Health Visitor 59(12):375–377, 1986

Riesch SK, Munns SK: Promoting awareness: The mother and her baby. Nurs Res 33:271, 1984

SUGGESTED READINGS

Anderson GC: Pacifers: The positive side. MCN 11:122–124, 1986

Censullo M, Lester B, Hoffman J: Rhythmic patterning in mother–newborn interaction. Nurs Res 34:342–346, 1985

Durham ML, Swanson B, Paulford N: Effect of tachypnea on oral temperature estimation: A replication. Nurs Res 35:211–214, 1986

Haddock B, Vincent P, Merrow D: Axillary and rectal temperatures of full-term neonates: Are they different? Neonatal Network 4:36–40, 1986

Karraker KH: Adult attention to infants in a newborn nursery. Nurs Res 35:358–363, 1986

Krozy RE, McColgan JJ: Auto safety. J Obstet Gynecol Neonatal Nurs 14:11–15, 1985

Rush J: Does routine newborn bathing reduce *Staphylococcus aureus* colonization rates? A randomized controlled trial. Birth 13(3):176–180, 1986

33 assessment of the at-risk neonate

LEARNING OBJECTIVES

After studying the materials in this chapter, the student should be able to

- Describe major goals and objectives in the assessment of neonatal risk factors

- Describe danger signals or signs in the neonate that indicate potential or actual problems

- Elaborate on the use of the Apgar score to assess the neonate's need for resuscitation after birth

- List the prescribed steps in resuscitation of the neonate

- Discuss nursing assessment of the high-risk family in terms of crisis theory

- Describe phases of the grieving process in parents of high-risk or sick neonates

- List significant signs of potential parenting disorders that may be observed in the assessment of parents of a high-risk or sick neonate

KEY TERMS

Apnea

Asphyxia

Crisis

Empathy

Hypoxemia

Hypoxia

Morbidity

Mortality

Neonatal Clinical Nurse Specialist

Neonatal Nurse Practitioner

Neonatology

Perinatal

Newborns who, in the past, would have died can now be saved by modern technologic methods. However, these newborns are at more risk for complications. Nurses have been challenged to create a new standard of care for the newborn at risk for developing complications. This is done by following assessment protocols and by using sophisticated equipment that enhances the nurse's ability to recognize illness early.

Neonatal nursing is an emerging speciality, which evolved as a direct result of the unique needs of high-risk infants. Although the care of healthy neonates is still within the realm of maternity nursing, the needs of sick infants and their families are more and more often being met by neonatal nurses. Neonatal nurses have advanced theoretical preparation and clinical training to function in this specialized role. The scope of practice, once narrowly defined by the walls of the neonatal intensive care unit, has expanded. Neonatal nurses provide professional outreach to clients' homes and to community hospitals requiring additional support and training in the identification and care of high-risk infants. They are also involved in long-distance transport of sick newborns to facilities offering specialized care and services.

The nurse's most valuable tool in the systematic identification of the high-risk and sick neonate is the nursing process. Assessment, problem identification, and nursing diagnosis form the cornerstone of nursing care for all newborns requiring continued monitoring and support after birth. The overall goals of risk assessment in the neonatal period are the identification of risk factors and the early recognition and treatment of illness.

This chapter defines the concept of risk assessment in the neonatal period, demonstrates how nursing assessment can be used systematically to identify potential or actual problems in the newborn, and also details the nurse's role in the resuscitation, stabilization, and support of the high-risk infant. The concepts of crisis and the grieving process are also discussed as they relate to the birth of a high-risk or sick neonate.

IDENTIFICATION OF PERINATAL RISK FACTORS

Identification of Prenatal Risk Factors

Optimal care can best be provided when the health care team is prepared for the birth of a sick neonate. The proper equipment and supplies needed for resuscitation of the infant can be assembled ahead of time, and essential members of the team can be present in the delivery room to begin immediate evaluation and support of the newborn. It is estimated that approximately 60% of in-

fants requiring special care and treatment at birth can be identified through careful evaluation of the mother's prenatal history.

Table 33–1 lists examples of prenatal maternal conditions and obstetric complications that place the fetus at risk for increased morbidity and mortality. It becomes evident, in studying this table, that the nurse caring for the neonate must have access to the prenatal history to fully appreciate the potential problems confronting the infant when the mother has experienced problems in the present or in a previous pregnancy. If a client is referred to a Level II or Level III perinatal regional center for prenatal care when complications arise, maternity and neonatal nurses can be alerted before the birth and will be prepared to meet the special needs of the infant.

Some prenatal risk factors, such as the hemoglobinopathies, are rarely seen and require nurses to consult with nurse specialists and physicians on the health team to identify potential problems and to plan care. Other disorders, such as maternal diabetes and chronic hypertension, are frequently encountered, and standardized care plans are available to assist nurses in identifying problems and in planning and implementing care.

Identification of Intrapartal Risk Factors

It is not possible to predict, with complete accuracy, from the prenatal history alone, which infants will require special assistance and care after birth. Approximately 10% to 20% of all women who experienced normal pregnancies will develop intrapartal problems that place the infant at increased risk for neonatal complications. Obstetric accidents, such as abruptio placentae and prolapse of the umbilical cord, can occur without warning. The administration of analgesia and anesthesia and the use of forceps or a vacuum extractor to assist in the delivery also place the infant at greater risk postnatally.

Electronic fetal monitoring is now used extensively to assess fetal wellbeing during the labor and delivery process. Periodic monitoring of maternal vital signs, evaluation of the progress of labor, and inspection of amniotic fluid after rupture of the membranes are all essential aspects of assessment and aid the nurse in identifying risk factors.

Table 33–2 lists major intrapartal factors that contribute to neonatal morbidity and mortality. Some of these factors, such as severe intrapartal hemorrhage or infection, can result in life-threatening complications that require immediate intervention, while others merely increase the risk of injury or illness. It is essential that the nurse attending the birth report all pertinent information

Table 33–1 **Prenatal Risk Factors and Potential Fetal and Neonatal Complications**

Risk Factors	Potential Complications
Demographic Factors	
Maternal age	
Under 16 or over 35 yr	Small for gestational age (SGA); genetic abnormalities
Primigravida over 30 yr	Labor dystocia; birth trauma
Parity	
Grand multiparity (Over five pregnancies)	Fetal malposition
Substance abuse	
Drug addiction	SGA; neonatal withdrawal syndrome; neonatal HIV
Alcoholism	Fetal alcohol syndrome
Smoking	SGA; polycythemia
Multiple sex partners, prostitution	Neonatal HIV
Sex partner IV drug abuser or bisexual	Neonatal HIV
Maternal Nutritional Status	
Maternal malnutrition	
Weight less than 100 lb	SGA
Weight more than 200 lb	SGA, LGA
Previous Pregnancy Complications	
Fetal loss at over 28 wk of gestation	Fetal loss
Premature delivery	Prematurity
Abnormal fetal position	Fetal malposition and potential birth trauma
Bleeding in second or third trimester	Recurrent bleeding in subsequent pregnancy
Pregnancy-induced hypertension	Recurrent hypertension
Rh sensitization	Erythroblastosis
Fetal distress of unknown origin	Fetal distress
Birth of an infant with anomalies	Congenital anomalies
Birth of infant over 10 lb	Birth of large for gestational age (LGA) infant
Birth of post-term infant	Post-term infant; intrauterine growth retardation (IUGR)
Neonatal death	Neonatal death
Central Nervous System Disorders	
Hereditary CNS disorders	Inherited CNS disorder
Seizure disorders requiring medication	Congenital anomalies (as a result of Dilantin use)
Cardiovascular Disease	
Chronic hypertension	IUGR; asphyxia
Congenital heart disease with congestive heart failure	Prematurity; inherited defects
Hematologic Disorders	
Anemia (Under 10 g)	Prematurity; low birth weight
Sickle cell disease	IUGR; fetal demise
Hemoglobinopathies	IUGR; inherited hemoglobinopathies
Idiopathic thrombocytopenic purpura (ITP)	Transient ITP
Renal Disease	
Chronic glomerulonephritis	IUGR; SGA; prematurity; asphyxia
Renal insufficiency	IUGR; SGA; prematurity; asphyxia
Reproductive Disorders	
Uterine malformation	Prematurity; fetal malposition
Cervical incompetence	Prematurity

(continued)

Table 33–1   **Prenatal Risk Factors and Potential Fetal and Neonatal Complications** (continued)

Risk Factors	Potential Complications
Metabolic Disorders	
Diabetes	LGA; hypoglycemia and hypocalcemia; anomalies; respiratory distress syndrome
Thyroid disease	Hypothyroidism; CNS defects
	Hyperthyroidism, goiter
Current Pregnancy Complications	
Pregnancy-induced hypertension	IUGR; SGA
Maternal infections:	
TORCH infections	IUGR; SGA; active infection; anomalies
Sexually transmitted disease	Ophthalmia neonatorum; congenital syphilis
Acute cystitis, pyelonephritis	Prematurity
Hepatitis	Hepatitis
AIDS or HIV seropositive	Neonatal HIV
Multiple gestation	Prematurity; asphyxia; IUGR; SGA
Fetal malposition	Prolapsed cord; asphyxia; birth trauma
Rh sensitization	Erythroblastosis fetalis
Prolonged pregnancy	Postmaturity; meconium aspiration; IUGR; asphyxia

about the delivery to the nurse assuming responsibility for the infant.

The Apgar score assigned the infant at 5 minutes after birth predicts potential complications as well as the long-term neurologic status of the neonate. A 5-minute Apgar score of 3 or less indicates that the infant is severely depressed. Neonatal depression has been associated with neurologic abnormalities in both low-birth-weight and full-term, appropriate-for-gestational-age infants. The nurse who cares for the newborn should be fully cognizant of the Apgar scores assigned at 1 and 5 minutes and of any resuscitation efforts employed to support the infant.

Identification of Neonatal Risk Factors

Another useful tool the nurse can employ to identify those infants at greatest risk for neonatal morbidity and mortality is the neonatal mortality rate chart (Fig. 33–1). The chart relates the mortality rate to the gestational age and birth weight of the infant. It is evident from the chart that the risk is greatest for premature infants whose weight and gestational age fall to the lower left corner of the graph. The causes of death in these infants are related to the extreme immaturity of all systems and include respiratory distress syndrome, intracranial hemorrhage, and infection. The presence of congenital anomalies is another major contributing factor to the high rate of morbidity and mortality in these infants.

INITIAL ASSESSMENT AND SUPPORT

The nurse and physician often collaborate in the initial assessment of the high-risk infant at birth. In Level II and Level III perinatal regional centers (discussed in Chapter 34), pediatricians and nurses skilled in the evaluation and stabilization of neonates are usually present at the birth of the infant identified as being at risk of complications. In Level I hospitals, where low-risk clients give birth, the nurse must be prepared to initiate resuscitation and provide immediate supportive care until help arrives.

Apgar Score

Evaluation begins with the assignment of the Apgar score (discussed in Chapters 24 and 31). Guidelines are available to assist nurses in determining appropriate interventions based on the 1-minute Apgar score (Table 33–3, page 1003) (Epstein 1985).

Neonates with Apgar Scores of 8 to 10. The infant who receives an Apgar score of 8 to 10 has a strong, regular heart rate of over 100 bpm, an adequate respiratory effort, and responds quickly to stimulation. Major interventions are unnecessary. The mouth and pharynx are suctioned with a bulb syringe, the skin is dried quickly, the infant is wrapped with warm blankets to

Table 33-2   **Intrapartal Risk Factors and Potential Fetal and Neonatal Complications**

Risk Factors	Potential Complications
UMBILICAL CORD	
Prolapsed umbilical cord	Asphyxia
True knot in cord	Asphyxia
Velamentous insertion	Intrauterine blood loss; shock; anemia
Vasa previa	Intrauterine blood loss; shock; anemia
Rupture or tearing of cord	Blood loss; shock; anemia
MEMBRANES	
Premature rupture of membranes	Infection; RDS; prolapsed cord; asphyxia
Prolonged rupture of membranes	Infection
Amnionitis	Infection
Oligohydramnios	Congenital anomalies
Polyhydramnios	Congenital anomalies; prolapsed cord
PLACENTA	
Placenta previa	Prematurity; asphyxia
Abruptio placentae	Prematurity; asphyxia
Placental insufficiency	IUGR; SGA
ABNORMAL FETAL PRESENTATIONS	
Breech delivery	Asphyxia; birth injuries (CNS, skeletal)
Face or brow presentation	Asphyxia; facial trauma
Transverse lie	Asphyxia; birth injuries; cesarean delivery
LABOR DYSTOCIAS	
Prolonged labor	Asphyxia; birth trauma; infection
Uterine inertia	Complications of prolonged labor
Uterine tetany	Asphyxia
Precipitate labor	Asphyxia; birth trauma
DELIVERY COMPLICATIONS	
Forceps-assisted delivery	CNS trauma; cephalhematoma; asphyxia
Vacuum extraction	Cephalhematoma
Manual version or extraction	Asphyxia; birth trauma; prolapsed cord
Shoulder dystocia	Asphyxia; brachial plexus injury; fractured clavicle
Precipitate delivery	Asphyxia; birth trauma (CNS)
Undiagnosed multiple gestation	Asphyxia; birth trauma
ADMINISTRATION OF DRUGS	
Oxytocin	Complications of uterine tetany (asphyxia)
Magnesium sulfate	Hypermagnesemia; CNS depression
Analgesics	CNS and respiratory depression
Anesthetics	CNS and respiratory depression; bradycardia

prevent hypothermia, and the infant is given to the parents as quickly as possible. The nurse continues to observe the infant closely for signs of maladaptations, but allows the new family to become acquainted, keeping distractions and interruptions to a minimum.

Neonates with Apgar Scores of 5 to 7.   The infant with an Apgar score of 5 to 7 is mildly depressed and requires immediate assistance to establish and maintain effective respirations. The neonate appears cyanotic, with a decreased muscle tone and diminished respiratory effort. Heart rate is usually above 100 bpm. A laryngoscope should be inserted by a skilled attendant and the larynx suctioned, if the amniotic fluid is meconium-stained, to clear the airway and prevent meconium aspiration. Gentle stimulation can then be accomplished by briskly drying the infant. An oxygen-enriched atmosphere should be provided by placing the mask of a bag-and-mask device with continuous flow over the infant's nose and mouth. The goal is to elevate arterial PO_2 by delivering more oxygen to the alveoli with each breath.

Neonates with Apgar Scores of 3 to 4.   The infant with an Apgar score of 3 to 4 is moderately depressed. The neonate appears cyanotic and flaccid, with weak, ineffectual respirations. The heart rate is under 100 bpm. Immediate support is necessary to reverse the infant's deteriorating condition. A laryngoscope should be inserted to suction meconium from the airway. Then, 100% oxygen is administered through a tightly fitting face mask attached to a flow-inflating bag.

Ventilation is initiated by compressing the bag 30 to 50 times per minute, using pressures of 25 to 35 cm H_2O. High pressures may be required initially to expand the lungs adequately, but continued application of excessive pressures may result in pneumothorax. Use of a ventilation bag with a pressure "pop off" valve reduces the risk of overinflation of the lungs. Generally, the moderately depressed infant will respond to these measures with an increased heart rate, an improvement in color, and spontaneous respirations. If there is no improvement, or the infant's condition deteriorates, the resuscitation team advances to the next stage of resuscitation, described below.

Neonates with Apgar Scores of 0 to 2.   The infant with an Apgar score of 0 to 2 is severely depressed and requires the maximum resuscitation effort and support. The neonate is cyanotic and flaccid. There may be no respiratory effort or heart rate. Stimulation will not effect an improvement in the infant's condition, and precious time should not be wasted flicking in the infant's soles.

A laryngoscope should be inserted and an endotracheal tube passed immediately after the airway is cleared by suctioning. A flow inflating bag is attached to the end of the endotracheal tube and 100% oxygen is administered utilizing the rate and pressure guidelines listed above.

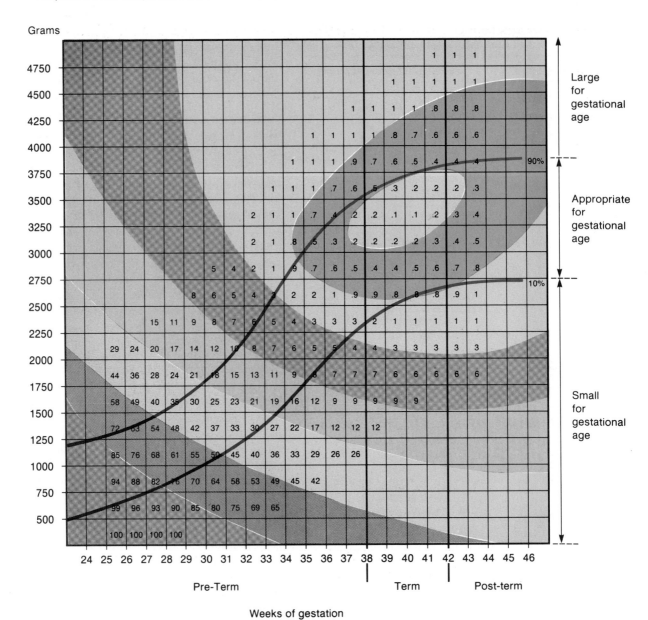

Grams

Figure 33–1. Neonatal mortality rate chart. The chart shows the relationship between neonatal mortality, shown in percentages by numbers in boxes, and birth weight and gestational age. Note the dramatic decrease in mortality as age and weight increase. Shaded zones are areas of similar mortality. (Original data from University of Colorado Medical Center. Redrawn from Mead Johnson Laboratories)

(Higher rates or pressures may be required with severe meconium aspiration.) If maternal overmedication with narcotics is identified as a contributing factor in the infant's depressed state, narcotic antagonists are administered.

If the heart beat is absent or the heart rate remains low (under 60 bpm) after a minute of ventilation, external cardiac massage is begun at a rate of 100 to 120 compressions per minute. Drugs may be administered to correct

metabolic acidosis (sodium bicarbonate), hypoglycemia (glucose), and bradycardia (epinephrine or atropine).

Managing Neonatal Resuscitation

Resuscitation efforts are conducted with a recognition of the unique anatomic and physiologic characteristics of the neonate, a knowledge of neonatal emergency drugs,

Table 33–3   **Management of Neonatal Resuscitation Based on the Infant's Condition and Assigned Apgar Score**

Apgar Score	Infant's Condition	Management
8 to 10 (No evidence of asphyxia)	Pink, active, responsive to stimuli, crying, heart rate over 100 bpm	Suction mouth and nares Dry thoroughly, including head Maintain body temperature Perform brief physical exam Unite with parents Assign 5-min Apgar score
5 to 7 (mild asphyxia)	Cyanotic, moving with decreased muscle tone, breathing shallow, decreased respiratory effort, heart rate above 100 bpm	Suction mouth, nares and larynx if amniotic fluid is meconium-stained Dry quickly Maintain body temperature Stimulate gently by rubbing body dry Provide 100% oxygen via bag and mask set-up by placing over infant's nose and mouth Call for help if alone in case infant's condition deteriorates
3 to 4 (moderate asphyxia)	Cyanotic, minimal movement, decreased muscle tone, breathing shallow, poor respiratory effort, heart rate below 100 bpm	Suction mouth, nares and larynx if amniotic fluid is meconium-stained Dry quickly Maintain body temperature Provide 100% oxygen via bag and mask Call for help if alone Continue ventilating at 30 to 50 times/min until heart rate is above 100 bpm, color is pink, and spontaneous respirations begin As soon as possible, assign someone to support parents
0 to 2 (severe asphyxia)	Deeply cyanotic, no muscle tone, absent respiratory effort or periodic gasps, heart rate slow or absent	Clear airway quickly; call for help Insert endotracheal tube Initiate bag ventilation with 100% oxygen at 40 to 60 breaths/min at pressures great enough to move chest wall Perform cardiac massage at a rate of 100 to 120 times/min If heart rate is under 100 bpm despite 2 min of adequate ventilation and cardiac massage, insert umbilical venous catheter and administer drugs (Table 33–4) As soon as additional personnel arrive, ensure maintenance of body temperature Assign someone to support parents

Adapted from Cloherty JP, Start AR: Manual of Neonatal Care, 2nd ed. Boston, Little, Brown, & Co, 1985

and an understanding of the special equipment required for infant resuscitation.

Airway Management

The infant is initially placed on a flat surface in a Trendelenburg position (15° to 30°) to facilitate mucus drainage. Once the airway is cleared and ventilation is established, the examining table is returned to a horizontal position (unless an injury or anomaly requires a different position). If ventilation is necessary, the infant's head is placed in a "sniffing position" (Fig. 33–2) to fully open the airway. A folded towel may be placed under the shoulders to bring the head into correct alignment, but care must be taken not to hyperextend the neck or the airway will be obstructed.

When the infant is placed in a supine position, the tongue does not usually fall back and obstruct the airway as it does in older children and adults. Many neonatologists skilled in resuscitation of the newborn believe that a pharyngeal airway is unnecessary. High-risk infants with chromosomal disorders, characterized by a large protruding tongue or those with congenital anomalies of the face and neck, may require airways.

Suctioning and Suction Equipment

Because the infant is an obligate nose breather, once the mouth and pharynx are suctioned, the nose should be

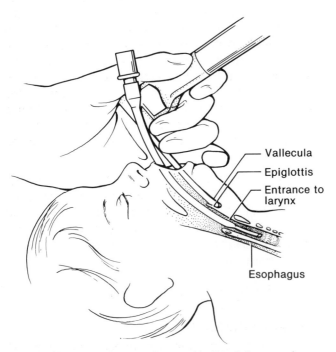

Figure 33–2. Infant in "sniffing position" to fully open airway for laryngoscopy. Laryngoscopy allows visualization and suctioning of meconium and mucus from the airway and is necessary for placement of an endotracheal tube if ventilation is required.

cleared. If the infant is moderately to severely depressed, a laryngoscope is inserted and the larynx is carefully suctioned (see Fig. 33–2). When there has been meconium passage *in utero,* a suction catheter is inserted past the vocal cords under direct visualization by the laryngoscope, and deep suctioning is employed to remove all meconium before it is inhaled into terminal bronchioles and alveoli.

Bulb Syringe. A bulb syringe is adequate only for removing secretions from the mouth and nose. It usually is used by the birth attendant after the head is delivered but before the thorax emerges from the birth canal. If the infant receives an Apgar score of 7 to 10 and no meconium was passed *in utero,* the nurse can complete the suctioning process with the bulb syringe after the infant is delivered. The bulb must be compressed fully before the syringe tip is inserted into the mouth or nares. Compressing the bulb after it is inserted will force fluids deeper into the airway.

Suction Catheter. With the introduction of universal body-substance precautions to prevent the transmission of HIV, the type of equipment and procedures recommended for suctioning have been revised. A 8F to 12F catheter is attached to a mechanical suction device to remove meconium from the mouth, oropharynx, and nares (see the accompanying display). A manually operated suction catheter with mucus trap (De Lee Mucus Trap) should no longer be used. The practitioner must apply negative mouth pressure to the end of these catheters to suction secretions from the infant's mouth and nares. The danger of accidentally aspirating contaminated body fluids into the operator's mouth has rendered this equipment unsafe for use today. Adapters are available for wall suction.

Ventilating the Neonate

The nurse must ventilate the neonate using the correct rate, pressures, oxygen concentration, and equipment. The use of improper technique or equipment can lead to injury or permanent damage.

Ventilation Rate. The normal ventilation rate is 30 to 50 times per minute. Exceptions to the rule exist: with severe meconium aspiration, higher rates may be necessary for the adequate exchange of gases.

Ventilation Pressures. The initial pressure required to inflate the lungs may be quite high (over 40 cm H_2O). Subsequent pressures of 25 cm H_2O to 35 cm H_2O or lower should be sufficient. The nurse should carefully note the rise and fall of the chest to make sure correct ventilation technique is being employed.

Hand Ventilation. In hand ventilation an inflatable bag is compressed to deliver a breath to the infant. The

NURSING ALERT

Care of the Infant Delivered Through Meconium

Evidence of the passage of meconium by the infant prior to delivery requires attendance of personnel at the delivery who are skilled at newborn intubation and resuscitation so that meconium aspiration can be avoided or limited. On delivery of the infant's head on the perineum (or in cesarean birth, at the level of the abdomen) and before delivery of the rest of the body, the infant's nares, mouth, and pharynx should be suctioned with an 8F to a 12F catheter attached to mechanical suction. This helps remove meconium the infant might possibly inhale with the first gasping respiration.

After delivery is complete, the infant should be placed quickly on the radiant warming table with as little stimulation as possible, in order to prevent vigorous crying, which could increase aspiration of meconium. The nursery nurse, nurse anesthetist, or physician skilled in intubation should then quickly intubate the infant orally.

A meconium aspirator is attached to the end of the tube and mechanical suction is applied to aspirate meconium present below the level of the vocal cords as the endotracheal tube is removed. Reintubation may be required several times for repeated suctioning until meconium is cleared but provides more efficient removal of very thick meconium than does the method using the suction catheter.

The practice of placing one's mouth directly over the end of an endotracheal tube to suction meconium from the trachea after intubation is no longer permissible and has been discarded with the institution of universal body precautions to prevent transmission of HIV.

Even if the infant appears quite asphyxiated with a heart rate as low as 40–60 bpm, at least one quick intubation with suctioning should be performed before the oxygen bag is applied to the endotracheal tube for further resuscitation efforts.

Immediately after endotracheal suctioning and resuscitation in the delivery room, the infant should be taken to the admission or intensive care nursery as the infant's condition warrants, for further care, including postural drainage, percussion, and other care directed at consequences of possible meconium aspiration.

tages, including the ability to deliver continuous positive airway pressure and 100% oxygen. Because this bag does not have a preset pop-off valve, the risk of pneumothorax is increased when the bag is used by a person inexperienced in hand ventilation.

A second type of resuscitation bag is self-inflating, and does not need to be attached to flowing oxygen in order to function. Many of these bags have a preset pop-off pressure limit that reduces the risk of pneumothorax. However, the concentration of oxygen delivered by this unit is limited to approximately 40%. A special adaptor may be attached to increase the concentration to 90% or slightly higher.

Administering Oxygen to the Neonate

During the initial resuscitation efforts, a 100% oxygen concentration is administered to the neonate. As soon as the infant's condition is stabilized, the concentration is adjusted to maintain the PaO$_2$ (partial pressure of oxygen in the blood determined by obtaining and analyzing arterial blood samples) within acceptable limits. This adjustment is essential, since elevated PaO$_2$ levels (caused by administration of oxygen in high concentrations) can cause irreparable damage to retinal vessels (retrolental fibroplasia). Furthermore, high oxygen concentrations can directly injure lung tissue.

Oxygen Mask.   Oxygen masks are used only as a temporary method for the delivery of oxygen to the neonate during resuscitative efforts. If an infant is mildly (Apgar 5 to 7) to moderately depressed at birth (Apgar 3 to 4), oxygen is administered through a tight-fitting mask specifically designed for infants. The nurse must be certain to use a mask of the correct size to avoid oxygen leaks. Care must be taken to prevent pressure on the infant's eyeballs, because this can cause tissue ischemia and blindness. The use of soft-edged masks to deliver oxygen will minimize the risk of trauma to the face and eyes.

Endotracheal Tube.   When the infant is severely depressed (Apgar 0 to 2), oxygen is administered through an uncuffed endotracheal tube (see Fig. 33–2). The end of the tube is attached to a ventilation bag or to a mechanical ventilator if the neonate requires extended ventilatory assistance.

Initiating and Supporting Cardiac Function

External Cardiac Massage

If the heart beat is absent or remains low (under 60 bpm) after breathing is established, external cardiac massage should be initiated.

1.   The infant is placed in a supine position on a flat, firm surface.

preferred ventilation bag is a flow-inflating anesthesia-type with a safety "pop-off" valve. This prevents the buildup of excessive pressures within the bag and decreases the risk of pneumothorax. A manometer should be attached to the ventilation system to assist the nurse in monitoring the pressures applied during hand ventilation.

The flow-inflating anesthesia bag has several advan-

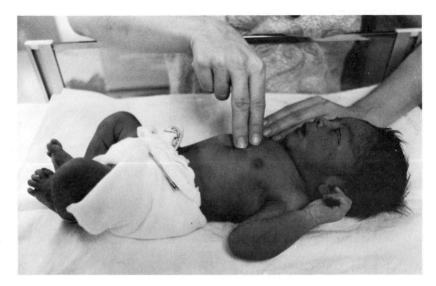

Figure 33-3. The two-finger method of external cardiac massage of the neonate. The fingertips are placed over the middle third of the sternum. The sternum is compressed 1 to 2 cm at a rate of 100 to 200 times per minute.

2. The index and middle finger are placed on the middle third of the sternum (Fig. 33-3). An alternative method is to stand at the foot of the infant and place both thumbs on the middle third of the sternum (Fig. 33-4).

3. The sternum is depressed 1 to 2 cm at a rate of 100 to 120 times per minute.

The effectiveness of massage is evaluated by palpating the femoral pulse or the umbilical cord.

A 3:1 ratio is recommended between heart beat and assisted breathing, but the ventilation rate may be increased, depending on the infant's response to resuscitation and the presence of other complicating factors (*e.g.,* meconium aspiration, congenital anomalies of the respiratory tract).

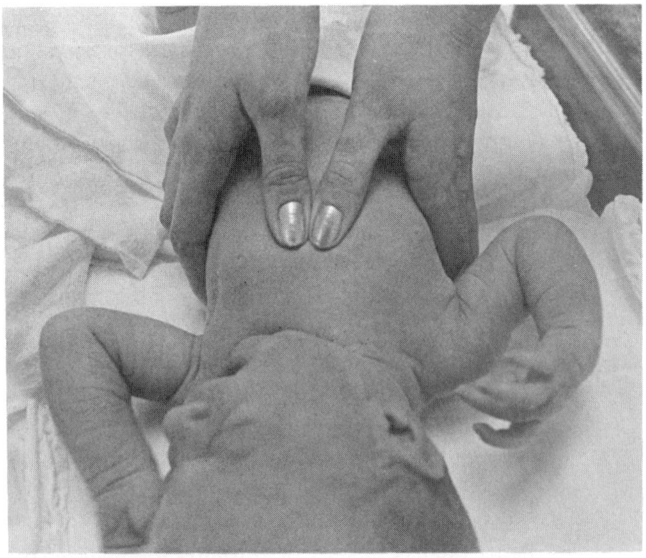

The pulse rate should be checked periodically and chest compression discontinued when the spontaneous heart rate reaches 80 bpm or greater. Compressions should always be accompanied by positive pressure ventilations with 100% oxygen at a rate of 40 to 60 per minute. There are currently no data to permit a recommendation regarding the coordination of ventilation and chest compressions (American Heart Association 1986).

Adjunctive Drug Therapy

If a spontaneous heart rate of at least 100 bpm has not been established after 5 minutes of cardiac massage, adjunctive drug therapy is administered via an umbilical venous catheter to correct metabolic acidosis, hypoglycemia, and poor cardiac output (Table 33-4).

ONGOING ASSESSMENT

Once the neonate's condition has stabilized after birth, it may be possible to reunite baby and parents and provide the new family with extended contact in a rooming-in arrangement. Ongoing assessment occurs at the mother's bedside and provides the nurse with opportunities for teaching and support. An infant who requires additional support and observation after delivery will be placed in an admission or observation nursery. The nurse should encourage parents to visit the infant as soon as possible, and the father can accompany the neonate to the nursery to provide emotional support during the admission procedures.

Figure 33-4. The two-thumb method of external cardiac massage requires the nurse to stand at the foot of the neonate and encircle the chest with her hands. Thumb placement and compression rate are similar to the two finger method shown in Figure 33-3.

Table 33-4   **Adjunctive Therapy to Support Cardiac Function**

Agent	Administration and Function
Sodium bicarbonate	2–3 mEq/kg diluted in a 1:1 solution with sterile water or a 10% dextrose solution infused slowly over 2 to 4 min via the umbilical vein to correct metabolic acidosis
Dextrose	2 ml/kg of 10% solution infused slowly via umbilical vein to correct hypoglycemia followed by 4 ml/kg/hr maintenance
Epinephrine	0.1 ml/kg of a 1:10,000 solution via direct injection into the heart or umbilical vein infusion or into the endotracheal tube to correct asystole or severe bradycardia
Calcium gluconate	1–2 ml/kg of a 10% solution by slow IV infusion to correct bradycardia and low cardiac output
Atropine	0.01–0.03 mg/kg IV infusion to correct bradycardia
Isoproterenol	1–2 mg/100 ml 5% dextrose infused at a rate sufficient to maintain heart rate (usually 1 ml/kg/hr is adequate)
Whole blood	10–20 ml/kg to correct blood loss and hypotension
Albumin	10–15 ml/kg of 5% solution to improve perfusion
Ringer's lactate	10 ml/kg to improve perfusion

Identifying Danger Signals

The neonate is usually placed in an isolette or under a radiant warmer to support thermoregulatory control and may be attached to a cardiorespiratory monitor and pulse oximeter for continuous assessment of cardiopulmonary function and blood oxygen saturation. Because the infant is unable to articulate problems and needs, the nurse must be alert for signs of change in neonatal condition. Subtle and barely perceptible clues are often the first sign of morbidity.

Because the infant is physiologically immature, many signs of illness are nonspecific. A thorough physical examination, laboratory analyses of body fluids, and other tests may be required to identify the exact cause of the problem. Major danger signals that may identify the high-risk neonate are shown in the Nursing Alert on page 1008.

Central Nervous System Signs

The neurologic system is particularly sensitive to both external and internal stressors. Chromosomal anomalies and chronic intrauterine infection associated with mental retardation are often characterized by central nervous system aberrations. Decreases in blood oxygen concentration and serum glucose levels result in central nervous system dysfunction, manifested by altered states of consciousness, seizure activity, or even coma. The nurse is frequently first alerted to illness in the neonate by alterations in CNS functioning. When physical assessment of the infant is conducted in a systematic manner, neurologic status is evaluated first.

Lethargy. A change in the infant's state of consciousness may be the first indication of illness. The neonate may become listless or lethargic and difficult to rouse

for feedings. The nurse must review the intrapartum record to determine if maternal analgesia or anesthesia could be a possible cause of sleepiness or lethargy in the infant. Persistent lethargy is a significant finding that must be documented and reported to the physician.

High-Pitched Cry. A high-pitched or shrill cry may be an indicator of CNS injury or abnormality in the newborn. It is often found in infants with brain defects caused by chromosomal abnormalities, such as *cri du chat* syndrome, in infants undergoing drug withdrawal, or with fetal alcohol syndrome.

Jitteriness. Transient jitteriness (fine motor tremors) is observed in normal infants when they are hungry or irritable, but when the brain has sustained injury, as in hemorrhage or with drug and alcohol withdrawal, persistent jitteriness is common. Jitteriness also occurs with hypoglycemia, hypocalcemia, and hypomagnesemia when brain cells are depleted of glucose, the essential fuel for metabolic activities. Infants of addicted mothers may demonstrate severe tremulousness during postnatal withdrawal from drugs the mother ingested prenatally.

Marked tremors are easily recognized by the experienced nurse. An immediate evaluation of the serum glucose level should be obtained, since untreated hypoglycemia can result in permanent neurologic injury. The nurse discusses observations and the results of the serum glucose test with the physician. If glucose levels are normal, further diagnostic tests are ordered to determine the cause of the jitteriness.

Seizure Activity. Seizure activity is also a nonspecific sign of disease and injury in the neonate and most frequently presents as subtle signs difficult for the untrained observer to recognize. The signs include nystagmus, repeated blinking, sucking motions, or tongue

NURSING ALERT

Major Danger Signs of Neonatal Morbidity

Central Nervous System Signs

- Lethargy (listlessness, difficulty in rousing for feedings)
- High pitched cry
- Jitteriness
- Seizure activity (nystagmus, repeated blinking, sucking motions, tongue thrusting, rhythmic rowing movements of upper extremities, bicycling motions of lower extremities, assumption of rigid posture)
- Abnormal fontanelle size or bulging fontanelles

Respiratory Signs

- Apnea (frequently preceded by "periodic breathing," which is a cyclic pattern of regular breathing for 10–15 sec followed by a similar period with no breathing, resulting in *no* cyanosis of heart rate change, with an average respiratory rate of 30–40/min)
- Tachypnea (rapid respiratory rate)
- Nasal flaring
- Chest retractions
- Asynchronous breathing movements (flattening of chest and protrusion of abdomen with each inspiration: seesaw respirations)
- Expiratory grunting

Cardiovascular Signs

- Abnormal rate and rhythm
- Murmurs (frequently associated with other cardiovascular findings)
- Alterations and differentials in pulses (variations in rate, regularity, amplitude, volume, rhythm, symmetry)
- Changes in perfusion and skin color

Gastrointestinal Signs

- Refusal of two or more feedings
- Absent or uncoordinated feeding reflexes (uncoordinated suck, swallow, or gag reflexes)
- Vomiting (projectile, occurring at any time, resulting in significant losses of body fluids and electrolytes)
- Abdominal distention (protuberant abdomen; taut, shiny skin; prominent superficial veins)
- Changes in stool patterns (diarrhea, absence of stools, bloody stools)

Metabolic Alterations

- Hypoglycemia
- Hypocalcemia
- Hyperbilirubinemia
- Temperature instability

thrusting. Vasomotor instability with mottling of skin and apnea have also been associated with seizures. More obvious indicators include rhythmic rowing movements of upper extremities, bicycling motions of lower extremities, and assumption of a rigid posture.

The nurse must distinguish jitteriness from seizure activity. Jitteriness can be dampened or stopped by holding the extremities or swaddling the infant, whereas seizures do not cease when the limbs are held. Infants at greater risk for developing seizures include those who sustained severe asphyxia or intracranial hemorrhage at birth and those who have meningitis. Neonates experiencing acute drug withdrawal are also susceptible. The nurse takes note of risk factors associated with the development of seizures and closely observes the infant for evidence of seizure activity.

Abnormal Fontanelle Size or Bulging Fontanelles.
The anterior fontanelle may normally pulsate or bulge slightly when the infant cries vigorously, especially in a supine or prone position. True bulging or palpable tenseness of the fontanelles is associated with increased intra-

cranial pressure resulting from hemorrhage or hydrocephalus (an abnormal accumulation of cerebrospinal fluid in the ventricles of the brain). Enlarged fontanelles are associated with chromosomal anomalies, such as trisomies; skeletal disorders, including osteogenesis imperfecta; and congenital hypothyroidism.

The nurse must report and document findings of abnormal fontanelle size or shape and obtain daily measurements of head circumference to determine the rate of head growth. Hydrocephalus may be obvious at birth or can develop rapidly within the first several months of life, and early detection will assist in the diagnosis and treatment of the disorder.

Respiratory Signs

Any alterations in cardiac or respiratory function will result in observable changes in respiratory effort. Early signs of distress, such as mild nasal flaring or an increased respiratory rate, may be missed if the nurse is not alert to these subtle signs of dysfunction. Marked respiratory distress is obvious and is manifested by cyanosis, tachypnea, chest retractions, or grunting. It may appear suddenly with acute airway obstruction or pneumothorax.

The infant may present with immediate signs of respiratory distress at the time of birth or develop symptoms at any time during the neonatal period. Close observation and frequent monitoring of respiratory function is essential to prevent life-threatening compromise in high-risk neonates. Prematurity, birth asphyxia, meconium aspiration, pneumonia, pneumothorax, and diaphragmatic hernia are associated with respiratory distress.

Apnea.   The neonate may experience episodes of apnea immediately after birth or at any time during the transition period. Premature infants may suffer from episodes of apnea for many weeks after birth until the central nervous system matures. True apnea is defined as a cessation of respiration for 15 seconds or longer (Epstein 1985). In addition to prematurity, it is associated with a variety of conditions, including hypoxia, upper airway obstruction, gastroesophageal reflux, seizures, and fatigue.

Apneic spells are frequently preceded by an episode of "periodic breathing," which consists of shorter periods of apnea lasting 5 to 15 seconds followed by rapid and often shallow respirations. The nurse must be alert to alterations in respiratory patterns and is assisted by the use of cardiorespiratory and transcutaneous oxygen monitors, which can document apnea and changes in oxygenation.

Primary apnea occurs immediately after delivery. A severely depressed infant will take several gasping breaths in an effort to initiate respirations and then stop breathing. After a pause ranging from several seconds to 1 to 2 minutes, weak and ineffectual breathing efforts begin again. Quick and correct management — which includes (1) maintenance of the airway, (2) oxygenation and ventilation, and (3) mild stimulation — generally results in improved respiratory effort and stabilization of the neonate.

If measures are not initiated to assist the severely depressed infant during the initial gasping and apnea episode, *secondary apnea* ensues, and progressive hypoxia and brainstem depression will make subsequent attempts to resuscitate the infant difficult. Tactile stimulation and blow-by oxygen (a flow of oxygen passed across the face) will not be sufficient to stimulate respirations. Immediate endotracheal intubation and ventilation with 100% oxygen is essential if the infant is to have any chance to survive.

Signs of respiratory distress are evident as the neonate struggles to improve oxygen intake. The degree of distress may be graded using the Silverman–Andersen Index, shown in Figure 33–5.

Tachypnea.   One of the earliest signs of illness in the neonate and a common indicator of respiratory distress is a rapid respiratory rate (over 60 breaths per minute).

Nasal Flaring.   The neonate is an obligate nose breather. With respiratory distress, the neonate will dilate the nares with each inspiration in an attempt to increase the inflow of air.

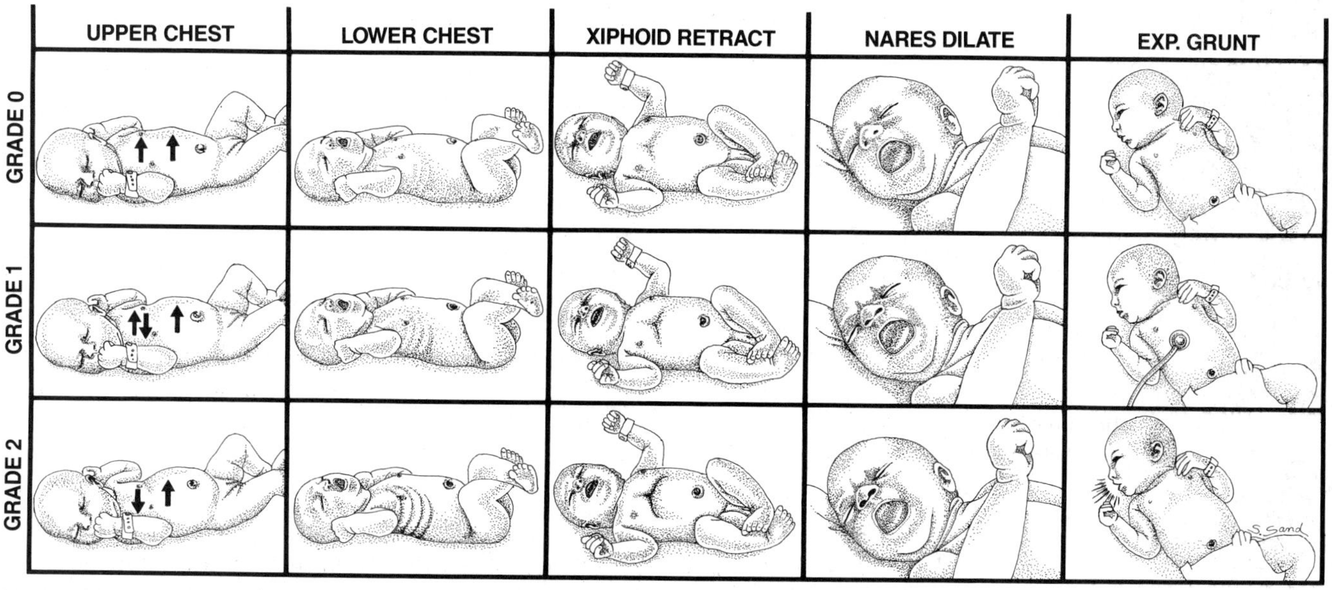

Figure 33–5. The Silverman–Andersen index of neonatal respiratory distress. Observation of retractions. An index of respiratory distress is determined by grading each of five arbitrary criteria. Grade 0 indicates no difficulty; grade 1 indicates moderate difficulty; and grade 2 indicates maximum respiratory difficulty. The retraction score is the sum of these values; a total score of 0 indicates no dyspnea, whereas a total score of 10 denotes maximal respiratory distress.

Chest Retractions.   Pulmonary atelectasis and non-compliant lung tissue increase the amount of negative intrathoracic pressure experienced on inspiration. As the rib cage expands with each inspiration, the soft tissues of the thorax and weak intercostal muscles are pulled in toward the spine, giving rise to intercostal retractions. Breathing is difficult and labored.

Asynchronous Breathing Movements.   As respiratory distress increases in severity, chest and abdominal breathing movements become asynchronous. The chest flattens and the abdomen protrudes with each inspiration. Respirations that follow this pattern are called *see-saw respirations.*

Expiratory Grunting.   The neonate in respiratory distress exhales against a closed glottis in an effort to increase intrapulmonary pressure and keep alveoli open during exhalation, thus preventing atelectasis. This effort produces a peeping noise, which may be audible without use of a stethoscope in severe respiratory distress.

Cardiovascular Signs

Congenital heart anomalies, pulmonary disease, and severe asphyxia affect cardiovascular function. The nurse assesses heart rate and rhythm, pulses, and skin perfusion for evidence of alteration in cardiovascular status. Because the nurses caring for the neonate conduct systematic evaluations of heart function at least once per shift, it is often the nurse who initially identifies cardiovascular abnormalities.

Abnormal Rate and Rhythm.   Dysrhythmias may be found in the normal newborn (sinus tachycardia, PAT, and ectopic beats) but also occur with cardiomyopathies, certain drug therapies, electrolyte imbalance, and congenital anomalies. The neonatal heart responds to mild-to-moderate stress with an increase in heart rate. Premature infants normally have a high baseline rate (above 160 bpm).

If stressors placed on the cardiovascular system are severe, such as profound hypoxia or massive brain hemorrhage, bradycardia will occur. Sinus bradycardia is found with congenital heart block and can be induced by stimulating the vagus nerve during suctioning or endotracheal intubation. Premature infants may also experience bradycardia in association with apnea or fatigue.

Cardiac monitors and pulse oximeters are frequently employed by the nurse today to assist in continuous monitoring of heart rate and rhythm and blood oxygen saturation in the high-risk or sick neonate. Alarms may be set on these electronic monitors to alert the nurse to episodes of tachycardia, bradycardia, and decreasing blood oxygen saturation. Electrocardiograph strips can be generated during periods of abnormal heart activity to assist physicians in diagnosing cardiac abnormalities.

Murmurs.   Murmurs can be heard in up to 60% of normal newborns after the first 2 hours of life. They result from the incomplete closure of fetal circulatory bypasses. Most are grade 1 and 2 systolic ejection murmurs, which are best auscultated at the second left intercostal space. Pathologic murmurs are frequently associated with other cardiovascular findings, such as cyanosis, diminished or bounding pulses, hypotension, hypertension, and abnormal cardiac size or shape. Holosystolic murmurs coupled with thrills or with an active precordium (easily palpated movement of the chest wall over the heart associated with systole) are also indicative of pathology. Pathologic murmurs are also associated with congenital heart anomalies, such as ventricular septal defect. Premature infants are at high risk for developing murmurs associated with persistent patent ductus arteriosus. It is suggested that lack of muscular development in ductal tissues in very immature infants contributes to persistent patent ductus. The ductus is extremely sensitive to blood oxygen concentrations and normally closes with rising arterial PO_2 levels after birth. Both preterm and full-term infants with severe hypoxia may develop murmurs with the reopening of the ductus arteriosus secondary to lowered arterial PO_2 levels.

Alterations and Differentials in Pulses.   Weak or thready pulses (charted as $1+$) are evident with hypovolemia and shock. Bounding ($3+$) pulses may be palpated with congestive heart failure. Differential pulses (that is, pulses in which there is a difference in amplitude or volume between left and right upper extremities or upper and lower extremities) may be found with shunting and with certain cardiac anomalies. The nurse palpates the peripheral pulses (brachial, femoral, dorsal pedal, and posterior tibial) at regular intervals to detect alterations in rate, regularity, amplitude, volume, rhythm, and symmetry.

Changes in Perfusion and Skin Color.   The nurse should evaluate skin perfusion and color in a well-lit environment; subtle color changes may be one of the first signs of illness in the neonate. A pale or gray color or circumoral cyanosis, particularly when associated with feeding or crying, may indicate a cardiac problem. Generalized mottling and poor peripheral perfusion (capillary filling time greater than 3 seconds) may be an early sign of disease or distress.

Gastrointestinal Signs

The feeding and elimination patterns of the healthy neonate are remarkably predictable. Many infants are alert and stable enough to breast-feed almost immediately after birth. The passage of meconium stools usually occurs in the first 24 hours of life and frequently within several hours of birth. The neonate who refuses two or more feedings is a sick infant; this is often an early sign of neonatal complications. The nurse observes the infant closely for deviations from these norms in behavior.

Absent or Uncoordinated Feeding Reflexes. An infant who feeds slowly with weak and uncoordinated suck, swallow, or gag reflexes is characterized as a "poor feeder." This pattern is encountered with prematurity, congenital cleft lip or palate, oral-pharyngeal trauma secondary to endotracheal intubation, and maternal overmedication in labor and delivery as a sequela of birth asphyxia or injury. The neonate with uncoordinated feeding reflexes is at risk for aspiration and pneumonia. Careful assessment of the infant's ability to suck and swallow effectively is essential to prevent major respiratory complications related to aspiration and to prevent calorie and fluid deficits.

Vomiting. Although some degree of regurgitation is normal in neonates because the neonatal cardiac sphincter is immature and weak, vomiting is an abnormal sign associated with overfeeding, sepsis, metabolic disorders such as galactosemia, increased intracranial pressure, and intestinal atresia and stenosis. It may also be a nonspecific indicator of illness in the neonate.

It is essential that the nurse differentiate between regurgitation and vomiting. Regurgitation most frequently occurs within the first hour after feeding and commonly occurs in conjunction with burping or spontaneous eructation of air. Simple regurgitation is not normally associated with disease and does not cause fluid and electrolyte imbalances. In contrast, vomiting is often projectile in nature, can occur at any time, and results in the loss of significant amounts of body fluids and electrolytes.

The nurse assesses the nature of the emesis. The vomitus may be mixed with a large amount of mucus, suggesting an obstruction proximal to the stomach, may be bile-stained, suggesting an obstruction distal to the ampulla, or fecal in nature, indicating a lower gastrointestinal tract obstruction. Hematemesis also occurs and may be caused by swallowed maternal blood during labor or organic disease in the neonate.

Abdominal Distention. An increase in abdominal girth is associated with a variety of neonatal complications, including necrotizing enterocolitis, meconium plug and ileus, and congenital atresia or stenosis of the bowel. Abdominal distention may be present at birth or can develop within the first 24 to 48 hours of life. The abdomen becomes tense and protuberant, the skin appears taut and shiny, and superficial veins become prominent over the abdomen. Respiratory distress occurs if distention becomes severe. Bowel sounds may be absent, or peristaltic waves strongly suggestive of obstruction may be visible.

The nurse must obtain serial measurements of abdominal girth when the infant is at risk for the development of gastrointestinal disorders, or when abdominal distention is suspected. Continued frequent inspection, palpation, and auscultation of the abdomen is an essential aspect of nursing assessment. Routine palpation is contraindicated if the abdomen is distended or tight.

Changes in Stool Patterns. Diarrhea may be a sign of intestinal infection or intolerance to cow's milk. An absence of stools after birth may indicate imperforate anus or congenital intestinal atresia or stenosis. Meconium ileus or meconium plug will also result in diminished or absent stooling and may be due to cystic fibrosis. Blood in the stools (gross or microscopic) occurs with necrotizing enterocolitis and is a grave sign. Altered stool patterns, including loose stools, can follow antibiotic therapy and can occur with an infant receiving phototherapy.

The nurse documents the passage of all stools, noting the amount, color, consistency, and odor. In high-risk or sick neonates, fecal material is tested for the presence of blood or glucose, both of which are early warning signs of gastrointestinal dysfunction.

Metabolic Alterations

The high-risk or sick neonate is at risk for a variety of metabolic disorders that can be lethal if left untreated. These disorders occur as a result of stressors that deplete the neonate's energy reserves and injure cells essential to major metabolic functions. Responsibility for early detection of these metabolic abnormalities lies primarily with the nurses who are caring for the infant.

Hypoglycemia. One of the major complications of disease or injury in the newborn is hypoglycemia. Hypoglycemia is defined as a glucose level of under 30 mg/dl of whole blood during the first 72 hours after birth in the full-term infant and under 40 mg/dl after the first 72 hours. Normal blood values are slightly lower in low-birth-weight infants (under 20 mg/dl of whole blood with two consecutive blood samples).

Many high-risk infants are born with limited or depleted stores of liver glucose, including small for gestational age, preterm, and post-term infants. Infants who are stressed at birth (from asphyxia or cold) quickly utilize all available glucose stores and become hypoglycemic. Infants of diabetic mothers may experience profound hypoglycemia shortly after birth as a result of hyperinsulinism.

Hypoglycemia is frequently manifested by jitteriness and lethargy. The nurse who identifies signs of hypoglycemia must determine the serum glucose level immediately. A glucose strip (Dextrostix or Chemstrip) test can be used to determine the blood glucose level in 60 seconds when a capillary blood sample is obtained by heel prick. A venous blood sample can also be drawn for a more accurate laboratory determination, but requires time for analysis. The glucose strip test can be used as a guide to immediate therapy, until laboratory results are obtained.

Hypocalcemia.   Hypocalcemia is defined as a calcium level of less than 7 mg/dl. It is found in preterm infants with immature parathyroid function, in infants of diabetic mothers, with hypertrophy of the parathyroid gland, and in infants who have sustained birth asphyxia. Any high-risk neonate who receives intravenous fluids containing low levels of calcium is also at risk for hypocalcemia. Signs of hypocalcemia include jitteriness, twitching, and heightened sensitivity to sensory stimuli. If untreated, the infant may develop carpopedal spasms, laryngospasm, and convulsions. Vomiting and hematemesis may occur. The nurse observes infants at risk for hypocalcemia for signs of increased neuromuscular irritability and monitors serum calcium levels closely.

Early neonatal hypocalcemia occurs within the first 2 to 3 days of life and is related to the above conditions. Late hypocalcemia occurs between the sixth and tenth day and results from the ingestion of formula with an inappropriate calcium-phosphorus ratio. With recent advances in the development of feeding formulas for preterm and high-risk neonates, late hypocalcemia is encountered less frequently.

Hyperbilirubinemia and Jaundice.   Many sick neonates are at risk for the development of hyperbilirubinemia and jaundice. Preterm neonates and infants of diabetic mothers have an immature liver enzyme system. Asphyxiated infants are at increased risk because acid metabolites compete with bilirubin for albumin binding sites. Other conditions predisposing to the development of jaundice are congenital obstruction of the intestinal tract, urinary tract infections, enclosed hemorrhage, hypoglycemia, hypothermia, and extreme ecchymosis secondary to traumatic delivery. The nurse examines the infant (in natural light if possible) for evidence of jaundice and closely monitors serum bilirubin levels.

Temperature Instability.   The elevation in temperature that normally accompanies bacterial infections in adults is absent in the newborn. Hypothermia and wide swings in temperature are more common and may be an early sign of sepsis. The rapid depletion of brown fat and liver glucose stores that often accompanies severe stress contributes to hypothermia in the high-risk neonate. Infants who have sustained severe head injuries and intracranial hemorrhage also suffer from temperature instability.

Because high-risk infants are so susceptible to temperature swings or hypothermia, they are frequently placed in an isolette or under a radiant warmer to support their thermoregulatory function. A temperature probe may be attached to the skin surface to assist the nurse in monitoring changes in skin temperature. When the probe senses changes in skin temperature, the heating element used to warm the infant is adjusted automatically to maintain the infant's body temperature within normal limits.

Identifying Behavioral Abnormalities in the High-Risk Neonate

The high-risk or sick neonate may have limited behavioral capacities during the stabilization period following birth. Internal and external stressors may render the infant incapable of organizing its responses into adaptive behavior patterns that support social interaction with care givers and parents. Attempts at stimulation may actually worsen the infant's condition if the attempts are improperly timed or inappropriate for the level of neurobehavioral development. Gorski (1979) identified three stages of behavioral organization unique to the high-risk neonate.

Physiologic Stage.   During the first critical days after birth, the high-risk infant may be unable to participate reciprocally with care givers or parents in establishing mutually satisfying interactions. All of the neonate's energies are focused inward, on the development of physiologic stability. The infant may lie motionless for long periods. Response to painful stimuli may range from a generalized startle response to uneven and intermittent focal reactions. It may be impossible to rouse the infant to the alert state of consciousness. The neonate is incapable of organizing behaviors for any type of social response.

First Active Response Stage.   As a state of physiologic stability is achieved, the infant is able to respond to external stimuli in an organized manner. The neonate is able to provide care givers with some indication of behavioral capacities and unique temperament and is capable of moving to an alert, awake state of consciousness for short periods.

It is during this stage that care-givers can significantly affect the physical and emotional wellbeing of the infant by responding appropriately to cues. Feeding schedules can be adjusted to emerging sleep/wake cycles. Eliminating nonessential noise from the environment and providing time for cuddling and eye-to-eye contact also have a positive impact on the infant's condition.

Reciprocity Stage.   The infant is now strong enough to respond to care giver behaviors in specific and predictable ways. Brazelton states that the developing relationship between parents and infant plays a key role in this final phase of development. A critical factor is the ability of parents to identify and respond to infant cues in an appropriate manner. Infants exposed to overstimulation or who are stimulated at the wrong time are at risk for both physical and emotional disorders. Nursing interventions are aimed at acquainting parents with the unique behavioral capacities of their infant and supporting appropriate reciprocal interactions. Some high-risk neonates continue to suffer from behavioral disorganization and do not provide consistent cues. Parents of these infants require additional assistance and support.

Identifying Parenting Risk Factors

An integral aspect of risk assessment is an ongoing evaluation of the parents' response to the birth of the high-risk or sick neonate. The nurse must be familiar with current theories regarding psychological reactions to this stressful event in order to understand observations and analyze the data collected about the new family. A brief review of crisis and grieving theory is presented in this section. The student is also referred to the previous chapters that have discussed the childbearing couple's response to high-risk pregnancy and to the references at the end of this chapter for further readings on parental reactions to the birth of a high-risk or sick infant.

Birth of a High-Risk Infant: A Potential Family Crisis

The birth of a less than perfect infant can be viewed as a potential crisis. The key word is "potential," because this unhappy event does not inevitably lead to disorganization within the family unit. It can result in growth for both parents and a restructuring of the family unit so that it is actually stronger than before the birth of the baby. The way in which the family responds to the period of stress is crucial in determining whether a crisis will develop. Environmental factors, such as family and professional support, will also influence the eventual outcome. Aguilera and Messick (1985) have identified major balancing factors that aid in the resolution of a potential crisis situation with the birth of a preterm infant (Fig. 33–6).

Three major balancing factors operate during a potential crisis:

- The parents' perception of the event
- The situational supports available to the parents
- The coping mechanisms used to deal with the stressful event

If parents have an accurate perception of their infant's problem and prognosis, problem-solving efforts will be focused on realistic solutions. If the parents have an adequate support system to help them solve their problems, their chances of avoiding a crisis are better. The support system can be composed of family, friends, and health

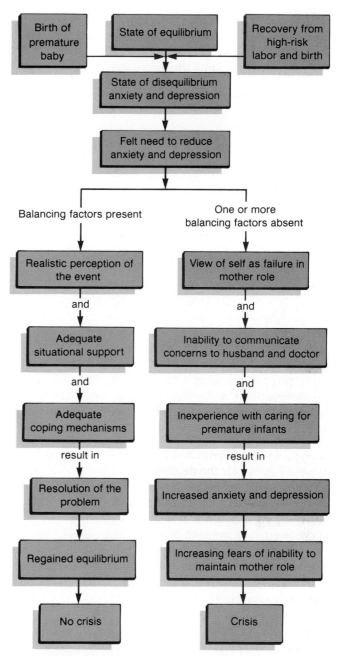

Figure 33–6. Environmental factors may balance the negative aspects of the birth of a high-risk infant so that parents adapt well. If these balancing factors are absent, the negative aspects of the situation may be intensified. The result then is likely to be difficulty in adaptation and crisis. (From Aguilera DC, Messick J: Crisis Intervention, 4th ed. St Louis, CV Mosby, 1982)

professionals. Recently, community support groups have been formed to help parents cope with the stressors surrounding the birth of a high-risk infant (*e.g.,* Parents of Premies). If defense mechanisms, such as denial or anger, are used constructively in the coping process, the parents have a better chance of resolving the potential crisis.

Family Considerations

Characteristics of the Early Stages of the Grieving Process

Shock

Stunned silence

Inability to verbalize

Inability to follow simple explanations or directions

Inability to give information

Inability to understand what is said about infant's condition

Physical reactions — pallor, tremors, nausea or vomiting, feedings of faintness or actual syncope

Denial/Disbelief

Withdrawal from infant or other family members

Physical abandonment of mother/infant by father of infant

Unrealistic optimism

Expressions of feelings of unreality: "I can't believe this is happening"

Refusal to speak about infant's condition

Refusal to see infant

Refusal to participate in decisions about treatment of child

Anger

Irritability

Use of profanity

Throwing objects

Hitting out at others in the environment

Verbal abuse of spouse, family members, or staff members

Angry requests to be left alone

Assignment of blame to staff or others

Verbalizations of anger

Guilt

Repeated reviews of course of pregnancy, labor, and delivery for causes of neonatal problems

Repeated questions about possible causes of problem

Verbalization of guilt: "It's my fault"

Statements such as "If only I had not done . . ."

Assignment of cause of problem to past actions, omissions, or "sins"

Statements that problem is "a punishment from God"

Sadness

Loss of appetite

Difficulty in sleeping

Crying

Restlessness

Other somatic complaints

Inability to focus attention

Verbalization of sadness or depression

Verbalization of sense of failure

Verbalization of wanting to be left alone

Parental Grieving Process

Birth of a sick or high-risk infant evokes a grief response in parents as they mourn the loss of the idealized child they fantasized about during pregnancy. The stages of grieving are essentially the same as those described by Kubler–Ross (1974).

Shock. Parents feel numb and unable to comprehend the full import of the problem. They may withdraw, showing no evidence of discomfort or sadness, in an effort to avoid the pain that will follow with full realization of the infant's condition. This period may last from minutes to days.

Denial and Disbelief. Parents cannot believe that the stressful event is really happening to them. If the defect or disorder is not observable, they may deny that any problem exists. This phase may also be characterized by unrealistic optimism in the face of a very poor prognosis. Parents may say that the situation seems "unreal."

The length of this period depends in part on the visibility of the defect or disease. It is more difficult for parents to continue denying the problem when there is a severe and obvious anomaly.

Anger. Once parents permit themselves a full realization of the problem, feelings of anger surface. A healthy response is to displace the anger outward on staff members, family, or friends. Feelings of anger may be verbalized or a parent may react physically by throwing things or hitting out at persons close by.

Sadness and Guilt. Painful feelings are now fully experienced. Physical symptoms of grief may be present, including tightness in the chest or epigastric distress. The parent may experience a feeling of emptiness. Self-recriminations and strong feelings of guilt also emerge: "What did I do to cause this to happen to my baby?" The parent will frequently review the entire course of pregnancy trying to pinpoint something he or she did to cause the problem.

Reorganization and Resolution.   After a prolonged period (sometimes months to years) the feelings of sadness are blunted, the guilt feelings are resolved, and the parent is able to reorganize his or her life. If long-term disabilities remain, parents may regress to previous stages of grieving when new, related problems occur.

In assessing the parents of the high-risk infant, the nurse should attempt to evaluate the success of coping mechanisms and to identify the stage of grief the parents are in. Parents will provide both verbal and nonverbal cues that will assist the nurse in identifying adaptive and maladaptive responses to the birth of the high-risk or sick neonate. Examples of both adaptive and maladaptive responses are shown in Figure 33–7. Characteristics of the early phases of the grieving process are listed in the accompanying display on the opposite page.

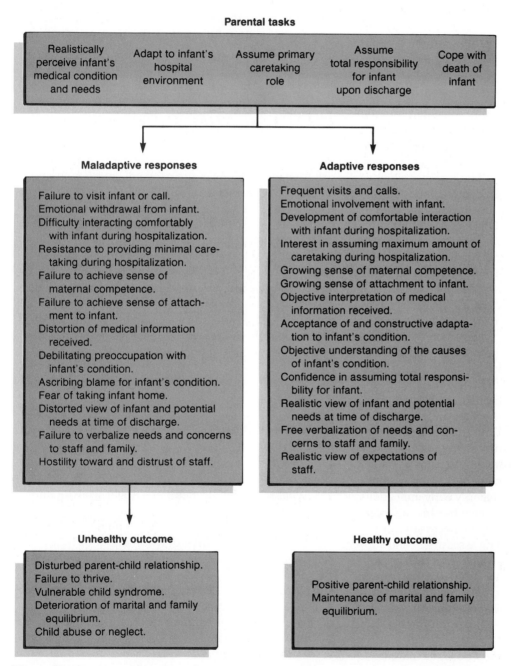

Parental tasks

| Realistically perceive infant's medical condition and needs | Adapt to infant's hospital environment | Assume primary caretaking role | Assume total responsibility for infant upon discharge | Cope with death of infant |

Maladaptive responses

Failure to visit infant or call.
Emotional withdrawal from infant.
Difficulty interacting comfortably with infant during hospitalization.
Resistance to providing minimal caretaking during hospitalization.
Failure to achieve sense of maternal competence.
Failure to achieve sense of attachment to infant.
Distortion of medical information received.
Debilitating preoccupation with infant's condition.
Ascribing blame for infant's condition.
Fear of taking infant home.
Distorted view of infant and potential needs at time of discharge.
Failure to verbalize needs and concerns to staff and family.
Hostility toward and distrust of staff.

Adaptive responses

Frequent visits and calls.
Emotional involvement with infant.
Development of comfortable interaction with infant during hospitalization.
Interest in assuming maximum amount of caretaking during hospitalization.
Growing sense of maternal competence.
Growing sense of attachment to infant.
Objective interpretation of medical information received.
Acceptance of and constructive adaptation to infant's condition.
Objective understanding of the causes of infant's condition.
Confidence in assuming total responsibility for infant.
Realistic view of infant and potential needs at time of discharge.
Free verbalization of needs and concerns to staff and family.
Realistic view of expectations of staff.

Unhealthy outcome

Disturbed parent-child relationship.
Failure to thrive.
Vulnerable child syndrome.
Deterioration of marital and family equilibrium.
Child abuse or neglect.

Healthy outcome

Positive parent-child relationship.
Maintenance of marital and family equilibrium.

Figure 33–7. Parents may show either adaptive or maladaptive responses to the tasks of parenting a high-risk newborn. The nurse should assess the quality of parental adaptation so that effective and appropriate intervention can be implemented. (Grant P: Psychosocial needs of families of high-risk infants. Fam Commun Health 11:93, 1978)

Indications of Positive Coping Behavior

The parents of a high-risk infant will need time to adjust to the birth of their infant. Separation of parent and child may lengthen the time it takes for adaptive responses to appear. Frequent visits or calls are one indicator of the beginning of attachment. Naming the child is another. A desire to assume increasing responsibility for the care of the neonate and demonstrations of increasing competency in his care over time are other positive signs. The parents should also develop a realistic perception of the infant's special problems and needs after repeated explanations and reinforcement by the nursing and medical staff.

Indications of Negative Coping Behavior

The nursing staff must gather sufficient data about the parents' past experiences with high-risk infants, their current living conditions, the distance they live from the hospital, their social networks, the transportation available to them, and their work and home responsibilities before determining whether a particular behavior is truly maladaptive. Danger signals include infrequent visits or calls, inability to develop confidence in parenting skills over time, unrealistic view of the infant's condition or needs, or an inability to name the infant.

Klaus and Kennell (1982) have done extensive research on parental reactions to the birth of a high-risk or sick neonate. They recommend that the nurse observe how much time new parents spend with their own infant when they visit the nursery and the type of comments they make about the baby. Do they move from isolette to isolette, apparently just as interested in the other infants' conditions as their own child's? Do they respond to the nurse's suggestions for care of the infant with appropriate efforts at parenting, or do they show growing withdrawal and detachment? As discharge time approaches, do they show increased confidence in their ability to care for the infant? Have they made adequate preparations at home?

It is essential that nurses document their assessment of parental coping behavior and identify early indications of parenting disorders so that the health team can intervene as quickly as possible. It may be necessary for the nursing staff to arrange for ongoing assessment and support for the new family after discharge from the hospital. Frequent distress telephone calls from the parents or more than one visit to the emergency room with an apparently healthy infant are indications that the infant's high-risk status may have contributed to difficulties in parental adaptation.

Nursing care to meet identified needs of parents is planned in collaboration with other members of the health team, such as social workers, psychologists, physicians, and members of support groups and community agencies that help parents of sick infants. Nursing interventions in the care of the high-risk infant and the family are based on systematic assessment and nursing diagnosis; nursing care of the high-risk neonate is presented in Chapter 34. The nurse must remember that nursing assessment, diagnosis, and planning must be a continuous process, since parental needs will change as the neonate's condition changes. The nurse is likely to be the health professional who has the most consistent contact with the infant and family; as such, the nurse is in a unique position to promote optimal health and adaptation after the stressful event of the birth of a high-risk infant.

CHAPTER SUMMARY

Nursing assessment and identification of the newborn at risk for complications in the neonatal period is an essential aspect of neonatal care. The nurse identifies health risks to the fetus during the prenatal period, assists in the immediate resuscitation and stabilization of the infant in the delivery room, and assumes responsibility for ongoing nursing assessment and diagnosis in the period after birth. This chapter has discussed the components of neonatal risk and has described how the nursing process begins with assessment to identify potential or actual problems and development of nursing diagnoses upon which subsequent care will be based. Chapter 34 focuses on nursing care of the high-risk neonate.

STUDY QUESTIONS

1. What is the purpose of identifying perinatal risk factors for the neonate?

2. What is the significance of the Apgar score for immediate and long-term neonatal outcome?

3. What is the role of the nurse in immediate stabilization and resuscitation of the infant at birth?

4. What are the normal steps in resuscitation of the neonate?

5. What drugs are commonly used in neonatal resuscitation and what is their therapeutic function?

6. What are danger signals of potential illness in the high-risk neonate?

7. What are the phases of behavioral reintegration in the high-risk or sick neonate?

8. What are signs of potential parenting disorders in parents of the high-risk or sick neonate?

REFERENCES/BIBLIOGRAPHY

Aguilera D, Messick J: Crisis Intervention: Theory and Methodology, 5th ed. St Louis, CV Mosby, 1985

American Heart Association: Neonatal advanced life support. JAMA 255(21):2969–2973, 1986

Epstein MF: Resuscitation in the delivery room. In Cloherty JP, Stark AR (eds). Manual of Neonatal Care. Boston, Little, Brown & Co, 1985

Gorski P, Davison M, Brazelton B: Stages of behavioral organization in the high-risk neonate: Theoretical and clinical considerations. Semin Perinatol 3(1):61, 1979

Klaus M, Kennell J: Maternal–Infant Bonding, 2nd ed. St Louis, CV Mosby, 1982

Korones S: High-risk Newborn Infants: The Basis For Intensive Nursing Care, 4th ed. St Louis, CV Mosby, 1986

Kubler–Ross E: Questions and Answers on Death and Dying. St Louis, CV Mosby, 1974

SUGGESTED READINGS

Garland KR: Unresolved grief. Neonat Network 4:29–37, 1986

Gunderson LP, Kenner C: Neonatal stress: Physiologic adaptation and nursing implications. Neonat Network 6(1):37–42, 1987

Lemons PM, Weaver DD: Beyond the birth of a defective child. Neonat Network 5(3):13–19, 1986

Sendak MJ, Harris AP: Neonatal pulse oximetry in the delivery room. Perinatol Neonatol 7(1):8–19, 1987

Stevenson DK, Frankel LR, Benitz WE: Immediate management of the asphyxiated infant. J Perinatol 7(3):221–226, 1987

34 nursing care of the high-risk neonate

LEARNING OBJECTIVES

After studying the material in this chapter, the student should be able to

- State nursing objectives in the care of the high-risk neonate

- Describe therapeutic interventions in the care of the neonate with alterations in cardiac and respiratory function

- Describe therapeutic interventions in the care of the neonate with fluid volume deficits

- Describe therapeutic interventions in the care of the neonate with alterations in nutrition

- List principles of infection control in the special care nursery

- Describe therapeutic interventions employed in the prevention of cold stress

- List nursing interventions that may be employed to support the parents of the high-risk neonate

- Describe therapeutic interventions employed in the prevention of hyperbilirubinemia and kernicterus

- Detail therapeutic interventions in the care of the infant who has been asphyxiated at birth

- Detail therapeutic interventions in the care of the neonate with problems related to gestational age

- Describe a nursing care plan for sensory stimulation of the high-risk neonate

- Discuss therapeutic interventions in the care of the infant who is born with a chronic intrauterine infection or who develops an infection in the neonatal period

- Describe nursing care of the neonate who has sustained trauma at birth

KEY TERMS

Apnea

Asphyxia

Intrauterine growth retardation

Large-for-gestational-age infant

Low-birth-weight infant

Post-term infant

Preterm infant

Respiratory distress syndrome

Rh incompatibility

Sepsis

Small-for-gestational-age infant

Just as the nurse caring for the childbearing family rejoices in the birth of a healthy infant, when complications arise the nurse shares in the family's sadness. Nevertheless, the challenge of creating a climate that will support the new parents during this crisis must be met. At the same time, the physical needs of the sick neonate must also be met, using an increasingly complex array of technologic devices.

Whether in a primary care or a tertiary care facility, the nurse must possess the basic skills and knowledge required to recognize major neonatal complications, initiate resuscitation, and assist in stabilizing the neonate's condition. As a result of the regionalization of perinatal care, infants with major complications (*e.g.,* severe anomalies or extreme prematurity) are frequently transported to tertiary care centers once they are in stable condition, but the eventual outcome is influenced by the care the infant receives in the referring hospital immediately after birth.

A major goal of nursing care of the high-risk neonate is to provide optimal family-centered care — that is, to recognize the inherent worth and unique characteristics of each infant, to support parents during the grieving process, and to facilitate parent-infant attachment. The nursing process can serve as a basis for meeting these needs in a rational and systematic manner.

This chapter describes major complications of the neonatal period and describes how the nursing process can be utilized to accomplish the goals of nursing care. Nursing interventions to meet the basic life-support needs of the high-risk neonate, as reflected in nursing diagnoses, are discussed in the first section of this chapter. Specific neonatal disorders and nursing care of neonates with these major complications are listed in the display and are discussed in the second half of this chapter. Legal/ethical dilemmas confronting the NICU nurse are explored. (Neonates with congenital anomalies are discussed in Chapter 35.)

SPECIALIZED NEONATAL CARE AND REGIONALIZATION

All nurses caring for the newborn should possess the knowledge and skills required to recognize neonatal risk factors and signs of illness and should be capable of functioning competently in emergency situations that require resuscitation and stabilization of a sick infant. Continuing care of the high-risk neonate, however, requires specialized services that only a limited number of health care professionals and facilities are capable of providing. There is often inequity in the distribution of these essential services. In rural and impoverished areas, health care facilities may be limited in their ability to provide the equipment and personnel necessary to care for high-risk

Major Complications of Neonates

Birth asphyxia
Birth injuries
    Fracture of clavicle
    Fracture of humerus or femur
    Skull fracture
Central nervous system injuries
    Intracranial hemorrhage
    Brachial plexus injury
    Facial nerve injury
    Phrenic nerve injury
Infection
    Bacterial infections
    Viral and protozoan infections
Hemolytic disease
    Rh incompatibility
    ABO incompatibilities
Complications related to gestational age
    Preterm status
    Small-for-gestational-age (SGA) status
    Large-for-gestational-age (LGA) status
    Post-term status
Maternal substance withdrawal

neonates. In large urban settings there may be unnecessary duplication of services. In an effort to solve these problems, a coordinated system for the provision of care within a designated area or region has been developed. Three levels of perinatal care have been defined and the functions and goals of each described. Table 34–1 describes the types of care provided and the roles and responsibilities of nurses at each level.

An additional goal of perinatal regionalization is to limit the spiraling rise in health care costs. The development of subspecialties within the field of neonatology and the use of complex technology have added to the ever-growing price tag for the care of high-risk infants. Perinatal regionalization helps to prevent needless duplication of services.

Level I Facilities

A Level I facility offers services to low-risk clients. It has three major functions:

Management and care of normal mothers and newborns

Early identification of high-risk pregnancies or neonates

Provision of emergency care during unanticipated obstetric or neonatal emergencies

This kind of facility is usually found in sparsely populated rural areas. Clients requiring more sophisticated care are referred or transported to Level II or Level III facilities.

Table 34–1 **Levels of Care, Functions, and Nursing Roles in Regionalization of Perinatal Care**

Level I	Level II	Level III
Management and care of low-risk clients	Management and care of low-risk clients using facility	Management and care of high-risk clients
Normal pregnancy, labor, delivery	Management and care of medium- and high-risk clients	Pregnancy, labor, and delivery
Normal newborns	Pregnancy, labor, and delivery	Fetal surgery
Identification of high-risk clients	High-risk or sick neonates	Neonatal care
Referral of high-risk clients to Level II or III facility	Emergency care and stabilization of clients	Neonatal surgery
Provision of emergency care and stabilization of client for transport to Level II or III facility	Referral to Level III facilities, of high-risk clients (clients requiring care beyond the facility's capability — e.g., fetal surgery, neonatal cardiac surgery)	Long-term care of high-risk infants with multiple medical problems who remain acutely ill (e.g., extreme prematurity)
		Provision of continuing education programs for staffs of Level I and Level II facilities
		Inhouse programs
		Community outreach
		Development and provision of both short- and long-distance transport system for high-risk clients

Staff Nurse

Level I	Level II	Level III
Assessment, diagnosis, planning, and implementation of care for low-risk families	Assessment, diagnosis, planning, and implementation of nursing care for low-risk clients (see Level I)	Assessment, diagnosis, planning, and implementation of nursing care for high-risk clients (see Level II)
Childbirth preparation	Assessment, diagnosis, planning, and implementation of nursing care for medium- and high-risk clients	
Discharge teaching and parent education	Provision of special education and orientation of clients with special health care needs (e.g., diabetes management)	
Identification of high-risk clients	Childbirth education	
Consultation with other health team members in planning care	Initial emergency care and stabilization of clients	
Referral of clients with special needs (to nutritionists, social workers, clinical nurse specialists)	Neonatal resuscitation	
Preparation of high-risk clients for referral to Level II or III facility	Use of electronic monitors and diagnostic devices to assist in assessment and care of clients	
Emergency care and stabilization of high-risk client prior to transport	Consultation with other health team members in planning care of clients with special needs (e.g., with nutritionists, respiratory therapists)	
	Referral of clients with special needs to appropriate resources: physical therapy, clergy, community agencies, financial counselor	
	Parenting education for parents of both normal and high-risk infants	

Clinical Nurse Specialist (CNS)

Level I	Level II	Level III
Clinical nursing consultation for patients with complex care needs; primary nursing care for selected patients.	Staff education and development	(See Level II)
Staff education and development	Consultation with nursing staff and other members of health team in planning care for clients with special needs	Development and implementation of educational programs for Level I and II staff nurses within the designated perinatal region
Consultation with nursing staff and other health team members in planning care for clients	Patient education for clients with special needs	Direct supervision and training of Level I and II nurses who are in training at the Level III facility
Client education	Referral of clients to Level III facilities	
Referral of clients to Level II or III facility	Nursing research	
Nursing research	Direct patient care of selected high-risk clients	
Assistance with emergency care and stabilization of high-risk clients for transport	Participation in transport of high-risk clients from Level I facility	
	Development and implementation of nursing care plans and procedures to meet the needs of high-risk clients	

(continued)

1021

Table 34–1   **Levels of Care, Functions, and Nursing Roles in Regionalization of Perinatal Care** (continued)

Level I	Level II	Level III
Pediatric, Neonatal or Women's Health Nurse Practitioner, or Certified Nurse Midwife		
Management and care of low-risk clients	Management and care of low-risk clients who use the facility	Management and care of low-risk clients who use the facility
Provision of prenatal care		
Childbirth education		
Management of labor, delivery, and postpartum care (CNM)		
Family planning		
Parenting education		
Newborn physical exams		
Parent education		
Nursing research		

Nurses in Level I facilities are prepared through basic nursing education to care for healthy mothers and infants and must be skilled in assessment of risk factors and the stabilization of sick clients for transport when unexpected complications arise.

Level II Facilities

A Level II facility offers services to medium-risk clients. Its major function is to be able to provide competent care in 75% to 90% of maternal or neonatal complications. It also provides services to low-risk clients who use the facility. Level II facilities are usually found in urban or subur-

ban areas. Clients requiring care beyond the capability of the facility are referred or transported to a Level III center. Nurses in Level II facilities have advanced training or graduate education in the care of high-risk and sick clients. They must be skilled in the use of electronic monitoring equipment and other devices designed to support the delivery of medical and nursing care (Fig. 34–1).

Level III Facilities

A Level III facility offers services to high-risk clients who require the most sophisticated level of care. Full-time specialists and state of the art equipment are avail-

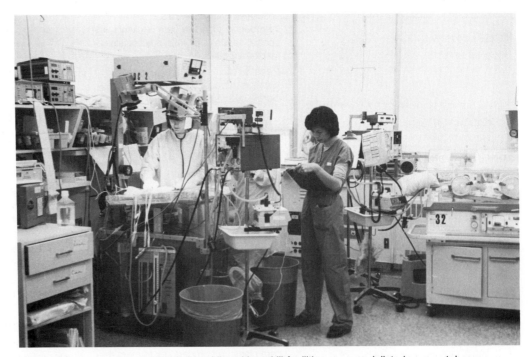

Figure 34–1. Nurses working in Level II and Level III facilities are specialists in neonatal care and are expert in managing complex nursing problems with the use of sophisticated technology. (Photo: Colleen Stainton, courtesy of University of California, San Francisco)

able to handle complex perinatal disorders. Additional functions of the Level III facility include continuing education for Level I and Level II health team members through perinatal outreach programs and the development of a system of referral and transport so that lower-level facilities can move high-risk clients to an appropriate high-risk center.

Depending on population density, only one or two facilities may be designated as Level III facilities in a particular region. Nurses in a Level III facility must have advanced training or graduate education in the care of clients with complex disorders. They must also be knowledgeable about community outreach and health education because preparation and support of the families of sick mothers and infants and continuing education of health care professionals are major parts of a Level III institution's function.

COMMON ELEMENTS IN CARE OF THE HIGH-RISK NEONATE

Many elements in the planning and implementation of nursing care for high-risk neonates are similar, regardless of the specific disorder. The following section discusses these common elements of high-risk neonatal nursing care as they relate to frequently used nursing diagnoses. This section is followed by a more detailed discussion of specific neonatal disorders and appropriate nursing care.

Assessment

Initial assessments of the neonate were discussed in Chapter 31, and further assessment of the high-risk neonate is discussed in Chapter 33. Data are gathered from the maternal and neonatal health histories, and a systematic physical and behavioral assessment is made. Appropriate nursing diagnoses and potential complications describe the infant's need for physiologic and behavioral support.

Diagnosis

Based on the initial assessment of neonatal status, the nurse formulates diagnoses that direct subsequent nursing care. Nursing diagnoses focus on continued support of physiologic functions and promote optimal family adaptations. The following possible nursing diagnoses are

LEGAL/ETHICAL CONSIDERATIONS

Preparation for the Birth of the High-Risk Neonate: Responsibilities of the Nursery Head Nurse or Charge Nurse

All nurses who care for women in labor must attempt to identify potential or actual problems that may result in the birth of a compromised infant. Delays in communication and response time during emergency situations can arise when the nursery is separate from the labor/delivery unit. Pediatricians and neonatal nurses may not be available immediately when needed to support and stabilize the sick newborn.

In cases of civil litigation, the courts have begun to scrutinize the response time of the nursery staff to the birth of a compromised infant. The nursery head nurse or charge nurse must implement a formal plan for ongoing communication with labor and delivery personnel. Hourly calls or rounds should be made to the unit to update nursery staff on the status of clients in labor. A list of all patients in labor and delivery should be maintained so that staff and equipment are prepared for the birth of a high-risk infant. It may even be appropriate to alert other personnel, such as radiologists, on-call neonatologists, and respiratory therapists, to ensure a rapid response when the infant is born.

Conversely, the labor/delivery head nurse or charge nurse must alert nursery personnel immediately when a patient is admitted in an advanced state of labor and the potential for infant compromise is identified. A list should also be developed, identifying all instances when nursery staff should be notified and present for the birth. If a woman has not received prenatal care prior to labor, it is advisable that at least one member of the nursery team be present to assist with the evaluation and support of the newborn, in case problems arise after birth.

applicable to direct independent nursing care of the high-risk neonate and family:

- Impaired gas exchange
- Fluid volume deficit
- Altered nutrition
- Potential for infection
- Potential altered body temperature
- Potential altered parenting

The nurse continues to monitor and provide care as indicated for complications in the high-risk neonate.

Planning and Implementation

Once nursing diagnoses have been established, the nurse plans and implements appropriate interventions to support physiologic functions and behavioral adaptations. Nursing interventions for the high-risk neonate are similar to those for the normal neonate but the possibility of complications is increased. Interventions include prevention and early identification of physical complications, assessment of extrauterine adaptation, establishing a feeding pattern, and support of parent-infant attachment.

The nurse, when planning care, takes into account the degree of seriousness of the newborn's condition, the level of care being given (as discussed at the beginning of this chapter), the emotional and physical status of family members, and the physiologic adaptations required of the newborn. When complications arise, regardless of the etiology of the disorder, the principles upon which care is based remain the same. Those common elements of care are discussed in this section. Nursing interventions are organized to minimize disturbance of the neonate and disruption of sleep patterns.

Promoting Physiologic Adaptation

Supporting Cardiopulmonary Adaptation

Because cold stress and unnecessary stimulation increase the infant's need for oxygen, the nurse must minimize energy requirements and support thermoregulatory function for the newborn. After initial resuscitation and stabilization at birth, infants requiring continuing respiratory and cardiac support will be placed in an isolette or under a radiant warmer. Equipment essential for cardiopulmonary support must be at hand. The nurse assists the neonate to maintain an adequate airway and, when indicated, provides an enriched oxygen atmosphere in conjunction with the medical team.

Maintaining the Airway

The potential for accidental aspiration is present in all newborns, since their weak neck muscles prevent quick repositioning of the head for drainage of fluids when regurgitation or vomiting occurs. A sick or compromised neonate can be at greater risk for airway obstruction as a result of the presence of mucus or meconium in the airways, congenital anomalies of the mouth, pharynx, and neck, or a weak or absent gag reflex.

Positioning

If not contraindicated, neonates should be positioned on their side to facilitate drainage of fluids from the mouth and nares. Many sick infants are placed in a supine position on an open bed to facilitate the administration of IV fluids through the umbilical artery or performance of such procedures as chest x-ray studies and ultrasonography. The nurse can tilt the mattress slightly to one side and turn the infant's head in the same direction to encourage drainage of fluids. When the infant is extremely flaccid or hypotonic, the nurse may need to place a small towel roll under the scapula to bring the head into proper alignment and to prevent airway obstruction. Oropharyngeal airways, although available in infant sizes, are rarely indicated or used in newborns.

Suctioning

Although a bulb syringe may be adequate for clearing the mouth and nares of the newborn with normal gag and swallow reflexes, the sick or compromised neonate often needs additional assistance. A suction catheter (5F to 10F) attached to a portable suction machine or a wall outlet can be employed to clear the airway of mucus. This method is most often used with infants receiving oxygen therapy or those who are attached to a mechanical ventilator and require intermittent suctioning.

For deep suctioning, sterile technique should be used. It should last no longer than 10 seconds with a low-pressure setting (less than 50 mmHg) to decrease the amount of oxygen removed from the airways. Negative pressure is applied only after the catheter has been fully inserted into the airway and is being withdrawn. Applying negative pressure while the catheter is being passed can cause trauma to the airway mucosa. The infant's heart rate must be monitored closely during suctioning of the oropharynx, nasopharynx, or trachea, because bradycardia can occur due to stimulation of the vagus nerve.

Chest Percussion and Drainage

Another method for facilitating the drainage of mucus and maintaining a patent airway involves chest percussion and postural (gravity) drainage.

Chest Percussion.   A dome-shaped cupping device is used manually to percuss the infant's chest over lung tissue to loosen pulmonary secretions (see Fig. 34-2).

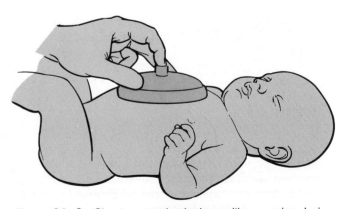

Figure 34-2. Chest percussion is done with a cupping device specially designed for neonatal care.

The nurse places the cup on the chest and begins with a rapid vibrating motion lasting several seconds, followed by chest percussion for 20 to 30 seconds. Quick, firm, downward strokes are essential to catch air within the dome of the cup and transmit the vibratory waves to the secretions within the lung.

Postural Drainage. The infant's position is changed frequently in order to prevent stasis of lung secretions (Fig. 34 – 3). The infant may be placed in the Trendelenburg position to promote drainage of secretions, but this position may be contraindicated in preterm infants who are at risk for intracranial hemorrhage.

Supporting Ventilation

The high-risk neonate may require assistance with ventilation in order to adequately oxygenate tissues. Infants with depressed central nervous system function or congenital anomalies of the chest or abdomen, and premature infants with respiratory distress syndrome, frequently need ventilatory assistance. The neonate will be intubated and placed on a mechanical ventilator. A variety of machines are available and operate on a volume-limit, pressure-limit, or timed-interval principle (Fig. 34 – 4).

Two additional forms of ventilatory assistance can be achieved utilizing the ventilator:

- *Continuous positive airway pressure (CPAP):* a continuous positive atmospheric pressure is applied to the lungs during the respiratory cycle in an effort to prevent alveolar collapse and atelectasis. Infants may be able to breathe without assistance and yet require CPAP in order to ease the work of breathing, which would be made more difficult if alveoli collapsed with each expiration. CPAP may be applied through a face mask, nasal prongs, nasopharyngeal tube or endotracheal tube attached to a mechanical ventilator.

- *Positive end expiratory pressure (PEEP):* a positive atmospheric pressure is applied to the lungs at the end of the expiratory phase of the breathing cycle to prevent collapse of the alveoli. It is frequently used for smaller infants who require ventilatory assistance.

High-Frequency Ventilation. A new technique of mechanical ventilation has recently been developed in an effort to reduce the barotrauma that occurs in infants who require assisted ventilation at high-mean airway pressures and tidal volumes. High-frequency ventilation (HFV) is a technique for delivering small volumes of gas at

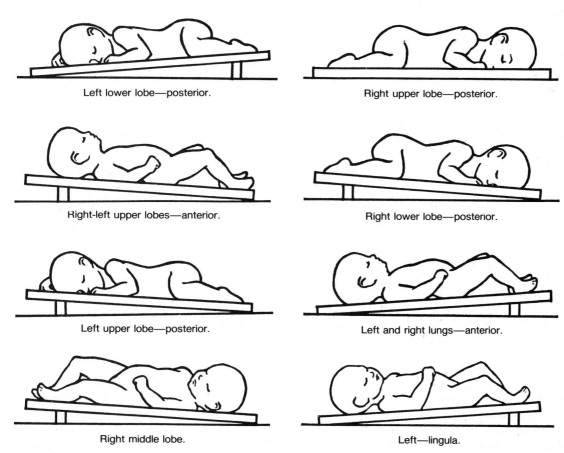

Left lower lobe—posterior.

Right upper lobe—posterior.

Right-left upper lobes—anterior.

Right lower lobe—posterior.

Left upper lobe—posterior.

Left and right lungs—anterior.

Right middle lobe.

Left—lingula.

Figure 34 – 3. Various positions for chest physiotherapy.

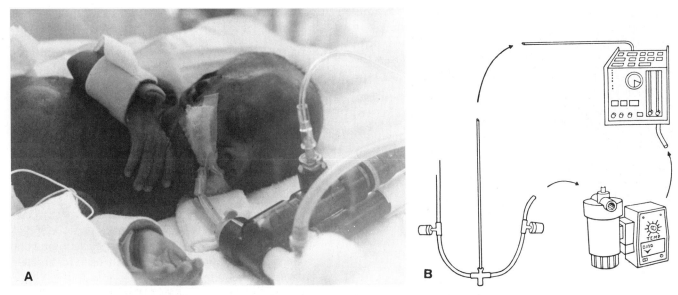

Figure 34–4. Mechanical ventilation assists the sick neonate by preventing collapse of alveoli with expiration and by reducing the work needed to maintain effective respiration. *(A)* Baby on ventilation. *(B)* Typical ventilator circuit used with neonates. (Photo: Colleen Stainton)

very high rates (150 breaths/minute up to 3000 cycles/minute). Several types of HFV are now available. It appears a promising mode of therapy in infants with severe hyaline membrane disease, but is currently used in only a small number of institutions (Richardson 1988).

Muscle Paralysis.   In some cases, adequate ventilation can be achieved only by inducing muscle paralysis. Full-term infants with normal muscle tone may struggle against the respiratory phases of the ventilator, disrupting gas exchange. Skeletal muscle paralysis is achieved by administration of a drug, such as Pavulon, which blocks transmission of acetylcholine across the neuromuscular synapse. Therefore, the infant remains fully conscious and perceptive to pain stimuli. Morphine is usually also administered.

The nurse must remain at the bedside at all times to assess significant changes in the neonate's respiratory status. He or she should also be prepared to initiate ventilation with a bag and mask, if the infant's condition suddenly deteriorates while on mechanical ventilation or if the ventilator fails.

Administering Oxygen

During the initial resuscitation efforts, a 100% oxygen concentration is administered to the neonate. As soon as the infant's condition is stabilized, the concentration is adjusted to maintain the PaO_2 (partial pressure of oxygen in the blood) within acceptable limits. This adjustment is essential, since elevated PaO_2 levels (caused by administration of oxygen in high concentrations) can cause irreparable damage to retinal vessels. Furthermore, high oxy-

gen concentrations can directly injure lung tissue. Premature infants with immature lungs and eye vessels are at particular risk for two conditions that are a direct result of oxygen toxicity: retrolental fibroplasia and bronchopulmonary dysplasia. These complications related to oxygen therapy are discussed later in this chapter.

Oxygen Mask.   An oxygen mask is only used as a temporary method for delivering oxygen to the neonate. If an infant is moderately depressed at birth (Apgar 4 to 6), oxygen is administered through a tight-fitting mask specifically designed for infants. The nurse must be certain to use the correct size to avoid oxygen leaks. Care must be taken to prevent pressure on the infant's eyeballs, as this can cause tissue ischemia and blindness.

Endotracheal Tube.   When the infant is severely depressed at birth (Apgar 0 to 2), oxygen is administered via an uncuffed endotracheal tube (Fig. 34–5). The end of the tube is attached to a ventilation bag or to a mechanical ventilator, if the neonate requires extended ventilatory assistance.

Oxygen Hood.   If the infant requires continuing oxygen therapy after the initial resuscitation but can breathe without assistance, a clear plastic oxygen hood is frequently used (Fig. 34–6). It fits over the infant's head and is connected to oxygen tubing. This delivery system has the advantage of leaving the rest of the infant's body exposed for essential procedures and treatments and allows the administration of very high concentrations of oxygen (up to 100%). Oxygen piped into an isolette can rarely be delivered in concentrations higher than 40% and

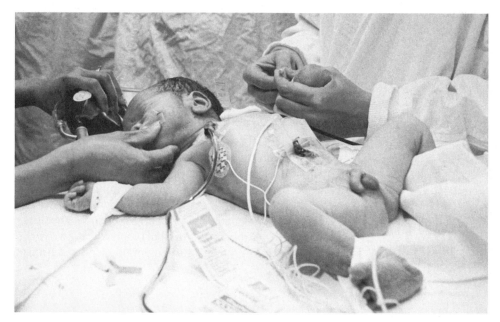

Figure 34–5. This neonate showed respiratory distress at birth and required ventilatory assistance. An endotracheal tube has been passed and connected to a ventilation bag. A transcutaneous oxygen monitor is in place (upper chest) as is an EKG lead and an umbilical artery catheter. (Photo: Kathy Sloane)

the concentration cannot be monitored adequately because of the large number of portholes located in the plastic walls.

Nasal Prongs. Nasal prongs may be used to deliver oxygen to the neonate who is fairly stable and breathing on his own but who requires an oxygen concentration higher than room air (21%) for extended periods of time. Growing preterm infants with bronchopulmonary dysplasia or infants with cardiac disease may be administered oxygen via nasal prongs. This method allows the infant to be placed in an open crib and greatly increases the spectrum of external stimuli available to the neonate. It also allows the parents and staff to hold and cuddle the infant for longer periods of time without disconnecting him from the source of oxygen.

Expected Outcomes: The neonate achieves and maintains normal cardiac output and adequate tissue perfusion as evidenced by:

- Heart rate between 100 to 160 bpm
- Sinus rhythm
- Stable blood pressure
- 1- to 2-sec capillary refill time
- Presence of symmetrical, normal peripheral pulses (+2)
- Quiet precordium
- Absence of peripheral edema
- Absence of pathologic murmurs

The neonate achieves and maintains an effective

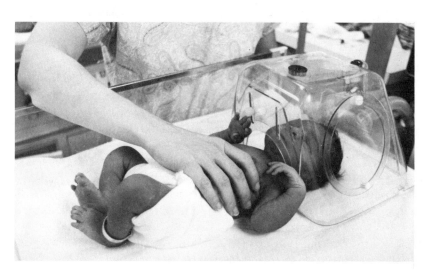

Figure 34–6. The oxygen hood is used for infants who require oxygen administration but who can breathe without mechanical assistance.

respiratory pattern and an adequate gas exchange as demonstrated by:

- Respiratory rate between 30 and 60 breaths/minute
- Breath sounds that are clear and equal bilaterally
- Symmetrical respiratory excursions
- Pink skin and mucous membranes
- Absence of flaring, grunting, or chest retraction

Promoting Fluid and Electrolyte Balance

The sick neonate is at special risk for fluid and electrolyte imbalances. Oral fluid intake is frequently limited or impossible as a result of anomalies, injury, or disease. Sick infants are often lethargic or poor feeders. Congenital anomalies of the face may interfere with the neonate's ability to suck and swallow, and preterm and small for gestational age infants have a limited stomach capacity. Oral intake may be absolutely contraindicated after severe asphyxia or with major congenital anomalies of the gastrointestinal or respiratory tracts.

Fluid losses may also be greater for the sick neonate. Vomiting, diarrhea, and drainage of body fluids from open wounds, cysts, or exposed organs deplete water and essential electrolytes. Insensible water loss is also greatly increased in infants with rapid respiratory rates and in those placed under radiant warmers or phototherapy lights. These factors are complicated by the immature kidney function normally present in the newborn, which limits the capacity to conserve fluids and electrolytes.

Nursing care focuses on both the prevention and correction of fluid volume deficits and electrolyte imbalances. Careful monitoring of fluid intake and output alerts the nurse to excessive losses. Placing the infant in a neutral thermal environment prevents the elevation in metabolic rate and minimizes the concomitant water loss that occur when cold stress activates nonshivering thermogenesis (see Neutral Thermal Environment later in this chapter). Because insensible water loss is greatly increased when the infant is placed under a radiant warmer, the infant's skin is frequently covered with a transparent barrier, such as plastic food wrap, to minimize the loss. The neonate should be placed in an incubator with a double wall or a heat shield as soon as possible. The nurse also carefully limits the amount of blood withdrawn to the absolute minimum necessary to obtain blood gas studies and other tests.

Intravenous (IV) Therapy

IV therapy may be instituted to meet the infant's basic fluid requirements when oral intake is limited. Fluid requirements during the first few days of life are approximately 60 to 75 ml/kg/day. This figure may be adjusted upward when there is excessive sensible and insensible water loss. The nurse must evaluate the infant carefully for signs of dehydration or fluid overload during IV therapy. Table 34–2 lists the major indicators of fluid imbalance in the neonate.

Peripheral Intravenous Lines. Peripheral veins may be used for the infusion of fluid and electrolytes and are preferred to the umbilical artery or central veins, since

---

Table 34–2   **Signs of Fluid Imbalance in the Neonate**

Dehydration	Overhydration
Early Signs	
Lower urine volume (less than 1 ml/kg/hr)	Higher urine volume (more than 3 ml/kg/hr)
Higher urine osmolality (more than 400 mOsm)	Lower urine osmolality (less than 10 mOsm)
Higher urine specific gravity (more than 1.012)	Lower urine specific gravity (less than 1.008)
Signs of Decompensation	
Weight loss (5%–15% a day)	Weight gain (5%–15% a day)
Higher serum sodium (more than 150 mEq/liter)	Lower serum sodium (less than 130 mEq/liter)
Higher serum osmolality (more than 300 mOsm)	Lower serum osmolality (less than 270 mOsm)
Dry mucous membranes	Subcutaneous edema
Sunken fontanelles	
Poor skin turgor	
Higher hematocrit (10% or more)	Lower hematocrit (≤ 10%)
Higher serum protein (>6 g/dl)	Lower serum protein (less than 4 g/dl)
Lower blood volume	Higher blood volume
Late Signs	
Shock	Pulmonary edema and rales
	Cardiac failure

the risk of serious complications is lower. Scalp veins are frequently chosen as sites for IV infusion of fluid in the infant (Fig. 34–7). It is often easier to restrain the movement of the head with sandbags than to extend and restrain the upper extremities when arm veins are used. However, recent research suggests that IV fluids infused through stainless steel scalp-vein needles tend to infiltrate much sooner than flexible Teflon catheters inserted into the extremities.

A variety of needles and catheters are available for peripheral IV infusions, and the type chosen depends on the infant's size, the purpose for which the line is to be used, and the sites available for insertion. As noted, Teflon angiocatheters are preferred to needles, since the risk of infiltration is less and the line can normally be maintained for a longer period.

The nurse is often responsible for inserting the IV line and should be skilled in proper venipuncture technique, securing the line, and restraining the infant's head or limbs. She must carefully restrain the infant prior to the procedure. Tightly swaddling the neonate is the most effective way of preventing him from moving during the insertion and accidentally dislodging the needle. If an arm vein is used, the limb should be restrained on a padded armboard prior to insertion of the line. A fiberoptic transilluminator may be held against the skin to locate veins and facilitate successful venipuncture.

Tape must be applied to secure the IV line, but the fragile condition of the neonate's skin and the need to observe the insertion site closely must be taken into account when applying adhesives. Clear, porous tape allows the nurse to inspect the site and is less adherent, thus minimizing injury to the skin when removed. Even clear porous tape may damage the skin of very premature infants, and special skin adhesives must be used with them (see Preventing Infections, later in this chapter). The application of tincture of benzoin to provide a protective layer between tape and skin is not recommended, since it may be absorbed (Kuller et al 1984).

Once the line is secured in place, the nurse must take care to control head movement with sandbags, if a scalp vein has been selected. The upper extremities may also need to be restrained to prevent the infant from acciden-

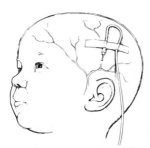

Figure 34–7. Peripheral intravenous infusion using a scalp vein.

tally grasping the tubing and pulling the IV line out. Special padded limb restraints, now available for infants, eliminate the need to create makeshift restraints and minimize the risk of circulatory impairment.

Because small amounts of fluid are administered to the infant at very slow rates (sometimes less than 1 ml/hour), a special infusion pump must be utilized, and many institutions heparinize the IV solutions to prevent clotting of the line. All solutions should be infused through minidrip tubing (60 drops/ml) attached to a fluid reservoir (Volutrol) that contains no more than several hours' worth of fluid. This prevents accidental infusion of a large and potentially lethal volume. Meticulous measurement of all fluid intake and output is essential with IV therapy, as is evaluation of urine specific gravity at least once per shift.

The nurse must examine the IV site hourly for signs of infiltration or irritation of the vein. Circulation distal to the site must also be evaluated. The infusion pump is checked for proper functioning and the tubing for kinks or obstruction. If the limbs are restrained, they should be released at least every 2 hours for passive range of motion exercises.

Central Intravenous Lines

Neonates requiring prolonged IV therapy or hyperalimentation may have a special central IV catheter inserted. The procedure is normally performed by a skilled practitioner utilizing sterile technique. The catheter may be introduced through a peripheral vein in the arm and then slowly threaded into a central vein (percutaneous insertion), or it may be inserted into the scalp, passed into the jugular vein and finally placed in the superior vena cava (Fig. 34–8). Clinical experience with both techniques suggests there is a lower incidence of thrombophlebitis with prolonged vessel catheterization when the distal cutaneous site is used (Shapiro 1986).

The nurse caring for the infant with a central IV line must be alert to common complications, including infiltration, phlebitis, and systemic infection, accidental fluid overload, and air embolus. All tubing and IV solution must be replaced every 24 hours using strict sterile technique. Care must be taken when disconnecting lines to prevent the accidental introduction of air into the system. The nurse must inspect the skin at the site of insertion for evidence of erythema, edema, or leakage of solution. She must observe for edema in the neck and chest area, which would suggest infiltration. The occurrence of sudden respiratory distress and cyanosis suggests infiltration of the central line, air embolus, or fluid overload.

Umbilical Artery Catheterization

The umbilical artery is frequently used for the administration of drugs and fluids in sick neonates. A radiopaque catheter is inserted into one of the arteries and passed into the abdominal aorta. Catheterization is considered a sur-

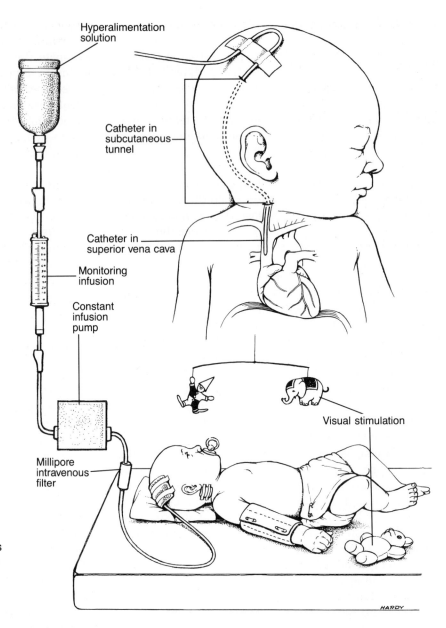

Hyperalimentation
solution

Catheter in
subcutaneous
tunnel

Catheter in
superior vena cava

Monitoring
infusion

Constant
infusion
pump

Millipore
intravenous
filter

Visual stimulation

HARDY

Figure 34–8. Placement of a central venous line for prolonged intravenous or hyperalimentation therapy. Catheter is inserted through scalp and threaded through the jugular vein and into the superior vena cava.

gical procedure requiring strict aseptic technique. Once placement of the catheter is confirmed by radiographic examination (either above or below the level of the renal arteries), it is secured in place with suture and tape. The catheter allows arterial blood samples to be obtained for blood gas analysis, and a special electronic monitor can be attached to the catheter to monitor systemic blood pressure.

Several major complications have been associated with umbilical artery (UA) catheterization: infection, thrombosis, vasospasm, and hemorrhage. The nurse caring for the neonate with a UA line must use scrupulous aseptic technique, when opening the system, to prevent infection and the introduction of air emboli. The nurse must also be alert to signs of compromised blood flow below the level

of the catheter, including blanching and coolness of the skin in the perineal area, over the buttocks, and in the lower extremities, and absence of femoral and pedal pulses. Hypertension is associated with infarcts of the renal arteries, and abdominal distention and bloody stools are associated with thrombosis of mesenteric arteries.

Electrolyte Supplementation

Electrolytes (sodium, chloride, potassium, and calcium) are frequently added to the IV solution and are essential if the infant remains unable to take food by mouth for more than 24 to 48 hours. Electrolyte values are monitored closely, and the nurse must be familiar with norms as well as daily maintenance requirements. Table 34–3 lists daily electrolyte requirements and nor-

Table 34–3   **Maintenance of Electrolyte Balance**

Electrolyte	Normal Blood Value*	Daily Requirement
Sodium	148 mEq/liter (134–160)	2–3 mEq/kg/day
Chloride	102 mEq/liter (92–114)	2 mEq/kg/day
Potassium	6.0 mEq/liter (5.2–7.3)	2 mEq/kg/day
Calcium	8.0 mg/100 ml (6.9–9.9)	150–200 mg/kg/day

* 24 to 48 hr after birth
(Cloherty J, Stark A: Manual of Neonatal Care. Boston, Little, Brown & Co, 1985)

mal blood values for the infant. When calcium and potassium are infused, it is essential that the infant be placed on a cardiac monitor because of their effect on myocardial function. Furthermore, because infiltration of calcium-containing solutions can cause severe sloughing of tissues, the IV site must be observed closely for evidence of infiltration.

Expected Outcomes: Neonate achieves fluid and electrolyte balance as evidenced by:

- Normal urine output: *Term infant:* 15–60 ml/24 hr in first few days of life to 200 ml/24 hr by 1 week or 6 to 7 wet diapers per day. *Preterm infant:* 1–3 ml/kg/hr in first week of life
- Normal skin turgor
- Moist mucous membranes
- Absence of peripheral or periorbital edema
- No greater than 5% to 10% weight loss with "physiologic diuresis" during first 5 to 6 days of life
- Urine specific gravity between 1.005 and 1.012
- Adequate fluid intake: *Term infant:* 105 ml/kg/day; *Preterm infant:* 60–100 ml/kg/day
- Absence of bulging or depressed anterior fontanelle

Providing for Nutrition Needs

Meeting the nutritional needs of the high-risk neonate and preventing caloric and nutrient deficits is a major challenge. Many complications make it difficult or impossible for the infant to breast-feed or bottle-feed or to digest the standard formulas prescribed for the healthy full-term newborn. A variety of formulas and solutions have been developed to provide calories and essential nutrients to the high-risk infant, and special equipment is available to deliver them via the gastrointestinal tract or IV routes.

The nurse must carefully monitor the responses of the sick infant to the substances ingested or infused. Vital signs are taken before each feeding, and the abdominal girth is measured if nutrients are given by the gastrointestinal tract. The urine is tested periodically for the presence of sugar and protein and the stools for blood. When nutrients are infused intravenously, the infant's blood is tested frequently for evidence of protein, carbohydrate, or fat intolerance.

Orogastric Feedings

If the infant can tolerate oral feedings, there are several ways to provide the necessary nutrients.

Nipple Feedings.   Special care and patience are required if the neonate is allowed to nipple-feed. The sick neonate is often characterized as a "poor feeder" who sucks weakly and has an uncoordinated suck-swallow reflex. Energy reserves may be low, and sucking efforts can easily exhaust the infant. The nurse must allot extra time for the feeding and carefully note the infant's response (heart, respiratory rate, and color). Breast-feeding may be possible, and the host-resistance factors contained in breast milk are especially beneficial to the sick neonate. When bottle-feeding is selected, special soft nipples can be used to assist the infant and decrease the work of feeding. There are also specially designed nipples for infants with cleft lip or palate (see Fig. 34–5).

Gavage Feedings.   Nipple-feeding is contraindicated for some high-risk neonates. Preterm infants born before 33 to 34 weeks of gestation lack a gag reflex and would aspirate the feeding if they attempted to suck from breast or bottle. Infants with very rapid respiratory rates (above 70 per minute) and those with severe cardiac disease may not tolerate nipple-feedings, because of their diminished energy reserves, and may experience increased respiratory distress when they attempt to suck. Gavage-feeding may be the method of choice in these circumstances.

An orogastric tube (5, 8, or 10 F) is passed, and milk flows into the stomach from a syringe or feeding funnel by gravity drainage (Fig. 34–9). The nurse must carefully restrain the infant and secure the tube prior to the procedure so that it is not accidentally pulled out during the feeding. Before beginning the gavage-feeding, proper placement must be confirmed (most commonly by aspirating stomach contents) to rule out passage of the tube into the trachea.

The amount of milk remaining in the stomach since the last feeding (gastric residual) is also measured at this time. Physicians' directives are often provided to guide the nurse in whether to subtract the residual amount from the next feeding. Stomach contents are rarely dis-

NURSING ALERT

Measurement and Insertion of the Gavage Tube

Two common methods of gavage tube measurement have been recommended to ensure accurate placement in the stomach.

Method A:

With the infant supine, the head positioned in the midline, the tip of the feeding tube is placed at the right corner of the right nostril or mouth and extended to the lobe of the right ear. It is then extended down to the termination of the xiphoid process. A strip of adhesive tape is wrapped around the tube and the tape then secured 2 cm beyond the point measured. After the tip is lubricated with sterile water, it is inserted and advanced nasally or orally until the tape marker is at the orifice, where it is secured to the skin.

Method B:

Placement differs only in the termination point of measurement. The tube tip is placed at the right corner of the mouth or nose, extended to the right earlobe, and then to a point midway between the termination of the xiphoid process and the umbilicus.

Weibley et al (1987) conducted a study to determine which of these methods resulted in more accurate placement in the stomachs of 30 preterm infants between 28 to 36 weeks' gestation. Incorrect placement rates of 55.6% (Method A) and 39.3% (Method B) were recorded. Tube slippage and improper technique were eliminated as possible causes.

Until a placement method is perfected, it is recommended that once the tube is passed using either method, the nurse should auscultate over the stomach while insufflating 0.5 cc of air through the tube. This is not an absolute indication of correct positioning as it is possible to hear air entering the stomach even when the tube orifice is above the gastroesophageal sphincter. The tube is properly placed if gastric contents are aspirated following air insufflation.

Weibley TT, Adamson M, Clinkscales N, et al: Gavage tube insertion in the premature infant. MCN 12:24–27, 1987

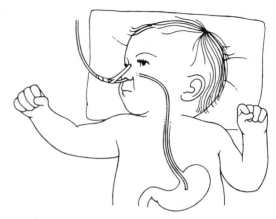

Figure 34–9. Gavage feeding of the neonate. The neonate's hands should be restrained and the neonate must be positioned on the side or prone before the procedure is begun.

litis, which is frequently encountered in very premature infants (see the section on this condition later in this chapter). For this reason the nurse reports unusual gastric residuals immediately.

When the feeding is begun, the milk reservoir is held no higher than 12 inches above the infant. Force should not be applied with a syringe plunger to speed the flow of the milk. This can lead to regurgitation of fluid and aspiration. The tube is clamped before it is withdrawn to prevent milk remaining in the tube from dripping into the pharynx and being aspirated. If not contraindicated by a gastrointestinal or respiratory anomaly, the infant may be offered a pacifier during and immediately after the gavage-feeding to satisfy nonnutritive sucking needs and to stimulate the flow of saliva and digestive juices. The infant is burped in the same manner as a breast-fed or bottle-fed infant after the feeding.

Continuous Nasogastric or Continuous Transpyloric Feeding

Less frequently used methods are continuous nasogastric and transpyloric feeding. These may be indicated in infants with problems of gastric retention or regurgitation and in very low birth weight infants. For continuous nasogastric feeding, a 5F polyethylene feeding tube is threaded slowly through the naris and passed until it enters the stomach. Formula is administered at a constant slow rate by a pump, after placement is confirmed.

If transpyloric feeding is desired, a silastic mercury-tipped feeding tube is threaded through the naris and allowed to pass through the pylorus into the jejunum or duodenum. Proper placement of the tube is tentatively verified by a *p*H reading of over 5 in aspirated contents and confirmed by radiographic examination. Formula or breast milk is then administered at a constant rate by infusion pump.

Gastric residuals are checked at least every 4 hours to

carded, as this would cause the loss of hydrochloric acid and lead to alkalosis. Increasing residuals or the sudden presence of a large residual may indicate intolerance of the food or the development of a severe and life-threatening intestinal disorder, known as necrotizing enteroco-

monitor emptying; presence of residuals may indicate malposition of the tube, intestinal obstruction, or ileus.

With continuous nasogastric or transpyloric feeding, the nurse must guard against bacterial growth in tubing or other equipment. For this reason, syringes and connector tubing should be changed every 4 to 8 hours, and the nasogastric tube itself changed every 24 hours to prevent bacterial growth and possible sepsis.

Total Parenteral Nutrition

If the introduction of nutrients via the gastrointestinal tract is contraindicated, they can be provided through IV infusion of specially prepared parenteral solutions. Total parenteral nutrition (TPN) is the delivery of fluid, calories, minerals, and vitamins by the IV route. Energy sources available for TPN include carbohydrates (dextrose), protein (protein hydrolysates and free amino acid solutions), and fats. Fats are delivered in a separate solution (intralipids) piggybacked to the TPN infusion. Intralipids can be administered only through a peripheral IV line. TPN may be infused peripherally or through a central venous catheter threaded through the right external jugular vein or subclavian vein into the superior vena cava. The central venous route requires surgical placement of the IV line and is used less frequently because of the risk of infection and mechanical complications.

The nurse must monitor the TPN infusion closely. The IV site should be examined at least every hour for evidence of infiltration or inflammation. TPN solution is an excellent medium for the growth of bacteria and will cause severe damage to tissues (necrosis, sloughing, and scarring) if infiltration occurs. If intralipids are administered, the neonate is observed for such complications of lipid infusion as respiratory distress, vomiting, and diarrhea.

Because of the high dextrose concentration found in TPN, the infant is at risk for hyperglycemia, osmotic diuresis, and dehydration. The nurse must be alert for signs of fluid imbalance, keep meticulous intake and output records, and test the urine for the presence of glucose and protein at least once every 8 to 12 hours. The specific gravity of the urine is also measured. The infant is also evaluated for potential hyperbilirubinemia secondary to cholestasis, a complication of TPN.

If hyperglycemia persists, the glucose concentration in the hyperalimentation solution is decreased. Continuous intravenous infusion of insulin may be initiated if plasma glucose levels remain higher than 250 mg/dl (Shannon 1988).

Expected Outcomes: The infant maintains nutritional requirements for growth and development as demonstrated by:

- Breast-feeding vigorously for 15 to 20 minutes every 2 to 3 hours
- Ingestion of 60 to 120 ml of formula every 3 to 4 hours/24 hours, or approximately 24 oz/day in full-term infant (120 kcal/kg/24 hours)
- Intake of at least 104–126 kcal/kg/24 hours in preterm infants
- Daily weight gain of at least 30 g or greater per day
- Blood glucose level of at least 45 mg/dl using Dextrostix or Chemstrip test

Preventing Infection

The high-risk infant is susceptible to infection in the neonatal period due to a variety of factors. The skin is the first line of defense against infection. If the neonate is born with an injury or anomaly that disrupts this natural barrier or is so premature that the skin is thin and permeable, pathogenic bacteria and viruses can gain entry to the body. Severe birth asphyxia, especially in preterm infants, can lead to ischemia and necrosis of intestinal tissue and invasion of the damaged mucosa by enteric bacteria, a condition known as necrotizing enterocolitis. Many life-sustaining procedures and diagnostic tests are invasive and thus become routes for the transmission of pathogens.

Handwashing

Handwashing is the single most important preventive measure against infection. Because hands are the most common vehicle for the spread of pathogens, it is essential that they be washed after contact with an infant before touching another infant or his equipment. Parents should be taught to wash their hands before holding their baby. The nurse must also monitor other health team members and remind them to observe good handwashing technique before they come in contact with the infant. Most neonatal intensive care nurseries also require an initial 2- to 3-minute wash, from fingertips to elbows, with an antibacterial detergent for nursing staff. Iodinated solutions are preferred because of their action against gram-positive cocci and gram-negative rods (Korones 1986).

Nursery Attire and Procedures

Attire.   Nurses caring for the sick neonate should wear scrub gowns with short sleeves, which allow them to wash up to the elbows. Parents or health team members who handle the infant should wear long-sleeved gowns that cover street clothes or other hospital attire. Research indicates that the use of caps, hairnets, or masks is not necessary.

Policies on Illness Among Staff and Visitors. A parent, health team member, or other hospital employee who experiences any of the following illnesses or signs of illness should not have contact with the infant:

- Cold, sore throat, or fever
- Infectious skin rash or lesions (*e.g.,* impetigo, herpesvirus)
- Diarrhea
- Hepatitis
- Other communicable diseases (*e.g.,* chickenpox, tuberculosis)

Isolation. Routine isolation of infants born out of asepsis (*e.g.,* precipitous home or automobile birth) or after prolonged rupture of membranes is no longer advocated. Even infants with bacterial meningitis, septicemia, or pneumonia need not be isolated (Korones 1986). Similarly, the routine separation of mother and baby when there is a postpartum infection is not always necessary, as many infections are not spread by maternal-infant contact. Only those neonates with diarrhea or draining infections must be moved to a separate nursery.

Neonates with disseminated herpes virus should also be handled with strict isolation. Placing them in an isolette is not adequate protection for other infants who are in open cribs in the same environment (Sessions et al 1985). The air circulating in the interior of the incubator is expelled into the room when ports are opened. The practice of observing universal body substance precautions with all infants is the most effective method for preventing transmission of pathogens.

Care of Equipment. The infant is exposed to numerous pieces of equipment that can serve as fomites for the transmission of pathogenic organisms. Care must be taken to clean all equipment coming in contact with the neonate. All IV bags and tubing and oxygen equipment must be changed every 24 hours. Periodic culturing of nursery equipment and plumbing fixtures to identify potential sources of contamination is an essential aspect of infection control.

Skin Care

Because the skin is the infant's first line of defense against infection, skin care practices are of special importance. The use of alkaline soaps has been found to temporarily disrupt the protective acid mantle of the skin; thus, infrequent baths, using only water, are recommended. When more thorough cleansing is necessary, a less alkaline soap (Neutrogena, Lowila, or Oilatum) should be used.

When adhesive tape is removed from the skin, the epidermis can be removed with it. Hollihesive, a porous adhesive described as a "skin blanket," can be applied first and the tape needed to secure equipment placed on top of it. This will help prevent denuding of skin surfaces. Alcohol, tincture of benzoin, and adhesive removers should be avoided. The skin can be adequately prepped for heel sticks and injections with sterile water and cotton balls. Iodinated solutions should be used sparingly when needed, to prepare the skin for drawing blood cultures or starting IV lines.

Expected Outcomes: Neonate remains free of infection as demonstrated by:

- Intact skin and mucous membranes
- Maintenance of temperature between 36.4° and 37.2°C
- Absence of erythema, streaking, or purulent discharge from base of umbilical cord or any intravenous insertion sites
- Absence of signs of neonatal sepsis, including lethargy, feeding intolerance, temperature instability, respiratory distress, apnea, bulging fontanelles, or seizures

Supporting Thermoregulation

Many of the interventions in this section disclose the importance of supporting the newborn's body temperature. This intervention begins immediately after birth and is important through the newborn period. It is especially important in the high-risk infant.

Prevention of Cold Stress

The effects of cold stress on the neonate have been well documented. They include an increase in the metabolic rate, an increase in oxygen consumption, a decrease in surfactant production, and hypoglycemia. Cold stress initiates the breakdown of brown fat stores for heat production, releasing acid metabolites into the blood stream. High-risk infants are particularly susceptible to cold stress because interventions, beginning with resuscitation in the delivery room, require exposing of body surfaces. The nurse's first step in resuscitation is to place the neonate under a radiant warmer and quickly dry the skin, as other health team members establish an airway.

The infant must be able to produce and conserve heat in order to maintain a normal body temperature and prevent hypothermia. The high-risk infant is at a distinct disadvantage. The neonate's ability to accomplish nonshivering thermogenesis depends upon his stores of brown fat tissue. Infants who are preterm and small for gestational age (SGA) have limited amounts of brown fat. They also lack the thermal insulation adipose tissue provides, thus experiencing a more rapid dissipation of heat from the blood vessels underlying skin surfaces. To some extent, a flexed posture decreases heat loss by decreasing the amount of skin surface exposed. Infants who are severely depressed and flaccid are at greater risk for heat loss.

Maintenance of a Neutral Thermal Environment

The high-risk neonate is initially placed in a neutral thermal environment, which minimizes the work of maintaining the body temperature. The radiant warmer is preferred when the infant requires frequent evaluations, tests, and procedures that require exposure (Fig. 34–10). An incubator is used when the infant can be left undisturbed for long periods of time and requires less intensive care (Fig. 34–11). The ambient temperature is adjusted to maintain the infant's temperature in the range of 36.4° to 37.0°C (97.7°–98.6°F).

Ideally, all oxygen administered to the neonate should be warmed. Cold air blown across the face can stimulate thermal receptors there and induce apnea. Wet towels or clothing should be replaced, and care should be taken to cover the infant's head (25% of the total body length) with

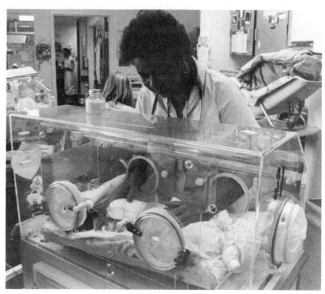

Figure 34–11. Use of an isolette for care of the sick neonate allows maintenance of a neutral thermal environment for those neonates not requiring minute-to-minute intervention. (Photo: Colleen Stainton)

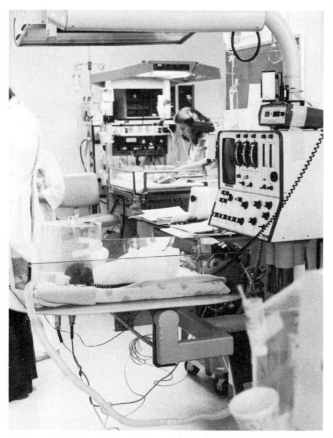

Figure 34–10. The neonate in the intensive care bed with overhead radiant warmer (in the foreground) can be examined periodically with ease.

a stockinette cap when it is feasible to do so. The hands of the nurse should be warmed before she handles the infant, especially a very low-birth-weight-infant, to decrease heat transfer by conduction. If the infant is in an isolette, the portholes should be kept closed between procedures, and work should be organized to minimize entry.

Rapid swings in temperature must be avoided. Infants who are hypothermic must be warmed slowly and cautiously, since a rapid rise in temperature may cause apnea. The infant who has been in a neutral thermal environment for an extended length of time must be weaned from it slowly to prevent hypothermia and cold stress. The infant's temperature-regulating center needs time to assume the total work of temperature maintenance.

Expected Outcomes: Neonate maintains a normal core temperature as evidenced by:

- An axillary temperature of 36.4° to 37.0°C
- Absence of temperature instability

Promoting Behavioral Adaptation
Supporting Parent–Newborn Attachment

The parent–newborn attachment process is seriously threatened when the infant is ill at birth. Parents and infant are separated when the infant is taken to the neonatal intensive care unit. The neonate may even be transported to a tertiary care center located many miles from the hospital where he was born, making visiting by parents difficult or impossible. The nurse caring for the infant must have an understanding of current theory regarding parental responses to the birth of a high-risk infant before she attempts to facilitate the attachment process.

The nurse can assist parents in developing realistic perceptions of the problem. When a complication arises at birth, it is essential that parents be informed as soon as possible about the nature and extent of the problem. A brief statement may be all that is possible if immediate resuscitation or emergency care is required: "Your baby is having difficulty breathing and the doctor is helping him. We will let you know how he is doing as soon as we can."

If the infant is stable but has an obvious congenital anomaly, the parents should be prepared for what they will see and given a simple explanation of what the anomaly is, how it will affect the infant, and what can be done about it. The physician is often the health professional who imparts this information in the delivery room. The nurse then reinforces the information and answers any questions the parents may have.

Once the infant has been transferred to the special care nursery, parents should be kept closely informed of the infant's condition and progress. Initially they may be overwhelmed by the intensive care nursery — the

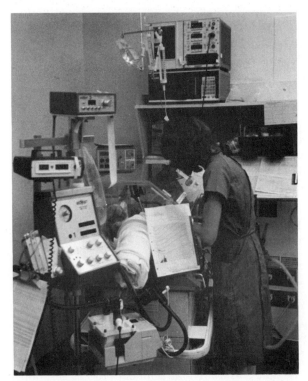

Figure 34–12. Parents may be overwhelmed by the sights, sounds, and busy staff in the intensive care nursery. (Photo: Colleen Stainton)

sounds, lights, and equipment (Fig. 34–12). They may not hear what is being said, so that information will have to be repeated. Explanations should be simple but complete. Nurses can encourage the parents to telephone the nursery when they have questions or want an update on the infant's condition.

The nurse who welcomes parents to the nursery and encourages their participation in the care of the infant becomes a part of their support system. She listens to their concerns, answers their questions, and makes appropriate referrals. She helps build a sense of confidence in their ability to recognize and meet their baby's special needs.

Supporting Coping and Grieving

When parents begin to care for the baby, the nurse is in an excellent position to observe coping mechanisms. She can alert the health team to potential or actual problems that arise as a result of ineffective coping. Many intensive care nurseries have clinical nurse specialists, social workers, or psychologists with expertise in family therapy to support and guide parents. A support group may be formed for all parents with infants in the special care unit. The sharing of experiences, fears, and frustrations can help parents realize they are not alone.

First and foremost the nurse must understand the dynamics of the grieving process and accept the parents' expression of grief, whether it is denial, anger, guilt, or sadness. Many health care professionals are uncomfortable about being with parents who have experienced the birth of a high-risk child. In some way they feel that they have also failed to produce the perfect baby. Avoidance and withdrawal by the staff only serve to reinforce the parents' feelings of lowered self-esteem, isolation, and failure.

Although parents must have privacy and time to be alone with their feelings of sadness and loss, they should also feel that a caring staff is available to support them. The nurse who hurries in and out of the mother's room, attending only to her physical needs, is failing to meet the equally important psychologic needs. It is important to avoid phrases such as "It's God's will" or "You're young and can have another baby." They convey a lack of understanding about the extent of the parents' grief at this time. A sincere expression of sorrow by the nurse, followed by silence and an opportunity for the parent to verbalize his or her feelings, is an appropriate therapeutic approach.

Staff should not be surprised if anger is directed toward them. Anger is a normal phase of the grieving process, and parents must be allowed to vent their feelings of frustration, disappointment, and helplessness. Tranquilizers and sedatives have limited therapeutic value at this time and should never take the place of supportive nurs-

FAMILY CONSIDERATIONS

Using Guilt Constructively to Affirm Parental Coping

Guilt is one of the primary and often most intense reactions of parents to the birth of a sick infant. Whetsell and Larrabee (1988) note that it is common practice for health care providers to attempt to diffuse guilt feelings, although they are a functional response to the shock of a negative birth experience and have the potential for stimulating positive family responses. While guilt may have destructive effects, the nurse can intervene therapeutically to foster positive outcomes.

Whetsell and Larrabee have developed an Affirmation Model, a strategy that assists parents to channel guilt feelings into constructive goal-setting. The nurse accomplishes this by (1) affirming the parents' experience; (2) exploring the negative outcomes of guilt; (3) negotiating a time for parental care giving; (4) redirecting the parents' focus to the present; (5) aiding parents in goal setting and care-taking plans; (6) implementing the parental care-taking plan; and (7) reinforcing parents' actions and encouraging self-evaluation.

Whetsell MV, Larrabee MJ: Using guilt constructively in the NICU to affirm parental coping. Neontatal Network 6(4):21–27, 1988

tachment process and allow parents to assume increasing responsibility for the infant's care. If this is accomplished by discharge time, they are more likely to feel capable of recognizing and meetings his needs.

The special care nursery should have open visiting hours. Even when the infant is critically ill, parents should be given an opportunity to touch and talk to him. As his condition stabilizes, they can be encouraged to spend an increasing amount of time caring for, feeding, bathing, and holding him. The parents may at first be afraid to handle the infant, especially the premature neonate, who appears extremely fragile. The nurse must reassure them, guide and support their initial efforts, and praise their successes. Patience is required of the skilled nurse who knows she could accomplish a task with greater speed and proficiency.

If possible, the infant should be assigned a primary care nurse, who then becomes the consistent contact between parents and the unit. They should have the nursery telephone number and be encouraged to call day or night with questions and concerns. Parents should be made to feel that they are the most important people in the infant's life, and the care they provide is most responsible for the baby's progress. They should also be actively involved in the infant-stimulation program and provide as much of the sensory stimuli as possible. A special care unit that attempts to implement these suggested interventions will effectively facilitate the parent-infant attachment process.

ing care. Crying also has therapeutic value, and parents should be given permission to cry, if they appear to be fighting back tears: "It's O.K. to cry. What's happening with your baby is very upsetting." Putting an arm around the parent and staying with him or her at this time conveys a sense of acceptance and caring.

Encouraging Parent – Newborn Interaction

Klaus and Kennell (1982) believe that there may be a critical period immediately after birth for the formation of bonds between parent and infant. Skin-to-skin contact appears to enhance the development of ties at this time, and interaction plays an important role. When parents are separated from their infant during this sensitive period because of illness, they may have difficulty in reestablishing a relationship with the baby at a later date, when he is well enough to go home.

However, Klaus and Kennell advise health professionals to interpret their findings with caution. Separation at birth does not result in an irreversible disruption in parent–infant ties. Humans are quite adaptable, and with proper support by nursing staff, parents can become acquainted with their infant at a later point. An individualized discharge plan can be developed to facilitate the at-

Expected Outcomes: Neonate achieves a state of behavioral stabilization and beginning organization as evidenced by:

- Establishing recognized sleep/awake states
- Developing habituation behaviors to environmental stimuli
- Demonstrating orienting behaviors toward parents and care-givers while maintaining physiologic stability
- Acquiring increasingly sophisticated self-quieting abilities
- Engaging in social behaviors with parents and care-givers including cuddling
- Developing increasing motor maturity in control of extremities

Monitoring for Complications

While performing independent interventions, the nurse is also responsible for preventing potential complications related to therapy. Oxygen toxicity is a major complication of oxygen therapy.

Potential Complications Related to Oxygen Toxicity

As a result of oxygen therapy, two conditions may arise: retinopathy of prematurity and bronchopulmonary dysplasia. The nurse should be aware of these conditions so she can monitor for toxicity.

Conditions of Hyperoxia

Retinopathy of Prematurity.   Retinopathy of prematurity, previously referred to as retrolental fibroplasia (RLF), is a disease of the eye that results from high PaO_2 levels. Hyperoxemia initially results in vasoconstriction of retinal arteries (primary stage). After oxygen therapy is terminated, arterial vessels dilate and proliferate rapidly (secondary stage). Hemorrhage from damaged vessels leads to scarring and detachment of the retina, causing permanent blindness. Although the incidence of RLF is highest in preterm infants with PaO_2 levels above 70 mmHg, the disease has been documented in full-term infants maintained at lower PaO_2 levels during oxygen therapy. Because the disease has also been documented in infants who have not received oxygen, it is difficult to determine a completely safe therapeutic PaO_2 range for all neonates.

The following risk factors have been associated with the development of RLF (Avery 1987):

- Very low birth weight/prematurity
- Exchange transfusions
- Intraventricular hemorrhages
- Apnea
- Sepsis
- Patent ductus arteriosus with indomethacin administration
- Vitamin E deficiency

A classification system has been developed to describe the extent of injury (staging or grading) and the location of the disease in the retina. Three methods of surgical treatment have been attempted in the treatment of RLF, with varying degrees of success:

1. Laser therapy to reattach the retina
2. Cryotherapy to freeze selected areas of the retina to prevent vasoproliferation
3. Cryotherapy with scleral buckling to support retinal reattachment

Bronchopulmonary Dysplasia.   Bronchopulmonary dysplasia (BPD) is a disease of the lungs associated with prolonged oxygen therapy (at least 3 to 4 days), positive-pressure mechanical ventilation, and oxygen concentrations above 70%. Injury to the lung is not due to a high blood oxygen tension as in RLF, but rather to the direct effect of high oxygen concentrations on lung tissue and to

changes caused by pressure (barotrauma). Oxygen toxicity results in thickening and necrosis of the alveolar walls and bronchiolar epithelial lining. The infant becomes oxygen- and ventilator-dependent, and weaning the neonate from oxygen therapy is prolonged and difficult. Respiratory acidosis and right heart failure secondary to pulmonary changes are common complications. The infant often remains in the hospital for months during the weaning process and may be discharged home with oxygen. A mortality rate as high as 38% has been documented in affected infants.

Monitoring Oxygen Therapy

In order to minimize the risk of oxygen therapy, it is essential that the nurse continuously assess the oxygen delivery system and prevent hyperoxia by monitoring arterial blood gases. The use of transcutaneous oxygen monitors and pulse oximeters (see following section) also enables the nurse to evaluate the neonate's blood oxygenation status.

Oxygen Analyzer.   The percentage of oxygen (FIO_2 = fraction of inspired oxygen) administered to a neonate is monitored by an *oxygen analyzer* (Fig. 34–13). The oxygen analyzer is placed within the infant's environment, as close to the airway as possible, to measure the concentration of oxygen the neonate inspires. If the newborn is placed on a mechanical ventilator, the oxygen analyzer is usually connected directly to the airway tubing through which the oxygen flows.

Infants receiving oxygen therapy also require frequent determinations of PaO_2 levels. Arterial oxygen levels can be measured directly by arterial blood gas (ABG) analysis or indirectly by transcutaneous oxygen monitoring.

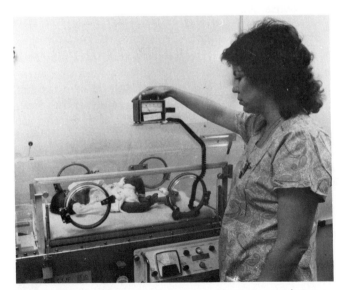

Figure 34–13. Infant in an incubator with oxygen analyzer.

Arterial Blood Gas Analysis. A small arterial blood sample (usually less than 1 ml) is obtained directly from the umbilical, temporal, brachial, or radial artery. The *p*H, PaO_2, and $PaCO_2$ can be measured as well as the HCO_3 (bicarbonate) level and base excess (amount of base buffer available to neutralize acid metabolites). The most accurate blood gas measurements are obtained by the invasive technique of withdrawing and analyzing arterial blood samples. Repeated withdrawal of blood, however, increases the risk of infection and anemia.

Transcutaneous (TC) Oxygen Monitoring. Transcutaneous oxygen ($PtcO_2$) monitoring is an indirect, noninvasive method for measuring PaO_2 levels in the neonate. An electrode attached to the infant's skin surface measures the oxygen tension of blood flowing past the skin site (Fig. 34–14). A constant "readout" or measurement of the PaO_2 is possible, allowing the nurse to evaluate the effects of nursing care and procedures on the infant's blood oxygen levels. For less critically ill infants, this method also eliminates the risks of invasive monitoring. For more seriously ill infants, for whom precise monitoring of blood gases is needed, $PtcO_2$ monitoring will be used in combination with intermittent ABG analysis, often using blood drawn from umbilical artery catheters.

A minor complication encountered with noninvasive monitoring is the development of skin blisters and pitting at the site of electrode placement. The electrode is heated (42°–44°C) to increase blood flow to the skin and may cause superficial injury if the site is not changed frequently (every 2–3 hours) or if the probe is too hot (premature infants cannot tolerate higher settings).

Pulse Oximetry. Another noninvasive method of assessing the blood oxygenation status of the neonate is pulse oximetry. The pulse oximeter sensor contains two light-emitting diodes (LED) and a photodetector. The sensor is wrapped around a finger or toe so that the LED is aligned directly opposite the photodetector. The tissue bed interposed between the two sides of the probe is transilluminated by the LED and the photodetector measures the heart rate and oxygen saturation of arterial hemoglobin (SpO_2).

Significant complications have not been reported with the use of pulse oximetry. The most notable problem is the potential for damage to the fragile skin of preterm infants from the adhesive tape used to secure the sensor to the extremity. This can be avoided by wrapping a small piece of gauze around the probe and securing it with tape. No adhesive need be attached to the skin.

The accuracy of SpO_2 readings is influenced by bright ambient light, movement of the extremity to which the sensor is applied, and the presence of abnormal hemoglobin. Finally, the accuracy of the pulse oximeter is not reliable at saturations above 90%. Hyperoxia may thus be missed. It is therefore imperative to simultaneously monitor the PO_2 with a transcutaneous oxygen monitor when oxygen is administered to the neonate. If an indwelling line, such as an umbilical artery catheter, is available, an indwelling arterial-oxygen electrode can be used.

Expected Outcomes: The infant demonstrates the absence of oxygen toxicity as evidenced by normal arterial blood gas values: *Term Infant:* 60 + mmHg; *Preterm Infant:* 50 – 80 mmHg.

Potential Complications: Hyperbilirubinemia and Kernicterus

General screening tests for such metabolic alterations as phenylketonuria (PKU), galactosemia, branched-chain amino acid defects (maple syrup urine disease), homocystinuria, and congenital hypothyroidism were discussed in Chapter 33. Care of the infant with such conditions is a specialized field and is not discussed in this text. This section pertains only to hyperbilirubinemia and kernicterus. For a review, the student is referred to Chapter 32 for a discussion of bilirubin conjugation and jaundice.

The sick or compromised infant is at greater risk for the development of hyperbilirubinemia and jaundice. Major disorders associated with pathologic jaundice are listed in the display, page 1040. The goal of therapeutic nursing interventions in the care of infants with hyperbilirubinemia is to prevent kernicterus, an encephalopathy caused by the deposition of unconjugated and unbound bilirubin in brain cells. Kernicterus has been associated with serum bilirubin levels approaching 20 mg/dl in the full-term infant and with much lower levels in the extremely premature neonate.

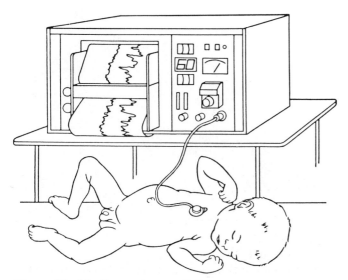

Figure 34–14. Transcutaneous PaO_2 monitoring system.

Major Disorders Associated with Pathologic Jaundice

- Intravascular hemolysis
  Hemolytic disease of the newborn
    Rh incompatibility
    ABO incompatibility
  Acquired hemolytic disorders secondary to infection
  Chemical hemolysis related to drugs
  Inherited defects of red cell metabolism
    Hereditary spherocytosis
    G6PD deficiency
    hemoglobinopathies
  Polycythemia
- Extravascular hemolysis (extravasation of blood)
  Petechiae
  Ecchymoses
  Hemorrhage
  Hematomas
- Swallowed blood
- Impaired hepatic function
  Glucoronyl transferase deficiency
    Familial nonhemolytic jaundice (Type I, II)
    Transient familial neonatal hyperbilirubinemia
      (Lucey–Driscoll syndrome)
  Sepsis
    Bacterial
    Nonbacterial (TORCH)
  Abnormal metabolic function
    Infants of diabetic mothers
    Galactosemia
    Hypothyroidism
    Hypopituitarism
    Tyrosinosis
    Cystic fibrosis
- Increased enterohepatic circulation of bilirubin
  Intestinal obstruction
  Pyloric stenosis
  Meconium ileus
  Paralytic ileus
  Hirschsprung's disease
- Biliary obstruction
  Biliary atresia

The classic signs of kernicterus, including lethargy, diminished reflexes, hypotonia, and seizures, are seen less frequently today as a result of advances in medical treatment and nursing care. Preterm neonates, weighing less than 1500 g, who are ill appear to be at greatest risk for developing kernicterus and sustaining permanent neurologic damage (deafness, cerebral palsy, or mental retardation). Other factors that appear to contribute to the development of kernicterus are hypothermia, asphyxia, acidosis, hypoalbuminemia, and sepsis.

When the infant develops pathologic jaundice, the nurse supports the conjugation and excretion of bilirubin by the following measures:

- Preventing hypothermia and reducing energy expenditures by placing the infant in a neutral thermal environment
- Supporting frequent feedings to facilitate adequate hydration and excretion of wastes (if oral feeding is not contraindicated)
- Supporting adequate caloric intake to meet energy requirements and maintain adequate serum albumin levels

The nurse will also initiate phototherapy when it is ordered by the physician.

Phototherapy

Phototherapy is the exposure of the infant's skin to high-intensity light. The process by which phototherapy reduces serum bilirubin involves the photoisomerization of unconjugated bilirubin deposited in the skin to a polarized compound. This compound diffuses into the blood stream, bound to albumin, and transported back to the liver where hepatic cells secrete it in unconjugated form into the biliary tract. The bilirubin is then excreted into the duodenum with bile salts and removed from the body with fecal wastes. Oxidation products are also formed in the skin when bilirubin is exposed to light, and these photodegradation products are excreted in the urine.

Several types of phototherapy lights are available today. A bank of eight to ten fluorescent lights (Fig. 34–15) with a wavelength of 420 to 550 nanometers (nm) can

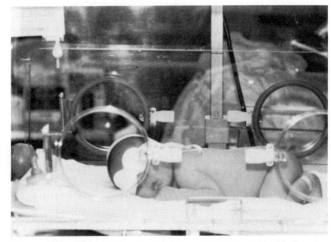

Figure 34–15. A full-term newborn receiving phototherapy in a closed isolette for hyperbilirubinemia. (Photo: BABES, Inc.)

FAMILY CONSIDERATIONS

Home Phototherapy

To reduce hospital costs and yet promote parent–infant attachment, home phototherapy has been instituted in some family-oriented maternity centers in the United States. Portable equipment is available and the American Academy of Pediatrics has developed guidelines to help health care providers establish a home phototherapy program. It is recommended that home phototherapy be limited to infants with the following characteristics: (1) term gestation, 48 hr old but otherwise healthy; (2) serum bilirubin levels greater than 14 mg/dl but less than 18 mg/dl; (3) no elevation in direct bilirubin levels; and (4) negative diagnostic evaluation.

Before phototherapy is instituted outside of the hospital setting, the home environment and the parents' ability to care for the infant and follow phototherapy guidelines should be evaluated. A visiting nurse, in collaboration with a physician, must be available to assess the neonate every 12 to 24 hr, check equipment, and measure serum bilirubin levels. Findings are documented and the physician contacted by phone or messenger service. Program evaluations have demonstrated the success of home therapy and its acceptance by families, nurses, and physicians.

Committee on the Fetus and Newborn: Home Phototherapy. American Academy of Pediatrics, 1984–1985
Dortch E, Spottiswoode P: New light on phototherapy: Home use. Neonatal Network 4:30–34, 1986

be used. Banks of daylight lamps, blue light, and high-intensity quartz lamps specifically designed for phototherapy are available to provide the proper irradiance.

The infant's clothes are removed and patches placed over the eyes to protect them from the light source. The infant is then placed in an isolette that provides a neutral thermal environment. The light source is positioned above the infant, and a photometer is used to measure the light intensity. Light flux should normally range between 6 to 8 μW/cm^2/nm. The distance of the light source from the infant should be based on the photometric reading. Light bulbs should be changed at preset intervals to ensure appropriate light output. It is suggested that Cavitron bulbs be changed after 150 hours of use and fluorescent lights before 2000 hours (Cloherty 1985). The infant is turned approximately every 2 hours in order to expose all body surfaces to the light. Phototherapy is continued until serum bilirubin levels fall to within normal limits.

Nursing care of the jaundiced infant who remains under the "bili lights" focuses on preventing complications of phototherapy, educating parents about this therapy, and providing emotional support and opportunities for them to hold and feed their infant. The nurse checks vital signs at least every 4 hours, since hyperthermia can occur under the lights. Because insensible water loss is increased with phototherapy and copious loose green "bili stools" are common sequelae of the treatment, the infant is also observed for signs of dehydration. Intake and output are monitored closely, and fluid intake is increased by at least 25% (10–15 ml/kg increase).

The skin is inspected for evidence of excoriation resulting from the passage of bili stools. Care must be taken to keep the skin clean and dry. Surgical face masks may be used as "bikini diapers" for infants who are urinating or stooling frequently and changed when soiled to prevent skin breakdown. A benign bronzing or tanning of the skin or the development of a diffuse malculopapular rash occurs in some infants as a response to phototherapy. No treatment is necessary, and no long-term adverse effects of bronzing or rashing have been documented.

Protection of the eyes is an essential aspect of care. The nurse should observe the infant frequently to be sure the patches are correctly positioned and the eyes remain closed. Phototherapy is discontinued and eye patches removed at least once every 4 to 8 hours so that the eyes can be inspected and the parents given an opportunity to hold and interact with their infant. Phototherapy lights must also be turned off each time a blood specimen is drawn for serum bilirubin determination (usually every 12 hours) to prevent photoisomerization of the specimen.

Exchange Transfusion

Another therapeutic modality employed in the treatment of severe hyperbilirubinemia is an exchange transfusion. In an exchange transfusion the neonate's blood is withdrawn to remove serum bilirubin and is replaced with donor's blood to maintain normal blood volume and provide free albumin-binding sites for bilirubin. Figure 34–16 illustrates guidelines for the management of hyperbilirubinemia and indicates when both phototherapy and exchange transfusions should be initiated to prevent kernicterus. Exchange transfusions are are also employed in the treatment of Rh isoimmunization to remove red blood cells that will be hemolyzed by maternal antibodies, thus elevating serum bilirubin levels, and to correct severe anemia caused by hemolysis of sensitized red blood cells. The reader is referred to the section on hemolytic disease of the newborn (later in this chapter) for further information on blood incompatibilities and their treatment.

In an exchange transfusion fresh blood, less than 24 hours old, that has been heparinized should be used. CPD (citrate-phosphate-dextrose) blood is preferred to ACD (acid-citrate-dextrose) because it has less than half the acid load and decreases the risk of a pH imbalance in the infant. The umbilical vein is usually cannulized (although

Serum bilirubin (mg/100 ml)	Birth weight	< 24 hrs	24–48 hrs	49–72 hrs	> 72 hrs
< 5					
5–9	All	Photo-therapy if hemolysis			
10–14	< 2500g	Exchange if hemolysis	Phototherapy		
	> 2500g			Investigate if bilirubin > 12 mg	
15–19	< 2500g	Exchange		Consider exchange	
	> 2500g			Phototherapy	
20 and +	All	Exchange			

☐ Observe   ▨ Investigate jaundice

Use phototherapy after any exchange

In presence of:

1. Perinatal asphyxia
2. Respiratory distress
3. Metabolic acidosis (pH 7.25 or below)
4. Hypothermia (temp below 35°C)
5. Low serum protein (5g/100 ml or less)
6. Birth weight < 1500 g
7. Signs of clinical or CNS deterioration

} Treat as in next higher bilirubin category

Figure 34–16. Guidelines for management of hyperbilirubinemia.

a central venous catheter can be used), and the blood is exchanged in 5- to 20-ml aliquots. The transfusion normally involves double the volume of the neonate's blood and is known as a "double volume exchange." Since the neonate's blood volume is approximately 80 ml/kg, the transfusion utilizes 160 ml/kg of blood and results in the removal of about 85% of the infant's red blood cells and their replacement with donor cells.

The nurse is an essential member of the exchange transfusion team. She prepares the neonate for the procedure, assembles essential equipment, and monitors physiologic responses during and after the transfusion. All feedings are stopped 4 hours before the transfusion to decrease the risk of aspiration during the procedure. The nurse places the infant on a procedure table, under a radiant warmer, and restrains his extremities. A cardiorespiratory monitor is attached for continuous monitoring of vital signs. Equipment required for emergency resuscitation is prepared and readily available.

When the transfusion is completed, the nurse continues to monitor the infant for complications of exchange transfusion. These include:

- Hemorrhage at the cannulization site
- Infection at the cannulization site
- Hypokalemia
- Hypoglycemia
- Thrombosis
- Necrotizing enterocolitis
- Cardiac failure secondary to fluid volume excess

Expected Outcomes:

- Neonate responds to phototherapy with reduction of hyperbilirubinemia as evidenced by (1) absence of observable jaundice and (2) reduction in serum bilirubin levels to within normal limits (usually 12% to 14% after 48 hours)

- The infant receiving exchange transfusion remains free of complications and maintains serum bilirubin levels within normal limits

Evaluation of Care of the High-Risk Infant

The quality of nursing care for the high-risk and sick neonate cannot necessarily be measured by complete recovery and discharge of the newborn to the care of his parents. Very premature infants and those with severe physiologic insults or congenital anomalies present medical and nursing problems of tremendous complexity.

NURSING ALERT

Caring for Care-givers: The Impact of the NICU Environment on the Nurse

Continuous responsibility for new life in a high-tech environment is a major stress factor neonatal nurses must confront daily. The sensory overload created by the vast array of equipment and personnel compound the potential for the depletion of the nurse's energies and eventual burnout. Other problems faced by the nurse in the NICU include lack of adequate staffing, the need to constantly acquire new knowledge, conflicts with physicians regarding treatment of infants, and dealing with distraught parents.

The neonatal nurse can engage in stress-reducing behaviors to prevent burnout. Simone (1984) suggests the following steps:

1. Identify personal stress factors
2. Develop a personal philosophy of life
3. Form realistic expectations regarding infant outcomes
4. Plan strategies to cope with stressful situations
5. Work as a member of the team and avoid isolation
6. Develop and use communication skills
7. Participate in ongoing professional education
8. Seek out positive role models
9. Plan appropriate withdrawals from the NICU environment

Simone JA: The intensity of newborn intensive care: Caring for caregivers. Neonatal Network 2(2):27–35, 1984

FAMILY CONSIDERATIONS

Discharge Planning and Home Health Care for the Impaired Neonate

Technologic advances have resulted in the survival of infants that require ongoing and intensive nursing care in the home for indefinite periods of time. They may require mechanical ventilation, oxygen therapy, frequent suctioning and gavage, or transpyloric feedings. The infant is often receiving multiple medications. Parents who make the decision to assume care for an impaired infant will require extensive support services.

Nurses frequently become case-managers for the discharge planning team. They coordinate the services of social workers, physical therapists, home health care nurses or aides, respiratory therapists, and other health professionals involved in ongoing treatment and care of the infant. Many institutions are now developing home health care programs to facilitate the transition for parents from hospital to home. Early evidence suggests these programs may reduce the incidence of re-hospitalization of the chronically ill infant, reducing hospital costs and family stress.

Of critical importance is the planning of respite care for parents. Care of the sick neonate may quickly exhaust the family's physical, emotional, and financial resources. It may divert parental energies from the siblings of the infant and result in family dysfunction. It may be impossible to find baby-sitters skilled in caring for the impaired infant. Some health care agencies are beginning to train home health aids in the care of sick newborns. For the very sickest infants, professional nurses may be needed to provide respite care. Home health care nursing for this population is a growing subspeciality, offering new opportunities for neonatal nurses.

Censullo M: Home care of the high-risk newborn. JOGN Nurse 15:146–153, 1986

Outcomes for many infants cannot be predicted with confidence, and nurses in the field of neonatal care must often intervene when knowledge and time are both limited. However, the nurse in neonatal care functions as part of an expert team of professionals; through the collaborative efforts of physicians, social workers, health science researchers, and others, the frontiers of knowledge are constantly being expanded (Fig. 34–17).

Evaluation of family-centered nursing care in the environment of the neonatal intensive care unit is also difficult. Nursing interventions to support parents and assist them in establishing a meaningful relationship with their newborn must take into account the conflicting forces of

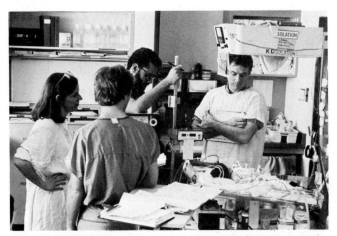

Figure 34–17. The nurse is an integral part of the neonatal intensive care unit staff. Often, expert nursing care makes the difference between a tragic outcome and a happy one. (Photo: Teresa Rodriguez)

hope and grief. The neonatal nurse may never see the results of her sensitive care for parents. The evidence of effective nursing care may only be apparent in the resolution of parental grief and the reintegration of family life. However, the most valued sign of expert and effective nursing care remains the "graduation" of a recovered and thriving infant to the care of happy parents, and the reunion of a new family.

The Neonate with Birth Asphyxia

Birth asphyxia is a condition characterized by hypoxemia (decreased PaO_2), hypercarbia (increased $PaCO_2$), and acidosis (lowered blood *p*H). Respiratory effort is minimal or absent as a result of brain stem hypoxia. With severe asphyxia, cardiac function is also depressed, caused by hypoxia of the myocardium.

Asphyxia is a progressive process that can be reversed in its initial stages with proper medical and nursing management. The initial drop in PaO_2 leads to a selective shunting of blood to the vital organs (brain and myocardium). The infant may be observed to gasp in an attempt to inflate the lungs. If efforts at ventilation fail and resuscitation is not initiated, the myocardium is eventually affected by the lowered PaO_2 level, and cardiac output decreases. Metabolic and respiratory acidosis occurs, decreasing the blood pH and causing vasoconstriction of pulmonary vasculature. The myocardium and brain rely on glucose for energy. Once glycogen stores are depleted, both brain and myocardial function deteriorate further. Unless vigorous resuscitation is started immediately, irreversible changes in brain and myocardial function will result, leading to permanent brain damage or death.

Etiologic Factors

A variety of maternal, fetal, and neonatal conditions can lead to asphyxia of the infant at birth.

Impaired Maternal Blood Flow Through the Placenta. Asphyxia occurs when the flow of oxygenated maternal blood to the intervillous spaces of the placenta is diminished. Any condition that leads to a decrease in the mother's blood pressure will impair blood flow to the intervillous spaces. Vena cava syndrome (supine hypotension) and conduction anesthesia are two common causes of maternal hypotension, but it may also result from hemorrhage and hypovolemic shock. Maternal vascular disease may also lead to birth asphyxia. The severe vasospasm found in pregnancy-induced hypertension leads to a decreased blood flow to the intervillous spaces. Vascular changes of chronic hypertension also interfere with placental perfusion. Placental accidents, such as infarcts and premature separation, also interrupt perfusion of the intervillous spaces.

Impaired Blood Flow Through the Umbilical Cord. Compression of the umbilical cord prevents oxygen transport through the fetal blood stream. Compression occurs when the cord is trapped between a fetal part and the maternal pelvis or cervix. Partial or total compression can also occur when the cord is tightly wrapped around a part of the fetal body, for example the neck (nuchal cord), or when there is a true knot in the cord.

Impaired Fetal Circulation. Any condition that decreases the efficiency of fetal circulation will lead to asphyxia. Trauma that produces fetal hemorrhage and hypovolemic shock, severe anemia (Rh disease), and congestive heart failure all diminish cardiac output and lead to fetal hypoxia.

Impaired Respiratory Effort. Whereas asphyxia leads to impaired respiratory effort, several conditions present at birth prevent the initiation of respiration and lead to asphyxia. Severe neonatal narcosis caused by maternal overmedication and an obstructed airway will both lead to asphyxia unless quickly corrected.

Implications for Nursing Care

During the first 60 seconds, the airway is cleared and the infant is quickly dried and stimulated. The heart rate, respiratory effort, color, muscle tone, and reflex irritability are all rapidly evaluated. Oxygen may be given, and ventilation and cardiac compression are begun if the infant is severely depressed (see Immediate Resuscitation of the Neonate in Chapter 33). By 1 minute, the type and extent of *continuing* support needed is determined by the Apgar score. A score of 7 or under indicates a need for ongoing intensive life support.

Once the infant's condition is stabilized, he is transferred to the special care unit, where nursing care is directed at supporting vital functions (cardiac, respiratory, and thermal regulation).

Potential Complication: Postasphyxial Syndrome

If resuscitation efforts are successful, the neonate who has suffered birth asphyxia is transferred to a special care unit for continuing observation. This is essential because hypoxia can lead to necrosis of tissues in major organ systems and profound metabolic alterations. *Postasphyxial syndrome* is the resultant condition and is characterized by a constellation of signs.

The neonate with postasphyxial syndrome usually exhibits seizure activity, resulting from brain edema, within the first 24 hours of birth. Edema is caused by the death of brain cells and the increased permeability of cerebral vessels secondary to increased $PaCO_2$ levels. Intracranial hemorrhage can also occur as a result of increased capillary fragility secondary to metabolic acidosis or the too rapid infusion of sodium bicarbonate during neonatal resuscitation.

Necrosis of both renal and intestinal tissues is a result of the protective shunting of blood to the brain and liver that occurs with hypoxia. Renal failure, characterized by either "high output" or "low output" urine volume, is observed. Hypoxic injury to the neonatal gut leads to a condition known as necrotizing enterocolitis (NEC). Patches of necrotic tissue in the intestinal lumen may perforate, spilling intestinal contents into the peritoneal cavity and causing peritonitis. Preterm infants are particularly susceptible to necrotizing enterocolitis, and the mortality rate remains very high.

Metabolic alterations are also associated with postasphyxial syndrome. Glucose stores are rapidly depleted during asphyxial episodes, and this leads to hypoglycemia. Hypocalcemia occurs, and although its etiology is unclear, changes in parathyroid function and increased cell permeability secondary to hypoxia appear to alter the calcium/phosphorus ratio. Potassium is also released into the vascular compartment from cells damaged by hypoxia and causes hyperkalemia.

The major concern after an asphyxial episode and oxygen deprivation to the neonate's brain is the long-term neurologic outcome. Recent research suggests that the Apgar score alone is not a reliable predictor of long-term neurologic sequelae. An Apgar score of 0 to 3 at 5 minutes is associated with an increased risk of cerebral palsy, but the increase is slight (0.3% to 1%) (Committee on Fetus and Newborn, AAP 1986). The correlation between the Apgar score and future impairment in neurologic functioning is clearer when the score is 0 to 3 at 10, 15, or 20 minutes. An even stronger indicator of eventual neurologic impairment appears to be the development of postasphyxial seizures in the neonate (Blackman 1988). Although statistical evidence is available to assist physicians in determining prognosis, it is often difficult to accurately predict an individual infant's eventual neurologic status.

The infant is monitored closely for signs of increased intracranial pressure, including bulging fontanelles, "setting sun" eyes (a condition in which the sclera are visible above the iris), decreased or absent reflexes, and seizures, as well as for myocardial ischemia (arrhythmias), intestinal ischemia, and necrotizing enterocolitis (absence of bowel sounds, increasing girth, and bloody stools).

Intake and output are meticulously recorded to evaluate renal function and rule out renal failure. The urine is checked with each voiding for the presence of blood and protein, an indication of renal injury, and the stools are also tested for heme, a danger sign suggesting the development of necrotizing enterocolitis. Serial blood glucose determinations are made by obtaining heel prick blood samples to detect hypoglycemia, and serum electrolytes are also checked once or twice each day for evidence of hypocalcemia and hyperkalemia.

The infant who experiences birth asphyxia ingests nothing by mouth for at least 24 to 48 hours after birth to rest the gut and prevent additional injury if intestinal ischemia and necrosis have occurred. Intravenous therapy is administered to meet immediate needs for fluid and calories (dextrose), and prophylactic antibiotic therapy may be instituted if invasive emergency care was started at birth. Antibiotic therapy will be discontinued if blood culture results prove negative (results usually take about 72 hours to become available). If seizure activity is noted, the infant will be placed on phenobarbital or Dilantin.

Most parents are well aware of the impact of asphyxia on mental functioning. The wait-and-see policy often maintained by physicians is extremely hard on parents. They may bombard the nurse with questions regarding signs of possible brain damage in their infant and press for concrete predictions regarding neurologic function. Parents will need ongoing support and counseling to deal with these uncertainties. Long-term follow-up of the infant will be necessary, and it may be years before the child's maximum neurologic capabilities can be determined.

THE NEONATE WITH COMPLICATIONS RELATED TO GESTATIONAL AGE

The Preterm Infant

The preterm or premature neonate is one born before 37 weeks of gestation. The etiology of preterm labor is

NURSING CARE PLAN

The Mildly Asphyxiated Newborn (Apgar at 1 Minute: 4–6)

Nursing Diagnosis (Patient Problem) and Assessment Data	Nursing Interventions	Rationale
Potential complications resulting from mild asphyxiation at birth:		
Asphyxia may predispose the neonate to: • Respiratory distress syndrome • Patent ductus arteriosus • Cardiogenic shock due to the effect of hypoxia on cardiovascular and pulmonary tissue • Pneumothorax due to ventilation by bag during resuscitation	Review the prenatal and labor and delivery records. Obtain a full report from the delivery room nurse regarding the delivery history, Apgar scores, perinatal complications, and resuscitative efforts required for the infant. Observe the infant for: • Pallor > 1° • Central cyanosis • Tachypnea, flaring, grunting, retracting • Tachycardia • Bounding or thready pulses • Heart murmur • Shift in point of maximal impulse • Decreased blood pressure Report signs and symptoms of the physician. Monitor vital signs every ½ hour for 2 hours, then every hour for 4 to 6 hours or until the infant is stable.	Information on the prenatal health of the mother and the course of her labor and delivery may help identify the cause.
Nursing Diagnosis: *ineffective breathing pattern*		
Exhibited by: • Central cyanosis • Grunting • Flaring • Retractions • Tachypnea • Apnea	Administer oxygen in the amount to relieve cyanosis until an ABG is done.	Oxygen should be treated like any medication and used with care. An arterial blood gas will accurately determine the amount of oxygen needed.
	Assist in obtaining an ABG by holding or positioning neonate.	Adequate restraining prevents additional needle sticks, thereby maintaining oxygenation.
	Notify physician if cyanosis persists; obtain further orders.	Persistent hypoxia can lead to patent ductus arteriosus and persistent fetal circulation.
	Place neonate on a cardiorespiratory monitor with alarm limits set at 100	Continuous monitoring is essential to validate changes in status. Alarms

(continued)

1046

NURSING CARE PLAN

The Mildly Asphyxiated Newborn (Apgar at 1 Minute: 4–6) (continued)

Nursing Diagnosis (Patient Problem) and Assessment Data	Nursing Interventions	Rationale
	BPM for low rate and 200 BPM for high rate.	set at these limits alert the nurse prior to the infant becoming severely compromised.
	Resuscitation bag and mask or CPAP (continuous positive airway pressure) bag and mask should be at the bedside.	Readily available resuscitation equipment will prevent further hypoxic episodes

Expected Outcome:

The neonate achieves and maintains effective respiratory pattern and adequate gas exchange as demonstrated by pink mucous membranes, nail beds, and skin color.

Nursing Diagnosis:
altered cardiac output, decreased

Exhibited by:	Assess capillary refill; impaired if greater than 3 sec.	Perfusion changes reflect the status of cardiac output.
• Inadequate perfusion		
• Hypotension	Check BP, preferably by arterial transducer monitoring; note changes in mean arterial pressure.	Hypotension, if present, may be treated with a cardiovascular preparation such as Dopamine. Dopamine produces an inotropic effect on the myocardium, resulting in increased cardiac output.
• Active precordium		
• Weak pulses		
• Cyanosis		
• Heart murmur		
	Assess the apical at the fifth intercostal space left of the midclavicular line for activity of the precordium, visually and through palpation.	An active precordium indicates an increased work load on the heart.
	Assess bilateral brachial and femoral pulses for equality and pressure.	Unequal pulses may indicate impaired blood flow. Weak pulses represent a decrease in pressure and/or cardiac output.
	If cyanosis is present, administer oxygen to keep color and mucous membranes pink.	Hypoxia can lead to patent ductus arteriosus (PDA).
	Place a pulse oximeter on infant to keep saturation greater than 90% until an ABG can be done.	Pulse oximeter gives a quick, noninvasive reliable indication of oxygen saturation. *Caution:* If peripheral perfusion is poor, saturation may not be accurate. Pulse oximetry does not replace the need for an ABG, which gives an accurate picture of the gas exchange ability.

(continued)

NURSING CARE PLAN

The Mildly Asphyxiated Newborn (Apgar at 1 Minute: 4–6) (continued)

Nursing Diagnosis (Patient Problem) and Assessment Data	Nursing Interventions	Rationale
	Auscultate for a heart murmur.	For a symptomatic PDA resulting in increased oxygen requirement and poor cardiac output, Indomethacin or PDA ligation may be indicated.

Expected Outcome:

The neonate achieves and maintains normal cardiac output and adequate tissue perfusion as evidenced by normal heart rate, rhythm, pressure, and pulses and absence of peripheral edema and murmurs.

Nursing Diagnosis:
hypothermia

	Take the infant's temperature every half hr for 2 hr, then every hr for 4 to 6 hr. Observe for temperature less than 36.4°C or 97.5°F, or wide fluctuations in temperature over short time period.	Thermoregulation in the asphyxiated newborn is poor. Temperature instability will cause further depletion of glucose stores.
	Place the infant in a radiant warmer for 4 to 6 hr	To maintain the newborn's temperature at 98°F (37°C).
	If on a radiant warmer:	
	• Set warmer on servo control with skin temp probe attached with plastic tape and probe cover. Never position infant on temp. probe.	Servo control enables accurate regulation of skin temperature. Positioning infant on probe will give false temperature readings.
	• Change wet diaper as soon as possible.	Dry diapers prevent heat loss by conduction and evaporation.

Expected Outcome:

The neonate maintains normal core temperature as evidenced by an axillary temperature of 36.4° to 37.2°C and absence of temperature instability.

Potential Complication:
hypoglycemia

	Observe the infant for signs of hypoglycemia: jitteriness, lethargy, irritability, tremors, hypotonia, cyanosis, apnea.	Hypoglycemia results from the stress of asphyxia at birth, which causes utilization of all available glucose stores, and can lead to CNS injury.
	Perform a Dextrostix (DS) or Chem-strip test on admission, then every	These tests provide an approximation of serum blood sugar levels.

(continued)

NURSING CARE PLAN

The Mildly Asphyxiated Newborn (Apgar at 1 Minute: 4–6)

Nursing Diagnosis (Patient Problem) and Assessment Data	Nursing Interventions	Rationale
	half hr for 2 hr, then every hr for 2 hr, then as appropriate until the infant is stable.	
	When the Dextrostix or Chemstrip level is <45 mg, give the infant oral 10% dextrose in water, 5 ml/kg body weight, by nipple or gavage. Repeat these tests in 15 min. Notify the physician.	The dextrose solution provides glucose to the newborn.

Expected Outcome:

Neonate maintains a stabilized metabolism as evidenced by normal serum glucose level in the first 24 hr after birth.

Potential Complication:
hyperbilirubinemia

	Observe newborn every 8 hr, monitoring for icterus progressing cephalocaudally. Notify the physician of jaundice or rising serum bilirubin levels present in the first 24 hr.	Metabolites that result from acidosis compete for bilirubin-binding sites, resulting in large amounts of free circulating indirect bilirubin.

Expected Outcome:

The newborn remains free of jaundice as evidenced by absence of observable jaundice and presence of serum bilirubin levels within normal limits (12% to 14%) after 48 hr. The infant maintains normal serum glucose and bilirubin levels in the first 24 hr after birth.

Nursing Diagnosis:
actual fluid volume deficit

Exhibited by:		
• Output greater than intake • Increased serum sodium • Dry skin and mucous membranes • Decreased urine output • Weight loss • Feeding intolerance	Assess for dehydration: increased pulse, increased respirations, decreased BP, decreased turgor, pale color, depressed fontanelles, sunken eyes.	Dehydration which results in a decreased blood volume causes an increased pulse and respirations. Decreased turgor, pale color, depressed fontanelles and sunken eyes result from shifting of water between body compartments as well as a decreased blood volume.
	Check urine output and specific gravity with each voiding.	Output is primarily regulated by the kidneys' ability to concentrate urine. Specific gravity measures this function. The greater the value, the

(continued)

NURSING CARE PLAN

The Mildly Asphyxiated Newborn (Apgar at 1 Minute: 4–6) (continued)

Nursing Diagnosis (Patient Problem) and Assessment Data	Nursing Interventions	Rationale
		greater the dehydration. Normal: 1.004–1.025. *Caution:* Neonatal urine may be falsely elevated by high molecular weight solutes such as radiographic dye, sugars, or protein. In these cases, osmolarity will best signify the kidneys' concentrating abilities.
	Weigh utilizing the same scale, time, and method.	Accurate weights are essential to the calculation of fluid requirements.

Expected Outcome:

Neonate achieves fluid/electrolyte balance as evidenced by urine specific gravity within normal limits and minimal daily weight loss within 5 to 6 days.

Nursing Diagnosis:
potential for injury: seizures

Exhibited by: • Tonic eye deviations • Blinking or eyelid fluttering • Sucking or mouthing movements • Smiling • Drooling • Tonic posture of single limb	Assess for signs and symptoms of seizures.	Early recognition of seizures facilitates prompt treatment, improving long-term prognosis.
	Be prepared to respond to the ABCs of CPR (establish a patent airway; assure adequate breathing; maintain circulation through heart rate/ rhythm status).	ABCs may be impaired due to altered neurologic function.
• Bicycling of the legs • Rowing movements of the arms • Apnea	Obtain Chemstrip or Dextrostix and serum glucose.	Hypoglycemia is a cause of seizures and dextrose may be needed as a treatment.
Caution: All behaviors can be normal. However, when the behavior is repetitive, associated with a change or deterioration in clinical condition, or interruption of the behavior is not possible, it is probably seizure activity.	Administer anticonvulsant medication as ordered.	There is a dramatic increase in metabolic rate during a seizure and glucose stores may be depleted. Control of seizures minimizes brain hypoxia.

Expected Outcome:

Neonate responds to treatment for seizure activity, as evidenced by normalization of neurologic and physiologic status and absence of recurrent seizure activity.

Table 34-4   **Causes of Prematurity**

Obstetric Complications	Medical Complications	Socioeconomic Factors
Uterine malformation	Maternal diabetes	Absence of prenatal care
Multiple gestation	Chronic hypertensive disease	Low socioeconomic status
Incompetent cervical os	Urinary tract infection	Malnutrition
Premature rupture of membranes and chorioamnionitis	Other acute illnesses	Early adolescent pregnancy
Pregnancy-induced hypertension		
Placenta previa		
History of previous premature birth		
Rh isoimmunization		

poorly understood, although variables associated with premature delivery have been identified (Table 34-4).

Preterm infants suffer from anatomic and physiologic immaturity in all systems, preventing them, in many instances, from making major adaptations without continuous medical and nursing care. It is no longer possible to describe a typical preterm infant. Although technologic advances have made it possible for infants under 500 g and between 24 to 26 weeks of gestation to survive very premature births, the mortality rate is highest among these neonates. Their physical characteristics and physiologic capabilities are quite different from those of the preterm neonate born at 36 weeks of gestation. Although a description of these differences is beyond the scope of this chapter, it is possible to discuss the problems and requirements for nursing care that preterm infants have in common.

Potential for Impaired Gas Exchange

The preterm infant is at risk for respiratory complications because the lungs and the regulatory centers of the central nervous system are immature at birth. Alveolar sacs begin to differentiate and increase in number at 24 weeks of gestation, but the surface for exchange of gases is limited, and air sacs tend to collapse because of minimal surfactant production. The regulatory center for respiration located in the brain is also immature, and the preterm infant can suffer from serious episodes of apnea and bradycardia.

Respiratory Distress Syndrome Type I (Hyaline Membrane Disease). Respiratory distress syndrome (RDS) is a disorder of the lungs characterized by pulmonary hypoperfusion, hypoxemia, metabolic and respiratory acidosis, and classic changes in lung tissue, including decreased compliance, capillary damage, and alveolar necrosis. RDS I (hyaline membrane disease) is primarily due to immaturity and inadequate surfactant production,

leading to progressive atelectasis and decreased perfusion of lung tissue.

The infant with RDS I exhibits rapid, labored respirations as he attempts to re-expand collapsed alveoli with each inspiration. Classic signs of distress, including cyanosis or pallor, retractions, nasal flaring, grunting, and see-saw breathing, are evident. The neonate is hypotonic and inactive, focusing all energy on the effort to sustain respiration. Mechanical ventilation is frequently used to assist the infant or breathe for him. If adaptations are successful, respiratory distress diminishes within 3 to 5 days as surfactant production increases and alveoli expand. Death is rare after 72 hours in cases of uncomplicated RDS I. Recent clinical trials evaluating the efficacy of surfactant replacement therapy offer hope for future improvements in the treatment and outcomes of RDS for the preterm infant (Jabe and Ikegami 1987).

Apnea. Preterm neonates may suffer from apneic episodes, even in the absence of identified disorders, as a result of immature neurologic and pulmonary function. Continued severe apnea will result in decreased PaO_2, increased $PaCO_2$, and acidosis. Apneic episodes can be decreased or eliminated in many preterm infants by nursing care aimed at maintaining body temperature, stimulating the neonate with a rocker bed or water bed, and placing him in a prone position to improve ventilation and oxygenation. Theophylline or caffeine, both respiratory stimulants and bronchodilators, are used in the treatment of apnea with good results.

Potential for Altered Cardiac Output

The major cardiovascular adaptation in both full-term and preterm infants is the change from fetal to neonatal circulation. Fetal circulatory bypasses close as a result of an increase in systemic blood pressure, lung expansion, and the shift in pressure gradients from the right side of the heart to the left. A rise in blood oxygen concentrations

NURSING ALERT

Umbilical Cord Blood Gas Analysis

In an effort to evaluate the severity of the asphyxial insult, the degree of metabolic aberration at birth, and the effectiveness of resuscitation efforts, cord blood gas and *p*H analyses have been instituted in many birthing units. The nurse is often responsible for obtaining the cord blood samples and sending them to the laboratory for analysis.

Immediately after the delivery of a compromised infant, a segment of umbilical cord is obtained and clamped at both ends. A sample of blood is collected from both the artery and the vein and placed in separate, plastic heparinized syringes. The samples are then transported to the lab in an ice-filled container. Acid–base and blood gas analyses are performed (preferably within 5 minutes) and *p*H, PO$_2$, PCO$_2$ and Base Excess determined.

Management of the asphyxiated infant in the immediate postresuscitation period will, in part, be based on the cord blood gas analysis in order to correct hypoxia, hypercarbia, and acidosis.

Normal *p*H and Blood Gas Values At Birth in The Term Infant

	Umbilical Vein	Umbilical Artery
*p*H	7.32	7.24
PO$_2$	27.5	16
PCO$_2$	39	49

also facilitates closure of the ductus arteriosus. Incomplete development of the pulmonary system in the preterm infant significantly affects major cardiovascular adaptations.

Persistent Fetal Circulation. The preterm infant may experience a persistent fetal circulation when the ductus arteriosus remains open after birth. In the full-term neonate the ductus is sensitive to oxygen and constricts with rising PaO$_2$ levels. It is hypothesized that immature muscular development of the ductus arteriosus in the preterm infant results in the incomplete constriction and closure of this fetal bypass. As systemic blood pressure rises and pressure in the right side of the heart decreases, left-to-right shunting occurs. Shunting results in an increased blood volume entering the pulmonary vessels and leads to pulmonary congestion, decreased lung compliance, and increased respiratory effort. Pulmonary congestion, in turn, impairs adequate gas exchange and results in hypoxia.

The vicious cycle initiated with persistent patent ductus arteriosus and shunting of blood is difficult to reverse. In some infants, patent ductus arteriosus can be managed successfully by fluid restriction. Indomethacin, a prostaglandin-inhibitor, has been used with limited success to constrict the ductus arteriosus, but it has severe side effects, including renal failure and gastrointestinal bleeding. Surgical ligation of the ductus is also employed in the treatment of persistent patent ductus, but surgery poses major risks for the unstable preterm infant.

Potential for Fluid Volume Deficits

Immaturity in the structure and function of the renal system produces fluid and electrolyte imbalances in the preterm neonate. The infant's diminished ability to concentrate urine or excrete fluids efficiently can result in fluid volume excess. There is an increased risk for metabolic acidosis because of excessive bicarbonate loss. The preterm infant is also susceptible to fluid volume deficits and dehydration as a result of increased frank and insensible fluid losses and the inability to conserve water.

Potential for Altered Nutrition

The preterm neonate's immature gastrointestinal tract prevents ingestion, digestion, and absorption of essential nutrients. Suck, swallow, and gag reflexes are often absent, requiring the delivery of nutrients by alternative routes (gavage tube, transpyloric feedings, or parenteral hyperalimentation). The stomach capacity is greatly reduced and requires that nutrients be introduced in very small volumes. Liver glycogen stores are minimal, so that the infant is at risk for development of hypoglycemia. Digestive enzymes and bile salts may also be deficient, resulting in inadequate digestion of nutrients. Infants who are capable of nipple feeding are easily exhausted by sucking efforts and may experience episodes of apnea, bradycardia, and cyanosis during feeding. Finally, commercial formulas available for the full-term infant do not provide sufficient calories and minerals for growth nor the appropriate proportions of casein and whey for the preterm neonate.

Potential for Complications

Necrotizing Enterocolitis. The preterm neonate is at great risk for the development of necrotizing enterocolitis, a disorder in which necrosis of the bowel results from an asphyxial insult. It is hypothesized that hypoxia leads to shunting of blood from the kidney, intestines, and muscles to the brain, heart, and liver to sustain essential metabolic, neurologic, and cardiac functioning. Cell death follows this "gut shunting," and ischemia and areas of necrosis develop in the bowel. Perforation of the intestinal wall can also occur. Localized infection and septicemia

NURSING RESEARCH

Benefits of Non-Nutritive Sucking in the Preterm Infant

Many preterm infants are unable to breast- or bottle-feed for extended periods of time after birth due to physiologic immaturity or illness. Nursing research has, however, recently demonstrated a number of significant benefits in allowing the infant to engage in non-nutritive sucking behaviors with a pacifier before oral feedings are initiated. Findings include a more rapid weight gain, earlier initiation of oral feedings, and earlier hospital discharge coupled with reduced hospital costs.

Further study is required with larger numbers of subjects and the evaluation of other outcome variables, such as energy expenditure, effects on oxygen levels, and neurobehavioral development. It appears appropriate, however, at this stage of knowledge development to recommend the clinical practice of initiating non-nutritive sucking for infants older than 28 weeks' gestation when gavage feedings are begun. The nurse should closely monitor the infant's physiologic responses during the process.

Schwartz R, Moody L, Yarandi H et al: A meta-analysis of critical outcome variables in non-nutritive sucking in preterm infants. Nurs Res 36;292–295, 1987

frequently complicate the condition. Figure 34–18 illustrates the possible etiology and consequences of necrotizing enterocolitis.

Classic signs of necrotizing enterocolitis include abdominal distention, increasing gastric residuals, vomiting, and blood in the stools. Temperature instability and apnea are commonly observed and are associated with infection. Surgical intervention is often necessary to remove necrotic sections of the bowel, and a temporary colostomy may be performed. A small percentage of infants develop "short bowel syndrome" following surgery. The infant suffers from chronic malnutrition and failure to thrive secondary to removal of large sections of the intestines and incomplete absorption of nutrients. The mortality rate for necrotizing enterocolitis is high, ranging between 20% and 75%, depending on the gestational age and condition of the neonate (Walsh 1986).

Intraventricular Hemorrhage. Intraventricular hemorrhage (IVH) is the most common type of brain bleed in preterm infants. It is closely associated with birth asphyxia and resultant hypoxia and hypercapnia as well as increased blood osmolality related to sodium bicarbonate administration (Cunningham 1987).

Hemorrhage occurs in tissue surrounding the ventricles. The blood then enters the brain cavities, circulating in the cerebrospinal fluid. The infant who sustains a catastrophic intraventricular hemorrhage experiences a sudden deterioration in his condition. There is shock with depressed or absent vital signs. Seizures may be evident. Bulging fontanelles, falling hematocrit, hypothermia, and hypotonia are also observed. Prognosis and long-term neurologic sequelae depend on the extent of the bleed. Grading (I through IV) is done by CT scan and ultrasonography. Infants with Grade I bleeds sustain the least injury and fare best. Those with Grade IV bleeds have the poorest prognosis.

Hypothermia. Preterm infants have little ability to generate heat or prevent heat loss. Heat production is limited by minimal brown fat and glycogen stores and the immaturity of the thermoregulatory center. Heat loss is greater than in the full-term infant because the preterm neonate has little subcutaneous fat, has a much larger ratio of body surface to mass, and remains in a more relaxed, less flexed posture.

Infection. Because maternal antibodies cross the placenta during the third trimester of pregnancy, the very premature infant is deprived of these immune globulins and susceptible to infection. Preterm infants are also at increased risk for infection because their immunity is depressed and the skin is immature. The invasive nature of diagnostic procedures and treatments, such as mechanical ventilation and the use of umbilical catheters, also place the neonate at risk for infection.

Hyperbilirubinemia. Because the liver is immature and the number of albumin-binding sites is decreased, the preterm neonate is at greater risk for hyperbilirubinemia and jaundice. Hemolysis associated with sepsis, acidosis, and bleeding disorders also increases the incidence of jaundice in preterm infants. Kernicterus and irreversible brain damage can occur at much lower blood levels of bilirubin than in the full-term infant. As a result, blood exchange transfusions and phototherapy are initiated earlier.

Impaired Mobility. Preterm infants are at risk for impaired mobility later in life as a result of postural problems and improper body mechanics in the nursery rather than from neurologic impairment. For instance, some infants eventually exhibit rigid posturing, arching of the back, and other abnormal motor patterns, such as "toe walking," the inability to place the heel of the foot flat on the floor later in life. Excessive hypotonia and muscle flexibility in the preterm neonate, coupled with improper positioning and handling by nursery personnel result in these nursery-acquired mobility problems.

Techniques for encouraging the development of proper posture have been recently developed by physical

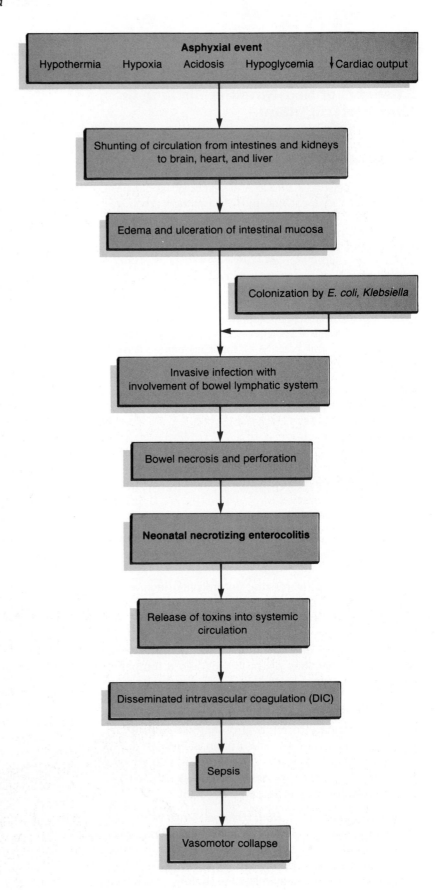

Figure 34–18. Possible causes and consequences of neonatal necrotizing enterocolitis.

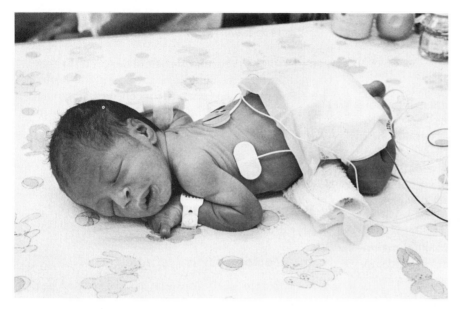

Figure 34–19. Correct flexion can be encouraged in the neonate by bringing knees up to the chest, placing arms close to the body, and placing a small roll under the hips when the neonate is in prone position. (Adapted from Fry M: The positive effect of positioning. Neonatal Network 6[5]:23–28, 1988)

therapists to minimize problems related to impaired mobility. Flexion is essential for the development of normal body movement and control in the infant. The majority of preterm neonates are born before physiologic flexion has developed. The goal of proper positioning is to promote flexion, avoid excessive extension, and maintain symmetrical positioning (Fig. 34–19).

Placing the infant in a prone position with its arms and legs flexed and close to the body is the optimum position.

If the infant must be supine to accommodate equipment and procedures, blanket rolls can be placed around the body to encourage as much flexion as possible and to prevent later arching behaviors. Providing the infant with boundaries that contain his movements also supports flexion, promotes comfort, and may assist in optimal neuromuscular development as the infant learns to control muscles and body parts by pushing against firm surfaces.

NURSING RESEARCH

Reexamining the Practice of Tactile Stimulation in Preterm and Sick Infants

The importance of touch and sensory stimulation for the neonate has resulted in the development of infant stimulation protocols to prevent developmental delays in premature infants. With the survival of extremely ill and very-low-birth-weight infants between 24 and 26 weeks' gestation, questions have been raised regarding the appropriateness of tactile stimulation for these infants. Very little research has been conducted to identify the full range of behavioral responses to touch and other forms of sensory stimulation in these two groups of high-risk infants or to determine which interventions elicit positive responses.

Oehler (1985) examined the preterm infant's capacity for responsiveness to social stimuli between 26 and 30 weeks' gestation. Results suggest that stimulation of immature and sick infants requires careful assessment and consideration. Some subjects demonstrated decreased ability to use stabilizing activities and experienced drops in oxygen levels when

talking was combined with touching. Avoidance behaviors were also noted.

Tactile stimulation interventions must be geared to each infant's changing needs and must be sensitive to his cues. They must take into account his tolerance levels for stimulation and nursing care should seek to normalize or modify the NICU environment to reduce noxious stimuli (*i.e.*, noise and intense light). Much more research is required before formalized interventions can be developed and recommended for clinical use with these infants.

Oehler JM: Examining the issue of tactile stimulation for preterm infants. Neonatal Network 3:25–33, 1985

VandenBerg KA: Revising the traditional model: An individualized approach to developmental interventions in the intensive care nursery. Neonatal Network 3:32–38, 1985

Potential for Altered Parenting

The preterm neonate is exposed to numerous environmental stimuli and even physical insults for a prolonged period in the neonatal intensive care unit. His premature birth separates him from the comforting world of the womb, and his immature state often prevents his parents from holding or comforting him for weeks or months. Once the neonate has achieved physiologic stability, he is placed in an isolette until adequate growth and development permit him to return home with his parents. Social isolation and further distortion of external stimuli occur in this environment. Under these conditions, the development of sensory-perceptual capabilities can be adversely affected.

Recent nursing research indicates that skillful manipulation of the environment to minimize stimuli and support developing sensory capabilities can actually accelerate physical growth and maturation and shorten the length of the infant's hospital stay. Ongoing research is exploring ways to foster the sensory and perceptual development of the high-risk neonate, including the preterm infant. Nurse researchers have created guidelines for infant stimulation in the intensive care nursery (Ludington–Hoe 1984, Anderson 1986). The accompanying display presents basic techniques for infant stimulation. Parents have a central role in any stimulation care plan, making this an extremely effective means of fostering parent-infant acquaintance.

The preterm infant will initially demonstrate periods of behavioral disorganization related to neurologic immaturity and illness. He will be unable to respond in predictable and appropriate ways to stimuli. Routine nursing care activities and interaction with the neonate can result in rapid physiologic deterioration. Sleep patterns are different from those demonstrated in the full-term neonate. As the infant's condition stabilizes, he will be able to engage in very short periods of reciprocal interaction with care-givers, but will become quickly exhausted by these encounters.

It may take many months before the preterm neonate begins to exhibit the behavioral patterns of full-term neonates. Parents may be unable to reconcile their fantasized image with the preterm newborn presented to them. They may become discouraged when their attempts to communicate with the infant do not produce the expected response. Furthermore, if the infant actually experiences physiologic decompensation during interaction with parents, they may become frightened and withdraw from future efforts at interaction.

Implications for Nursing Care

Nursing care of the preterm neonate is focused on supporting major physiologic adaptations, preventing complications, and supporting the parents. See the accompanying Nursing Care Plan for the Preterm Infant.

The Small-for-Gestational-Age (SGA) Neonate

Although the SGA infant resembles the preterm infant in size, his physical characteristics and physiologic capabilities are quite different. The SGA infant is any infant whose weight falls below the tenth percentile or is 2 standard deviations below the mean. The low birth weight and subsequent physiologic adaptations are a result of intrauterine growth retardation (IUGR) caused by a variety of prenatal conditions, including maternal malnutrition, premature placental aging secondary to diabetes mellitus or other vascular conditions, placental infarcts, congenital

(text continued on page 1063)

Sensory Stimulation Techniques For Stable Preterm Infants

Sensory Modality	Appropriate Nursing Intervention
Touch	Gently stroke skin in head-to-toe direction at a rate of approximately 12 strokes per minute. Expose to a variety of textures, including cotton, satin, and silk.
Taste	Allow infant to suck on a pacifier (if not contraindicated by a gastrointestinal or respiratory anomaly) to stimulate salivary glands and digestive enzymes.
Vision	Place black and white schematic faces in an *en face* position within visual range (19 to 22 cm). Provide time for eye-to-eye contact. Periodically reduce intensity of lights.
Smell	Introduce different pleasant-smelling odors, including the smell of the mother's breast milk if she intends to breast-feed the baby.
Hearing	Play a tape recording of the parents' voices. Play soft classical music. Eliminate loud and unnecessary noises.
Kinesthetics	Place the infant on an oscillating waterbed. Periodically rock the neonate or place him in a swing.

NURSING CARE PLAN

The Preterm Neonate

Nursing Diagnosis (Patient Problem) and Assessment Data	Nursing Interventions	Rationale
Nursing Diagnosis: *ineffective airway clearance*		
• Tachypnea • Grunting • Flaring • Retracting • Cyanosis	Suction infant as needed. Position infant on abdomen, side, or with small roll under head and shoulders to maintain airway. Position infant to facilitate drainage of mucus or regurgitated milk. Ascertain that gag and suck reflexes are intact before initiating oral feedings.	Mucus will obstruct airway. Preterm infant has weak neck muscles and cannot control head movement. Hyperflexed or hyperextended neck causes airway obstruction. Weak or absent gag reflex increases the risk of aspiration. To prevent aspiration.
Nursing Diagnosis: *ineffective breathing patterns*		
• Tachypnea • Apnea	Monitor breathing and HR with cardiorespiratory monitor. Position infant to facilitate chest expansion (prone position is best).	To alert nurse to alterations in cardiorespiratory function. Preterm infant with weak chest and abdominal muscles, has difficulty with chest expansion in supine position.
Nursing Diagnosis: *impaired gas exchange*		
• Cyanosis • Decreased oxygen saturation • Decreased oxygen levels • Abnormal arterial blood gases	Prevent stomach distention by • Aspirating air before gavage feedings • Avoiding overfeeding Discontinue oral feedings if signs of respiratory distress occur. Administer oxygen concentrations to keep PO_2 between 50–80 mmHg on ABGs. Monitor oxygen concentration with oxygen analyzer. Use $TcPO_2$ monitor and/or oxygen saturation monitor.	Preterm infant has small stomach capacity. Stomach distention prevents full respiratory excursion and may lead to respiratory distress. To prevent aspiration and allow infant to rest and focus energies on respiratory effort. Hypoxia can lead to opening of ductus arteriosus of metabolic acidosis. Hyperoxemia increases potential for retrolental fibroplasia. Mechanical ventilation and intensive monitoring of respiratory status may be needed.

Expected Outcome:

The preterm neonate establishes effective respiratory function, as evidenced by successful weaning from mechanical support by time of discharge.

(continued)

NURSING CARE PLAN

The Preterm Neonate (continued)

Nursing Diagnosis (Patient Problem) and Assessment Data	Nursing Interventions	Rationale
Nursing Diagnosis: *alteration in nutrition: less than body requirements*		
• Decreased gag, suck, and swallow reflexes	Administer correct formula in correct amounts.	To ensure adequate growth and development. Incorrect solute load leads to fluid and electrolyte imbalances.
• Gastric reflux		
• Vomiting	Check stomach for formula residual before gavage feeding.	Undigested formula $<$ 72 cc/kg may indicate formula intolerance or early stage of necrotizing enterocolitis (NEC).
• Gastric residuals		
• Weight loss		
• Failure to gain 10–15 gm per day		
	Measure abdominal girth every 4 h.	Abnormal increase in girth may indicate obstruction or early stage of NEC.
	Evaluate for evidence of exhaustion during feeding.	Excessive expenditure of calories when infant is exhausted during feeding prevents weight gain and prolongs hospital stay.
	Obtain weight daily, and plot on growth chart.	Weight loss or poor weight gain may indicate • Inadequate caloric intake • Excessive energy expenditure
	Maintain normal body temperature.	Excessive expenditure of calories to maintain temperature results in poor weight gain.
	Test all stools for presence of glucose.	Presence of glucose may indicate excessive glucose hyperalimentation or intolerance of formula.
	Observe for bradycardia after feedings and associated with emesis.	Gastric reflux causes vasovagal response.

Expected Outcome:

The preterm neonate gains weight and shows no sign of gastrointestinal complications.

Potential Complication:
necrotizing enterocolitis (NEC)

	Test all stools for presence of occult blood.	Presence of blood may indicate NEC.
	Position infant on right side of abdomen after feeding.	To promote stomach emptying.

(continued)

NURSING CARE PLAN

The Preterm Neonate (continued)

Nursing Diagnosis (Patient Problem) and Assessment Data	Nursing Interventions	Rationale
	Avoid disturbing infant for at least 1 hr after feeding.	Disturbance slows stomach emptying and decreases absorption of nutrients.

Expected Outcome:

Preterm neonate gains weight and shows no sign of gastrointestinal complications.

Nursing Diagnosis:
fluid volume excess

• Edema • Congestive heart failure	Strictly monitor all intake/output.	Early identification of fluid imbalance permits timely intervention.
	Administer diuretics.	To prevent CHF.
	Maintain all IV infusions with IV infusion pumps.	
	Administer correct solutions and formulas.	To prevent accidental volume overload.

fluid volume deficit

• Tachycardia • Poor skin turgor • Decreased urine output • Abnormal electrolyte levels • Increased urine osmolarity • Decreased blood pressure	Obtain daily sodium, chloride, potassium levels.	To prevent electrolyte imbalance and dehydration.
	Minimize insensible water losses:	To decrease water loss through skin.
	• Cover infant with heat shield	To decrease water loss through respiratory tract.
	• Humidify oxygen	
	• Closed isolette	
	Minimize withdrawal of blood for laboratory analysis.	To avoid fluid volume deficit.
	Test urine for pH and specific gravity.	To alert nurse to dehydration, alteration in pH balance.

Expected Outcome:

Preterm neonate achieves fluid and electrolyte balance, as evidenced by output of 1 to 3 ml/kg/hr in first week of life.

Possible Complication:
physiologic anemia

• Tachycardia • Pallor	Minimize withdrawal of blood for laboratory analysis.	To avoid exacerbating physiologic anemia.

(continued)

NURSING CARE PLAN

The Preterm Neonate (continued)

Nursing Diagnosis (Patient Problem) and Assessment Data	Nursing Interventions	Rationale
• Decreased blood pressure • Apnea • Failure to gain weight	Administer vitamin K.	To prevent hemorrhagic disease of newborn.
	Place infant in neutral thermal environment.	To decrease energy requirements in cases of severe anemia.
	Obtain hematocrit at birth and periodically thereafter.	To alert nurse to falling hematocrit and anemia.
	Transfer to ICN for further treatment of anemia, if necessary.	To provide specialized care and treatments, including blood transfusion and exchange transfusion that removes sensitized cells and prevents hemolysis.

Expected Outcome:

The neonate maintains normal hematocrit of 10 g/dl.

[handwritten annotation: Hbg circled around "hematocrit"]

Nursing Diagnosis:

infection related to immature immunologic function

• Temperature instability • Hypothermia, apnea • Cyanosis • Decreased oxygen saturation • Decreased oxygen levels • Poor feeding, gastric residuals	Observe strict handwashing protocols.	To avoid exposure of infant to pathogens.
	Maintain strict surgical asepsis when administering parenteral fluids, changing IV tubing and solutions, and assisting with sterile procedures.	Invasive procedure increases risk of infection.
	Change IV solutions and tubing every 24 hours.	To minimize bacterial growth in IV solutions and lines.
	Avoid excessive use of chemical skin preparations (benzoin, Betadine) and tapes.	To prevent chemical or mechanical skin trauma and decrease risk of infection.
	Restrict visitors.	To avoid exposure of infants to pathogens.
	Change isolettes weekly.	To minimize risk of exposure to pathogens.

Expected Outcome:

The preterm neonate maintains intact skin free of infection.

Possible Complication:

alteration in metabolic processes related to hypoglycemia/hyperglycemia

• Jitteriness • Lethargy	Check Dextrostix or Chemstrip for evidence of hypoglycemia:	Preterm infant is at increased risk for hypoglycemia.

(continued)

NURSING CARE PLAN

The Preterm Neonate (continued)

Nursing Diagnosis (Patient Problem) and Assessment Data	Nursing Interventions	Rationale
• Cyanosis • Apnea	• At birth • Every hr until stable • Before feeds • Periodically with hyperalimentation • Administer IV insulin	The risk for *hyperglycemia* increases with hyperalimentation.

Expected Outcome:

The preterm neonate remains free of metabolic alterations.

Nursing Diagnosis:
hypothermia

	Place infant in neutral thermal environment.	To prevent cold stress and promote growth by decreasing calories expended on maintaining body temperature.
	Place infant in double-walled isolette; use heat shield over infant's body and warm hands before handling infant.	To prevent heat transfer by convection and conduction.
	Place isolettes away from windows and outside walls.	To prevent heat transfer by radiation.
	Place cap on infant's head.	The head makes up 25% of total body size.
	Warm and humidify oxygen; keep skin dry.	To prevent heat loss by evaporation.
	Use skin temperature probe to monitor temperature variation.	To alert nurse to temperature swings, hypothermia, or hyperthermia.

Expected Outcome:

The preterm neonate maintains a normal core temperature, as evidenced by an axillary temperature of 36.4° to 37.2°C.

Possible Complication:
hyperbilirubinemia and kernicterus (bilirubin encephalopathy)

• Jaundice • Decreased tone • Lethargy • Poor feeding	Observe skin for jaundice. Observe for signs and symptoms of bilirubin encephalopathy. Apply phototherapy as ordered.	To alert nurse to development of hyperbilirubinemia. To prevent bilirubin encephalopathy.

(continued)

NURSING CARE PLAN

The Preterm Neonate (continued)

Nursing Diagnosis (Patient Problem) and Assessment Data	Nursing Interventions	Rationale
• Decreased Moro • High-pitched cry • Seizures • Rigidity	Assist with exchange transfusions. Administer phenobarbital.	To decrease levels of bilirubin. Increases bilirubin conjugation and excretion.

Expected Outcome:

The preterm neonate remains free of signs of hyperbilirubinemia or encephalopathy.

Nursing Diagnosis:
impaired mobility related to decreased neuromuscular development

• Arching behaviors • Hyperextension of extremities • Resistance to cuddling	Place infant in prone position with flexed extremities close to body. Encourage flexion in supine position by use of blanket rolls.	Encourages physiologic flexion, comfort and security, and prevents abnormal neuromuscular development.
	Provide infant with body boundaries through swaddling or use of blanket rolls against body and feet.	Provides comfort and encourages flexion.
	Minimize use of waterbeds before 34 wk gestation.	To encourage muscle development and strength.
	Develop appropriate infant stimulation plan based on gestational age, physiologic limitations, and presence of disease.	To promote and enhance growth and support organized patterns of behavior.

Expected Outcome:

The preterm neonate develops increasingly organized patterns of behavior and demonstrates age-appropriate growth and development parameters.

Nursing Diagnosis:
possible altered parenting

• Decreased or absent visits by parents • Resistance/refusal of parents to participate in infant care • Denial of severity of infant illness • Resistance/refusal to touch infant • Persistent verbalization of guilt	Encourage early and frequent visits by parents. Place infant's name on isolette. Give parents the unit phone number and names of contact people who can provide support and information.	To facilitate acquaintance process. To identify infant as a real person with a unique identity. To allow parents to obtain information about infant at any time.

(continued)

NURSING CARE PLAN

<table>
<tr><td colspan="3">The Preterm Neonate (continued)</td></tr>
<tr><td>Nursing Diagnosis (Patient Problem) and Assessment Data</td><td>Nursing Interventions</td><td>Rationale</td></tr>
<tr><td></td><td>Provide parents with simple care task initially and progress to more complex skills.</td><td>Early successes will build in parenting ability.</td></tr>
<tr><td></td><td>Encourage parents to spend a good deal of time just before discharge caring for infant and familiarizing themselves with his behavior patterns.</td><td>To prepare for home care and establish realistic expectations.</td></tr>
<tr><td></td><td>Point out the infant's unique characteristics and behaviors.</td><td>To assist parents in identifying infant cues.</td></tr>
<tr><td></td><td>Provide parents with appropriate referrals to health professionals and parent groups in the community upon discharge.</td><td>To provide ongoing support.</td></tr>
<tr><td></td><td>Encourage rooming in of parent before discharge.</td><td>Familiarizes parent with medicine, treatment, and equipment to be used at home.</td></tr>
</table>

Expected Outcome:

The parents of the preterm neonate show appropriate and progressive attachment behaviors, such as frequent visits or calls, interest and growing confidence in providing care, and identification of the neonate as their own.

infections, and environmental hazards (teratogens and maternal substance abuse). Table 34–6 provides an expanded list of disorders and other factors associated with IUGR. (See the material in Chapter 20 on chronic maternal disease, especially diabetes, and its effects on placental functioning.)

Intrauterine Growth Retardation (IUGR)

Two types of IUGR have been identified. These affect both the general appearance of the neonate and his potential for normal growth and mental development after birth.

Symmetrical Intrauterine Growth Retardation. Symmetrical IUGR occurs when the fetus has experienced early and prolonged nutritional deprivation caused by severe chronic maternal malnutrition, placental insufficiency, intrauterine infection, or fetal chromosomal

anomalies. Hypoplastic cell growth and development occurs, and there is a generalized deficiency in cell numbers throughout the body and in all organ systems. The neonate's body and head both appear small (proportional growth retardation). Head circumference often falls below the tenth percentile. This condition is associated with diminished brain size and permanent mental retardation. The infant never "catches up" with other infants of the same gestational age whose birth weights fall within the mean.

Asymmetrical Intrauterine Growth Retardation. Asymmetrical IUGR, in contrast, results from nutritional deficits and placental insufficiency in late pregnancy. Atrophy of preexisting cells occurs, resulting in diminished cell size, but cell numbers are not reduced. The neonate appears to have a disproportionately large head in relation to his body (disproportional growth retardation). The body

(text continued on page 1067)

NURSING CARE PLAN

The Small-for-Gestational-Age (SGA) Neonate

Nursing Diagnosis (Patient Problem) and Assessment Data	Nursing Interventions	Rationale
Nursing Diagnosis: *Ineffective airway clearance* • Tachypnea • Grunting • Flaring • Retracting • Cyanosis	Suction infant as needed. Position infant on side or abdomen to maintain airway. Administer ultrasonic mist therapy or aerosol via oxygen hood. Place infant in Trendelenburg position for chest physiotherapy. Perform chest physiotherapy (percussion and drainage).	Mucus will obstruct airway. Muscle wasting and large head in SGA infant diminish head control; incorrect alignment of head and neck may lead to airway obstruction. Liquefaction of mucus and meconium facilitates removal of secretions from airway. To facilitate drainage of secretions. To facilitate drainage and mobilize secretions from all lobes.
Nursing Diagnosis: *ineffective breathing pattern* • Tachypnea • Apnea	Monitor respiration with cardiorespiratory monitor. Position infant to facilitate chest expansion. Prevent stomach distention. Aspirate air before gavage feedings. Avoid overfeeding. Discontinue oral feedings at first sign of respiratory distress.	To alert nurse to alterations in cardiotherapy function. SGA infant with weak chest muscles may have difficulty in supine position. Infant's stomach capacity is small. Distention prevents full respiratory excursion and may lead to respiratory distress. To prevent aspiration and allow infant to rest and focus energy on respiratory effort.
Nursing Diagnosis: *ineffective gas exchange* • Cyanosis • Decreased oxygen saturation • Abnormal arterial blood gases	Administer oxygen concentrations to maintain PO_2 60–80 mmHg on ABGs. Monitor oxygen concentrations with oxygen analyzer. Use $PtcO_2$ monitor or O_2 saturation monitor. If alterations persist, transfer to ICN as needed.	Hypoxia can lead to opening of ductus arteriosus or metabolic acidosis. Hyperoxemia can predispose to retrolental fibroplasia and chronic lung changes.

Expected Outcome:

The SGA neonate maintains optimal respiratory and cardiac function.

(continued)

NURSING CARE PLAN

The Small-for-Gestational-Age (SGA) Neonate (continued)

Nursing Diagnosis (Patient Problem) and Assessment Data	Nursing Interventions	Rationale
Nursing Diagnosis: *altered growth and development secondary to intrauterine infection or maternal substance abuse*		
• Dysmorphic features	Obtain IgM level	If elevated, can denote infection *in utero* and will require further follow-up.
• Wasting of trunk and extremities		
• Rough, dry skin		
• Large anterior fontanelle	Obtain maternal history concerning possible TORCH infections during pregnancy.	Infection and substance abuse during pregnancy can affect growth and development of fetus.
	Obtain history of maternal substance abuse.	
	Obtain development follow-up by neonatal physical therapists during hospitalization and first year of life.	Impaired fetal growth and development of brain can cause developmental delays and behavioral/learning disorders

Expected Outcome:

The SGA neonate demonstrates age-appropriate growth and development behaviors by discharge.

Nursing Diagnosis: *altered nutrition: less than body requirements*		
• Gastric reflux	Administer formula per doctor's order: 150 cc/kg/day or 100–120 Kcal/kg/day in small, frequent feedings.	SGA infant has small stomach capacity and may need more frequent feedings.
• Weight loss		
• Failure to gain weight (10–15 gm per day)	Obtain weight daily, and plot on growth chart.	Weight loss or poor weight gain may indicate: • Inadequate caloric intake • Excessive energy expenditures
	Maintain normal body temperature.	Excessive expenditure of calories in maintaining body temperature results in poor weight gain.

Possible Complication: *hypoglycemia*		
• Jitteriness	Check Dextrostix or Chemstrip for evidence of hypoglycemia	SGA infant has limited liver glycogen stores.
• Lethargy	• At birth	
• Cyanosis	• Every hour until stable	
• Apnea	• Before feedings	
• Dextrostix or Chemstrip ≦ 45 mg/dl		

(continued)

NURSING CARE PLAN

The Small-for-Gestational-Age (SGA) Neonate (continued)

Nursing Diagnosis (Patient Problem) and Assessment Data	Nursing Interventions	Rationale
Possible Complication: *polycythemia*		
• Hct >65%	Obtain central hematocrit at birth.	Polycythemia can result in hyperviscosity and ischemia of organs, thrombus formation, hypoglycemia, and respiratory distress.
• Plethora		
• Cyanosis		
• Respiratory distress		
• Tachypnea		
• Flaring		
• Grunting		
• CNS Signs		
• Lethargy		
• Poor feeding		
• Convulsions		
• Hypotonia		
• Hypoglycemia		

Expected Outcome:

The SGA neonate will begin to gain weight and size and to approximate normal newborn parameters.

Nursing Diagnosis: *hypothermia*		
• Swings in temperature	Place infant in a neutral thermal environment.	To prevent cold stress (SGA infant has minimal adipose tissue) and promote optimal environment for growth by decreasing calories expended on maintaining body temperature.
• Temperature ≦ 36.4°C		
	Place infant in double-walled isolette, use heat shield over infant's body, and warm hands before handling infant.	To prevent heat transfer by convection and conduction.
	Place isolettes away from windows and outside walls.	To prevent heat transfer by radiation.
	Place a cap on infant's head.	Head makes up 25% of total body size.
	Warm and humidify oxygen; keep infant dry.	To prevent heat loss by evaporation.
	Use a skin temperature probe to monitor skin temperature variations.	To alert nurse to temperature swings or hypothermia.

Expected Outcome:

The SGA newborn maintains a normal core temperature, as evidenced by an axillary temperature of 36.4° to 37.2°C.

Table 34–5   **Maternal Factors Associated With Intrauterine Growth Retardation**

Obstetric Complications	Medical Complications	Socioeconomic Factors	Environmental Factors

History of infertility
History of abortions
Grand multiparity
Pregnancy-induced hypertension
	Heart disease
	Renal disease
	Chronic hypertension
	Sickle cell disease
	Phenylketonuria
	Diabetes mellitus (class D, E, F, or R)
	Other chronic diseases
		Low socioeconomic status
		Maternal age (extremes of youth and age)
		Absence of prenatal care
		Marital status (single)
			Poor living conditions
			High altitude
			Use of therapeutic drugs:
			   Antimetabolites
			   Anticonvulsants
			Substance abuse
			   Alcohol
			   Drugs
			   Cigarettes
			Malnutrition

is long and emaciated, with little subcutaneous fat. There is evidence of generalized muscle wasting, and the abdomen is wrinkled and scaphoid in shape. The skin has very poor turgor, the hair on the scalp is coarse and sparse, and underlying sutures are widely separated. Although these infants fall below the tenth percentile for birth weight, head circumference approaches the norm on the growth curve. Postnatal growth and development are rapid, and the potential for normal intellectual functioning is excellent.

Potential for Impaired Gas Exchange

There is an increased incidence of perinatal asphyxia in the SGA infant secondary to sudden interruptions in uteroplacental blood flow. Aspiration of meconium *in utero* is associated with asphyxia and results from relaxation of the anal sphincter and respiratory gasping secondary to hypoxia. The presence of meconium in the airways and alveoli at birth prevents adequate gas exchange after birth (see Meconium Aspiration Syndrome later in this chapter).

Potential Complications: Hypoglycemia, Hypothermia, Polycythemia

IUGR results in minimal stores of liver glycogen. The SGA infant is therefore at risk for hypoglycemia in the period immediately after birth.

All low-birth-weight infants are at risk for hypothermia because limited stores of brown fat and liver glycogen prevent adequate heat production. Heat loss is increased as a result of the SGA infant's large surface area in relation to mass and the lack of adipose tissue to serve as insulation.

Chronic intrauterine hypoxia appears to cause increased RBC production (polycythemia). When the neonate's hematocrit rises above 65% to 70%, problems related to increased blood viscosity (thick blood syndrome),

including respiratory distress, cyanosis, renal vein thrombosis, hypoglycemia, and congestive heart failure occur. A partial exchange transfusion is performed to remove some of the RBCs. The RBCs are replaced with fresh frozen plasma or 5% albumin.

Implications for Nursing Care

Nursing care of the SGA infant is aimed at supporting physiologic adaptations after birth and preventing the major complications associated with this disorder. Because IUGR is frequently associated with maternal disease or lifestyle (*e.g.,* alcoholism, smoking, or absence of prenatal care), the mother may experience overwhelming feelings of failure and guilt and will require ongoing emotional support. Infants frequently require referrals for continued care and evaluation upon discharge. See the accompanying Nursing Care Plan for the SGA Infant.

The Large-for-Gestational-Age (LGA) Neonate

The LGA neonate belies the maxim "The fat baby is a healthy baby." LGA infants are at risk for a variety of complications. Birth injuries, including fractures and intracranial hemorrhage, are more common, as are hypoglycemia and polycythemia (Spellacy et al 1985). Major physiologic adaptations are related to these complications. The predisposing factors for excessive size (over 4000 g above the 90th percentile, or two standard deviations above the mean) include genetic predisposition, excessive maternal weight gain during pregnancy, and maternal gestational diabetes.

The infant of a diabetic mother (IDM) is often LGA as a result of the high levels of maternal glucose that cross the placenta during pregnancy and the effect of fetal hyperinsulinism on cell growth. (Mothers with severe or long-

(text continued on page 1073)

NURSING CARE PLAN

The Infant of a Diabetic Mother (IDM)

Nursing Diagnosis (Patient Problem) and Assessment Data	Nursing Interventions	Rationale
Possible Complication: *hypoglycemia*		
• Prenatal history reveals maternal diabetes (DM class A through R)	Review the prenatal record for information regarding the mother's physical condition and insulin control of diabetes mellitus. Observe the infant for jitteriness.	Maternal physical status and insulin control affect the condition of the fetus and the postnatal stabilization of the infant.
These are signs and symptoms of hypoglycemia: • Dextrostix or Chemstrip value ≦ 45 mg/dl • Tremors • Hypotonia • Lethargy • Irritability • Sweating • Apnea • Seizures	Check Dextrostix or Chemstrip: • Every 30 min four times • Every hr until feedings are started • Then before feedings until infant is stable Give D₁₀W 5 ml/kg by mouth via nipple or gavage. Retest blood glucose less than 15 min after feeding. Notify the physician of decreased blood glucose readings. Begin oral formula or breast-feeding as soon as possible. When the blood glucose reading remains low or there is a pattern of rebounding readings in relation to feedings, prepare to transfer the infant to the intensive care nursery (ICN) for continuous IV dextrose infusion.	To quickly evaluate the infant's serum glucose and permit rapid intervention to prevent depletion of glucose from the central nervous system which could result in death. To maintain the infant's glucose level. Formula and breast milk help in stabilizing the blood sugar because of the longer period of digestion. Continuous IV infusion of dextrose may be needed to stabilize the infant.
Potential Complication: *small-for-gestational-age status secondary to placental insufficiency*		
• Infant weight falls below the 10th percentile or 2 standard deviations below the mean.	See Nursing Care Plan for SGA Neonate	
Potential Complication: *large-for-gestational-age status secondary to intrauterine hyperglycemia*		

(continued)

NURSING CARE PLAN

The Infant of a Diabetic Mother (IDM) (continued)

Nursing Diagnosis (Patient Problem) and Assessment Data	Nursing Interventions	Rationale
• Infant weight is over 4,000 gm, above the 90th percentile or two standard deviations above the mean.	See Nursing Care Plan for LGA Newborn	

Possible Complication: *hypocalcemia*

Total serum calcium less than 7.0 mg/dl • Jitteriness • Irritability • Seizures • Apnea • Chvostek's sign	Observe for signs and symptoms for hypoglycemia; check calcium level if ordered. Notify the physician if calcium level is below 7 mg/dl. If the level is low, prepare the infant for transfer to the ICN for IV administration of calcium.	Signs and symptoms of hypocalcemia are clinically indistinguishable from those of hypoglycemia. To restore normal calcium metabolism.

Possible Complication: *respiratory distress syndrome*

• Tachypnea • Grunting • Flaring • Retraction • Breath sound changes • Cyanosis	Closely observe respiratory status and check vital signs every 4 hr. Check for signs of respiratory distress. Transfer infant to ICN if symptoms develop.	IDM is at higher risk because of slower surfactant production. To permit rapid intervention if pulmonary problems develop.

Potential Complication: *polycythemia*

• Hemocrit greater than 65%	Observe for plethora. Check heelstick hematocrit (Hct) as needed or ordered. If peripheral Hct is 65%–70%, notify the physician. Draw central Hct (venous) as ordered. If the central Hct is over 68% or 70%, prepare infant for possible transfer to ICN for partial exchange transfusion with albuminated saline or lactated Ringer's.	An elevated Hct can indicate thickening of the blood. Respiratory distress or cerebral thrombosis may result. To restore normal blood values.

(continued)

NURSING CARE PLAN

The Infant of a Diabetic Mother (IDM) (continued)

Nursing Diagnosis (Patient Problem) and Assessment Data	Nursing Interventions	Rationale
Potential Complication: undiagnosed congenital anomalies or heart murmur	Carefully assess the infant for the presence of physical anomalies, especially cardiac or neural tube defects.	IDMs have a high incidence of congenital anomalies, such as cardiac defect and artrial–septal hypertrophy.
Potential Complication: hyperbilirubinemia		
• Appearance of jaundice within first 24 hr of life.	Observe for development of jaundice and check the bilirubin level as ordered; report symptoms to the physician if necessary.	To identify condition and permit intervention.

Expected Outcome:

The infant's metabolic and physical processes will be stabilized unless congenital anomalies exist and recovery proceeds without sequelae by discharge.

Nursing Diagnosis: *altered parenting related to infant condition*		
• Parents verbalize anxiety • Parents resist or refuse to touch/care for infant • Absence of parent visits	Keep the parents apprised of the infant's condition. Explain the need for Dextrostix or Chemstrip and other laboratory diagnostic studies. Carefully explain the infant's treatment and its rationale.	To promote parental understanding of their infant's physical problems and treatment, and to address their anxieties.
	As soon as the infant's condition permits, the parents should be allowed to spend time with their baby.	To promote parent–infant attachment.

Expected Outcome:

Parents respond to nursing teaching by touching infant, visiting as often as possible, and participating in infant care.

NURSING CARE PLAN

The Large-for-Gestational-Age (LGA) Neonate

Nursing Diagnosis (Patient Problem) and Assessment Data	Nursing Interventions	Rationale
Potential Complication: *hypoglycemia*		
• Infant above the 90th percentile or more than 2 standard deviations above the mean for weight and/or height and head circumference according to the Dubowitz assessment. • Serum glucose ≦ 45 mg/dl	Observe for signs and symptoms of hypoglycemia (see Nursing Care Plan for the IDM). Check Dextrostix or Chemstrip regularly (see protocol in Nursing Care Plan for the IDM).	Infants of Class A, B, or C diabetic mothers are frequently LGA. The stress of LGA delivery may result in infant hypoglycemia. Stress from delivery of a large presenting part may lead to hypoglycemia.

Expected Outcome:

Unanticipated infant of diabetic mother responds to appropriate support after identification and demonstrates no signs of hypoglycemia.

Possible Complication: *birth injury: fracture of the clavicle*		
• Crepitus • Hematoma or deformity over clavicle • Decreased movement of arm on affected side • Asymmetrical or absent Moro	Notify the physician of signs of fracture, and assist with X-ray filming when ordered. Keep infant positioned on unaffected side. Pin shirt sleeve on the affected side to the opposite shoulder.	The clavicle is the bone most commonly fractured because of its perpendicular angle in relation to the birth canal, especially when there is shoulder dystocia. To diagnose fracture. To promote comfort and healing of the fracture. Callus forms and pain subsides in 7–10 days.
Bell's palsy		
• Facial hemiparesis evidenced by drooping of lip to normal side, no wrinkling of forehead on affected side.	Observe the infant for difficulty sucking or swallowing. Assist mother and infant if necessary by placing fingers under the infant's chin to keep the lips closed around the nipple.	Bell's palsy may result from pressure on the facial nerve during delivery. Lip droop may make sucking and swallowing difficult.
Erb–Duchenne palsy, or brachial plexus paralysis		
• One arm weakness, or paralysis • Weak or absent grip	Pin the shirt sleeve and position the infant as in cases of fractured clavicle.	Erb–Duchenne palsy can result from difficult shoulder delivery.

(continued)

NURSING CARE PLAN

The Large-for-Gestational-Age (LGA) Neonate (continued)

Nursing Diagnosis (Patient Problem) and Assessment Data	Nursing Interventions	Rationale
	Begin passive range of motion exercises with the affected arm every 4 hr for 7–10 days.	To support the affected arm; avoid early ROM due to painful neuritis. To maintain muscle tone, increase circulation, and prevent stiffness.
phrenic nerve palsy		
• Weakness of the diaphragm with possible dyspnea, decreased breath sounds in lower lobes, and poor to absent rise of the abdomen with inspiration.	Position the infant on the affected side. Keep the head of the bed elevated.	To allow expansion of the affected lung. Phrenic nerve palsy may decrease innervation of the diaphragm after difficult delivery of the neck and shoulder. To reduce the pressure of the diaphragm on the thoracic cavity.
	Support respiratory function and transfer to intensive care nursery if respiratory distress develops.	To permit stabilization of the infant's condition.
possible skull fracture		
• Soft tissue swelling over site of fracture.	Observe infant for signs of intracranial hemorrhage.	Neurologic injury can occur with skull fracture.
• Visible indentation in scalp.	Transfer to intensive care nursery.	To permit close observation for CNS signs
• Cephalhematoma		
• Positive skull X-ray		
• CNS signs with intracranial hemorrhage:		
• Lethargy		
• Seizures		
• Apnea		
• Hypotonia		
• Cranial nerve		

Expected Outcome:

The LGA newborn makes the transition to extrauterine life without sequelae or with resolution of sequelae within a few days or weeks after birth.

Nursing Diagnosis:
  hyperthermia

	Observe infant every hr while under radiant warmer to check for possible hyperthermia ($\geqq 37.2°C$).	Hyperthermia may occur in the LGA infant because of increased amount of fatty tissue.

(continued)

NURSING CARE PLAN

The Large-for-Gestational-Age (LGA) Neonate (continued)

Nursing Diagnosis (Patient Problem) and Assessment Data	Nursing Interventions	Rationale

Expected Outcome:

The LGA neonate maintains a normal core temperature as evidenced by an axillary temperature of 36.4°C to 37.2°C.

Nursing Diagnosis:
anxiety related to parental concerns

(See Nursing Care Plan for Infant of Diabetic Mother)	Discuss with the parents the birth sequelae affecting their infant. Explain that nerve palsies are usually transient and resolve in a few days or fractures will heal in a short time. Describe the infant's treatment.	To keep the parents informed, help to allay their anxiety, and facilitate attachment.

Expected Outcome:

Parents of LGA neonate demonstrate signs of growing attachment to the newborn as evidenced by their participation in care and growing ease in touching and handling the infant.

---

standing diabetes with vascular changes may also deliver infants who are growth-retarded or SGA caused by decreased placental functioning.) The IDM is at risk for the classic complications of the LGA infant.

Potential for Impaired Gas Exchange
Respiratory Distress Syndrome Type II

RDS II (transient tachypnea of the newborn) may be related to the IDM's decreased level of surfactant production and to retained fetal lung fluid. Some theorize that insulin may interfere with the production of lecithin, a major constituent of surfactant.

Potential Complications

Hypoglycemia. The IDM's blood sugar levels are high at birth because of maternal hyperglycemia. Pancreatic insulin production is also high because islet cells are hypertrophied. The infant's blood sugar level begins to drop before the first feeding, but pancreatic activity remains high. Severe hypoglycemia can ensue rapidly unless glucose supplementation is given.

Polycythemia. The exact etiology of increased numbers of RBCs is not clearly understood, but IDMs are at greater risk than other infants for polycythemia. Hypocalcemia in the IDM may be related to depressed parathyroid function in the neonate, secondary to higher calcium levels in the pregnant diabetic. Hyperbilirubinemia and jaundice are related to the increased incidence of prematurity in the LGA infant, who may be delivered several weeks early to prevent fetal demise or complications related to excessive size. They are also related to polycythemia, which results in an increased hemolysis of RBCs.

Implications for Nursing Care

Nursing care of the LGA infant is aimed at preventing hypoglycemia and hypocalcemia by periodic monitoring of blood glucose and calcium levels. Heel prick samples may be obtained for glucose determination. Early oral feeding or an IV glucose infusion is initiated to maintain blood sugar levels. The nurse monitors the infant closely for signs and symptoms of hypoglycemia, hypocalcemia, RDS, and hyperbilirubinemia. The infant is assessed carefully at birth for signs of birth trauma. (See accompanying Nursing Care Plans for the IDM and the LGA Infant.)

The Post-term Neonate

The post-term neonate is born after 42 weeks of gestation. Many of this infant's problems are related to the compromised placental functioning and starvation associated with prolonged pregnancy. The infant is long and very thin. The head appears disproportionately large because of the wasted appearance of the body. The skin is thick, wrinkled, and parchment-like, and there may be generalized peeling of the epidermis. There may be meconium staining of the skin, nails, and umbilical cord as a result of intrauterine hypoxia. The neonate has a wide-eyed, alert look and may suck hungrily at his hands.

The etiology of postmaturity is poorly understood. Fetal and maternal factors associated with postmaturity are listed in the accompanying display. The mortality rate for post-term neonates is more than twice as great as that for full-term infants, and they are at risk for the development of complications related to compromised uteroplacental perfusion and hypoxia.

Potential for Impaired Gas Exchange
Meconium Aspiration Syndrome

Intrauterine hypoxia leads to relaxation of the anal sphincter and passage of meconium *in utero*. The asphyxiated fetus engages in gasping movements, which draw meconium into the large airways. At birth, meconium is inhaled into the distal airways and alveoli when the infant takes the first breath. The thick, viscous meconium creates a ball-valve effect in the alveolus. Inspired air is trapped in the alveolus by the meconium plug, distending the alveolar sac but preventing adequate gas exchange. This condition is known as *meconium aspiration syndrome* (MAS). Chemical pneumonitis occurs as a response to meconium aspiration and leads to thickening of alveolar walls and interstitial tissues. This rigid, noncompliant lung tissue also prevents adequate gas exchange. MAS is often characterized by pulmonary hypertension. Vasoconstriction and vasospasm occur in pulmonary vessels in response to hypoxia. The resultant pulmonary vascular hypertension leads to elevated pressures in the right side of the heart, reopening of fetal bypasses, and right-to-left shunting of blood. Blood exiting the right side of the heart bypasses the lungs, increasing systemic hypoxemia and exacerbating pulmonary vasoconstriction (Fig. 34–20).

Mechanical ventilation at very high rates and pressures is often necessary to ventilate the lungs adequately, but even very high concentrations of oxygen may not correct the hypoxemia that occurs with hypertension and shunting. Currently, many tertiary care centers are using a

Factors Associated with Postmaturity

- First pregnancies
- Grand multiparity (five or more pregnancies)
- History of prolonged pregnancy
- Anencephaly (congenital absence of cranial vault and underlying cerebral hemispheres)
- Trisomy 16–18 (chromosomal anomaly)
- Seckel's dwarfism

potent vasodilator, tolazoline, in an attempt to correct pulmonary hypertension. Its significant side-effects, including gastrointestinal hemorrhage and severe hypotension, limit the use of the drug to select groups of neonates.

One of the newest therapies proposed to treat the neonate suffering from persistent pulmonary hypertension secondary to meconium aspiration is extracorporeal membrane oxygenation (ECMO). ECMO is an invasive treatment in which a cardiopulmonary bypass is established to allow the lungs to rest and heal. The infant's blood is rerouted to a machine that functions as a lung, removing carbon dioxide and reoxygenating the blood. Further research must be conducted before the long-term value of this treatment is established.

Pneumothorax. Pneumothorax is a major complication of MAS secondary to the pathologic changes in lung tissue and the high ventilator pressures required to treat the disease. Sudden, acute respiratory distress is the classic sign of pneumothorax, but a constellation of systemic signs and symptoms are often evident (see the display, page 1076). With rupture of alveoli, air enters the pleural space, causing lung tissue to collapse. Breath sounds may be diminished on the affected side, and as air accumulates in the pleural space, mediastinal shifting toward the uninvolved side of the chest occurs. The point of maximal impulse (PMI) of cardiac activity may also shift to the unaffected side.

Once pneumothorax is suspected, transillumination of the chest wall with a high-intensity fiberoptic light source can be performed immediately to assist the physician in a correct diagnosis. With pneumothorax, there will be increased transmission of light across the affected side of the chest. Diagnosis is confirmed by chest x-ray. Because pneumothorax is a life-threatening complication, immediate intervention may be required before a chest x-ray study is performed. A small-gauged scalp-vein needle connected to a stopclock and a 20-ml syringe is inserted through the chest wall into the pleural space, and air is aspirated. Emergency aspiration itself is associated with

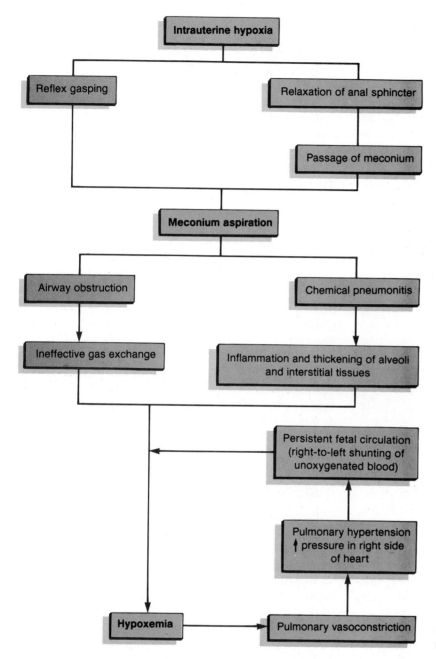

Figure 34–20. Causes and consequences of meconium aspiration syndrome.

complications, including hemorrhage, lung perforation, and phrenic nerve injury (Oellrich 1985), and must be performed by a skilled practitioner.

Chest tubes are inserted to remove air and fluid from the pleural space and to allow the collapsed lung to re-expand. The tubes are connected to a closed-drainage system, which prevents air from reentering the pleural space. The system is then connected to a suction source to aid in the removal of air and fluid from the chest cavity.

Continuous monitoring of the neonate who sustained a pneumothorax is essential. The nurse must also be familiar with the closed-drainage system used in the evacuation of fluid and air from the pleural space.

Potential Complications: Hypoglycemia, Polycythemia, Hypothermia

The post-term infant is at increased risk for the development of hypoglycemia as a result of depletion of liver glycogen stores. Polycythemia, the production of an abnormal number of RBCs, is hypothesized to occur in the post-term infant in response to intrauterine hypoxia. The neonate may be born with a hematocrit of 65% or higher and is at risk for the development of complications associated with hyperviscosity, including hypoglycemia, cerebral ischemia, thrombus formation, and respiratory distress.

Signs and Symptoms of Pneumothorax

Sudden acute respiratory distress:
    Tachypnea
    Flaring
    Grunting
    Retraction
Cyanosis or pallor
Mottling of the skin
Decreased PaO_2
Decreased *p*H
Possible diminished breath sounds on affected side
Asymmetric chest expansion
Hyperresonance with chest percussion
Cardiovascular changes:
    Tachycardia (initially)
    Bradycardia
    Arrhythmias
    Distant heart sounds
    Shift in heart sounds
    Shift in point of maximal impulse (PMI)
    Decreased arterial blood pressure
    Pressure in right side of heart
    Right-to-left shunting of unoxygenated blood

The loss of subcutaneous tissue in the last weeks of a prolonged pregnancy deprives the post-term infant of insulating adipose tissue and puts the neonate at risk for hypothermia.

Implications for Nursing Care

An immediate and essential aspect of nursing care when assisting at the birth of a post-term neonate with meconium-stained amniotic fluid is to aid the physician in suctioning the trachea to remove any meconium present in the airway. As soon as the infant is delivered, an endotracheal tube is passed and deep tracheal suctioning is performed by the pediatrician until the infant's airway is clear. The infant's chest may be swaddled to prevent him from taking the first breath until the airway is adequately suctioned. (See Chapter 33 for discussion of delivery room management of the infant delivered through meconium.)

Ongoing nursing care focuses on support of respiratory function and prevention of complications associated with postmaturity (the Nursing Care Plan for the respiratory care of the SGA infant is also applicable to the post-term neonate with potential MAS). A hematocrit is obtained immediately after birth to determine whether polycythemia is a complicating factor. A partial exchange transfusion may be necessary to prevent such adverse

sequelae as hyperviscosity. Serial glucose determinations are made to monitor blood glucose levels. Post-term neonates can be voracious eaters, and early feedings are often initiated (if not contraindicated by respiratory complications) to prevent hypoglycemia. Although the infant may possess little adipose tissue and thus may be at risk for hypothermia, the thermoregulatory center is mature, and careful attention to bundling and avoiding drafts is usually adequate to prevent cold stress. When meconium aspiration complicates the postnatal course, the post-term neonate will be placed in a neutral thermal environment.

THE NEONATE WITH INFECTION

The neonate is susceptible to infection as a result of immature immunologic functioning at birth. Susceptibility is increased when the infant is preterm or is suffering from other complications, such as asphyxia or trauma. Infection can be the result of maternal disease during pregnancy (*e.g.*, rubella, syphilis, or chlamydia). The infant can also come in contact with pathogens during passage through the birth canal (*e.g.*, herpesvirus, gonococci, or β-hemolytic streptococci). The increasing use of invasive procedures and diagnostic tests places the infant at risk for iatrogenic infection during the neonatal period.

Signs of Infection

Early signs and symptoms of infection in the neonate are often nonspecific. The infant may become lethargic, refuse feedings, or vomit. Temperature instability and hypothermia are other indicators. Subtle color changes (cyanosis, mottling, or grayish tone) may be noted by the nurse. Less frequently, apnea may occur as a sign of infection. Other signs may indicate the location of the infection. Jitteriness and seizure activity are observed with a disease of the central nervous system, respiratory distress with pulmonary infection, and diarrhea with intestinal disease. Once an infection occurs, it can quickly spread via the blood stream, and generalized sepsis will ensue.

The neonate may also demonstrate signs of viral infection transmitted during the prenatal period from mother to fetus. Evidence of chronic intrauterine infection at birth includes growth retardation, microcephaly, and hepatosplenomegaly. Central nervous system involvement is common (microcephaly, cerebral calcification, and mental retardation). The infant is frequently SGA and suffers from problems common to this group of infants (see Small-for-Gestational-Age Neonate elsewhere in this chapter), including hypoglycemia and hypothermia.

Once infection is suspected, a "septic workup" is performed. Blood, spinal fluid, and urine cultures are obtained. A Gram stain of gastric aspirate may be done immediately after birth, and cultures of the axilla, groin, rectum, and nasopharynx are performed when amnionitis is suspected following prolonged rupture of the membranes or delivery through purulent amniotic fluid. A complete blood count with differential and a chest x-ray study are also obtained.

Viral studies may be included in the evaluation of infants suspected of suffering from intrauterine or postnatal viral infection. The level of immune globulin M (IgM) is measured in the neonate's serum. IgM does not cross the placenta, and elevated levels (over 20 mg/100 ml) are indicative of intrauterine infection. TORCH screening and antibody tests can also be performed on the infant's serum to determine the presence of this group of prenatal viral infections (see Viral and Protozoan Infections later in this chapter). Viral cultures for cytomegalovirus (CMV) and herpesvirus and a urine sample for CMV may also be obtained.

Implications for Nursing Care

The nurse caring for the infant with an infection places him in a neutral thermal environment to support thermoregulatory function and decrease energy expenditures. Antibiotic therapy is normally instituted immediately when bacterial infection is suspected and will be discontinued if septic workup results prove negative. An IV infusion is normally started to provide a route for the administration of antibiotics, since they are poorly absorbed by the gastrointestinal tract or muscle. An enriched oxygen atmosphere may be provided if the lung is the site of infection.

The infant's vital signs are monitored closely, and a cardiorespiratory monitor is attached to assist the nurse in continuous evaluation of cardiopulmonary function. If diarrhea or vomiting occurs or if respiratory distress is evident, oral feedings are discontinued and fluids and electrolytes are provided intravenously until the neonate's condition is stabilized. If the disease is infectious, the infant will be placed in isolation.

Because the infant with an infection may be separated from his parents, the nurse must provide him with special loving support and comfort when they are not present. Parents should be encouraged to visit the nursery frequently and at any time convenient for them. They should be made to feel that their presence is particularly important for the infant's care and recovery. If the infant is in isolation, the nurse should instruct the parents in proper techniques for handling and caring for him; they should not be discouraged from touching him.

To prevent the transmission of neonatal infections to other infants or staff members, universal body-substance precautions are observed with *every* infant. This procedure eliminates the need for the isolation category "Blood

and Body Fluid Precautions" previously recommended for patients infected with blood-borne pathogens. Each unit should also have established policies and procedures for the care and treatment of infants with specific infectious diseases, such as herpesvirus or tuberculosis.

Bacterial Infections

Bacterial infection in the neonate can result in permanent disability and still accounts for 10% to 20% of all infant mortality (Sessions et al 1985). Most bacterial infections are acquired prenatally (by movement of microorganisms through the mother's vagina and cervix) and during passage of the fetus through the birth canal at the time of delivery. The most significant bacterial infections are discussed in the following sections.

Group B Beta-Hemolytic Streptococcus

The Group B beta-hemolytic streptococcal microorganism is the most common cause of neonatal infection today. Many pregnant women are silent carriers of the potentially lethal pathogen, harboring the bacteria in the cervix or vagina. The neonate is colonized with the microorganism during labor and delivery and may develop infection in the neonatal period. Although preterm infants are at greatest risk for developing Group B streptococcal infections, it is not possible at present to identify all infants at risk. Even apparently healthy full-term neonates develop infections.

Two varieties of Group B streptococcal infection occur in the infant. The *early onset form* develops within the first 24 hours of life and is often fatal. The neonate is hypotonic and hypothermic and presents with acute respiratory distress and pneumonia. Cardiovascular collapse and death can occur within hours of the first indication of infection. The *late onset form* usually occurs after the first 2 weeks of life as a meningeal infection. The infant presents with fever, lethargy, and signs of increased intracranial pressure (bulging fontanelle, nuchal rigidity, and high-pitched cry). The late onset form is associated with a much lower mortality rate than early onset strep infection, but permanent neurologic disability secondary to meningitis can be a complicating factor. Both forms of the disease are treated with antibiotics (gentamicin, ampicillin, or penicillin) administered intravenously.

Listeria

Listeria, a gram-positive organism, is an intracellular parasite recently implicated in the etiology of neonatal sepsis. It appears that most affected newborns contract the disease during passage through a maternal birth canal colonized with the organism. Both an early onset and a late onset form have been identified. The neonate with an *early onset* Listeria infection frequently demonstrates diffuse granulomatous skin papules over the trunk and on the pharynx. The infant appears very ill and may experience respiratory distress and cyanosis.

As with Group B streptococcal infection, the *late onset* form of Listeria infection usually occurs around the second week of life. The disease is usually manifest as a meningitis that appears to be associated with a different strain of the organism (Type IV B) found in the environment. Ampicillin and gentamicin (or kanamycin) are recommended for treatment of both forms of the disease.

Escherichia coli

One strain of *E. coli* (K1 antigen-positive) is an extremely virulent gram-negative organism recognized as a major cause of neonatal meningitis and septicemia. *E. coli* is transferred from mother to infant in a manner similar to the transmission of Group B streptococcus. The neonate is colonized during labor and delivery and develops signs of infection within several days. *E. coli* infections can also be acquired from nursery personnel who are colonized with the pathogen. It has been suggested that infants susceptible to this pathogen have a decreased circulating antibody level against *E. coli* K1 antigen (Oellrich 1985). Treatment consists of IV antibiotic administration.

Neisseria gonococcus

Ophthalmia neonatorum is a severe infection of the conjunctiva caused by the pathogen *Neisseria gonococcus*. The mother who has gonorrhea transmits the microorganism to her infant as he passes through the birth canal during labor and delivery. The instillation of a 1% silver nitrate solution or erythromycin ointment into the neonate's eyes will prevent gonococcal conjunctivitis. An untreated neonate will exhibit signs of eye infection (copious purulent discharge) by the third or fourth day of life. Corneal ulceration and blindness occur rapidly, if appropriate treatment is not initiated. Therapy consists of saline eye irrigations followed by topical and systemic administration of penicillin. In rare cases the gonococcal organism will invade joint capsules, causing a septic arthritis that requires prolonged systemic antimicrobial therapy for 4 weeks or more.

Tuberculosis

Congenital tuberculosis is rare and is seen only when the mother has advanced, untreated pulmonary disease. The tubercle bacillus is transmitted via the placenta and umbilical vein. The focus of the disease is usually the liver, although tuberculosis meningitis has been diagnosed in newborns. The neonate is lethargic, may be febrile, and is a poor feeder. Hepatomegaly and splenomegaly are often evident. The chest x-ray study may be normal. Treatment

of active disease consists of the administration of isoniazid (INH) with rifampin for 1 year.

The infant can also acquire tuberculosis during birth by aspiration of infected secretions or during the neonatal period through contact with infected parents. The infant is separated from the mother until she is no longer contagious. Prophylaxis for the newborn is a 1-year course of INH administration. If evaluation of the family and home environment indicate a high probability of noncompliance with INH therapy, BCG (bacillus Calmette-Guerine) vaccine may be administered.

If the mother has an inactive infection at birth, is receiving treatment, and has negative sputum and a negative x-ray study, the mother-infant dyad is not separated. The nursery should have a carefully delineated policy and procedure regarding care of the infant when tuberculosis is suspected in the mother or infant.

The incidence of tuberculosis is high among recent immigrants from Southeast Asia and is increasing in the United States as a result of the rise in homelessness and HIV. When mother and infant are separated at birth, intense anxiety may be generated in parents who suffer from language barriers, lack of understanding regarding the disease, or who fear that the neonate is being taken away from them because they lack living accomodations. The nurse must reassure parents that the separation is temporary and use social services, interpreters, and child welfare workers to assist supporting the new family and in discharge planning.

Viral and Protozoan Infections

The neonate is also susceptible to over a dozen known viral infections contracted either *in utero* or in the postnatal period. *TORCH* is an acronym for a group of infections that can attack the fetus and result in permanent physical disability or mental retardation in the neonate: *T*—toxoplasmosis; *O*—other viruses known to attack the fetus, including syphilis; *R*—rubella; *C*—cytomegalovirus; and *H*—herpesvirus type 2 (Modlin 1985).

Toxoplasmosis

Toxoplasmosis is a protozoan infection caused by *Toxoplasma gondii*. Raw meat and infected feces appear to be the vehicles for transmission of the infection. The cat is the most common carrier of the pathogen in the United States. The pregnant woman may have a "silent infection" that is undiagnosed and untreated. Placental transmission of the organism occurs, and the neonate is born with serious disease. Signs characteristic of toxoplasmosis include microcephaly, cerebral calcifications, chorioretinitis, hepatosplenomegaly, and jaundice.

Treatment consists of drug therapy, which appears to

(text continued on page 1084)

NURSING CARE PLAN

The Newborn With Bacterial Sepsis

Nursing Diagnosis (Patient Problem) and Assessment Data	Nursing Interventions	Rationale
Nursing Diagnosis: *potential for infection related to immature immune system*		
• Transmission from maternal, contact, or vector-borne source	Review the prenatal, labor, and delivery records to identify predisposing factors.	To document possible risk to the infant on the problem list, and to alert all staff that close observation and prompt reporting of beginning symptoms is crucial.
Risk Factors: *Maternal*	Notify physician when predisposition to infection exists.	Rapid identification of infant at risk or overtly infected infant is important.
• Premature rupture of membranes (>24 hr before delivery)	Monitor CBC and blood cultures	Because of the relatively low cellular and humoral immunologic response
• Elevation of maternal temperature during labor		of the neonate to infection, early intervention is essential.
• Diagnosed amnionitis or chorionitis		
• Bleeding during pregnancy		
• Infection before delivery		
Infant		Slight WBC elevation indicates viral etiology. Large elevation indicates bacteria source. Positive blood cultures require initiation of appropriate antibiotics.
• Foul odor at delivery		
• Traumatic delivery		
• Invasive procedure performed at delivery		
• Meconium staining	Check Dextrostix or Chemstrips every 4 hr	Blood sugars may be low with stress. During sepsis there will be an increased basal metabolic rate that will cause hyperglycemia. As compensatory mechanisms are depleted, blood sugar will be low as glycolysis occurs.
• Respiratory distress		
	Use meticulous handwashing when caring for compromised newborns.	Handwashing reduces nosocomial infections

Expected Outcome:

The newborn predisposed to sepsis will be asymptomatic for infection following prophylactic administration of a 72-hr or 7- to 10-day course of antibiotic.

Nursing Diagnosis:
ineffective thermoregulation

• Temperature less than 36.4°C axillary or greater than 37.2°C.	Monitor temperature for instability.	Unstable temperature is a common sign of sepsis.

(continued)

NURSING CARE PLAN

The Newborn With Bacterial Sepsis (continued)

Nursing Diagnosis (Patient Problem) and Assessment Data	Nursing Interventions	Rationale
• Decreased perfusion	Monitor capillary refill, which should be less than 3 sec.	Poor perfusion may indicate sepsis.
	Monitor for subnormal or elevated temperature that does not respond or responds slowly to increase or decrease in ambient heat.	Ambient temperature can mask temperature instability common with sepsis.
	Alert physician to signs of temperature instability.	

Expected Outcome:

The newborn predisposed to sepsis maintains a normal axillary temperature and remains pink and well perfused.

Probable Complication:
infection

• Maternal or neonatal infection due to known pathogen, or strong suspicion of neonatal infection from laboratory reports. White blood cell count >25,000 or <5,000. Platelet count <150,000. Positive cerebrospinal fluid Gram stain.	Assist with laboratory and radiologic evaluation for a septic work-up ordered by the physician:	To provide diagnostic evidence of infection directly, by identification of pathogens in culture and Gram stain, or indirectly, by cellular or metabolic response to infection.
	• Complete blood count and differential work-up.	
• Growth on blood culture.	• Platelet count	
• Elevated IgM level	• Blood culture	
• Chest x-ray film reveals evidence of pneumonia	• Urine culture	
	• Gastric aspirate culture	
	• Lumbar puncture for Gram stain and culture, protein, glucose, cell count	
	• IgM level	
	• Chest x-ray	
	Notify physician of laboratory results and developing signs or symptoms of infection.	
	Administer prophylactic antibiotics as ordered intramuscularly in the anterior thigh muscle.	Due to rapid and overwhelming infection of neonatal sepsis, some physicians choose to treat prophylactically for 72 hr pending culture reports.
	Place infant in isolation.	To prevent spread of pathogens to other infants.
	Administer antibiotic as ordered. Double-check ordered dosages of	To provide more effective treatment, antibiotics may be ordered by

(continued)

NURSING CARE PLAN

The Newborn With Bacterial Sepsis (continued)

Nursing Diagnosis (Patient Problem) and Assessment Data	Nursing Interventions	Rationale
	antibiotic. Note infant response to antibiotic.	intermittent intravenous push.
	Transfer infant to intensive care nursery if continuous intravenous infusion is needed for instilling medications.	

Expected Outcome:

The newborn with diagnosed sepsis and clinical signs and symptoms of infection responds to intensive nursing care and a 7- to 10-day course of antibiotics with no residual physiologic sequelae.

Potential Complication Secondary to Infection:
CNS aberrations

• Hypotonia • Lethargy • Irritability • Shrill or weak cry • Bulging fontanelle • Labile temperature, especially hypothermia	Assess for signs of increased intracranial pressure (shrill cry, bulging fontanelle, irritability).	Meningitis and pneumonia are the most common manifestations or overwhelming bacterial septicemia in the neonate, as demonstrated by central nervous system and respiratory symptoms.
	Assess for seizure activity (blinking or eyelid fluttering, sucking, drooling, tonic posture of a single limb, and apnea).	Seizures may result from septicemia, meningitis, or metabolic abnormalities. Appropriate treatment will prevent hypoxemia, which can lead to brain injury.
	Keep environment calm, quiet with minimal light.	Infant will be more calm/less irritable.

cardiovascular aberrations

• Low blood pressure • Slow pulse • Pallor/mottling • Tachycardia or bradycardia	Place infant on cardiorespiratory monitor for continuous evaluation if respiratory or cardiac aberrations appear.	To identify the document alterations in pulmonary and cardiac functioning.
	Apply pulse oximeter for continuous evaluation of oxygen saturation.	These symptoms may indicate septic shock.
	Evaluate heart and breath sounds q 1 hr.	

respiratory aberrations

• Cyanosis • Diminished or moist breath sounds	Apply transcutaneous oxygen monitor as ordered.	To reduce energy and oxygen demands.

(continued)

NURSING CARE PLAN

The Newborn With Bacterial Sepsis (continued)

Nursing Diagnosis (Patient Problem) and Assessment Data	Nursing Interventions	Rationale
• Tachypnea • Grunting • Flaring • Retracting • Episodes of apnea	Assist with radiologic exam, chest x-ray filming. Assist with arterial puncture for arterial blood analysis. Administer oxygen by hood as ordered. Place infant in neutral thermal environment.	
gastrointestinal aberrations		
• Poor suck • Poor appetite and oral intake • Vomiting • Diarrhea	Observe for gastrointestinal aberrations. Notify physician of GI aberrations.	Poor suck and appetite are early signs of sepsis.
hematologic aberrations		
• Jaundice before age of 24 hr • Petechiae, ecchymosis on other than presenting part • Hepatosplenomegaly	Observe for hematologic aberrations. Notify physician of aberrations. Assist with laboratory evaluations of bilirubin levels and clotting factors.	Clotting disorders may result from platelet destruction secondary to sepsis. Enlarged liver and spleen are indicators of sepsis. Hemolysis secondary to sepsis may lead to hyperbilirubinemia and jaundice.
Nursing Diagnosis:		
Transient responses to stimulation: • Bradycardia • Tachypnea • Cyanosis	Assess severity of intolerance by monitoring vital signs and color with stimulation.	Baseline intolerance level is necessary to plan nursing care. Bradycardia, tachypnea, pale or cyanotic color change frequently occurs with intolerable stress. Decreased cardiac output results in vasoconstriction and oxygenated blood is delivered to

(continued)

NURSING CARE PLAN

The Newborn With Bacterial Sepsis (continued)

Nursing Diagnosis (Patient Problem) and Assessment Data	Nursing Interventions	Rationale
		the vital organs, resulting in generalized pale or cyanotic color.
	Utilize minimal stimulation during acute phase.	Minimal stimulation promotes normal cardiac output, maintaining perfusion.

Expected Outcome:

Newborn maintains normal cardiac output and tolerates progressive stimulation.

Nursing Diagnosis:
altered nutrition: less than body requirements related to poor feeding ability

Exhibited by: • Poor suck reflex • Gastric residual • Vomiting • Diarrhea	Monitor feeding ability by bottle. Tube feed if oral feedings take longer than 30 min. Check residuals before NG/OG feedings. Assess stools for amount, type, frequency, consistency. Test all stools for blood. Check abdominal girth before feedings.	Weak suck reflex may cause aspiration. Excessive time bottle feeding will expend calories, causing weight loss. Residuals are an early sign of feeding intolerance. Diarrhea indicates feeding intolerance and causes loss of fluid and electrolytes. Increasing girth indicates delayed emptying and/or air resulting from release of bacterial toxins.
	Observe for hypoglycemia: • Jitteriness • Lethargy • Irritability • Tremors • Hypothermia • Cyanosis • Apnea	This sign occurs due to stress of infection, and/or poor feeding.
	Monitor Dextrostix or Chemstrip for hypoglycemia (<45 mg). Notify physician of hypoglycemia. Draw blood glucose as ordered. Withhold oral feedings as ordered. Start IV therapy as ordered.	To determine blood glucose level. To decrease energy requirements. To prevent aspiration of vomitus. To maintain fluid and electrolyte balance.

(continued)

NURSING CARE PLAN

The Newborn With Bacterial Sepsis (continued)

Nursing Diagnosis (Patient Problem) and Assessment Data	Nursing Interventions	Rationale
Expected Outcome:		
Newborn tolerates feedings, maintains normal blood glucose levels with gastric residuals, forms stools that are negative for blood, and stabilizes abdominal girth.		
Nursing Diagnosis: *altered parenting*		
Exhibited by: • Projection of anger • Crying • Decreased visitation • Inability to touch infant.	Explain policies and procedures to parents in terms they understand. Encourage family visits. Encourage parental participation in neonate's care.	Keeping parents well-informed will decrease anxiety and reduce the risk of fear of the unknown. Normal parent–infant acquaintance is more likely to occur with frequent visits. Parental confidence will be reinforced.
Expected Outcome:		
Parental–neonate acquaintance proceeds normally as evidenced by parents demonstrating knowledge and confidence in caring for the neonate.		

limit further central nervous system injury but does not reverse the prenatal damage already sustained by the neonate. Repeated courses of pyrimethamine, an antimalarial drug, sulfadiazine, and folinic acid are administered within the first year of life. Corticosteroids may also be administered to infants with chorioretinitis.

Syphilis

Transmission of the organism responsible for syphilis (*Treponema pallidum*) can occur during the second half of pregnancy. If the mother does not receive treatment for this sexually transmitted disease, the neonate will be born with congenital syphilis and is usually infectious. Clinical signs of the disease include intrauterine growth retardation (IUGR), ascites (fluid in the peritoneal cavity), persistent rhinitis (snuffles), jaundice, anemia, hepatosplenomegaly, and lymphadenopathy. The classic chancre observed in adult first-stage syphilis does not appear in the neonate, but a copper-colored rash may develop over the face, the palms of the hands, and the soles of the feet within the first week of life.

A fluorescent-labeled immune globulin M specific for antitreponemal IgM antibodies is available as a diagnostic tool. A positive serologic test necessitates immediate treatment with procaine penicillin G for 10 to 14 days. Nasal secretions and open syphilitic lesions are extremely infectious; the infant is, therefore, initially placed in isolation. After 24 hours of penicillin therapy, the neonate is no longer infectious.

Nursing care includes support of physiologic adaptations and administration of antimicrobial therapy.

Rubella

The rubella virus is another pathogen that attacks the fetus *in utero*. The severity of damage apparent in the neonate born with congenital rubella reflects the length of intrauterine infection and the time of first exposure to the virus. Approximately 30% to 50% of fetuses who acquire rubella in the first month of gestation suffer cardiac anomalies. Neural deafness is a common sequela when infection occurs in the second gestational month. Other signs of rubella infection in the neonate include congenital cataracts, glaucoma, microphthalmia, and blindness. The infant may exhibit other signs of chronic infection, such as IUGR and hepatosplenomegaly. Central nervous system involvement is reflected in microcephaly and mental retardation.

The neonate born with congenital rubella is often highly infectious and should be isolated and cared for only by nursery personnel with immunity to the disease. It is possible to isolate the mother and infant together, if the neonate does not require special care. No specific drug therapy is effective in limiting the disease process postnatally, and the infant may continue to shed the virus for a year or longer. He remains a source of infection during this time.

Cytomegalovirus

Cytomegalovirus (CMV) disease is a poorly understood infection that causes severe central nervous system injury in neonates who acquire the infection prenatally. The infant is born with a constellation of signs characteristic of many other intrauterine viral infections (microcephaly, IUGR, cerebral calcifications, and hepatosplenomegaly). The diagnosis can be confirmed by isolating the virus in the urine. Recently, more sophisticated tests allow identification of specific CMV antibodies in serum. Frustratingly, many neonates who harbor the virus are asymptomatic, but develop central nervous system injury (*e.g.*, blindness and mental retardation) later in childhood. Neonates with a symptomatic CMV infection have a very poor prognosis. Approximately 30% die in infancy and 90% of survivors will suffer from CNS, visual, and auditory handicaps (Modlin 1985). At present, there is no effective means of preventing or treating CMV. Nursing care of the infant with this infection is supportive.

Herpesvirus Type 2

The neonate with herpesvirus type 2 infection usually contracts the disease during passage through the birth canal. Prenatal infection is rare. The risk of developing a neonatal infection after vaginal delivery when the mother has an active genital lesion is as high as 50% (Cloherty 1985). Infants born to mothers with primary herpes infections develop a more severe, systemic form of the disease (hepatitis, pneumonia, encephalitis, and disseminated intravascular coagulopathy). Death can occur within hours of birth. The mortality rate approaches 50% to 60%.

Infants born to mothers with recurrent infections often have a milder disease process. Vesicular skin lesions, lethargy, hypothermia, and hypotonia are frequently present, but severe systemic infection does not occur. Viral cultures are obtained and blood samples are drawn to identify specific IgM antibodies. The infant is highly contagious and is isolated. Treatment with antiviral drugs such as acyclovir or vidarabine has been attempted but with limited success. Nursing care in the milder form of the disease is primarily supportive. Life support systems are employed in the care of critically ill neonates, and intensive nursing care is required 24 hours a day.

Hepatitis B

The transmission of hepatitis B virus, as well as surface antigen (HBsAg) occurs transplacentally during pregnancy and during passage through the birth canal when mothers have a hepatitis B infection of either a chronic (carrier-state) or acute nature. Although the neonate rarely presents with classic signs of the disease, prematurity and low birth weight are frequently observed. Jaundice, hepatomegaly, abdominal distention, and a poor feeding pattern develop some time (usually 4 to 6 weeks) after birth. Significantly, most infants who become HBsAg-positive due to transmission of the virus in the perinatal period suffer from the chronic (carrier-state) form of the disease and never demonstrate signs and symptoms of acute infection.

Infants at risk for the development of hepatitis B include those born to mothers who are intravenous drug users, and refugees from Southeast Asia and the Far East, where the incidence of the disease is very high. Currently, recommended prophylaxis for the neonate born to the mother found to be positive for hepatitis B antigen (HBsAg) consists of the intramuscular (IM) administration of 0.5 ml of hepatitis B immune globulin (HBIG) intramuscularly as soon as possible after birth (at least within 12 hours). Hepatitis B vaccine (HBV), 0.5 ml is given intramuscularly within 7 days of birth, at 1 month, and at 6 months of age.

Nursing care normally includes administration of the HBIG and HBV and scrupulous but gentle removal of all maternal blood, mucus, and amniotic fluid from the infant's skin as soon as possible after birth. Care is taken to remove excess secretions from the nares and oropharynx. Stomach contents may also be aspirated to remove maternal body fluids swallowed during passage through the birth canal. If the neonate is born with problems, immediate supportive care is provided (Withers and Bradshaw 1986).

When the infant's condition has stabilized and his temperature is within normal limits, he may remain with the mother. She is instructed in proper handwashing techniques, and reinforcement is provided as needed. There is currently some controversy about breast-feeding. Hepatitis B virus is found in breast milk, but many experts believe that this route of contamination is rare and nursing should be allowed. Other neonatologists suggest that breast-feeding should be discouraged when the mother has the acute form of the disease.

Chlamydia

Chlamydia is an intracellular parasite found in the vaginas of 2% to 13% of women in this country. It has only recently been identified as a causative agent in neonatal infection. It is the most frequently occurring sexually transmitted disease in the United States today (approximately three times as common as gonorrhea) and is the most common cause of blindness in the world (Larson 1984). Chlamydia is transmitted from mother to infant during the passage through the birth canal and can result in neonatal conjunctivitis, pneumonia, and otitis media. It may also infect the genital tract.

Prenatal diagnosis of chlamydia is possible, and screening of pregnant women is recommended to aid in the identification of *Chlamydia trachomatis* and to prevent infection in the neonate. A simplified technique for culturing the parasite has been developed and may assist in the prenatal detection of the disease in the near future. Unfortunately, at present, it is not generally available in most hospitals in the United States.

Chlamydial Conjunctivitis (Inclusion Blennorrhea). An infection of the neonate's eyes, chlamydial conjunctivitis results in inflammation of the conjunctiva, edema of the eyelids, and copious purulent discharge. A pseudomembrane may form over the eye. The disease is usually bilateral. It is important to note that instillation of a 1% silver nitrate ophthalmic solution does *not* provide prophylaxis against chlamydial conjunctivitis. Treatment consists of the topical application of erythromycin ointment or tetracycline combined with the systemic administration of oral erythromycin. The nurse caring for the neonate with chlamydial conjunctivitis must observe scrupulous aseptic technique, since the disease is highly contagious.

Chlamydial Pneumonia. Chlamydial infection of the lungs results in the development of a late onset pneumonia. The infant is usually afebrile and presents with a severe, often paroxysmal cough. Diffuse lung involvement is common, and rales can often be auscultated. The pneumonia is frequently preceded by a chlamydial conjunctivitis that has been ineffectively treated with topical antibiotics alone. Treatment with systemic antibiotics, including erythromycin, is recommended. Recovery is often slow and may take up to 2 months.

Neonatal HIV Infection and Acquired Immune Deficiency Syndrome (AIDS)

AIDS is an immune disorder that destroys the infant's defenses against infection. The etiologic agent is a retrovirus, human immunodeficiency virus (HIV), that infects T lymphocytes. The virus is able to replicate by altering the T cell's genetic makeup. Immunologic evidence of the disease includes B-cell abnormality and elevated immunoglobulins (IgG, IgA, and IgM). The infant is unable to develop antibodies in response to infection or immunization.

The exact mode of perinatal HIV transmission is unknown. Possible modes of infection include transplacental transmission, intrapartum contact with contaminated maternal secretions, or postnatal contact with parents who have HIV. The virus has also been isolated from the breast milk of women with HIV or ARC, and it is currently suggested that breast-feeding be avoided. While the exact risk of perinatal transmission is unknown, in one study 65% of the infants born to infected mothers had serologic or clinical evidence of HIV within several months of birth (Centers for Disease Control 1985).

The classic signs and symptoms of HIV in adults may not be present in neonates. Infants exhibit chronic lymphadenopathy, hepatosplenomegaly, recurrent salivary gland enlargement, oral candidiasis, bacterial infections, and failure to thrive. Several studies have described craniofacial abnormalities similar to those observed in fetal alcohol syndrome. Many infants with HIV are premature or small for gestational age, with microcephaly. Fever, diarrhea, dehydration, lethargy, encephalitis, spasticity, and recurrent eczema are also frequently observed (Grippi et al 1988).

There is currently no cure for HIV, and the prognosis is very poor. All treatment modalities are experimental. Intravenous gamma globulin with HIV specific or anti-CMV antibody, interleukin-2, and acyclovir have been used with varying degrees of success. The major focus of nursing care is supportive. A nursing care plan for the infant with HIV delineates major problems and interventions.

Nurses caring for infants with HIV should observe universal body substance precautions; these are listed as a Nursing Alert in Chapter 32. Current data indicate that occupational exposure to patients with HIV poses little threat to health care workers if CDC guidelines are observed. Edmondson (1988) notes that there is a tendency to avoid infants with HIV and their parents. This places the baby at risk for sensory deprivation. Daily sensory stimulation and interaction with nurturing care-givers is essential. Special support services (social workers, counselors, *(text continued on page 1090)*

NURSING CARE PLAN

The Neonate With HIV Infection

Nursing Diagnosis (Patient Problem) and Assessment Data	Nursing Interventions	Rationale
Nursing Diagnosis: *potential for infection related to abnormal immunoregulation*		
• Temperature instability	Monitor temperature for instability.	Temperature instability indicates an infectious process.
• Hepatosplenomegaly		
• Decreased serum antibodies	Palpate liver and spleen once a day for enlargement. The liver is palpable 1–2 cm below the right costal margin. The spleen is palpable along the lateral aspect of the left upper quadrant.	Enlarged liver and spleen suggests inflammation.
• Increased IgB and IgM		
• Poor feeding		
• Lethargy		
• Skin mottling		
	Monitor immunoglobulins and serum antibodies.	IgB is transferred to the neonate through the placenta and affects the infant's ability to fight infection. IgM elevation indicates infection; however, can be elevated in a maternal–fetal blood link such as an abruption. For this reason an IgM may need to be repeated. An increased antibody level indicates a response to an invading antigen.
	Monitor feeding ability.	Inability to suck with feeding may be present with an altered level of consciousness.
	Assess activity level.	Lethargy and decreased spontaneous movement is a sign of sepsis.
	Assess skin color and perfusion. Capillary refill should be less than 3 sec.	Circulatory changes also indicate an infectious process.

Expected Outcome:

The neonate remains free of infection as demonstrated by normal thermoregulation, normal serum antibody levels, alert response, and pink, well-perfused skin.

Nursing Diagnosis:
impaired gas exchange related to invasion of the immune system through infecting helper T cells.

• Grunting	Assess breath sounds bilaterally for equality and aeration.	Unequal breath sounds indicate partial pneumothorax, increased congestion, or atelectasis.
• Flaring		
• Retractions		
• Tachypnea	Assess respiratory rate and use of accessory muscles.	Increasing distress may indicate the need for assisted mechanical ventilation.
• Cyanosis		

(continued)

NURSING CARE PLAN

The Neonate With HIV Infection (continued)

Nursing Diagnosis (Patient Problem) and Assessment Data	Nursing Interventions	Rationale
• Abnormal acid–base balance	Elevate head of bed.	There will be less pressure on the diaphragm promoting lung expansion. Gastric emptying will be facilitated.
	Administer oxygen to relieve cyanosis or until an arterial blood gas (ABG) is drawn.	Hypoxia can lead to acidosis and opening of fetal shunt pathways, promoting fetal circulation. ABG evaluates acid–base balance and indicates infant's ability to exchange oxygen and carbon dioxide at the pulmonary–capillary bed.
	Suction as necessary.	Secretions will obstruct the airway, increasing respiratory distress.

Expected Outcome:

Newborn remains pink and well perfused with normal ABGs and equal and clear breath sounds.

Nursing Diagnosis:
altered nutrition: less than body requirements related to poor feeding and/or formula intolerance

• Gastric residuals • Vomiting • Abdominal distention • Diarrhea • Failure to thrive • Anemia	Check for residuals and abdominal girth before feedings.	Residuals are an early sign of feeding intolerance. Abdominal distention is a result of gas and/or inflammation in the bowel and may be a sign of an infectious process.
	Obtain accurate intake and output (weigh diapers).	This is essential in evaluating feeding tolerance.
	Monitor stools for amount, type, consistency, and change in pattern. Check all stools.	Stool changes may show feeding intolerance infection or inflammation. Blood may be present with irritation or ulceration.
	Weigh every day.	Weight loss may necessitate IV fluids or total parenteral nutrition.
	Monitor CBC.	Increase in WBC may indicate sepsis. Decrease in HGB/HCT indicates a blood loss or the body's inability to produce new RBCs.

Expected Outcome:

Newborn maintains balanced nutrition as evidenced by well-tolerated feedings and normal bowel function, weight loss of no more than 10%–15% since birth followed by a steady weight gain, and normal CBC.

(continued)

NURSING CARE PLAN

The Neonate With HIV Infection (continued)

Nursing Diagnosis (Patient Problem) and Assessment Data	Nursing Interventions	Rationale

Nursing Diagnosis:
sensory/perceptual alteration: visual, auditory, tactile related to inadequate stimulation and CNS changes

• Failure to thrive • Irritability • Growth retardation • Decreased alertness • Decreased response to visual and auditory stimuli.	Assess and document growth pattern (height, weight, and head circumference). Assess infant's response to stimuli and degree of irritability Provide visual and auditory stimulation with a mobile, musical toy or mirror. Utilize consistent care-givers.	Impaired growth detected early is less difficult to correct. Lack of response may indicate CNS or systemic virus invasion. Sensory stimulation promotes normal growth and development. Primary care-givers learn the idiosyncrasies of the infant and will be able to detect behavioral changes immediately.

Expected Outcome:

Newborn demonstrates growth pattern appropriate for gestational age and alert response to stimulation.

Nursing Diagnosis:
altered parenting related to diagnosis

• Lack of parental visits • Decreased interest in infant's care • Impaired bonding • Fear of infant outcome	Encourage visitation and active participation in newborn's care. Educate the family on the disease process, etiology, pathophysiology, signs and symptoms, risks, and preventive measures. Encourage questions and verbalization of misgivings. Contact social service agency to follow family through discharge to home.	Visitation promotes bonding and decreases fears of infant care. Parents will be prepared for home care upon discharge. Education may reduce the fear of contracting the disease. The knowledge can be relayed to friends and family, thereby increasing their social support system. Decreasing fears will promote parent–infant bonding. Ongoing support is essential for effective coping. Community resources can assist in adjusting to life change brought about by HIV infection.

Expected Outcome:

Parents exhibit effective coping as demonstrated by verbalization of fear and understanding of HIV infection and its outcome and beginning of parent–infant attachment.

and child welfare agencies) should be used to support parents and assist the nurse with discharge planning.

Fungal Infections

In recent years, there has been an increase in the incidence of fungal infections in neonates. At particular risk are very low birth weight, preterm infants. The most common fungal organism implicated in topical and systemic infections is *Candida albicans,* but *Candida tropicalis, Aspergillus,* and *Cryptococcus* are other species implicated in neonatal sepsis. Colonization may occur during birth with passage of the infant through infected vaginal secretions. Candidal infection is also spread by direct contact with infected persons.

Impaired host factors in preterm infants, including impaired cellular and humoral immune responses and poor skin and gastrointestinal mucosal barriers, predispose the neonate to fungal infections. Iatrogenic causes contributing to Candida sepsis include the administration of broad-spectrum antibiotics, which inhibit normal microbial flora, the use of central indwelling arterial or venous catheters, and total parenteral nutrition.

While the most common neonatal Candida infections are cutaneous (thrush and diaper dermatitis), disseminated systemic infections are estimated to occur in up to 10% of infants weighing under 1000 g. Infants may present with nonspecific signs of deterioration, including temperature instability, episodes of apnea, feeding intolerance, carbohydrate intolerance, and generalized erythematous rash. Diagnosis is often difficult. Sites of infections include the urinary tract, central nervous system, heart, lungs, joints, and eyes.

Nursing care is directed first and foremost at preventing infection by scrupulous handwashing, maintenance of aseptic technique when handling equipment and TPN solution, and during blood-drawing procedures. Preventing skin trauma is also critical. The drug of choice in the treatment of candidiasis is amphotericin B. Other agents used with limited effectiveness include fluorocytosine and miconazole nitrate. Because of the potentially toxic side-effects of these drugs, close monitoring of vital signs and the infant's general response to the infusion of these agents is essential.

THE NEONATE WITH FRACTURES

Some birth injuries may be visibly or easily identified by the nurse during the assessment of the neonate. Other injuries may be internal or so minor at birth that they are missed until the infant shows evidence of trauma. The nurse who is aware of the major types of trauma to which the neonate is susceptible during labor and delivery can more quickly recognize them and implement appropriate care.

Fractures occur in the neonate as a result of traction, manipulation, or compression of body parts during delivery or from the use of forceps. Certain infants are at greater risk for fractures. The increased chest circumference of infants who are large for gestational age (LGA) may lead to shoulder dystocia at the time of birth. Neonates with abnormal presentations at delivery, such as breech or arm presentations are also at increased risk for skeletal injury. Preterm infants, whose bones are especially fragile, may sustain fractures with very little manipulation at birth.

Both complete fractures of the bone and "green stick" fractures, in which one side of the bone is broken while the other side is intact or slightly bent, may occur. When fractures occur in the long bones (clavicle, humerus, ulna, and femur), edema, erythema, or ecchymosis may be evident over the injury. There may be diminished movement or "guarding" of the affected extremity, and if nerve damage accompanies the fracture, partial or complete flaccidity of the extremity may be observed. Skull fractures and fractures of the vertebrae may have more serious sequelae because they can result in injury to the central nervous system and permanent impairment in function.

Fracture of the Clavicle

Clavicular fracture is the most common fracture during vaginal birth. It can result in the development of ecchymosis or hematoma over the injured site and diminished movement of the extremity on the affected side. The Moro reflex may be asymmetrical. A snapping noise or crepitus (a crackling sound produced by the rubbing together of bone fragments) may sometimes be heard with movement. Fracture of the clavicle is painful, and guarding of the extremity on the affected side will often be noted.

Implications for Nursing Care

A fractured clavicle normally heals quickly and without special treatment. Nursing interventions are aimed at minimizing pain. This is accomplished by gentle handling and positioning the neonate on the abdomen or the unaffected side as much as possible. The sleeve can be pinned to the infant's shirt to stabilize the arm on the affected side, but the use of splints is not recommended.

Fracture of the Humerus or Femur

Fractures of the humerus or femur occur less frequently and are often associated with assisted breech deliveries. Edema, ecchymosis, hematoma, and even hemorrhage can occur over the fracture site, and marked restriction of the extremity is noted. It may be necessary to manipulate the bone to accomplish realignment; and casts, slings, or splints may be indicated to maintain correct positioning of the extremity.

Implications for Nursing Care

If a cast is applied, the nurse must carefully assess the tissues for adequate circulation by blanching the fingers or toes. If the tissue does not blanch, congestion may be present; if blanching persists for more than 3 seconds, circulation may be impaired. Either finding should be documented and reported to the physician. The nurse must be sure there is adequate room around the edges of the cast to prevent pressure sores. The condition of the skin must also be evaluated frequently. The rough edges of the cast can excoriate the skin, and moleskin should be placed along the edges to prevent trauma.

Because a plaster cast is porous and will absorb urine and liquid stools, it is important that it be waterproofed once it has completely dried. Diapers should be changed frequently to prevent excessive soiling of the cast. The infant should not be lifted by the legs to change diapers when a leg has been casted, since this can place pressure on the tissue surrounding the cast edges and can distort bone alignment or place undue tension on leg ligaments above the level of the cast.

Nursing interventions are also aimed at minimizing pain by gentle handling of the infant and immobilization of the extremity. Pain medications are not normally prescribed, since they will make the infant lethargic, depress feeding reflexes, and increase the risk of aspiration. Support of the parents and preparation for discharge are essential aspects of care when the infant will go home with a splint or cast or will require special swaddling. Parents should be provided with ample opportunities to handle and care for the infant in the hospital so that they will feel comfortable and confident about their ability to meet the infant's needs. Appointments for follow-up care should be made before discharge, and parents should be given the names and telephone numbers of health professionals to contact if questions or problems arise at home.

Skull Fracture

Because the neonate's skull is quite pliable at birth as a result of incomplete mineralization, skull fractures are less common than those involving long bones. Skull fractures may, however, occur during labor or delivery, and infants delivered by forceps are at increased risk for this type of birth injury. The two types of skull fracture seen are linear and depressed. Simple linear fractures are frequently benign and normally heal without treatment.

They may be associated with cephalhematoma and are discovered when an x-ray study is performed.

Depressed skull fractures may be palpated under the scalp as a depression in the bone. They may result in an actual break in the bone and can cause tears in the meninges, rupture of blood vessels, and damage to brain tissue underlying the fracture. If brain tissue is injured, neurologic signs and symptoms, including increased intracranial pressure and seizures, may be evident, and permanent neurologic impairment can occur. Depressed fractures, sometimes called "pingpong ball" fractures because of their configuration, may require surgical elevation.

Implications for Nursing Care

The infant suspected of or diagnosed as having a skull fracture is assessed closely for evidence of increased intracranial pressure secondary to hemorrhage or brain edema. Such evidence includes seizure activity, hypotonia, bulging fontanelles, unusual posturing, depressed cardiac or respiratory function, and hypothermia. A cardiorespiratory monitor is attached for continuous evaluation of vital signs, and the neonate is placed in an isolette to support thermoregulatory function and minimize energy requirements.

Because the neonate who has sustained neurologic injury as a result of skull fracture is at risk for the development of seizures, oral feedings are normally discontinued, and an IV fluid is infused until the infant's condition stabilizes. If hypotonia or paralysis is present, the infant is positioned to maintain a patent airway and to correctly align extremities so that contractures may be prevented. Sandbags, mattress rolls, and hand rolls will aid the nurse in positioning the infant. A sheepskin mattress pad is placed beneath the neonate, who is turned frequently to prevent the breakdown of skin. Anticonvulsants will be administered to control seizure activity.

As with asphyxia, the parents are usually primarily concerned about the long-term neurologic sequelae of the injury. It is impossible at present to accurately predict the eventual intellectual capacity and neuromuscular function of a child in the neonatal period. Physicians are encouraged to be truthful with parents about the extent of the injury but to remain hopeful about the eventual outcome. Klaus and Kennell (1982) suggest that the physician refrain from discussing the possibility of mental retardation in the period immediately following the diagnosis of brain injury or hemorrhage, since this may profoundly influence parental perceptions of the infant.

Nurses should be supportive of parents, taking time to answer questions about the infant's current condition and to reinforce information that the physician has imparted. Even when the infant is totally unresponsive or comatose, the parents should be allowed to spend as much time as they desire and, as is possible at the bedside, touching him and talking to him. Allowing them to participate in skin care and range of motion exercises can help dispel some of the sense of helplessness and hopelessness parents experience and support the early attachment process.

THE NEONATE WITH CENTRAL NERVOUS SYSTEM INJURIES

Intracranial Hemorrhage

Rupture of cerebral vessels resulting in intracranial hemorrhage is one of the most serious complications of the neonate. It may result in permanent neurologic impairment or death.

Intracranial hemorrhage can occur with prolonged labor and severe molding of the fetal skull; a difficult vaginal birth that requires rotation of the fetal head or forceps extraction; or a precipitous labor or delivery that causes a sudden, severe increase in intracranial pressure. Tears in the dura mater may cause hemorrhage and an accumulation of blood in the subdural space (subdural hematoma).

The type and extent of neurologic injury depends on the location of the hemorrhage. Hemorrhage within the posterior fossa results in compression of the fourth ventricle and obstruction in the flow of cerebrospinal fluid. Signs of increased intracranial pressure will occur, including seizures, decreased or absent reflexes; hypotonia; bulging fontanelles; enlarged head circumference; "setting sun eyes"; a high, shrill cry; hypothermia; and episodes of apnea or bradycardia. Hemorrhage is confirmed by computed tomography (CT) scan.

The outcome of intracranial hemorrhage will depend on the extent and location of the hemorrhage. In severe hemorrhage, when minimal brain activity is recorded by electroencephalogram and decerebrate posturing occurs, the prognosis is very guarded. With milder hemorrhages, minimal neurologic dysfunction is evident in later years.

Implications for Nursing Care

Nursing interventions are aimed at supporting vital functions and reducing the neonate's energy requirements to a minimum. The infant is placed in a neutral thermal environment, and, using a cardiorespiratory monitor, vital signs are observed constantly. The head is elevated slightly above the hips, and its circumference is measured daily to determine the presence and extent of head enlargement. If flaccidity or paralysis is evident, care is taken to maintain a patent airway, correctly align extremities, and turn the infant routinely to prevent skin breakdown.

Because the infant may demonstrate depressed reflexes and diminished responsiveness, oral feedings are suspended and IV therapy is instituted. The nurse keeps an accurate intake and output record. Anticonvulsants may be administered to control seizure activity. Emotional support of the parents is the same as for the infant who has sustained brain injury secondary to skull fracture (see the nursing interventions described under Skull Fracture earlier in this chapter).

Nerve Injury

A variety of nerve injuries can result from excessive pressure or traction on areas of the neonate's head and neck, or in association with fractures.

Brachial Plexus Injury

The brachial plexus is a major network of nerves that arises from the spinal column (C-5 through T-7). The plexus is located in the base of the neck above the clavicle. The nerves in the plexus innervate the muscles of the arm and upper extremities. The plexus may be injured as a result of the stretching or torsion of the neck or extremities during a difficult delivery (breech or vertex). Nerve trauma can also occur in conjunction with fractures. The resultant limitation in movement may be a transient phenomenon or a permanent disability.

In approximately 80% of affected neonates, injury to the brachial plexus involves the nerves emanating from the upper spinal roots (C-5 and C-6) and leads to a loss of motor function in the upper arm. In Erb–Duchenne palsy the arm assumes a characteristic position, tightly adducted with internal rotation of the shoulder, extension of the elbow, and pronation of the forearm. The Moro reflex cannot be elicited on the affected side. There is usually no loss of sensory function. If injury to the plexus involves nerves emanating from the lower spinal roots (C-7 and T-1), the muscles of the lower arm are affected. There is a rare injury that leads to loss of motor function in the muscles of the hand (Klumpke's paralysis). The grasp reflex cannot be elicited. The entire brachial plexus can also be damaged, resulting in complete paralysis of the arm and hand.

Implications for Nursing Care

The primary nursing responsibility in the care of a neonate with brachial plexus injury is to prevent contractures of the affected muscles by placing the arm in a neutral position and performing passive range of motion exercises. Rigid immobilization of the extremity and corrective positioning (external rotation of the shoulder, flexion of the elbow, and supination of the forearm) are no longer recommended, since they may actually result in contractures and deformities. The arm is immobilized in a natural position by pinning the sleeve to the shirt or by swaddling the infant. After approximately 7 to 10 days, gentle passive range of motion exercises are initiated. Before the infant is ready for discharge, the parents are instructed in the correct positioning of the arm and range of motion exercises and should be given ample time and opportunities to practice care.

Phrenic Nerve Injury

Paralysis of the diaphragm occurs when the phrenic nerve is injured. It is most frequently associated with brachial plexus injury when lateral hyperextension of the neck occurs during delivery. The diaphragm on the affected side is elevated and fixed (eventration). Lung tissue is displaced upward and fails to expand completely, resulting in diminished respiratory excursion on the affected side. The infant is tachypneic and evidences signs of respiratory distress. Atelectasis and pneumonia are common complications. The diagnosis of diaphragmatic paralysis is confirmed by fluoroscopy or ultrasonography. Often the condition is temporary, with eventual complete return of function.

Implications for Nursing Care

Nursing care is aimed initially at alleviating respiratory distress. The neonate is placed in a neutral thermal environment, and an enriched oxygen atmosphere is frequently ordered by the physician. The infant is placed on the affected side to allow for full expansion of the opposite lung.

Oral feedings may be withheld initially to decrease energy expenditures and prevent the risk of aspiration. Gavage feedings may be performed, but as the infant's condition stabilizes, he will be allowed to breast-feed or bottle-feed. Parents will need encouragement and support in their efforts to feed and hold the infant and must feel fully competent to care for him before discharge.

Facial Nerve Injury

Facial paralysis frequently occurs when pressure is applied to the facial nerve by the blade of the obstetric forceps during delivery. The affected side of the face remains flaccid when the infant cries. The eyelid on the affected side may not close completely, and the lips do not grasp the nipple effectively for sucking. Facial paralysis is usually transient.

Implications for Nursing Care

Nursing responsibilities include protecting the eye on the affected side by applying artificial tears and keeping the eyelid closed with a dressing until the paralysis disappears. The infant may also need additional support during feeding to prevent drooling of formula or aspiration. Spe-

cial support and teaching parents so that they will feel comfortable about caring for the newborn at home will be necessary.

THE NEONATE WITH HEMOLYTIC DISEASE OF THE NEWBORN

Hemolytic disease of the newborn is a disorder in which the infant's red blood cells (RBCs) are destroyed or hemolyzed with resultant hyperbilirubinemia and jaundice. It may be caused by maternal antibodies that cross the placenta and enter the fetal blood stream. Other causes of RBC hemolysis include infection and enzymatic deficiencies in the RBC (*e.g.,* glucose-6-phosphate-dehydrogenase deficiency, or G6PD). Two of the most frequently occurring hemolytic diseases of the newborn are ABO incompatibility and Rh disease. (The student may find it helpful to review related material in Chapter 19.)

At birth, the neonate with Rh incompatibility has a positive direct Coombs' test, indicating the presence of circulating maternal antibodies in his blood stream. The infant is anemic and has a falling hematocrit, and there are an increased number of circulating immature RBCs. A rapidly rising serum bilirubin level occurs with continued hemolysis of RBCs, and jaundice develops soon after birth. Phototherapy is initiated, and an exchange transfusion may be performed to prevent kernicterus when serum bilirubin reaches dangerously high levels.

Rh Incompatibility (Erythroblastosis Fetalis)

Rh disease occurs when the mother is Rh-negative and the fetus is Rh-positive. When fetal Rh-positive RBCs gain access to the maternal blood stream, which contains Rh-negative RBCs, an antigen-antibody response is stimulated. Conditions that increase the likelihood of fetal RBCs from a previous pregnancy, having passed into the mother's blood stream, include previous abortions, placental accidents, amniocentesis, and separation of the placenta at birth. Rh-positive antibodies are produced, pass through the placenta, attach to the fetal RBCs, and destroy them. The fetus reacts by producing large numbers of immature RBCs to replace those that were hemolyzed (thus the name *erythroblastosis fetalis*).

Hydrops Fetalis

In the most severe form of the disease, known as *hydrops fetalis,* the fetus becomes severely anemic. Hepatosplenomegaly is evident at birth. Fluid leaks out of the intravascular compartment, resulting in hydrothorax (fluid in the pleural space) and ascites. Generalized edema is also evident. Eventually, severe cardiomegaly and hypoxia lead to cardiac failure and death if the fetus is not treated by intrauterine transfusion of RBCs and delivered early.

ABO Incompatibility

ABO incompatibility is a much milder form of hemolytic disease. It involves group A or B infants born to group O mothers and, less frequently, group B infants born to group A mothers. Because anti-A and anti-B antibodies naturally exist in the blood stream of group O mothers, senitization can occur with the first pregnancy. Stillbirths and the severe hydrops seen in the Rh disease almost never occur. The infant becomes jaundiced after birth, but massive hemolysis and resultant anemia are rare.

Implications for Nursing Care

When hyperbilirubinemia is a result of blood incompatibility and isoimmunization, the following guidelines for blood type and Rh factor are followed when exchange transfusions are performed:

- Rh incompatibility (mother Rh-negative; infant Rh-positive): group O, Rh-negative whole blood or packed cells. The RBCs in this type of blood contain no Rh antigens and will not be hemolyzed by any maternal antibodies remaining in the infant's blood stream.
- ABO incompatibility (mother group O; infant group A, B, or AB): group O, Rh-specific whole blood with low titers of anti-A and anti-B antibodies. The RBCs in this type of blood contain no antigens that will be hemolyzed by maternal antibodies.

If the neonate with a blood incompatibility develops pathologic jaundice, phototherapy is instituted. The nurse initiates the therapy and monitors the neonate closely for common complications of the procedure, including hyperthermia, dehydration, skin excoriation, rashes, and bronzing. An exchange transfusion may be performed to remove sensitized RBCs and serum bilirubin and correct severe anemia, but because of the risk of transmission of hepatitis and HIV with blood transfusion, lower RBC and hematocrit levels may be tolerated in neonates today. (See Hyperbilirubinemia and Kernicterus earlier in this chapter.)

Nursing care is organized to allow extended periods of rest for the anemic neonate who is hemolyzing RBCs and is jaundiced. The infant is placed in a neutral thermal environment to reduce energy expenditures until his condition stabilizes. Vital signs are monitored frequently. Tachycardia may be evident with severe anemia. Parents are encouraged to visit the infant frequently and are given

the opportunity to hold and care for him each day. Phototherapy should be discontinued (even if only for short periods of time) to allow parents to have eye-to-eye contact with their infant.

THE NEONATE WITH EFFECTS OF MATERNAL SUBSTANCE ABUSE

The infant born to the mother who is addicted to drugs or alcohol presents with many physical characteristics and anomalies that reflect the direct effect of the substance on fetal growth and development. The infant of an addicted mother (IAM) is also likely to suffer from the effects of maternal malnutrition (*i.e.*, to be SGA) and from disease processes associated with drug abuse (*e.g.*, sexually transmitted diseases and hepatitis).

Infants of mothers who ingest more than 3 oz of 100% alcohol per day are at risk for being born with *fetal alcohol syndrome* (FAS). Affected infants present with a number of physical signs that aid in the diagnosis of the disorder:

- Microcephaly
- Facial anomalies: short palpebral fissure; epicanthal folds; short, upturned nose, micrognathia; thin upper lip
- Cardiac defects (primarily septal)
- Minor joint and limb anomalies, especially joint malformations
- Altered palmar crease patterns

The infants also demonstrate postnatal growth retardation and mental retardation and experience withdrawal symptoms similar to those of infants of drug-dependent mothers.

Neonatal Withdrawal

The neonate begins to experience acute withdrawal from the substances in his system shortly after birth. The severity and length of withdrawal depend on the type and amount of drug the mother was addicted to during pregnancy, and the time of the last dose before delivery.

Withdrawal symptoms primarily involve the central nervous system, the respiratory system, and the gastrointestinal tract. The infant is irritable, jittery, and hypertonic and has a high-pitched cry. Constant activity leads to excoriation of the skin at pressure points over bony prominences. Seizure activity may be demonstrated with severe withdrawal. Tachypnea and tachycardia are common, and the infant may be incapable of nipple-feeding at the height of the withdrawal. Nasal stuffiness, which results from vasomotor instability, exacerbates the infant's tachypnea and can lead to respiratory distress.

NURSING ALERT

Flandermeyer AA: A comparison of the effects of heroin and cocaine abuse upon the neonate. Neonatal Network 5:42–47, 1987

Cocaine Abuse and the Neonate

Cocaine abuse crosses all socioeconomic and ethnic lines, and the incidence of cocaine use in pregnancy is increasing at an alarming rate. The availability of a purer and more potent form of cocaine (crack), which is smoked, may precipitate life-threatening cardiovascular or CNS complications in the mother, fetus, and neonate.

Cocaine causes peripheral and placental vascular constriction, increased heart rate, elevated blood pressure, and can result in ventricular arrhythmia, acute myocardial infarction, cerebral vascular accident, pulmonary edema, and sudden death. Taken in the first trimester it has been linked to congenital anomalies. Chronic use during pregnancy causes fetal intrauterine growth retardation, intolerance to labor, and low birth weight. The most serious consequences of cocaine use for the neonate include cerebral infarction, sudden abruption of the placenta, and preterm labor and birth. The infant is often very immature and suffers from hypovolemic shock.

Unlike heroin, cocaine-addicted infants do not demonstrate a predictable sequence of physical withdrawal. Tachycardia and hypertension may be observed until the drug is metabolized and excreted, but some infants may remain asymptomatic or suffer from subtle behavioral problems that only become evident later in life. If cocaine abuse is suspected, a urine specimen should be obtained from the infant as soon as possible after birth for toxicology screening. The nurse observes the neonate for danger signals and supports adaptations to extrauterine life.

If cocaine metabolites are detected in the urine, social service, child welfare, and law-enforcement agencies will be involved in plans for placing the infant upon discharge. Substance abuse is a value-laden diagnosis, but the nurse must attempt to provide nonjudgmental care and offer parents the information and support necessary for the formation of parent–infant bonds.

Gastrointestinal signs and symptoms are often marked and interfere with ingestion of adequate calories and fluid. Although the infant has an unusually strong, hyperactive suck, he is a very poor feeder with an uncoordinated suck–swallow reflex. Persistent vomiting may lead to severe fluid and electrolyte imbalances, and it is often necessary to discontinue feedings until the crisis has passed.

Hyperthermia frequently accompanies other symptoms and is related to increased physical activity, dehydration, and central nervous system involvement. The infant also experiences vasomotor instability as reflected by sweating, flushing, and stuffy nose.

Implications for Nursing Care

Nursing care of the IAM requires great patience and skill. The infants may cry for hours in a shrill, high-pitched tone that is extremely unpleasant to listen to for long periods. They are hypertonic and resist cuddling or holding; they are most comfortable when tightly swaddled and left undisturbed in a quiet, dimly lit environment. Seizures are common, and the infant will require anticonvulsants if they occur. Valium may be administered for several days to diminish the intensity of withdrawal if the infant experiences extreme irritability, respiratory distress, hyperthermia, and vomiting.

Extra time is required during feedings, since the infant is often a poor feeder who gags, regurgitates, or vomits the milk. Intravenous therapy may be initiated when fluid and electrolyte imbalances occur. Because of the constant rubbing of extremities against the mattress and increased incidence of diarrhea, meticulous care of the skin is required to prevent its breakdown.

The nurse must monitor vital signs closely and observe for evidence of seizure activity, respiratory distress, and hyperthermia. Cardiorespiratory monitors may be attached to assist the nurse in the continuous surveillance of cardiopulmonary function. Fluid intake and output are measured. Skin turgor and the condition of mucous membranes are evaluated frequently to alert the nurse to signs of dehydration.

Many mothers with addiction disorders are actively involved in methadone maintenance programs during pregnancy and begin the withdrawal phase after delivery. They will need extra support and encouragement in caring for their infants during the early stressful period of detoxification. Other mothers are unable to find the resources to conquer their addiction after the infant's birth. Nurses working with the parents of withdrawing infants must meet the challenge of maintaining an accepting, nonjudgmental attitude in the face of life-styles that they may find objectionable.

The nurse should focus her energies on supporting appropriate efforts at parenting, allowing mothers to ventilate feelings of guilt and anxiety, and answering questions about the infant's condition as they arise. Before the infant is discharged, the parents should be given every opportunity to care for him so that they are confident of their ability to recognize and meet his special needs. Signs of central nervous system disturbance may persist for many months after the acute phase of withdrawal, and the family will need concrete suggestions for dealing with a hyperactive, irritable infant who is easily aroused and difficult to soothe. Referrals for follow-up by a social service agency and a visiting nurse or a public health nurse are essential.

Sometimes the infant is placed temporarily in foster care, if conditions in the home are hazardous to his health or if the parents are unable to care for him because of their own frequent substance abuse. The final decisions made by the court regarding parental rights and placement of the infant are often based, in part, on nursing documentation. It is essential that the nurse document all telephone calls and visits made by the parents, and chart subjective and objective data regarding maternal–infant interactions. Regardless of the ultimate disposition of the infant, his parents should have every opportunity to visit the nursery and care for him until he is discharged.

CHAPTER SUMMARY

The nurse must face the challenge of providing family-centered care in less than ideal circumstances when complications occur in the neonatal period. Innovative approaches to care must be devised to support infant and parents. This can best be accomplished using the nursing process in assessing needs, diagnosing problems, planning interventions, and evaluating outcomes of care. The nurse must also possess a comprehensive knowledge of theories about attachment, parental grieving, and crisis to support the new family. This chapter has reviewed major neonatal complications, common parental reactions to the birth of an infant with problems, and appropriate nursing interventions to support the high-risk family. It provides the maternal-infant nurse with a basic foundation for practice. The reader is referred to the References and Suggested Readings for further information about the high-risk and sick neonate.

STUDY QUESTIONS

1. What therapeutic techniques can be employed to maintain a patent airway in the high-risk neonate?
2. What is the purpose of chest percussion and drainage for the neonate with alterations in respiratory function?
3. What are the major risks of oxygen therapy for the neonate?
4. Why is the high-risk or sick neonate at risk for fluid volume deficits and electrolyte imbalance?
5. What are the major complications of umbilical artery catheterization?
6. What are the major risks of IV therapy in the neonate?

7. What are the major risks of total parenteral nutrition for the neonate?
8. Why is the high-risk neonate susceptible to infection?
9. What is the primary preventive measure against infection in the nursery?
10. What is the significance of a "neutral thermal environment" for the high-risk or sick neonate?
11. How can the nurse prevent alterations in parenting for a neonate in the intensive care nursery?
12. By what mechanism does phototherapy reduce serum bilirubin levels?
13. What are the major complications of phototherapy?
14. What are the purposes of exchange tranfusions in the high-risk neonate?
15. What are the major causes of birth asphyxia?
16. What pathophysiologic changes are responsible for postasphyxial syndrome in the infant?
17. What nursing interventions may be employed in the prevention of apnea of prematurity?
18. Why is the preterm infant at increased risk for persistent fetal circulation?
19. What are the major complications of the SGA infant?
20. What are the major implications of symmetric growth retardation in the SGA infant?
21. Why is the infant of a diabetic mother at increased risk for the development of hypoglycemia?
22. What is meconium aspiration syndrome, and which groups of infants are at increased risk for the development of this complication?
23. What are the major nursing interventions in the care of the neonate with an infection?
24. What are TORCH infections?
25. What are the major nursing interventions in the care of the neonate who has been casted after a long bone fracture at birth?
26. What are the major signs of increased intracranial pressure in the neonate?
27. What is the mechanism for hemolysis in isoimmunization in the neonate?
28. What are the major signs and symptoms of pneumothorax in the neonate?
29. How can the nurse best support the infant experiencing drug withdrawal?

REFERENCES/BIBLIOGRAPHY

Anderson J: Sensory intervention with the preterm infant in the neonatal intensive care unit. J Occup Ther 40(1):19–26, 1986

Avery GB: Neonatology, 3rd ed. Philadelphia, JB Lippincott, 1987

Bishop AH, Scudder JR: Nursing ethics in an age of controversy. Adv Nurs Sci 9(3):34–43, 1987

Blackman JA: The value of Apgar scores in predicting development outcome at age five. J Perinatol 7(3): 204–210, 1988

Centers for Disease Control: Recommendations for assisting in the prevention of perinatal transmission of human T-lymphotropic virus Type III lymphadenopathy associated virus and acquired immunodeficiency syndrome. MMWR 34(48): 721–732, 1985

Chaze B, Luddington–Hoe S: sensory stimulation in the NICU. Am J Nurs 84:68, 1984

Cloherty JP: Neonatal hyperbilirubinemia. In Cloherty JP, Stark AR (eds): Manual of Neonatal Care, 2nd ed. Boston, Little, Brown & Co, 1985

Committee on the Fetus and Newborn, American Academy of Pediatrics. Use and abuse of the Apgar score. Pediatrics 78:1148, 1986

Cunningham M: Intraventricular hemorrhage in the premature. Dimens Crit Care Nurs 6(1):20–27, 1987

Edmondson KS: Acquired immune deficiency syndrome in the neonate. Neonat Network 6(4):7–12, 1988

Gordon PC: Candida infection in the very low birth weight infant. J Perinat Neonat Nurs 1(4):47–55, 1988

Grippi C, Wand L, Roncoli M: The case of baby Alice: AIDS/ARC in infancy. Neonatal Network 6(5):9–14, 1988

Jobe A, Ikegami M: Surfactant for the treatment of respiratory distress syndrome. Am Rev Respir Dis 136:1256–1275, 1987

Klaus M, Kennell J: Parent–Infant Bonding, 2nd ed. St Louis, CV Mosby, 1982

Korones S: High-risk Newborn Infants: The Basis For Intensive Care Nursing, 4th ed. St Louis, CV Mosby, 1986

Kuller J, Lund C, Tobin C: Improved skin care for premature infants. MCN 8:200–207, 1984

Marecki MA: Chlamydia trachomatis: A developing perinatal problem. J Perinat Neonat Nurs 1(4):1–11, 1988

Modlin JF: Perinatal Viral Infections and Toxoplasmosis. In Cloherty JP, Stark AR (eds). Manual of Neonatal Care, 2nd ed. Boston, Little, Brown & Co, 1985

Oellrick R: Pneumothorax, chest tubes and the neonate. MCN 10:29–34, 1985

Richardson C: Hyaline membrane disease: Future treatment modalities. J Perinat Neonat Nurs 2(1):78–88, 1988

Riedel K: Pulse oximetry: A new technology to assess patient oxygen needs in the neonatal intensive care. J Perinat Neonat Nurs 1(1):49–57, 1987

Sessions FC, Cloherty JP: Infection: Prevention and Treatment. In Cloherty JP, Stark AR (eds): Manual of Neonatal Care. Boston, Little, Brown & Co, 1985

Shannon LF: Insulin usage in the neonate. Neonatal Network 6(5):31–39, 1988

Shapiro C: Retrolental fibroplasia: What we know and what we don't know. Neonatal Network 4:33–43, 1986

Spellacy W, Miler S, Winegar A, et al: Macrosomia — Maternal characteristics and infant complications. Obstet Gynecol 66:158–161, 1985

Walsh MD, Kleigman RM: Necrotizing enterocolitis: Treatment based on staging criteria. Pediatr Clin North Am 33(1):179–201, 1986

Withers J, Bradshaw E: Preventing neonatal hepatitis-B infection. MCN 11:270–272, 1986

SUGGESTED READINGS

Arenson J: Discharge teaching in the NICU: The changing needs of NICU graduates and their families. Neonatal Network 6(4):47–52, 1988

Brown L: Physiologic responses to cutaneous pain in neonates. Neonatal Network 6(3):18–22, 1987

Franck LS: A new method to quantitatively describe pain behavior in infants. Nurs Res 35:28–31, 1986

Lagner SM: Preparing a family for home monitoring. Neonatal Network 6(5):57–60, 1988

Lynch TM: Invasive and noninvasive pressure monitoring in neonates. J Perinat Neonat Nurs 1(1):58–71, 1987

Gunderson LP, Kenner CK: Neonatal stress: Physiologic adaptation and nursing implications. Neonatal Network 6(1):37–42, 1987

Novak J: An ethical decision-making model for the neonatal intensive care unit. J Perinat Neonat Nurs 1(3):57–67, 1988

35 congenital anomalies in the neonate

LEARNING OBJECTIVES

After studying the material in this chapter, the student should be able to

- Describe the current state of perinatal regionalization and implications for the family of a neonate with a congenital anomaly

- Identify the most common types of congenital anomalies detected in the neonatal period

- Discuss nursing responsibilities in the stabilization and preparation for transport of an infant born with a major congenital anomaly

KEY TERMS

Anomaly

Atresia

Congenital

Dysplasia

Hereditary

Stenosis

One of the most distressing situations health team members must face is the birth of an infant with a congenital anomaly. In most instances it is an undiagnosed and, therefore, unexpected problem. It is very difficult to inform parents their newborn baby has a physical defect. Parents may view even a minor anomaly, which poses no threat to the infant's health, a major crisis, especially when the defect involves the face or genitalia.

Parents are extremely sensitive to nonverbal cues from staff members involved in the birth of their baby. When an infant is born with an anomaly, there is a sudden change in the behavior of staff members. Communication patterns are altered, and silence often ensues. It is essential the birth attendant inform the parents at once that there is a problem. If the infant requires immediate emergency care, a member of the health team should be available to support the parents and provide them with basic information about the infant's condition, until the pediatrician can speak with them.

Although parents differ in their responses to the birth of a child with a defect, the health team should be prepared for reactions commonly observed in the early stages of the grieving process, including shock, denial, and anger. The father, in particular, may be overwhelmed if the mother is also ill or has had a cesarean delivery. He is often the parent who accompanies the sick neonate to the intensive care nursery and is asked to sign consent forms and to make immediate decisions about life-sustaining procedures while the mother is incapacitated. This places a heavy burden of responsibility on him during a time of disorganization and potential crisis.

NEONATAL TRANSPORT

Not only is the birth of a neonate with an anomaly distressing in and of itself, but the subsequent immediate medical and nursing management may require the neonate be moved to another facility for treatment. The three levels in regionalizing perinatal care were discussed in the previous chapter. The development of perinatal regionalization has made it possible to transport the neonate with major congenital anomalies to a Level III facility for surgical correction of the defect and specialized nursing care. Highly skilled physician–nurse transport teams are on call 24 hours a day to move the sick neonate from the place of birth. A telephone call or radio message from the referring physician or nurse midwife activates the transport system. A specially designed mobile transport unit (ambulance, helicopter, or airplane), containing all the equipment required to support the infant, can be dispatched within a matter of minutes. Telephone consultation with neonatologists and nurses at the Level III facility will assist the staff at the referring hospital to stabilize the

---

Responsibilities of Maternal – Infant Nurses Practicing in Level I and II Referring Hospitals

- Immediate resuscitation and support of the compromised neonate
- Postnatal stabilization of the neonate until the transport team arrives:
  1. Maintaining a patent airway
  2. Supporting ventilation and oxygenation
  3. Correcting acidosis and preventing fluid and electrolyte imbalances
  4. Providing a neutral thermal environment and preventing cold stress
  5. Protecting exposed organs and internal structures from injury and infection
- Preparation of parents for the transport of the neonate
- Taking pictures of the infant for parents unable to travel immediately to the Level III facility
- Coordinating efforts with delivery room or postpartum nursing staff so that the mother can see the infant, if at all possible, before transport
- Completing essential paperwork for transport, including arrangements to have all infant records duplicated for the Level III facility

---

infant and prepare him for transport as soon as possible after the team arrives.

As a result of this neonatal transport system, most maternal – infant nurses working in Level I and II hospitals in the United States today rarely care for the infant born with a major congenital defect for an extended period of time. In many states, in fact, *all* infants requiring cardiac surgery or repair of other significant anomalies (*e.g.*, craniofacial or spinal defects and limb malformations) are normally transported to a designated Level III hospital within the state. Only a few dozen neonatal nurses in a huge geographic area may be trained to provide specialized nursing care to these infants. Therefore, the types of sick infants cared for at Level I and II facilities are changing, as is the focus of newborn nursing within these hospitals.

In light of this change in nursing roles and responsibilities for most maternal – infant nurses, this chapter provides only basic information about major congenital anomalies. All nurses caring for these high-risk infants in Level I and II facilities must be familiar with major categories of defects. They must have a basic understanding of how the neonate is affected, the types of treatment available, immediate nursing interventions required, and prognosis, in order to care for the infant's immediate needs after birth and to support the parents. The student is referred to comprehensive pediatric or neonatal nursing texts for in depth treatment of the ongoing medical and nursing care of the infant with a serious congenital anomaly.

CONGENITAL ANOMALIES

This chapter outlines the most common anomalies found in neonates and summarizes appropriate nursing care. The chapter closes with a brief discussion of legal and ethical issues in the care of neonates with congenital anomalies.

Central Nervous System Anomalies

Neural Tube Defects
Spina Bifida Occulta

Spina bifida occulta is the absence or incomplete closure of one or more of the vertebral arches. The skin covering the defect may be dimpled or covered with a tuft of hair. If there is no extrusion of meninges or spinal cord

through the opening, the condition is usually asymptomatic and repair may not be required.

Meningocele and Myelomeningocele

A meningocele is a cyst outpouching of the meninges and cerebrospinal fluid, through a defect in the vertebral column, without associated anomalies of the spinal cord (Fig. 35–1). Because the sac may rupture and infection can occur, surgical repair is usually indicated. The prognosis is quite good when the spinal cord is not involved.

A myelomeningocele is a cystic outpouching of the meninges, cerebrospinal fluid, and spinal cord through a defect in the posterior wall of the vertebral column (Fig. 35–1). The neonate has no motor or sensory function below the level of the defect. Surgical repair can be done to prevent rupture of the cyst and infection. Prognosis depends on the degree of spinal cord involvement and the level of the defect. The higher the defect, the greater the degree of neurologic impairment the neonate will sustain. Even with surgical correction, the infant may never be able to walk and may suffer from incontinence of both urine and stool.

Congenital Anomalies

Central Nervous System Anomalies

Neural Tube Defects
- Spina bifida occulta
- Meningocele and myelomeningocele
- Anencephaly

Hydrocephalus

Respiratory Tract Anomalies

Choanal atresia
Diaphragmatic hernia
Pulmonary hypoplasia/agenesis

Cardiac Anomalies

Acyanotic heart disease
- Atrial septal defect
- Ventricular septal defect
- Patent ductus arteriosus
- Coarctation of the aorta

Cyanotic heart disease
- Pulmonary stenosis
- Tetralogy of Fallot
- Transposition of the great vessels

Gastrointestinal Anomalies

Cleft lip and palate
Esophageal atresia and tracheoesophageal fisula
Omphalocele
Intestinal obstruction and imperforate anus

Genitourinary Anomalies

Ambiguous genitalia
Exstrophy of the bladder and patent urachus

Musculoskeletal Anomalies

Congenital hip dysplasia
Talipes equinovarus

Chromosomal Abnormalities

Trisomies (including Down syndrome)
Inborn errors of metabolism:
- Phenylketonuria
- Maple syrup urine disease
- Homocystinuria
- Galactosemia
- Congenital hypothyroidism

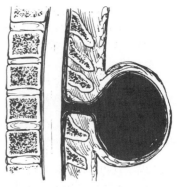

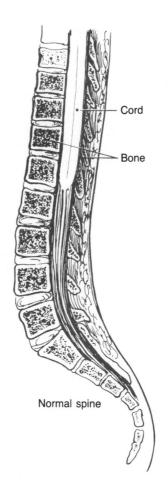

Cord

Bone

Spina bifida with meningocele

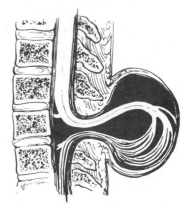

Normal spine

Spina bifida with meningomyelocele

Figure 35–1. Transverse section of a normal spine compared to a meningocele and myelomeningocele. In the meningocele, the meninges have protruded through the vertebral column and are filled with cerebrospinal fluid. In a myelomeningocele, the meninges and spinal cord have protruded through the vertebral column and have joined the meningocele filled with cerebrospinal fluid.

Primary nursing responsibility when a cyst is present is to prevent rupture and subsequent central nervous system infection. The infant is positioned on the side to eliminate pressure on the defect. If leakage of cerebrospinal fluid is evident, the sac should be covered with a sterile pad and strict asepsis maintained when the dressing is being changed. There must be meticulous attention to skin care to prevent breakdown of delicate tissues. The bladder may need to be emptied by Credé massage at regular intervals.

Anencephaly

Anencephaly is the congenital absence of part of the cranial vault and underlying brain tissue. It is incompatible with life. The infant may be born with a heart rate and respiration, but dies shortly after birth.

Hydrocephalus

Hydrocephalus is an abnormal accumulation of cerebrospinal fluid in the ventricles of the brain. It is frequently associated with myelomeningocele due to blockage in the flow of fluid. The infant's head circumference increases with the accumulation of fluid. Suture lines in

the cranium separate, and the fontanelles bulge and feel tense. The infant exhibits "setting sun eyes" and has a high-pitched cry. If the buildup of fluid has been extensive prenatally, the infant may suffer permanent brain damage. Surgical repair involves placing a polyethylene shunt to drain excess fluid from the ventricles. Prognosis depends on the success of the shunt procedure and the degree of brain damage sustained prior to surgery.

The nurse must support the neonate's head carefully when handling him and position the infant so as to maintain a patent airway. A waterbed and sheepskin mattress pad can be used to prevent the skin from breaking down when the head is very large and neurologic impairment is present. The head circumference is measured daily. If the infant is fed orally, care must be taken to prevent aspiration and to watch for projectile vomiting, which may occur with increased intracranial pressure.

Respiratory Tract Anomalies

Choanal Atresia

Choanal atresia is the unilateral or bilateral blockage of the posterior nares. Because the neonate is an obligate nose breather, he will suffer from immediate respiratory distress at birth if both nares are occluded. Surgical intervention is essential, and the prognosis is excellent if there are no associated anomalies.

Diaphragmatic Hernia

Diaphragmatic hernia is a congenital defect in the diaphragm, which allows herniation of abdominal contents into the thoracic cavity and displacement of the heart and lung tissue. The infant has a scaphoid-shaped abdomen, and bowel sounds may be heard over the chest wall. Birth asphyxia and respiratory distress are common with severe herniation. Surgical intervention is essential to remove abdominal organs from the thoracic cavity and relieve pressure on the lungs. The prognosis depends on the adequacy of ventilation and support before surgery and the extent of the herniation. If the defect is large, severe herniation prenatally leads to incomplete development of lung tissue, which is incompatible with extrauterine life.

Immediate endotracheal intubation and hand ventilation are essential to establish respiration. The nurse assists the physician with resuscitation efforts. The infant's head is elevated, and he is placed on the affected side to let the normal lung expand fully. The gastric contents are aspirated to decompress the stomach, and an orogastric tube is passed to prevent distention of the gastrointestinal tract with air. An umbilical artery catheter is inserted, and the nurse administers the IV drugs and fluids required to stabilize the infant. If assisted ventilation is required, the infant is intubated and placed on a mechanical ventilator. Small tidal volumes and a rapid respiratory rate are preferred to reduce the risk of pneumothorax. Surgery to repair the herniation is done as soon as possible.

Pulmonary Agenesis

Pulmonary agenesis, the underdevelopment or complete absence of one or both lungs, is a rare but often fatal congenital defect. One third of infants die within the first year of life, often secondary to recurrent pulmonary infections. Approximately 50% of cases are associated with anomalies of the cardiovascular, gastrointestinal, urogenital, and skeletal systems. This defect may result when a diaphragmatic hernia occurs, caused by the limited space available for growth and development of the lung. Pulmonary agenesis has also been associated with oligohydramnios, and it is postulated that lack of amniotic fluid in the fetal alveoli prevents normal lung expansion and growth *in utero*.

The neonate with pulmonary agenesis may exhibit signs of acute respiratory distress, including dyspnea, tachypnea, stridor, diminished breath sounds and chest asymmetry, and respiratory lag on the affected side. However, in some instances, the infant may be asymptomatic at birth. Chest x-ray films will demonstrate a homogeneous density or complete opacification on the involved side.

Maintaining a patent airway and supporting pulmonary function are critical aspects of nursing care. The neonate's oropharynx or endotracheal tube may need to be suctioned frequently. Preventing pulmonary infection is another objective of care, and scrupulous sterile technique as well as frequently turning and repositioning the infant to prevent stasis and drainage of pulmonary secretions is essential.

Oral feedings are initiated only after the infant is stabilized, and the nurse proceeds slowly to prevent respiratory distress or aspiration of formula. Breast-feeding may be permitted if the neonate tolerates nipple feedings. Discharge planning must begin early. Parents will require extensive teaching regarding pulmonary toilet and suctioning. The infant may be discharged home with an apnea monitor, and families must understand how to apply the monitor and respond to system alarms. A visiting nurse referral is essential (Brenner 1987).

Cardiac Anomalies

Cardiac anomalies are a significant cause of neonatal morbidity and mortality. They are responsible for over 30% of all deaths caused by anomalies in the first year of life. Anomalies of the heart are frequently categorized on the basis of the presence or absence of cyanosis (see Figs. 35–2 and 35–3).

Acyanotic Heart Disease

Atrial Septal Defect.   An atrial septal defect (ASD) is an opening in the septum between the atria of the heart (see Fig. 35–2). Because of the higher pressure in the left side of the heart, blood is shunted from left to right. Blood is able to circulate through the pulmonary vasculature, and thus there is no cyanosis. ASD is most frequently asymptomatic. The defect is closed by a surgical procedure to prevent possible development of subacute bacterial endocarditis later in life.

Ventricular Septal Defect.   A ventricular septal defect (VSD) is an opening in the septum between the ventricles of the heart (see Fig. 35–2). It is the most frequently occurring cardiac anomaly, accounting for over 20% of all defects. A VSD may be totally asymptomatic or may be severe enough to cause pulmonary edema and congestive heart failure. When the opening between the left and right ventricles is large, blood is shunted into the right ventricle, increasing its workload and eventually leading to right heart failure. Pulmonary congestion is also seen and is the result of the increased amount of blood flowing from the right ventricle into the pulmonary vasculature. Surgical correction is possible using a Da-

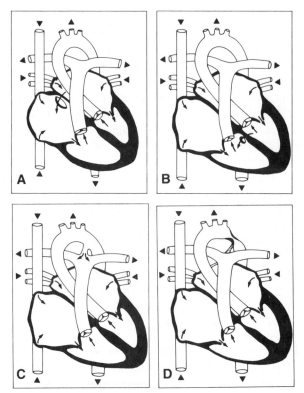

Figure 35-2. Major congenital anomalies resulting in acyanotic heart disease. *(A)* Atrial septal defect, which is an abnormal opening between the left and right atria that leads to left-to-right shunting of blood. *(B)* Ventricular septal defect, a condition in which there are abnormal openings between the right and left ventricles. *(C)* Patent ductus arteriosus, which is the abnormal persistence of a vascular connection that, during fetal life, short circuits the pulmonary vascular bed and directs blood from the pulmonary artery to the aorta. *(D)* Coarctation of the aorta, which is an abnormal narrowing of the lumen of the aorta, causes an increased left ventricular pressure and workload. (Courtesy of Ross Laboratories)

cron patch. Prognosis is good if the VSD is not associated with other cardiac anomalies.

Patent Ductus Arteriosus. Patent ductus arteriosus (PDA) is the persistent opening of the fetal bypass that connects the aorta to the pulmonary artery (see Fig. 35-2). Any infant who suffers from hypoxemia and preterm infants under 1500 g may experience a reopening of the ductus. A PDA is often diagnosed by a harsh grade 2 or 3 systolic murmur auscultated at the upper left sternal border. A left-to-right shunting of blood occurs and can lead to right heart failure and pulmonary congestion. For many infants, medical management of the condition, including oxygen therapy and blood transfusions to maintain adequate oxygenation of tissue, is sufficient to prevent problems. Fluid restriction and the administration of cardiotonics and diuretics may also be necessary. Indomethacin, a prostaglandin inhibitor, has been used with

limited success to close the bypass medically. The ductus can be ligated surgically if medical management fails.

Coarctation of the Aorta. Coarctation is a narrowing of that section of the aorta that causes the backup of blood above the stricture and results in increased pressure in the left side of the heart (see Fig. 35-2). If the extent of stenosis is minimal, the anomaly may be asymptomatic except for diminished femoral pulses. Surgical intervention is required but may be postponed for several months if there are no immediate problems. The prognosis is very good if the coarctation is not associated with other cardiac defects.

Cyanotic Heart Disease

Pulmonary Stenosis. Pulmonary stenosis is a stricture or narrowing of the pulmonary artery that prevents blood from leaving the right ventricle and entering the lungs. If the stenosis is severe, pressure will build in the right side of the heart, reopening the foramen ovale and causing a right-to-left shunt with mild cyanosis. Surgical intervention to remove the stricture is possible. Prognosis is good if the stenosis is not associated with other anomalies.

Tetralogy of Fallot. Tetralogy of Fallot (Fig. 35-3) is an anomaly composed of four separate defects: (1) pulmonary stenosis; (2) a VSD; (3) an overriding aorta; and (4) hypertrophy of the right ventricle. The pulmonary stenosis prevents blood from leaving the right ventricle and entering the lungs. Pressure builds up in the right side of the heart, leading to right ventricular hypertrophy and shunting the blood to the left side of the heart through the ventricular septal defect. Cyanosis occurs with the left-to-

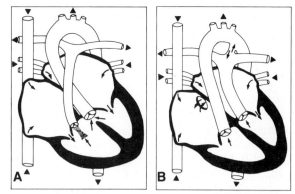

Figure 35-3. Major congenital anomalies resulting in cyanotic heart disease. *(A)* Tetralogy of Fallot, which is characterized by the combination of four defects: pulmonary stenosis, ventricular septal defect, overriding aorta, and hypertrophy of right ventricle. *(B)* Transposition of the great vessels, a condition in which the aorta originates from the right ventricle and the pulmonary artery from the left ventricle. (Courtesy of Ross Laboratories)

right shunt because blood does not circulate through the pulmonary vascular system. Any stressors placed on the infant, such as crying or feeding, cause an increase in cyanosis and respiratory distress. Surgical intervention to correct the defects is possible.

Transposition of the Great Vessels.   In transposition of the great vessels (see Fig. 35–3), the aorta arises from the right ventricle and the pulmonary artery from the left ventricle. Blood enters the right side of the heart, exits the right ventricle, and enters the aorta. It then circulates through the body, completely bypassing the lungs and the oxygenation process. Blood entering the left side of the heart passes through the atrium, the ventricle, and then the pulmonary artery, where it enters the pulmonary vascular bed. It circulates through the pulmonary vasculature and then returns to the left side of the heart. There are two totally separate and nonfunctional circulatory systems. Unless there is a congenital opening between the right and left sides of the heart or one is created surgically, this defect is incompatible with life. Surgery is done as soon as possible to create an opening if none exists, and major repairs are completed later. The prognosis is poor because of the nature of the defect and the current limitations of the surgical procedure.

Tricuspid Atresia.   Tricuspid atresia is a cardiac anomaly characterized by VSD, hypoplastic right ventricle, and enlarged left ventricle. It may be associated with transposition of the great arteries, pulmonary stenosis, or both. It results from the failure of the right atrioventricular valve to develop. Blood entering the right atrium cannot pass into the right ventricle, and both a patent foramen ovale and some type of passage between the right side of the heart and the lungs are necessary for survival. The infant is usually very cyanotic shortly after birth, and surgery is required to construct an adequate shunt from the right heart to the lungs (Blalock-Taussig shunt). With surgery, a 50% survival rate at 1 year has been demonstrated in some infants (Avery 1987).

Truncus Arteriosus.   The truncus arteriosus is an embryonic arterial structure that normally divides, during fetal growth and development, into the aorta and pulmonary artery. Failure of septation results in the presence of a single great artery, originating from the base of the heart, which supplies both the systemic and pulmonary circulation. A VSD is also associated with this defect. Pulmonary congestion and congestive heart failure develop within the first month of life, and prognosis is very poor without medical and surgical treatment. Recent advances in pediatric cardiac surgery, however, have greatly improved the outcome and long-term survival for many of these infants.

Anomalous Venous Return.   In anomalous venous return, one or more pulmonary veins empty into the right atrium. The infant is frequently cyanotic shortly after birth. If all pulmonary veins return to the right side of the heart, surgical correction to permit an arterial connection is essential to provide the systemic circulation with adequate amounts of oxygenated blood.

The primary goal of nursing care of the neonate with a cardiac anomaly is to decrease the workload of the heart. The infant may be placed in a neutral thermal environment. Oxygen is administered, as indicated, to reduce cyanosis and maintain an adequate blood oxygen tension. The infant may be given cardiotonics and diuretics. Feeding can be stressful and tiring. Gavage feedings may be ordered to decrease the infant's energy requirements, and small frequent feedings are given to prevent overdistention of the stomach and respiratory embarrassment. Care is taken to calm the infant if crying episodes increase cyanosis. Positioning the infant in a cardiac chair with the head and shoulders elevated can help to alleviate respiratory distress. Prevention of infection is also essential to reduce stress on the heart.

Although the prognosis for infants with congenital heart disease has improved over the years, parents may be overwhelmed with feelings of anxiety and guilt when informed that the infant has a heart defect. Nursing interventions are focused on repeating necessary explanations as needed, promoting initial interactions, and encouraging parental care giving as it becomes feasible. Parents may become particularly anxious when infants with cyanotic heart disease turn blue. Parents are taught specific techniques that may alleviate the cyanotic episode. CPR training is also provided. A discharge planning team should meet with parents well in advance of discharge to prepare them for home care (Brenner 1987, Higgins 1986).

Gastrointestinal Anomalies
Cleft Lip and Cleft Palate

Cleft lip is a result of the incomplete fusion of the nasomedical or intermaxillary process. The extent of the defect ranges from a slight dimpling in the lip area to the large bilateral clefts associated with cleft palate. With recent advances in facial cosmetic surgery, cleft lip repairs are very successful. Surgery may now be done soon after birth, which greatly improves the infant's ability to nipple-feed and gain weight.

Cleft palate results from incomplete fusion of the palatal process. The extent of the defect ranges from a small unilateral groove on the uvula to bilateral clefts that extend the entire length of the hard and soft palates and involve the nasal cavity (Fig. 35–4). Because there is an opening in the palate, the infant cannot create a vacuum in the mouth when sucking on a nipple. When the infant feeds, milk is often forced upward into the nasal cavity

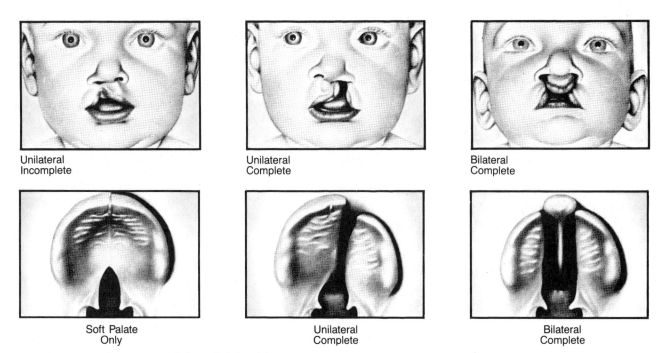

Unilateral
Incomplete

Unilateral
Complete

Bilateral
Complete

Soft Palate
Only

Unilateral
Complete

Bilateral
Complete

Figure 35–4. Variations in cleft lip and cleft palate.

and regurgitated through the nose. There may be problems with speech development and dentition if the defect is extensive. Surgical repair is undertaken between 12 and 18 months of age, when further development of the palate and jaw has occurred. Current techniques can produce excellent results, but several surgical procedures and orthodontia may be necessary before the repair is completed.

Immediately after birth, nursing care of the neonate with a cleft lip or palate is focused on assisting the infant to ingest nutrients without aspirating the milk or regurgitating it through the nose. Infants differ in their ability to feed. Some will be able to breast feed or take formula from a bottle with little difficulty. Others will require special equipment. A variety of special nipples are available (Fig. 35–5). Some have special phalanges that fit over the opening in the palate and improve the neonate's ability to suck. A small percentage of infants will fare better when fed with a spoon or a syringe with a soft tip. Once a satisfactory method is found, the nurse helps the parents become comfortable with feeding the infant before he is discharged home.

Esophageal Atresia and Tracheoesophageal Fistula

A variety of defects involving the trachea and esophagus occur when the two structures do not develop normally. The most frequently occurring anomaly results in the esophagus ending in a blind pouch (atresia) with a fistula that connects it to the trachea. The infant experi-

ences episodes of cyanosis and drooling of saliva. If he is fed sterile water or milk, the blind pouch will fill up, fluid will enter the trachea via the fistula, and the neonate will suffer acute respiratory distress and cyanosis. Immediate surgical intervention is essential. Although aspiration pneumonia is a frequent sequela, prognosis is excellent if the defect is not associated with other major anomalies.

Nursing care is aimed at preventing aspiration until surgery is performed. The infant ingests nothing by mouth, and a nasogastric catheter is passed into the blind pouch and attached to suction to prevent the accumulation of mucus in the esophagus. The nurse supports the infant's vital functions in a neutral thermal environment and administers IV fluids to prevent hypoglycemia.

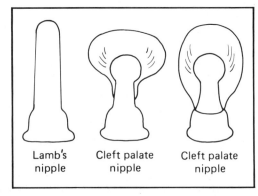

Lamb's
nipple

Cleft palate
nipple

Cleft palate
nipple

Figure 35–5. Cleft palate nipples. Lamb's nipple carries milk beyond palate defect to back of nasopharynx. Flange nipples can be trimmed to cover and fit palate defect.

Pyloric Stenosis

Pyloric stenosis is the congenital obstruction of the pylorus, the distal opening of the stomach through which gastric contents empty into the duodenum. Male infants are affected three to four times more frequently than females. The classic signs of this anomaly include vomiting, observable gastric peristaltic waves, and constipation. The condition is rarely diagnosed in the newborn nursery, unless the infant has an extended stay as a result of other problems experienced at birth. Most infants with pyloric stenosis begin to vomit in the third to fifth week of life. Surgical correction is indicated and consists of incision of the muscles of the pylorus. Today the prognosis is excellent after the defect is corrected.

Omphalocele/Gastroschisis

Omphalocele is the protrusion of abdominal contents through a defect in the ventral abdominal wall with herniation of abdominal viscera through an open umbilical ring. The protruding bowel is normally covered by a thin membrane composed of amnion and peritoneum. The umbilical cord inserts into this membrane with the umbilical arteries and vein contained within the sac. Omphalocele occurs in approximately 1 in 6000 live births. The protruding sac may contain small and large intestine, stomach, liver, spleen, bladder, uterus, and ovaries. Many other anomalies and syndromes are associated with omphalocele (*i.e.*, meningomyelocele, intracardiac defects, and trisomy syndromes) and complicate treatment and prognosis.

Gastroschisis is a much rarer anomaly, occurring in approximately 1 in 30,000 to 50,000 live births. The neonate is frequently premature. The disorder is characterized by evisceration of abdominal contents (intestines, stomach, gallbladder, uterus, fallopian tubes, bladder, undescended testes, and liver) through a full-thickness defect in the abdominal wall, usually located to the right of the umbilical cord. Associated anomalies are rare (Brentner 1987).

Immediate emergency surgery is required to reduce the bowel. If the defect is large, it may be impossible to reduce abdominal contents all at once. Several repairs may be needed over time. Prognosis is guarded if the defect is associated with other congenital anomalies or is very large and includes all major abdominal organs.

Immediately after birth, nursing interventions are aimed at protecting abdominal contents. The abdominal contents are covered with a sterile gauze moistened with warm sterile saline. A nasogastric tube is passed and attached to suction to prevent the intestines from becoming distended with air. The infant receives no nourishment by mouth, and intravenous therapy is initiated to prevent fluid and electrolyte imbalance and to supply needed calories for metabolic activity. The prevention of hypother-

mia, strict sterile technique to prevent infection, and maintenance of fluid and electrolyte balance are major nursing goals.

The physical appearance of the anomaly and the life-threatening nature of omphalocele or gastroschisis may result in shock and disbelief in parents. They may hesitate to form initial bonds with the neonate because of the guarded prognosis. Nursing interventions are aimed at reinforcing information provided by physicians, identifying grief responses, and functioning as a liaison between parents and the tertiary level hospital where the infant is transported. Before the neonate is transferred, the nurse may take photographs of the infant for the mother to keep, until she is well enough to be discharged home.

Intestinal Obstructions and Imperforate Anus

Intestinal obstructions in the neonate may range from a narrowing of the lumen to complete atresia. Twisting of a part of the intestine (volvulus) can also occur and will result in obstruction. The neonate may fail to pass meconium and experiences increasing abdominal distention. Vomiting occurs and may be bilious or fecal in nature. Surgical intervention is essential. If the obstruction is due to a simple defect, prognosis is good.

Imperforate anus is an anomaly of the lower rectum or anus. The extent of the defect ranges from a transparent membrane at the anal opening, which can be surgically incised, to a major obstruction in which the rectum ends in a blind pouch some distance from the anal orifice. Fistulas connecting the intestine with the bladder or vagina are frequently associated with imperforate anus. Surgical repair is essential and may require a temporary colostomy if the defect is some distance from the perineum. Prognosis is good.

Signs of intestinal obstruction are not immediately evident. When obstruction is suspected, nursing care is focused on the assessment of gastrointestinal function and supportive care that diminishes energy requirements for the neonate. The abdominal girth is measured frequently. Bowel sounds are auscultated. The infant's stooling pattern is monitored closely, and the nature and amount of vomitus is assessed. The infant is given nothing by mouth, and an orogastric tube is passed and attached to suction or gravity drainage. Intravenous therapy is administered to prevent fluid and electrolyte depletion and to meet the infant's energy requirements.

Genitourinary Anomalies
Hypospadias and Epispadias

Hypospadias is a condition in which the urethral opening is found on the ventral side, or underside, of the penis or on the perineum in males. In females born with hypospadias, the meatal urethra opens in the vagina. It is a fairly common anomaly in males (1 in 700 are born with some degree of the defect) and is usually corrected surgically shortly after the first year of life. Nurses should be aware that circumcision is not recommended when the male has hypospadias, because the foreskin is frequently useful in the later surgical correction of this anomaly.

Epispadias, a rare anomaly, is the congenital absence of the anterior wall of the urethra. It is more common in males and ranges in severity from a small meatal opening on the dorsal surface of the penis to a deep furrow or groove that extends its entire length. Epispadias is often associated with other major genitourinary anomalies, including exstrophy of the bladder. Surgical repair is also indicated with this defect.

Ambiguous Genitalia

A small proportion of infants are born with anomalies of the genitalia, which make it impossible to identify their sex. These anomalies may be associated with defects in the internal reproductive organs. Chromosomal studies are done to determine the infant's biologic sex, and reconstructive surgery is done as soon as possible to prevent gender identity problems. Because of their concerns about sexuality, gender identity, and reproductive functioning, parents of infants with ambiguous genitalia and other genitourinary anomalies require special support and counseling. Health team members skilled in the repair and treatment of these anomalies are best prepared to discuss the long-term consequences of the particular defect.

Exstrophy of the Bladder and Patent Urachus

Exstrophy of the bladder results from incomplete closure of the abdominal wall and pubic arch. The bladder is exposed on the surface of the abdomen, and the anterior wall of the bladder is absent, exposing its inner surface. As urine enters the bladder, it drains directly onto the skin surface surrounding the defect. Surgical repair is essential. Results are often poor because of associated anomalies of the ureters, and an ileal conduit may have to be constructed connecting the ureters to the small intestine.

Patent urachus is the persistence of a fetal opening between the bladder and the base of the umbilical cord. Urine constantly drains onto the surface of the abdomen. Surgical repair is done early.

Nursing care of infants with anomalies of the bladder is aimed at preventing infection. With exstrophy of the bladder, a sterile covering is placed over the bladder to protect it. Meticulous skin care is essential to prevent breakdown from the constant drainage of urine.

Musculoskeletal Anomalies
Congenital Hip Dysplasia

The infant born with congenital hip dysplasia has an abnormally formed acetabulum. The acetabulum is most often shallow and imperfectly rimmed with cartilage so that the head of the femur does not fit snugly into the hip capsule. The femoral head may ride on the lateral edge of the acetabulum in a state of partial dislocation (subluxation), or it may be completely dislocated above the acetabular rim (luxation). This anomaly is found approximately six times more frequently in female infants than in males and is a potentially crippling disorder associated with degenerative arthritis in adult life.

Congenital hip dysplasia is detected by inspecting the dorsal gluteal folds for asymmetry in appearance and performing Ortolani's maneuver (see Chapter 31) to identify hip instability. A significant "clunking" noise may be heard or an appreciable sudden movement or "jerk" in the upper thigh can be felt when it is abducted and when the dislocated femoral head is reduced and moves back into the acetabulum.

Treatment consists of reducing the femoral head into the acetabulum and maintaining its position while muscle and cartilage develop and a stable hip capsule forms. This is accomplished through use of an appliance that causes abduction and external rotation of the femur, such as a Frejka pillow splint or Pavlik harness. In some cases the use of triple diapers may be sufficient to reduce the head of the femur into the acetabulum.

Prognosis is good if the anomaly is identified and treated in the neonatal period. A delay of even several months may necessitate surgical reduction of the femur and some permanent limitation in function.

A thorough assessment of hip stability by the nurse will aid in the early diagnosis of the anomaly. Once the infant is fitted with the appropriate orthopedic device, care is directed toward preparing the parents for home care, and helping them to feel comfortable holding and caring for the infant while he remains in the appliance.

Talipes Equinovarus

Talipes, commonly known as "clubfoot," is a congenital deformity of the ankle and foot. A variety of talipes deformities occur, and their characteristic appearance is determined by the degree and extent to which the muscles and tendons of the foot, ankle, and leg are shortened or atrophied. In the most common form (talipes equinovarus), the heel is turned toward the midline of the body (inversion) and the foot is fixed in a position of plantar flexion. In valgus deformities the heel is turned outward from the midline of the body.

Treatment of talipes deformity consists of correcting the position of the foot and heel by applying successive plaster casts during infancy. Denis-Browne splints may also be used. The device consists of foot plates attached to a rigid crossbar. When the child begins to walk, he is fitted with specially designed orthopedic shoes to maintain the foot in the correct position. Prognosis is quite favorable if treatment is initiated in the neonatal period.

Nursing care is directed toward supporting the parents and educating them about the anomaly. Most infants with talipes are placed in plaster casts before they are discharged from the nursery. The nurse prepares the parent for home care, explaining why the cast is applied, how to keep it clean, and what signs of complication (*i.e.,* compromised circulation and pressure sores) to watch for. Many parents may be afraid to hold or cuddle the infant in a cast, and the nurse must demonstrate proper handling and support parents in their initial attempts to hold their infant.

Chromosomal Abnormalities

The student may find it helpful to review Chapter 9, Genetics and Genetic Counseling.

Trisomies (Including Down Syndrome)

The normal neonate is born with 46 chromosomes in 23 pairs. The presence of a third chromosome results in a trisomy. The extra chromosome can be found attached to different chromosome pairs and results in identifiable syndromes frequently associated with mental retardation and multiple congenital anomalies.

Down syndrome (formerly known as Mongolism) results from the presence of an extra chromosome at pair 21 or 22 or a translocation usually involving pairs 15 and 21. Infants with Down syndrome present with a variety of signs that aid in the initial tentative diagnosis, which is confirmed by chromosomal studies. The infant may have close-set, slanting eyes with narrow palpebral fissures. The nose is flat, and the tongue appears large and protrudes from the mouth. The fingers are short and thick, and there is incurving of the little finger. A simian crease may be apparent on the palmar surfaces. The infant's mental capacity is impaired, and the multiple congenital anomalies frequently associated with the syndrome include cardiac and gastrointestinal tract defects. Recent advances in surgical repair of cardiac and gastrointestinal anomalies have improved the life expectancy of infants with Down syndrome, but mental capacity is still limited.

Some infants with Down syndrome will be stable at birth and free of life-threatening anomalies. In such cases nursing interventions are aimed at supporting parents and helping them work through the grieving process. If major anomalies are evident, nursing care is focused on providing the specific support required by the congenital defects. Genetic counseling is indicated to assist parents

in understanding the extent of the anomaly and the probability of recurrence with future pregnancies. A social worker may be involved in discharge planning to assist parents who chose to place the infant in a special care facility. If the infant is discharged home to the parents, referrals to a public health nurse or visiting nurse will be made.

Inborn Errors of Metabolism

The neonate with an inborn error in metabolism has an enzyme deficiency that results in aberrations in protein, fat, or carbohydrate metabolism. Accumulation of toxic metabolites may cause permanent brain damage or death in the severest forms of this disorder. An inborn error of metabolism is an inherited defect usually transmitted by an autosomal recessive gene (two heterozygous parents who carry the trait produce a homozygous infant with the disease). Recent advances in detection make it possible to screen neonates for many of the disorders within several days of birth before the abnormal metabolites in the blood stream and brain reach toxic levels.

Phenylketonuria

One of the first inborn errors in metabolism to be recognized and treated was phenylketonuria (PKU). Infants with PKU lack the enzyme phenylalanine hydroxylase and are unable to convert the amino acid phenylalanine to tyrosine. Phenylalanine is an essential amino acid found in breast milk and most formulas. Once the infant with PKU ingests milk, phenylpyruvic acid and phenylacetic acid, abnormal metabolites of phenylalanine, begin to accumulate in the body. If untreated, the infant will show symptoms of failure to thrive, including vomiting, listlessness, and poor weight gain. Signs of central nervous system damage and mental retardation are evident as early as 6 months of age.

The incidence of PKU is estimated at 1 in 1500 live births and is highest in white populations in the United States and in people of northern European descent. Most states require a neonatal screening test for PKU in all newborn nurseries. Because screening equipment may not detect the disorder when abnormal metabolites are present in very low concentrations in the neonate's blood stream, it is essential that the test be delayed for at least 24 hours after milk feedings are initiated.

Treatment and Prognosis. Treatment of PKU consists of the dietary restriction of foods high in phenylalanine. The infant with PKU is placed on a special formula, low in this essential amino acid. As phenylalanine is found in most animal and vegetable products, parents require ongoing support and instruction regarding food restrictions and the preparation of meals for the growing child with PKU.

There is controversy over how long a child with PKU

should remain on a low phenylalanine diet. Because brain growth slows after age 6, some clinicians advocate lifting the severest dietary restrictions at this time. Other practitioners contend that myelination of brain cells continues through early adult life, and dietary restriction of foods high in phenylalanine should continue. Recent evidence has confirmed that infants born to women with PKU who have not limited their phenylalanine intake during pregnancy have an increased risk for central nervous system damage and mental retardation.

The risk of permanent neurologic impairment is minimized if treatment of PKU is started before the infant is 3 months old. The long-term prognosis for normal brain growth and development is excellent if PKU is detected and treatment is begun in the neonatal period. For optimum effectiveness, the diet should be started before 3 weeks of life.

Nursing Intervention.   Nursing intervention in the detection of PKU involves careful notation regarding the initiation of feeding so that screening tests can be performed at the proper time. Nurses also perform the screening test; thus it is essential that the nurse collect the blood specimen accurately. Parent education is particularly important today as an increasing number of families are involved in early discharge programs and infants are sent home before the neonatal screening tests can be performed. The nurse must be sure that parents understand the importance of returning to the hospital, clinic, or pediatrician's office for the test after milk feedings are established.

Branched-Chain Ketoaciduria (Maple Syrup Urine Disease)

Recent research has led to the discovery and understanding of other metabolic disorders in which aberrations in enzyme pathways lead to the accumulation of toxic metabolites. Two rare disorders of protein metabolism that can now be detected by neonatal screening tests are maple syrup urine disease and homocystinuria. Infants with maple syrup urine disease (MSUD) have an enzyme defect that prevents the metabolism of three amino acids: leucine, isoleucine, and valine. The untreated infant shows signs of central nervous system injury within several days after milk feedings have been started. The urine of an untreated infant has a characteristic maple syrup odor. A special formula (MSUD Formula) low in the three amino acids has recently been developed. Dietary restrictions are observed throughout early childhood, as in cases of PKU. The prognosis for normal neurologic development of the child in whom MSUD is diagnosed and treated within the first weeks of life appears promising.

Homocystinuria

Homocystinuria is a rare metabolic disorder in which an enzyme defect prevents the conversion of the amino acid methionine to cystine. The infant with homocystinuria exhibits signs of central nervous system damage, which, if untreated results in mental retardation. Dietary restriction of methionine is the required treatment for this inborn error in metabolism. Long-term neurologic prognosis is good when the disorder is detected early and treated promptly.

Galactosemia

Galactosemia is an inborn error of carbohydrate metabolism, which can be detected by neonatal screening tests. The neonate with galactosemia is unable to convert galactose into glucose. As galactose levels rise in the blood stream, signs of central nervous system involvement appear (lethargy, poor feeding, seizures). The early diagnosis and treatment of galactosemia (removal of galactose from the diet) reverses the central nervous system signs. Prognosis for normal neurologic development is excellent.

Congenital Hypothyroidism

One cause of congenital hypothyroidism is an inherited enzymatic deficiency that prevents the normal synthesis of thyroid hormone. The infant may appear normal at birth but soon develops early signs of thyroid insufficiency, including failure to thrive (poor feeding, poor weight gain, and lethargy), neonatal jaundice, and constipation. If untreated, the infant will demonstrate an arrested growth pattern and mental retardation. Neonatal screening tests can now detect congenital hypothyroidism. Prompt treatment with the appropriate dosage of thyroid medication reverses early signs and prevents retardation.

LEGAL/ETHICAL ISSUES

Today, ethical concerns related to quality of life and financial concerns, including the need to contain spiraling health care costs, are involved in the decision to provide or withhold care from the infant born with a congenital defect. Tertiary care centers have ethics committees to help parents and health team members deal with the problems surrounding the birth of an infant with a defect. Genetic counselors are also available to discuss with the family the known causes of the defect and the probability the anomaly will recur in subsequent pregnancies.

Recently, the federal government has become involved in the decision-making process through the so-called "Baby Doe" regulations intended to ensure that infants

LEGAL/ETHICAL CONSIDERATION

Ethical Dilemmas and Decision Making in the Nursing Care of Sick Infants

As survival rates for smaller and sicker neonates improve each year, neonatal intensive care nurses are confronted with greater numbers of complex moral and ethical dilemmas. Some of the most commonly faced issues include resuscitation of very-low-birth-weight infants, withdrawal of life support systems, hydration and feeding of severely handicapped neonates, parent participation in treatment decisions and the rights of infants as research subjects.

The American Nurses' Association Code for Nurses (1976) provides a mandate for nursing participation in ethical decision making and several bioethical decision-making models have been developed to facilitate moral reasoning in nursing practice. Thompson and Thompson (1985) list ten steps, which may be employed to explore an ethical issue:

1. Review the situation to determine the ethical dilemma, decisions to be made, and individuals involved
2. Gather any additional data needed to clarify the issue
3. Identify the key ethical issue
4. Define the professional moral responsibilities
5. Identify the moral values of the individuals involved
6. Identify value conflicts
7. Determine who should be responsible for decision-making
8. Identify a range of actions and possible outcomes
9. Decide on a course of action and carry it out
10. Evaluate the results

Thompson JE, Thompson HO: Bioethical Decision-Making for Nurses. Norwalk, CT, Appleton-Century-Crofts, 1985

with serious congenital anomalies receive needed care, even if there are doubts as to their viability and expected quality of life. The United States Supreme Court has since struck down the "Baby Doe" rules, stating that the federal government cannot force hospitals to treat severely handicapped infants over the objections of their parents.

Presently, what the appropriate roles are for parents, health care professionals, and the government in the decision-making process concerning the treatment of the impaired child is being heatedly debated. The Supreme Court decision does leave intact the traditional role of states in regulating these matters. State courts can appoint guardians when parents make decisions the court considers "against the best interests of the child." All hospitals are encouraged to establish review committees composed of medical, legal, and ethics specialists. Nursing professionals must take their place on these committees to provide input and sustain excellence in practice.

Nurses caring for the neonate must examine and understand their own values and belief system before they attempt to care for families with high-risk infants. There are no easy answers to the questions being raised. Our current technologic capabilities have pushed us beyond the current legal and moral codes, which were established by society during an era when most critically ill babies simply died because there were no medical solutions to their problems.

Regardless of personal convictions, the nurse must convey respect for the acceptance of the parents' feelings and beliefs. The major objective of care should be to provide the neonate with the highest level of nursing care possible regardless of the elected course of medical treatment or prognosis.

IMPLICATIONS FOR NURSING CARE

The nurse involved in the care of a family whose neonates are found to have congenital anomalies must be prepared for a complex situation with emotional, ethical, technologic, medical, and nursing factors that influence outcomes. Such families are often in need of the most technologically sophisticated medical and nursing care as well as the most sensitive emotional care. In addition to providing necessary care for the neonate, the nurse must provide caring and knowledgeable support as parents come to grips with the perceived threat to their newborn's health and well-being. This field is increasingly specialized; the nurse who provided labor and birth care is not only responsible for providing initial nursing care but also for interacting effectively with a team of neonatal care providers to ensure that family needs are met.

CHAPTER SUMMARY

While the birth of a neonate with a congenital anomaly remains relatively rare, when it occurs, knowledgeable and sensitive nursing care is needed for both the neonate and the parents. Perinatal regionalization has made it possible for such families to receive specialized care for major congenital anomalies. However, initial nursing care for the neonate must be based on an understanding of the nature of the anomaly in order to provide the necessary physical support in preparation for transport to a referral hospital. Further, nurses involved in perinatal care must examine and understand their own beliefs and values because technologic advances in the care of compromised neonates have created ethical dilemmas for providers and parents alike.

STUDY QUESTIONS

1. How can the nurse best support parents immediately after the birth of an infant with a congenital anomaly?
2. What is the major goal of nursing care of the neonate with a cardiac anomaly?
3. What is the primary form of treatment for all neonates who have inborn errors of metabolism?
4. What strategies can the neonatal nurse employ to deal effectively with legal-ethical dilemmas?

REFERENCES/BIBLIOGRAPHY

Avery GB: Neonatology: Pathophysiology and Management of the Newborn, 3rd ed. Philadelphia, JB Lippincott, 1987
Brenner VM: Unilateral pulmonary hypoplasia/agenesis in the neonate. Neonat Network 6(3):49–57, 1987
Brentner S: Abdominal wall defects: Omphalocele and gastroschisis. Neonat Network 6(3):29–41, 1987
Higgins SS, Kashani IA: The cyanotic child: Heart defects and parental learning needs. MCN 11:259–262, 1986

SUGGESTED READINGS

Penticuff JH: Neonatal nursing ethics: Toward a consensus. Neonat Network 5(6):7–15, 1987
Raff B: The use of homemaker–home health aides, perinatal care of high-risk infants. J Obstet Gynecol Neonate Nurs 15:142–145, 1986

36 individual and family adaptation in the fourth trimester

LEARNING OBJECTIVES

After studying the material in this chapter the student should be able to

- Identify nursing goals and objectives for families during the fourth trimester

- Describe expanding family developmental tasks

- Describe frequent and unanticipated stressors experienced by parents and families in the fourth trimester

- Discuss myths about parenthood

- Cite two components of parental role taking

- Describe three factors that affect parental role taking

- Discuss nursing actions that promote parental role taking

- Assess family adaptation during the fourth trimester

- Identify families at risk for healthy adaptation during the fourth trimester

- Discuss approaches to nursing care in the fourth trimester

- Initiate intervention strategies to foster healthy adaptation in the fourth trimester

- Develop a fourth-trimester teaching plan that fosters self-care within the family

KEY TERMS

Acquaintance

Adaptation

Adaptive demand

Attachment

Bonding

Cues

Fourth trimester

Infant behavioral assessment

Parent–infant interaction

Parental role taking

Stress

Developmental Tasks for Families

Expectancy Phase

Anticipates providing for the physical care of the expected baby

Adapts family financial pattern

Defines evolving role patterns

Adjusts patterns of sexual expression to pregnancy

Expands communication systems to meet present and anticipated emotional needs

Reorients relationships with relatives

Adapts relationships with friends and community at large to realities of pregnancy

Acquires knowledge and plans for specifics of pregnancy, childbirth, and parenthood

Maintains morale and philosophy of life

Expanding Phase

Reconciles conflicting concepts of roles
  Demonstrates parental role taking
  Reconciles fantasized expectations with reality

Accepts and adjusts to the strains and pressures of parenthood
  Exhibits intrafamily cooperation
  Demonstrates mutual parental support by sharing infant caretaking and family maintenance tasks
  Describes realistic perception of stressors
  Demonstrates appropriate active problem-solving behavior
  Mobilizes support systems to augment family resources

Learns to care for infant with confidence and competence
  Demonstrates appropriate identification of infant cues
  Demonstrates appropriate caretaking behaviors
  Expresses positive regard for characteristics of infant and pleasure in his or her thriving

Establishes and maintains a family wellness lifestyle
  Demonstrates appropriate postpartum physiologic restoration
  Demonstrates awareness of and compliance with basic health concepts of nutrition, hydration, rest, hygiene, exercise, recreation, and stress reduction

Nurtures development of infant and young child
  Demonstrates appropriate verbal and tactile communication
  Provides appropriate sensory stimulation
  Demonstrates knowledge of age-specific safety hazards and realistic protection of infant
  Exhibits awareness of unique temperament of child and modifies nurturing behavior accordingly

Promotes marital relationship
  Reestablishes satisfactory sexual, emotional, and recreational interaction
  Maintains open, effective patterns of communication

Adjusts to practical realities of expanding family life
  Adapts to limits of time, space, and privacy
  Develops appropriate priorities for utilization of family resources

Maintains personal autonomy of family members
  Encourages expression of sense of self with personal values and interests
  Promotes expression of and respect for individuality of members
  Promotes individual growth and development of members

Explores and develops sense of family identity
  Establishes sense of family cohesion, affection, and shared goals
  Demonstrates positive regard for peer group and community at large
  Exhibits traditions and values reflecting cultural heritage and family identity

After Duvall E: In Donaldson NE: The postpartum follow-up clinician role—a design for extending the scope of nursing practice. Master's project, 1979, California State University at Los Angeles

The traditional emphasis on care during pregnancy limits one's appreciation of the major adaptations required immediately after birth and during the puerperium. This unique period in the family life cycle is surely the "fourth trimester" of the childbearing year.

Nursing care, defined by the ANA in its Social Policy Statement as *the diagnosis and treatment of human responses to actual or potential health problems,* is critical to families trying to adapt to life with a new infant. Well into the first year of parenthood, nursing care should focus on the complex adaptive demands facing mothers, fathers, infants, and siblings.

Support of families during the fourth trimester is enhanced by the nurse's ability to establish a therapeutic rapport. Focusing on the unique strengths and stresses of each family enables the nurse to reinforce and nurture healthy adaptation, as well as further assess and monitor potentially maladaptive responses. Because families may be quite receptive to even minimal intervention during periods of disequilibrium or crisis, the nurse has a unique opportunity to monitor and support healthy adaptive outcomes.

This chapter discusses adaptations the family makes to the new family member and the nurse's role in seeing that the transition is positive and healthy. Developmental tasks, stressors, and role taking in the family are all discussed in this chapter. The chapter also follows the nurse's role in assessment and care planning during the fourth trimester, considering former problems of the family; assessment of current family roles and behaviors; and various strategies that can be used to facilitate optimal family adaptation.

THE FOURTH TRIMESTER

Required adaptations in the fourth trimester are both physiologic and psychosocial. The normal processes of involution and restoration following pregnancy and birth occur while the mother and father must also reorganize their life style and routines to meet the needs of their infant and maintain an environment that meets their own needs and those of their other children. This unique transition in the family life cycle has received attention from researchers in the social sciences for well over two decades.

The period following the birth of a child has been described as a "normal crisis," a "moderate or severe crisis," or the "transition to parenthood." Regardless of the terminology used, there is ample evidence that the birth of a child makes major adaptive demands on the family and that current modes of health care delivery may not be meeting the needs of the childbearing family. Most families see health care providers during the intrapartum and immediate postpartum period but may not have regular contact again until the routine well-baby check and the routine postpartum check. The initial 2-week period is a critical time for maternal restoration, infant adaptation, and establishment of feeding and sleeping patterns. By 2 weeks, and certainly by 6 weeks, the family has made major adjustments for better or worse.

A review of the changes that occur in family relationships during the fourth trimester illustrates the complex nature of this period. Childbirth leads a couple to reassess their roles as spouses and then as mother and father. Each parent must establish a relationship with the infant. Children must also renegotiate their "standing" in the family and begin to relate to the new infant as a sibling. Each set of family relationships must be reestablished or renegotiated after the birth of an infant. Thus, the fourth trimester is a period of reorganization and adaptation by all members of the family and by the family as a whole.

This process of family adaptation and reorganization may create turbulence and disequilibrium. The accompanying stress, although an essential ingredient of healthy reorganization, is a stimulus for crisis and potential maladaptation. A family's inability to adapt during the fourth trimester may reflect maternal physiologic complications, marital discord, sibling distress, or infant health and development trauma. Families having trouble adapting can benefit from a continuity of care during the months after birth; during this period, the nurse can monitor the family's progress, provide needed support, and initiate intervention.

Family Development: The Expanding Family

The transition of parenthood is typically defined as encompassing two phases; the *expectancy phase,* which involves the developmental tasks inherent in the process of pregnancy and birth, and the *expanding phase,* which encompasses the developmental demands of integrating the new family member, initial adaptation in the postpartum period, and continuing growth in the first years of child-rearing. As discussed in Chapter 12, the tasks the family faces during the expectancy phase are biologically triggered and urgent to the extent that pregnancy is time limited. The tasks of the expanding phase are initiated following birth and continue over a longer period. Expectancy-phase tasks are reviewed in the accompanying display, opposite page.

The nurse can use family development theory with its concept of developmental tasks as a basis for nursing care during the childbearing year. Developmental task attainment, as reflected in observable behaviors, can guide the clinician in her assessment of the family. Data about family adaptation can be collected from health care records, through personal contact, or from telephone interviews. When they come in contact with health care providers, mothers often describe their own efforts to deal with these developmental challenges, thus providing the nurse with valuable information for assessing family status.

Parental Role Taking

CLASSIFIED ADVERTISING
WANTED: Infant Care-giver

Infant seeks relaxed, easy-going, loving type. Should enjoy holding, cuddling, and comforting. Be able to hold baby patiently for feedings every 2 to 4 hours without fidgeting. Light sleeper, early riser desired. Must be willing to work all shifts, 7-day week. No degree necessary. No vacation unless can arrange substitute TLC.

How many new parents are adequately prepared for the reality of parenthood? Myths about parenthood are fueled by media distortions, old wives' tales, and folklore. Expectant parents are bombarded with information about the miracle of birth and the romance of parenthood. Research shows that new parents' expectations of their newborns vary widely and are usually unrealistic with respect to behavioral, developmental, and interactional capacities. The newborn is known to be an active individual with unique characteristics and able to influence the environment. Table 36–1 lists common myths about newborns, as well as facts about newborn behavior and capabilities.

The Process of Parental Role Taking

Parents adopt their roles within a framework of complex beliefs and expectations. Perhaps the ultimate truth about parenthood is that it requires continuous growth and adaptation. Parenting is learned by doing; taking on the parental role means plunging into new territory, and that territory is different with every child. Furthermore, the transition into parenthood is abrupt and irrevocable.

Much study has been devoted to the process of mater-nal role taking and mother–infant interaction. Much less is known about the father. The nurse must recognize that parental role taking may vary between fathers and mothers. Most current scientific knowledge on attachment has come from research on mothers and should therefore be applied cautiously to father–infant relationships. However, there is evidence that the processes of acquaintance, bonding, and attachment are similar in fathers and mothers, although they may be demonstrated in slightly different ways and to different degrees.

Acquaintance

Acquaintance, the natural beginning of all human relationships, begins when the new parents gather information about and form impressions of their infant. This involves comparing the "real" infant to the expected or fantasized newborn with respect to such characteristics as gender and size. These first impressions form the basis for later attachment. Continued acquaintance provides the opportunity for the parents to reinforce or change their initial views of the infant. The parents may then celebrate the realization of their expectations or grieve at the loss of a fantasized child.

Table 36–1 **Folklore and Facts About Infants**

Folklore	Facts
Infants are sweet and cute.	Every infant has a unique inborn temperament.
Newborn infants can't see.	Newborn infants are visually responsive and demonstrate intense visual interest in the human face.
Newborn infants can't hear.	Newborn infants have acute hearing; they will quiet, try visually to locate a sound, and move their extremities in response to rhythmic speech patterns.
Between feedings, newborn infants sleep all the time.	Newborn infants display six states of consciousness, including deep sleep, crying, and quiet alertness. Every infant establishes a unique sleep-activity pattern.
Newborn infant smiles are no more than a response to intestinal gas.	Many newborns demonstrate the ability to smile in response to caretaker smiles.
Newborn infants are helpless and oblivious to their surroundings.	Newborn infants demonstrate a full repertoire of adaptive behaviors, including the ability to shut out noxious stimuli, to withdraw from painful stimuli, and to console themselves with hand-to-mouth activity.
Girls are harder to rear than boys (or vice versa)	Gender is not a major determinant of temperamental characteristics; it is the *clustering* of temperamental characteristics that results in some infants being more difficult to care for than others.
Infants aren't capable of learning.	Infants explore their environment through sight and sound, become bored with repetitious stimuli, differentiate among sensory stimuli, and respond accordingly; they learn from an environment that is sensitive to their cues and responds appropriately.
Infants can't communicate.	Infants demonstrate a full range of visual, verbal, and motor behaviors that reflect pleasure, pain, fatigue, and hunger and that should serve as cues for care-givers.
Infant behavior and development are determined by the love and parenting ability of the caretakers.	Infant behavior and development are the result of a complex interaction among the innate characteristics of the infant, the environment, and the caretakers.

After Erickson M: Trends in assessing the newborn and his parents. MCN 3:99, 1978

Bonding and Attachment

Bonding and attachment are two components of parental role taking. *Bonding* is unidirectional, from parent to child; it has been described as "a rapid process occurring immediately after birth, which reflects mother-to-infant attachment. Bonding is facilitated by skin-to-skin contact, suckling, and mutual visual regard" (Campbell 1979). *Attachment* is bidirectional, or reciprocal, between parent and infant. Attachment is the tie of affection and mutual devotion between infant and parents, which grows during the first year (Campbell 1979).

The research of Klaus and Kennell in the 1970s on early parent–neonate contact significantly altered perinatal health care by focusing attention on the importance of early interaction (Klaus 1982). The researchers hypothesized the existence of a "sensitive period" immediately following birth, during which time bonding is facilitated. Many investigators explored the effects of changes in traditional postpartum practices (usually early or extended mother–infant contact) on later breast-feeding, child health, and child development. A link between high-risk birth, which interferes with early mother–infant contact, and child neglect and abuse was proposed; however, debate continues about the validity of the conclusions drawn, with some researchers questioning whether the effects of early mother–newborn contact are strong enough to overcome other, more damaging risk factors. Suffice it to say that parent–infant bonding and later attachment are a result of the complex interaction of variables among parents, infant, and environment. The early parent–infant relationship forms the foundation of later child health and development.

Factors Affecting Parental Role Taking

Research suggests that background factors, infant characteristics, and perinatal hospital experiences affect the process of acquaintance. The accompanying display summarizes variables in maternal and family background that affect maternal adaptation and, ultimately, maternal role taking. Although much less is known about the factors that affect fathers, some are likely to be the same.

The Powerful Newborn

Infant characteristics can be described in terms of temperament and capacity for interaction, both of which affect parental confidence and feelings of competence in parenting. Brazelton's Newborn Behavioral Assessment Scale measures the unique response repertoire of the infant to animate and inanimate environmental stimuli. Clarity of cues, responsiveness to care-giver, consolability, and smile are some of the factors assessed by the scale. (For a more detailed discussion of this scale, see Chapter 31.) Infant characteristics cluster to make each infant uniquely "easy" or "difficult" from the perspective of the care-giver.

The Hospital Environment

The perinatal hospital setting is usually where parent–infant acquaintance begins. When the hospital environment promotes opportunities for parents to identify, explore, and interact with their infant, and to discover their ability to successfully care for their infant, acquaintance thrives. Numerous studies have examined strategies that foster early parent–infant relationships. The results suggest that individualized family-centered care, continuity of care, and minimal parent–infant separation support the development of healthy early parent–infant relationships. During the first part of the fourth trimester the primary task of the mother is to establish a suitable meshing of mothering activities with the baby's cues. The

---

Factors Affecting Maternal Role Taking

Self Concept and Personality Traits
  Ego strength, adaptability, hostility, self-esteem, age
Support System
  Relationships with mate, family; friendship patterns
  Confidence in adequacy of support if needed
Perceptions of Birth Experience
  Definition of pregnancy (wanted/desired); affiliation with fetus
  Impact of events on expectations, self-worth, and early mother–infant interactions
Early Mother–Infant Separation
  Opportunities for infant identification, acquaintance, and care giving
  Amount and quality of contact with infant
Maternal Illness
  Severity of, duration of, and impact on self-worth and parent–infant interaction
Social Stress
  Presence and mutuality with significant other
  Frequency and intensity of life-change events during pregnancy and postbirth period
Infant's Behavioral Style
  Impact of clustered temperament traits, responsiveness, clarity of cues, and sleep–wake patterns
Childrearing Beliefs
  Knowledge, experience, expectations, and interpersonal style

After Mercer R: A theoretical framework for studying factors that impact on the maternal role. Nurs Res 30(2):73–77, 1981

process of acquaintance sets the stage for achieving this task.

Frequent and Unanticipated Stressors

Numerous studies have identified the adaptive demands placed on the mother during the postpartum period. Stressors frequently cited include the following:

- Physiologic restoration
- Changes in body image
- Fatigue/sleep deprivation
- Role conflict (parent, spouse, worker)
- Understanding and meeting infant needs

Additional studies have explored and described additional, unanticipated maternal stressors:

- Preterm birth
- Cesarean birth
- Infant birth defects
- Maternal complications

Although research on new fathers is much less extensive, many of these stressors logically affect the father as well. While parents each cope with their individual stressors, they must also adapt to the changing spousal subsystem. Communication, roles, and sexuality evolve significantly between adult partners following the birth of a child. Maintaining adult intimacy and nurturing each other is a continuing challenge to the couple.

In addition, parenthood is the 1990's presents opportunities and involves vulnerabilities unknown to previous generations. Expanding career options for women, increased access to education, and rapid social change have resulted in conflicting priorities for men and women in their adult roles. Family mobility and suburban/metropolitan living have reduced access to supportive extended family. This often means that the advice and practical assistance traditionally provided to new parents by supportive friends and relatives may no longer be forthcoming.

The presence of multiple stressors, including the need for family reorganization, contributes to the sense of crisis felt by many in the fourth trimester.

When new parents confront a problem and discover their initial attempts to solve it are inadequate, they feel anxious and stressed. When further attempts to resolve the problem continue to be unsuccessful, a stressor may precipitate a crisis.

Although expectant parents may be aware that unanticipated stressors do occur, most are not prepared to meet them. Preterm birth, cesarean birth, birth defects, and maternal and infant trauma all affect the family's adaptation in the fourth trimester. The impact of unanticipated events is individual to each family, according to their definition of the events and their emotional, social,

and physical resources. Nursing care of families experiencing unanticipated stressors, in addition to the common stressors of the fourth trimester, must be a priority. Figure 36-1 shows the effects of stressors on the family during the transition to parenthood and how postpartum clinical nursing care may help.

Maternal Adaptation. Maternal physiologic adaptations are complex. During the first weeks following birth, restorative processes related to maternal involution are underway; these include endometrial healing (lochial drainage and accompanying uterine contractions), perineal healing, endocrine shifts, lactation initiation or suppression, and reestablishment of normal bowel and bladder function. Additional physiologic concerns may include lingering headaches and assorted neuromuscular discomforts. Thus, the mother must deal with the psychosocial adaptive demands of the fourth trimester while also experiencing significant postpartum physiologic changes.

Although pregnancy only gradually alters the appearance of the mother's body, it is common for mothers to expect an instant return to their prepregnant physical appearance immediately after birth. Mothers often measure their postpartum progress in terms of their return to a desired physical dimension. Does the dress fit? Can the jeans be zipped? Will the blouse button? Helping mothers to accept involution as a gradual process of restoration and healing and not to turn to fad diets or panic fasting is a common nursing intervention. Realistic planning to achieve their desired physical appearance between 6 months and 1 year after birth helps mothers gain control of their bodies without compromising their health during the fourth trimester.

In addition to physiologic changes, acute and chronic fatigue is a universal stressor of the fourth trimester. Because infants are not neurologically mature enough to sustain a sleep state comparable to that of adults, new parents suffer from sleep interruption or deprivation for several weeks. Fatigue will exacerbate postpartum anemia, infection, or other physiologic stress. The new mother who attempts to resume her normal roles and full activities too soon may also suffer from extraordinary fatigue. Mothers find their psychic energy often exceeds their physical energy during the postpartum period. Healthy adaptation requires setting priorities, reorganizing, and using supports and help resources. Anticipating fatigue and planning for adequate rest are essential both in the last trimester of pregnancy and immediately postpartum.

Role conflict is often triggered by fatigue. Inability to fulfill previous roles and ambivalence about new roles frustrate new parents. Expectations confront reality during the postpartum period. Parents must deal with the loss of autonomy, privacy, and spontaneity and must re-

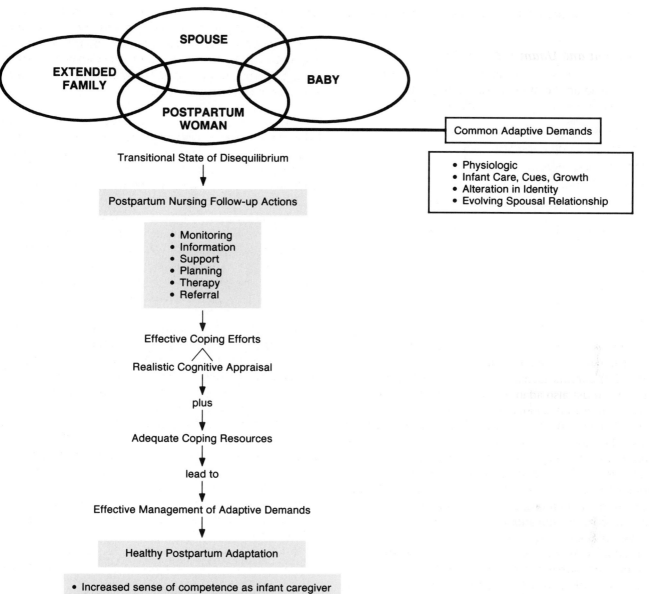

Figure 36–1. Effect of nursing services on maternal adaptation during the postpartum period. (Redrawn from Donaldson N: Effect of Telephone Postpartum Follow-up: A Clinical Trial. Doctoral Dissertation, University of California, San Francisco, 1988)

negotiate their roles. Finally, as parents move through the fourth trimester, they develop growing confidence and feelings of competence in their roles as partners and parents.

Perhaps the key to the perceived confidence of the new mother is her ability to meet the needs of her infant and obtain feedback that her care is adequate. Reading infant cues and successfully feeding and comforting her infant are her primary concerns, which are relieved or worsened through the "reactive" tasks of feeding, bathing, and diapering. Feedback from the infant, such as allowing himself or herself to be comforted, periods of quiet alertness,

and appropriate sleep patterns, encourages the mother in her efforts. Mastering the basics of infant care requires information, reinforcement, practice, and feedback; the mother can discover the unique behavioral capacity of her infant by meeting the child's physical needs. Reassurance by health care providers that the infant is gaining weight and "looking good" affirms the mother's feelings of adequacy (Fig. 36–2).

Paternal Adaptation. The father also experiences a variety of stressors during the fourth trimester. However, because the father rarely has contact with health profes-

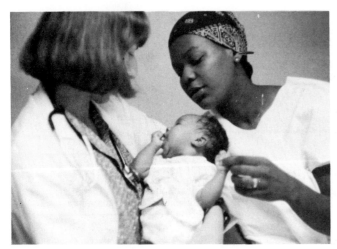

Figure 36–2. Nurse with mother and baby at well-baby check. The nurse has an excellent opportunity to assess the adaptation of mother and infant at the well-baby check, and to reassure the mother that her care-giving is satisfactory. (Courtesy of John B. Franklin Maternity Hospital, formerly Booth Maternity Center, Philadelphia, PA)

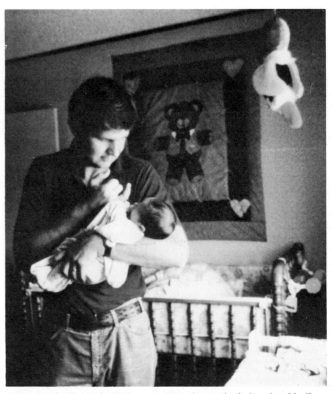

Figure 36–3. Most fathers want to be actively involved in the care of their newborn but may need extra encouragement and teaching to feel confident in their new role. (Photo: BABES, Inc.)

sionals after the birth of his infant and is less likely than the mother to attend support groups and parenting classes, he may find himself under significant stress without adequate support.

Most men identify their spouses as their primary support persons; in the case of a couple coping with a newborn, the spouse may be unable to support him as in the past, or he may be unable to ask for support for fear of making her burden greater than it already is. Although the father does not undergo the physiologic restoration the woman experiences after childbirth, his physical health may still deteriorate because of sleep deprivation and fatigue, which may be compounded by the emotional and physical energy expended during the birth, lingering worries about the wellbeing of his spouse and newborn, missed meals, increased household responsibilities, and ongoing job commitments.

Most men feel both gratified and burdened by parenthood (Fig. 36–3). Participation in childbirth classes and the birth itself may be positive experiences for the father, but they do not adequately prepare him for the level of reorganization and adjustment required once the couple is home with their new baby. Factors that appear to affect the new father's adjustment are his preparation for parenting, support from other family members, support from his workplace, and agreement with his spouse about their respective parental roles.

Many men are unable to take time off work after the birth of a child; some may even work more to bring in additional needed income. Some men welcome the time away from the demands of home life, whereas others, especially those who were intensely involved in the preg-

nancy and birth experience, resent their enforced separation from their spouses and infants. Time spent away from home and the new infant usually leads to decreased father involvement as infant caretaker. Most men feel unprepared to assist with child care and defer to the mother because she is (or appears to be) more competent. Breast-feeding may seem to limit the time a father can participate in infant care and may create or exacerbate his feelings of being left out.

Sibling Adaptation. Just as parents must adjust to the changes of the fourth trimester, so must older children. The nurse can be a valuable resource to parents as they help their older children adapt to the new baby. The responses of older children to the birth of a new sibling will vary according to age, level of preparation, and sex. Responses may range from hostility and aggression to overaffectionate displays toward the new baby (Fig. 36–4). Regardless of how well prepared an older child is, the disruption of family routines caused by the birth (separation from parents, temporary caretakers, etc.), the newborn being the focus of attention, and the reality of having to share the parents with another child combine to make some sibling jealousy inevitable. Jealously tends to be most intense among children less than 3 years apart and among those of the same sex. The first born child may

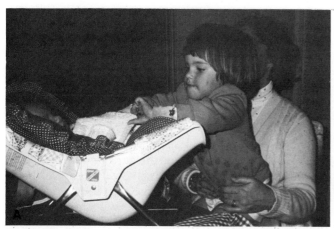 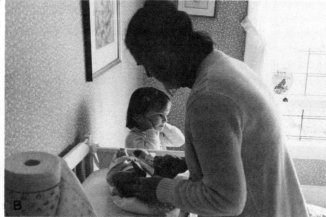

Figure 36–4. Older siblings must also adapt to the presence of a newborn in the family. *(A)* The older child may at times want to help in the care of the infant, and should be assisted to do so in a way that is age-appropriate and safe. *(B)* Other times, the older child will normally respond to the newborn's crying or immaturity with disappointment. (Photo: Colleen Stainton)

have a more difficult adjustment than subsequent children, who have always shared their parents with other siblings. Younger children may regress to more infantile behavior to gain attention and love. Prenatal preparation probably cannot prevent such responses totally. Because pregnancy is a lengthy event and is quite abstract to young children, they do not express ambivalent or negative feelings about the arrival of a sibling, until the baby actually comes home. Sibling jealousy reflects competition for parental love and is considered by most authorities to be an inevitable occurrence (Fox 1984).

Assessment

During history-taking, the nurse can collect information about previous experiences or personal traits suggesting a parent might be at particular risk for a difficult adjustment after birth. The nurse can also note current family circumstances that might enhance or inhibit parental attachment to the newborn. If circumstances are likely to inhibit attachment, the nurse is in a unique position to recommend and initiate interventions to foster positive parent–infant interaction. Appropriate interventions include encouraging such parental behaviors as identification, caretaking, and interaction; teaching and modeling appropriate care-giving; and planning for aggressive postpartum support, including the use of community resources.

The nurse should remember that while the infant's need for mothering is absolute, the need of an individual woman to mother is relative. In an early study, Yarrow and Goodwin (1965) identified maternal feelings of *emotional*

involvement, individualization, and *acceptance* as major components of mother–infant interaction. Emotional involvement is feeling the significance of the infant in the mother's life. Individualization is awareness of the unique characteristics of the infant, as well as the mother's differentiation of her infant as a being separate from herself. Acceptance is an integration of emotional involvement and individualization in which the mother accepts her infant without reservation.

Sugarman (1977) summed up many of the attributes of attachment when she noted that

> Attachment is the strong affectional bond causing the mother to make the unusual sacrifices necessary for the care of her infant day in and day out, night after night; to protect, nurture, fondle, kiss, cuddle, gaze at, and comfort her infant; to recognize her own infant's cry and smell; to know its needs and signals; and to vigorously resist separation from her baby for any reason.

Objective assessment of maternal role taking helps the nurse view each mother–infant dyad individually while striving to minimize bias related to cultural, behavioral, or value differences. A "high" level of mother–infant attachment is indicated when the mother

- Feels the baby is hers soon after delivery
- Is confident in caring for her baby
- Seeks and maintains close contact with the infant
- Accepts caring for the infant in the middle of the night without excessive resentment or anger toward the infant
- Responds to the baby's cry, usually knowing what the cry is a request for, within 1 or 2 minutes

Attachment is thus an observable, active, sensual, specific, affective, reciprocal process in which the unique characteristics of the infant interact with the genetic and acquired capacities of the parent. This relationship forms the foundation on which the subsequent health and development of the child and the entire family are built.

Behavioral expressions of the early parent–infant relationship can be observed and noted during the provision of nursing care. Maternal delivery room behaviors may be important indices of attachment. An initial lack of positive verbal, visual, and tactile responses by the mother after the birth of her baby may be predictive of later accidents, neglect, and abuse. Thus, depending on their initial responses to their infants, some mothers may benefit from further observations of bonding and attachment behaviors and close postpartum follow-up.

Assessing Maternal Behaviors

Several researchers have described specific maternal behaviors that reflect attachment to the infant. Rubin described the progression of maternal touch and related behaviors, which are indicators of the maternal processes of "taking in," "taking hold," and "letting go" (Rubin 1961). Ludington (1977) proposed nine behaviors that should be observed in every mother as indicators of her developing attachment to her infant (see accompanying display). Such observational assessment provides a framework for an objective appraisal of the process of mother–infant attachment and for the identification of

---

Specific Maternal Behaviors Reflecting Attachment to Infant

- Initial identifying behaviors before and after delivery
- Active and passive reaching behaviors
- Touch progression — fingertip to palmar to hand; hand to arm embrace
- Positioning of infant to left of sternum; *en face* positioning
- Eye-to-eye contact
- Verbal identifying behaviors — association and pronoun identification (referring to the baby as "he" or "she" rather than "it")
- Postpartum phases — "taking in" phase of dependency, "taking hold" phase of task mastery, "letting go" of predelivery expectations
- Rhythm/reciprocity patterns
- Cooing behaviors

After Ludington S: Postpartum development of maternicity. Am J Nurs 77(7):1171–1174, 1977

---

mothers who need further assessment and supportive intervention.

Assessing Paternal Behaviors

Assessment of paternal behaviors in the postbirth period is hampered by the relative lack of research on early fathering. There is no convincing evidence that father attendance at birth or early father–neonate interaction enhances father–infant attachment (Toney 1983). However, early evidence indicated the father who attends the birth of his child and has early contact with the newborn may report feeling intensely close and being engrossed with the infant (Greenberg 1974). Some attachment behaviors observed in mothers are also readily observable among fathers, especially in situations in which fathers are alone with their newborns.

Father–infant interaction is similar to mother–infant interaction, although the mother usually engages in more caretaking activities, while the father is more likely to play with his child, hold the infant passively, or transport the infant somewhere. Father–infant interaction may be limited and sporadic owing to the father's insecurity about his caretaking skills, an early return after the birth to his job, or performance of most tasks by the mother. The best predictor of the father's level of involvement in caretaking is the mother's attitude about the value of father involvement; the more the mother values his participation, the more likely the father is to be actively involved in care taking activities.

Assessing Sibling Behaviors

The nurse can help parents assess the level of disruption older children in the family may be feeling during the fourth trimester; she may also help them deal with sibling jealousy. Parents should be reminded that the older child cannot be expected to accept and love the new baby automatically and that young children should be observed closely when interacting with the newborn. The nurse can help parents identify patterns in the older child's behavior, which are attempts to get more attention and love, and help parents meet the older child's needs for such attention; strategies include planning special outings for the child with one parent, displaying the child's baby pictures prominently in the house, encouraging the child to verbalize feelings of resentment, and avoid comparing the children with one another. Older children should be invited to participate in infant care but should not be pressured to do so. Regression in young children usually resolves itself in 4 to 6 weeks; regressive behavior should be handled in a matter-of-fact way, and the child's need for more love and attention should be acknowledged. Children usually accept a newborn without much difficulty, and jealous behaviors usually diminish after 3 to 4 months, at about the same time the infant becomes more social and interesting to the older child. Parents should be reminded that some sibling competition is normal and will persist as the children grow.

Assessing Parent–Infant Interaction

Barnard (1980), a leading researcher in the field of maternal–child health, examined the efficacy and predictive value of multiple nursing strategies with respect to child health and development. The Nursing Child Assessment Project (NCAP) in Seattle examined screening and assessment variables, and stability of high-risk characteristics over time, and other factors predictive of later child health and development. The study population was assessed prenatally and at intervals throughout the first year of each child's life.

The NCAP study identified variables related to the mother as primary care-giver, to the infant, and to the environment; these variables were placed on a continuum of optimal circumtances during the first year of parenthood. This "Optimal Profile," shown in the assessment tool, page 1124, provides the nurse with the opportunity to screen families, to determine the status of their profile circumstances, and to initiate further in-depth assessment and a variety of follow-up options.

During the NCAP study, new nursing assessment tools were tested, refined, and validated. Nurses working with parents and infants can be trained to use the following tools:

- The Nursing Child Assessment Sleep/Activity Record
- The Nursing Child Assessment Feeding Scale
- The Nursing Child Assessment Teaching Scale
- The Home Observation of the Environment

The NCAP assessment tools are among the most sophisticated nursing strategies for the systematic assessment of parents, infants, and family environments. This type of standardized assessment can guide nursing interventions to maximize healthy child development.

Diagnosis

Based on data gathered through the assessment process, the nurse involved in fourth-trimester care must also formulate diagnoses that will help to direct specific interventions to meet family needs. In addition to nursing diagnoses related to the biophysical processes of involution (discussed in Chapter 29), the following are nursing diagnoses that reflect possible problems that may arise and be addressed independently in the care of families during the fourth trimester:

- Sleep pattern disturbance related to infant night waking

- Activity intolerance related to anemia and fatigue
- Parental role conflict related to changes in role functioning, crises, or unmet needs
- Altered family process related to impact of parenting
- Knowledge deficit related to lack of experience or preparation for demands of parenting
- Potential altered parenting related to inadequate role models or inadequate support
- Ineffective breast-feeding related to lack of knowledge or anxiety

Priorities in care may be established from these. The latter nursing diagnosis is discussed in the next chapter.

Complications requiring collaboration with other members of the health care team may arise during the postpartum. If the nurse has ongoing contact with the family during the fourth trimester, it is important to monitor for the following potential complications:

- Late postpartum hemorrhage
- Postpartum mood disturbance/postpartum depression
- Mastitis
- Failure-to-thrive syndrome

Monitoring these complications is discussed at the end of the section on Planning and Implementation. Further discussion of care is found in Chapters 29 and 30.

Planning and Implementation

In order to plan effectively, the postpartum nurse must view the family as a unit during the fourth trimester. If family history and current assessments suggest preexisting crises, excessive life change, coping difficulties, ineffective communication and cooperation, or inadequate support systems, continuity of care is crucial. Health threats to families in the fourth trimester can be diagnosed and care planned and implemented within the scope of independent and interdependent nursing practice. A challenge facing maternity nurses is to plan nursing care that is cost effective and produces documentable positive health outcomes.

Promoting Adaptation in the Fourth Trimester

Nursing literature contains evidence that postpartum women have benefitted from a number of postpartum structured teaching and supportive counseling nursing interventions specifically related to their needs, concerns,

(text continued on page 1126)

ASSESSMENT TOOL

Optimal Parent–Infant Profile — Nursing Child Assessment Project

	Prenatal	Newborn	1 Month	4 Months	8 Months	12 Months
Mother's Psychosocial Assets	Is pleased about pregnancy	←—————————— Is satisfied with marriage ——————————→				
	Has someone to share concerns with	←———————— Has positive feelings about motherhood ————————→				
		←————— Is satisfied with father's involvement in child care ————→				
	Has enough physical and emotional help	←———————— Has positive experiences with motherhood ————————→				
	Planned the pregnancy	←————————— Has adequate help in home —————————→				
	Little disruption in plans					
Father's Involvement		←——————————————————————— Living with family ——————————→				
	Is pleased about pregnancy	←———————— Moderate or high participation in child care ————————→				
	Gives physical and emotional help	←———— Participates in teaching child ——→				
	Shares mother's concerns	←————— Is concerned about child's welfare and development ————→				
Parental Mutuality		←——————————————————— Make decisions jointly ——————————→				
		←————————————— Agree on childrearing —————————→				
		←————————————— Agree on discipline —————————→				
Life Change		←——————————————————————— Low ——————————————→				
Parents' Developmental Expectations	Are realistic about when infant sees, hears, is aware, etc.					
	Attend antepartum classes	←– Recognize increasing social responsiveness ——→		←–Expect increasing child mobility, curiosity, and independence ————→		
Mother's Health	Has no perinatal complications					
	Follows recommended antepartum and postpartum care					
		←————————————— Few health problems —————————→				
Infant's Health	Has no perinatal complications					
		←————————— Shows normal growth pattern ————————→				
		←————————————— Has little illness —————————→				
		←————————Has few accidents, none serious ————————→				
		←————————— Receives recommended well-child care ————————→				

The timing for specific entries is determined by the age of most importance and by the age at which the dimension was measured in this study.

Barnard K: Nursing Child Assessment Overview. Child Assessment Training Instructor's Manual. Seattle, Washington, University of Washington: Nursing Child Assessment Satellite Training

(continued)

ASSESSMENT TOOL (continued)

	Prenatal	Newborn	1 Month	4 Months	8 Months	12 Months
Mother's Perception of Infant	Shows pleased anticipation	←----Perceives infant positively compared with other children----→				
Infant's Behavior		Is alert for good inter-action Shows smooth, co-ordinated motor be-havior Habituates to repeti-tive stimuli Cuddly Consolable	Responds with look-ing, move-ment, or sounds Attends to mother's presence, especially voice	Engages in socially modulated behavior	Initiates be-havioral in-teractions more fre-quently More ver-bal Increased mobility, such as crawling	Exhibits more ex-ploratory behavior Uses move-ment, look-ing, listen-ing for a purpose
		←-------------- Motor activity is moderate --------------→				
		←---- Shows low irritability, is predominantly in a good mood ----→				
			←---- Attends to specific stimuli ----→			
Infant's Sleep–Activity Patterns		Shows pro-gressively regular pat-terns of sleeping and eating Has at least four feed-ings a day	Sleeps through the night		Begins to have night awakening again, but frequency not proble-matic to parents	
			←-------------- Regularity of night sleep ----→			
			←-------------- Infant can adapt to changes in daily routine --------→			
Mother–Infant Interaction		←---------Mother is comfortable during interaction ---------→				
		←------------- Mother facilitates learning --------------→				
		←-- Mother encourages exploration of toys and objects				
		←----------- Mother provides positive feedback ------------→				
		←-- Mother does not use forcing/controlling techniques --------------------→				
		←---- Infant demonstrates readiness to learn and involvement----→				
		←---- Mutuality and adaptation of mother and infant behaviors in routine caretaking activities such as feeding--------→				
		← Infant becomes more adaptive ------------------→				
Stimulation in the Home		(not measured)	←----High emotional and verbal responsivity to child --------------→			
			←----Low restriction and punishment------→			
			←----Temporal environment organized --------------------→			
			←----Appropriate play materials provided -------------------→			
			←----High maternal involvement with child-------------------→			

and role (Brooten 1986). It also suggests that nursing interventions that enhance the mother's knowledge, skill, and growth-fostering interaction with her baby, do influence the infant's growth, development, and health outcomes (Fig. 36–5).

Factors to consider when planning to extend nursing services to postpartum women during the fourth trimester include: general characteristics of the population being served, timing of the first contact, number of nursing contacts possible, types of contacts (*i.e.,* telephone-based or home visit), and the duration of care. In addition, it is important to consider whether the nursing assessment and intervention approach will be highly structured or flexible, allowing for individualized care.

Teaching for Effective Self-Care

Preparation for self-care during the fourth trimester must begin early in pregnancy and be expanded during the perinatal hospital stay. Postpartum follow-up is an opportunity for the nurse to reinforce discharge teaching, provide additional information to enhance self-care, and evaluate the efficacy of the self-care regimen.

Maternal self-care teaching should initially focus on the five Bs — breasts, bladder, bowels, bleeding, and bottom. Basic hygiene and comfort measures should be taught, and the mother should understand potential portals of infection and principles of personal hygiene related to breast care, elimination, perineal care, and showering.

A review of dietary and fluid requirements related to lactation and involution should emphasize balanced meals, prenatal and postnatal vitamins, and adequate fluids. A specific nutritional intake (calories, protein, carbohydrate, etc.), milk and juices with meals, and a full glass of water during each breast-feeding session should be recommended. Foods that serve as dietary laxatives should be eaten to reestablish regular bowel movements following birth.

Self-care related to physical exercise and sexual activity must also be explored. Gradual resumption of full physical activity during the fourth trimester and vaginal rest until lochial discharge ceases are common guidelines. It is important that the nurse clarify misconceptions about potential postpartum conception. Family planning options need to be considered before the mother resumes full sexual activity.

The nurse should teach the parents about infant care, cues, states, and behavioral characteristics. She should first explore parental observations, expectations, and perceptions; this provides a database for teaching-learning assessment. The fundamentals of infant care taught should include hygiene; bathing; cleansing of eyes, ears, umbilicus, and perineum; feeding frequency, duration, position, and amount, as well as post feeding "bubbling"; and normal physical appearance, vital signs, and reflexes. Finally, information of sleep–wake patterns, state-related behaviors, consolability, self-comforting, and sen-

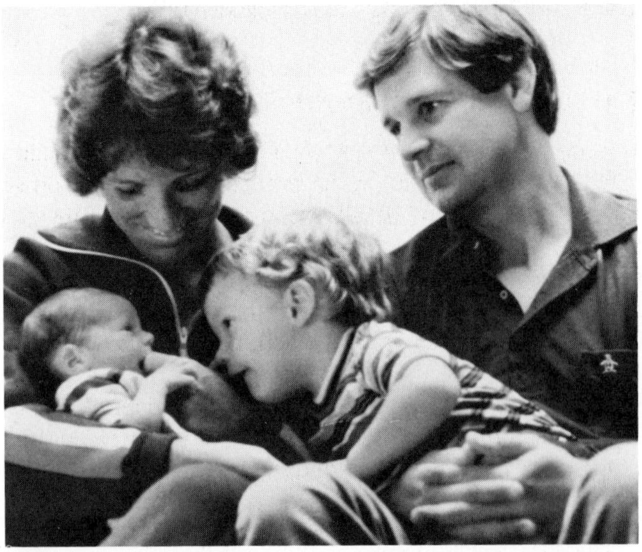

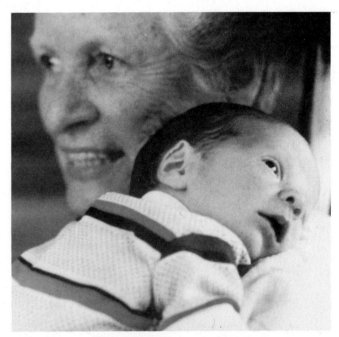

Figure 36–6. The nurse should encourage new parents to use supports and resources already available to them in the fourth trimester. Grandparents are often an excellent source of help with older children and with newborn care. (Photo: BABES, Inc.)

Figure 36–5. The integration of a thriving newborn into a healthy, happy family: the goal of nursing in the fourth trimester. (Photo: BABES, Inc.)

sory capacities helps parents develop an awareness of the unique needs of their baby.

Comprehensive self-care teaching includes a discussion of family developmental tasks and anticipatory guidance. The nurse should discuss how family roles, relationships, and communication necessarily change following the birth of a baby. Parents who already have children are especially appreciative of information related to sibling adaptation to the newborn.

The nurse should remember that a critical aspect of self-care is the use of appropriate supportive resources during times of stress. By discussing the myths and realities surrounding the fourth trimester and emphasizing the practical and supportive assistance of extended family, friends, and other resources, the nurse promotes realistic expectations and coping behaviors (Fig. 36–6).

NURSING RESEARCH

Early Discharge and Transitional Care

In response to pressures for cost containment as well as because of consumer demand, hospital stays for childbearing have decreased substantially in recent years, and early discharge is becoming more commonplace, even for families experiencing some perinatal complication, such as cesarean birth or low birth weight.

A team of nurse researchers at Univerity of Pennsylvania (Brooten et al 1986) demonstrated that very low birth weight infants could be safely discharged an average of 11 days earlier with home follow-up by a perinatal nurse specialist. This home followup program resulted in an average savings of $18,506 per infant without any increased risk to the infant, such as rehospitalization, acute return visits or losses in physical or mental growth.

This same team is now testing the applicability and effectiveness of this model of nurse home followup on women who experienced unplanned cesarean birth, women with diabetes in the perinatal period and women who experienced hysterectomies. This model includes telephone contacts, home visits and telephone availability by nurse specialists, and provides for comparison of normal discharge and early-discharge/home follow-up patients on specific expected patient outcomes as well as cost of care.

Brooten D, Kumar S, Brown L et al: A randomized clinical trial of early hospital discharge and home followup of very low birth weight infants. New Engl J Med 315:934–939, 1986

Brooten D, Brown L, Munro B et al: Early discharge and specialist transitional care. Image 20:65–68, 1988

Providing Home Visits

In an attempt to show the impact of home-based nursing interventions, studies have focused on the effects of home nursing care on maternal and infant health (see accompanying Nursing Research display). Findings suggest the need to include and strengthen the documentation of assessment and the intervention content of home nursing services. Implementing and evaluating specific nursing actions facilitates drawing conclusions that demonstrate the outcomes of nursing actions.

Home-based postpartum follow-up services have traditionally been delivered by public health nurses to high-risk populations. When economic and consumer pressures led to the establishment of short-stay or alternative birth centers, from which mother and infant go home after only a short stay, home-visit postpartum follow-up services were developed. "Early discharge" is generally defined as occurring between 8 and 48 hours postpartum. With early discharge, health care providers realized that some form of outreach strategy would be necessary to provide services usually given during the 3- to 5-day postpartum hospital stay. Systematic physical assessment of the mother and newborn, as well as comprehensive discharge planning and follow-up teaching, is provided in home-visit programs. Nursing follow-up care requires specialized tools for assessment and documentation.

A useful clinical tool for tracing the content and nature of nursing actions during postpartum nursing care has been developed by Donaldson (1988). This guide for nursing assessment and intervention may assist the nurse in systematically following the adaptive course of new mothers and promote comprehensive, yet individualized care (see accompanying display, next page).

Providing Telephone Follow-up

Clinicians have explored the effectiveness of postpartum follow-up nursing care services using telephone-based contacts with families during the fourth trimester. One advantage of telephone-based contact is the reduced travel time and costs may result in more frequent contact with a larger population of postpartum families. An important drawback of this approach, however, is the obvious limitations of only verbal contact.

Donaldson (1988) has described such a hospital-based telephone contact postpartum follow-up program. In this program, based on crisis theory, the nurse focuses on supporting "crisis-balancing factors." Nursing actions include clarifying stressors, providing ego support, monitoring for appropriate modification of the environment, and initiating anticipatory guidance. These actions are intended to support or strengthen cognitive perception, mobilize supports, and enhance coping abilities. Support or strengthening of these crisis-balancing factors is intended to help the individual or family regain a sense of balance and adapt to their new situation in the midst of stressors that cannot easily be resolved and may otherwise precipitate crisis.

Planning Parent Classes and Support Groups

In recent years a variety of self-help mechanisms have evolved to meet the needs of families during the transition to parenthood. Educational programs include postpartum and parenting classes. Self-help programs, especially support groups and baby-care cooperatives, link new parents to one another to share the joys and frustrations of the fourth trimester.

Such experiences expand the practical knowledge and supportive resources of the participants. Expanding family centers developed and operated by nurses provide many individualized services to help new parents become more effective in their self-care. The nurse can conduct an inventory of her geographic area to determine which official and voluntary services are available to meet the needs of childbearing and early child-rearing families.

Meleis and colleagues (1978) tested role supplementation as a nursing strategy to provide new parents with information and experiences geared to support mastery of their new roles. Role-supplementation group meet-

ings, home visits, role modeling, rehearsal, and clarification are structured so as to provide individual support. The desired outcome of role supplementation is the ability to function in the parental role with confidence and competence.

Expected Outcomes:

- Parents state they are getting more sleep by supporting each other in caring for the neonate at night.
- Mother demonstrates more energy as a result of rest periods and eating nutritious foods.
- Parents display initial adaptations to role taking by showing affection for each other and the newborn.
- Parents communicate to each other their needs and concerns for themselves and family and begin the process of helping each other meet needs.
- Parents in turn demonstrate skills they learned in parenting classes.
- Parents respond to nurse and others in class as role models.
- Parents state they acquired adequate help at home for support.

ASSESSMENT TOOL

Postpartum Nursing Follow-up Tool

Introduction:

Describe initial contact _____

_____

Review of pertinent data (hx this pregnancy, response to birth, special problems) _____

_____

_____

Vital family developmental hx (including cultural orientation) _____

_____

Nursing Assessment

General Family State:

By _____

"I'm _____ "

Family name _____

Mother _____

Father _____

Infant _____

Date birth _____

Date DC _____

Date initial FU _____

Date DCFU _____

Physicians _____

_____

FU Nurse _____

_____

Family Phone # _____

PHYSIOLOGIC SELF-CARE

01 Breasts
02 Vagina
03 Perineum
04 Elimination
05 Fundus/Abdomen
06 Cesarean incision
07 Breast care
08 Peri-care
09 Physical hygiene
10 Postpartum activity
11 Postpartum exercises
12 Fatigue/Rest
13 Sexual relations
14 Family planning
15 Basic four food groups tid
16 Fluid intake
17 Prenatal vitamins/Medications
18 Postpartum check appt.

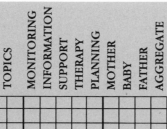
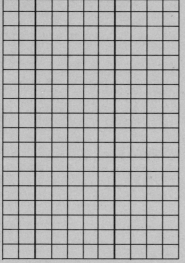

INFANT CARE-GIVING

19 Infant feeding frequency
20 Infant feeding behaviors
21 Mother's response to feeding
22 Bath
23 Cord/Circ care
24 Diapering skin care
25 Clothing/swaddling
26 Comforting
27 Sleep/Activity
28 Infant cue clarity
29 Interaction during care-giving
30 Pediatric check appt.
31 Safety: Care-giving/Vehicular
32 Signs of illness
33 CPR
34 Father involvement

INFANT DEVELOPMENT

35 Infant states
36 Infant state related behaviors
37 Engagement/Disengagement cues
38 Reciprocity
39 Distress
40 Sensory capacities
41 Sensory stimulation
42 Infant play
43 Infant toy safety
44 Temperament
45 Fostering growth in care-giving

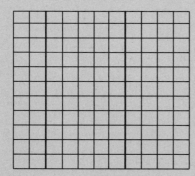

POSTPARTUM ADAPTATION

46 Expectations
47 Concerns
48 Stressors/Demands/Threats
49 Problem solving
50 Personal development issues
51 Spousal relationship issues
52 Parent development issues
53 Family development issues
54 Mood disturbance
55 Self-esteem
56 Role conflict
57 Stress reduction strategies
58 Use of supports
59 Exploring resources
60 Expectations
61 Anticipatory guidance
62 Bibliotherapy

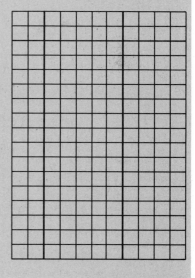

(Column headers for all grids: TOPICS, MONITORING, INFORMATION, SUPPORT, THERAPY, PLANNING, MOTHER, BABY, FATHER, AGGREGATE)

(continued)

*Continuing Nursing Care Plan

Assessment of Problem	Goals:	Intervention/Date	Evaluation

(Nursing Diagnosis)

(*Continue as needed on attached pages _____)

Discontinue Follow-up:

Referral re: _____ Agency/professional _____

Referral feedback: Family _____

Agency/professional _____

Discontinue follow-up date: _____ Report to: _____

Signed _____ Follow-up nurse _____

Donaldson N: Effect of Telephone Postpartum Follow-up: A Clinical Trial. Doctoral dissertation, University of California, San Francisco, 1988

Focus

1. *Mother:* the major care-giver for this infant.
2. *Baby:* this is used when specific action is for baby only.
3. *Father:* any male taking role of father consistently, with the action specifically for him only.
4. *Aggregate:* action focused on more than one person.

Type of Nursing Act

1. *Monitoring:* collecting information; keeping track of events; making diagnosis; formulating problems; identifying concerns; subsumed in information, support, therapy, and planning.
2. *Information:* providing verbal, written, or behavioral guidance to client; role modeling, demonstration, discussion, showing; mass media (pamphlets, books).
3. *Support:* validating behaviors, reinforcing, praising, encouraging of *ongoing* behavior; listening; giving resources, supplies (diapers, etc.).
4. *Therapy:* providing methods for correcting an identified problem, *i.e.,* information, discussion, problem solving.
5. *Planning:* a program of action to achieve goal; subject of recording must be planner, *i.e.,* nurse gives information to client to plan.

Monitoring for Complications

Throughout the nursing-care modalities discussed in the previous section, the emphasis on assessment and diagnosis of potential or actual complications is clear. The nurse in contact with families during the fourth trimester must be alert to signs of deviation from normal recovery, and determine the most appropriate form of care, given the family's needs. The process of monitoring for complications is especially important in families already known to be at risk.

While the stressors and adaptive demands of the fourth trimester put a strain on most families, some families are at especially great risk. Termed *high-risk* or *multiproblem families,* they present a challenge to the health care delivery system and to the individual professionals involved with them. The infant who is already at risk, owing to the circumstances of his or her birth, and is part of a multiproblem family as well, is doubly vulnerable during the first year of life.

Helfer and Wilson (1982) introduced the idea of the perinatal coaching role, which is based on the premise "that most new parents have limited understanding of the methods used to communicate with their new infant." The coach is a specially trained nonprofessional who uses home-based visits to teach, model, motivate, and celebrate skilled parent–infant interaction and resulting care-giving. In collaboration with professionals, the coach can provide early intervention for potentially maladaptive parent–infant relationships and initiate referrals, as needed, to professional resources.

Barnard and coworkers (1982) examined two postpartum nursing care delivery models designed to meet the needs of multiproblem families. Using a structured educational model, they focused on fostering "the mutual adaptation process between the care-giver and the infant." Goal-oriented home-based services provided information and support based on the common concerns of parents during the fourth trimester.

A second model involved direct supportive services, including services to meet a wide spectrum of parent and infant needs (Barnard 1982). One outcome of this project was the identification of supportive acts within the scope of nursing practice in postbirth care. Some of these are listed in the accompanying display.

Expected Outcomes:

- Mother demonstrates she has followed recommended care by experiencing no postpartum complications.
- Parents demonstrate concern about child's welfare and development.
- Infant demonstrates increasing social responsiveness, normal growth pattern, and few illnesses.

Supportive Actions for Multiproblem Families

Self-disclosure	Input regarding personal experiences; use self as therapeutic entity
Mutual sharing	Easy give and take, generally on emotional level; dialogue; focus on client
Social sharing	Interaction that emphasizes other family members, pets, sports/activities outside context of program goals, such as offering tea, coffee, showing house, conversing with grandmother
Active listening	Response to emotional message, reflection, clarification, restatement of ideas, and so on
Information exchange	Interactive conversation about infant, mother, family, or problems; nurse or client initiation; client an active participant
Sounding board	"Being there," taking in, listening, but not necessarily responding
Validation	Praise, encouragement, positive reinforcement or feedback (common words: *admired, reassured,* and so on)
Information giving	Program content, pamphlets, resources, anticipatory guidance, teaching, suggestions, advice, discussion, instructions, demonstration of Brazelton behaviors; client passive receiver of information
Doing for	Demonstrating infant care skills, arranging resources (calling agencies), grocery shopping, watching sibs, running errands with mother, bringing reading materials, cutting nails, and so on
Baby and mother touch	Any nonverbal gesture that results in contact between nurse and mother or infant

Barnard K, Synder C, Spietz A: Supportive acts for high risk infants and families. Paper presented at the Conference on Social Support for Families of Vulnerable Infants, University of Washington, Seattle, October 1982. Used with permission.

Evaluation

Since the needs of families during the fourth trimester are at once unique and universal, nursing care is best evaluated against expected outcomes that are rather general, but which can be made much more specific, depending on the particular needs presented by each family. The knowledge base related to maternal adaptation during the fourth trimester is much better developed, and most nursing care will be directed to the mother-infant dyad. Objectives for maternal outcomes can be derived from existing knowledge and used to evaluate the effectiveness of nursing care for a particular mother and her family as she moves through this period of adaptation. For instance, upon completion of the fourth trimester during which nursing services are provided, a first-time mother could be expected to accomplish the following behaviors:

- Apply knowledge of normal postpartum physical restoration by establishing an appropriate pattern of self-care, including recognizing and reporting abnormal signs and symptoms,
- Apply knowledge of basic infant needs, states, and state-related behaviors through increasingly confident and competent contingent care-giving,
- Apply knowledge of appropriate expectations of infant growth through care-giving that fosters the infant's physical, emotional, social, and cognitive growth,
- Apply knowledge of common individual and marital changes triggered by taking on the parental role through coping strategies that nurture individual autonomy and the spousal relationship.

CHAPTER SUMMARY

Follow-up care in the fourth trimester is an area in which nursing can make a unique, valuable contribution to the health and wellbeing of child-bearing families. The traditional gap between obstetric and pediatric care has been lengthened by short postpartum hospital stays; early discharge programs should be associated with home follow-up for assessment of maternal and newborn well-being. In addition, the family faces many stressors in the fourth trimester as the members strive to recover from childbirth, to learn about each other in their new roles, to meet their infant's needs, and to sustain and establish loving relationships. The nurse can assess individual family members' adjustments to these stressors, clarify the situation, support coping mechanisms, and offer factual information, anticipatory guidance, and emotional support. Nursing follow-up care contributes to the overall health of the family and may be especially helpful to multiproblem families.

The fourth trimester is a vulnerable period in the family life cycle. Ideally, mastery of the adaptive demands of this period will strengthen the overall health and well-being of the family. Integration of the newborn into the family and achievement of the developmental tasks facing the family are the long-term goals of nurses who seek to fill a major gap in health care delivery in the fourth trimester.

STUDY QUESTIONS

1. What are six developmental tasks of the expanding family? What nursing interventions can promote achievement of those tasks?
2. List your own beliefs about parenthood, and compare them with the myths about parenthood presented in this chapter.
3. Describe nursing actions that can support parental role taking in the first two weeks after birth.
4. What are some factors that may place mothers and their families at risk for problems in adapting during the fourth trimester? Why do these factors place families at risk?
5. Identify programs, in your community, geared toward promoting healthy family adaptation in the fourth trimester.
6. What are the advantages and disadvantages of telephone-based postbirth nursing follow-up and home-visit nursing follow-up in the postpartum period?

REFERENCES/BIBLIOGRAPHY

Barnard K: Nursing child assessment overview. Child Assessment Training Instructor's Manual. Seattle, Washington, University of Washington: Nursing Child Assessment Satellite Training, 1980

Barnard K: Newborn Nursing Models. First report of project supported by Grant Number R01 NU-00719. Seattle, Washington, University of Washington School of Nursing, Department of Parent and Child Nursing, 1983

Barnard K, Elsas T, Johnson–Crowley N: Description of nursing support for biobehavioral program. Grant research report, 1982

Barnard K, Snyder C, Spietz A: Supportive acts for high-risk infants and families. Paper presented at the Conference On Social Support for Families of Vulnerable Infants, University of Washington, Seattle, October 1982

Brooten D, Kumar S, Brown L et al: A randomized clinical trial of early hospital discharge and home follow-up of very-low birth weight infants. New Engl J Med 315:934–939, 1986

Campbell S, Taylor P: Bonding and attachment: Theoretical issues. Semin Perinatol 3:1, 1979

Donaldson N: Effect of Telephone Postpartum Followup: A Clinical Trial. Doctoral dissertation, University of California, San Francisco, 1988

Fox N: Who's that sleeping in my crib? Genesis (ASPO/Lamaze) 6(3):23, 1984

Greenberg M, Morris N: Engrossment: The newborn's impact upon the father. Am J Orthopsychiatry 41:520, 1974

Helfer R, Wilson A: The parent–infant relationship: Promoting a positive beginning through perinatal coaching. Pediatr Clin North Am 29(2):249, 1982

Klaus M, Kennell J: Parent–Infant Bonding. St. Louis, CV Mosby, 1982

Ludington S: Postpartum development of maternicity. Am J Nurs 77(7):1171, 1977

Meleis A, Swensen L, Jones D: Role supplementation for new parents—A role master plan. MCN 3:84, 1978

Rubin R: Basic maternal behavior. Nurs Outlook 9:683, 1961

Sugarman M: Perinatal influences on maternal–infant attachment. Am J Orthopsychiatry 47(3):407, 1977

Toney L: The effects of holding the newborn at delivery on paternal bonding. Nurs Res 32(1):16, 1983

Yarrow L, Goodwin M: Some conceptual issues in the study of mother–infant interaction. Am J Orthopsychiatry 35:473, 1965

SUGGESTED READINGS

Cronenwett L: Parental network structure and perceived support after birth of first child. Nurs Res 34(6):347–352, 1985

Dahlberg N: A perinatal based antepartum home care program. J Obstet Gynecol Neonatal Nurs 17(1):30–34, 1988

Golas G, Parks P: Effect of early postpartum teaching on primaparas' knowledge of infant behavior and degree of confidence. Res Nurs Health 9:209–214, 1986

Mercer R: The process of maternal role attainment over the first year. Nurs Res 34:198–204, 1985

Mercer R: First-time Motherhood: Experiences From Teens to Forties. New York, Springer Publishing Co, 1986

37 maternal and infant nutrition in the fourth trimester

LEARNING OBJECTIVES

After studying the material in this chapter, the student should be able to

- Explain the nutritional requirements of the lactating and nonlactating mother during the fourth trimester

- Discuss the effects of nutrition on the quality and quantity of breast milk produced

- Discuss the advantages and disadvantages of breast-feeding and formula-feeding

- Explain the nutritional requirements of the infant from birth to 6 months of age

- Advise mothers about dietary recommendations for themselves and their infants during the fourth trimester

- Describe nursing interventions to promote optimal infant feeding practices

KEY TERMS

Areola

Casein

Colostrum

Engorgement

Kwashiorkor

Lactalbumin

Let-down reflex

Marasmus

Renal solute load

Weaning

Whey

The maternity nurse is in a unique position to assess the nutritional status of the woman in the fourth trimester and also support optimal infant feeding practices. New parents require information and support as they take over the responsibility for infant feeding. Mothers who choose to breast-feed require special support and teaching as they learn the necessary skills.

New mothers are also motivated to return to their non-pregnant physical state as quickly as possible and are open to suggestions about nutrition and exercise that will expedite the process. The nurse can carry out an important function of patient care by educating new mothers about nutrition.

The postpartum nurse is in a position to assess the concerns, eating habits, and activities of her patients. Her observations of her patients' behaviors provide insight into individual needs for counseling, teaching, self-help, and financial or social services. In the area of nutrition, one of the most important parameters of health, the nurse — in conjunction with the nutritionist — can have a significant effect on the comprehensive care of patients in the fourth trimester.

This chapter provides the information necessary to carry out this function. Breast feeding versus formula-feeding, nutritional requirements for lactating and non-lactating women, and nutrition for infant health are discussed. In addition, nursing diagnosis, intervention, planning, and evaluation are presented to guide the student in her clinical practice in the nutritional care of mothers and infants in the postpartum setting.

REDISCOVERY OF BREAST-FEEDING

Throughout most of human history, breast-feeding was the only means of feeding newborns. If biologic mothers were unable to nurse their infants, other lactating mothers (called *wet nurses*) took over the feeding. In the 20th century, however, the baby bottle became a symbol of women's freedom and of the "modern" way of child-rearing. The popularity of formula-feeding was helped by the availability of a number of "ready-to-feed" infant formulas, which made formula preparation easy and safe.

In the 1950s and 1960s, formula-feeding became quite common and well accepted in the United States. Breast-feeding was largely forgotten in a culture in which women's breasts were either hidden or displayed as sexual objects. The woman who modestly nursed her infant was often considered a source of embarrassment and was hidden in a bedroom or ladies room, whereas the woman who dressed provocatively to reveal most of her breasts was considered socially acceptable.

However, the trend away from breast-feeding has been reversed. A resurgence of breast-feeding practices began in 1971 and has continued through the present. Estimates indicate that over 60% of babies are now breast-fed. There also appears to be an increase in the period of time over which women breast-feed. At the same time, the use of whole cow's milk or evaporated milk for 5- to 6-month-old infants dropped and the use of prepared formula rose. This reflects current pediatric practice, in which whole cow's milk and evaporated milk for infant feeding has been discouraged; the American Academy of Pediatrics recommends iron-fortified commercial formula as the best alternative to breast milk.

Scientific investigation has demonstrated that formula-feeding is not as good as breast-feeding with respect to nutritional value or immunologic advantages. Although babies have thrived on formula for several generations and will continue to do so, many lay people and most health professionals feel that breast-feeding is optimal for the normal mother and baby. The American Academy of Pediatrics suggests all mothers should be urged to breast-feed.

MATERNAL-INFANT FOURTH-TRIMESTER NUTRITIONAL NEEDS

Nutritional Comparison of Breast- and Formula-Feeding

The positive effects of feeding a baby breast milk include health benefits and often psychologic benefits for the infant and the mother. Human milk is ideally suited to the human infant; it contains the nutrients, minerals, and other substances needed for optimal growth. When the digestibility, absorption, and metabolism of human and cow's milk are compared, human milk is found to be superior for infant feeding in all respects. In addition to its biochemical, nutritional, antibacterial, and immunologic value, breast-feeding also maximizes physical interaction between mother and infant and may thereby enhance the infant's long-term emotional well-being.

Production of infant formulas has reached a high degree of sophistication. There are many different types of formula in use, some based on cow's milk protein and others on protein from sources such as soybeans. The fat in commercial formulas may be cow's milk fat or vegetable fat. Various carbohydrates are used, including lactose, sucrose, glucose, and corn starch; some formulas contain combinations of these ingredients. Specific vitamins and minerals may also be added. Some formulas come very close to breast milk in content and are called *humanized* by their manufacturers. However, even these formulas are not equivalent to breast milk. Nutritional information on commonly used commercial infant formulas is given in Table 37–1.

Protein, Fat, and Carbohydrate Comparison

The protein in breast milk is more easily digested and more readily absorbed than the protein in any other infant food. Cow's milk has more protein than human milk, but 80% of cow's milk protein is in the form of *casein*. This

milk protein forms a large, tough curd in the human stomach, is poorly digested by infants, and may cause intestinal obstruction. Cow's milk must, therefore, be treated chemically or mechanically to reduce the curd tension so that it can be digested readily by human babies. The whey protein *lactalbumin* constitutes the other 20% of cow's milk protein; in contrast, it constitutes

Table 37–1   **Nutritional Information for Commonly Used Commercial Infant Formulas**

	Enfamil	Similac	SMA	Soy Isolates*
Components				
Protein	Nonfat milk	Nonfat milk	Whey and nonfat milk	Soy isolate
Fat	Vegetable oils	Vegetable oils	Vegetable and oleo oils	Vegetable oils
Carbohydrate	Lactose	Lactose	Lactose	Corn syrup and/or sucrose
Major Constituents				
Protein	1.5	1.55	1.5	1.8–2.5
Fat	3.7	3.6	3.6	3–3.6
Carbohydrates	7.0	7.1	7.2	6.4–6.8
Ash (minerals)	0.36	0.37	0.3	0.4–0.5
Cal per oz[†]	20	20	20	20
Percent of Calories				
Protein	9	9	9	12–15
Fat	50	48	48	45–48
Carbohydrate	41	43	43	39–40
Minerals per Liter				
Sodium (mEq)	11	11	6.5	9–24
Potassium (mEq)	19	19	14.3	15–28
Chloride (mEq)	12	17	10	7–15
Calcium (mg)	536	600	445	700–950
Phosphorus (mg)	454	440	300	500–690
Magnesium (mg)	46	40	53	50–80
Copper (mg)	0.6	0.4	0.4	0.4–0.6
Zinc (mg)	4.1	5	3.2	2–5.3
Iodine (µg)	67	40	69	70–160
Iron (mg)[‡]	1.5	Trace	12.7	8.5–12.7
Vitamins per Liter				
A (IU)	1650	2500	2650	2100–2500
D (IU)	413	400	423	400–423
E (IU)	12.4	15	9.5	9–11
K (mg)	—[§]	—[§]	—[§]	0.09–0.15
C (mg)	52	55	58	50–55
Thiamine (mcg)	510	650	710	400–700
Riboflavin (mcg)	620	1000	1060	600–1060
Niacin (mg)	8.25	7	7	5–8.4
Pyridoxine (mcg)	410	400	423	400–530
Folacin (mcg)	100	50	32	50–100
B$_{12}$ (mcg)	2	1.5	1.1	2–3
Pantothenate (mg)	3.1	3	2.1	2.6–5

* Prosobee, Isomil, Nursoy, Neo-mulsoy, i-soyalac (contains tapioca starch).
† Diluted per manufacturer's specifications.
‡ Enfamil with iron contains 12.7 mg; Similac with iron, 12 mg/liter.
§ Vitamin K not added because milk base supplies ample amounts.

60% of human milk protein. Whey proteins such as lactalbumin form a small, soft, easily digestible curd in the stomach.

Human milk contains enzymes that, when activated by bile salts in the intestine, help digestion of the *lipid,* or fat component of milk. Human milk fat is better absorbed than cow's milk fat; as a result, the calcium in human milk has a higher rate of absorption as well. Excess dietary fat (or poor fat absorption) results in an excess of fat in the intestine. This causes the formation of insoluble calcium soaps, which are excreted with the consequent loss of incorporated calcium. Despite the fact that cow's milk is higher in calcium than human milk, only 17% of cow's milk calcium is absorbed, in contrast to the 51% absorption rate of calcium from human milk.

The carbohydrate content of human milk is 7%; that of cow's milk is 4.8%. The higher carbohydrate content of human milk provides a favorable intestinal environment for the growth of beneficial microorganisms and is thought to enhance the absorption of calcium, magnesium, and other minerals. With respect to the metabolism and utilization of nutrients, the high protein, calcium, phosphorus, magnesium, sodium, potassium, and chloride levels of cow's milk result in a *renal solute load* about two thirds greater than that resulting from the ingestion of human milk. The renal solute load consists of metabolic end products, especially nitrogenous compounds and electrolytes, that must be excreted by the kidneys. Young infants have a limited ability to concentrate urine; depending on its composition, cow's milk formula can place a strain on an infant's immature kidneys because the solutes it contains may require 3 to 4 times as much water for excretion as the solutes in human milk.

Human milk is a rich source of cholesterol, and infants who consume breast milk develop serum cholesterol levels similar to or slightly higher than the levels found in infants fed formulas containing fat from vegetable sources. Because high serum cholesterol levels have been associated with coronary heart disease, there has been interest in lowering serum cholesterol levels for all groups including infants. However, current questions evolve around whether limiting dietary cholesterol in infants may be harmful rather than beneficial. Cholesterol is used in the synthesis of myelin, bile salts, and steroid hormones, and ingestion of cholesterol early in life may be necessary to trigger the enzyme systems that regulate the biosynthesis and catabolism of cholesterol later on.

Immunologic and Biochemical Properties of Breast Milk

Another major benefit of breast-feeding is the protection human milk gives infants against infections and allergies.

Prevention of Infection

Because of the immunologic value of breast milk, breast-fed infants have lower rates of infection than formula-fed infants. The incidence of necrotizing enterocolitis, diarrhea, respiratory infections, and gastroenteritis is very low in breast-fed infants. This suggests that breast-feeding in the early months of life offers protection against infections.

Prevention of Allergies

In addition to protecting against infections, breast-feeding may also help protect against the development of allergies. It is believed that prolonged breast-feeding may be associated with a low incidence of obvious allergic disease, particularly in babies with a family history of allergies. Specifically, prolonged breast-feeding decreases the incidence of allergic dermatitis (eczema) in babies with and without a family history of allergies up to 1 year of age. Breast-feeding also decreases the incidence of food allergies in babies with a family history of such allergies.

Growth-Promoting Factors

As more sophisticated methods became available to analyze the composition of breast milk, it was discovered that the milk contains a substance with growth-promoting activity. This substance, a polypeptide called *epidermal growth factor* (EGF), has been found in breast milk as well as in human plasma, serum, urine, and amniotic fluid. This growth factor has significant biologic effects in mammals, particularly in the fetus and newborn. Effects on the fetus and neonate include enhanced proliferation and differentiation of the epidermis, increased growth and maturation of fetal pulmonary epithelium, and stimulation of DNA synthesis in the digestive tract. Researchers have concluded that the demonstrated ability of breast milk to stimulate DNA synthesis and cell multiplication in cell cultures is probably due to the presence of EGF. In fact, breast milk is more potent in producing this effect than is purified EGF itself, leading to speculation that milk may contain substances that enhance the effect of EGF.

Potency of EGF in breast milk appears to be highest shortly after birth and decreases thereafter. Colostrum (the precursor of breast milk, a clear, yellow fluid that contains more protein and less fat and lactose than either transitional or mature breast milk) has the most marked EGF activity, about 15 times that of third-day breast milk, which in turn has EGF activity 10 times greater than 57th-day breast milk.

Psychophysiologic Advantages

Psychologic advantages of breast-feeding are more difficult to document clinically than immunologic or nutritional advantages. Breast-feeding provides a synchronous reciprocal interaction, with mother and infant simultaneously giving and receiving physical and emotional pleasure. If the infant associates the comfort of suckling and feeding with the mother, a strong infant-to-mother attachment may develop. This is not to say that the formula-feeding mother cannot develop strong feelings of attachment to and high levels of interaction with her infant; however, breast-feeding seems to enhance such an attachment.

Breast-feeding is also beneficial to the mother's physical restoration after birth; suckling stimulates the production of oxytocin, which causes the uterus to contract, thereby promoting good uterine tone, and the high energy demands of lactation lead to the utilization of fat reserves, which helps the mother regain her prepregnant figure. (See later section in this chapter for a more complete discussion of the process and management of lactation.)

However, the nurse must remember that breast-feeding will not be successful if the mother does not want to breast-feed. The nurse can answer the mother's questions, discuss any concerns the mother may have, and provide encouragement for breast-feeding if the mother has not made a firm decision about how to feed her infant. However, if the mother has considered her own feelings and situation and decided to formula-feed, the nurse should support her decision. Reasons mothers may not want to breast-feed and counseling about breast-feeding are dealt with later in this chapter.

Infant Nutritional Needs in the First Year of Life

The physical growth and development of an infant are largely dependent on the nutritional status of the mother before, during, and after (if she is breast-feeding) pregnancy, as well as on the adequacy of the infant's diet. Hereditary and environmental factors also play a role and must be considered in any evaluation of an infant's nutritional status. Generally, the characteristics listed in the

accompanying display are considered to be indications of a well-nourished infant.

The infant undergoes more rapid growth during the first year of life than in any other period. Most infants double their birth weight by 4 to 6 months and triple their birth weight by the end of the first year. During the first 6 months, the weekly weight gain normally averages 5 to 8 oz; in the second 6 months it decreases to 4 to 5 oz. A baby whose birth length is 20 to 22 inches adds another 9 to 10 inches in the first year of life.

In general, as the infant grows, the number of daily feedings decreases and the volume of feedings increases. A typical pattern of feedings for the first year of life is shown in Table 37–2. This pattern may be disrupted during growth spurts, which commonly occur at 6 and 12 weeks of age, at which time the infant may demand more frequent feedings.

A variety of factors affect the physical growth and development of the infant; these include heredity, nutritional status of the mother before and during pregnancy, and breast-feeding postpartum. A child who does not receive minimal levels of each needed nutrient will not reach his or her full physical and intellectual potential. Brain growth is not complete until the child reaches the age of 2. It has been postulated that malnutrition during this period of brain growth decreases the number of brain cells, causing permanent impairment of brain development.

Breast milk is sufficient to meet the nutritional needs of the infant for the first 4 to 6 months of life, although some supplementation for particular nutrients is necessary for the breast-fed infant, as discussed in the following section. After 6 months, the nutrients from human milk are insufficient, and the infant's diet should be supplemented with other foods.

Commercially prepared infant formulas are also sufficient to meet the infant's nutritional needs for the first months of life. Infants receiving an iron-fortified commercial formula need no nutritional supplementation during the first 6 months. If a formula without iron is used, iron supplementation or a change to an iron-fortified formula is indicated at around 4 months of age.

After 6 months to the end of the first year, breast milk or formula continues to be the most important part of the

General Characteristics of a Well-Nourished Infant

- Steady increase in weight and height
- Regular sleeping and elimination patterns
- Vigorous activity and generally happy disposition
- Firm muscles and moderate amount of subcutaneous fat
- Teething at 5 to 6 mo

Table 37–2   **Typical Pattern of Infant Feedings**

Age of Baby	Number of Feedings	Volume per Feeding	Total
Birth–2 wk	6–10	2–3 oz	12–30 oz
2 wk to 1 mo	6–8	3–4 oz	18–32 oz
1–3 mo	5–6	5–6 oz	25–36 oz
3–7 mo	4–5	6–7 oz	25–36 oz
7–12 mo	3–4	7–8 oz	25–36 oz

infant's diet. However, solid foods in the form of cereals, fruits, vegetables, and meats should be introduced during this period to help meet the infant's increasing demands, as well as to provide the infant with the opportunity to learn about different flavors and textures and to begin establishing healthy food habits. Dietary requirements for infants up to 1 year of age are listed in Table 37–3.

Nutritional Supplementation for Breast-fed Infants

The breast-fed infant's nutritional needs are met quite well by breast milk for the first 3 to 4 months of life. However, supplements of vitamin D, iron, and fluoride are recommended.

With the increased incidence of breast-feeding, the composition of breast milk is being studied more carefully. Recent studies show that breast milk contains inadequate amounts of fat- and water-soluble forms of vitamin D. Supplementation with 400 IU of vitamin D is considered prudent for the breast-fed infant; however, the specific age at which supplementation is started depends on many factors, including the amount of exposure to sunshine and skin color.

The term infant's iron stores last about 4 months. The concentration of iron in human milk is approximately 0.5 mg/liter, only 50% of which is absorbed by the infant. The average 4- to 5-month old infant consumes about 1 liter of breast milk a day and, therefore, receives about 0.25 mg of iron daily. The recommended daily iron requirement for infants from birth to age 5 months is 10 mg/day and from age 6 months to age 12 months, is 15 mg/day. (Thus, human milk does not provide the infant with an adequate supply of iron.) Iron can be provided to the older infant through supplements or, more often, through food sources such as iron-fortified infant cereals.

The amount of fluoride in breast milk does not appear to be influenced by the mother's fluoride intake. If the infant is not taking substantial amounts of water from a source providing 0.3 ppm (parts per million) of fluoride, the baby's diet should be supplemented with 0.25 mg of fluoride a day.

Maternal Nutritional Needs in the Fourth Trimester

The nutritional status of the mother in the fourth trimester is important to her own as well as to her infant's well-being. All new mothers need adequate nutrients to promote healing of tissues traumatized by labor and delivery. The mother's body chemistry and fluid and elec-

Table 37–3   Recommended Dietary Allowances for Infants

Nutrient	Recommended Dietary Allowance	
	Birth to 6 Mo	6 Mo to 1 Yr
Calories	kg × 115	kg × 105
*Protein (g)	kg × 2.2	kg × 2
Vitamin A (μg RE)[†]	420	400
*Vitamin D (μg, cholecalciferol)	10	10
Vitamin E (mg, α TE)[‡]	3	4
*Vitamin C (mg)	35	35
Folacin (μg)	30	45
Niacin (mg, NE)[§]	6	8
Riboflavin (mg)	0.4	0.6
Thiamin (mg)	0.3	0.5
*Vitamin B_6 (mg)	0.3	0.6
Vitamin B_{12} (μg)	0.5	1.5
*Calcium (mg)	360	540
*Phosphorus (mg)	240	360
Iodine (μg)	40	50
Magnesium (mg)	50	70
Zinc (mg)	3	5
*Iron (mg)	10	15

* Only these nutrients have been discussed in this chapter.
† RE = retinol equivalents
‡ TE = tocopherol equivalents
§ NE = niacin equivalents
National Academy of Sciences, National Research Council: Recommended Dietary Allowances, 9th ed. Washington, DC, Government Printing Office, 1980

trolyte balances have been altered dramatically and need time and proper nourishment to return to homeostasis. The breast-feeding woman has an increased need for fluids, nutrients, and calories to produce sufficient amounts of milk for her baby.

The woman who has a chronic illness, such as diabetes or heart disease, or the woman who experienced complications during pregnancy or delivery may have special dietary needs. These needs are best evaluated by a nutritionist. It is the nurse's responsibility to recommend the intervention of a nutritionist when appropriate and to ensure that all postpartum women receive nutritional counseling appropriate to their needs.

Nutritional Requirements of Lactating Mothers

Lactation is a physiologic part of the reproductive process and may be influenced by maternal nutrition during pregnancy and after childbirth. The weight gain recommended during pregnancy, approximately 12.5 kg, is thought to provide adequately for fetal growth and the accumulation of maternal reserves. In some respects lactation makes even greater demands on the maternal organism than does pregnancy. Nutritional requirements for pregnant women, lactating women, and nonlactating women are shown in Table 37–4.

Calorie and Protein Requirements

A lactating woman can meet the energy costs of milk production through an adequate dietary intake of calories and protein, and through the catabolism of body tissue (fat or lean tissue). Lactating mothers produce 850 ml of breast milk per day on the average. The average fat reserve accumulated during pregnancy is 2 to 4 kg, which can provide an additional 200 to 300 kcal per day for 100 days to assist in breast-milk production.

These factors, and the efficiency with which breast milk is produced, were considered when the current RDA for energy for lactating women was proposed, that is: *an additional 500 kcal per day* above the normal dietary intake level is recommended. Women with low weight gain during pregnancy have less energy reserve and therefore may require more than this additional 500 kcal a day to meet their energy needs without causing the catabolism of lean tissue. Women who engage in heavy activity or who breast-feed beyond 6 months will also require a higher calorie intake than do other lactating women.

Vitamin and Mineral Requirements

The lactating woman needs extra amounts of most vitamins and minerals for milk production, as shown in Table 37–1. It is believed that the content of water-soluble vitamins in human milk is directly related to the ma-

Table 37–4   **Recommended Dietary Allowances for Adult Women**

Nutrients	Woman's Condition		
	Pregnant	*Lactating*	*Nonlactating*
Calories	2300	2500	2000
Protein (g)	74	64	44
Vitamin A (μg RE)*	1000	1200	800
Vitamin D (μg cholecalciferol)	10	10	5
Vitamin E (mg α TE)†	10	11	8
Vitamin C (mg)	80	100	60
Folacin (mg)	800	500	400
Niacin (mg NE)‡	15	18	13
Riboflavin (mg)	1.5	1.7	1.2
Thiamine (mg)	1.4	1.5	1
Vitamin B_6 (mg)	2.6	2.5	2
Vitamin B_{12} (μg)	4	4	3
Calcium (mg)	1200	1200	800
Phosphorus (mg)	1200	1200	800
Iodine (μg)	175	200	150
Iron (mg)	18+	18+	18
Magnesium (mg)	450	450	300
Zinc (mg)	20	25	15

* RE = retinol equivalents
† TE = tocopherol equivalents
‡ NE = niacin equivalents
National Research Council, National Academy of Sciences: Recommended Dietary Allowances, 9th ed. Washington, DC, 1980

ternal intake of those vitamins. In contrast, concentrations of fat-soluble vitamins and minerals in human milk appear to be unrelated to maternal diet. If calcium is not ingested by the mother in sufficient quantities for breast-milk production, the needed amount will be mobilized from her bone stores.

Effects of Maternal Nutrition on Lactation

It was once thought that the process of lactation was unaffected by nutritional deficits. However, there is increasing evidence that suboptimal maternal nutrition adversely affects lactation. The problem of maternal depletion has not been well researched. Milk production and infant wellbeing have been of greater interest, so that studies have usually emphasized three criteria in the evaluation of lactational performance: milk volume, milk composition, and rate of infant growth.

Most women are unaware of the extra energy demands imposed by lactation. However, studies of well-nourished women indicate that successful lactation is associated with increased food intake. One classic study compared lactating and nonlactating women with respect to dietary pattern and weight loss. Both groups lost an average of 3 kg during the first 3 months postpartum. The lactating women ingested an average of 2930 kcal per day, whereas the nonlactating women ingested an average of 2070 kcal per day (Whichelow 1975).

The same study observed that the intake of women who were successfully breast-feeding ranged from 2460 to 3060 kcal a day. All of the women studied were losing weight at a modest rate, except for those whose intakes exceeded 2950 kcal a day. Women who consciously restricted their intake to 1950 kcal a day did not produce sufficient milk for their infants and had to use supplemental feedings. This study also reported two cases of lactational failure, both of which were attributed to inadequate weight gain during pregnancy (4.5 and 5 kg respectively). These women failed to produce a sufficient volume of milk despite dietary intakes of 2400 kcal a day or more. This suggests that mobilization of body fat and catabolism of lean tissue to support lactation may be more limited than was previously believed, and that nutritional status during pregnancy may be of some importance in determining lactational success.

Lactational failure in poor women may be caused by substandard diets but may also be related to the combined stresses of maternal disease, chronic undernutrition, and difficult living conditions. In general, lactational performance in undernourished women is less than optimal. Milk composition may be normal because maternal stores of essential nutrients, such as iron and calcium, are used. However, milk volume is often less than 500 ml per day, resulting in poor infant growth. When the diets of undernourished women are supplemented with protein and additional calories, milk production increases and is sustained for a longer period.

Dietary Recommendations for the Breast-feeding Mother

The lactating mother has an increased need for energy, protein, minerals, and vitamins to replenish nutrients used by the infant, to provide the necessary calories to produce milk, and as protection against a nutritional deficit. Energy requirements vary depending on the amount of milk being produced. An 11-lb infant needs 600 kcal per day, which requires 850 ml of milk. As the amount of milk needed for the infant increases, so does the need for additional calories in the mother's diet. Women who gain sufficient weight during pregnancy have body fat reserves that can be mobilized for extra milk production. This fat store is also of benefit during the first few weeks postpartum, when the mother is busy and may not be eating enough to meet her needs.

The amounts of essential nutrients required during lactation are greater than those needed in pregnancy. The breast-feeding mother's diet should contain at least 1 quart of milk or its equivalent in cheese or yogurt per day. Adequate milk intake protects against calcium and phosphorus drain. When maternal calcium intake is low, calcium supplements should be provided. Large amounts of fluid are essential for providing water to the breast milk in addition to meeting the mother's needs for fluid. Two to three quarts of various liquids should be consumed each day; vegetable and fruit juices (which provide vitamins and minerals), water, and milk are good choices. Table 37–5 shows suggested servings of food groups for both lactating and nonlactating mothers.

The nursing mother should continue taking her prenatal vitamin pills and one iron pill per day. Since many substances pass into her milk, the mother should avoid ingesting alcohol, artificially sweetened products, and drugs such as aspirin, laxatives, sedatives, oral contraceptives, and street drugs.

As mentioned, breast-feeding requires extra energy, so that the lactating woman needs to ingest 500 kcal over her normal maintenance diet to sustain adequate milk production.

Dietary Recommendations for the Formula-Feeding Mother

The nutritional status of a woman affects not only her own health but also that of her family. A woman of reproductive age, who already has children, usually has a basic knowledge of and understanding about the need for specific nutrients, food groups, and a well-rounded diet. If the family plans their meals with these concepts in mind, they will benefit from the positive effects of good nutri-

Table 37–5   Food Guide for the Fourth Trimester

Food Group	Breast-feeding Dairy	Breast-feeding No Dairy*	Not Breast-feeding	Lower-Calorie Food Choices
Protein foods (vegetable or animal) 1 serving = 2 oz cooked meat, poultry, fish 2 eggs 2 tbsp to ¼ cup nutbutter ½ cup nuts or seeds 1 cup cooked beans, peas ½ cup low-fat cottage cheese	4	6–8	3	Trim fat from all meats. Use more fish and poultry (white meat) than red meat. Remove poultry skin. Use water-packed canned fish. Limit luncheon meats (high in fat). Use dry-roasted nuts and old-fashioned style peanut butter.
Dairy products 1 serving = 1 cup milk, yogurt ⅓ cup dry milk powder 1 cup tofu or soymilk 1½ oz hard cheese 1⅓ cup ice cream 1 cup soft frozen yogurt	4	0–1†	2	Nonfat milk or a mixture of nonfat and low-fat. Nonfat or plain yogurt. Limit ice cream. Use yogurt in place of sour cream. Cook with nonfat milk.
Grains (whole grains are best) 1 serving = 1 slice bread 1 oz cereal (cold) ½ cup cooked hot cereal ½ cup cooked pasta or rice 1 tsp wheat germ 1 tortilla	6	6	5	Limit amount of fat (margarine, butter, mayonnaise), sauces, and sweets (jam) you add to grains. Limit sweet rolls, donuts, cookies, croissants, rich crackers (look for fat listed toward the front of the ingredient list). Use cereals without added oil, shortening, sugar, or honey.
Vitamin-C-rich vegetables 1 serving = ½ to ¾ cup citrus juice or broccoli, cabbage, peppers, cantaloupe, tomato, strawberries	2+	2+	1+	Overcooking destroys vitamin C. Use fresh fruits or those canned without added sugar. Drink fruit fizzes (juice and water) in place of full-strength juice.
Leafy green vegetables 1 serving = 1 cup, raw or cooked	1+	1+	1+	Steam or stir-fry or eat raw. Avoid sauces, added fat, etc. Use low-fat salad dressing.
Other fruits and vegetables 1 serving = ½ cup to ¾ cup	3	3	3	Snack on fruits and vegetables often. Limit avocados (high in calories).

* Plus supplemented calcium (1000 mg/day)
† Only for mothers who must avoid milk products because of allergy or lactase deficiency
Adapted from California Department of Health Services, Maternal and Child Health Branch: Nutrition During Pregnancy and the Postpartum Period: A Manual for Health Care Professionals, 1988

tion. However, the nurse cannot assume that every woman has this knowledge.

A formula-feeding mother has special dietary needs. While adjusting to her new baby and her higher than normal energy requirements, the mother should be particularly aware of her own nutrient intake. Her nutrient stores may have been lost during pregnancy and must be replaced to provide the energy and stamina she requires for her physical and mental health. Table 37–5 gives a fourth-trimester food guide for the breast-feeding and nonbreast-feeding mother. If the new infant is not her first child and her pregnancies have been close together, the store of nutrients expended during the previous pregnancy may not have been fully replenished; this is particularly likely to be the case if the pregnancies occurred within a year of one another.

Dietary Recommendations for the Adolescent Mother

When the postpartum mother is an adolescent, her nutritional deficits are compounded. Adolescence is a period of rapid growth, when nutritional needs for body metabolism are greatly increased. The pregnant adolescent must consume an unusually large number of calories to meet her own growth requirements as well as the nutrient demands of her fetus. The needs for increased amounts of protein, iron, calcium, and other essential nutrients is important. During pregnancy, when her nutritional status is closely monitored to assure proper weight gain and dietary intake, the adolescent may become relatively well nourished. However, her only postpartum contact with a health professional will probably occur at her 6-week checkup or when she seeks contraception. Therefore, adolescent mothers should be given special attention by the nurse, who must be realistic in developing a nutritional plan. Adolescents generally are very active, may be dependent financially, are subject to peer pressure, and will feel the urgent need to get their bodies back in shape. Early postpartum referral to a public health nurse may be helpful in following the adolescent at home; this nurse can reinforce and encourage good eating habits and also offer support if the young mother is feeling stressed.

Women should be conscious of the need to improve their nutritional status during the postpartum and interconceptual periods. The woman who follows the recommended dietary allowances shown in Table 37–5 with careful food purchasing and meal planning can be assured of adequate nourishment that will benefit not only her health but also that of her family.

HORMONAL SUPPORT OF LACTATION

With the baby's birth and expulsion of the placenta, changes occur in hormonal control by the hypothalamus. The following section discusses the hormonal support of lactation and resulting mechanisms. Nurses must understand the anatomy and physiology of the lactating breasts, not only for their own knowledge base but also to educate the new mother.

The mammary glands are modified exocrine glands that undergo numerous anatomic and physiologic changes during pregnancy and immediately following birth. The breast is composed of glandular tissue surrounded by adipose tissue and is separated from the underlying chest muscles and ribs by connective tissue.

Lactogenesis, the initiation of milk flow, requires fully developed mammary glands. The hormones necessary for milk production include prolactin, growth hormone, glucocorticoids, insulin, and parathyroid hormone. These hormones supply the amino acids, fatty acids, glucose, and calcium required for milk formation.

During pregnancy, estrogen and progesterone produce specific effects in the breasts. The ductal system proliferates and differentiates under the influence of estrogen, and progesterone promotes an increase in the size of lobes, lobules, and alveoli (Fig. 37–1). Colostrum, the

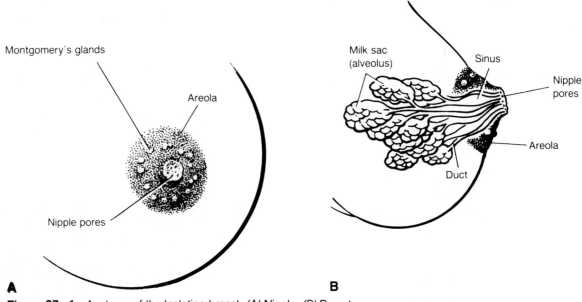

Figure 37–1. Anatomy of the lactating breast. *(A)* Nipple. *(B)* Breast.

clear, yellow-colored "first milk," is secreted from the lining of the alveoli and ductules. Colostrum is the major component of breast milk in the first 1 or 2 days and contains antibodies important to the vulnerable newborn.

Placental and ovarian estrogens decrease after birth, and the hypothalamus stimulates the anterior and posterior pituitary glands to activate prolactin and oxytocin (Fig. 37–2).

Prolactin

Prolactin is the single most important hormone for the normal production of milk. Its secretion is regulated by the hypothalamic control of prolactin inhibitory factor

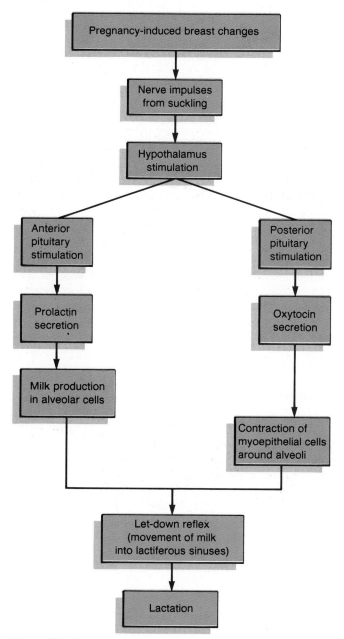

Figure 37–2. Milk production and let-down reflex.

(PIF) and thyrotropin-releasing factor. The suckling of the infant at the breast inhibits the PIF, and prolactin is released. When the concentration of prolactin in the blood stream is high, the hypothalamus responds by secreting PIF.

The sucking of the infant at the mother's breast is necessary to maintain lactation. It not only removes milk from the glands, but it also causes the release of prolactin, which is essential for the continuous secretion of milk. During breast-feeding, plasma prolactin levels rise, with normal levels rising and declining in 3-hour periods. This means that frequent nursing is essential to maintain plasma prolactin levels over a 24-hour period. Frequent nursing is also vital to continuation of the pituitary responsiveness necessary to maintain the suckling response at an optimal level. As intervals between nursing are lengthened, the pituitary prolactin release prompted by the baby's sucking is diminished. To establish lactation, the infant should be put to the breast as soon as possible after delivery. To maintain optimum lactation, a regular breast-feeding pattern should be established.

Oxytocin

Oxytocin is released by a neurohumoral reflex called the *milk-ejection* (or *let-down*) reflex. Sensory nerve endings located in the areola of the nipple are stimulated by the baby's sucking. Impulses are transmitted through the spinal column to the hypothalamus, which stimulates the posterior pituitary to release oxytocin. The blood stream carries the oxytocin to the mammary gland receptors located in the myoepithelial cells, which respond by contracting.

Oxytocin is released over several minutes during each breast-feeding. In some women the milk-ejection reflex may become conditioned, and a stimulus from the baby, such as crying, may trigger the release of milk before the baby has even begun to nurse. The mother may experience the let-down reflex as a tingling sensation. Also, when breast-feeding their infants, many mothers experience uterine contractions that are probably related to oxytocin secretion. The reflex becomes more coordinated as breast-feeding is well established. In the early days of breast-feeding, the reflex may be so strong that while the baby nurses at one breast, the other breast may leak milk. The mother may also experience milk let-down upon hearing another new baby cry or in situations where she cannot nurse her baby. The nurse should show the mother how she can cross her arms and discreetly place firm pressure on her nipples to stop the leaking.

The mother who is anxious or in pain may experience difficulty in establishing this reflex, thereby making less milk available to the newborn. This may have one of two causes: the effect of stress on the hypothalamus, or the release of adrenalin, which blocks the effects of oxytocin on the myoepithelial cells at the local level.

The nurse can assist by providing a relaxed and supportive atmosphere and contributing to a sense of maternal well-being.

Insulin

Insulin has an important role in the synthesis and metabolism of nutrients for both the mother and baby during lactation. Its three primary functions are: (1) to promote glucose uptake from the maternal blood stream; (2) to induce synthesis of enzymes needed for carbohydrate metabolism; and (3) to help in stimulating the production of proteins and lipids in the active mammary gland.

Glucocorticoids

The glucocorticoids, adrenal steroid hormones, regulate water transport across the cell membranes during lactation.

Parathyroid Hormone

The parathyroid hormone limits the calcium content of the mother's milk and adjusts the iron content to the needs of the infant. It also protects the mother against hypocalcemia and excessive calcium depletion.

IMPLICATIONS FOR NURSING CARE

Promoting optimal maternal–infant nutrition is a significant part of the nursing care of childbearing families. The following sections address briefly the process of assessment, identification of potential and actual problems in relation to maternal–infant nutrition, and the nurse's role in providing care.

Assessment

Initial assessment of maternal nutritional status in the postpartum period is based on data regarding maternal prepregnant and pregnant weight, evidence of adequate iron stores, an adequate dietary history or profile, as well as the recognition of any complicating factors, such as unusual blood loss during delivery. The assessment of infant nutritional status is usually carried out in routine pediatric care and thus is not an area of responsibility of the maternity nurse. However, the maternity nurse is directly responsible for assessing the parents' knowledge and skill related to infant feeding, and for providing essential patient teaching in the early postpartum period. This teaching is detailed in the following sections on promoting maternal–infant nutrition.

Diagnosis

Problems related to maternal–infant nutrition in the first 3 months after birth are usually diagnosed by standard indicators, such as infant weight gain and feeding patterns, maternal weight loss or gain, restoration of maternal iron stores, maternal energy levels, and maternal patterns of elimination. The maternity nurse's most consistent contact with childbearing women and their infants usually occurs in too short a time frame to pick up such problems.

However, the postpartum nurse can anticipate common concerns among new mothers about infant feeding and self-care, and may identify particular patient needs for teaching and support. The following are some nursing diagnoses that may be useful in providing nursing care related to maternal-infant nutrition:

- Potential for altered bowel elimination: diarrhea
- Ineffective breast-feeding
- Altered health maintenance
- Altered nutrition: more or less than body requirements

Planning and Implementation

The most important implications for nursing care center around promoting optimal maternal–infant nutrition in the fourth trimester. The following sections address the nurse's role in promoting maternal nutrition and optimal infant-feeding practices. The maternity nurse is responsible for early instruction regarding breast-feeding and formula-feeding and for assisting parents in their first attempts to feed their infant.

Promoting Optimal Maternal Nutrition

The nurse can anticipate that the new mother will have concerns about reestablishing her normal patterns quickly in the postpartum period, and may need nutritional guidance in relation to her own physical restoration. Major concerns shared by most new mothers include weight loss and reestablishing prepregnant weight, maintaining energy levels, and establishing and maintaining breast-milk supply if the mother chooses to breast-feed.

Weight Loss

One of the primary concerns of the new mother is her weight; she would like to get rid of her flabby abdomen and return to her prepregnant shape. Delivery causes a weight loss of approximately 12 to 17 lb due to expulsion

SELF-CARE TEACHING

Nutritional Recommendations for Optimal Maternal Health

The nurse should review the following recommendations with new mothers:

Maintain an adequate diet by eating a variety of foods daily. These foods should include

- Fruits
- Vegetables
- Whole-grain and enriched breads, cereals, and grain products
- Milk, cheese, and yogurt
- Meats, poultry, fish, and eggs

Avoid too much fat, saturated fat, and cholesterol

- Choose lean meat, fish, poultry, dry beans, and peas as good protein sources
- Use egg yolks and organ meats such as liver in moderation
- Limit intake of butter, cream, hydrogenated margarines, shortenings, coconut oil, and foods made from such products
- Trim excess fat from meats
- Broil, bake, or boil rather than fry
- Read labels carefully to determine the amounts and types of fat contained in food
- Eat more meatless or low-meat meals
- Use nonfat or low-fat dairy products

Eat more complex carbohydrates daily

- Substitute starches for fats and sugars
- Select foods that are good sources of fiber and starch, such as whole-grain breads and cereals, fruits and vegetables, beans, peas, and nuts

Avoid excessive sugar

- Use less of all sugars, including white sugar, brown sugar, raw sugar, honey, and syrups
- Eat less foods containing these sugars, such as candy, soft drinks, ice cream, cakes, and cookies
- Eat fresh fruits or fruits canned without sugar or light syrup rather than fruits canned with heavy syrup
- Read food labels for clues on sugar content; if an "-ose" word—sucrose, glucose, maltose, dextrose, lactose, fructose—or the word *syrup* appears first, the food contains a large amount of sugar
- Remember that how often you eat sugar is as important as how much sugar you eat

Avoid too much sodium

- Learn to enjoy the unsalted flavors of foods
- Cook with only small amounts of added salt
- Add little or no salt to food at the table
- Limit your intake of salty foods such as potato chips, pretzels, salted nuts and popcorn, condiments (soy sauce, steak sauce, garlic salt), cheese, pickled foods, and cured meats
- Read food labels carefully to determine the amounts of sodium present in processed foods and snack items
- If you crave salt during pregnancy, salt your food to taste and tell your health care provider you are doing so

Get regular exercise
Assure your baby an adequate diet

- Breast-feed unless there are special problems
- Delay other foods until the baby is 4 to 6 mo old
- Do not add salt or sugar to the baby's food

Copyright, Abrams B: Department of OB/GYN and Reproductive Sciences, University of California, San Francisco. Reprinted with permission

of the infant, placenta, amniotic fluid, and, to some degree, other body fluid. Another small weight loss occurs during the first 2 to 5 days postpartum, when fluid accumulated in the body during the prenatal period is passed through diuresis and diaphoresis. The postpartum nurse should reassure the mother that by her 6-week checkup she will have lost a total of 20 to 25 lb and should not attempt a weight-loss diet until after this visit.

The nursing mother should be advised not to try to lose weight until her baby is weaned. To avoid fatigue and anemia she needs to reestablish and maintain her nutri-

tional reserves. Not all mothers need to lose weight; some merely need to tighten up their muscles with an exercise regimen after 6 weeks.

Energy Level

During the immediate postpartum period, the new mother's energy level is low, and she needs to know that this is normal. Labor and delivery are physically and emotionally exhausting. It may have been hours since the mother has had an extended, comfortable period of sleep, and she may have missed some meals. Although very hungry after delivery, the mother may be unable to eat and may need reassurance that she will be able to do so soon. If she has not received intravenous fluids, she may also be dehydrated and thirsty. The mother should be urged to rest as much as possible between her meals and her baby's feedings in preparation for going home.

The postpartum nurse should explain to the new mother that going home with a new baby can be exhausting, especially with family and friends flocking to visit the newcomer. The mother will have more demands than usual placed on her and may well find it difficult to rest, particularly if she has other youngsters who need attention and care. She should be made to realize that, because of her increased activity level and the need for her body to heal, it is important she eat nutritious meals and drink quantities of fluids. Without proper nourishment, she will soon become exhausted.

The nurse should reassure the mother that by her 6-week checkup she and her baby will have their feeding and sleep schedules established. Her body will be back to a more normal state, and she will be more rested and adjusted to her new routine. An anemic woman may need longer to regain her former energy level.

Replacement of Iron Stores

Many woman have iron deficiency anemia when they become pregnant. This means that iron stores in the body have been depleted owing to an iron-poor diet, a previous pregnancy, loss of blood through hemorrhage, or excessive loss of blood during menstrual periods. Iron deficiency anemia reduces the oxygen-carrying capacity of the blood. It may produce a variety of symptoms, including paleness of the skin, weakness, shortness of breath, lack of appetite, and a general slowdown of vital body functions.

Pregnancy may also precipitate anemia because iron needs may be increased due to the iron requirements of fetal blood and the buildup of a store of iron in the placenta and fetal liver for use in the first 3 to 6 months of life.

The nurse should explain to the postpartum woman some of the possible causes of her iron deficiency anemia. Once she learns the cause of the disorder or experiences symptoms, she may realize the importance of replenishing her iron stores and become consistent about pill-taking, if she hasn't been in the past.

The patient should be counseled about iron-rich foods to include in her daily diet and should be given a prescription for supplemental iron to be taken daily. The nurse should be sure to explain that reversing iron deficiency is a slow process and iron pills must be taken daily; when diet alone, without supplementation, is used to treat iron deficiency anemia, it takes 2 years to replace the iron lost during pregnancy.

Hydration and Elimination

Large quantities of fluids are lost from the mother's body during labor and delivery. The administration of intravenous fluids diminishes the problem, but fluids by mouth are still indicated. If she does not feel nauseated after delivery, the mother should be encouraged to drink quantities of water and nourishing liquids to help restore her body's fluid balance. When "forcing" fluids, she will want to void often and may need help to the bathroom.

Constipation may be a problem a day or two after delivery. The patient may have had little to eat in the interim and have little bulk in her gut. Stool softeners, which add moisture and bulk to the stool, make defecation easier and reduce straining. When large quantities of fluid have been ingested, constipation is less of a problem.

Promoting Successful Breast-feeding

The advantages of breast-feeding are well recognized and breast-feeding is increasing in popularity in the United States. Mothers frequently require information and support in their efforts to establish breast-feeding, and the nurse in the postpartum setting plays an especially important role in this process (Fig. 37–3).

The optimal time for initiating breast-feeding depends on the mother's physical and psychologic status and on her wishes. Mothers vary in their desire to breast-feed and their knowledge about it. The nurse must be knowledgeable about the basic anatomy and physiology of breast-feeding and its practical aspects in order to assist the new mother.

The newborn's suckling stimulates milk production on a supply-and-demand basis. Since there is a temporary lag in milk production, breast-fed infants may be offered plain water feedings after breast-feedings until breast milk has come in and the newborn no longer needs the extra fluid. However, healthy full-term newborns may not require additional fluids, and the mother should consult her pediatrician about this practice.

Separation of the mother and baby, rigid feeding schedules, substitutions of other liquids for breast milk, and delaying feedings will gradually decrease the supply of milk. The mother's milk supply will increase if she puts the baby to breast more frequently and on demand and does not give the baby substitutes for breast milk.

Assisting with Breast-feeding

The first step in assisting the mother with breast-feeding is to assess her feelings about it. The nurse might ask the mother how she made her decision and how she feels about it. A decision to breast-feed, made at the time of delivery without prenatal preparation or support from

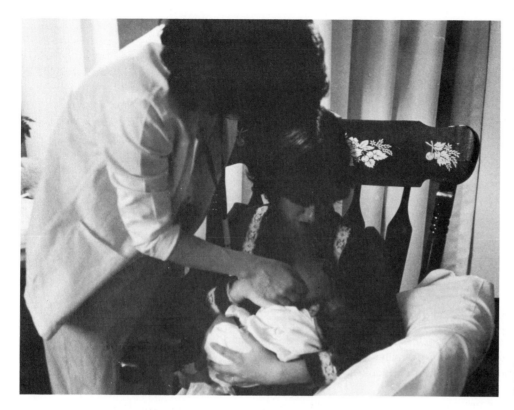

Figure 37–3. The maternity nurse provides knowledgeable and sensitive support to the breast-feeding mother. (Photo: Colleen Stainton)

family members, may predispose the mother to failure. Some women receive undue pressure to breast-feed and may not have explored their own feelings about it. Classic research in this area shows that parents who had negative feelings about breast-feeding were successful only 26% of the time, whereas those who were ambivalent were successful 35% of the time, and those who were positive had a 74% success rate under the same hospital management (Newton et al 1950). The nurse should be sensitive to what a mother is saying, and help eliminate unnecessary feelings of guilt and failure by supporting the woman in making the best decision for herself and her newborn.

The infant, as well as the father, is important to the promotion of breast-feeding. The nurse should assess the newborn's behavior to help the mother understand her baby. The nurse can also help by encouraging frequent interaction with the newborn and include the father in breast-feeding assessment and teaching. A recent study of Mexican and Mexican-American women found the only significant interpersonal influence on the feeding decision was that of the husband or partner (Sweeney and Gulino 1987). If the grandmother is an important family figure, she also should be included in teaching. In this way, important people who may significantly affect the course of breast-feeding can gain information and confidence. This may subsequently lead to more available support for the nursing mother.

Assessment of the Breasts and Nipples

Helping the mother assess her breasts in preparation for breast-feeding is an important step. The breast tissue should be checked for lumps and cysts that may require further medical evaluation. The nurse should remind the mother that regular breast self-examination is an important part of self-care, especially during the postpartum period.

Assessment includes inspection and palpation. Breast size, shape, and symmetry vary among women and have little affect on lactation. The size of the breast does not correlate with the amount of mammary tissue and its ability to produce milk. The nurse may need to reassure the mother with small breasts that she will be able to breast-feed and produce sufficient amounts of milk.

The elasticity of breast tissue also varies. Inelastic tissue feels firmly knitted together, and the overlying skin is taut, firm, and cannot easily be picked up. The elastic breast is looser, and the overlying skin is free and readily picked up (Fig. 37–4). Inelastic breasts are more prone to engorgement, which can be managed by massage, application of heat, and preventive measures.

Examination of the areola and nipple is especially important. Early detection and intervention for nipple flatness or inversion will help prevent future feeding problems. The normal and most common nipple type is the

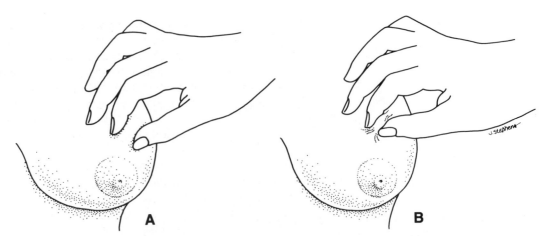

Figure 37–4. Assessing for elasticity of breast tissue. *(A)* Inelastic tissue. *(B)* Elastic tissue. (Childbirth Graphics)

erect everted nipple. This nipple is easiest for the baby to draw into its mouth and position properly against the hard palate. The *flat nipple* is smooth and may protrude little or not at all. The *inverted nipple* may partially or completely disappear inside the overlying skin and look like a fold in the skin (Fig. 37–5).

When appearance suggests that protraction of the nipple may be a problem, it is assessed by compressing the areola between the forefinger and thumb just behind the base of the nipple. If the nipple can be made to protrude manually, the flatness and inversion will probably correct itself when the newborn suckles; a truly inverted nipple will stay flat or retract further inward. The mother with complete nipple inversion should be given plastic nipple shields to wear under her bra, as shown in Figure 37–6. These cause gentle pressure at the edge of the areola, gradually forcing the nipple through the center opening of the shield, and help to increase nipple protractility. When wearing nipple shields, the mother should be re-

minded that milk may leak into the shields but should not be fed to the infant. Body warmth fosters rapid bacterial growth; nipples and nipple shields should be kept clean and dry.

Factors Affecting Milk Production

Successful breast-feeding depends upon the balance between milk production and emptying of the breast. This balance can be enhanced by a number of factors, including an adequate diet and fluid intake, adequate rest and relaxation, and the newborn's skill at suckling.

Diet

An adequate diet for a breast-feeding woman includes foods from the four major food groups and a high intake of protein and calcium (see section later in this chapter for a more detailed discussion of nutritional needs during lactation). The mother should avoid intentional weight

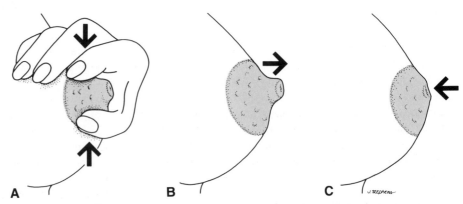

Figure 37–5. Assessing for nipple flatness or inversion. The nipple should be assessed before breast-feeding is begun by compressing the areola *(A)*. Normally, the nipple will protrude *(B)*; if it remains flat or turns in *(C)*, special attention may be required to facilitate breast-feeding. (Childbirth Graphics)

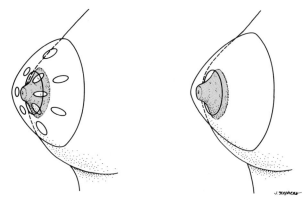

Figure 37 – 6. Plastic breast shields used to correct inverted nipples. (Childbirth Graphics)

reduction at this time because an additional 500 kcal over maintenance levels are needed for optimal milk production. The mother should drink 2 quarts of fluids per day, preferably water, milk, and unsweetened juice. Drinking a glass of water with each feeding will ensure an adequate fluid intake. Breast milk reflects the substances the mother takes into her system. Care-providers usually recommend that prenatal vitamin supplements be continued during lactation. Smoking, caffeine, alcohol, and many drugs should be avoided, since most substances ingested by the mother are excreted in breast milk.

Rest. *Adequate rest and relaxation* are essential to successful breast-feeding. The nurse should stress this and encourage the mother to nap or rest while the baby is sleeping. Limiting visitors and letting others do household chores will also help to reduce fatigue. The father's support is important here, as he can encourage her to relax and rest, eat and drink properly, and set limits on family activities. The nurse might encourage the father to bring the baby to the mother for late night feedings and handle diaper changes at that time, or to ''take over'' a feeding with a bottle of expressed and properly stored breast milk.

Newborn's Sucking Ability. *The infant's skill at emptying the breast* also affects milk supply. Although breast-feeding is thought to be an instinctive activity, only the newborn's sucking reflex is, in fact, instinctive. Many newborns must learn how to suck properly to empty the breast effectively. That process may take time for some infants, and the mother should not be overly discouraged if her newborn requires more time and practice than others.

Putting the Baby to Breast

The mother should hold the baby in a comfortable position with its arms and legs tightly wrapped and out of the way. The mother holds the breast, placing her thumb

above the nipple and the remaining four fingers on the lower part of the breast. She should then tickle the baby's cheek or bottom lip with her nipple to stimulate the rooting reflex. Once the baby's mouth opens widely, the mother centers the nipple in it and pulls the baby toward her to ensure that it takes a large portion of the areola into its mouth. The baby must compress about an inch of tissue behind the nipple with sucking pressure to empty the lactiferous sinuses, stimulate the milk ejection reflex, and avoid nipple abrasion. Figure 37 – 7 shows the good position, with the infant's sucking pressure exerted on the areola and compressing the sinuses, and the poor position, where suckling pressure is primarily exerted on the nipple itself.

The newborn generates considerable suction when nursing. Breast-feeding requires about 60 times more effort than feeding from a bottle (Coulter et al 1984). The mother should be taught to observe her newborn's sucking pattern. Usually, the baby starts with very rapid movements as it positions the nipple against its hard palate. Soon, sucking movements become rhythmic and slow down, and a soft sighing sound or a click maybe heard as the baby swallows. This signals effective or ''nutritive'' sucking.

The nurse should remind the mother that the newborn must breathe through its nose; if its breathing is impeded by clothing or by the side of the mother's breast, it will stop nursing. The nurse should show the mother how to use her free hand to push her breast away from the baby's nose, as shown in Figure 37 – 8.

The mother should be reminded never to pull the nipple from the baby's mouth once strong suction has been established. Pulling away without breaking this suction will cause her pain and can abrade the nipple. To break the suction, the mother should put a clean fingertip into the corner of the baby's mouth and pull back slightly; once the suction is broken, she can move the baby off the nipple without difficulty, as shown in Figure 37 – 9. Abrasion can also be caused by persistent pressure on one part of the nipple; thus, the mother should be encouraged to vary the baby's positions for nursing.

The baby should be nursed on both breasts at each feeding, beginning with a different breast each time. Alternating breasts is important because the baby usually sucks longer on the first breast. The nurse can advise the mother to wear a small safety pin on her bra strap to remind her which breast should be used first for the next feeding.

Babies also need ''nonnutritive'' sucking, some babies more than others. Often, this will occur at the end of a feeding when the baby resumes a more rapid pattern or swallows only with every two or three jaw movements. The mother will have to learn her baby's own pattern, and may provide the baby with a soft, solid pacifier to help meet the baby's need for sucking.

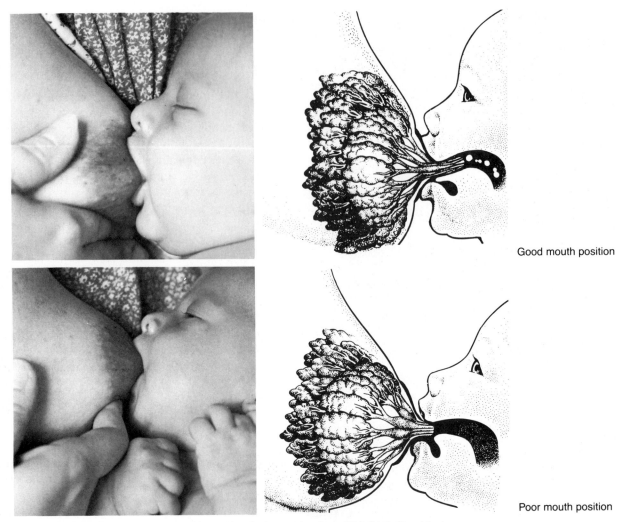

Good mouth position

Poor mouth position

Figure 37-7. Good and poor mouth position for breast-feeding. (Childbirth Graphics)

Routine Care of Breasts and Nipples

The nurse should stress the importance of good nipple care to promote successful breast-feeding. She should discuss the use of a nursing bra; many women feel more comfortable with the support and convenience of a nursing bra, but others may choose not to use them. Even if a mother does not purchase special nursing bras with flaps that can be let down for nursing, she may still want to purchase nipple pads or a supply of cotton handkerchiefs that can be used as nipple pads and easily laundered. These prevent clothing from being stained by leaking breast milk, which is a common occurrence in the early weeks of breast-feeding.

The mother should wash the breasts and nipples with warm water daily; soap may be excessively drying and may predispose the nipples to cracking. The breasts should then be dried; the mother may wish to buff her nipples for a few seconds to help decrease their sensitivity, thereby increasing her tolerance of the newborn's

strong initial sucking. The nurse can also encourage the mother to expose her nipples to the air for 5 minutes after each feeding to promote drying and healing of any early irritation. Wearing the flaps of the nursing bra down allows the nipples to rub against clothing and will also help decrease their sensitivity.

The mother should be advised to avoid putting any substances on the areola or nipple. Many commercial breast creams contain alcohol, which may irritate the skin. Vitamin E or aloe vera may be used in very small amounts if the nipples seem excessively dry, but must be removed before feeding. Nipples should be kept dry between feedings; wet nipple pads should be changed promptly.

Positions for Breast-feeding

The nurse should assist the mother in finding comfortable and effective positions for nursing. The mother should try several positions, both to prevent nipple irrita-

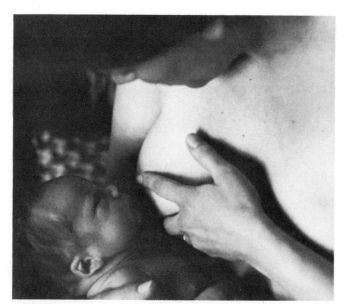

Figure 37–8. The nurse can assist the mother in establishing early breast-feeding by reminding the mother that the newborn is an obligate nose-breather and that the infant will stop nursing if its nose is obstructed by her breast. The mother can prevent this by placing her finger as shown and pressing her breast away from the infant. (Photo: BABES, Inc.)

NURSING RESEARCH

Prevention of Postpartum Nipple Tenderness and Breast Engorgement

A study reported in the Journal of Obstetrical and Gynecological Neonatal Nursing indicated that prenatal preparation may decrease nipple tenderness in the postpartal period, and early postpartum breast massage may decrease engorgement. The study of 25 women who prepared one nipple and massaged one breast but not the other, found significantly less nipple soreness and engorgement in the prepared breast. Nipple preparation consisted of nipple rolling for 30 seconds twice daily, beginning at 34 weeks of gestation. Breast massage was done after each feeding for the first 4 days postpartum. Although previous studies found no significant benefit in nipple preparation, this study suggests that nipple preparation and massage may be helpful to breast-feeding women.

Storr GB: Prevention of nipple tenderness and breast engorgement in the postpartum period. J Obstet Gynecol Neonatal Nurs 17:203, 1988

tion and to enable the baby to become accustomed to different positions. Figure 37–10 shows side-lying, sitting, and back-lying (or Australian) positions.

The most common position is the *cradle* position (Fig. 37–10D). The mother should be seated comfortably; a pillow can be placed on her lap to help support the infant's

weight, an especially helpful tip for mothers recovering from a cesarean birth, since this helps avoid pressure on the abdominal incision.

Another common position is the *football hold* (Fig. 37–10E), so called because the baby is tucked under the mother's arm on the side on which it is nursing. This position may also be comfortable for cesarean mothers and will vary the position of the infant's mouth on the nipple when used alternately with other positions.

The *side-lying* position (Fig. 37–10F) is often comfortable in the early hours after birth and is especially useful at night. Some infants fall asleep easily if cuddled and kept warm, and this position may keep the baby alert enough to nurse.

The *Australian* or *back-lying* position (Fig. 37–10G), in which the mother lies on her back holding the infant on her abdomen, may be useful for mothers whose milk flows more quickly than the infant can swallow, causing choking. This position allows the infant to better control the flow of milk to the back of the mouth.

Feeding Schedules

Mothers are sometimes advised to limit the amount of time the baby nurses during the first few days to prevent sore nipples. However, this may only delay soreness until after the mother goes home and may even interfere with

(text continued on page 1156)

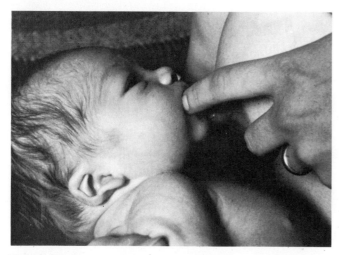

Figure 37–9. The nurse should explain that the nursing infant creates suction on the nipple and that a finger should be inserted in the corner of the infant's mouth to release this suction before removing the infant from the breast. This prevents the nipple from becoming sore. (Photo: BABES, Inc.)

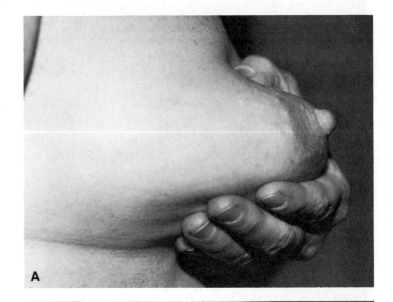

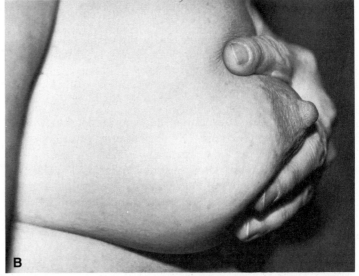

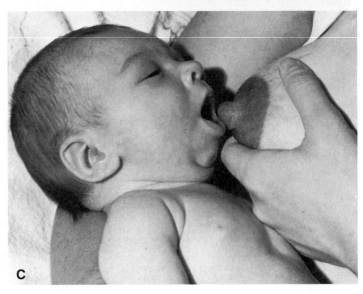

Figure 37–10. The breast should be well supported with the fingers from below, while the thumb compresses slightly to evert the nipple so that the baby can latch on effectively *(A)*. Compressing the nipple between two fingers *(B)* does not support the breast well and keeps the baby from easily latching on to the nipple. *(C)* Correct hand position makes it easier for the mother to elicit the baby's rooting reflex and place the nipple well back in the baby's mouth.

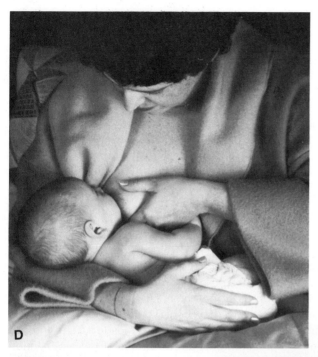

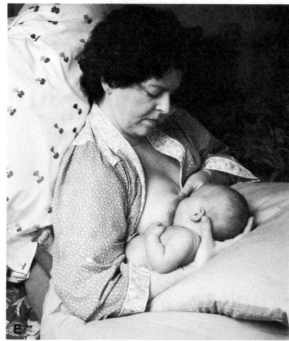

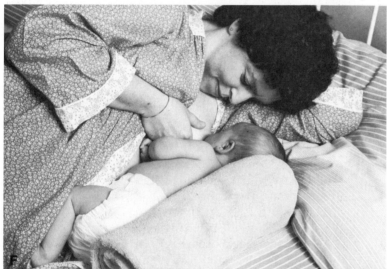

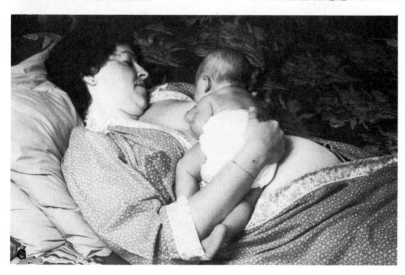

Figure 37–10 (continued). *(D)* The cradle position, with the baby on its side and tucked close to the mother. *(E)* The football hold. *(F)* The side-lying position. Note the rolled towel used to support the baby, freeing the mother's hand. *(G)* The Australian position. (Childbirth Graphics)

early breast-feeding by delaying the establishment of the let-down reflex and encouraging engorgement from clogged ducts and ductules. The mother should be advised to breast-feed the baby as soon after delivery as possible, and then to feed it on demand.

The first 5 to 7 minutes of nursing empty 90% of the milk in the breast; nursing beyond 10 minutes helps satisfy the baby's sucking needs. To increase the milk supply, the mother should be encouraged to nurse more frequently for periods of 10 minutes on each breast, rather than nurse for progressively longer periods and at longer intervals.

Concerns About the Adequacy of Milk Supply

A common concern of breast-feeding mothers, and often of other family members, is whether the baby is getting enough milk. Women frequently stop breast-feeding because of this concern, but lactational failure is rare in healthy women. If the baby is sleeping in a fairly predictable pattern, has a satisfactory weight gain, wets six or more diapers a day with colorless urine, and has a soft stool after most feedings, it is receiving enough milk (Neifert et al 1986).

Offering a breast-fed baby a supplemental bottle after a feeding is not an accurate test of whether the baby is receiving enough milk. Most breast-fed infants will not refuse an offered bottle; getting milk from a bottle is much easier than getting it from the breast, and the baby may take the feeding without really needing it.

The nurse should advise the mother that if she becomes concerned her infant is not getting enough milk, she should contact her pediatrician or an experienced lactation counselor, who can advise her on practices that can increase her milk production. These include increasing fluids and rest, nursing the baby more frequently than usual, and manual expression of the breasts after the baby has nursed.

Manual Expression and Breast Pumping

The nurse may wish to teach the mother the technique of manual expression of breast milk and alert her to the availability of breast pumps. Manual expression and breast pumping are ways to empty the breast at times when the infant cannot be nursed, to provide breast milk that can later be bottle-fed, or to provide breast milk for an infant who cannot nurse. Manual expression is gentler on breast tissue but slower than hand or electric pumps.

Manual expression of milk involves emptying the sinuses by compressing the areola and squeezing milk from the nipple, as shown in Figure 37–11. The nurse can teach the mother this technique before a feeding. The mother should be instructed to grasp the breast between the thumb and forefinger just behind the areola so that she can feel the distended ducts between her thumb and

finger. She presses her thumb and forefinger together with a rapid and gentle movement, then releases quickly. The force of compression should be directed inward toward the body. Massage and compression is repeated 10 to 12 times, rotating around the breast to compress all the sinuses. Milk should squirt out in several thin streams from the many openings in the nipple. The mother should express from one breast until the stream slows to drops, then move to the other breast. Milk in that breast will "let down" in response to the stimulation of the other. If compression is intended to empty the breast, it may be necessary to continue for as long as an hour before no more milk is expressed. About 20 to 30 minutes may be required to express the amount of milk usually emptied in an average feeding. For this reason, hand or electric breast pumps are often useful. Figure 37–12 shows a hand and an electric breast pump in use.

Hand pumps empty the breast faster than manual expression because they operate by suction rather than compression. Electric pumps are most efficient and can empty a breast in only a few minutes. However, suction from breast pumps may be more traumatic to breast tissue and may be more uncomfortable at first. Directions for using breast pumps vary. If pumping is intended to empty the breast, it should be continued until the flow of milk has stopped and the breasts are soft.

One common reason for manually expressing or pumping the breasts is to store breast milk for bottle-feeding. This can be done safely if some guidelines are followed. First, the milk should be expressed into a container that has been sterilized by immersion in boiling water for 5 minutes. Breast milk can then be poured into sterilized bottles and refrigerated up to 24 hours or it can be frozen, in which case it will last up to 4 months.

Breast-feeding and Sexuality

Lactation has consequences for the woman's sexuality, and the nurse should alert the mother to these effects so that she will recognize them as normal. In the early weeks of breast-feeding, the mother may experience either an increased or a decreased libido. Both partners should understand that this is a normal, temporary pattern and should be encouraged to discuss their feelings openly with each other.

Breast-feeding mothers should make a special effort to allow themselves uninterrupted time with their mates to maintain the couple relationship. A breast-feeding mother and her infant establish an intense, uniquely close relationship, one that may unintentionally seem to exclude the father. The father may not know how to "break in" to this closeness and may feel that his partner's decreased sexual interest is more evidence he is unneeded. On the other hand, the mother may have her body contact and sensual needs met in large part by breast-feeding and thus have less interest in sexual contact with her mate.

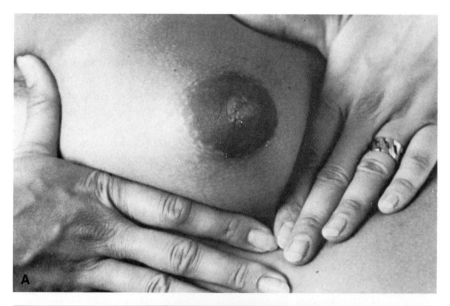

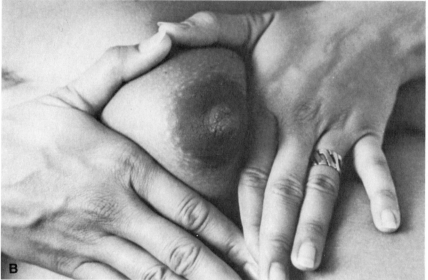

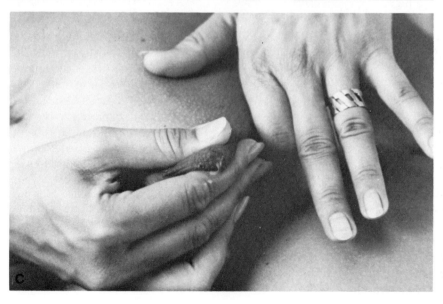

Figure 37–11. Manual expression of breast milk. *(A)* The thumb and fingers massage from the edges of the breast toward the nipple. *(B)* The thumb and forefinger are placed just outside the areola and press in toward the chest to move milk into the sinuses lying just behind the areola. *(C)* The thumb and forefinger compress the outer edge of the areola (not the nipple itself), pushing together and backward against the breast to express milk. The entire procedure is repeated until as much milk as desired has been expressed. (Photo: BABES, Inc.)

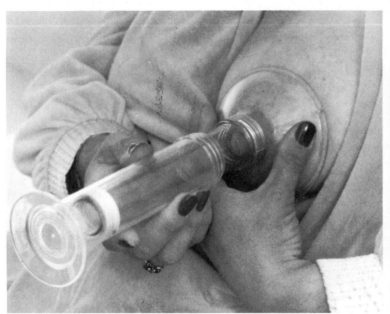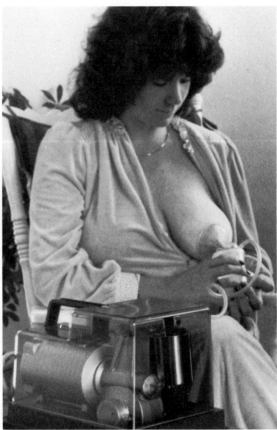

Figure 37–12. Breasts can be emptied using hand pumps or electric breast pumps. (Photo: BABES, Inc.)

Parents may also find the presence of the baby nearby quite distracting. Although it may seem that the baby wakes and cries whenever parents begin to become sexually involved, the fact is that breast-feeding infants may feed as often as every 2 hours, so that the likelihood of *any* activity's being interrupted by crying is quite high. The nurse can alert parents to the fact that these feelings are common and quite normal. Open communication and nurturance of the couple relationship is the treatment of choice.

Nursing mothers and new fathers may also find that they are frequently very tired and uninterested in sexual activity. The nurse can encourage them to substitute other forms of closeness and intimacy that include the baby and to think of their bedroom as a focal point for cuddling, breast-feeding, and playing with the baby, a haven for comfort, sleep, and privacy.

Lactation also has some direct physiologic effects on the woman's sexuality. The relative estrogen depletion in lactating women results in a dry vaginal mucosa, which may lead to some discomfort during sexual intercourse. The nurse should advise the mother to use a water-soluble lubricant (personal lubricant or contraceptive cream) or light vegetable oil to increase her comfort (Riordan et al

1980). The mother should also expect to experience some milk leakage from her breasts with sexual stimulation and orgasm; this can be minimized by nursing the baby before sexual activity or simply by keeping towels handy to keep bedding dry.

Common Breast-feeding Problems

In the postpartum setting, the nurse may not actually see breast-feeding problems develop. Most mothers and their newborns are discharged before breast-feeding is well established, and problems usually arise at home. The nurse should encourage the mother to consult a lactation specialist or health professional with expertise in breast-feeding, or a lactation support group should a problem develop. The postpartum nurse may also provide some anticipatory guidance about these common problems.

Engorgement

Engorgement is caused by the accumulation of colostrum or milk. Mild engorgement is characterized by overfilled sinuses so that the breasts become distended. The baby may not be able to grasp the firm, flat areola and will probably compress only the nipple. The mother should express some milk from the sinuses to soften this area, thereby allowing the baby to compress it and nurse properly. *Peripheral engorgement* involves the entire breast, causing physical discomfort or pain from the hardness and overdistention of the breasts. If this condition continues for 3 to 4 days without emptying of the sinuses, retrogression of the secretory tissue occurs and may cause lactation to cease.

Treatment of engorgement should include the application of heat, breast massage, and expression of milk. A hot, wet washcloth applied to the breast or a hot shower before massaging the breast decreases the discomfort. The mother should massage by making several gentle but firm stroking movements with the fingertips along the swollen ducts, moving toward the nipple. This should be done around the entire surface of the breast. After massaging, milk should be expressed or pumped until it flows freely. The baby should then be allowed to nurse from both breasts.

Sore Nipples

Sore nipples are usually caused by the improper position of the baby on the nipple. The mother should ensure that the baby is grasping the areola when sucking and not just the nipple. If nipples become sore or cracked, as shown in Figure 37–13, the mother should start feedings on the less affected breast. After feedings, she should air-dry the breasts and expose them to dry heat. Drying the breasts with a hair dryer on low setting, or exposing them to an electric lamp with a 60-watt bulb at a distance of 2 to 3 feet for 20 minutes two or three times a day, helps to promote healing. Applications of vitamin E, pure aloe vera, or lanolin may be soothing, but these substances should be removed before feeding. Nipple shields or applications of ice just before a feeding may be used if nipples are extremely sensitive.

Mastitis

Mastitis is an infectious process in the breast, producing localized tenderness, redness, and warmth. The symptoms include fever, malaise, and nausea. Mastitis is usually not seen in the early postpartum period. The mother should be advised to consult her health care provider if these symptoms occur. Treatment may include an antibiotic that is safe to use with breast-feeding and expression of milk from the affected breast. The mother should continue to breast-feed, although she should be

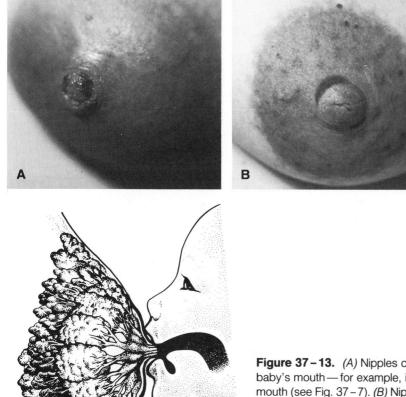

Figure 37–13. *(A)* Nipples can become sore from improper positioning of the baby's mouth—for example, if the baby does not take the entire nipple into the mouth (see Fig. 37–7). *(B)* Nipples can become cracked and sore because of uneven or repetitive pressure on one area. This can be prevented by varying the position used for nursing. *(C)* Nipples may also become sore because the breasts are overfull (engorged) and the baby cannot latch on to the nipple because the breast tissue is too firm. (Compare Fig. 37–7). (Childbirth Graphics)

advised to nurse the baby on the unaffected side first. Bed rest, fluids, warm or cold packs, and analgesics should be recommended. (See Chapter 30 for further discussion.)

Cessation of Breast-feeding (Weaning)

Mothers breast-feed for variable amounts of time, depending on their motivation to continue, their babies' responses, their work schedules, continued milk production, and a variety of other reasons. The mother who chooses to breast-feed should be encouraged to do so for at least the first 5 to 6 months of her infant's life. By this time semisolid foods have been introduced and the baby is learning to drink from a cup. The mother who introduces solid food into her baby's diet before the infant is 5 or 6 months old finds that her milk production decreases, her baby sucks less vigorously than before, and weaning occurs earlier than desired.

When the mother decides to wean her baby, she should do so gradually to minimize her discomfort. If she tries to wean abruptly, her breasts swell with milk and become extremely uncomfortable. Extracting milk from the breasts for relief eases the discomfort but also causes milk production to continue. Additionally, the infant is not prepared for an abrupt change in feeding pattern and will protest if weaned suddenly. The mother should eliminate one feeding each week or every two weeks, depending on her eagerness to wean. This will cause a gradual reduction in her milk supply. A bottle or cup should be substituted for the deleted feeding, and other foods slowly introduced. Weaning the child from the breast in this gradual way causes the mother little or no discomfort and provides time for the child to adapt to changes in the feeding pattern.

In general terms, the effectiveness of nursing support for breast-feeding in the postpartum period can be evaluated by the duration of breast-feeding. If the mother sustains breast-feeding for at least 2 to 3 months and feels satisfied with the level of nursing support she received, with her own knowledge about breast-feeding, and with her own and her infant's performance, this suggests effective nursing care (Fig. 37–14). Unfortunately, the nurse in the postpartum setting rarely sees these outcomes. However, breast-feeding success stories are becoming more common, and the maternity nurse must be knowledgeable in this area to provide complete care to the postpartum patient and her family.

Promoting Optimal Formula-Feeding

The ideal food for the infant is breast milk. When the mother chooses not to breast-feed, commercial formulas can be used to meet the infant's nutritional needs. Current attitudes toward the value of breast-feeding are strongly positive; many pediatricians feel that all full-

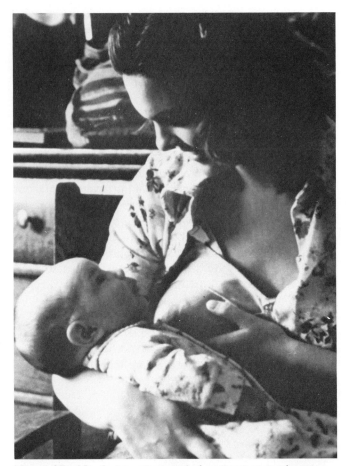

Figure 37–14. An important goal of postpartum nursing care is to promote establishment of effective and satisfying breast-feeding for infant and mother in the early months of life. (Photo: BABES, Inc.)

term infants should be breast-fed when no contraindications exist.

However, the mother may be ambivalent about breast-feeding for a multitude of reasons. She may be afraid her breasts are too small to produce sufficient milk; she may be embarrassed at the prospect of putting the baby to her breast; she may feel the need to see that her infant is taking in enough food; her partner may view her breasts as sexual objects and resent the infant's priority; the mother may feel that her work schedule precludes breast-feeding; or the mother may be afraid that breast-feeding will cause her to gain weight. The nurse should explore with the woman her motivation for breast-feeding, respecting her decision and giving support as needed.

When a mother chooses to feed her child formula, she should receive guidance from pediatric health personnel about which formula is best for her infant. However, the maternity nurse should have some understanding of the characteristics of commercial formulas and be prepared to advise the mother in the basics of formula-preparation and feeding.

A variety of commercial formulas are available; most are manufactured to contain levels of nutrients and calories similar to those found in breast milk. However, several types of formula, such as soy protein formulas and a range of caloric-content formulas, are manufactured for infants with special needs. The nurse should find out whether a specific type of formula has been recommended for an infant and advise the parents to be careful to purchase the correct type.

As discussed earlier in this chapter, most commercial formulas are prepared from nonfat cow's milk that has been modified so it can be readily metabolized by an infant. The protein and mineral content is reduced to reduce the solute load and thus the demands placed on the infant's kidneys. The curd is homogenized to make it more easily digestible. Vegetable oils, carbohydrates, vitamins, and minerals are then added so that the formula more closely matches the nutritive value of breast milk.

Most commercial formulas come in a variety of forms (see the accompanying display). Selection of a brand and form of formula should be based on the pediatrician's recommendations, cost, convenience, and the parents' ability to prepare the formula accurately and safely.

If she is planning to use a powdered or concentrated formula, the mother should be cautioned to follow directions carefully to prevent overdilution or underdilution. Both are hazardous to the infant. Underdilution of formula results in an increased solute load and may lead to dehydration. Overdilution reduces the calories and nutrients available to the infant and thereby prevents optimal growth.

Evaporated milk mixtures, widely used for infant feeding before commercial formulas were available, are not generally recommended. Mixtures consisting of evaporated milk, water, and corn syrup present a higher risk of bacterial contamination and improper measurement of ingredients than do commercial formulas. Infants fed on evaporated milk mixtures also require regular supplements of vitamin C and iron.

The nurse should remind the mother that an infant fed

iron-fortified commercial formula generally does not require other supplementation. If the formula used is not supplemented with iron, the infant will need additional dietary iron after 4 months of age. This can be provided by an iron-fortified infant cereal when the baby is developmentally ready for solid foods. Infants show their readiness for solid foods from about 4 months, when they have enough head control to facilitate feeding, have more coordinated swallowing patterns than before, can transfer food from the front of the tongue to the back, and use more rotating tongue movements than sucking movements.

Teaching About Safe Infant-Feeding Practices

There is a wide variety of teaching aids and instructional materials available on infant feeding; many are available in languages other than English. The nurse should identify and have available printed materials that may be helpful to parents with questions on infant feeding. These materials need not be expensive or difficult to produce. An example of a "tip sheet" produced for use in an obstetric clinic is shown in the display on page 1162; it contains helpful information, answers most commonly asked questions, and gives important safety tips about infant feeding. The nurse should be knowledgeable about these points and should reinforce them in her patient teaching.

The nurse should make sure that the parents understand principles of safety in infant feeding. Cleanliness in the preparation of infant foods is important. It may not be necessary for parents to sterilize bottles or equipment used to prepare infant formula, if they have a clean water source and wash bottles and nipples thoroughly, storing them away from sources of contamination. Mothers interested in preparing their own baby foods should obtain current information about safe methods of preparation, either from printed materials provided by a clinic or hospital, or from a knowledgeable health professional.

The nurse must assess whether parents understand precautions against choking and aspiration in relation to infant feeding. Practices to reduce the risk of regurgitation and aspiration are particularly important. The nurse should explain that the bottle nipple should be kept full of milk during feeding to reduce the amount of air the baby swallows. Putting an infant on his or her right side after feeding, perhaps with the head of the cot slightly elevated, facilitates gastric emptying and allows air to rise through the esophagus without causing regurgitation.

The nurse should stress that "propping" the bottle is an unwise practice. In very young babies the nipple can become lodged in the back of the throat and block respiration or cause regurgitation and aspiration of fluid, which may cause aspiration pneumonia or even death. In older

Forms of Commerical Formulas

- Concentrated (liquid) — requires dilution with equal amounts of water
- Powdered form — requires mixing with water according to directions
- Ready-to-use — requires measuring into individual bottles for feeding
- Ready-to-use, prepackaged — ready to feed in disposable bottles

SELF-CARE TEACHING

Tips on Infant Feeding

The nurse should review the following points with parents:

- Breast milk or formula is sufficient for the first 4 to 6 mo of life for most babies.
- Many babies show signs of readiness for solid food by the age of 6 mos. When you are certain your baby is ready for baby food:
  a. Introduce the simplest foods first.
  b. Add only one new food at a time (no mixtures) and wait 5 to 7 days to see how your baby adjusts to that food. If your baby shows an allergic reaction, discontinue that food and discuss the reaction with your baby's health care provider.
  c. Allergy symptoms are vomiting, diarrhea, colic, skin rash, eczema, wheezing, and runny nose. Usually symptoms occur 2 to 3 days after you introduce the food.
  d. Foods most likely to cause allergies are cow's milk, egg white, wheat, peanuts, corn, soybeans, citrus, strawberries, tomatoes, chocolate, and fish.
  e. At first, offer small amounts (1 tbsp. or less) of food from a spoon. Make the food thin and smooth by mixing it with a little breast milk or formula.
  f. As your baby grows older, remember to vary the textures of the foods you provide. A 6-mo-old needs strained (very thin) food; by 8 mo most babies do well with mashed, lumpy foods; by 10 mo give the baby bits of tender, well-cooked foods to feed himself or herself.
- Store-bought or homemade baby food?
  a. It is easy and fun to make food for your baby at home. Ask your nurse or nutritionist for information on making baby food. Your kitchen must be very clean, and you will need some inexpensive kitchen equipment.
  b. Store-bought baby food is nutritious, if you follow these suggestions:
     (1) Buy only single foods (there is as much protein in 1 jar of strained chicken as in 4.3 jars of chicken and noodles).
     (2) Read labels to avoid sugars, salt, and starches.
     (3) Check the date on the top of the jar for freshness and make sure the vacuum pop-top has not been broken.
     (4) Do not feed your baby directly from the jar, unless she or he can eat the entire portion in one sitting; refrigerated leftovers eaten later can cause food poisoning.
  c. Better bottle-feeding
     (1) Bottles are for water, formula, or breast milk *only*.
        - No solids (cereals, etc.) should be put in bottles; feed solids with a spoon.
        - Powdered drinks, sodas, and even juices can give a baby cavities when fed from a bottle. Juices should be fed from a cup. Powdered drinks and sodas should be avoided; they provide only empty calories.
        - Always hold your baby when giving a bottle. Your love is as important as the food. "Propping" the bottle can cause problems such as choking, cavities, and ear infections.
  d. Never force your baby to finish food or milk she or he doesn't want. Overfeeding can lead to weight problems.
  e. Do not give your baby the following foods during the first year or two of life: nuts, raw carrots, popcorn, seeds and other foods that might cause choking, or honey in any form (honey can cause food poisoning).

babies, sucking in the horizontal position from a propped bottle has been shown to contribute to otitis media, or infection of the middle ear. This is because the eustachian tube opens during swallowing, allowing mucus from the nose to drain into the opening of the tube and obstruct it. Falling asleep while sucking a bottle of juice or milk contributes to early dental caries, because bacterial action on tooth enamel is increased by the continuous presence of sugar in the mouth; older babies, at bedtime, should therefore not be allowed bottles that contain any liquid other than clear water.

The mother needs to be informed that any drug that can enter the maternal blood stream can also enter breast milk. If the mother requires medical treatment, the physician should consider altering doses, changing the schedule of doses, or substituting an alternative drug so as to minimize the ingestion of medication by the nursing infant.

Occasionally, even healthy infants develop feeding problems. Problems may involve feeding itself (*e.g.*, type of formula, amount, and method of feeding) or the environment (*e.g.*, relationships within the family). The nurse

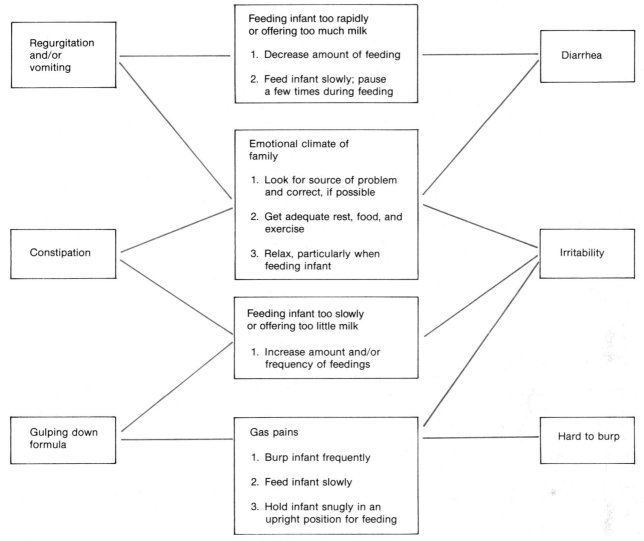

Figure 37–15. Common infant feeding problems and corrective measures.

can help the mother understand these signs and symptoms and help her develop steps to correct the problem (Fig. 37–15).

Evaluation

Evaluation of the effectiveness of nursing care in regard to maternal–infant nutrition is sometimes difficult, because outcomes can only be observed after discharge when most maternity nurses no longer have contact with families. Evaluation of care, by necessity, focuses on the consistency and quality of patient teaching in the early postpartum period, and on the adequacy and responsiveness of nursing support for problems parents encounter in learning to feed their infants and in reestablishing ma-

ternal health and wellbeing. Outcomes of effective nursing care in the postpartum period may include a rising incidence of successful early breast-feeding, which continues up to and beyond 6 months, and evidence of maternal physical restoration, such as satisfactory weight loss and adequate iron stores and energy levels.

CHAPTER SUMMARY

Breast feeding of infants is currently favored over formula-feeding in the United States. Advances in the field of infant feeding and nutrition have revealed that breast feeding has many advantages, both nutritional and immunologic.

Early infant feeding is a potentially critical period that may determine the success of later breast-feeding. The postpartum nurse can offer support and advice during this time, until the mother becomes confident about her ability to breast-feed. The nurse should also stress the mother's need for additional nutrients and fluids to maintain the quantity and quality of her milk.

The formula-feeding mother needs the nurse's support in the preparation of her infant's formula. The mother may need to be told the most comfortable positions for infant feeding; she may also need information about feeding schedules, and use of iron and vitamins, and when to begin supplemental feedings.

Teaching mothers about infant nutrition and feeding is an important nursing role. The well-informed mother will know when and how to feed her baby and will be able to establish an early and comfortable pattern of feeding without undue stress to herself or her infant.

STUDY QUESTIONS

1. Why is breast-feeding nutritionally desirable for both infant and mother?
2. What nutritional supplementation is recommended for breast-fed and formula-fed infants, and at what age(s)?
3. Explain how the human milk of poorly-nourished populations differs from that of well-nourished groups. What implications does this have for infant growth?
4. How does the recommended dietary intake of calories and protein for the lactating mother compare with that for the nonlactating mother? What are good

sources of these nutrients for the mother who is breast-feeding?
5. What kind of nutritional advice should the nurse give to a lactating mother who complains of constant fatigue?

REFERENCES

Coulter S, Cerruti E: Nursing Your Baby Beyond the First Days. New York, Childbirth Graphics, 1984

Neifert M, Seacat J: A guide to successful breastfeeding. Contemp Pediatr 3:26, 1986

Newton N, Newton M: Relationship of ability to breastfeed and the maternal attitudes toward breastfeeding. Pediatrics 5:869, 1950

Riordan J, Countryman B: Preparation for breastfeeding and early optimal functioning. J Obstet Gynecol Neonat Nurs 9:210, 1950

Sweeney MA, Gulino C: The health belief model as an explanation for breast-feeding practices in a Hispanic population. Adv Nurs Sci 9(4):35–40, 1987

Whichelow M: Calorie requirements for successful breastfeeding. Arch Dis Child 50:669, 1975

SUGGESTED READINGS

Graef P: Postpartum concerns of breastfeeding mothers. J Nurse Midwif 33(2)62–66, 1988

Radius SM, Joffe A: Understanding adolescent mothers' feelings about breastfeeding. J Adol Health Care 9(2):156–160, 1988

appendixes, glossary, and index

appendix A

Normal Values and Reference Tables

A-1 Normal Peripheral Blood Values at Different Ages

Age	Hemoglobin (g/dl)	Hematocrit (%)	MCV (fl)	WBC (10^3/mm³)	Neutrophils (%)	Lymphocytes (%)	Platelets (10^3/mm³)
Birth	13.5–21	42–65	100–140	9–30	60	30	100–300
1 wk	13.5–21	42–65	95–135	5–21	40	50	100–300
1 mo	10–16	30–48	85–125	5–21	35	55	100–300
Adult:							
Male	14–18	42–54	80–100	4–11	0	30	100–300
Female	12–16	36–48	80–100	4–11	60	30	100–300
Pregnancy	11.5–12.3	32–46	80–95	15–18	60 ± 10	34 ± 10	100–300

A-2 Blood Chemistries

Determination	Specimen	Age/Sex	Normal Value
Acetone	Serum/plasma		
Qualitative			Negative
Quantitative (acetone and acetoacetic acid)			0.3–2.0 mg/dl
Albumin (see Protein Electrophoresis)			
Aldolase	Serum	Newborn	4 × adult value
		Adult	<11 IU/liter
Alpha fetoprotein	Serum		<10 mg/dl
Amylase	Serum	Newborn	5–65 U/liter
		>1 yr	25–125
Ascorbic acid	Serum		0.6–2.0 mg/dl
Bicarbonate	Serum	Arterial	21–28 mmol/liter
		Venous	22–29
	Serum	Pregnancy	20.5–26
Base excess	Whole blood	Newborn	(−10)–(−2) mmol/liter
		Adult	(−3)–(+3)

(continued)

A-2   **Blood Chemistries** — (continued)

Determination	Specimen	Age/Sex	Normal Value	
			Premature (mg/dl)	*Full-term (mg/dl)*
Bilirubin, total	Serum	Cord	<2	<2
		0–1 day	<8	<6
		1–2 days	<12	<8
		2–5 days	<16	<12
		Adult	<2	0.2–1.0
		Pregnancy	Unchanged	
Bilirubin, direct (conjugated)	Serum		0.8–0.2 mg/dl	
Calcium, ionized	Serum, plasma, whole blood	Cord, newborn	5.5 ± 0.3 mg/dl	
		3–24 hr	4.3–5.1	
		24–48 hr	4.0–4.7	
		Adult	4.48–4.92	
Calcium, total	Serum	Cord, newborn	9–11.5 mg/dl	
		3–24 hr	9–10.6 mg/dl	
		24–48 hr	7–12	
		4–7 days	9–10.9	
		Adult	8.4–10.2	
		Pregnancy	7.8–9.3	
Carbon dioxide, partial pressure, PCO_2	Whole blood, arterial	Newborn	27–40 mm Hg	
		Infant	27–40	
		Pregnancy	27–32	
		Female adult	32–45	
Carbon dioxide (total CO_2)	Serum, venous	Cord	14–22 mmol/liter	
		Premature (1 wk)	14–27	
		Newborn	13–22	
		Infant	20–28	
		Adult	23–30	
		Pregnancy	23–30 at term	
Carbon monoxide	Whole blood		0.5–1.5% saturation of Hgb (children and nonsmokers); symptoms > 20%	
Carboxyhemoglobin (See carbon monoxide)				
β-Carotene	Serum	Infant	20–70 mcg/dl	
		Adult	60–200	
Chloride	Serum or plasma	Cord	96–104 mmol/liter	
		Newborn	97–110	
		Adult	98–106	
		Pregnancy	slight elevation	
	Sweat	Normal	0–35 mmol/liter	
		Marginal	30–60	
		Cystic fibrosis	60–200	
Cholesterol, total	Serum	Cord	45–100 mg/dl	
		Newborn	53–135	
		Infant	70–175	
		Adult	140–310	
		Pregnancy	Elevated	
Copper	Serum	Newborn–6 mo	20–70 mcg/dl	
		Adult: M	70–140	
		F	80–155	
Cortisol	Plasma or serum	8 AM specimen	5–23 mcg/dl	
		4 PM specimen	3–15	
Creatine kinase, CK (creatine phosphokinase, CPK; 30°C)	Serum	Newborn	68–580 U/liter	
		Adult: M	12–70	
		F	10–55	
			(higher after exercise)	
Creatinine	Serum or plasma	Cord	0.6–1.2 mg/dl	
		Infant	0.2–0.4	
		Adult: M	0.6–1.2	

(continued)

A–2   **Blood Chemistries** (continued)

Determination	Specimen	Age/Sex	Normal Value		
Creatinine clearance (endogenous)*	Serum or plasma and timed urine	F Pregnancy Newborn Under 40 yr M F Pregnancy	0.5–1.1 (0.47–0.7) 40–65 ml/min/1.73 m² 97–137 88–128 (decreases 6.5 ml/min/decade) decreased		
Disaccharide tolerance (dose: twice oral glucose tolerance test dose)	Serum		>20 mg/dl change in glucose concentration		
Ethanol	Blood		0.0% Toxic: 50–100 mg/dl; CNS depression: >100 mg/dl		
Fatty acids, free	Serum or plasma	Adults Children and obese adults	8–25 mg/dl <31		
Fibrinogen	Whole blood	Newborn Adult Pregnancy	125–300 mg/dl 200–400 450		
Folate	Serum	Newborn Adult Pregnancy	7–32 ng/ml 1.8–9 ng/ml 1.9–14		
Follicle-stimulating hormone (FSH)	Serum/plasma	Birth–1 yr M F Adult F Premenopause Midcycle peak	<1–12 mU/ml <1–20 5–30 4–30 10–90		
Galactose	Serum	Newborn/Infant Adult	0–20 mg/dl <5		
Glucose	Serum	Cord Premature Neonate Newborn, 1 day Newborn, >1 day Adult	45–96 mg/dl 20–60 30–60 40–60 50–90 70–105		
	Blood Urine	Adult	65–95 <0.5 g/d		

Glucose tolerance — Serum

Dosages:	Time	Normal	Diabetic
Child 1.75 g/kg of ideal weight, maximum 75 g Adult 75 g total dose	Fasting 60 min 90 min 120 min	70–105 120–170 100–140 70–120	>115 ≥200 ≥200 ≥140

Determination	Specimen	Age/Sex	Normal Value		
Growth hormone (HGH), fasting	Serum or plasma	Cord Newborn Adult: M F	10–50 ng/ml 10–40 <5 <8		

Immunoglobulin levels	Serum		*IgA* *(mg/dl)*	*IgC* *(mg/dl)†*	*IgM* *(mg/dl)*
		Cord Newborn Adult	0–5 0–2.2 60–380	760–1700 700–1480 600–1600	4–24 5–30 40–345
IgD	Serum	Newborn Adult	None detected 0–8 mg/dl		
IgE	Serum	M F	0–230 IU/ml 0–170		
Insulin (12 hr, fasting)	Serum, plasma	Newborn Adult	3–20 mcIU/ml 7–24		

(continued)

A–2   **Blood Chemistries** — (continued)

Determination	Specimen	Age/Sex	Normal Value		
			IgA (mg/dl)	IgC (mg/dl)†	IgM (mg/dl)
Insulin with oral glucose tolerance test	Serum			0 min: 7–24 mcIU/ml 60 min: 18–276 120 min: 16–166 180 min: 4–38	
Iron-binding capacity (TIBC)	Serum	Infant	100–400 mcg/dl		
		Adult	250–400		
		Pregnancy	300–450		
Iron	Serum	Newborn	100–250 mcg/dl		
		Infant	40–100		
		Adult: M	50–160		
		F	40–150		
		Pregnancy	decreased		
Lactate	Whole blood, venous		0.50–2.2 mmol/liter		
	Whole blood, arterial		0.50–1.6		
Lactate dehydrogenase (LDH)	Serum	Newborn	160–450 U/liter		
		Infant	100–250		
			60–170		
		Adult	45–90		
Lead	Whole blood	Child	<30 mcg/dl		
		Adult	<40		
		Acceptable for industrial exposure	<60		
		Toxic	≥100		
Lipase (Tietz method; 37°C)	Serum		0.1–1.0 U/ml		
		Child	1–6 mIU/ml		
		Adult:	4–14		
		F, premenopause	4–25		
		F, midcycle	25–250		
		F, postmenopause	25–200		
Magnesium	Serum	Newborn	1.2–1.8 mEq/liter		
		Adult	1.3–2.1		
Methemoglobin	Whole blood		0.06–0.24 g/dl		
Osmolality	Serum		275–295 mOsm/kg H₂O		
Oxygen capacity	Whole blood, arterial		1.34 ml/g hemoglobin		
Oxygen partial pressure (PO₂)	Whole blood, arterial	Birth	8–24 mm Hg		
		5–10 min	33–75		
		30 min	31–85		
		>1 hr	55–80		
		1 day	54–95		
		Adult	83–108 decreases with age		
Oxygen, % saturation	Whole blood, arterial	Newborn	40–90%		
		Thereafter	95–99%		
pH (37°C)	Whole blood, arterial	Premature (48 hr)	7.35–7.50		
		Birth, full term	7.11–7.36		
		5–10 min	7.09–7.30		
		30 min	7.21–7.38		
		>1 hr	7.26–7.49		
		1 day	7.29–7.45		
		Mid Pregnancy	7.40–7.45		
Phenylalanine	Serum	Premature/low birth weight	2.0–7.5 mg/dl		
		Full-term newborn	1.2–3.4		
		Adult	0.8–1.8		
Phosphatase, acid prostatic, 37°C	Serum		<3.0 ng/ml		
			0.11–0.60 U/liter		
Phosphatase, alkaline SKI method		Infant	50–155 U/liter		
		Child	20–150		
		Adult	20–70		

(continued)

A-2   **Blood Chemistries**—(continued)

Determination	Specimen	Age/Sex	Normal Value
Phospholipids (lipids P × 25)	Serum and plasma	Pregnancy > 50% rise Newborn Infant Adult	75–170 mg /dl 100–275 125–275
Phosphorus, inorganic	Serum	Cord Premature (1 wk) Newborn Adult Pregnancy	3.7–8.1 mg/dl 5.4–10.9 4.3–9.3 3.0–4.5 unchanged
Potassium	Serum	Newborn Infant Adult Pregnancy	3.9–5.9 mmol/liter 4.1–5.3 3.5–5.1 3.5–5.3
Protein, total	Serum	Premature Newborn Adult, recumbent –0.5 g higher in ambulatory patients	4.3–7.6 g/dl 4.6–7.4 6.0–7.8
Protein, electrophoresis, (cellulose acetate)	Serum	Total	

		Protein (g/dl)	Albumin (g/dl)	α_1-glob (g/dl)	α_2-glob (g/dl)	β-glob (g/dl)	γ-glob[†] (g/dl)
	Premature	4.3–7.6	3.0–4.2	0.1–0.5	0.3–0.7	0.3–1.2	0.3–1.4 g/dl
	Newborn	4.6–7.4	3.6–5.4	0.1–0.3	0.3–0.5	0.2–0.6	0.2–1.0
	Infant	6.2–8.0	4.0–5.0	0.2–0.4	0.5–0.8	0.5–0.8	0.3–1.2
		6.0–7.8	3.5–5.0	0.2–0.3	0.4–1.0	0.5–1.1	0.7–1.2
	Pregnancy		decreased 2nd and 3rd trimester	increased 2nd trimester	increased 2nd trimester	increased 2nd trimester	decreased 3rd trimester

Determination	Specimen	Age/Sex	Normal Value
Salicylates	Serum, plasma		Negative: <2.0 mg/dl Therapeutic: 15–30 Toxic: >30
Sodium	Serum	Newborn Infant Adult Pregnancy	134–146 mmol/liter 139–146 136–146 increased retention > 500 over normal
T₃ resin uptake (T₃RU)	Serum	Newborn Adult Pregnancy	26–36% 26–35 decreased
Testosterone	Serum	Adult: M F	572 ± 135 37 ± 10
Thiamine (vitamin B₁)	Serum		2.0 mcg/dl
Thyroid-stimulating hormone (TSH)	Serum, plasma	Cord Newborn Adult	3–12 mcU/liter 3–18 2–10
Transferrin	Serum	Newborn Adult	130–275 mg/dl 200–400

Determination	Specimen		*mg/dl*	
			Male	Female
Triglycerides (TG)	Serum, after 12-hr fast	Cord blood	10–98	10–98
		0–5 yr	30–86	32–99
		6–11	31–108	35–114
		12–15	36–138	41–138
		16–19	40–163	40–128
		20–29	44–185	40–128

(continued)

A–2   **Blood Chemistries** (continued)

Determination	Specimen	Age/Sex	Normal Value
Tyrosine	Serum	Recommended (desirable) levels for adults:	Male 40–160
			Female 35–135
		Premature	7.0–24.0 mg/dl
		Newborn	1.6–3.7
		Adult	0.8–1.3
Urea nitrogen	Serum/plasma	Cord	21–40 mg/dl
		Premature (1 wk)	3–25
		Newborn	3–12
		Adult	7–18
Uric acid	Serum	Child	2.0–5.5 mg/dl
		Adult: M	3.5–7.2
		F	2.6–6.0
Vitamin A	Serum	Newborn	35–75 mcg/dl
		Adult	30–65
Vitamin B$_{12}$	Serum	Newborn	175–800 pg/ml
		Adult	140–700
Vitamin C	Plasma		0.6–2.0 mg/ml
Vitamin E	Serum		5–20 mcg/ml
Volume	Whole blood	Premature	90–108 ml/kg
		Newborn	80–110
		Adult	72–100
	Plasma	Adult	49–59

* Endogenous creatinine clearance is expressed in ml per minute and is corrected to average adult surface area of 1.73 m².

$$\frac{UV}{P} \times \frac{1.73}{A} = ml/min$$

† Higher in blacks.

A–3   **Urine Chemistries**

Determination	Age/Sex	Normal Value
Catecholamines (24 hr)	Infant	
	Norepinephrine	0–10 mcg/day
	Epinephrine	0–2.5
	Adult	
	Norepinephrine	15–80
	Epinephrine	0.5–20
Chloride (24 hr)	Infant	2–10 mmol/day
	Adult	110–250
	(varies greatly with Cl intake)	
Creatinine (24 hr)	Infant	8–20 mg/kg/day
	Adult	14–26
	Pregnancy	elevated
Homovanillic acid (HVA) (24 hr)	Child	3–16 mcg/mg creatinine
	Adult	<15 mg/day
17-Hydroxycorticosteroids (24 hr)	0–1 yr	0.5–1.0 mg/24 hr
	Adult: M	3.0–10.0
	F	2.0–8.0
17-Ketogenic steroids (17-KGS) (24 hr)	0–1 yr	<1 mg/day
	Adult: M	5–23
	F	3–15
17-Ketosteroids (17-KS) (24 hr)		
Zimmerman reaction	Infant	<1 mg/day
	Adult: M 18–30 yr	9–22
	>30 yr	8–20
	F	6–15

(continued)

A-3 **Urine Chemistries** (continued)

Determination	Age/Sex	Normal Value
	(decreases with age)	
Lead (24 hr)		$<80\ \mu g/L$
Osmolality (random)		50–1400 mOsmol/kg H_2O depending on fluid intake. After 12 hr fluid restriction >850 mOsmol/kg H_2O
Porphyrins		34–234 mcg/day
Coproporphyrin (24 hr)		0–2.0 mg/day
Porphobilinogen (24 hr)		1–14 mg/dl
Protein, total 24 hr		50–80 mg/day (at rest)
		<250 mg/day after intense exercise
Reducing substances		<150 mg/dl (as glucose)
Specific gravity		
Random void		1.002–1.030
After 12-hr fluid restriction		>1.025
24 hr		1.015–1.025
Vanillylmandelic acid	Newborn	<1.0 mg/day
VMA	Infant	<2.0
(24 hr)	Adult	2–7

A–4 Weight Conversion Table (Pounds and Ounces to Grams)

Lbs.	Ounces															
	0	1	2	3	4	5	6	7	8	9	10	11	12	13	14	15
0	—	28	57	85	113	142	170	198	227	255	283	312	340	369	397	425
1	454	482	510	539	567	595	624	652	680	709	737	765	794	822	850	879
2	907	936	964	992	1021	1049	1077	1106	1134	1162	1191	1219	1247	1276	1304	1332
3	1361	1389	1417	1446	1474	1503	1531	1559	1588	1616	1644	1673	1701	1729	1758	1786
4	1814	1843	1871	1899	1928	1956	1984	2013	2041	2070	2098	2126	2155	2183	2211	2240
5	2268	2296	2325	2353	2381	2410	2438	2466	2495	2523	2551	2580	2608	2637	2665	2693
6	2722	2750	2778	2807	2835	2863	2892	2920	2948	2977	3005	3033	3062	3090	3118	3147
7	3175	3203	3232	3260	3289	3317	3345	3374	3402	3430	3459	3487	3515	3544	3572	3600
8	3629	3657	3685	3714	3742	3770	3799	3827	3856	3884	3912	3941	3969	3997	4026	4054
9	4082	4111	4139	4167	4196	4224	4252	4281	4309	4337	4363	4394	4423	4451	4479	4508
10	4536	4564	4593	4621	4649	4678	4706	4734	4763	4791	4819	4848	4876	4904	4933	4961
11	4990	5018	5046	5075	5103	5131	5160	5188	5216	5245	5273	5301	5330	5358	5386	5414
12	5443	5471	5500	5528	5557	5585	5613	5642	5670	5698	5727	5755	5783	5812	5840	5868
13	5897	5925	5953	5982	6010	6038	6067	6095	6123	6152	6180	6209	6237	6265	6294	6322
14	6350	6379	6407	6435	6464	6492	6520	6549	6577	6605	6634	6662	6690	6719	6747	6776
15	6804	6832	6860	6889	6917	6945	6973	7002	7030	7059	7087	7115	7144	7172	7201	7228
16	7257	7286	7313	7342	7371	7399	7427	7456	7484	7512	7541	7569	7597	7626	7654	7682
17	7711	7739	7768	7796	7824	7853	7881	7909	7938	7966	7994	8023	8051	8079	8108	8136
18	8165	8192	8221	8249	8278	8306	8335	8363	8391	8420	8448	8476	8504	8533	8561	8590
19	8618	8646	8675	8703	8731	8760	8788	8816	8845	8873	8902	8930	8958	8987	9015	9043
20	9072	9100	9128	9157	9185	9213	9242	9270	9298	9327	9355	9383	9412	9440	9469	9497
21	9525	9554	9582	9610	9639	9667	9695	9724	9752	9780	9809	9837	9865	9894	9922	9950
22	9979	10007	10036	10064	10092	10120	10149	10177	10206	10234	10262	10291	10319	10347	10376	10404

A-5   **Temperature Conversion Table (Centigrade to Fahrenheit)**

Celsius (C°)	Fahrenheit (F°)	Celsius (C°)	Fahrenheit (F°)
34.0	93.2	38.6	101.4
34.2	93.6	38.8	101.8
34.4	93.9	39.0	102.2
34.6	94.3	39.2	102.5
34.8	94.6	39.4	102.9
35.0	95.0	39.6	103.2
35.2	95.4	39.8	103.6
35.4	95.7	40.0	104.0
35.6	96.1	40.2	104.3
35.8	96.4	40.4	104.7
36.0	96.8	40.6	105.1
36.2	97.1	40.8	105.4
36.4	97.5	41.0	105.8
36.6	97.8	41.2	106.1
36.8	98.2	41.4	106.5
37.0	98.6	41.6	106.8
37.2	98.9	41.8	107.2
37.4	99.3	42.0	107.6
37.6	99.6	42.2	108.0
37.8	100.0	42.4	108.3
38.0	100.4	42.6	108.7
38.2	100.7	42.8	109.0
38.4	101.0	43.0	109.4

Conversion of Celsius (Centigrade) to Fahrenheit: $(9/5 \times \text{temperature}) + 32$
Conversion of Fahrenheit to Celsius (Centigrade): $(\text{Temperature} - 32) \times 5/9$

appendix B

Laboratory Data and Procedures to Assess the Prenatal Patient

Laboratory Test	Normal Nonpregnant Value	Normal Pregnant Value	Comments
Blood Tests			
Complete Blood Count (CBC)			
White blood cell count (WBC)	4,500 to 10,000/mm^3	15,000 to 18,000/mm^3 (during pregnancy); 18,000 to 25,000/mm^3 (during delivery and immediate postpartum period)	WBCs are elevated during an infectious process, eclampsia, following hemorrhage, and in response in physiologic stress. Additional tests to detect infection should be performed to avoid unnecessary antibiotic therapy.
Red blood cell count (ml/mm^3)	4,000,000 to 5,000,000 ml/mm^3	Increased 25% to 30%	By 6 to 8 wk of gestation there is progressive increase in blood plasma and red blood cell volume. It peaks at 28 to 32 wk and remains constant until delivery. Plasma volume increases 40% to 50% whereas red cell mass increases only 25% to 30%, resulting in dilutional (physiologic) anemia of pregnancy.
Hemoglobin	12 to 16 g/100 ml	11.5 g/100 ml mean in midpregnancy; 12.3 g/100 ml mean in late pregnancy	Hemoglobin value measures the body's capacity to transport oxygen. Anemia is diagnosed when the form value is 10.5 g/100 ml or under. The commonest form is iron deficiency anemia.
Hematocrit	36% to 46%	32% to 46%	The percentage expresses the portion of the total blood volume occupied by the red blood cells. This test is also used in the detection of anemia; a value of under 32% indicates anemia.

(continued)

Laboratory Data and Procedures to Assess the Prenatal Patient (continued)

Laboratory Test	Normal Nonpregnant Value	Normal Pregnant Value	Comments
Red Cell Indices			
Mean corpuscular volume	80 to 95 μm^3	Same	This index describes the size of the cell. A value under 80 is *microcytic*, or smaller than normal, as found in iron deficiency anemia, parasite infestaton, or thalassemia. A value over 95 is *macrocytic*, or larger than normal.
Mean corpuscular hemoglobin concentration	32 to 36 g/dl	Same	This test measures the portion of each cell occupied by hemoglobin. A reading of over 39 g/dl occurs in only one condition, hereditary spherocytosis, a congenital abnormality of the cell wall. A decreased reading may indicate anemia.
Red cell morphology			This test measures variability in cell size and shape; the amount of blueness in the cells (amount of retained RNA); the presence of central pallor in the cells; other cells such as sickle cells, spherocytes, cells seen in thalassemia
Platelets	140,000 to 450,000/mm^3	Same	
Coagulation Factors Fibrinogen Factor (I)	300 mg/dl	450 mg/dl	
Factors II, VII, VIII, IX, and X Factors XI and XIII		Increased Decreased	Platelet counts are unchanged, but certain coagulation factors are altered as shown. Also called thrombocytes, the platelets contribute to hemostasis by forming platelet plugs at bleeding sites and promoting thrombin formation. They are formed in the bone marrow. A decrease in their production is never benign. Low levels are found in leukemia, disseminated intravascular coagulation (DIC), uremia, severe systemic infection, and bone marrow hypofunction.
Prothrombin time Bleeding time	11 to 12 sec 1 to 5 min	Same Same	Despite alterations in blood Factors II, VII, VIII, IX, X, XI, and XIII, prothrombin and bleeding times remain within the normal nonpregnant range.
Reticulocytes	0.5% to 1.5%	Increased	Reticulocytes are immature red blood cells that are released from the bone marrow in response to hemolysis, hemorrhage, or iron therapy for anemia. Reticulocytosis (increased production) may reach 3% in response to iron therapy in anemic pregnant women.
Erythrocyte sedimentation rate (ESR)	0 to 15 mm/hr	Not valid in pregnancy	ESR is elevated during infection and helps to document chronic inflamma-

(continued)

Laboratory Data and Procedures to Assess the Prenatal Patient (continued)

Laboratory Test	Normal Nonpregnant Value	Normal Pregnant Value	Comments
			tory processes in patients with vague symptoms. Higher levels of fibrinogen and plasma globulins in pregnancy make this test invalid.
Iron			
Serum iron	50 to 150 mcg/dl	Same	Low serum values usually result from insufficient intake of iron (iron deficiency anemia).
			Causes include repeated pregnancies, low-iron diet (especially in adolescents), heavy menses, pregnancy (600 to 900 mg iron are drained from the mother by the fetus), and IUD use.
Total iron-binding capacity (TIBC)	280 to 400 mcg/dl	300 to 450 mcg/dl	The ability of the red blood cells to bind iron is increased in pregnancy because of maternal and fetal needs for iron. A simple formula to rule out iron deficiency anemia is: Serum iron ÷ TIBC = % saturation A result of 16% or less is diagnostic of iron deficiency anemia; such a result, in conjunction with mean corpuscular volume less than 80, requires further study.
Serum Folate	1.9 to 14.0 ng/ml		Folate is essential for production of RNA and DNA. The fetus parasitizes large quantities from the mother. Combined iron and folate deficiency is common in pregnancy. Most prenatal vitamins now supply a folate supplemental dose of 1 mg.
Electrolytes Sodium	135 to 148 mEq/liter	Increase in retention of 500 to 900 mEq/liter over the norm	Aldosterone is the sodium-conserving hormone of the adrenal cortex. Its excretion is increased throughout pregnancy, causing cumulative total sodium retention. Urinary loss of sodium in late pregnancy is normal.
Potassium	3.5 to 5.3 mEq/dl	Same	Aldosterone is also potassium-depleting. However, the increase in its production during pregnancy does not cause potassium wastage.
Chloride	102.7 to 107.0 mEq/liter	98 to 108 mEq/liter	There is no significant change.
Calcium	3.5 to 5.0 mg/dl	Increased	Increased intake is necessary to meet fetal requirements along with increased vitamin D to promote intestinal calcium absorption.
Phosphorus	2.5 to 4.5 mg/dl	Same	

(continued)

Laboratory Data and Procedures to Assess the Prenatal Patient (continued)

Laboratory Test	Normal Nonpregnant Value	Normal Pregnant Value	Comments
Blood Chemistry			
Albumin	3.5 to 5.0 g/dl	3.0 to 4.2 g/dl	Albumin concentration falls quickly in the first 3 mo, then more slowly until late pregnancy. Decline in serum albumin below normal pregnancy levels is associated with preeclampsia.
Human chorionic gonadotropin (HCG)	None (placental hormone of pregnancy)	50,000 to 100,000 mIU/ml (early); 10,000 to 20,000 mIU/ml (late)	Concentration peaks at 10 wk of gestation, then declines and remains at this lower level until delivery. HCG sustains progesterone secretion in early pregnancy and is necessary for growth and preparation of endometrium for implantation. Levels that far exceed normal in conjunction with exaggerated pregnancy symptoms, large-for-dates uterus, bleeding, and absent fetal heart tones may indicate trophoblastic disease.
Serum creatinine	0.8 to 1.4 mg/dl	0.9 to 2.0 mg/dl	Elevated levels may indicate kidney disease or preeclampsia.
Thyroid hormone T_3	100 to 200 ng/dl	25% to 35% decrease	T_3 is in lower concentrations than T_4 but is biologically more active and has a shorter serum half-life.
Thyroid hormone T_4	5.0 to 12.0 mcg/dl	5% to 10% increase	T_4 levels directly measure the thyroxine in serum. Increased T_3 levels and decreased T_4 levels may indicate hyper- or hypoactivity of the thyroid gland.
Hemoglobin electrophoresis (% of total hemoglobin)	Hgb A 95% to 97% Hgb A_2 2.0% to 3.5% Hgb F less than 2%	Same	This test identifies hemoglobinopathies, such as sickle cell trait or disease, hemoglobin C disease, and thalassemia, by the changed ratios of the three types of normal hemoglobin. (*E.g.*, Hgb A_2 level over 3.5% is diagnostic of thalassemia.)
Glucose-6-phosphate dehydrogenase (G6PD) (IU/g)			G6PD is an enzyme that protects hemoglobin from denaturation. When activity of this enzyme is less than 25% of normal, hemolysis occurs. Drugs that can precipitate anemia are acetaminophen, aspirin, sulfa drugs, vitamin K, thiazides, Furadantin, and Macrodantin, and patients should be warned against their use. In pregnancy, when serum iron is normal but the patient is anemic, G6PD disease must be ruled out. Pregnancy complications include urinary tract infections, neonatal jaundice, hydrops fetalis, anemia.
Blood Sugar Levels			
Fasting 2-hr postprandial	75 mg/100 ml 120 mg/100 ml (upper limit)	65 mg/100 ml 145 mg/100 ml (upper limit)	Screening for diabetes mellitus is done in pregnancy for all patients and is especially important when

(continued)

Laboratory Data and Procedures to Assess the Prenatal Patient — (continued)

Laboratory Test	Normal Nonpregnant Value				Normal Pregnant Value	Comments

The normal values for this test are as follows:

Oral glucose tolerance test	*Hour*	*Whole Blood (mg/dl)*	*Plasma (mg/dl)*	*Serum (mg/dl)*
	0	90	103	100
	1	165	188	200
	2	145	165	150
	3	125	143	130

Comments (Oral glucose tolerance test): there is consistent spilling of glucose in the urine (glucosuria) or there is a family history of the disease or some other indicator of diabetes.

Values that are abnormal in any two specimens constitute a positive test.

Laboratory Test	Normal Nonpregnant Value	Normal Pregnant Value	Comments
Blood Group and Rh Factor	O, A, B, AB Rh+ Rh−	Same Same Same	If the mother has type O blood and her partner has type A, B, or AB, an ABO incompatibility may exist in the infant. The incidence of clinically significant incompatibility resulting in hemolytic disease in the infant is small. To prevent Rh immunization, screening will identify that 15% of the population that is Rh−. The presence of anti-D serum identifies the Rh-immunized woman. All Rh-negative women are given anti-D globulin after abortion, amniocentesis, or delivery of an Rh+ infant and, prophylactically, in pregnancy in unsensitized women.
Rubella Titer	Depends on sensitization	Same	A result of less than 1.8 indicates that the patient is *not* immune to rubella. Such a patient should be advised to avoid exposure to the disease. If she is exposed, a titer should be obtained in 3 to 4 wk.
Serology or VDRL Test	Negative	Negative	A serology test is done to detect syphilis in the pregnant woman at the first prenatal visit. When positive, the VDRL screen is confirmed by an FTA-ABS test specific for syphilis.

Urine Tests

Urinalysis

Laboratory Test	Normal Nonpregnant Value	Normal Pregnant Value	Comments
pH Color Specific gravity	4.5 to 7.5 Yellow 1.010 to 1.020	Same Same Same	The *pH* test measures acidity or alkalinity of the urine. Levels below the norm indicate high fluid intake; levels above the norm indicate inadequate fluids and dehydration.
Protein	Negative	Negative	Small amounts may occur from vaginal contamination and dehydration. Amounts of 2+ to 4+ may indicate urinary tract or kidney infection or preeclampsia.
Glucose	Negative	Negative or 1+	Urine that registers 1+ may result from decreased renal threshold and increased glomerular filtration rate in pregnancy. High levels of glucose may indicate high levels of blood sugar, gestational diabetes, or diabetes mellitus.

(continued)

Laboratory Data and Procedures to Assess the Prenatal Patient — (continued)

Laboratory Test	Normal Nonpregnant Value	Normal Pregnant Value	Comments
Ketones	Negative	Negative	Ketone bodies are products of fatty acids and fat metabolism. Fasting causes breakdown of fat when carbohydrates and protein are not available. Ketones may be deleterious to the fetus and should be avoided in pregnancy by regular eating habits.
Bilirubin	Negative	Negative	Bilirubin is a product of red blood cell destruction. Its presence in urine suggests liver or gallbladder disease.
Blood	Negative	Negative	Blood in urine suggests urinary tract infection, kidney disease, or vaginal contamination.
White Blood Cells	Negative	Negative	Greater than 5 to 10 per high power field (HPF) may indicate urinary tract or vaginal infection.
Bacteria	Negative	Negative	Trace = rare; 1+ = 1 to 10/HPF; 2+ = 10 to 12/HPF; 3+ = innumerable; and 4+ = closely packed. Result greater than 4/HPF indicates urinary tract infection.
Casts	Negative	Negative	Casts are molds of the kidney tubules and may indicate kidney disease or excessive exercise.
Crystals	Few	Few	These compounds of various chemicals are found in most specimens.
Epithelial Cells	None	None	These are found when the specimen is contaminated by vaginal discharge. A clean-catch specimen should be obtained.
Urine Culture and Sensitivity	Negative	Negative	Specimens for urine cultures should be obtained by clean catch only. The test cannot be accurately read and reported when contaminated with vaginal secretions. A colony count over 100,000 (10^5) represents a positive culture and indicates urinary tract infection. The sensitivity of the infecting organism to various antibiotics is also reported.

appendix C

Known Teratogens That Cause Human Malformations

Teratogen	Classification	Effects on Embryo/Fetus
DRUGS		
Testosterone	Male hormone	• May cause virilization of female fetus; ambiguous genitalia with hypertrophy of clitoris and fusion of labia
Estrogens diethylstilbestrol (DES), stilbestrol	Female hormone	• Cause a variety of genital malformations in female fetuses and some possible changes in males. Genital cancer may occur in female offspring of mothers who took DES during their pregnancy.
Cyclophosphamide (Cytoxan, Endoxana)	Antineoplast and immunosuppressant (folic acid antagonist)	• Blocks synthesis of DNA, RNA, and protein. During first trimester of pregnancy, it is used only when potential benefits to mother outweigh hazards to fetus, since it causes many major congenital deformities.
Busulfan (Myleran)	Antineoplast (tumor-inhibiting)	• May cause skeletal deformities, corneal opacities, cleft palate, hypoplasia of organs, and stunted growth
Methotrexate (Amethopterin, Mexate)	Antineoplast	• Multiple skeletal deformities of face, skull, limbs, and vertebral column
Aminopterin	Antineoplast	• May result in death of conceptus during embryonic period. Multiple skeletal and other congenital malformations may occur if fetus survives.
Phenytoin (Dilantin)	Anticonvulsant	• Causes fetal hydantoin syndrome: IUGR, mental retardation, microcephaly, inner epicanthic folds, ptosis of the eyelids, depressed nasal bridge, phalangeal hypoplasia
Warfarin (Coumadin)	Anticoagulant	• Nasal hypoplasia, mental retardation, microcephaly, optic atrophy, chondroplasia punctata
Lithium carbonate (Cibalith, Eskalith, Lithane, Lithobid)	Psychotropic drug (used to control manic episodes of manic-depressive psychosis)	• May cause a variety of malformations, particularly involving heart and great vessels
Thalidomide	Antiemetic in early pregnancy (no longer available)	• Absence of one or more limbs, meromelia and other limb deformities; and malformations of heart, gastrointestinal system, and external ear
Alcohol	Drug	• Fetal alcohol syndrome (FAS): IUGR, mental retardation, microcephaly, ocular anomalies, joint abnormalities, short palpebral fissures

(continued)

Known Teratogens That Cause Human Malformations — (continued)

Teratogen	Classification	Effects on Embryo/Fetus
MATERNAL DISEASE		
Herpesvirus	Infection	• Microcephaly, microphthalmia, retinal dysplasia, mental retardation
Rubella virus (German measles)	Infection	• Cataracts, cardiac malformations, deafness, glaucoma, chorioretinitis
Cytomegalovirus	Infection	• Abortion during embryonic period, IUGR, microphthalmia, chorioretinitis, blindness, microcephaly, mental retardation, deafness, cerebral palsy, cerebral calcifications, hepatosplenomegaly (enlargement of liver and spleen)
Toxoplasma gondii (contracted by eating raw or poorly cooked meat; infects cats; causes toxoplasmosis)	Protozoan infection (intracellular parasite)	• Oocyst of contaminated cat crosses human placenta, causing microcephaly, microphthalmia, hydrocephaly
Treponema pallidum (causes syphilis)	Spirochete infection	• Hydrocephaly, deafness, mental retardation, Hutchinson's teeth, saddlenose, poorly developed maxilla
RADIATION		
High-level radiation therapy, radioiodine, atomic weapons	Radiation	• Microcephaly, mental retardation, skeletal deformities

appendix D

Appendix D **Common Treatable Sexually Transmitted Diseases**

Disease and Etiologic Agent	Clinical Features	Diagnosis	Therapy	Complications	Nursing Implications
Chlamydia trachomatis A microbe with properties of a virus (lives within cells) and bacteria (maintains its own cellular identity) susceptible to antibiotics	*Women:* • May be asymptomatic -or- • Inflamed cervix • Mucopurulent endocervical exudate *Men:* • May be asymptomatic -or- • Dysuria, frequency • Mucoid, purulent urethral discharge	• Growth of cells in special medium • Sample endocervical exudate -or- • Sample urethral discharge	• Tetracycline hydrochloride (HCl) 500 mg by mouth, daily for 7 days; OR • Doxycycline 100 mg by mouth, twice daily for 7 days. *Alternative Regimens* (for patients in whom tetracyclines are contraindicated or not tolerated) • Erythromycin base or stearate: 500 mg daily for 7 days; OR • Erythromycin ethylsuccinate 800 mg by mouth, 4 times daily for 7 days *Treatment During Pregnancy* Erythromycin base or stearate: 500 mg by mouth, 4 times daily for 7 days on an empty stomach; OR erythromycin ethylsuccinate 800 mg by mouth, 4 times daily for 7 days *Alternative regimen* (for women who cannot tolerate these regimens) Erythromycin base or stearate: 250 mg by mouth, 4 times daily for at least 14 days; OR erythromycin ethylsuccinate 400 mg by mouth, 4 times daily for at least 14 days *Note:* The optimal dose and duration of antibiotic therapy for pregnant women has not been established.	*Women:* Ascending infections may lead to symptomatic or asymptomatic endometritis and salpingitis and subsequent infertility. *Pregnancy:* Ascending infections may lead to adverse obstetric outcomes. *Men:* • Prostatitis • Epididymitis *Newborn:* • Infected by direct contact with maternal genital tract at birth • Conjunctivitis, pneumonia	Explain how to take any prescribed oral medications. If tetracycline is prescribed, it should be taken 1 hr before or 2 hr after meals and dairy products, antacids, iron or other mineral-containing preparations, and sunlight should be avoided. Advise the patient to return for test-of-cure or evaluation 4–7 days after completion of therapy, or earlier if symptoms persist or recur. Refer sexual partner(s) for examination and treatment. Encourage condoms use to prevent future infections. Encourage patient and partner to abstain from sex until both are cured.

Genital warts	Presents as single or multiple soft, fleshy, papillary or sessile, painless growths around the anus, vulvovaginal area, penis, urethra, or perineum	A pap smear of cervical lesions shows typical cytologic changes.	Newborn: Confirmed disease:	Although some of the HPV produce benign warts, 2 types — 16 and 18 — are found in 95% of squamous cell cancers of the cervix.	Discuss current available information on HPV as indicated.
Human papilloma viruses (HPV) are a family of more than 50 viruses with an affinity for mucocutaneous tissue		A biopsy is required to make a definitive diagnosis. Very atypical lesions, where neoplasia is a consideration, should be biopsied before initiating therapy.	• Conjunctivitis and/or • Pneumonia: oral erythromycin syrup, 50 mg/kg/day in 4 divided doses for 2 wk Newborn Prophylaxis Erythromycin 0.5% ophthalmic ointment applied to eyes within 1 hr of birth	Evidence currently suggests one or several "cofactors" must be present to cause neoplastic transformation.	Urge all sexually active clients to have Pap smears at least every 2 yr.
	-or- Flat, discoid lesions; may not be visible to naked eye, on cervix or vaginal walls		No treatment is completely satisfactory to eliminate the virus. • Chemical ablation – Cryotherapy, e.g. direct application of liquid nitrogen or oxygen (dry ice) – Podophyllin 10% in tincture, painted on external warts; repeated until cleared • Surgical excision • Carbon dioxide laser (under anesthesia) • Pharmacologic treatment: – 5 fluorouracil, 5% topical cream to intravaginal lesions – Interferon, an anti-infective protein; injected or applied; FDA approved, 1988	Neonate: Transmission of the virus at birth may cause laryngeal papillomas, usually benign; rarely become malignant; current data are not sufficient to set cesarean birth as a standard.	If a Pap is abnormal, showing koilocytes, refer patient for further testing. Encourage all partners to be examined for warts
			Pregnancy: Cryotherapy and laser may be used in some centers; other therapies contraindicated. Neonate/Infant: Surgical excision, but recurrence is frequent		

(continued)

Appendix D **Common Treatable Sexually Transmitted Diseases** (continued)

Disease and Etiologic Agent	Clinical Features	Diagnosis	Therapy	Complications	Nursing Implications
Gonorrhea *Neisseria gonorrhoeae*, a gram negative, anaerobic diplococcus	• May be asymptomatic. -or- • Women may have abnormal vaginal discharge, abnormal menses, dysuria, or be asymptomatic. Anorectal and pharyngeal infections are common. These may be symptomatic or asymptomatic. • When symptomatic, men usually have dysuria, frequency, and purulent urethral discharge.	*Screening:* • Obtain specimen from endocervix suspected infection • Add specimens from rectum and/or nasopharynx as indicated. • *Laboratory report:* Growth on selective medium demonstrating typical colonial morphology, positive oxidase reaction, and typical Gram's stain morphology.	*All adults:* Amoxicillin 3.0 g by mouth; OR Ampicillin 3.5 g by mouth; OR Aqueous procaine penicillin G (APPG) 4.8 million units IM; OR ceftriaxone 250 mg IM *NOTE:* Amoxicillin, ampicillin, and penicillin (but not ceftriaxone) are accompanied by probenecid 1 g by mouth. *Special Considerations:* In women with rectal infection, the above regimens are effective. Homosexual men with rectal gonococcal infection should be treated with ceftriaxone 250 mg IM or aqueous procaine penicillin G 4.8 million units IM plus probenecid 1.0 g by mouth. For those allergic to penicillin, use spectinomycin 2.0 g IM. Patients allergic to penicillins, cephalosporins, or probenecid should be treated with tetracycline 500 mg by mouth 4 times daily for 7 days or doxycycline 100 mg by mouth twice daily for 7 days. Those patients who cannot tolerate tetracyclines may be treated with spectinomycin 2.0 g IM followed by erythromycin (except for homosexual men). Plus treatment for	10%–20% of women develop pelvic inflammatory disease (PID) and are at risk for its sequelae (see below). Men are at risk for epididymitis, sterility, urethral stricture, and infertility. Newborns are at risk for ophthalmia neonatorum, scalp abscess at the site of fetal monitors, rhinitis, pneumonia, or anorectal infections. All infected, untreated persons are at risk for disseminated gonococcal infection (includes septicemia, arthritis, dermatitis, meningitis, and endocarditis).	• Explain how to take oral medications. • Encourage discussion of transmission and importance of prompt therapy with sexual partner(s). Advise return for test-of-cure 4–7 days after completing therapy. Refer sexual partners for examination and treatment. Encourage patient to avoid sex until patient and partner(s) are cured. Have her return early if symptoms persist or recur. Encourage condoms use to prevent future infections.

Herpes Genitalis
Herpes Simplex virus (HSV) types 1 and 2.

Types 1 and 2 cannot be distinguished clinically. Single or multiple vesicles appear anywhere on the genitalia. Vesicles spontaneously rupture to form shallow ulcers that may be very painful. Lesions resolve spontaneously without scarring. The first occurrence is termed initial infection (mean duration 12 days). Subsequent, usually milder, occurrences are termed recurrent infections (mean duration 4.5 days). The interval between clinical episodes is termed latency. Viral shedding occurs intermittently during latency. Prodromal symptoms may precede recurrent infections.

- Vesicular fluid is collected on a cotton swab
- Inoculate a tissue culture sample with the swab.
- Tissue culture demonstrates HSV infection after 7 days' incubation.

presumptive chlamydia infection (see Therapy, Chlamydia chart)
Special Considerations
Newborn Prophylaxis:
- Erythromycin 0.6% ophthalmic ointment OR
- Tetracycline 1% ointment OR
- Silver Nitrate, 1 drop to each eye

-ALL-
administered within 1 hr of birth
Note: Some strains of *Neisseria Gonorrheoae* are resistant to penicillins; use ceftriaxone OR spectinomycin.

There is no known cure.
First Clinical Episode:
To reduce the signs and symptoms, use acyclovir 200 mg by mouth, 5 times daily for 7 to 10 days, initiated within 6 days of onset of lesions. For patients who have severe symptoms or complications that necessitate hospitalization, an alternative regimen is acyclovir 5 mg/kg of body weight IV every 8 hr for 5 to 7 days.
Recurrent Genital Herpes
Acyclovir 200 mg by mouth, 5 times daily for 5 days initiated within 2 days of onset.
Pregnancy:
None available; safety of oral acyclovir has not been established.

Males and females:
Neuralgia, meningitis, ascending myelitis, urethral strictures, and lymphatic suppuration may occur.
Females: There is a possible increased risk for cervical cancer and fetal wastage.
Neonates: Virus from an active genital infection may be transmitted during vaginal delivery, causing neonatal herpes infection. Neonatal herpes ranges in severity from clinically inapparent infections to local infections of the eyes, skin, or mucous membranes to severe disseminated infection that may involve the central nervous system. The infection has a high case fatality rate and many survivors have oc-

Discuss the following self-care:
- Keep involved area clean and dry.
- Since both initial and recurrent lesions shed high concentrations of virus, patients should abstain from sex while symptomatic.
- An undetermined but presumably small risk of transmission also exists during asymptomatic intervals. Condoms may offer some protection.
- Annual Pap smears are recommended.
- Pregnant women should make their providers aware of any history of herpes, and report any symptoms.
- Discuss conditions that would necessitate cesarean birth; encourage questions,

(continued)

Disease and Etiologic Agent	Clinical Features	Diagnosis	Therapy	Complications	Nursing Implications
				ular or neurologic sequelae. *NOTE:* Neonatal risk is greatest with initial maternal infection. Cesarean section is indicated for documented, active infection at the time of birth.	assist with planning as needed. • Offer ongoing support during recurring infections.
Syphilis *Treponema pallidum,* a motile spirochete	*Primary:* The classical chancre is painless, indurated, and located at the site of exposure. All genital lesions should be suspected to be syphilitic. *Secondary:* Patients may have a highly variable skin rash, mucous patches, *condylomata lata,* lymphadenopathy, or other signs. *Latent:* Patients are without clinical signs.	*Screening: General* • Serologic test for syphilis is positive; (several types used: RPR, VDRL most common). • To rule out false positive serology, test all patients with positive serology with the specific treponemal antibody test, either FTA-ABS or MHA-TP. *Note:* Once a patient has a positive serology, it will not return to negative after treatment. Primary and secondary syphilis are definitely diagnosed by demonstrating *T. pallidum* with darkfield microscopy in material from a chancre, regional lymph node, or other lesion. A definitive diagnosis of latent syphilis cannot be made under usual circumstances.	Primary, secondary, or early syphilis of less than 1 yr duration: Benzathine penicillin G. 2.4 million units IM. Syphilis of indeterminate length or of more than 1 yr duration: Benzathine penicillin G. 7.2 million units total; 2.4 million units IM, weekly, for 3 successive wk. Patients allergic to penicillin: Tetracycline HCl 500 mg by mouth, 4 times daily.* For penicillin-allergic pregnant patients or tetracycline-intolerant patients only: Erythromycin (stearate, ethylsuccinate or base) 500 mg by mouth, 4 times daily.* * Duration of therapy based upon estimated duration of infection. If less than 1 yr, treat for 15 days; otherwise, treat for 30 days.	Both late syphilis and congenital syphilis are complications since they are preventable with prompt diagnosis and treatment of early syphilis. Sequelae of late syphilis include neurosyphilis (general paresis, tabes dorsalis and focal neurologic signs), cardiovascular syphilis (thoracic aortic aneurism, and aortic insufficiency).	Teach how to take any prescribed oral medications. If tetracycline is given, it should be taken 1 hr before or 2 hr after meals, and dairy products, antacids, iron or other mineral-containing preparations, and sunlight should be avoided. The patient should return for follow-up serologies 3, 6, 12, and 24 mo after therapy. Refer sexual partner(s) for evaluation and treatment. Have patient avoid sexual activity until patient and partner(s) are cured. Encourage condoms use to prevent future infections.
Vaginitis *Trichomonas vaginalis vaginitis:* A motile protozoan with an undulating membrane and four flagella *Bacterial vaginosis* (also	Presentations vary from no signs or symptoms to erythema, edema, and pruritus of the external genitalia. Excessive and/or malodorous discharge are common	*Trichomonas vaginalis vaginitis:* Mobile trichomonads are identified in a saline wet mount of vaginal discharge. *Bacterial vaginosis:* The	*Trichomonas vaginalis vaginitis:* Metronidazole 2.0 g by mouth, 3 times daily for 7 days *Alternative regimen:* Metronidazole 250 mg by mouth, 3 times daily	Secondary excoriations. Recurrent infections are common. *Bacterial vaginosis* may be associated with infectious complications of pregnancy, and with	Teach how to take or use any prescribed medications. Advise patient to avoid alcohol until 3 days following completion of metronidazole therapy.

called nonspecific vaginitis or Gardnerella vaginalis–associated vaginitis): An infection of uncertain etiology: Gardnerella vaginalis (a small gram-negative pleomorphic coccobacillus), Mobiluncus spp. (motile, curved anaerobic rods), and other anerobes have been implicated. Fungal vaginitis (predominantly Candida albicans): Dimorphic fungi that grow as oval budding yeast cells and as chains of cells (hyphae). Other vaginitides: Other infectious, chemical, allergenic, and physical agents can cause vaginitis.

findings
Male sexual partners may develop urethritis, balanitis, or cutaneous lesions on penis.

most practical confirmatory microbiologic test is the demonstration of characteristic changes in vaginal flora by Gram's stain of vaginal fluid; few or no lactobacilli, with predominance of G. vaginalis plus other organisms resembling gram-negative Bacteroides sp., anaerobic gram-positive cocci, and/or curved rods
Fungal vaginitis: Microscopic identification of yeast forms (budding cells or hyphae) in Gram's stain or KOH wet mount preparation of vaginal discharge.

for 7 days
Bacterial vaginosis: Metronidazole 500 mg by mouth, twice daily for 7 days
Alternative regimen: Ampicillin or amoxicillin 500 mg by mouth, 4 times daily for 7 days is less effective but may be used for pregnant patients or individuals for whom metronidazole is contraindicated
NOTE: Treatment is not recommended for male or female asymptomatic carriers of Gardnerella vaginalis.
Fungal vaginitis: Miconazole nitrate or clotrimazole 100 mg intravaginally daily for 7 days. The medication is available as cream or tablets, and the forms are equally effective.
Pregnancy: Metronidazole may be used after the first trimester. All other therapies are considered safe throughout.

upper genital tract infections in nonpregnant women, such as endometritis and salpingitis.
Fungal vaginitis in pregnancy increases the risk of neonatal oral thrush.

Teach patient to continue taking vaginally-administered medications even during menses.
Advise patient to return if problem not cured or if it recurs.
Encourage condoms use to prevent reinfection.

Adapted from Tennessee Department of Health and Environment: Sexually Transmitted Disease Summary, September 1986

appendix E

Medications in Breast Milk

Drug or Agent	Contra-indicated	Prescribe With Caution	No Apparent Harm	Insufficient Information	Comment
Analgesics					
Acetaminophen			X		Small amounts excreted
Aspirin			X		Infant salicylate plasma level should be monitored if mother is on high chronic doses
Codeine			X		Small amount excreted
Propoxyphene (Darvon)			X		Small amount secreted
Morphine			X		Small amount secreted
Meperidine			X		Small amount secreted
Oxycodone			X		Small amount secreted
Methadone			X		Avoid breast-feeding 3–4 hr after dose during peak level
Anticoagulants					
Ethyl biscoumacetate	X				Bleeding in infant
Phenindione	X				Bleeding in infant
Heparin			X		No passage into milk
Warfarin sodium (Coumadin)			X		
Bishydroxycoumarin (dicumarol)		X			
Anticonvulsants					
Ethosuximide (Zarontin)			X		Milk levels close to maternal serum level. Do infant level
Phenobarbital			X		Accumulation may occur. Infant levels should be done
Primidone (Mysoline)			X		Possible drowsiness
Carbamazepine			X		Possible drowsiness; significant infant levels: no reported effects
Diphenylhydantoin (phenytoin, Dilantin)			X		Low levels in infant Methemoglobinemia, one case
Valproic acid			X		Small amounts excreted

(continued)

Medications in Breast Milk (continued)

Drug or Agent	Contrain-dicated	Prescribe With Caution	No Apparent Harm	Insufficient Information	Comment
Antihistamines					
Diphenylhydantoin (Benadryl)		X			Small amounts excreted; increased sensitivity of newborn to antihistamines
Trimeprazine (Temaril)			X		Small amounts secreted
Tripelennamine (Pyribenzamine)			X		Small amounts secreted
Anti-Infective Agents					
Most anti-infective agents can cause (1) modification of bowel flora, (2) possible allergic sensitization, (3) interference with culture results, and (4) potential drug accumulation owing to infant's immature liver enzymes systems and renal elimination pathways.					
Aminoglycosides (Kanamycin Gentamicin)			X		Significant secretion in milk; not absorbed
Chloramphenicol	X				Bone marrow depression; gastrointestinal and behavioral effects
Erythromycin			X No adverse effects		
Penicillins and Cephalo-sporins			X		Possible sensitization
Sulfonamides		X			Hemolysis, G6PD deficiency; bilirubin displacement, avoid premature infants
Tetracyclines			X		Limited absorption by infant
Nalidixic acid		X			Hemolysis in G6PD; low levels in milk
Nitrofurantoin		X			Possible G6PD hemolysis
Metronidazole (Flagyl)		X			Give single 2-g dose got trichomonas and continue breast-feeding for 24–48 hr. Low absorption but potentially toxic
Isoniazid		X			High levels in milk, possible toxicity
Pyramethamine	X				Vomiting, marrow depression, convulsions
Chloroquine			X		Not excreted
Trimethoprim		X			Thrombocytopenia; avoid in G6PD deficiency
Aspirin			X		Perform infant salicylate plasma levels if mother is on high chronic doses
Indomethacin		X			Seizures, 1 case
Phenylbutazone		X			Low levels, possible blood dyscrasia
Gold	X				Found in baby: nephritis, hepatitis, hematologic changes
Ibuprofen			X		Small amounts secreted
Naproxen			X		Small amounts secreted
Naproxen Sodium			X		Small amounts secreted
Steroids				X	Low levels with prednisone and prednisolone; avoid feeding for 4 hr after the dose
Antineoplastic Agents					
Azathioprine		X			Low levels of mercaptopurine in milk when mothers took 75–100 mg in 3 infants
Cyclophosphamide	X				Neutropenia
Methotrexate	X				Very small excretion; may accumulate
Antithyroid Agents					
Radioactive iodine	X				Thyroid suppression
Propylthiouracil	X				Thyroid suppression

(continued)

Medications in Breast Milk (continued)

Drug or Agent	Contrain-dicated	Prescribe With Caution	No Apparent Harm	Insufficient Information	Comment
Methimazole	X				Thyroid suppression
Bronchodilators					
Aminophylline (Theophylline)			X		Irritability, one case; rapidly absorbed
Iodides	X				Thyroid suppression
Sympathomimetics				X	Inhalers probably safe
Cardiovascular Agents					
Digoxin			X		Insignificant levels
Propranolol			X		Insignificant levels
Reserpine	X				Nasal stuffiness, lethargy
Guanethidine (Ismelin)			X		Insignificant levels
Methyldopa (Aldomet)				X	
Quinidine				X	Insignificant levels; potential accumulation and thrombocytopenia
Cathartics					
Anthraquinones	X				Diarrhea, cramps
Aloe, senna		X			Safe in moderate doses
Bulk agent, softeners			X		
Contraceptives, Oral					
Diethylstilbestrol	X				Possible vaginal cancer
Depo-provera		X			May affect lactation at 300 mg IM, not at 150 mg
Noresthisterone		X			May affect lactation
Ethyl estradiol		X			May affect lactation
Diuretics					
Chlorthalidone				X	Low levels, but may accumulate
Thiazides		X			May affect lactation; low levels in milk
Spironolactone			X		Insignificant levels
					Avoid in first month of lactation
Ergot Alkaloids					
Bromocriptine	X				Lactation suppressed
Ergot	X				Vomiting, diarrhea, seizures
Ergotamine				X	
Ergonovine	X				Brief postpartum course may be safe; insignificant levels
Methylergonovine	X				Brief postpartum course may be safe, insignificant levels
Hormones					
Corticosteroids				X	Low levels with short-term prednisone or prednisolone
					Avoid feeding for 4 hr after dose
Sex hormones (see Contraceptives, Oral above)					
Thyroid (T_3, T_4)			X		Levels too low to interfere with neonatal thyroid screening; excreted in milk
Insulin			X		Not absorbed in breast milk
ACTH			X		Not absorbed in breast milk
Epinephrine			X		Not absorbed in breast milk

(continued)

Medications in Breast Milk (continued)

Drug or Agent	Contrain-dicated	Prescribe With Caution	No Apparent Harm	Insufficient Information	Comment
Narcotics					
Codeine			X		In usual doses
Meperidine (Demerol)			X		Small amounts excreted
Morphine			X		Low infant levels on usual dosage
Heroin	X				Addiction and withdrawal in infants
Methadone		X			Minimal levels
Oxycodone			X		Small amount excreted
Psychotherapeutic Agents					
Lithium	X				High levels in milk (40% of maternal serum level)
Phenothiazines		X			Drowsiness; chronic effects uncertain
Tricyclic Antidepressants				X	Low levels; effects uncertain
Diazepam (Valium)	X				Lethargy, weight loss, EEG changes; may accumulate
Meprobamate (Equanil)	X				High levels in milk; two to four times that of maternal plasma
Chlordiazepoxide (Librium)	X				Low levels in milk but but can accumulate, especially in neonates
Radiopharmaceuticals					
131I	X				No breast-feeding for 72 hr
Technetium (Tc-99M)	X				No breast-feeding for 48 hr
131I albumin	X				No breast-feeding for 10 days
Sedatives – Hypnotics					
Barbiturates		X			Short-acting, some drowsiness
Chloral hydrate		X			Drowsiness; 50% – 100% of maternal blood level
Bromides	X				Depression, rash
Diazepam (Valium)	X				Depression, weight loss
Flurazepam	X			X	Chemically related to diazepam
Nitrazepam				X	
Social-Recreational Drugs					
Alcohol			X		Milk levels equal plasma; moderate consumption apparently safe; high levels inhibit lactation
Caffeine			X		Jitteriness with very high intakes
Nicotine			X		Low levels in milk
Marijuana (dronabinol)			X		Minimal passage in milk; THC can reach high levels with heavy use
Phencyclipine	X				Concentrates in milk
Cocaine	X				One case of cocaine intoxication
Miscellaneous					
Atropine		X			May cause constipation or inhibit lactation
Dihydrotachysterol		X			Renal calcification in animals; hypercalcemia in infant
Etretinate	X				Manufacturer considers use contraindicated owing to potential adverse effects
Isotretinoin (Accutane)	X				Manufacturer considers use contraindicated owing to potential adverse effects
Tretinoin (Retin-A)				X	Minimal topical absorption

Briggs GG, Freeman RK, Yaffe SJ (eds): Drugs in Pregnancy and Lactation, 2nd ed. Baltimore, Williams & Wilkins, 1986; Briggs GG, Freeman RK, Yaffe SJ (eds): Drugs in Pregnancy and Lactation Update 1:3. Baltimore, Williams & Wilkins, 1988; Knoben JE, Anderson PG (eds): Handbook of Clinical Drug Data, 6th ed. Hamilton, IL, Drugs Intelligence Publications, 1988

glossary

abortion: Termination of pregnancy prior to viability of the fetus (which begins between 20 and 24 weeks)

    complete: Abortion in which all the products of conception have been expelled

    incomplete: Abortion in which some portions of the products of conception are retained in the uterus

    criminal: Illegal abortion

    habitual: Spontaneous abortion occurring in third or subsequent consecutive pregnancies

    inevitable: Impending abortion in presence of bleeding, pain, and dilatation and effacement of the cervix

    induced: Intentional abortion by consumption of drugs, removal of the products of conception by suction, or injection of drugs into the amniotic sac

    missed: Condition in which the embryo dies *in utero* and the products of conception are retained in the uterus

    septic: Infected abortion in which infective organisms disseminate into the maternal circulatory system

    spontaneous: Spontaneous expulsion of the products of conception before the 20th week of gestation

    therapeutic: Legally and medically sanctioned interruption of pregnancy before the 20th week of gestation

    threatened: Condition in which intrauterine bleeding occurs in early pregnancy; the cervix does not dilate and the products of conception are not necessarily expelled

abortus: A fetus that spontaneously delivers at less than 21 weeks gestational age and is less than 600 g

abruptio placentae: Complete or partial separation of the normally implanted placenta from the uterine wall

abscess: Localized collection of pus resulting from disintegration of tissue in any part of the body

abstinence: Abstention from sexual intercourse

accouchement: Act of childbirth

accoucheur: Obstetrician

accoucheuse: Midwife

accountability: Public or social responsibility for services delivered

acculturation: .Changes in customary practices in one group through extended contact with other groups that result in greater similarity with the dominant culture

acetonuria: Presence of acetone bodies in the urine from ketosis of diabetes or starvation

acetylcholine: Neurotransmitter at the myoneural junction

acidosis: Excessive acidity of body fluids due to accumulation of acids or loss of bicarbonate, resulting in lowered pH

acini cells: Milk-secreting cells of the breast

acquaintance: Process of getting to know the newborn; includes bonding and initial attachment

acrocyanosis: Cyanosis of the extremities in most infants at birth; may persist for 7–10 days

acrosome: Head of the spermatozoon

active management of labor: Intervention by birth attendants to control and improve on the body's own mechanisms

active phase of labor: Period from 5 centimeters of cervical dilatation through complete (10 cm) dilatation

adaptation: Process of responding to internal or environmental stimuli; implies modification of previous responses

adaptive demand: Internal or environmental stimulus that cannot be easily avoided and that requires behavioral response from an individual or family group

adipose: Pertaining to body fat

adnexa: Accessory parts of the uterus: fallopian tubes and ovaries

adolescence: Period of physical, social, and emotional transition between childhood and adulthood

adrenarche: Pubertal changes that result from effects of increased secretion of adrenocortical hormones

adrenocorticotropic hormone (ACTH): Pituitary hormone that stimulates the adrenal cortex

aerobes: Microorganisms that live and grow in oxygen

afibrinogenemia: A blood disorder that results from the absence or decrease of fibrinogen in the blood plasma, which becomes incoagulable; the acquired type may occur in obstetrical practice when abruptio placentae or retention of a dead fetus occurs

afterbirth: Placenta and membranes that are expelled after birth of a child

afterpains: Uterine contractions that cause pain during the first few days after childbirth

AGA: Appropriate (weight) for gestational age

agenesis: Absence of an organ

AIDS: Acquired immune deficiency syndrome; see *HIV*

albuminuria: Presence of albumin in the urine

alkalosis: Increase in *p*H of the body fluids

alleles: Different forms of a gene that can occupy the same locus on homologous chromosomes

alveolar surface tension: Cohesive force exerted by intermolecular attraction in the surface layer of fluid lining the alveolar walls; the force exerted results in a constant tendency for contraction of the surface fluid layer and collapse of alveoli

amenorrhea: Absence of menstruation, primary or secondary

amniocentesis: Insertion of a needle through the abdominal wall into the uterus and amniotic cavity in order to withdraw amniotic fluid by syringe

amnion: Membrane that forms the lining of the amniotic sac; fetal membranes

amnionitis: Inflammation of the inner layer of the fetal membranes

amnioscope: Optical device that allows direct visualization of the amniotic cavity

amniotic fluid: Transparent fluid contained in the amnion that protects the fetus and maintains its temperature

amniotomy: Artificial rupture of the amniotic sac, or bag of waters

anabolism: Synthetic or building-up reaction of the metabolic process

anaerobic: Pertaining to microorganisms that can live and grow in the absence of oxygen

androgen: Male hormone; the substance that produces or stimulates male characteristics

android pelvis: Male type of the bony pelvis

anemia: Condition in which number of red blood cells and hemoglobin concentration are reduced

anencephaly: Congenital absence of brain and spinal cord

anesthesia: Partial or complete loss of sensation with or without loss of consciousness

  general anesthesia: Pharmacologic pain relief measures that produce progressive central nervous system depression, loss of consciousness, and thus loss of sensation from the entire body

  local anesthesia: Pharmacologic pain relief measures that block sensory nerve pathways at the organ level, producing loss of sensation in that organ only

  regional anesthesia: Pharmacologic pain relief measures that block sensory nerve pathways along large sensory nerves from an organ and surrounding tissue, providing loss of sensation in that organ and the surrounding area

anomaly: Marked deviation from the norm; a malformation in an organ or structure

anorexia: Loss of appetite

anovulatory cycle: Menstrual cycle in which menstrual flow was not preceded by discharge of an ovum

anoxia: Deficiency of oxygen

anteflexion: Bending forward of the uterus

antenatal: Occurring before birth

antepartal: Occurring before the onset of labor

antibody: Protein substance formed by the body in response to presence of an antigen

antibody titer: Level of circulating antibody, measured per designated volume

anticipatory guidance: Nursing assessment of patient needs and planning for appropriate nursing interventions and patient actions to meet those needs

antidiuresis: Suppression of urine secretion

antiemetic: Substance that prevents or alleviates nausea and vomiting

antigen: Foreign substance introduced into the body that stimulates the immune system to form antibodies

antineoplastic: Substance that prevents the growth or proliferation of malignant cells

antipyretic: Agent that reduces fever

antiseptic: Agent that prevents the growth or arrests the development of microorganisms

antitoxin: Substance specifically antagonistic to a particular toxin

anuria: Failure of the kidney to produce urine

anus: Distal end of the large intestine and the outlet of the rectum

Apgar scale: System of numerical evaluation of neonate's condition at 1 minute and 5 minutes after birth; the maximum score is ten, and the higher the score the better the condition of the infant

apnea: Cessation of respirations

appendicular: Pertaining to the extremities, as opposed to axial, which pertains to the trunk

ARC: AIDS Related Complex; a cluster of severe physical

symptoms that may occur in individuals who have been infected by HIV

areola: Ring of dark pigment surrounding the nipple

arrest of descent: Lack of progress for 1 or more hours in the active phase of second-stage labor

arteriosclerosis: Thickening, hardening, and loss of elasticity in the walls of the arteries, resulting in altered functions of organs and tissues

arteriosclerosis obliterans: Complete occlusion of the lumen of the artery

ascites: Accumulation of serous fluid within the abdominal cavity

asepsis: Absence of infective organisms

aseptic technique: Method used to prevent transmission of pathogenic organisms

asphyxia: Condition caused by a lack of oxygen in the blood

asphyxia neonatorum: Delayed onset of breathing at the time of birth

aspiration: Act of inhaling; in the neonate, aspiration of mucus, meconium, or stomach contents into the lungs may result in atelectasis or pneumonia

atelectasis: Incomplete expansion of the lung or a portion of the lung

atony: Lack of normal muscle tone or strength (e.g., in uterine musculature)

atresia: Congenital absence or closure of a normal body opening

atrial septal defect: Congenital cardiac defect in which there is an abnormal opening between the atria of the heart

attachment: Affiliative tie formed after a period of mutual stimulation and response

attitude: Relationship of fetal parts to each other; the most common fetal attitude in utero is flexion, where the fetal head is bent onto the chest, the back is curved forward, and the arms and legs are folded in front of the body (fetal position)

auscultation: Listening for sounds within the body; e.g., listening for fetal heart tones with a fetoscope

autosome: Any of the 22 ordinary paired chromosomes; i.e., chromosome other than either of the two sex chromosomes

azoospermia: Absence of spermatozoa in the semen

bacteremia: Presence of bacteria in the blood

bacteria: Microorganisms of the class *Schizomycetes;* there are many varieties that may produce disease in man

bactericide: Agent that destroys bacteria

bacteriuria: Presence of bacteria in the urine

bag of waters: Amnion, or the membranes enclosing the amniotic fluid and the fetus

ballottement: Technique of palpation used to detect a floating object in the body; in pregnancy it is the rebound of a fetal part when displaced by a light tap of the finger through the abdominal wall or vagina

Bandl's ring: Abnormal, ringlike thickening at the junction of the upper and lower uterine segment that may obstruct delivery of the infant

Barr body: Material in the inactivated one of the two female (x) chromosomes in each body cell of normal females

Bartholin's glands: Small, mucus-secreting glands located at either side of the base of the vagina

basal body temperature: Temperature when body metabolism is at its lowest; used as an indirect method of determining whether ovulation has occurred (measurement in tenths of degrees is used in order to determine slight differences in temperature)

basal metabolism: Amount of energy needed to maintain life in a person completely at rest

baseline fetal heart rate: Average fetal heart rate within a 10-minute interval in the absence of or between contractions; normal baseline rate is 120–160 beats per minute

bearing down: Reflex effort on the part of the mother to coordinate activity of the abdominal muscles with the uterine contractions

bicornuate uterus: Uterus in which the fundus is divided into two parts

bilirubin: Yellowish pigment in bile produced from the hemoglobin of the red blood cells

bilirubinemia: Presence of an abnormal amount of bilirubin in the blood when red blood cells are broken down from a pathologic cause

bimanual examination: Pelvic examination performed with both hands; the first two fingers of one hand are placed in the vagina while the other hand is placed on the abdomen

biophysical profile: Antepartum surveillance of the fetus at risk by use of tests of fetal well-being, *i.e.,* nonstress test, contraction stress test, fetal movement

biparietal diameter: Largest transverse diameter of the fetal head; usually about 9.5 cm

birth: Passage of the infant from the uterus

birth defect: Congenital anomaly

birth rate: Number of live births per year for each 1000 individuals in the population

birthing room: Labor/delivery room, usually with a homelike decor, in which families labor, give birth, and recover; often adjacent to a more traditional labor and delivery unit with shared staff

bisexuality: Sexual attraction to members of both sexes

blastocyst: Structure that results when fluid accumulates within the morula, producing a cavity with the inner cell mass at one pole

blastomere: Cell that results from the cleavage of a fertilized ovum

blastula: Stage of the fertilized ovum in which the cells are arranged in a hollow ball

blighted ovum: Ovum with abnormal development

bloody show: Blood-tinged mucus discharge from the vagina that accompanies dilatation of the cervix in early labor

boggy uterus: Soft, spongy uterus that contracts inadequately in the early postpartum period

bonding: Initial phase in a relationship characterized by strong attraction and desire to interact

bony pelvis: Ring of bone containing the sacrum, coccyx, and two innominate bones

brachial palsy: Paralysis of the arm from injury to the brachial plexus during birth

bradycardia: Heart beat slower than 60 beats per minute

Braxton Hicks contractions: Painless intermittent contraction of the uterus during pregnancy that may be noticeable on abdominal palpation; may be perceived by the pregnant woman as painless tightening of the uterus

breakthrough bleeding: Vaginal bleeding or spotting occurring between periods in women using oral contraceptives; a result of the estrogen in the pill being inadequate to maintain the endometrium

breast pump: Electric or manual pump used to extract milk from the lactating breast

breech birth: Birth in which the buttocks or feet present first

broad ligament: Fibrous sheath covered by peritoneum extending from each side of the uterus to the lateral wall of the pelvis

bulbourethral glands: Two small glands lying along the membranous urethra of the male, just above the bulb of the corpus spongiosum (synonym: Cowper's glands)

Caldwell–Moloy classification: Classification of pelves into four types: anthropoid, gynecoid, android, and platypelloid

calorie: Unit of heat

canalization: Formation of channels within tissues

Candida: Yeastlike fungus that is common inhabitant of the skin, nails, mouth, and vagina; susceptibility to vaginal candidiasis increases during pregnancy because of changes in vaginal pH and increased levels of glycogen in the vaginal epithelium

capacitation: Process in which the surface characteristics of sperm cells change and enzymes are released, particularly hyaluronidase; these surface changes contribute to the sperm's ability to penetrate the ovum

caput succedaneum: Swelling produced on the fetal head during labor

carcinogen: Substance that can produce or incite cancer

cardiac output: Amount of blood that is ejected from the right or left ventricle per minute; in the average adult at rest, cardiac output is about 3 liters per square meter of body surface per minute

cardinal: Of primary importance; e.g., the cardinal symptoms are temperature, pulse, and respiration

cardiomegaly: Pathologic enlargement of the heart

carotene: Yellow pigment present in various plant and animal tissues; it is abundant in yellow vegetables (carrots, squash, corn)

carrier: Person who has two different forms of a particular gene (one normal and one mutant) at a given locus on a pair of homologous chromosomes (synonym: heterozygote)

catabolism: Destructive or breaking-down reaction of the metabolic process

catamenia: Menses, menstruation

caudad: Toward the tail; in a posterior or inferior position

caudal: Pertaining to a taillike structure

caul: Portions of the membranes or amnion covering the head of the fetus at birth

cell: Mass of protoplasm containing a nucleus and its nuclear material

    adipose: Fat cell

    basal: Cell in the basal layer of the epidermis

    columnar: Epithelial cell that is taller than it is wide

    daughter: Cell formed from the division of the mother cell

    Leydig's: Interstitial cells of the testes

    lutein: Cell of the corpus luteum of the ovary after ovulation

    mucous: Cell that secretes mucus

    sickle: Abnormal red blood cell shaped like a sickle

    squamous: Flat, scalelike, epithelial cell

cellulitis: Inflammation of the cellular tissue

central venous pressure (CVP) monitoring: Measurement of the pressure within the superior vena cava by means of an indwelling catheter and manometer; evaluates right atrial function by measuring its filling pressure and the capacity of its blood vessels; a high CVP indicates circulatory overload; a low CVP indicates reduced blood volume and circulatory depletion

cephalad: Toward the head

cephalhematoma: Localized collection of blood beneath the periosteum of the newborn skull caused by disruption of blood vessels during birth

cephalic: Pertaining to the head, or directed toward the head

cephalopelvic disproportion (CPD): Condition in which the infant's head is of a shape, size, or position that prevents it from passing through the mother's pelvis; the most common indication for cesarean delivery

cerclage: Encircling of the cervix with a suture

cervical mucus: Secretion of the columnar cells lining the endocervical canal

cervicitis: Inflammation of the uterine cervix

cervix: Lower portion of the uterus extending from the internal to the external cervical os

cesarean delivery: Extraction of the fetus, placenta, and membranes through an incision in the abdominal wall

Chadwick's sign: Bluish discoloration of the vaginal wall and vestibule; a presumptive sign of pregnancy

cheilosis: Reddened appearance and fissures at the angles of the lips; seen frequently in vitamin B deficiency

chlamydia: Caused by the organism *C.trachomatis* this sexually transmitted disease is the most prevalent STD in the US; as a sexual pathogen it is associated with a wide variety of adverse reproductive consequences

chloasma: Skin change in pregnancy characterized by the appearance of irregular brownish patches on the face (synonym: mask of pregnancy)

cholesterol: A sterol found widely in animal tissue, egg yolk, and various fats; important in metabolism as a precursor of steroid hormones, such as sex hormones and adrenal corticoids

chorioamnionitis: Inflammation of the chorion and amnion

chorion: Outer wall of the amniotic sac; composed of trophoblast and mesenchyme

chorionic plate: The portion of the chorion attached to the placenta

chorionic villi: Slender, branching projections of the chorion containing capillaries that are the means by which all substances (nutrients, gases, waste products) are exchanged between the maternal and fetal circulation

chorionic villi sampling (CVS): Aspiration of chorionic villi from the uterus during the first trimester for testing of chromosomal and medical disorders

chorioretinitis: Inflammation of the choroid and retina of the eye

chromosome: One of several microscopic rod-shaped bodies within the nucleus of a dividing cell that contain the hereditary material (genes) of the organism; the total chromosome number in humans is 46: females have 44 autosomes plus two X chromosomes; males have 44 autosomes plus one X and one Y chromosome

chromosome disorder: Abnormality of chromosome number or structure

cilia of fallopian tube: Hairlike processes lining the cell of the tubal mucosa that promote movement of the ova through the tube

circumcision: Removal of all or part of the prepuce, or foreskin, in the male infant

claudication: Severe pain in calf muscles while walking, resulting from inadequate blood supply that may be due to arterial spasm, atherosclerosis, arteriosclerosis, or an occlusion of vessels

cleavage: Process by which the zygote divides into blastomeres

cleft lip: Congenital fissure of the lip

cleft palate: Congenital deformity caused by the failure of the bones of the roof of the mouth to fuse

clinical nurse specialist: A registered nurse who has become expert at the graduate level in a defined area of knowledge and practice in nursing

clitoris: Small, cylindrical, erectile body in the female that is homologus to the male penis

clonus: Spasmodic contraction and relaxation

coagulation time: Time required for blood to clot

cognitive processes: Processes involved in perceiving, interpreting, organizing, storing, retrieving, coordinating, and using stimuli received from the internal and external environment

coitus: Sexual intercourse, copulation

collagen: A protein found in connective tissue, skin, bone, ligaments, and cartilage; constitutes about 30% of total body protein

collagenous: Pertaining to fibrous protein found in connective tissue, such as bone, ligaments, and cartilage

colostrum: Breast fluid secreted 2 or 3 days after childbirth and before the onset of true lactation

colposcope: Magnifying instrument inserted into the vagina to view the tissues of the vagina and cervix

colpotomy: Incision into the wall of the vagina

conception: Fertilization of the ovum by the sperm

conceptus: Products of conception

conditioned response: Response acquired as a result of training and repetition

condom: Thin, flexible sheath worn over the penis during sexual intercourse to prevent deposition of sperm into the vagina

condyloma: Sexually transmitted, viral, wartlike growth on the skin of the genitals

confidentiality: Implies that a private and personal relationship exists between the provider and the client

congenital: Present at birth

congenital anomaly: Abnormality present at birth

consanguinity: Blood relationship to another person

consent: Implies that the client has received adequate information to understand the risk/benefit ratio, alternatives to treatment (to include no treatment), and expected outcome

constipation: Difficult defecation

contraception: Prevention of conception

contraction: Periodic, rhythmic tightening of the uterine musculature during labor that effaces and dilates the cervix and, in concert with maternal pushing effort, expels the fetus

contraction stress test: Stimulation of the uterine muscles by use of oxytocin to assess fetal oxygen reserves prior to labor

contracture of the pelvis: Reduction in size of the bony pelvis so that a fetus of normal size cannot pass through; contracture may be general or at the inlet, midpelvis, or outlet

convulsion: Paroxysm of involuntary muscle contractions and relaxations

Coombs' test: Test used to detect sensitized red blood cells in erythroblastosis fetalis

copulation: Sexual intercourse

cor pulmonale: Abnormal cardiac condition characterized by hypertrophy of the right ventricle of the heart and resulting from hypertension of the pulmonary circulation

cord prolapse: Obstetric emergency in which the umbilical cord descends into or through the cervix ahead of the presenting fetal part, making it vulnerable to compression and resulting in diminished fetal oxygenation

coronal suture: Membrane-occupied spaces between the bones of the infant's head that extend transversely from the anterior fontanelle and lie between the parietal and frontal bones

corpus luteum: Solid yellow body that develops within a ruptured ovarian follicle; an endocrine structure, it primarily secretes progesterone

cotyledon: Segment or subdivision of the uterine surface of the placenta

Couvelaire uterus: Uterus with blood forced within the uterine walls between the muscle fibers; the condition may accompany premature separation of the placenta

Cowper's glands: Two small glands lying along the membraneous urethra of the male, just above the bulb of the corpus spongiosum (synonym: bulbourethral glands)

cradle cap: Seborrheic dermatitis of the newborn that appears on the head, scalp, and face of the newborn

crisis: Sudden change in condition; a turning point during which disorganization occurs because normal coping mechanisms fail

crowning: Distention of the perineum by the largest diameter of the presenting part; in a normal vertex presentation, this would be the biparietal diameter

crown-rump length: An estimate of fetal gestational age based on measurement from the top of the head (crown) to the buttocks

cryptorchidism: Condition in which testicles are undescended

cues: Signals expressed behaviorally and verbally

cul-de-sac: Extension of the peritoneal cavity lying between the rectum and the posterior wall of the uterus (synonym: pouch of Douglas, rectouterine pouch)

culdocentesis: Aspiration of fluid from the pouch of Douglas by puncture of the posterior vaginal fornix

culdoscopy: Visual examination of the female pelvic viscera through the posterior vaginal fornix by means of an endoscope

cultural relativism: Practice of judging a group or its traits by its own or similar standards

cunnilingus: Oral sexual stimulation of the female genitals

curettage: Scraping of the inner surface of the uterus with a curette to remove its lining or contents

cystitis: Infection of the urinary bladder

cystocele: Bladder hernia protruding into the vagina; usually occurs after repeated childbirth

cytomegalovirus: Group of herpesviruses that may cause disease in the newborn if the mother is infected

cytotrophoblast: Inner layer of trophoblast cells that is bathed in maternal blood for passage of nutrients, oxygen, and gases to the fetus and for removal of its waste products

decidua: Endometrium of the uterus enveloping the impregnated ovum

delivery: Expulsion of the infant, placenta, and membranes at birth

demand feeding: Practice of allowing the infant to determine the frequency of feeding and amount of milk ingested, as opposed to the imposition of rigid time schedules for feeding by adult care-givers

deoxyribonucleic acid (DNA): Chemical forming the genetic code; occurs as a double-stranded helix within chromosomes

dermatosis: Any disease of the skin in which inflammation is not usually a feature

descent: Passage of the presenting part of the fetus into and through the birth canal; begins at the onset of labor and proceeds during effacement and dilatation of the cervix

development: Gradual advance in the process of total human growth with emphasis on behavioral aspects of functioning

developmental task: Step, stage, or phase in the process of growth that is sequential and prerequisite to further growth

dextroversion: Deviation of the uterus from its normal position to the right side

diabetes mellitus: Endocrine disorder in which normal carbohydrate metabolism is disrupted because of a deficiency of insulin; the course of diabetes changes significantly when pregnancy intervenes and the prenatal care of a diabetic gravida must be closely supervised

diagonal conjugate measurement: Chief internal pelvic measurement made to determine the approximate diameter of the pelvic passage; it is the distance between the sacral promontory and the lower margin of the symphysis pubis

diaphoresis: Profuse perspiration

diaphragm, pelvic: Muscles and fascia providing primary support to the pelvic viscera

diastasis recti: Separation of the abdominal recti muscles; may occur during pregnancy because of stretching of the abdominal wall

dilatation: Opening or enlargement; the cervical canal dilates from a few centimeters to 10 centimeters in diameter during labor; synonymous with dilation

dilatation and curettage: Procedure in which the uterine cervix is dilated and the endometrium of the uterus is scraped away; performed for diagnostic or therapeutic purposes, to remove the products of conception after incomplete abortion, and for therapeutic abortion

dipping: Point in labor at which the presenting part of the fetus has passed through the plane of the inlet but engagement has not occurred

diuresis: Increased secretion of urine

diurnal rhythm: Patterns of physiologic functioning occurring with predictable frequency on a daily basis

diverticulum: Sac or pouch located in the wall of an organ or canal

dizygotic twins: Twins resulting from two fertilized ova; dizygotic twins have different genetic constitutions and may be of the same or different sex

Döderlein's bacillus: Normal inhabitant of the vagina that helps to maintain its acidic pH (synonym: Lactobacillus acidophilus)

dominant trait: Trait that is clinically expressed in both homozygous and heterozygous individuals

Doppler ultrasound sensor: Device used to monitor fetal heart rate

Down syndrome: Congenital condition characterized by mental retardation and multiple physiologic defects

Dubowitz tool: Method of estimating gestational age of a newborn based on 21 strictly defined clinical signs

ductus arteriosus: Channel between the fetal aorta and the main pulmonary artery; it is usually closed by normal neonatal respiratory function and may be medically or surgically treated if it remains open after birth

ductus venosus: Fetal blood vessel that connects the umbilical vein and the inferior vena cava

dysgenesis: Abnormal or defective development of the embryo

dysmenorrhea: Painful menstruation

dyspareunia: Painful intercourse

dysphagia: Inability or difficulty with swallowing

dysplasia: Abnormal development of tissue

dyspnea: Labored breathing

dystocia: Difficult labor resulting from fetal or maternal causes

dysuria: Painful urination

early extended parent–infant contact: Organization of care that facilitates parent–infant contact immediately after birth and throughout the first few hours of life

early withdrawal bleeding: Vaginal bleeding or spotting associated with oral contraceptives that begins during active pill taking and continues into the inactive or pill-free interval

ecchymosis: A form of macula that appears in large, irregularly formed hemorrhagic areas of the skin and results from extravasation of blood into the skin's mucous membrane; a bruise

eclampsia: Toxemia of pregnancy accompanied by high blood pressure, albuminuria, oliguria, tonic and clonic convulsions, and coma; may occur before, during, or after childbirth

ectoderm: Outer layer of the embryo; it develops into the epidermis and neural tube

ectopic pregnancy: Implantation of the ovum outside of the uterine cavity, e.g., in the fallopian tube or abdomen

ectopy: Displacement or placement in an abnormal position

eczema: Superficial dermatitis of unknown cause

edema: Excessive accumulation of fluid in the tissues

effacement: Softening, thinning, and shortening of the cervical canal as it is drawn up into the body of the uterus by labor contractions

effleurage: Light, rhythmic stroking of the abdomen during labor; useful for enhancing relaxation

egocentric: Pertains to a withdrawal from the external world with concentration on the inner self

ejaculation: Sudden emission of semen from the urethra that occurs during sexual intercourse or masturbation

embolus: Clot or other plug carried by a blood vessel and blocking a smaller one

embryo: Stage of human development occurring between the ovum and the fetal stages, or from 2–8 weeks after conception

emesis: Vomiting

empathy: Objective awareness or recognition of another person's feelings

en face: Position in which mother and infant are face-to-face with eye-to-eye contact

endemic disease: Disease with a low mortality rate occurring continuously in a particular population

endocervix: Membrane lining the canal of the uterine cervix

endocrine: Pertaining to an organ or gland that secretes a hormone into the bloodstream in order to induce a specific effect on another organ

endogenous: Pertaining to anything produced by or arising from within a cell or organism

endometrial biopsy: Diagnostic procedure in which a sample of endometrial tissue is obtained

endometrial cycle: An integrated evolutionary process of endometrial growth and regression that is repeated up to 300–400 times during a woman's adult life

endometriosis: Pathologic condition in which normal tissue that lines the uterus (endometrial tissue) grows outside of the uterus, often around the fallopian tubes, contributing to infertility

endometritis: Inflammation of the endometrium

endometrium: Mucous membrane lining the uterus (during pregnancy it is known as the decidua)

endoscope: Illuminated optical instrument used to visualize the interior of a body cavity or hollow organ

endotoxin: Toxin confined within bacteria and freed when the bacteria are broken down

engagement: Point in labor at which the widest diameter of the fetal presenting part passes through the pelvic inlet

engorgement: Hyperemia; local congestion; excessive fullness, *e.g.,* of the breast

epididymis: Organ made up of long, coiled seminiferous tubules; it provides for storage, transit, and maturation of sperm

epidural anesthesia: Anesthesia of the pelvis, abdomen, or genital area achieved by injection of a local anesthetic into the epidural space of the spinal column

epigastrium: Upper portion of the abdomen lying over the stomach

episiotomy: Incision into the perineum and vagina during delivery to enlarge the vaginal opening to prevent tearing of the underlying fascia and muscle as the infant's head is born

epithelioma: A malignant tumor originating in the epidermis of the skin or mucous membrane

Erb's palsy: Partial paralysis of the upper brachial plexus caused by traumatic injury during childbirth, often from forcible traction during delivery

erectile tissue: Vascular tissue, such as that in the penis, clitoris, and nipples, that becomes erect when filled with blood

erotic: Tending to arouse sexual desire

erythema: Inflammation of the skin or mucous membrane resulting from the dilatation and congestion of superficial capillaries

erythroblastosis fetalis: Hemolytic anemia of the fetus and newborn occurring when the blood of the fetus is Rh-positive and the blood of the mother is Rh-negative

escutcheon: Pattern of hair growth over the genitalia and lower abdomen; considered a secondary sexual characteristic

esophageal atresia: Condition in which the esophagus ends in a blind pouch or narrows into a thin cord, usually between the upper and middle third of the esophagus

essential hypertension: Blood pressure higher than normal for age that develops in the absence of kidney disease

estrogen: Female hormone that promotes development of female secondary sexual characteristics, affects the menstrual cycle, and prepares the female genital tract for fertilization and implantation of a fertilized ovum each month

ethnocentrism: Belief in the natural superiority of the group to which one belongs; tendency to judge a group by standards appropriate to another group

etiology: Study of the factors involved in the development of a disease

euthyroid: Normal thyroid function

exogenous: Anything originating outside an organ or part

exsanguination: Extensive, severe blood loss that is so extreme that it is incompatible with life

extragenital: Outside or unrelated to genital sexual organs

extraperitoneal cesarean delivery: Surgical delivery of an infant through an incision in the lower uterine segment, which avoids entry into the peritoneal cavity

extrinsic coagulation factors: Blood Factors V, VII, and X

fallopian tube: Oviduct

false labor: Irregular uterine contractions felt in late pregnancy that do not cause dilatation or effacement of the cervix (synonym: Braxton Hicks contractions)

family life cycle: Continuum of changes in a family over time; specifically, changes in the growth, development, and structure of the family group

fecundity: Ability to produce offspring (synonym: fertility)

ferning: Fernlike pattern seen microscopically when cervical mucus is thinly applied to a glass slide and allowed to dry; the pattern, which results from crystallization of the sodium chloride in the mucus, confirms the presence of estrogen at midcycle

ferritin: Iron–phosphorus protein containing iron; it is the form of iron stored in the liver, spleen, and bone marrow and is essential for hematopoiesis

ferrous: Containing iron

fertilization: Union of the male sperm and the female ovum to form a zygote, from which the embryo develops

fetal age: Age of the fetus, calculated from the time of conception

fetal alcohol syndrome: Set of birth defects in infants whose mothers ingest excessive amounts of alcohol during pregnancy

fetal dystocia: Difficulty in labor caused by fetal size, malposition, or abnormality or by a multiple pregnancy

fetal heart rate (FHR): Number of fetal heartbeats in a given time; normal FHR is 120 to 160 beats per minute

fetal heart rate fluctuations: Bradycardia, tachycardia, accelerations, decelerations, or changes in variability in the fetal heart rate

fetal heart tones (FHT): Beat of the fetal heart that can be heard through the maternal abdomen

fetal hydrops: Extreme edema of the fetus or newborn occurring in severe hemolytic disease (synonym: hydrops fetalis)

fetal membranes: Membranes consisting of an outer chorionic and an inner amniotic membrane that adhere to each other during the fifth month of fetal life and form the amniotic sac

fetal souffle: Sound of blood racing through the umbilical artery that is synchronous with the fetal heartbeat (synonym: funic souffle)

fetopelvic disproportion: Inability of the fetus to pass through the maternal pelvis

fetoscope: Stethoscope used for auscultating the fetal heartbeat through the mother's abdomen

fetus: Infant in utero after completion of the embryonic stage at 8 weeks of gestation; major development occurs from this time until birth

fetus papyraceus: A dead fetus pressed flat by the growth of a living twin

fibrinogen: Blood protein that becomes converted to fibrin, which is essential for blood clotting (synonym: Factor I)

fimbria: Finger-like projections of the infundibular portion of the fallopian tube

fixation of fetal head: Descent of the fetal head through the pelvic inlet to a point where it cannot move freely when pushed by both hands positioned over the lower pelvis

flaccid: Flabby, soft, lacking normal muscle tone

flexion: Normal bending forward of the fetal head in the uterus or birth canal

fluctuance: Wavy impulse felt during palpation of a fluid-filled space that is produced by vibration of body fluid

focal: Pertaining to focus

folic acid (folacin): Member of the vitamin B complex

fontanelle: Unfused areas between fetal skull bones that are covered with strong connective tissue, which allows movement of bones and molding of fetal head during birth

football hold: Method of holding a newborn, which is known as the safety hold in nurseries; the baby's back is supported on the nurse's lower arm, while its bottom is tucked securely between the elbow/upper arm of the nurse and its head rests in nurse's hand

foramen ovale: Opening between atria in fetal heart that normally closes within hours after birth; when the opening remains patent it can be closed surgically

forceps: Two-bladed instrument used to assist delivery of the infant after the cervix is fully dilated and the fetal head is engaged

foreskin: Prepuce, or loose fold of skin, covering the penis or clitoris

fornices: Anterior and posterior spaces into which the upper vagina is divided

fossa: Furrow or shallow depression

fourchette: Fold of mucous membrane at the posterior junction of the labia minora

fourth trimester: Final three months of the childbearing year; the 12-week period that begins immediately following birth and includes the puerperium

free-standing birth center: Homelike facility for labor, birth, and postbirth recovery outside of a hospital setting

frenulum linguae: Fold of mucous membrane extending from the floor of the mouth to the inferior portion of the tongue and restraining its movement

friable: Easily broken, e.g., blood vessels of the cervix

Friedman curve: Graph showing the progress of labor that facilitates detection of dysfunctional labor

full-term infant: Infant born between 38 and 42 weeks of gestation

functional residual capacity: Volume of gas that remains in the lung after a normal exhalation

fundus: Upper portion of the uterus lying between the points of insertion of the fallopian tubes

galactorrhea: Lactation or flow of milk not associated with childbirth or nursing; may be a symptom of a pituitary gland tumor

gamete: Mature male or female germ cell; a spermatozoon or ovum

gametogenesis: Maturation of gametes through the process of meiosis

gamma globulin: Blood protein that has the ability to resist infection

gastroenteritis: Inflammation of the stomach and intestines that accompanies many gastrointestinal disorders

gavage: The feeding of liquid nutrients through a tube passed into the stomach through the nose or mouth

gene: Segment of a DNA molecule that codes for the synthesis of a single product; the smallest unit of heredity

genetics: Study of heredity

genitalia: Organs of reproduction

genitourinary: Pertaining to the genital and urinary organs

genome: The complete set of chromosomes of an organism

genotype: Fundamental, hereditary makeup of a person's genes

germ layers: Three primary cell layers of the embryo that develop into organs and tissues: ectoderm, mesoderm, and endoderm

German measles: Acute contagious viral disease that has a rash of short duration; it may cause congenital anomalies in infants of mothers who contract the disease early in pregnancy (synonym: rubella)

gestagen: Natural or synthetic steroid hormone that produces progestational effects

gestation: Time from conception to birth, approximately 280 days

gestational age: Estimated age of the fetus calculated in weeks from the first day of the last menstrual period

gestational sac: Amnion and its contents (products of conception)

gingivitis: Condition in which the gums become inflamed and spongy and bleed easily; common in pregnancy, but with good oral hygiene and a balanced diet, will clear shortly after delivery

glomerular filtration rate (GFR): Amount of plasma filtered by the glomeruli of both kidneys per minute

glucocorticoids: Adrenal hormones that are active in protecting against stress and also affect protein and carbohydrate metabolism

glucogenesis: Formation of glucose in the liver from sources that are not carbohydrates, such as fatty or amino acids

glucose-6-phosphate dehydrogenase: Enzyme of the liver and kidney that plays an important role in the conversion of glycerol to glucose; a hereditary deficiency of the enzyme causes hemolytic anemia in persons who ingest certain drugs

glucosuria: Presence of glucose in the urine

goiter: Enlargement of the thyroid gland

gonadotropins: Hormones having a stimulating effect on the gonads; FSH (follicle stimulating hormone) causes ovarian follicles to grow and secrete estrogen, and LH (luteinizing hormone) causes formation of the corpus luteum following ovulation and produces progesterone during the second half of the menstrual cycle

gonads: Male and female sex organs (testes and ovaries)

gonorrhea: A sexually transmitted infection of the genital mucous membrane of the male and female

Goodell's sign: Softening of the cervix and vagina as determined by bimanual examination; an indication of pregnancy

graafian follicle: Ovarian sac that contains an ovum

gravida: Woman who is or has been pregnant, regardless of pregnancy outcome

grief process: Painful withdrawal of attachment to a lost object or wish during which memories that bind the individual to the lost object are reviewed and relived

G6PD: See glucose-6-phosphate dehydrogenase

GTPAL: Method of summarizing obstetric history; Gravida, Term pregnancies, Preterm birth, Abortions, Living children

gynecoid pelvis: Type of pelvis that is characteristic of the normal female and is the ideal pelvic type for childbirth

gynecologic examination: An examination including assessment of weight and blood pressure and palpation of the breasts, abdomen, vagina, and rectum

gynecology: Branch of medicine specializing in the health care of women, especially their sexual and reproductive functions and the diseases thereof

habitual abortion: Three or more consecutive spontaneous abortions

haploid cell: Cell containing only one member of each pair of homologous chromosomes; the haploid number in humans is 23

heel stick: A pin or lancet prick performed on an infant's heel to assess the blood for hematocrit, glucose levels, or other tests as indicated

Hegar's sign: Softening of the lower uterine segment felt on bimanual examination; a probable sign of pregnancy

hematocrit: Volume percentage of red blood cells in whole blood; the normal range in women is between 38% and 46%

hematoma, puerperal: Collection of blood in the soft tissue of the pelvis caused by the trauma of childbirth

hematuria: Blood in the urine

hemoconcentration: Decrease in plasma volume, resulting in increased concentration of red blood cells

hemodilution: Increase in blood plasma volume, resulting in reduced concentration of red blood cells

hemoglobinopathy: Disease caused by or associated with forms of abnormal hemoglobin

hemolysis: Destruction of red blood cells

hemolytic anemia: Anemia due to the premature destruction of red blood cells

hemorrhage: Rapid loss of large amounts of venous or arterial blood; bleeding may be external or internal

hemorrhoid: Dilatation of one or more of the hemorrhoidal plexus of veins; an external hemorrhoid is the dilatation of rectal veins beneath the skin of the anal canal; it may occur during labor due to pushing and distention of the anal tissues

hepatosplenomegaly: Pathologic enlargement of the liver and spleen

hereditary: Genetically transmitted from parent to offspring

herpesvirus: Family of viruses causing herpes simplex, herpes zoster, and varicella (chicken pox)

heterozygote: Person who has two different alleles, at a given locus on a pair of homologous chromosomes

hiatal hernia: Protrusion of the stomach upward into the mediastinal cavity through the esophageal hiatus of the diaphragm

high-density lipoproteins (HDL): Plasma proteins that carry cholesterol in plasma and decrease the possibility of coronary artery disease when their levels are high

histology: Study of the microscopic structure of tissue

HIV: Human immunodeficiency virus; causes AIDS, a virulent infection that causes collapse of the body's immune system and eventual death from opportunistic infection

Homans' sign: Pain in the calf on dorsiflexion of the foot; an indicator of thrombosis or thrombophlebitis

homeostasis: State of equilibrium in the internal environment of the body that is naturally maintained by adaptive body responses

homologous chromosomes: Matched pair of chromosomes, one from each parent, having the same gene loci in the same order

homosexuality: Sexual attraction to members of the same sex

homozygote: Individual who has two matching alleles at a given locus on a pair of homologous chromosomes

hot flush (flash): A characteristic symptom of menopause directly related to decreased circulating estrogen

human papillomavirus (HPV): A sexually related infection that may play a role in the development of cervical cancer

hydramnios: Excessive amniotic fluid inside the uterus leading to overdistention

hydrocephaly: Accumulation of cerebrospinal fluid within the ventricles of the brain

hydrops fetalis: Extreme edema of a fetus or newborn; usually caused by Rh incompatibility (erythroblastosis)

hygroscopic: Pertaining to a substance that readily absorbs moisture

hymen: Fold of mucous membrane that partially covers the vaginal orifice

hyperbilirubinemia: Excessive concentrations of bilirubin in the blood that may lead to jaundice

hypercalcemia: Excessive calcium in the blood

hypercapnia: Excessive carbon dioxide in the blood

hyperemesis gravidarum: Abnormal condition of pregnancy where protracted vomiting, weight loss, and fluid and electrolyte imbalance occurs

hyperemia: Increased blood flow to a part as evidenced by redness of the skin

hyperglycemia: Excessive glucose in the blood

hyperkeratosis: Overgrowth of the horny layer of the epidermis

hyperplasia: Excessive proliferation of normal cells in the normal arrangement of a structure or organ

hyperreflexia: Increased action of the reflexes

hypertension: Common disorder characterized by persistent blood pressure greater than 140/90 mm Hg

hyperthyroidism: Excessive secretion of the thyroid gland

hypertonicity: State of greater than normal muscle tension

hypertrophy: Increase in size of an organ or structure not resulting from an increase in the number of cells

hyperventilation: Increased, forced respiration that may induce dizziness or fainting

hypervolemia: Abnormal increase in the volume of circulating blood

hypocalcemia: Below-normal calcium levels

hypochromia: Condition in which red blood cells have reduced hemoglobin content and less color

hypofibrinogenemia: Deficiency of fibrin in the blood

hypogalactia: Decreased breast secretion of milk

hypoglycemia: Abnormally low blood glucose

hypokalemia: Extreme potassium depletion in the blood

hyponatremia: Extreme sodium depletion in the blood

hypoplasia: Defective tissue development

hypospadias: Developmental anomaly in which the male urethra opens on the undersurface of the penis

hypotension: Abnormally low blood pressure

hypothalamus: Structure within the brain that controls metabolic activities, one of which is the releasing of factors that control gonadotropin hormone secretion in the pituitary

hypothermia: Abnormally low body temperature

hypothyroidism: Diminished secretion of the thyroid gland

hypotonia, uterine: Failure of the uterine muscles to contract and retract with normal strength and frequency

hypovolemia: Diminished blood volume

hypoxemia: Deficiency of oxygen in the blood

hypoxia: Reduction to below physiologic levels in the supply of oxygen to tissues

hysterectomy: Surgical removal of the uterus

hysterosalpingogram: Diagnostic procedure in which radiopaque dye is injected into the cervix, uterus, and fallopian tubes to determine their patency

iatrogenic: Pertaining to any adverse mental or physical condition unintentionally induced by treatment by a physician or surgeon

icteric: Pertaining to jaundice

icterus neonatorum: Physiologic jaundice in the newborn

idiopathic respiratory distress syndrome (IRDS): Severe respiratory condition found primarily in preterm infants (synonym: hyaline membrane disease)

iliopectineal line: Ridge on the pubis and ilium marking the brim of the true pelvis

immune response: Reaction of the body to foreign substances or substances interpreted as being foreign

immunized: Protected or exempted from the effects of a foreign protein

immunosuppressant: Substance interfering with or suppressing the normal immune response

imperforate hymen: Hymen with no opening

implantation: Process by which the conceptus attaches to the uterine wall and penetrates both the uterine endometrium and the maternal circulatory system

implantation bleeding: Slight endometrial oozing of blood at implantation; may be noted as "spotting" by the woman

impotence: Inability of the male to achieve or maintain an erection

impregnation: Fertilization of an ovum

inborn error of metabolism: Hereditary disease caused by deficiency of a specific enzyme

incest: Sexual intercourse between those of near relationship

incontinence: Inability to control the excretion of urine or feces

incubator: Enclosed crib in which the temperature can be controlled; used in caring for premature infants

induction of labor: Deliberate initiation of uterine contractions

inertia, uterine: Sluggish uterine contractions

infant: Child under 1 year of age

infant behavioral assessment: Systematic survey of unique interactional and neuromuscular responses of newborn during the first 4 to 6 weeks of life

infant mortality rate: Number of deaths in the first year of life per 1000 live births

infertility: Inability to produce offspring

Inhospital (alternative) birth center: Room or cluster of rooms with homelike decor for labor, birth, and postbirth recovery; may be administratively separate from traditional labor and delivery unit; similar to or synonymous with birthing room

innominate bone: Hip bone, composed of the ilium, ischium, and pubis; it is united with the sacrum and coccyx by ligaments to form the pelvis

in situ: In position

insulin: Hormone secreted by the beta cells of the islets of Langerhans of the pancreas

intermenstrual: Between menstrual periods

internal rotation: Mechanism of labor characterized by rotation of the presenting part of the fetus within the birth canal

international unit (IU): Internationally accepted amount of a substance; the form in which quantities of fat-soluble vitamins, some hormones, enzymes, and vaccines are expressed

interstitial: Referring to spaces within a tissue or organ

intractable: Unrelenting

intrapartal: Occurring during labor or birth

intrauterine: Within the uterus

intrauterine growth curve: Line on a standardized graph that represents the mean weight of the fetus for gestational age through pregnancy to term; it is a method of classifying infants according to maturity and state of development

intrauterine growth retardation (IUGR): Fetal condition characterized by failure to grow at the expected rate

introitus: Vaginal opening

invaginate: To insert one part of a structure within a part of the same structure, or to ensheathe (synonym: intussusception)

inverted nipple: Deformity of the nipple that causes it to recede rather than erect when stimulated

in vitro fertilization: Process whereby ova are extracted surgically from a woman, fertilized in a test tube, and implanted in the uterus

involution: Reduction in the size of the uterus following delivery (total involution takes six weeks)

ischemia: Temporary obstruction of circulation to a part

isthmus: Constriction on the uterine surface between the uterine body and the cervix

jaundice: Yellow discoloration of the skin, whites of the eyes, mucous membranes, and body fluids caused by excessive bilirubin in the blood.

joule: Work done in 1 second by current of ampere against a resistance of 1 ohm; 1 kilo calorie is equal to 4185.5 joules

Kegel exercise: Conscious tightening and relaxing of the pubococcygeal muscles, which strengthens the muscles of the vagina and perineum

kernicterus: Abnormal toxic accumulation of bilirubin in the brain due to hyperbilirubinemia

ketoacidosis: Acidosis accompanied by excessive ketones in the body and resulting from faulty carbohydrate metabolism; primarily a complication of diabetes mellitus

ketones: End products of fat metabolism

ketosis: Accumulation of abnormal amounts of ketones in the body resulting from inadequate ingestion of carbohydrates; seen in starvation, in diabetes, and, rarely, in pregnancy

karyotype: Chromosomal makeup of the nucleus of a human cell; also, the photomicrograph of chromosomes arranged in an organized way

kick count: A maternal check of fetal health after 38 weeks by counting the number of times the baby kicks each day

kilocalorie (kcal): Unit of measure for heat; in nutrition it is known as a large calorie and written with a capital C

kilogram (kg): 1000 grams or 2.2 pounds

kwashiorkor: Disease of malnutrition caused by severe

protein deficiency, usually occurring when the child is weaned from the breast; primarily affects children in underdeveloped countries

labor: Rhythmic contraction and relaxation of the uterine muscles with progressive effacement and dilatation of the cervix (synonym: parturition)

labor stimulation: Augmentation of uterine contractions with drugs

laceration: Tearing; during delivery, tearing of the vulvar, vaginal, and, possibly, rectal tissue as the infant is born

lactalbumin: Important constituent of whey

lactation: Postpartum production of milk

Lamaze method of delivery: Psychoprophylactic method of prepared childbirth, in which in late pregnancy parents are taught the physiology of pregnancy and childbirth, exercises to strengthen abdominal, vaginal, and perineal muscles, and techniques of breathing to be used during labor and delivery

Laminaria: Genus of moisture-absorbing seaweed used to dilate the cervix before abortion; it is placed in the cervix at least 12 hours prior to the procedure and is used as a physiologic means of cervical dilatation

lanugo: Downy hair that covers the body of the fetus, especially preterm

laparoscopy: Examination of the abdominal cavity by the introduction of a laparoscope through a small abdominal incision; organs of the abdomen and pelvis can be visualized and such procedures as sterilization performed

laparotomy: Surgical incision into the abdominal cavity

large-for-gestational-age (LGA) infant: Infant of any weight who falls above the 90th percentile on the intrauterine growth curve

latent phase of labor: Period from initiation of true labor contraction through 3–4 centimeters of cervical dilatation

Leboyer method of delivery: Approach to delivery formulated by Charles Leboyer, a French obstetrician; delivery is gentle and controlled, the atmosphere quiet and dim, overstimulation of the newborn is avoided, and the infant is gently supported in a tub of warm water

lecithin/sphingomyelin (L/S) ratio: Ratio of lecithin to sphingomyelin in the amniotic fluid; a ratio of 2 : 1 is used as an indicator of fetal lung maturity

let-down: A reflex caused by increased oxytocin from the pituitary gland in the brain and resulting in contractions of muscles of the breasts that force milk into the ducts leading to the nipple

leukocytosis: Increase in number of leukocytes (white blood cells) to over 10,000/mm³

leukorrhea: White or yellowish mucous discharge that normally drains from the cervix or vagina

LGA: See large for gestational age infant

libido: Sexual drive

lie: Relationship of the long axis of the fetus to the long axis of the mother

lightening: Descent of the uterus into the pelvis occurring 2 to 3 weeks before labor in primigravidas, just before or during labor in multigravidas

linea nigra: Dark line of pigmentation extending from the pubis to the umbilicus during pregnancy

lipids: Easily stored fats that serve as a source of fuel for the body

lithotomy position: Position in which the patient lies on her back with thighs flexed on the abdomen and legs abducted on the thighs

lochia: Discharge of blood, mucus, and tissue that flows from the uterus in the postpartum period

locus: Location of a gene on a chromosome

longevity: Long duration of life

low-birth-weight-infant: Infant weighing 2500 g or less at birth, regardless of gestational age

low-density lipoproteins (LDL): Plasma proteins that carry cholesterol in plasma; high levels are associated with coronary heart disease

lumen: Space within a tube, such as an artery, vein, intestine

lunar month: 28 days

lung compliance: Elasticity of lung tissue that allows for expansion of airways during inhalation and recoil of tissues during exhalation

lymphadenopathy: Disease involving the lymph nodes

macrophage: Body cell that ingests dead tissue

macrosomia: Unusually large body, as in infants of diabetic mothers

maculopapular: Skin eruption with reddened, elevated patches

magnesium sulfate: Anticonvulsant used in preterm labor; also needed as an electrolyte source

malnutrition: Lack of necessary food substances within the body or their improper absorption and distribution

malpresentation: Faulty or abnormal fetal presentation

mammogram: An x-ray study of breast tissue used in the diagnosis of breast disease or cancer

manual rotation: Obstetric maneuver that is used to turn the fetal head by hand from a transverse to an anteroposterior position to facilitate delivery

marasmus: Emaciation and wasting due to malnutrition in an infant

mastitis: Acute inflammation of the breast caused by bacteria entering a cracked nipple during lactation

mastodynia: Breast pain

masturbation: Induction of sexual excitement to self through manipulation of the genitals or other body parts

maternal depletion: Nutritional deficits that adversely affect the volume and composition of mother's milk

maternal mortality rate: Number of maternal deaths from any cause during the pregnancy and postpartum period per 100,000 live births

mature minor doctrine: Position that adult competency of the adolescent is based on an arbitrary age limit or on a case-by-case review of maturity by the provider

meconium: Fecal material discharged by the newborn, green black in color and consisting of mucus, bile, and epithelial shreds; its presence in amniotic fluid during labor may indicate fetal distress

megadose: Amount of a substance (vitamin) that is at least 10 times greater than the RDA

megaloblastic anemia: Pernicious anemia characterized by megaloblasts, or large abnormal red blood corpuscles

meiosis: Cell division occurring in germ cells and leading to the production of gametes containing half the usual number of chromosomes, *i.e.*, one chromosome of each pair and one sex chromosome

menarche: First menstruation that marks the beginning of cyclic menstrual function

meningoencephalitis: Inflammation of the membranes of the spinal cord and brain

menopause: Cessation of menstruation; it is considered complete when menses has not occurred for a year

menstrual cycle: A hallmark of reproductive function in females associated with endocrine changes and cyclical menstruation

menstruation: Physiologic cyclic bleeding that, in the absence of pregnancy, normally occurs monthly in women of reproductive age

metabolism: Sum of all chemical and physical changes that take place in an organism

metabolite: Any product of metabolism

metritis: Inflammation of the uterus

microcephaly: Abnormal smallness of the head with underdevelopment of the brain

microcyte: Abnormally small red blood cell that is often seen in iron deficiency and other anemias

microphthalmia: Abnormally small size of one or both eyes

milia: Minute white cysts on the skin of newborns caused by obstruction of hair follicles; milia are commonly facial, appear over the bridge of the nose, chin, and cheeks, and disappear within a few weeks

miscarriage: Lay term for abortion

mitosis: Cell division leading to the production of two daughter cells, each containing the same chromosomal makeup as the parent cell

mittelschmertz: Abdominal pain on the side of ovulation that some women experience in the middle of the menstrual cycle

molar pregnancy: Abnormal condition in which cells forming the placenta continue to invade the uterine lining after the fetus has died (synonym: hydatidiform mole)

molding: Normal process by which a baby's head is shaped during labor as it passes through the tight birth canal; the head often becomes elongated and the bones of the head may overlap slightly at the suture lines

mongolian spots: Benign bluish pigmentation over the lower back and buttocks that may be present at birth, especially in dark-skinned races

monitrice: Labor coach especially trained in the psychoprophylactic (Lamaze) method of childbirth

mononucleated: Blood cells, such as lymphocytes or monocytes, that have only one nucleus

monosomy: Chromosome disorder in which one chromosome of a pair is missing

monozygous twins: Two offspring originating from a single fertilized ovum; the offspring are of the same sex and have identical genetic characteristics

mons veneris: Pad of fatty tissue lying over the symphysis pubis, which becomes covered with short, curly hair after puberty

Montgomery's glands: Sebaceous glands in the areola; they secrete a lubricant that protects the nipple during nursing

morbidity: The condition of being diseased or sick; pertaining to the sickness rate

morning sickness: Symptoms of nausea and vomiting occurring in some women in early pregnancy; it usually clears after the third month but may continue to some degree through pregnancy

Moro reflex: Defensive reflex present from birth to 3 months of age that causes the infant to draw its arms across the chest in an embracing manner when startled

morphology: Science of structure and forms of organisms

mortality: Condition of being mortal; pertaining to the death rate

mosaicism: Condition of an individual with at least two cell lines with differing karyotype

mucous plug: Plug developing in the endocervical canal during pregnancy that blocks the entrance of substances or bacteria into the uterus; the mucous plug becomes the "bloody show" in early labor when it breaks loose from its capillaries and is expelled

mucus-trap suction apparatus: Apparatus used to aspirate the nasopharynx and trachea of a newborn infant; it consists of a catheter with a trap that prevents mucus from the baby from being drawn into the operator's mouth

müllerian duct: One of a pair of embryonic ducts that become the fallopian tubes, uterus, and vagina

multifactorial: Pertaining to the interaction of genetic and nongenetic (*i.e.,* environmental) factors

multigravida: Woman who is pregnant and has been pregnant before

multipara: Woman who has completed two or more pregnancies to the stage of viability

mutagen: Agent that causes permanent genetic variation

mutation: Permanent change in the genetic code

myelin: Fatty substance that constitutes the sheaths of various nerve fibers throughout the body

myelomeningocele: Spina bifida with protrusion of the cord and membranes

myocarditis: Inflammation of heart muscle tissue

myotonia: Tension or spasm of a muscle

Nägele's rule: Method of estimating the expected date of confinement; add 7 days to the last menstrual period and count back 3 months

nanogram (ng): One thousandth of a microgram, or one billionth of a gram (synonym: millimicrogram)

narcosis: State of profound unconsciousness produced by a drug

natal: Pertaining to birth

natality: Birth rate in a community

nausea: Sensation that usually leads to the urge to vomit

navel: Umbilicus

neck webbing: Presence of a membrane connecting the lateral aspect of the neck with the shoulder

necrosis: Death of areas of tissue, surrounded by healthy tissue

necrotizing enterocolitis: Acute inflammatory bowel disorder that may occur in preterm or low birth weight neonates

neonate: Infant from birth through the first 28 days of life

neonatology: Art and science of diagnosis and treatment of disorders of the neonate

neonatologist: Physician with special training in the care of the neonate

neural tube defect: Group of congenital malformations that involves defects of the spinal column caused by failure of the neural tube to close during embryonic development

neurohumoral substances: Chemicals liberated at nerve endings that excite adjacent structures

neurohypophysis: Posterior lobe of the pituitary gland, which secretes antidiuretic hormone (ADH) and oxytocin

neuropathy: Abnormal condition characterized by inflammation and degeneration of peripheral nerves

neutrophil: Polymorphonuclear leukocyte, a circulating white blood cell that phagocytizes bacteria and other foreign particles gaining entrance into the body

newborn intrapartal care: Care of the newborn in the delivery room just after birth and before transfer to the postpartum unit

niacin (nicotinic acid): Antipellagra principle of the vitamin B complex

nidation: Implantation of a fertilized ovum into the endometrium

nipple shield: Soft latex shield used to protect the nipples of lactating women when they become sore and cracked from infant nursing; the infant nurses from the nipple of the shield

nocturia: Excessive urination during the night

noncompliance: Informed decision not to adhere to therapeutic advice or suggestions

nonstress test: Evaluation performed late in pregnancy of fetal heart rate as it relates to fetal movement

nonviable fetus: Immature fetus that is incapable of surviving outside the uterus

normotensive: Normal blood pressure

nosocomial: Pertaining to a hospital

noxious: Harmful or detrimental to health

nulligravida: Woman who is not now and never has been pregnant

nullipara: Woman who has never carried a pregnancy to the age of viability

nurse midwife: Certified nurse midwife (CNM), who holds a license as a registered nurse and has completed a specialized course of training accredited by the American College of Nurse Midwives in the care of the woman and her family during pregnancy, childbirth, and the postbirth and interconceptional periods

nursing diagnosis: Name or conceptual summary referring to an actual or potential health problem that falls within the scope of nursing intervention

nursing intervention: Nursing action taken to prevent a potential problem or to treat an actual health problem

nursing process: Application of systematic problem solving to the delivery of nursing care

nutrient: Food or substance that supplies the body with elements necessary for metabolism

nutrition: Processes involved in the ingestion and utilization of food substances responsible for growth, repair, and maintenance of the body and its parts

nutritional requirements: Foods necessary for good health, including a variety and amount necessary to maintain ideal weight, with adequate starch and fiber and an avoidance of excessive fat, cholesterol, excessive sugar, salt, and alcohol

nutritive: Pertaining to nutrition

obstetric forceps: Metal forceps that may be used to assist in the delivery of the fetal head

occipital bone: Bone in the lower back portion of the head

oligohydramnios: Abnormal decrease in the amount of amniotic fluid within the uterus

oligomenorrhea: Scanty or infrequent menstrual flow

oliguria: Diminished production of urine

omphalic: Pertaining to the umbilicus

omphalocele: Congenital herniation of the abdominal viscera through a defect in the abdominal wall at the umbilicus; surgical closure is performed after birth

onset of labor: Establishment of regular uterine contractions in conjunction with dilatation of the cervix

oocyte: Early primitive ovum before it has completely developed

oogenesis: Formation and development of the ovum

ophthalmia neonatorum: Purulent conjunctivitis of the newborn; gonorrheal conjunctivitis

organogenesis: Formation of body organs from embryonic tissue

orgasm: Culmination of sexual excitement; in females, contractions of the outer third of the vagina at the apex of sexual arousal

orgasm restriction: Specific direction not to have orgasm by any means because it is deemed threatening to the pregnancy

os: Any opening in the body, but particularly the cervical opening

ossification: Formation of bone or conversion of other tissue into bone

osteoblast: A cell that helps to form bone

osteomalacia: A disease marked by softening and deformity of the bone

osteopenia: Diminished amounts of bone tissue

osteoporosis: A serious disorder, partly due to estrogen decline, that increases porosity of bone as women age

outlet contracture: Abnormally small pelvic outlet that may impede or prevent passage of the fetus through the birth canal

ovarian cycle: A series of events controlled by the hypophysial hormones in which the ovaries produce reproductive cells and female hormones, maintain the secondary sexual characteristics, prepare the uterus for pregnancy, and stimulate the mammary glands

ovulation: Periodic ripening and rupture of the mature ovarian follicle with discharge of the ovum into the abdomen near the fallopian tube; occurs approximately 14 days before the beginning of the next menstrual period

ovum: Female germ cell

oxidizing agent: Agent in a chemical reaction that loses electrons

oxytocics: Drugs used to stimulate uterine contractions to assist childbirth and prevent postdelivery hemorrhage; during lactation they increase the let-down reflex

oxytocin challenge test (OCT): Tests the response of the fetus to uterine contractility stimulated by oxytocin (Pitocin) and assesses placental function

palpation: Examination by application of the hands or fingers to the outer body surfaces to detect evidence of disease or abnormalities of the organs

Papanicolaou smear: Cytologic test of cervical cells used as a screening test for cervical cancer (synonym: Pap smear)

paracervical block: Injection of local anesthetic into the paracervical nerve for pain relief in active labor

parametritis: Inflammation of the parametrium (synonym: pelvic cellulitis)

parametrium: Connective tissue around the uterus

parent–infant bonding: Process by which a tie develops between parents and infant

parity: Number of pregnancies reaching viability—not the number of fetuses delivered (synonym: para)

parturient: Woman in labor

parturition: Act of giving birth (synonyms: childbirth, delivery)

patent ductus arteriosus: Congenital abnormal opening between the pulmonary artery and the aorta that does not close after birth; the defect allows recirculation of arterial blood through the lungs, increasing the workload of the left side of the heart

pelvic inflammatory disease (PID): Bacterial infection of the pelvic organs, often caused by the presence of an IUD or venereal disease; a common cause of tubal adhesions, scar tissue, and consequent infertility

pelvic inlet: Inlet to the true pelvis, bounded by the sacral promontory, the rami of the pubic bone, and the superior rim of the symphysis pubis

pelvic tilt: Postural exercise done to align the pelvic girdle for proper support of the spinal column

pelvimetry: Clinical measurement of the pelvis to determine its adequacy for passage of the fetus during labor and delivery

perinatal period: Period from the 28th week of gestation through the 28th day after birth

perinatologist: Obstetrician with special interest and experience in the perinatal period, particularly with high-risk mothers and infants

perineal massage: Rhythmic massage and stretching of the perineum and lower vaginal walls to soften the tissues and promote relaxation of the pelvic floor

perineum: Floor of the pelvis; the tissues between the lower end of the vagina and the anal canal and lower rectum

periodic fetal heart rate: Fluctuations in the FHR baseline associated with uterine contractions

peritonitis: Inflammation of the peritoneum

petechiae: Small, purplish hemorrhagic spots on the skin

phagocyte: Cell that has the ability to ingest and destroy foreign matter or organisms that gain entrance into the body

phagocytosis: Ingestion of bacteria and particles by phagocytes

phenotype: Physical appearance of a person

phenylketonuria: Congenital disease caused by defective metabolism of the amino acid phenylalanine; if early treatment is not instituted, severe mental retardation will result

phlebitis: Inflammation of a vein

phototherapy: Therapeutic measure using light to treat hyperbilirubinemia and jaundice in the newborn

physiologic management of labor: Maintenance and support of spontaneous labor and birth processes

pica: Craving during pregnancy to eat substances that are not food, such as chalk, clay, starch, glue, toothpaste

placenta: Oval, flat, vascular structure in the uterus through which the fetus derives its nourishment

placenta previa: A placenta that is implanted in the lower uterine segment; there are three types:
centralis — the placenta is implanted over the lower uterine segment and covers the internal os
lateralis — the placenta lies within the lower uterine segment
marginalis — the placenta partially covers the internal cervical os

podalic version: Internal manual version of the fetus: the infant's feet are grasped inside the uterus and turned to a footling breech; version is complete when the feet are brought through the introitus

polycythemia: Excessive number of red blood cells

polyhydramnios: Excessive amount of amniotic fluid

polymicrobial infection: Infection caused by two or more microorganisms

polymorphism: The capacity for appearing in many different forms

position: Relation of the fetal presenting part to the maternal pelvis

postcoital test: Diagnostic procedure in which a sample of cervical mucus is extracted within about 6 hours of sexual intercourse at the presumed time of ovulation; the mucus is examined microscopically for the presence of live, motile sperm as well as for adequate ferning (indicating that the mucus is well estrogenated)

postpartum: After the birth

postpartum hemorrhage: Loss of 500 ml or more of blood from the uterus after completion of the third stage of labor

postpartum period: Period from birth to 6 weeks (42 days) after birth

postprandial: Following a meal

post-term infant: Infant born after the onset of the 42nd week of gestation

Potter's syndrome: Failure of the kidneys to develop or grow

precipitate labor: Labor that terminates in delivery of the infant in less than 3 hours

precursor: Substance that precedes the production of another substance

preeclampsia: Disorder of pregnancy or the puerperium characterized by hypertension, edema, and proteinuria

premature infant: Infant born before the end of the 37th week of gestation (synonym: preterm infant)

premature rupture of membranes: Rupture of the amniotic sac before the onset of uterine contractions

prenatal diagnosis: Diagnostic tests that determine whether a developing fetus is affected by a genetic disorder or other abnormality

presbycusis: Impairment of hearing in older age

presbyopia: Defect of vision in advancing years

presentation: Position of the fetus as described by the fetal part that appears first at the pelvic outlet, e.g., vertex (head), breech, arm, or face

preterm infant: Premature infant

preterm labor: Labor that occurs prior to the 37th week of gestation

primary infertility: Inability to conceive or carry a pregnancy to viability with no previous history of pregnancy carried to live birth

primigravida: Woman pregnant for the first time (synonym: gravida 1)

primipara: Woman who has delivered one fetus who reached the stage of viability

proband: A person presenting with a mental or physical disorder whose heredity is studied to determine if other members of the family have had the same disease or are carriers

prodromal labor: Period preceding labor when lightening occurs and increased pressure in the pelvis is felt

professionalism: Spirit or activities of a group emphasizing or aspiring to ideals of a profession, including career commitment, accountability, self-regulation, and independent functioning

progesterone: Hormone secreted by the corpus luteum that prepares the endometrium to receive the fertilized ovum

prolactin: Pituitary hormone that in association with estrogen and progesterone promotes breast development and the formation of milk during pregnancy and lactation

prolonged labor: Active labor that continues more than 20 hours

prolonged rupture of membranes: Rupture of the amniotic sac that occurs 24 hours or more before the onset of labor

prophylaxis: Protection from or prevention of a disease or event

prostaglandin (PG): Fatty acid found in many body tissues that affects smooth muscles and the cardiovascular system; one of its properties is to stimulate the uterus to contract

prosthesis: Replacement of a missing body part by an artificial substitute, *e.g.,* an artificial limb

protein: Class of complex nitrogenous compounds occurring naturally in plants and animals and containing amino acids essential for the growth and repair of animal tissue; proteins in milk are classified into two major categories: (1) casein is the protein in the curd; human milk contains 40% curd whereas cow's milk contains 82% curd; (2) whey is the protein in the watery portion after milk is coagulated; human milk contains 60% whey whereas cow's milk contains 18%

proteinuria: Presence of protein in the urine

prothrombin time: Test of clotting time used to evaluate the effect of anticoagulant therapy

pruritus: Intense itching

pseudocyesis: False pregnancy

psychosocial responses: Intrapersonal and interpersonal responses to external events

ptosis: Drooping of a part or organ, e.g., eyelid

puberty: Point at which a person is first capable of reproduction; also the phase marked by first development of secondary sex characteristics

pubescence: State of being at which a person of either sex becomes functionally capable of reproduction

puerpera: A woman who has just given birth

puerperal sepsis: Infection during the puerperium originating in the pelvic organs

puerperium: Period of 42 days following childbirth

purulence: State of containing pus (synonym: suppuration)

quickening: Perception of the first fetal movements by the mother, generally between the 18th and 20th weeks of pregnancy

radioimmunoassay: Test for pregnancy based on an antigen–antibody reaction and measured by sensitive radioisotope technique

rales: Abnormal respiratory sound auscultated over the chest during inspiration

RDA (recommended daily allowances): Standards by age and sex group for intake of major nutrients; serve as guidelines for maintaining health through nutrition

reactivity: Progression by neonate in the period immediately after birth through a series of predictable behavior patterns

recessive: Trait or gene that is clinically expressed only when homozygous

rectocele: Protrusion of the posterior vaginal wall from pressure of the anterior wall of the rectum against the vagina

rectouterine pouch (pouch of Douglas): Pouch formed from the parietal peritoneum, bounded anteriorly by the posterior fornix of the vagina and posteriorly by the rectum

recurrence risk: Mathematical probability that a genetic disorder present in a family will recur in a specified family member

reflex: Neurobehavioral response that occurs without conscious thought

regurgitation: Backward flowing of undigested food or fluid from the stomach: common in the neonate owing to the immaturity of the cardiac sphincter of the stomach

relapse: Recurrence of a disease or symptoms after apparent recovery

renal solute load: Metabolic end products, especially nitrogenous compounds and electrolytes, that must be excreted by the kidneys

respiratory distress syndrome (RDS): Disease of the newborn who is delivered before full lung maturity has occurred; symptoms include cyanosis, grunting, abnormal respiratory pattern, and retraction of the chest wall during inspiration

restitution: Spontaneous return of the fetal head to the normal position in relation to the fetal body after delivery of the head

retraction ring: Physiologic area of constriction at the junction of the upper, or contracting, portion and the lower, or dilating, portion of the uterus; Bandl's ring is pathologic constriction of the retraction ring

Rh (D) immune globulin: Passive immunizing solution of gamma globulin that contains anti-Rh; when given within 72 hours after delivery of an Rh+ infant to an Rh− mother, it acts to prevent the maternal Rh immune response

riboflavin: Water-soluble member of the vitamin B group; found in milk and milk products, leafy green vegetables, liver, beef, fish, and dry yeast

rickets: A vitamin D deficiency in children that causes abnormalities of the shape and structure of the bones

role: Pattern of behavior that is socially assigned or adopted

rooming-in: Hospital policy in which the infant stays with the mother after delivery and during the postpartum period

round ligaments: Fibromuscular bands extending from the superior lateral surface of the uterus down and forward through the inguinal canal to terminate in the

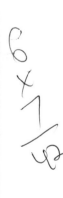

labia major; they stretch during pregnancy and may cause discomfort

rubella: Acute infectious disease (synonym: German measles)

Rubin's test: Insufflation of the fallopian tubes with carbon dioxide to test their patency

rupture of membranes: Breaking of the amniotic sac spontaneously or mechanically before or during labor

saddle block anesthesia: Injection of an anesthetic agent into a spinal subarachnoid space

sagittal suture: Suture between the parietal bones

salpingitis: Inflammation of the fallopian tubes

salpinx: Fallopian tube

Schultze's mechanism: Expulsion of the placenta in which the fetal surface appears first at the vulva

scotoma: Blind spot in the visual field

sebum: Fatty secretion of sebaceous glands

secondary infertility: Inability to conceive or carry a pregnancy to a live birth after one or more successful pregnancies

secundigravida: Woman pregnant for the second time (synonym: gravida 2)

semen: Viscid, sperm-containing secretion that passes from the male urethra at sexual climax

semen analysis: Diagnostic test in which semen is examined to determine count, motility, and morphology of the spermatozoa

sensitized: Having developed a susceptibility to a specific substance

separation of the placenta: Detachment of the placenta from the uterine wall

sepsis: Presence of pathogenic microorganisms or their toxins in blood or other tissues

septum: Wall dividing two cavities

Sertoli's cells: Cells of the seminiferous tubules that nourish spermatids

sex chromosome: Chromosome responsible for sex determination; in humans, females have two X chromosomes (XX), males have one X and one Y (XY)

sexual activity: Any activity that is arousing, such as manual or oral stimulation (not just intercourse)

SGA: A small-for-gestational-age infant weighing less than 2500 g but not premature by calculation of dates

Sheehan's syndrome: Hypopituitarism caused by infarct of the pituitary gland following postpartum shock or hemorrhage

Shirodkar cerclage: Operative procedure that sutures an incompetent cervix to ensure that it cannot dilate until removal of sutures in early labor

shunt: Passage that diverts flow from one main route to another

sinusoids: Small blood vessels found in the liver, spleen, and adrenal glands

Skene's glands: Glands whose ducts open into the female urethra; in gonorrheal infections these glands are always infected

small-for-gestational-age infant: Infant of any weight who falls below the tenth percentile on the intrauterine growth curve; infant weighing less than 2500 g at term

somatic: Pertaining to the body, in contrast to structures associated with viscera

spermatogenesis: Formation of mature, functional spermatozoa

spermicide: Agent that kills spermatozoa

spina bifida: Congenital defect in which the spinal canal fails to close at the lumbar region; protrusion of the cord and meninges occurs

spinnbarkeit: Cervical mucus that has the property of elasticity at the time of ovulation

spontaneous rupture of the membranes: Rupture of the amniotic sac without medical interference

spotting: Spotting of blood from the vagina between periods or during pregnancy

squamocolumnar junction: Location on the endocervix or on the ectocervix where transition from squamous to columnar epithelium occurs

standards of nursing practice: Agreed-upon levels of care that provide guidance in achieving excellence in nursing services to clients

stasis: Stagnation of the normal flow of fluids

static: Without movement; obstruction of the normal flow of fluids

station: Measurement of fetal descent into the bony pelvis in relation to the ischial spines

stenosis: Narrowing or stricture of a duct or canal

sterilization: (1) Complete removal or destruction of all microorganisms; (2) Process rendering a person unable to produce children

steroid hormones: Sex hormones and hormones of the adrenal cortex

steroidogenesis: Formation of steroid hormones

sterol: One of a group of substances related to fats and belonging to the liquid oils

stilbestrol: Diethylstilbestrol, an estrogenic compound

stillbirth: Birth of a dead fetus

stimulation of labor: Augmentation of labor; the process of improving contraction intensity, frequency, or duration

stress: Internal or environmental stimulus requiring a response that is not readily available and that arouses anxiety

striae gravidarum: Whitish or reddish lines seen on parts of the body where skin has been stretched; in pregnancy, they occur primarily on the abdomen, thighs, and breasts

stroma: Foundation or supporting tissues of an organ

subinvolution: Incomplete return of a body part to its normal size after physiologic hypertrophy; may occur in the uterus following childbirth as an abnormal condition

supine hypotensive syndrome: Lowered blood pressure and bradycardia in the supine position due to compression of the inferior vena cava by the weight of the pregnant uterus

suppository: Semisolid substance used as a vehicle for introduction of medicine into the rectum, vagina, or urethra, where it dissolves

suppuration: Process of pus formation

surfactant: Substance that lowers surface tension in the lungs and maintains expansion of its small air sacs; abnormalities in surfactant in premature infants cause respiratory distress syndrome

sympathomimetics: Drugs that mimic the stimulation of the sympathetic nervous system

syncytiotrophoblast: Outer layer of cells covering the chorionic villi of the placenta that is in contact with the maternal blood

synthesis: Formation of a complex substance from simpler elements or compounds

syphilis: A sexually transmitted disease that is transmitted by the spirochete *Treponema pallidum;* it is characterized by lesions that may involve any organ or tissue and may exist without symptoms for many years

tachycardia, fetal: Fetal heart rate of 160 beats or more per minute

Tanner staging: A standard method for measuring and classifying the development of sexual characteristics of the maturing reproductive system; stages progress from 1 to 5

teratogen: Substance that causes abnormal development of embryonic structures

term: Normal end period of pregnancy, occurring between 38 and 42 weeks

testes: Two male reproductive glands, located in the scrotum, that produce testosterone, the male hormone, and spermatozoa, the male reproductive cells

tetanic contraction: Abnormally long uterine contraction, lasting more than 70 seconds; usually in response to hyperstimulation from oxytocin infusion

thalassemia: A genetic disorder that affects hemoglobin in red blood cells and causes chronic anemia; it primarily affects people of Mediterranean, Asian, and African ancestry

thelarche: The beginning of breast development at puberty

thermoregulation, neonatal: Regulation of the body temperature of the newborn

thiamine: Vitamin B, essential for normal body metabolism of carbohydrates and fats

thrombocytopenia: Abnormal decrease in the number of platelets in the blood

thrombophlebitis: Formation of a thrombus in conjunction with inflammation of a vein

thromboplastin: Substance in blood and tissues that promotes blood clotting

thrombosis: Formation of a blood clot

thyroxine: Hormone produced by the thyroid gland

titer: Standard of strength per volume of test solution

tocolytic agent: Drug that alters the force of uterine contractions

tocopherol: Generic term for vitamin E

tonic contraction: Sustained muscular tension or contraction

TORCH infections: Group of infections that may affect the mother or fetus: Toxoplasmosis, Other (includes syphilis), Rubella, Cytomegalovirus, and Herpesvirus

total birth rate: Number of liveborn and stillborn infants per 1000 population

toxemia: Complication of pregnancy of unknown cause characterized by elevation of the blood pressure, proteinuria, and edema (preeclampsia); when convulsions occur, the condition is called eclampsia

transition: (1) Experience of passing from one phase or stage of living to another, involving letting go of attitudes and behaviors from the previous stage and taking on new attitudes and behaviors; (2) The last segment of active phase of labor from 8 – 10 centimeters of cervical dilatation, which may be characterized by particularly intense maternal discomfort

transplacental: Across the placenta; refers to the exchange of nutrients, waste products, and hormones between mother and fetus

trichomoniasis: Vaginal infection caused by the parasite Trichomonas vaginalis

triglyceride: A combination of glycerol with three fatty acids; most animal and vegetable fats are triglycerides

trimester: One of three periods into which pregnancy is divided; the first trimester is from the first day of the LMP until 12 weeks; second trimester is 13 weeks to 27 weeks; third trimester is 28 weeks to 40 weeks or delivery

trisomy: Chromosome disorder in which three copies of homologous chromosomes are present rather than two

tubercle: Solid elevation of the skin or mucous membrane

ultrasound: Use of sound waves to produce an outline of the shape of body organs and tissues; used in fetal assessment

umbilical cord: Cord containing two arteries and one vein that connects the fetus with the placenta

uterine inertia: Failure of the uterine muscles to contract and retract with normal strength and frequency (synonym: uterine dysfunction)

uterine prolapse: Downward displacement of the uterus that sometimes causes it to protrude from the vagina

uterus: Hollow, pear-shaped internal female organ of reproduction in which the embryo and fetus develop

vacuole: Clear, fluid-filled space within the cell protoplasm

vacuum aspiration: Method of first-trimester abortion in which the products of conception are extracted from the uterus by suction

vaginitis: Infection of the vaginal mucosa, usually accompanied by itching, increased discharge, and burning

values clarification: Process in which one identifies and examines the values that give meaning and direction to one's life, with the goal of increasing self-understanding

varicocele: Varicose vein of the spermatic cord, more often the left; a common cause of male infertility

vasa previa: Anomaly of insertion of the umbilical cord in which the umbilical blood vessels traverse the lower uterine segment and present at delivery in advance of the head

vasectomy: Method of male sterilization in which the vasa deferens are cut and ligated to prevent sperm from entering the ejaculate

vasocongestion: Congestion of blood vessels

VDRL: Venereal Disease Research Laboratory

velamentous insertion: Insertion of the umbilical cord where the blood vessels leave the placenta, course between the amnion and chorion, and unite to form the umbilical cord at some distance from the edge of the placenta

vernix caseosa: Grey white, cheeselike sebaceous material that covers the skin of the fetus to protect it from the amniotic fluid

version: Manipulation to alter presentation of the fetus

vertex presentation: Cephalic presentation

viable: Capable of living outside the uterus; the age of viability was previously considered to be 28 weeks, but many states now prepare birth certifications for pregnancy at 20 weeks of gestation or more, or for a fetus weighing 500 g or more

viscosity of lung fluid: Cohesiveness of pulmonary secretions that results in a resistance to flow of fluid through lung passages

vulva: External genitalia of the female, including the mons veneris, labia majora, labia minora, clitoris, and vestibule

weaning: Discontinuing breast milk and substituting other nourishment for the infant

whey: Liquid that remains after the cream and curd are separated from the milk

witches' milk: Milk secreted by the newborn infant's breast as a result of stimulation by circulating prolactin in the mother

withdrawal bleeding: Vaginal bleeding that occurs after the last oral contraceptive pill of the cycle has been taken

X-linked transmission: Transmission of characteristics by genes on the X chromosome

zygote: Cell produced by union of the sperm and egg; the fertilized egg

index

Page numbers followed by f indicate figures; those followed by t indicate tabular material; those followed by b indicate boxed material.